Nursing Actions

Clinical Drug Therapy

SIXTH EDITION

RATIONALES FOR NURSING PRACTICE

Anne Collins Abrams, RN, MSN
Associate Professor, Emeritus
Department of Baccalaureate and Graduate Nursing
College of Health Sciences
Eastern Kentucky University
Richmond, Kentucky

CONSULTANT

Tracey L. Goldsmith, PharmD
Clinical Manager
Department of Pharmacy Services
Hermann Hospital
Houston, Texas

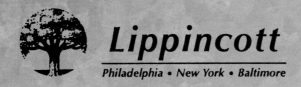

Lippincott

Philadelphia • New York • Baltimore

Acquisitions Editor: Margaret Zuccarini
Managing Editor: Lisa Popeck
Editorial Assistant: Helen Kogut
Project Editor: Debra Schiff
Senior Production Manager: Helen Ewan
Senior Production Coordinator: Michael Carcel
Art Director: Doug Smock
Indexer: Alexandra Nickerson
Manufacturing Manager: William Alberti
Sixth Edition

9 8 7 6 5 4 3 2

Library of Congress Cataloging-in-Publication Data

Abrams, Anne Collins.
    Clinical drug therapy : rationales for nursing practice / Anne Collins Abrams ;
consultant, Tracey L. Goldsmith.—6th ed.
      p. ; cm.
    Includes bibliographical references and index.
    ISBN 0-7817-2121-0 (alk. paper)
      1. Chemotherapy. 2. Drugs. 3. Nursing. I. Goldsmith, Tracey L. II. Title.
    [DNLM: 1. Pharmaceutical Preparations. 2. Drug Therapy—Nurses' Instruction. 3.
    Nursing Process. QV 55 A161c 2000]
    RM262 .A27 2000
    615.5'8—dc21   00-032736

Care has been taken to confirm the accuracy of the information presented and to describe generally accepted practices. However, the authors, editors, and publisher are not responsible for errors or omissions or for any consequences from application of the information in this book and make no warranty, express or implied, with respect to the contents of the publication.

The authors, editors, and publisher have exerted every effort to ensure that drug selection and dosage set forth in this text are in accordance with current recommendations and practice at the time of publication. However, in view of ongoing research, changes in government regulations, and the constant flow of information relating to drug therapy and drug reactions, the reader is urged to check the package insert for each drug for any change in indications and dosage and for added warnings and precautions. This is particularly important when the recommended agent is a new or infrequently employed drug.

Some drugs and medical devices presented in this publication have Food and Drug Administration (FDA) clearance for limited use in restricted research settings. It is the responsibility of the health care provider to ascertain the FDA status of each drug or device planned for use in his or her clinical practice.

CONTRIBUTORS

Constance J. Hirnle, RN, MN
Assistant Professor, School of Nursing
Seattle University
Seattle, Washington
*Chapter Opening Patient Care Scenarios, Nursing Notes:
  Apply Your Knowledge, How Can You Avoid This
  Medication Error?, Nursing Notes: Ethical/Legal
  Dilemma*

Carol Ann Barnett Lammon, RN, BSN, MSN
Assistant Professor of Nursing
University of Alabama
Tuscaloosa, Alabama
Chapter 17: Physiology of the Autonomic Nervous System
Chapter 18: Adrenergic Drugs
Chapter 19: Antiadrenergic Drugs
Chapter 20: Cholinergic Drugs
Chapter 21: Anticholinergic Drugs

Mary Jo McClure, RNC, MSN
Associate Professor, Emeritus
Clinical Instructor
Department of Baccalaureate and Graduate Nursing
College of Health Sciences
Eastern Kentucky University
Richmond, Kentucky
Chapter 67: Drug Use During Pregnancy and Lactation

Cynthia K. Perkins, RN, MSN, CEN, FNP
Instructor
Capstone College of Nursing, University of Alabama
Tuscaloosa, Alabama
Chapter 54: Drugs Used in Hypotension and Shock

REVIEWERS

Patricia A. Dickman, RN, BA
Nursing Instructor
BM Spur School of Practical Nursing
Colen Dale, West Virginia

Mervin R. Helmuth, RN, MN
Associate Professor of Nursing
Goshen College
Goshen, Indiana

Barbara D. Kinsman, MSN
Associate Professor
Corning Community College
Corning, New York

Sallie Kelly, RN, BSN, MSN
Assistant Professor
Grambling State University
Grambling, Louisiana

Carol Ann Barnett Lammon, RN, BSN, MSN
Assistant Professor of Nursing
University of Alabama
Tuscaloosa, Alabama

Renee Lewis, RN, MS, CCRN
Professor of Nursing Science
Rose State College
Midwest City, Oklahoma

PREFACE

The basic precepts underlying previous editions of *Clinical Drug Therapy* continued to guide the writing of this sixth edition. The overall purpose is to promote safe, effective, and rational drug therapy by:

- Providing essential information that accurately reflects current practices in drug therapy.
- Facilitating the acquisition, comprehension, and application of knowledge related to drug therapy. Application requires knowledge about the drug and the client receiving it.
- Identifying knowledge and skills the nurse can use to smooth the interface between a drug and the client receiving it.

GOALS AND RESPONSIBILITIES OF NURSING CARE RELATED TO DRUG THERAPY

- Preventing the need for drug therapy, when possible, by promoting health and preventing conditions that require drug therapy.
- Using appropriate and effective nonpharmacologic interventions instead of, or in conjunction with, drug therapy when indicated. When used with drug therapy, such interventions may promote lower drug dosage, less frequent administration, and fewer adverse effects.
- Enhancing therapeutic effects by administering drugs accurately and considering clients' individual characteristics that influence responses to drug therapy.
- Preventing or minimizing adverse drug effects by knowing the major adverse effects associated with particular drugs, identifying clients with characteristics that may increase risks of experiencing adverse effects, and actively monitoring for the occurrence of adverse effects. When adverse effects occur, early recognition allows interventions to minimize their severity. Because all drugs may cause adverse effects, nurses must maintain a high index of suspicion that symptoms, especially new ones, may be drug-induced.
- Teaching clients and caregivers about accurate administration of medications, nonpharmacologic treatments to use with or instead of pharmacologic treatments, and when to contact a health care provider.

ORGANIZATIONAL FRAMEWORK

The content of *Clinical Drug Therapy* is organized in 11 sections, primarily by therapeutic drug groups and their effects on particular body systems. This approach helps the student make logical connections between major drug groups and the conditions for which they are used. It also provides a foundation for learning about new drugs, most of which fit into known groups.

The first section contains the basic information required to learn, understand, and apply drug knowledge in patient care. The chapters in this section include drug names, laws and standards, schedules of controlled substances, cellular physiology, and cellular response to injury (Chapter 1); pharmacokinetics, the receptor theory of drug action, and factors that influence drug effects on body tissues (Chapter 2); dosage forms and routes and methods of accurate drug administration (Chapter 3); and guidelines for using the nursing process in drug therapy and general principles of drug therapy (Chapter 4).

Most drug sections include an initial chapter that reviews the physiology of a body system followed by several chapters that discuss drug groups used to treat disorders of that body system. The seven physiology review chapters are designed to facilitate understanding of drug effects on a body system. These include the central nervous system; the autonomic nervous system; and the endocrine, hematopoietic, immune, respiratory, cardiovascular, and digestive systems. The chapters within each section emphasize therapeutic classes of drugs and prototypical or commonly used individual drugs, those used to treat common disorders, and those likely to be encountered in clinical nursing practice. Drug chapter content is presented in a consistent format and includes a description of a condition for which a drug group is used; a general description of a drug group, including mechanism(s) of action, indications for use, and contraindications; and monographs or tables of individual drugs, with recommended dosages and routes of administration.

Additional clinically relevant information is presented under the headings of **Nursing Process, Principles of Therapy,** and **Nursing Actions.**

The **Nursing Process** section emphasizes the importance of the nursing process in drug therapy, including assessment of the client's condition in relation to the drug group, nursing diagnoses, expected outcomes in terms of client characteristics, needed interventions, and evaluation of the client's progress toward expected outcomes. Client teaching guidelines are separated from other interventions to emphasize their importance.

The **Principles of Therapy** section presents guidelines for individualizing drug therapy in specific populations, including children and older adults. General principles about drug usage in children and older adults are included in Chapter 4; specific principles related to drug groups are included in the chapters where those drug groups are discussed. This approach, rather than separate chapters on pediatric and geriatric pharmacology, was chosen because knowledge about a drug is required before that knowledge can be applied to a specific population with distinctive characteristics and needs in relation to drug therapy.

Each drug chapter includes a **Nursing Actions** display that provides specific nursing responsibilities related to drug administration and client observation.

Other drug sections include products used to treat nutritional, infectious, oncologic, ophthalmic, and dermatologic disorders.

NEW FEATURES

- **Vibrant Four-Color Design.** The striking design enhances liveliness of the text and promotes student interest and interactivity.
- **Interactive Displays.** Presented in consistent formats and colors throughout the text, these displays heighten student attention and emphasize critical thinking and clinical decision-making skills. Drug-related chapters contain two or more of the following displays: an opening patient care scenario, a knowledge application situation, a medication error prevention exercise, and an ethical/legal dilemma. The solutions to the knowledge application situations and the medication error prevention exercises appear at the ends of chapters.
- **Client Teaching Guidelines.** This feature has been designed to meet several goals. One is to highlight the importance of teaching clients and caregivers how to manage drug therapy at home, where most medications are taken. This is done by separating teaching from other nursing interventions in a consistent format and an easily recognizable color display. Another goal is to promote active and knowledgeable client participation in drug therapy regimens, which helps to maximize therapeutic effects and minimize adverse effects. In addition, written guidelines allow clients and caregivers to

have a source of reference when questions arise in the home setting. A third goal is to make client teaching easier and less time consuming. Using the guidelines as a foundation, the nurse can simply add or delete information according to a client's individual needs. To assist both the nurse and client further, the guidelines contain minimal medical jargon.

- **New Illustrations and Tables.** Fifteen new illustrations and 19 new tables have been designed to enhance understanding of drug actions.

IMPORTANT RECURRING FEATURES

- **Readability.** Since the first edition of *Clinical Drug Therapy* was published in 1983, many students and faculty have commented about the book's clear presentation style.
- **Organizational Framework.** The book's organizational framework allows it to be used effectively as both a textbook and as a reference. As a textbook, students can read chapters in their entirety to learn the characteristics of major drug classes, their prototypical drugs or commonly used representatives, their uses and effects in prevention or treatment of disease processes, and their implications for nursing practice. As a reference book, students can readily review selected topics for clinical laboratory practice or clinical nursing courses. Facilitating such uses are a consistent format and frequent headings that allow the reader to identify topics at a glance.
- **Chapter Objectives.** Learning objectives at the beginning of each chapter focus the student's attention on important chapter content.
- **Home Care.** Highlighted by an attractive icon and included in many of the drug chapters, this section discusses the nursing role related to drug therapy in clients' homes, an expanding area of nursing practice and responsibility.
- **Nursing Actions Displays.** These displays emphasize nursing interventions during drug therapy within the following categories: Administer accurately, Observe for therapeutic effects, Observe for adverse effects, and Observe for drug interactions. The inclusion of rationales for interventions provides a strong knowledge base and scientific foundation.
- **Review and Application Exercises.** Located at the end of each chapter, these questions encourage students to rehearse clinical application strategies in a nonclinical, nonstressful, nondistracting environment. They also promote self-testing in chapter content and can be used to promote classroom discussion.
- **Appendices.** These include recently approved and miscellaneous drugs, the International System of Units, therapeutic serum drug concentrations for selected drugs, Canadian drug laws and standards, and Canadian drug names.
- **Extensive Index.** Listings of generic and trade names of drugs, nursing process, and other topics provide rapid access to desired information.

NEW CONTENT IN THE SIXTH EDITION

- **Updated Drug Information.** Numerous new drugs have been added. Some are additions to well-known drug groups, such as the fluoroquinolones (Chapter 35) and the angiotensin II receptor antagonists (Chapter 55). Others represent advances in the drug therapy of some disease processes, such as newer oral agents for treatment of type 2 diabetes mellitus (Chapter 27). Still others represent new drug groups, such as the cyclooxygenase-2 (COX-2) inhibitors (Chapter 7) and newer antiplatelet drugs (Chapter 57).
- **Updated Physiology Information.** Of particular importance is the revision of several chapters in Section IX, Drugs Affecting the Cardiovascular System, to reflect current knowledge about the vital metabolic functions of vascular endothelium and the chemical mediators it produces (eg, nitric oxide). Overall, endothelial mediators regulate vasomotor tone, blood coagulation, cell growth, and inflammation. Endothelial dysfunction is important in major cardiovascular disorders, including atherosclerosis, angina pectoris, myocardial infarction, hypertension, hemostasis, and thrombosis.

- **Major Revision of Most Chapters.** Chapter revisions reflect current practices in drug therapy, integrate new drugs, explain the major characteristics of new drug groups, and present content in a clear, meaningful, and visually interesting way. For example:
  - ○ Chapter 1 differentiates the anti-inflammatory effects of corticosteroids (Chapter 24), nonsteroidal anti-inflammatory drugs (NSAIDS) (Chapter 7), and leukotriene inhibitors (Chapter 47).
  - ○ Chapter 7 differentiates the effects of traditional NSAIDs from those of the newer COX-2 inhibitors (eg, celecoxib).
  - ○ Chapter 26 has increased information about bone metabolism and drugs used to treat osteoporosis.
  - ○ Chapter 27 includes new types of oral drugs and combinations of drugs for the treatment of type 2 diabetes mellitus.
  - ○ Chapter 57 has increased information about platelet functions and the actions of newer types of antiplatelet drugs.
  - ○ Chapter 67 includes information about selected infections and their treatment, recommended and contraindicated vaccines, and home care during pregnancy.
- **Updated Principles of Therapy.** New content related to drug use in clients with renal or hepatic impairment is presented in most chapters. In selected chapters, drug use in clients with critical illness is also described.

ANCILLARY PACKAGE

Nursing students must develop skills in critical thinking, information processing, decision making, collaboration, and problem solving. How can a teacher assist students to develop these skills in relation to drug therapy? The goal of the ancillary package is to assist both student and teacher in this development.

The **student manual** engages the student's interest and active participation by providing a variety of learning exercises and opportunities to practice cognitive skills. Worksheets related to each chapter of the text (eg, matching and completion exercises) promote initial learning and a review of concepts, principles, and characteristics and uses of major drug groups. The worksheets can be completed independently, by a small group as an in-class learning activity, or by the instructor, with answers elicited from the class as a whole. Clinical scenarios and case studies promote appropriate data collection, critical analysis of both drug-related and client-related data, and application of the data in patient care.

The **instructor's manual** facilitates use of the text in designing and implementing courses of study, whether in separate pharmacology courses or in nursing courses with integrated pharmacology. To fulfill this purpose, the manual contains the following elements: a sample course syllabus with course objectives, general teaching strategies, strategies for classroom and clinical teaching of content in each chapter, and multiple-choice test items in NCLEX format for each chapter. In the back of the instructor's manual is a disk containing additional multiple-choice NCLEX-style questions.

In a separate package are 55 **overhead transparencies** (34 four-color illustrations and 21 black-and-white text).

These varied materials allow each instructor to choose or adapt those relevant to his or her circumstances. The test bank portion assists the instructor in evaluating students' knowledge of drug information and their ability to apply that information in client care.

Anne Collins Abrams, RN, MSN

ACKNOWLEDGMENTS

Sincere appreciation is expressed to the following people who assisted in the preparation of this book:

Margaret Belcher Zuccarini, Senior Nursing Editor at Lippincott Williams & Wilkins, who has encouraged and inspired the development of this edition.

Tracey Goldsmith, PharmD, who reviewed all chapters and made helpful suggestions. This is the fifth edition for which Tracey has served as consultant, and her continuing efforts are greatly appreciated.

Gail Ropelewski-Ryan, RN, MSN, who authored the Student Study Guide and the test bank portion of the Instructor's Manual.

Connie Hirnle, RN, MN, who prepared the interactive displays.

Contributors Carol Lammon, RN, BSN, MSN; Mary Jo McClure, RNC, MSN; and Cindy Perkins, RN, MSN, CEN, FNP, who revised a total of seven chapters.

All editors, staff assistants, artists, and others at Lippincott Williams & Wilkins who participated in this project. Special thanks to Helen Kogut, Lisa Popeck, and Debra Schiff.

CONTENTS

SECTION III
Drugs Affecting the Autonomic Nervous System 247

SECTION IV
Drugs Affecting the Endocrine System 307

Clinical Drug Therapy
RATIONALES FOR NURSING PRACTICE

Introduction to Drug Therapy

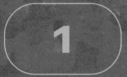

1

Introduction to Pharmacology

Objectives

After studying this chapter, the student will be able to:

1. Differentiate between pharmacology and drug therapy.

2. Differentiate between generic and trade names of drugs.

3. Define a prototypical drug.

4. Select authoritative sources of drug information.

5. Differentiate the main categories of controlled substances in relation to therapeutic use and potential for abuse.

6. Discuss the role of the Food and Drug Administration.

7. Describe characteristics of normal cells in relation to drug therapy.

8. Describe cellular responses to injury, including inflammation.

This is your first semester of clinical nursing. You are excited yet apprehensive about your ability to do well in the difficult nursing curriculum. This quarter, you will be taking a basic nursing theory course, a skills laboratory, and pharmacology. You have heard from senior students that pharmacology is very demanding.

Reflect on:

▶ What factors might contribute to your feelings of anxiety? Write them down.

▶ List successful strategies you have used in the past to learn difficult material. Reflect on which strategies might be helpful this semester.

▶ Assess support for your learning at your school (eg, learning center, peer tutors, student study groups) and develop a plan to use them.

▶ Review your course syllabus and pharmacology text. Develop a learning plan (eg, readings, assignments, study time for major tests) and enter this plan in your calendar.

Pharmacology is the study of drugs (chemicals) that alter functions of living organisms. Drug therapy is the use of drugs to prevent, diagnose, or cure disease processes or to relieve signs and symptoms. When prevention or cure is not a reasonable goal, relief of symptoms can greatly improve quality of life and ability to function in activities of daily living. Drugs given for therapeutic purposes are usually called *medications*.

Drugs may be given for local or systemic effects. Drugs with local effects, such as dermatologic preparations and local anesthetics, act mainly at the site of application. Those with systemic effects are absorbed into the bloodstream and circulated through the body. Most drugs are given for their systemic effects.

SOURCES OF DRUGS

Historically, drugs were mainly derived from plants (eg, morphine), animals (eg, insulin), and minerals (eg, iron). Now, most drugs are synthetic chemical compounds manufactured in laboratories. Technologic advances have enabled the production of synthetic versions of many drugs originally derived from plants and animals, as well as new drugs. Synthetic drugs are more standardized in their chemical characteristics, more consistent in their effects, and less likely to produce allergic reactions. Semisynthetic drugs (eg, many antibiotics) are naturally occurring substances that have been chemically modified.

Biotechnology is also an important source of drugs. This technology involves manipulating DNA and ribonucleic acid (RNA) and recombining genes into hybrid molecules that can be inserted into living organisms (*Escherichia coli* bacteria are often used) and repeatedly reproduced. Each hybrid molecule produces a genetically identical molecule, called a clone. Cloning makes it possible to identify the DNA sequence in a gene and produce the protein product encoded by a gene, including insulin and several other body proteins. Cloning also allows production of adequate amounts of the drug for therapeutic or research purposes.

DRUG NOMENCLATURE

Drugs are classified according to their effects on particular body systems, their therapeutic uses, and their chemical characteristics. For example, morphine can be classified as a central nervous system depressant, a narcotic analgesic, and an opiate. Individual drugs that represent groups of drugs are called *prototypes*. Morphine is the prototype of opioid analgesics and is the standard with which other opioid analgesics are compared. Drug classifications and prototypes are quite stable, and most new drugs can be assigned to a group and compared with an established prototype.

Individual drugs may have several different names, but the two most commonly used are the generic name and the trade name. The *generic name* (eg, amoxicillin) is related to the chemical or official name and is independent of the manufacturer. The generic name often indicates the drug group (eg, drugs with generic names ending in "cillin" are penicillins). The *trade* or *brand name* is designated and patented by the manufacturer. For example, amoxicillin is manufactured by several pharmaceutical companies, each of which assigns a specific trade name, such as Amoxil or Polymox. (Trade names are capitalized; generic names are lowercase.) Drugs may be prescribed and dispensed by generic or trade name.

SOURCES OF DRUG INFORMATION

There are many sources of drug data, including pharmacology textbooks, drug reference books, journal articles, and Internet sites. For the beginning student of pharmacology, a textbook is usually the best source of information because it describes groups of drugs in relation to therapeutic uses. Thus, the student can get an overview of the major drug classifications and their effects.

Drug reference books are most helpful in relation to individual drugs. Two authoritative sources are the *American Hospital Formulary Service* and *Drug Facts and Comparisons*. The former is published by the American Society of Health-System Pharmacists and updated periodically. The latter is published by the Facts and Comparisons division of Lippincott Williams & Wilkins and updated monthly (looseleaf edition) or annually (hardbound edition). A widely available but less authoritative source is the *Physicians' Desk Reference* (PDR). The PDR, published yearly, is a compilation of manufacturers' package inserts for selected drugs.

Numerous drug handbooks and pharmacologic, medical, and nursing journals also contain information about drugs. Journal articles often present information about drug therapy for clients with specific disease processes and may thereby facilitate application of drug knowledge in clinical practice. Helpful Internet sites include Medscape (http://www.medscape.com), Food and Drug Administration (http://www.fda.gov), PharmInfo (http://pharminfo.com), and RxMed (http://www.rxmed.com).

FEDERAL DRUG LAWS AND STANDARDS

Current drug laws and standards have evolved over many years. The first federal law, the Pure Food and Drug Act of 1906, established official standards and requirements for accurate labeling of drug products. This law was amended in 1912 (Sherley Amendment) to prohibit fraudulent claims of efficacy and in 1914 (Harrison Narcotic

Act) to restrict and regulate the importation, manufacture, sale, and use of opium, cocaine, marijuana, and other drugs that the act defined as narcotics.

The next major legal development was the Food, Drug, and Cosmetic Act of 1938, the first law to require proof of safety before a new drug could be marketed. One amendment in 1945 required governmental certification of biologic products, such as insulin and antibiotics. A second amendment in 1952 (Durham-Humphrey Amendment) designated drugs that must be prescribed by a physician and dispensed by a pharmacist (prescription drugs). A third amendment in 1962 (Kefauver-Harris Amendment) required proof of effectiveness for drugs to remain commercially available and gave the federal government the authority to standardize drug names. Overall, this law and its amendments regulate the manufacture, distribution, advertising, and labeling of drugs in an attempt to ensure safety and effectiveness. It also confers official status on drugs listed in *The United States Pharmacopeia*. The names of these drugs may be followed by the letters *USP*. Official drugs must meet standards of purity and strength as determined by chemical analysis or animal response to specified doses (bioassay). The Food and Drug Administration (FDA) is charged with enforcing the law. In addition, the Public Health Service regulates vaccines and other biologic products, and the Federal Trade Commission can suppress misleading advertisements of nonprescription drugs.

In 1970, the Comprehensive Drug Abuse Prevention and Control Act was passed. Title II of this law, called the Controlled Substances Act, regulates distribution of narcotics and other drugs of abuse and categorizes these drugs according to therapeutic usefulness and potential for abuse. These categories are described in Box 1-1. In addition to federal laws, state laws also regulate the sale and distribution of controlled drugs.

Additional developments include the Drug Regulation Reform Act of 1978, which shortened the time required for developing and marketing new drugs; the Orphan Drug Act of 1983, which provided incentives to manufacturers (decreased taxes and competition) for producing drugs to treat certain serious disorders affecting relatively few people; and 1992 changes that require pharmaceutical companies to pay a user fee each time they file a new drug application—the fees pay for FDA staff and equipment to accelerate the FDA drug approval process. The most recent legislation, the FDA Modernization Act of 1997, changes the regulation of food, medical devices, and cosmetics. Its major provisions include continuation of the user fee, updated regulation of biologic products, increased patient access to experimental drugs and medical devices, and accelerated review of important new medications, and it allows drug companies to disseminate information about off-label (ie, non-FDA–approved) uses of drugs and costs of drugs.

Drug Approval Processes

The FDA is responsible for approving new drugs and certain other aspects of drug use. The FDA reviews research studies (usually conducted or sponsored by a pharmaceutical company) about proposed new drugs; the organization does not test the drugs.

Before passage of the Food, Drug, and Cosmetic Act and its amendments, many drugs were marketed without

---

BOX 1–1   CATEGORIES OF CONTROLLED SUBSTANCES

Schedule I

Drugs that are not approved for medical use and have high abuse potentials: heroin, lysergic acid diethylamide (LSD), peyote, mescaline, tetrahydrocannabinol, marijuana.

Schedule II

Drugs that are used medically and have high abuse potentials: opioid analgesics (eg, codeine, hydromorphone, methadone, meperidine, morphine, oxycodone, oxymorphone), central nervous system (CNS) stimulants (eg, cocaine, methamphetamine, methylphenidate), and barbiturate sedative-hypnotics (amobarbital, pentobarbital, secobarbital).

Schedule III

Drugs with less potential for abuse than those in Schedules I and II, but abuse may lead to psychological or physical dependence: androgens and anabolic steroids, some CNS stimulants (eg, benzphetamine), and mixtures containing small amounts of controlled substances (eg, codeine, barbiturates not listed in other schedules).

Schedule IV

Drugs with some potential for abuse: benzodiazepines (eg, diazepam, lorazepam, temazepam), other sedative-hypnotics (eg, phenobarbital, chloral hydrate), and some prescription appetite suppressants (eg, mazindol, phentermine).

Schedule V

Products containing moderate amounts of controlled substances. They may be dispensed by the pharmacist without a physician's prescription but with some restrictions regarding amount, record keeping, and other safeguards. Included are antidiarrheal drugs, such as diphenoxylate and atropine (Lomotil).

confirmation of safety or efficacy. Since 1962, however, newly developed drugs have been extensively tested before being marketed for general use. The drugs are carefully evaluated at each step. Testing usually proceeds if there is evidence of safety and effectiveness but may be stopped at any time for inadequate effectiveness or excessive toxicity. Many potential drugs are discarded and never marketed; a few drugs are marketed but later withdrawn, usually because of adverse effects that become evident only when the drug is used in a large, diverse population.

Testing and Clinical Trials

The testing process begins with animal studies to determine potential uses and effects. The next step involves FDA review of the data obtained in the animal studies. The drug then undergoes clinical trials in humans. Most clinical trials use a randomized, controlled experimental design that involves selection of subjects according to established criteria, random assignment of subjects to experimental groups, and administration of the test drug to one group and a control substance to another group.

In Phase I, a few doses are given to a few healthy volunteers to determine safe dosages, routes of administration, absorption, metabolism, excretion, and toxicity. In Phase II, a few doses are given to a few subjects with the disease or symptom for which the drug is being studied, and responses are compared with those of healthy subjects. In Phase III, the drug is given to a larger and more representative group of subjects. In double-blind, placebo-controlled designs, half the patients receive the new drug and half receive a placebo, with neither patients nor researchers knowing who receives which formulation. In crossover studies, subjects serve as their own controls; each subject receives the experimental drug during half the study and a placebo during the other half. Other research methods include control studies, in which some patients receive a known drug rather than a placebo, and subject matching, in which patients are paired with others of similar characteristics. Phase III studies help to determine whether the potential benefits of the drug outweigh the risks.

In Phase IV, the FDA evaluates the data from the first three phases for drug safety and effectiveness, allows the drug to be marketed for general use, and requires manufacturers to continue monitoring the drug's effects. Some adverse drug effects may become evident during the post-marketing phase as the drug is more widely used.

Food and Drug Administration Approval

The FDA approves many new drugs annually. In 1992, procedures were changed to accelerate the approval process, especially for drugs used to treat acquired immunodeficiency syndrome. Since then, new drugs are categorized according to their review priority and therapeutic potential. "1P" status indicates a new drug reviewed on a priority basis and with some therapeutic advantages over similar drugs already available; "1S" status indicates standard review and drugs with few, if any, therapeutic advantages (ie, the new drug is similar to one already available).

The FDA also approves transfer of drugs from prescription to nonprescription (over-the-counter or OTC) status. For drugs taken orally, indications for use may be different, and recommended doses are usually lower for nonprescription products.

CELLULAR PHYSIOLOGY

Because all body functions and disease processes and most drug actions take place at the cellular level, cellular physiology is reviewed. Each body cell has the capacity to function and respond to injury. Although cells differ in various tissues according to location and function, they have common characteristics as well. For example, all cells normally can exchange materials with their immediate environment to obtain energy from nutrients, synthesize complex molecules, and duplicate themselves. They also can communicate with each other through various biologic chemicals, such as neurotransmitters and hormones.

Cells (Fig. 1-1) are composed of *protoplasm*, which, in turn, is composed of water, proteins, lipids, carbohydrates, and electrolytes (potassium, magnesium, phosphate, sulfate, and bicarbonate). The protoplasm contains several structures. The *nucleus* directs cellular activities by determining the type and amount of proteins, enzymes, and other substances to be produced. The *cytoplasm* surrounds the nucleus and contains the working units of the cell. The *endoplasmic reticulum* (ER) contains ribosomes, which synthesize enzymes and other proteins. These include enzymes that synthesize glycogen, triglycerides, and steroids and those that detoxify drugs and other chemicals. Overall, the ER is important in the production of hormones by glandular cells and the production of plasma proteins and drug-metabolizing enzymes by liver cells.

The *Golgi complex* stores hormones and other substances produced by the ER. It also packages these substances into secretory granules, which then move out of the Golgi complex into the cytoplasm and, after an appropriate stimulus, are released from the cell through the process of exocytosis (see below).

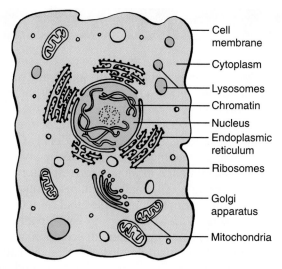

FIGURE 1–1 Schematic diagram of cell highlighting cytoplasmic organelles.

Mitochondria generate energy for cellular activities and require oxygen. *Lysosomes* are membrane-enclosed vesicles that contain enzymes capable of breaking down nutrients (proteins, carbohydrates, fats), foreign substances, and the cell itself. During phagocytosis, or when a cell becomes worn out or damaged, the membrane around the lysosome breaks and the enzymes are released. Thus, lysosomal enzymes are important in the digestion of cellular debris and phagocytized antigens. However, lysosomal contents also are released into extracellular spaces, destroying surrounding cells. They may cause the tissue destruction that sometimes accompanies inflammatory reactions. In addition, the enzymes act on complement to produce component C5a and on kinins to produce bradykinin, both of which are inflammatory mediators (Box 1-2). Normally, the enzymes (proteases) are inactivated by enzyme inhibitors (antiproteases) in serum and synovial fluids, and excessive tissue destruction is prevented.

The *cell membrane* separates intracellular contents from the extracellular environment, provides receptors for hormones and other biologically active substances, participates in electrical events that occur in nerve and muscle cells, and helps regulate growth and proliferation.

Substances enter and leave the cell by several transport mechanisms. In addition to the basic mechanisms (ie, diffusion, osmosis, facilitated diffusion, and active transport),

pinocytosis, phagocytosis, and exocytosis are important in inflammatory and immune processes. *Pinocytosis* involves the ingestion of small amounts of extracellular fluid and dissolved particles and is an important mechanism for the transport of proteins and electrolytes into cells. In this process, the cell membrane engulfs particles and forms a vesicle; the contents are eventually freed by lysosomal or other cytoplasmic enzymes. *Phagocytosis* resembles pinocytosis except that larger indentations occur in the cell membrane; these allow the cell to ingest large particles such as bacteria and cell debris. Microorganisms and particles become attached to phagocytic cells, where they are engulfed and killed or digested. *Exocytosis* is a mechanism for secreting intracellular substances into extracellular spaces. In this process, a fluid-filled sac fuses to the inner side of the cell membrane and opens to the external cell surface, where the contents are released into the extracellular fluid. Exocytosis allows the removal of cellular debris and the release of hormones and other substances synthesized inside the cell.

CELLULAR INJURY AND RESPONSE TO INJURY

Cellular injury may be caused by hypoxia, ischemia, microorganisms, chemicals, excessive heat or cold, radiation, and nutritional deficiencies or excesses. Chemicals, including therapeutic drugs, may injure the cell membrane and other cell structures, block enzymatic pathways, coagulate cell proteins, and disrupt the osmotic and ionic balance of the cell. Such injuries may result from the parent chemical or its metabolites. When a cell is injured, it accumulates water, fats, and other normal components and excessive amounts or abnormal types of products synthesized within the cell. These reversible changes lead to edema and impaired cellular function. If the damage continues long enough or is not repaired, the changes become irreversible and result in cell death and tissue necrosis.

Inflammatory and Immune Responses

Cellular response to injury involves inflammation, a generalized reaction to any tissue damage. Inflammation is

---

BOX 1–2   CHEMICAL MEDIATORS OF INFLAMMATION AND IMMUNITY

Bradykinin is a kinin in body fluids that becomes physiologically active with tissue injury. When tissue cells are damaged, white blood cells (WBCs) increase in the area and ingest damaged cells to remove them from the area. When the WBCs die, they release enzymes that activate kinins. The activated kinins increase and

prolong the vasodilation and increased vascular permeability caused by histamine. They also cause pain by stimulating nerve endings for pain in the area. Thus, bradykinin may aggravate and prolong the erythema, heat, and pain of local inflammatory reactions. It also increases mucous gland secretion.

(continued)

BOX 1–2 CHEMICAL MEDIATORS OF INFLAMMATION AND IMMUNITY (*continued*)

Complement is a group of plasma proteins essential to normal inflammatory and immunologic processes. More specifically, complement destroys cell membranes of body cells (eg, red blood cells, lymphocytes, platelets) and pathogenic microorganisms (eg, bacteria, viruses). The system is initiated by an antigen–antibody reaction or by tissue injury. Components of the system (called C1 through C9) are activated in a cascade type of reaction in which each component becomes a proteolytic enzyme that splits the next component in the series. Activation yields products with profound inflammatory effects. C3a and C5a, also called anaphylatoxins, act mainly by liberating histamine from mast cells and platelets, and their effects are therefore similar to those of histamine. C3a causes or increases smooth muscle contraction, vasodilation, vascular permeability, degranulation of mast cells and basophils, and secretion of lysosomal enzymes by leukocytes. C5a performs the same functions as C3a and also promotes movement of WBCs into the injured area (chemotaxis). In addition, it activates the lipoxygenase pathway of arachidonic acid metabolism (see leukotrienes, below) in neutrophils and macrophages, thereby inducing formation of even more substances that increase vascular permeability and chemotaxis.

In the immune response, the complement system breaks down antigen–antibody complexes, especially those in which the antigen is a microbial agent. It enables the body to produce inflammation and localize an infective agent. More specific reactions include increased vascular permeability, chemotaxis, and opsonization (coating a microbe or other antigen so it can be more readily phagocytized).

Cytokines may act on the cells that produce them, on surrounding cells, or on distant cells if sufficient amounts reach the bloodstream. Thus, cytokines act locally and systemically to produce inflammatory and immune responses, including increased vascular permeability and chemotaxis of macrophages, neutrophils, and basophils. Two major types of cytokines are interleukins (produced by leukocytes) and interferons (produced by T lymphocytes or fibroblasts). Interleukin-1 (IL-1) mediates several inflammatory responses, including fever, and IL-2 (also called T-cell growth factor) is required for the growth and function of T lymphocytes. Interferons are cytokines that protect nearby cells from invasion by intracellular microorganisms, such as viruses and rickettsiae. They also limit the growth of some cancer cells.

Histamine is formed (from the amino acid histidine) and stored in most body tissue, with high concentrations in mast cells, basophils, and platelets. Mast cells, which are abundant in skin and connective tissue, release his-

tamine into the vascular system in response to stimuli (eg, antigen–antibody reaction, tissue injury, and some drugs). Once released, histamine is highly vasoactive, causing vasodilation (increasing blood flow to the area and producing hypotension) and increasing permeability of capillaries and venules (producing edema). Other effects include contracting smooth muscles in the bronchi (producing bronchoconstriction and respiratory distress), gastrointestinal (GI) tract, and uterus; stimulating salivary, gastric, bronchial, and intestinal secretions; stimulating sensory nerve endings to cause pain and itching; and stimulating movement of eosinophils into injured tissue. Histamine is the first chemical mediator released in the inflammatory response and immediate hypersensitivity reactions (anaphylaxis).

When histamine is released from mast cells and basophils, it diffuses rapidly into other tissues. It then acts on target tissues through both histamine-1 (H_1) and histamine-2 (H_2) receptors. H_1 receptors are located mainly on smooth muscle cells in blood vessels and the respiratory and GI tracts. When histamine binds with these receptors, resulting events include contraction of smooth muscle, increased vascular permeability, production of nasal mucus, stimulation of sensory nerves, pruritus, and dilation of capillaries in the skin. H_2 receptors are also located in the airways, GI tract, and other tissues. When histamine binds to these receptors, there is increased secretion of gastric acid by parietal cells in the stomach mucosal lining, increased mucus secretion and bronchodilation in the airways, contraction of esophageal muscles, tachycardia, inhibition of lymphocyte function, and degranulation of basophils (with additional release of histamine and other mediators) in the bloodstream. In allergic reactions, both types of receptors mediate hypotension (in anaphylaxis), skin flushing, and headache. The peak effects of histamine occur within 1 to 2 minutes of its release and may last as long as 10 minutes, after which it is inactivated by histaminase (produced by eosinophils) or *N*-methyltransferase.

Platelet-activating factor (PAF), like prostaglandins and leukotrienes, is derived from arachidonic acid metabolism and has multiple inflammatory activities. It is produced by mast cells, neutrophils, monocytes, and platelets. Because these cells are widely distributed, PAF effects can occur in virtually every organ and tissue. Besides causing platelet aggregation, PAF activates neutrophils, attracts eosinophils, increases vascular permeability, causes vasodilation, and causes IL-1 and tumor necrosis factor-alpha (TNF-alpha) to be released. PAF, IL-1, and TNF-alpha can induce each other's release.

an attempt to remove the damaging agent and repair the damaged tissue. The hemodynamic aspect of inflammation includes vasodilation, which increases blood supply to the injured area, and increased capillary permeability, which allows fluid to leak into tissue spaces. The cellular aspect involves the movement of leukocytes (white blood cells [WBCs]) into the area of injury. WBCs are attracted to the injured area by bacteria, tissue debris, plasma protein fractions (complement; see Box 1-2), and other substances in a process called *chemotaxis*. Once they reach the area, they phagocytize causative agents and tissue debris.

White Blood Cells

Specific WBCs are granulocytes (neutrophils, eosinophils, and basophils) and nongranulocytes (monocytes and lymphocytes). Granulocytes often contain inflammatory mediators or digestive enzymes in their cytoplasm. *Neutrophils*, the body's main defense against pathogenic bacteria, are the major leukocytes in the bloodstream. Substances (eg, complement) released from infected or inflamed tissue cause neutrophils to migrate to the affected tissue. There, they localize the area of injury and phagocytize organisms or particles by releasing digestive enzymes and oxidative metabolites that kill engulfed pathogens or destroy other types of foreign particles. Neutrophils usually arrive within 90 minutes of injury, and their numbers increase greatly during the inflammatory process. They have a life span of approximately 10 hours.

Eosinophils increase during allergic reactions and parasitic infections. In parasitic infections, they bind to and kill the parasites. In hypersensitivity reactions, they produce enzymes that inactivate histamine and leukotrienes (see Box 1-2) and may produce other enzymes that destroy antigen–antibody complexes. Despite these generally beneficial effects, eosinophils also may aggravate tissue damage by releasing cytotoxic substances. *Basophils* release histamine, a major chemical mediator in inflammatory and immediate hypersensitivity reactions.

Nongranulocytes arrive several hours after injury, and monocytes usually replace neutrophils as the predominant WBC within 48 hours. Monocytes are the largest WBCs, and their life span is much longer than that of the granulocytes. Monocytes can phagocytize larger sizes and amounts of foreign material than neutrophils. In addition to their activity in the bloodstream, monocytes can leave blood vessels and enter tissue spaces (and then are called fixed tissue macrophages), although they can again become mobile and reenter the bloodstream in some circumstances. Tissue macrophages are widely distributed in connective tissue and other areas (eg, Kupffer's cells in the liver, alveolar macrophages in the lungs, others in the lymph nodes and spleen) and form the mononuclear phagocyte system. Both mobile and fixed monocytes are important in inflammatory and immune processes as the phagocytic cells digest or encapsulate foreign material and cellular debris. *Lymphocytes* include B cells, which are involved in antibody formation (humoral immunity), and T cells, which are involved in both cell-mediated and humoral immunity. Both types of lymphocytes play major roles in the immune response.

Chemical Mediators of Inflammation

Inflammatory (and immune) responses produce their effects indirectly, through complex interactions among cytokines and other chemical mediators. Cytokines are produced by WBCs and induce WBC replication, phagocytosis, antibody production, fever, inflammation, and tissue repair (see Box 1-2 and Chap. 42). Other chemical mediators are synthesized or released by mast cells, basophils, and other cells. Once activated, mediators may exert their effects on tissues locally or at distant target sites. They also may induce or enhance other mediators.

Prostaglandins and leukotrienes, mediators produced by the metabolism of arachidonic acid, play major roles in inflammation. When cellular injury occurs, phospholipase enzymes cause the phospholipids in cell membranes to release arachidonic acid. Arachidonic acid is then metabolized by cyclooxygenase enzymes (COX-1 and COX-2) to produce prostaglandins or lipoxygenase enzymes to produce leukotrienes (Fig. 1-2). Prostaglandins and leukotrienes are discussed in the following paragraphs; histamine and other important mediators are described in Box 1-2.

Prostaglandins are designated by PG, the letter E, F, G, or I, and the number of chemical bonds in their structure (eg, PGE_2). They are found in virtually all body tissues and act in the area where they are produced to regulate many cellular functions before being rapidly inactivated. The specific type of prostaglandin and its effects depend on the tissue involved, the stimulus, the type and amount of cyclooxygenase available, and the presence of receptors on tissue cells. For example, the lung and spleen are able to synthesize several prostaglandins. However, platelets form thromboxane A_2 because platelets mainly contain thromboxane synthase, and the endothelial cells that line blood vessels form prostacyclin (I_2) because they mainly contain prostacyclin synthase.

In the inflammatory process, prostaglandins cause or potentiate the vasodilation, vascular permeability, pain, and edema caused by other mediators (eg, bradykinin, histamine) in areas of tissue damage. They also regulate smooth muscle in blood vessels and the gastrointestinal (GI), respiratory, and reproductive systems; they protect GI mucosa from the erosive effects of gastric acid; they regulate the amount and distribution of renal blood flow; they control platelet function; and they maintain a patent ductus arteriosus in the fetus. Thus, prostaglandins exert various and opposing effects in different body tissues. Those produced by COX-1 enzymes are associated with platelet activation and protective effects on gastric mucosa and renal blood flow; those produced by COX-2 enzymes are associated with pain and inflammation.

Leukotrienes are formed by the lipoxygenase pathway of arachidonic acid metabolism and help regulate cellular

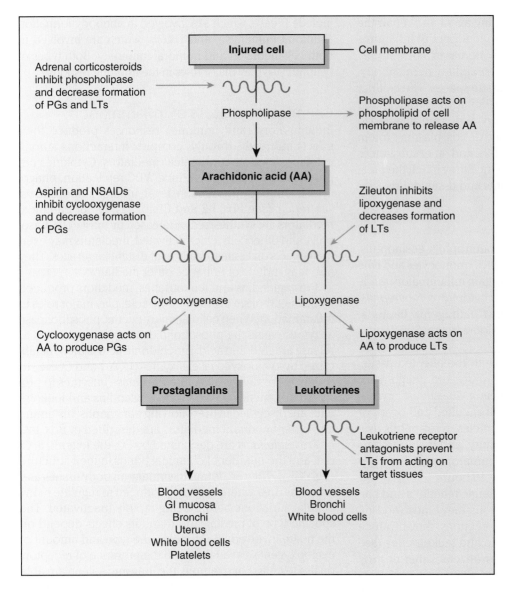

Adrenal corticosteroids inhibit phospholipase and decrease formation of PGs and LTs

Cell membrane

Injured cell

Phospholipase acts on phospholipid of cell membrane to release AA

Phospholipase

Arachidonic acid (AA)

Aspirin and NSAIDs inhibit cyclooxygenase and decrease formation of PGs

Zileuton inhibits lipoxygenase and decreases formation of LTs

Cyclooxygenase

Lipoxygenase

Cyclooxygenase acts on AA to produce PGs

Lipoxygenase acts on AA to produce LTs

Prostaglandins

Leukotrienes

Leukotriene receptor antagonists prevent LTs from acting on target tissues

Blood vessels
GI mucosa
Bronchi
Uterus
White blood cells
Platelets

Blood vessels
Bronchi
White blood cells

FIGURE 1–2 Production of prostaglandins (PGs) and leukotrienes (LTs): actions of anti-inflammatory drugs.

When a cell is injured, phospholipase acts on cell membrane phospholipid to release arachidonic acid. Metabolism of arachidonic acid produces the inflammatory mediators, prostaglandins and leukotrienes. Most anti-inflammatory drugs act to inhibit production of prostaglandins and/or leukotrienes. Leukotriene receptor antagonists occupy receptor sites on target tissues and prevent leukotrienes from acting on those tissues.

responses to injury, including inflammation. Leukotrienes are designated by LT, the letter B, C, D, or E, and the number of chemical bonds in their structure (eg, LTB_4). LTC_4, LTD_4, and LTE_4 (also called slow-releasing substances of anaphylaxis or SRS-A because they are released more slowly than histamine) cause sustained constriction of the bronchioles and are important mediators in bronchial asthma and immediate hypersensitivity reactions (anaphylaxis). The leukotrienes also may increase vascular permeability and movement of WBCs in injured tissues.

Characteristics of the Inflammatory Response

Local manifestations of inflammation include erythema, heat, edema, and pain. The erythema and heat result from vasodilation and increased blood supply, and edema results from leakage of blood plasma into the area. Pain is produced by the pressure of edema and secretions on

nerve endings and by the chemical irritation of bradykinin, histamine, and other substances released by the damaged cells. Prostaglandins increase the pain and edema caused by other mediators. Systemic manifestations include leukocytosis, increased erythrocyte sedimentation rate, fever, headache, loss of appetite, lethargy, and weakness. Both local and systemic manifestations vary according to the cause and extent of tissue damage. Skeletal muscle may be broken down to provide the amino acids required for the synthesis of substances used to repair injured tissue, such as lymphokines, immunoglobulins, fibroblasts, and collagen.

Inflammation may be acute or chronic. Acute inflammation involves the hemodynamic and cellular responses to injury described previously. It is often precipitated by a self-limited stimulus, such as infection, which may be controlled by host defenses. The inflamed area may heal completely, with the injured tissue returning to normal or near-normal appearance and function; it may progress and develop a purulent exudate composed of WBCs, proteins, and tissue debris; or it may become chronic.

Chronic inflammation may result from recurrent or progressive episodes of acute inflammation or from a low-grade, smoldering type of tissue response to persistent irritants (eg, foreign bodies; some viruses and bacteria, such as tuberculosis bacilli; and injured or altered tissue around a tumor or healing fracture). It follows a less consistent pattern, lasts longer (often months or years), and involves fewer neutrophils and more monocytes and lymphocytes in the affected area. It also produces more scar tissue, deformities, and impaired function. Little information is available about the chemical mediators of chronic inflammation, but immunologic mechanisms are thought to play an important role.

Characteristics of Anti-Inflammatory Drugs

Just as the inflammatory process needs to be activated appropriately to heal tissue injury, it also needs to be "turned off" appropriately. The strong chemical mediators must be deactivated to prevent further damage to injured tissue or damage to normal tissue. Deactivation is regulated largely by enzymes that metabolize the chemical mediators. For example, eosinophils produce enzymes that break down histamine (histaminase) and leukotrienes (arylsulfatase B). In most cases, inflammation eventually subsides. Anti-inflammatory drugs are needed when the inflammatory response is inappropriate, abnormal, or persistent, or destroys tissue.

Because inflammation may be a component of virtually any illness, anti-inflammatory drugs are extremely important in drug therapy. The main anti-inflammatory drugs are the adrenal corticosteroids (see Chap. 24), aspirin and other nonsteroidal anti-inflammatory drugs (NSAIDs; see Chap. 7), and leukotriene antagonists (see Chap. 47). The drugs' major mechanism of action is blocking arachidonic acid metabolism and decreasing production of prostaglandins or leukotrienes (see Fig. 1-2). In addition, two drugs (zafirlukast, montelukast) occupy leukotriene receptors on target tissues to prevent leukotrienes from exerting their effects. They are called leukotriene receptor antagonists (LTRAs).

Nursing Notes: Apply Your Knowledge

Answer: Meperidine (Demerol) is an opioid analgesic that is used to manage severe pain. Its abuse potential is high and it is therefore given a Schedule II classification. Diazepam (Valium) is an antianxiety agent that has some potential for abuse, so it is listed as a Schedule IV drug. Different references give you dif-

ferent information and are organized differently. A nursing textbook of pharmacology is comprehensive and gives you enough information to understand how drugs work. It is the best resource to use when you are first learning about drugs. Drug handbooks are helpful when you are trying to research specific information about a specific drug. They are arranged alphabetically and assume you have a basic understanding of pharmacology. The PDR is available in many health care facilities. It provides the reader with drug inserts from the manufacturer and color photographs of many medications. It is published annually, so it is a good resource for new drugs. Much information is provided, but without prioritization (eg, any reported side effect is given rather than identifying the most common or most serious side effects), which can make it difficult for a beginning student to use effectively.

 REVIEW AND APPLICATION EXERCISES

1. What is the difference between local and systemic effects of drugs?

2. Can a client experience systemic effects of local drugs and local effects of systemic drugs? Why or why not?

3. Why is it helpful for nurses to know the generic names of commonly used medications?

4. Why must nurses understand cellular physiology in relation to drug therapy?

5. How do body cells respond to injury?

6. What roles do histamine and prostaglandins play in the inflammatory process?

7. How do various anti-inflammatory drugs act to decrease inflammation?

SELECTED REFERENCES

Brestel, E.P. & Van Dyke, K. (1997). Antiinflammatory and antirheumatic drugs. In C.R. Craig & R.E. Stitzel (Eds.), *Modern pharmacology with clinical applications*, 5th ed., pp. 455–469. Boston: Little, Brown and Company.

Campbell, W.B. & Halushka, P.V. (1996). Lipid-derived autacoids. In J.G. Hardman, L.E. Limbird, P.B. Molinoff, & R.W. Ruddon (Eds.), *Goodman & Gilman's The pharmacological basis of therapeutics*, 9th ed., pp. 601–616. New York: McGraw-Hill.

Dayer, J.M. & Chizzolini, C. (1997). Inflammation: Cells, cytokines, and other mediators. In W.N. Kelley (Ed.), *Textbook of internal medicine*, 3rd ed., pp. 25–30. Philadelphia: Lippincott-Raven.

Guyton, A.C. & Hall, J.E. (1996). *Textbook of medical physiology*, 9th ed. Philadelphia: W.B. Saunders.

Nies, A.S. & Spielberg, S.P. (1996). Principles of therapeutics. In J.G. Hardman, L.E. Limbird, P.B. Molinoff, & R.W. Ruddon (Eds.), *Goodman & Gilman's The pharmacological basis of therapeutics*, 9th ed., pp. 43–62. New York: McGraw-Hill.

Sommers, C. (1998). Immunity and inflammation. In C.M. Porth (Ed.), *Pathophysiology: Concepts of altered health states*, 5th ed., pp. 189–212. Philadelphia: Lippincott Williams & Wilkins.

2

Basic Concepts and Processes

Objectives

After studying this chapter, the student will be able to:

1. Describe the main mechanisms by which drugs cross biologic membranes and move through the body.

2. Define each process of pharmacokinetics.

3. Describe drug-related factors that influence each pharmacokinetic process.

4. Describe client-related factors that influence each pharmacokinetic process.

5. Discuss drug actions at the cellular level (pharmacodynamics).

6. Describe major characteristics of the receptor theory of drug action.

7. Differentiate between agonist drugs and antagonist drugs.

8. Identify signs and symptoms that may occur with adverse drug effects on major body systems.

Mrs. Green, an 89-year-old widow, lives alone and has recently started taking many heart medications. She prides herself on being independent and able to manage on her own despite failing memory and failing health. When you visit as a home health nurse, you assess therapeutic and adverse effects of her medications.

Reflect on:

▶ Considering Mrs. Green's age, what factors might alter the pharmacokinetics (absorption, distribution, metabolism, excretion) of the drugs she takes? What data will you collect to determine her risk?

▶ What psychosocial factors could affect the therapeutic and adverse effects of Mrs. Green's medications? What data will be important to collect before developing a plan for Mrs. Green?

▶ When clients are taking many medications, the risk for drug interactions and toxicity increases. Describe how you will develop a plan to research possible drug interactions for any client.

Drugs are chemicals that alter basic physiochemical processes in body cells. They can stimulate or inhibit normal cellular functions. To act on body cells, drugs given for systemic effects must reach adequate concentrations in blood and other tissue fluids surrounding the cells. Thus, they must enter the body and be circulated in the bloodstream. After they act on cells, they must be eliminated from the body. This chapter describes the concepts and processes essential to understanding drug effects.

MECHANISMS OF DRUG MOVEMENT

The mechanisms of drug movement are passive diffusion, facilitated diffusion, and active transport.

Passive diffusion, the most common mechanism, involves movement of a drug from an area of higher concentration to one of lower concentration. For example, after oral administration, the initial concentration of a drug is higher in the gastrointestinal tract than in the blood. This promotes movement of the drug into the bloodstream. When the drug is circulated, the concentration is higher in the blood than in body cells, so that the drug moves into the fluids surrounding the cells or into the cells themselves. Passive diffusion continues until a state of equilibrium is reached between the amount of drug in the tissues and the amount in the blood.

Facilitated diffusion is a similar process, except that drug molecules combine with a carrier substance, such as an enzyme or other protein.

In *active transport*, drug molecules are moved from an area of lower concentration to one of higher concentration. This process requires a carrier substance and the release of cellular energy.

Drug movement, and therefore drug action, is affected by a drug's ability to cross cell membranes. For example, a drug given orally must pass through the cell membranes that line the intestinal tract, lymphatic vessels, and capillary walls to reach the bloodstream and circulate through the body. Cell membranes are complex structures composed of lipid and protein. Lipid-soluble drugs cross cell membranes by dissolving in the lipid layer; water-soluble drugs cross cell membranes through pores or channel openings. Lipid-soluble drugs can cross cell membranes more easily than water-soluble ones, and most drugs therefore are lipid soluble.

PHARMACOKINETICS

Pharmacokinetics involves drug movement through the body (ie, "what the body does to the drug"). Specific processes are absorption, distribution, metabolism (biotransformation), and excretion.

Absorption

Absorption is the process that occurs between the time a drug enters the body and the time it enters the bloodstream to be circulated. The rate and extent of absorption are affected by the dosage form of the drug, its route of administration, gastrointestinal function, and other variables. Dosage form is a major determinant of a drug's bioavailability (the portion of a dose that reaches the systemic circulation and is available to act on body cells).

Most oral drugs must be swallowed, dissolved in gastric fluid, and delivered to the small intestine before they are absorbed. Liquid medications are absorbed faster than tablets or capsules because they need not be dissolved. Increases in gastric emptying time and intestinal motility may increase drug absorption by promoting contact with absorptive mucous membrane. However, they also may decrease absorption because some drugs may move through the intestinal tract too rapidly to be absorbed. For most drugs, the presence of food in the stomach slows the rate of absorption and may decrease the amount of drug absorbed.

Drugs injected into subcutaneous or intramuscular tissues are usually absorbed more rapidly than oral drugs because they move directly from the injection site to the bloodstream. Absorption is rapid from intramuscular sites because muscle tissue has an abundant blood supply. Drugs injected intravenously do not need to be absorbed because they are placed directly into the bloodstream.

Other absorptive sites include the skin, mucous membranes, and lungs. Most drugs applied to the skin are given for local effects (eg, sunscreens). Systemic absorption is minimal from intact skin but may be considerable when the skin is inflamed or damaged. Also, a number of drugs have been formulated in adhesive skin patches for absorption through the skin (eg, clonidine, estrogen, fentanyl, nitroglycerin, scopolamine). Some drugs applied to mucous membranes also are given for local effects. However, systemic absorption occurs from the mucosa of the oral cavity, nose, eye, vagina, and rectum. Drugs absorbed through mucous membranes pass directly into the bloodstream. The lungs have a large surface area for absorption of anesthetic gases and a few other drugs.

Distribution

Distribution involves the transport of drug molecules within the body. Once a drug is injected or absorbed into the bloodstream, it is carried by the blood and tissue fluids to its sites of pharmacologic action, metabolism, and excretion. Drug molecules enter and leave the bloodstream through the capillaries. Distribution depends largely on the adequacy of blood circulation. Drugs are distributed rapidly to organs receiving a large blood supply, such as the heart, liver, and kidneys. Distribution to other internal organs, muscle, fat, and skin is usually slower.

An important factor in drug distribution is *protein binding* (Fig. 2-1). Most drugs form a complex with plasma proteins, mainly albumin, which act as carriers. Drug molecules bound to plasma proteins are pharmacologically inactive because the large size of the complex prevents their leaving the bloodstream through the small openings in capillary walls and reaching their sites of action, metabolism, and excretion. *Only the free or unbound portion of a drug acts on body cells.* As the free drug acts on cells, the decrease in plasma drug levels causes some of the bound drug to be released. Protein binding allows part of a drug dose to be stored and released as needed. This, in turn, maintains more even blood levels and reduces the risk of drug toxicity.

Protein binding is also the basis for some important drug–drug interactions. A drug with a strong attraction to protein-binding sites may displace a less tightly bound drug. The displaced drug then becomes pharmacologically active, and the overall effect is the same as taking a larger dose of the displaced drug.

Plasma protein binding is a method by which the body stores drugs. Some drugs also are stored in muscle, fat, or other body tissues and released gradually when plasma drug levels fall. Drugs that are highly bound to plasma proteins or stored extensively in other tissues have a long duration of action.

Drug distribution into the central nervous system (CNS) is limited because many drugs cannot pass the blood–brain barrier. The blood–brain barrier is composed of capillaries with tight walls that regulate diffusion of drug molecules from the bloodstream into brain tissue. This barrier usually acts as a selectively permeable membrane to protect the CNS. However, it also can make drug therapy of CNS disorders more difficult.

Drug distribution during pregnancy and lactation is also unique (see Chap. 67). During pregnancy, most drugs cross the placenta and may affect the fetus. During lactation, many drugs enter breast milk and may affect the nursing infant.

Metabolism

Metabolism is the method by which drugs are inactivated or biotransformed by the body. Most often, an active drug is changed into one or more inactive metabolites, which are then excreted. Some active drugs yield metabolites that are also active and that continue to exert their effects on body cells until they are metabolized further or excreted. Other drugs (called prodrugs) are initially inactive and exert no pharmacologic effects until they are metabolized.

Most drugs are lipid soluble, a characteristic that aids their movement across cell membranes. However, the kidneys, which are the primary excretory organs, can excrete only water-soluble substances. Therefore, one function of metabolism is to convert fat-soluble drugs into water-soluble metabolites.

Most drugs are metabolized by enzymes in the liver (called the cytochrome P450 enzyme system); red blood cells, plasma, kidneys, lungs, and gastrointestinal mucosa also contain drug-metabolizing enzymes. These enzymes, which are structurally complex proteins, catalyze the chemical reactions of oxidation, reduction, hydrolysis, and conjugation with endogenous substances, such as glucuronic acid or sulfate. With chronic administration, some drugs activate the hepatic enzymes, thereby accelerating drug metabolism. In a process called *enzyme induction*, the drugs stimulate liver cells to produce larger amounts of drug-metabolizing enzymes. Larger amounts of the enzymes then allow larger amounts of a drug to be metabolized during a given time. As a result, larger doses of the rapidly metabolized drug may be required to produce therapeutic effects.

Drugs that induce enzyme activity also may increase the rate of metabolism for endogenous steroidal hormones (eg, cortisol, estrogens, testosterone, and vitamin D). Metabolism also can be decreased or delayed in a process called *enzyme inhibition*, which most often occurs with concurrent administration of two or more drugs that compete for the same metabolizing enzymes. In this case, smaller doses of the slowly metabolized drug may be needed to avoid adverse reactions and toxicity from drug accumulation. The rate of drug metabolism also is reduced in infants because their hepatic enzyme system is immature, in people with impaired blood flow to the liver or severe hepatic or cardiovascular disease, and in people on low-protein diets.

When drugs are given orally, they are absorbed from the gastrointestinal tract and carried to the liver through the portal circulation. Some drugs are extensively metabolized in the liver, with only part of a drug dose reaching the systemic circulation for distribution to sites of action. This is called the *first-pass effect*.

Bloodstream

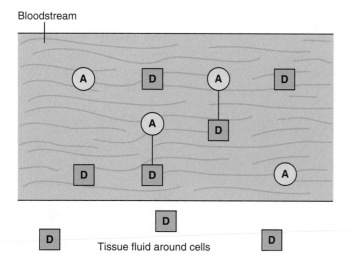

FIGURE 2–1   Plasma proteins, mainly albumin (A), act as carriers for drug molecules (D). Bound drug (A–D) stays in bloodstream and is pharmacologically inactive. Free drug (D) can leave the bloodstream and act on body cells.

Excretion

Excretion refers to elimination of a drug from the body. Effective excretion requires adequate functioning of the circulatory system and of the organs of excretion (kidneys, bowel, lungs, and skin). Most drugs are excreted by the kidneys and eliminated unchanged or as metabolites in the urine. Some drugs or metabolites are excreted in bile, then eliminated in feces; others are excreted in bile, re-absorbed from the small intestine, returned to the liver (called *enterohepatic recirculation*), metabolized, and eventually excreted in urine. Some oral drugs are not absorbed and are excreted in the feces. The lungs mainly remove volatile substances, such as anesthetic gases. The skin has minimal excretory function. Factors impairing excretion, especially severe renal disease, lead to drug accumulation and potentially severe adverse reactions if dosage is not reduced.

Serum Half-Life

Serum half-life, also called *elimination half-time*, is the time required for the serum concentration of a drug to decrease by 50%. It is determined primarily by the drug's rates of metabolism and excretion. A drug with a short half-life requires more frequent administration than one with a long half-life.

When a drug is given at a stable dose, approximately four or five half-lives are required to achieve steady-state concentrations and develop equilibrium between tissue and serum concentrations. Because maximal therapeutic effects do not occur until equilibrium is established, some drugs are not fully effective for days or weeks. To maintain steady-state conditions, the amount of drug given must equal the amount eliminated from the body. When a drug dose is changed, an additional four to five half-lives are required to re-establish equilibrium; when a drug is discontinued, it is eliminated gradually over several half-lives.

PHARMACODYNAMICS

Pharmacodynamics involves drug actions on target cells and the resulting alterations in cellular biochemical reactions and functions (ie, "what the drug does to the body").

Nursing Notes: Apply Your Knowledge

A client has a drug level of 100 units/mL. The drug's half-life is 1 hour. If concentrations above 25 units/mL are toxic and no more drug is given, how long will it take for the blood level to reach the nontoxic range?

Receptor Theory of Drug Action

Like the physiologic substances (eg, hormones and neurotransmitters) that normally regulate cell functions, most drugs exert their effects by chemically binding with receptors at the cellular level (Fig. 2-2). Receptors are mainly proteins located on the surfaces of cell membranes or within cells. Specific receptors include *enzymes* involved in essential metabolic or regulatory processes (eg, dihydrofolate reductase, acetylcholinesterase); *proteins* involved in transport (eg, sodium-potassium adenosine triphosphatase) or structural processes (eg, tubulin); and *nucleic acids* (eg, DNA) involved in cellular protein synthesis, reproduction, and other metabolic activities.

When drug molecules bind with receptor molecules, the resulting drug–receptor complex initiates physiochemical reactions that stimulate or inhibit normal cellular functions. One type of reaction involves activation, inactivation, or other alterations of intracellular enzymes. Because almost all cellular functions are catalyzed by enzymes, drug-induced changes can markedly increase or decrease the rate of cellular metabolism. For example, an epinephrine–receptor complex increases the activity of the intracellular enzyme adenyl cyclase, which then causes the formation of cyclic adenosine monophosphate (cAMP). cAMP, in turn, can initiate any one of many different intracellular actions, the exact effect depending on the type of cell.

A second type of reaction involves changes in the permeability of cell membranes to one or more ions. The receptor protein is a structural component of the cell membrane, and its binding to a drug molecule may open or close ion channels. In nerve cells, for example, sodium or

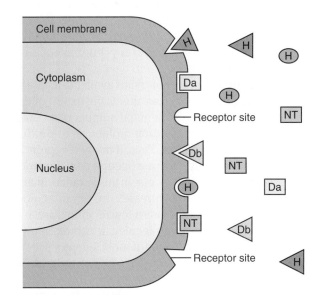

FIGURE 2–2 Cell membrane contains receptors for physiologic substances such as hormones (H) and neurotransmitters (NT). These substances stimulate or inhibit cellular function. Drug molecules (Da and Db) also interact with receptors to stimulate or inhibit cellular function.

calcium ion channels may open and allow movement of ions into the cell. This usually causes the cell membrane to depolarize and excite the cell. At other times, potassium channels may open and allow movement of potassium ions out of the cell. This action inhibits neuronal excitability and function. In muscle cells, movement of the ions into the cells may alter intracellular functions, such as the direct effect of calcium ions in stimulating muscle contraction.

A third reaction may modify the synthesis, release, or inactivation of the neurohormones (eg, acetylcholine, norepinephrine, serotonin) that regulate many physiologic processes.

Additional elements and characteristics of the receptor theory include:

1. The site and extent of drug action on body cells are determined primarily by specific characteristics of receptors and drugs. Receptors vary in type, location, number, and functional capacity. For example, many different types of receptors have been identified. Most types occur in most body tissues, such as receptors for epinephrine and norepinephrine (whether received from stimulation of the sympathetic nervous system or administration of drug formulations) and receptors for hormones, including growth hormone, thyroid hormone, and insulin. Some occur in fewer body tissues, such as receptors for opiates and benzodiazepines in the brain and subgroups of receptors for epinephrine in the heart (beta$_1$-adrenergic receptors) and lungs (beta$_2$-adrenergic receptors). Receptor type and location influence drug action. The receptor is often described as a lock into which the drug molecule fits as a key, and only those drugs able to bond chemically to the receptors in a particular body tissue can exert pharmacologic effects on that tissue. Thus, all body cells do not respond to all drugs, even though virtually all cell receptors are exposed to any drug molecules circulating in the bloodstream.

   The number of receptor sites available to interact with drug molecules also affects the extent of drug action. Presumably, a minimal number of receptors must be occupied by drug molecules to produce pharmacologic effects. Thus, if many receptors are available but only a few are occupied by drug molecules, few drug effects occur. In this instance, increasing the drug dosage increases the pharmacologic effects. Conversely, if only a few receptors are available for many drug molecules, receptors may be saturated. In this instance, if most receptor sites are occupied, increasing the drug dosage produces no additional pharmacologic effect.

   Drugs vary even more widely than receptors. Because all drugs are chemical substances, chemical characteristics determine drug actions and pharmacologic effects. For example, a drug's chemical structure affects its ability to reach tissue fluids around a cell and bind with its cell receptors. Minor changes in drug structure may produce major changes in pharmacologic effects. Another major factor is the concentration of drug molecules that reach receptor sites in body tissues. Drug- and client-related variables that affect drug actions are further described below.

2. When drug molecules chemically bind with cell receptors, the pharmacologic effects are those due to either agonism or antagonism. *Agonists* are drugs that produce effects similar to those produced by naturally occurring hormones, neurotransmitters, and other substances. Agonists may accelerate or slow normal cellular processes, depending on the type of receptor activated. For example, epinephrine-like drugs act on the heart to increase the heart rate, and acetylcholine-like drugs act on the heart to slow the heart rate; both are agonists. *Antagonists* are drugs that inhibit cell function by occupying receptor sites. This prevents natural body substances or other drugs from occupying the receptor sites and activating cell functions. Once drug action occurs, drug molecules may detach from receptor molecules (ie, the chemical binding is reversible), return to the bloodstream, and circulate to the liver for metabolism and the kidneys for excretion.

3. Receptors are dynamic cellular components that can be synthesized by body cells and altered by endogenous substances and exogenous drugs. For example, prolonged stimulation of body cells with an excitatory agonist usually reduces the number or sensitivity of receptors. As a result, the cell becomes less responsive to the agonist (a process called receptor desensitization or down-regulation). Prolonged inhibition of normal cellular functions with an antagonist may increase receptor number or sensitivity. If the antagonist is suddenly reduced or stopped, the cell becomes excessively responsive to an agonist (a process called receptor up-regulation). These changes in receptors may explain why some drugs must be tapered in dosage and discontinued gradually if withdrawal symptoms are to be avoided.

Nonreceptor Drug Actions

Relatively few drugs act by mechanisms other than combination with receptor sites on cells. These include:

1. Antacids, which act chemically to neutralize the hydrochloric acid produced by gastric parietal cells and thereby raise the pH of gastric fluid
2. Osmotic diuretics (eg, mannitol), which increase the osmolarity of plasma and pull water out of tissues into the bloodstream

3. Drugs that are structurally similar to nutrients required by body cells (eg, purines, pyrimidines) and that can be incorporated into cellular constituents, such as nucleic acids. This interferes with normal cell functioning. Several anticancer drugs act by this mechanism.
4. Metal chelating agents, which combine with toxic metals (eg, lead) to form a complex that can be more readily excreted

VARIABLES THAT AFFECT DRUG ACTIONS

Expected responses to drugs are largely based on those occurring when a particular drug is given to healthy adult men (18 to 65 years of age) of average weight (150 lb [70 kg]). However, other groups of people (eg, women, children, the elderly, different ethnic or racial groups, and clients with diseases or symptoms for which the drugs are designed to treat) receive drugs and respond differently than healthy adult men. Therefore, some authorities propose that these other groups be included in clinical trials. In any client, however, responses may be altered by both drug- and client-related variables, some of which are described in the following sections.

Drug-Related Variables

Dosage

Although the terms *dose* and *dosage* are often used interchangeably, dose usually indicates the amount to be given at one time and dosage refers to the frequency, size, and number of doses. Dosage is a major determinant of drug actions and responses, both therapeutic and adverse. If the amount is too small or administered infrequently, no pharmacologic action occurs because the drug does not reach an adequate concentration at cellular receptor sites. If the amount is too large or administered too often, toxicity (poisoning) may occur. Because dosage includes the amount of the drug and the frequency of administration, overdosage may occur with a single large dose or with chronic ingestion of smaller amounts. Doses that produce signs and symptoms of toxicity are called *toxic doses.* Doses that cause death are called *lethal doses.*

Dosages recommended in drug literature are usually those that produce particular responses in 50% of the people tested. These dosages usually produce a mixture of therapeutic and adverse effects. The dosage of a particular drug depends on many characteristics of the drug (reason for use, potency, pharmacokinetics, route of administration, dosage form, and others) and of the recipient (age, weight, state of health, and function of cardiovascular, renal, and hepatic systems). Thus, the recommended dosages are intended only as guidelines for individualizing dosages.

Route of Administration

Routes of administration affect drug actions and responses largely by influencing absorption and distribution. For rapid drug action and response, the intravenous route is most effective because the drug is injected directly into the bloodstream. For many drugs, the intramuscular route also produces drug action within a few minutes because muscles have a large blood supply. The oral route usually produces slower drug action than parenteral routes. Absorption and action of topical drugs vary according to the drug formulation, whether the drug is applied to skin or mucous membranes, and other factors.

Drug–Diet Interactions

Food may alter the absorption of oral drugs. In many instances, food slows the absorption of oral drugs by slowing gastric emptying time and altering gastrointestinal secretions and motility. When tablets or capsules are taken with or soon after food, they dissolve more slowly; therefore, drug molecules are delivered to absorptive sites in the intestine more slowly. Food also may decrease absorption by combining with a drug to form an insoluble drug–food complex. In other instances, however, certain drugs or dosage forms demonstrate enhanced absorption with certain types of meals. For example, a fatty meal increases the absorption of some sustained-release forms of theophylline. Interactions that alter drug absorption can be minimized by spacing food and medications.

In addition, some foods contain substances that react with certain drugs. One such interaction occurs between tyramine-containing foods and monoamine oxidase (MAO) inhibitor drugs. Tyramine causes the release of norepinephrine, a potent vasoconstrictive agent, from the adrenal medulla and sympathetic neurons. Normally, norepinephrine is active for only a few milliseconds before it is inactivated by MAO. However, because MAO inhibitors prevent inactivation of norepinephrine, ingesting tyramine-containing foods with an MAO inhibitor may produce severe hypertension or intracranial hemorrhage. MAO inhibitors include the antidepressants isocarboxazid (Marplan) and phenelzine (Nardil) and the antineoplastic procarbazine (Matulane). Tyramine-rich foods to be avoided by clients taking MAO inhibitors include beer, wine, aged cheeses, yeast products, chicken livers, and pickled herring.

An interaction may occur between oral anticoagulants, such as warfarin (Coumadin), and foods containing vitamin K. Because vitamin K antagonizes the action of oral anticoagulants, large amounts of green leafy vegetables, such as spinach and other greens, may offset the anticoagulant effects and predispose the person to thromboembolic disorders.

A third interaction occurs between tetracycline, an antibiotic, and dairy products, such as milk and cheese. The drug combines with the calcium in milk products to form an insoluble, unabsorbable compound that is excreted in the feces.

Drug–Drug Interactions

The action of a drug may be increased or decreased by its interaction with another drug in the body. Most interactions occur whenever the interacting drugs are present in the body; some, especially those affecting the absorption of oral drugs, occur when the interacting drugs are given at or near the same time.

Interactions that can increase the therapeutic or adverse effects of drugs are as follows:

1. *Additive effects* occur when two drugs with similar pharmacologic actions are taken.
   Example: alcohol + sedative drug → increased sedation

2. *Synergism or potentiation* occurs when two drugs with different sites or mechanisms of action produce greater effects when taken together than either does when taken alone.
   Example: acetaminophen (non-narcotic analgesic) + codeine (narcotic analgesic) → increased analgesia

3. *Interference* by one drug with the metabolism or elimination of a second drug may result in intensified effects of the second drug.
   Example: cimetidine (Tagamet) inhibits drug-metabolizing enzymes in the liver and therefore interferes with the metabolism of many drugs (eg, benzodiazepine antianxiety and hypnotic drugs, calcium channel blockers, tricyclic antidepressants, some antiarrhythmics, beta blockers and anticonvulsants, theophylline, and warfarin). When these drugs are given concurrently with cimetidine, they are more likely to cause adverse reactions and toxic effects. Cimetidine is a prescription drug for peptic ulcer disease and a nonprescription drug for heartburn.

4. *Displacement* of one drug from plasma protein-binding sites by a second drug increases the effects of the displaced drug. This increase occurs because the molecules of the displaced drug, freed from their bound form, become pharmacologically active.
   Example: aspirin (an anti-inflammatory/analgesic/antipyretic agent) + warfarin (an anticoagulant) → increased anticoagulant effect

Interactions in which drug effects are decreased are grouped under the term *antagonism*. Examples of such interactions are as follows:

1. In some situations, a drug that is a specific antidote is given to antagonize the toxic effects of another drug.
   Example: naloxone (a narcotic antagonist) + morphine (a narcotic analgesic) → relief of narcotic-induced respiratory depression. Naloxone molecules displace morphine molecules from their receptor sites on nerve cells so that the morphine molecules cannot continue to exert their depressant effects.

2. Decreased intestinal absorption of oral drugs occurs when drugs combine to produce nonabsorbable compounds.
   Example: aluminum or magnesium hydroxide (antacids) + oral tetracycline (an antibiotic) → binding of tetracycline to aluminum or magnesium, causing decreased absorption and decreased antibiotic effect of tetracycline

3. Activation of drug-metabolizing enzymes in the liver increases the metabolism rate of any drug metabolized primarily by that group of enzymes. Some anticonvulsants, antitubercular drugs, barbiturates, and antihistamines are known *enzyme inducers*.
   Example: phenobarbital (a barbiturate) + warfarin (an anticoagulant) → decreased effects of warfarin

4. Increased excretion occurs when urinary pH is changed and renal reabsorption is blocked.
   Example: sodium bicarbonate + phenobarbital → increased excretion of phenobarbital. The sodium bicarbonate alkalinizes the urine, raising the number of barbiturate ions in the renal filtrate. The ionized particles cannot pass easily through renal tubular membranes. Therefore, less drug is reabsorbed into the blood and more is excreted by the kidneys.

Client-Related Variables

Age

The effects of age on drug action are most pronounced in neonates, infants, and older adults. In children, drug action depends largely on age and developmental stage. During pregnancy, drugs cross the placenta and may harm the fetus. Fetuses have no effective mechanisms for metabolizing or eliminating drugs because their liver and kidney functions are immature. Newborn infants (birth to 1 month) also handle drugs inefficiently. Drug distribution, metabolism, and excretion differ markedly in neo-

---

How Can You Avoid This Medication Error?

Mr. Jones is a 69-year-old man who is taking warfarin, an anticoagulant. When warfarin was started, he was told not to take aspirin. Three weeks later, Mr. Jones experienced symptoms of a cold and started taking an over-the-counter (OTC) cold remedy. One week later, Mr. Jones noted large bruises on his arms and called his physician. What caused this adverse effect and how might it be avoided?

nates, especially premature infants, because their organ systems are not fully developed. Older infants (1 month to 1 year) reach approximately adult levels of protein binding and kidney function, but liver function and the blood–brain barrier are still immature.

Children (1 to 12 years) experience a period of increased activity of drug-metabolizing enzymes so that some drugs are rapidly metabolized and eliminated. Although the onset and duration of this period are unclear, a few studies have been done with particular drugs. Theophylline, for example, is cleared much faster in a 7-year-old child than in a neonate or adult (18 to 65 years). After approximately 12 years of age, healthy children handle drugs similarly to healthy adults.

In older adults (65 years and older), physiologic changes may alter all pharmacokinetic processes. Changes in the gastrointestinal tract include decreased gastric acidity, decreased blood flow, and decreased motility. Despite these changes, however, there is little difference in absorption. Changes in the cardiovascular system include decreased cardiac output and therefore slower distribution of drug molecules to their sites of action, metabolism, and excretion. In the liver, blood flow and metabolizing enzymes are decreased. Thus, many drugs are metabolized more slowly, have a longer action, and are more likely to accumulate with chronic administration. In the kidneys, there is decreased blood flow, decreased glomerular filtration rate, and decreased tubular secretion of drugs. All of these changes tend to slow excretion and promote accumulation of drugs in the body. Impaired kidney and liver function greatly increase the risks of adverse drug effects. In addition, older adults are more likely to have acute and chronic illnesses that require multiple drugs or long-term drug therapy. Thus, possibilities for interactions among drugs and between drugs and diseased organs are greatly multiplied.

Body Weight

Body weight affects drug action mainly in relation to dose. The ratio between the amount of drug given and body weight influences drug distribution and concentration at sites of action. In general, people heavier than average need larger doses, provided that their renal, hepatic, and cardiovascular functions are adequate. Recommended doses for many drugs are listed in terms of grams or milligrams per kilogram of body weight.

Genetic and Ethnic Characteristics

Drugs are given to elicit certain responses that are relatively predictable for most drug recipients. However, some people experience inadequate therapeutic effects, and others experience unusual or exaggerated effects, including increased toxicity. These interindividual variations in drug response are often attributed to genetic or ethnic differences in drug pharmacokinetics or pharmacodynamics.

As a result, there is increased awareness that genetic and ethnic characteristics are important factors and that diverse groups must be included in clinical trials.

Pharmacogenetics

Pharmacogenetics is concerned with genetically related variability in responses to drugs. A person's genetic characteristics may influence drug action in several ways. For example, genes determine the types and amounts of proteins produced in the body. When most drugs enter the body, they interact with proteins (eg, in plasma, tissues, cell membranes, and drug receptor sites) to reach their sites of action, and with other proteins (eg, drug-metabolizing enzymes in the liver and other organs) to be biotransformed and eliminated from the body. Genetic characteristics that alter any of these proteins can alter drug pharmacokinetics or pharmacodynamics.

One of the earliest pharmacokinetic genetic variations to be identified derived from the observation that some people taking usual doses of isoniazid (an antitubercular drug), hydralazine (an antihypertensive agent), or procainamide (an antiarrhythmic) showed no therapeutic effects, whereas toxicity developed in other people. Research established that these drugs are normally metabolized by acetylation, a chemical conjugation process in which the drug molecule combines with an acetyl group of acetyl coenzyme A. The reaction is catalyzed by a hepatic drug-metabolizing enzyme called acetyltransferase. It was further established that humans may acetylate the drug rapidly or slowly, depending largely on genetically controlled differences in acetyltransferase activity. Clinically, rapid acetylators may need larger-than-usual doses to achieve therapeutic effects, and slow acetylators may need smaller-than-usual doses to avoid toxic effects. In addition, several genetic variations of the cytochrome P450 drug-metabolizing system have been identified. Specific variations may influence any of the chemical processes by which drugs are metabolized.

As another example of genetic variation in drug metabolism, some people lack the plasma pseudocholinesterase enzyme that normally inactivates succinylcholine, a potent muscle relaxant used in major surgical procedures. These people may experience prolonged paralysis and apnea if given succinylcholine.

Other people are deficient in glucose-6-phosphate dehydrogenase, an enzyme normally found in red blood cells and other body tissues. These people may have hemolytic anemia when given antimalarial drugs, sulfonamides, analgesics, antipyretics, and other drugs.

Pharmacoanthropology

Pharmacoanthropology is concerned with racial and ethnic differences in responses to drugs. Most drug information has been derived from clinical drug trials using white men; few, if any, subjects of other ethnic groups are included. Interethnic variations became evident when drugs and dosages developed for white people produced unexpected responses, including toxicity, when given to other ethnic groups.

One common interethnic variation is that African Americans are less responsive to some antihypertensive drugs than are white people. For example, angiotensin-converting enzyme (ACE) inhibitors and beta-adrenergic blocking drugs are less effective as single-drug therapy. In general, African-American hypertensive clients respond better to diuretics or calcium channel blockers than to ACE inhibitors and beta blockers. Another interethnic variation is that Asians usually require much smaller doses of some commonly used drugs, including beta blockers and several psychotropic drugs (eg, alprazolam, an anti-anxiety agent, and haloperidol, an antipsychotic). Some documented interethnic variations are included in later chapters.

Gender

Except during pregnancy and lactation, gender has been considered a minor influence on drug action. Almost all research studies related to drugs have involved men, and clinicians have extrapolated the findings to women. Several reasons have been advanced for excluding women from clinical drug trials, including the risks to a fetus if a woman becomes pregnant and the greater complexity in sample size and data analysis. However, because differences between men and women in responses to drug therapy are being identified, the need to include women in drug studies is evident.

Some gender-related differences in responses to drugs may stem from hormonal fluctuations in women during the menstrual cycle. Although this area has received little attention in research studies and clinical practice, altered responses have been demonstrated in some women taking clonidine, an antihypertensive; lithium, a mood-stabilizing agent; phenytoin, an anticonvulsant; propranolol, a beta-adrenergic blocking drug used in the management of hypertension, angina pectoris, and migraine; and anti-depressants. For example, women with clinical depression may need higher doses of antidepressant medications premenstrually, when symptoms may be exacerbated, and lower doses during the rest of the menstrual cycle.

Another example is that women with schizophrenia require lower dosages of antipsychotic medications than men. If given the higher doses required by men, women are likely to have adverse drug reactions.

Pathologic Conditions

Pathologic conditions may alter pharmacokinetic processes (Table 2-1). In general, all pharmacokinetic processes are decreased in cardiovascular disorders characterized by decreased blood flow to tissues, such as heart failure. In addition, the absorption of oral drugs is decreased with various gastrointestinal disorders. Distribu-

tion is altered in liver or kidney disease and other conditions that alter plasma proteins. Metabolism is decreased in malnutrition (eg, inadequate protein to synthesize drug-metabolizing enzymes) and severe liver disease; it may be increased in conditions that generally increase body metabolism, such as hyperthyroidism and fever. Excretion is decreased in kidney disease.

Psychological Considerations

Psychological considerations influence individual responses to drug administration, although specific mechanisms are unknown. An example is the *placebo response*. A placebo is a pharmacologically inactive substance. Placebos are used in clinical drug trials to compare the medication being tested with a "dummy" medication. Interestingly, recipients often report both therapeutic and adverse effects from placebos.

Attitudes and expectations related to drugs in general, a particular drug, or a placebo influence client response. They also influence compliance or the willingness to carry out the prescribed drug regimen, especially with long-term drug therapy.

ADVERSE EFFECTS OF DRUGS

As used in this book, the term *adverse effects* refers to any undesired responses to drug administration, as opposed to *therapeutic effects*, which are desired responses. Most drugs produce a mixture of therapeutic and adverse effects; all drugs can produce adverse effects. Adverse effects may produce essentially any sign, symptom, or disease process and may involve any body system or tissue. They may be common or rare, mild or severe, localized or widespread, depending on the drug and the recipient.

Some adverse effects occur with usual therapeutic doses of drugs (often called side effects); others are more likely to occur and to be more severe with high doses. Common or serious adverse effects include the following:

1. *CNS effects* may result from CNS stimulation (eg, agitation, confusion, delirium, disorientation, hallucinations, psychosis, seizures) or CNS depression (dizziness, drowsiness, impaired level of consciousness, sedation, coma, impaired respiration and circulation). CNS effects may occur with many drugs, including most therapeutic groups, substances of abuse, and over-the-counter preparations.

2. *Gastrointestinal effects* (anorexia, nausea, vomiting, constipation, diarrhea) are among the most common adverse reactions to drugs. Nausea and vomiting occur with many drugs from local irritation of the gastrointestinal tract or stimulation of the vomiting center in the brain. Diarrhea occurs with drugs that cause local irritation or increase peristalsis.

(text continues on page 23)

TABLE 2-1	Effects of Pathologic Conditions on Drug Pharmacokinetics

Pathologic Conditions	Pharmacokinetic Consequences
Cardiovascular disorders that impair the pumping ability of the heart, decrease cardiac output, or impair blood flow to body tissues (eg, acute myocardial infarction, heart failure, hypotension, and shock)	*Absorption* of oral, subcutaneous, intramuscular, and topical drugs is erratic because of decreased blood flow to sites of drug administration. *Distribution* is impaired because of decreased blood flow to body tissues and thus to sites of drug action. *Metabolism* and *excretion* are impaired because of decreased blood flow to the liver and kidneys.
Central nervous system (CNS) disorders that alter respiration or circulation (eg, brain trauma or injury, brain ischemia from inadequate cerebral blood flow, drugs that depress or stimulate brain function)	CNS impairment may alter pharmacokinetics indirectly by causing hypo- or hyperventilation and acid–base imbalances. Also, cerebral irritation may occur with head injuries and lead to stimulation of the sympathetic nervous system and increased cardiac output. Increased blood flow may accelerate all pharmacokinetic processes. With faster absorption and distribution, drug action may be more rapid, but faster metabolism and excretion may shorten duration of action.

Gastrointestinal (GI) disorders that interfere with GI function or blood flow (eg, trauma or surgery of the GI tract, abdominal infection, paralytic ileus, pancreatitis)	Symptoms of impaired GI function commonly occur with both GI and non-GI disorders. As a result, many patients cannot take oral medications. Those who are able to take oral drugs may experience impaired *absorption* because of:
	    Vomiting or diarrhea.
	    Concurrent administration of drugs that raise the pH of gastric fluids (eg, antacids, histamine-2 blockers, proton pump inhibitors).
	    Concurrent administration of foods or tube feeding solutions that decrease drug absorption.
	    Crushing tablets or opening capsules to give a drug through a GI tube.

Inflammatory bowel disorders (eg, Crohn's disease, ulcerative colitis)	*Absorption* of oral drugs is variable. It may be increased because GI hypermotility rapidly delivers drug molecules to sites of absorption in the small intestine and the drugs tend to be absorbed more rapidly from inflamed tissue. It may be decreased because hypermotility and diarrhea may move the drug through the GI tract too rapidly to be adequately absorbed.
Endocrine disorders that impair function or change hormonal balance Diabetes-induced cardiovascular disorders	Impaired circulation may decrease all pharmacokinetic processes, as described previously.
Thyroid disorders	The main effect is on *metabolism*. Hypothyroidism slows metabolism, which prolongs drug action and slows elimination from the body. Hyperthyroidism accelerates metabolism, producing a shorter duration of action and a faster elimination rate. As a thyroid disorder is treated and thyroid function returns to normal, the rate of drug metabolism also returns to normal. Thus, dosages of drugs that are extensively metabolized need adjustments according to the level of thyroid function.
Adrenal disorders resulting from the underlying illness or the stress response that accompanies illness	Increased adrenal function (ie, increased amounts of circulating catecholamines and cortisol) affects drug action by increasing cardiac output, redistributing cardiac output (more blood flow to the heart and brain, less to kidneys, liver, and GI tract), causing fluid retention, and increasing blood volume. Stress also changes plasma protein levels, which can affect the unbound portion of a drug dose. Decreased adrenal function causes hypotension and shock, which impairs all pharmacokinetic processes.
Hepatic disorders that impair hepatic function and blood flow (eg, hepatitis, cirrhosis)	Most drugs are eliminated from the body by hepatic metabolism, renal excretion or both. Hepatic metabolism depends on hepatic blood flow, hepatic enzyme activity, and plasma protein binding. Increased hepatic blood flow increases delivery of drug molecules to hepatocytes, where metabolism occurs, and thereby accelerates drug metabolism. Decreased hepatic blood flow slows metabolism. Severe liver disease or cirrhosis may impair all pharmacokinetic processes. *Absorption* of oral drugs may be decreased in cirrhosis because of edema in the GI tract. *Distribution* may be altered by changes in plasma proteins. The impaired liver may be unable to synthesize adequate amounts of plasma proteins, especially albumin. Also, liver impairment leads to inadequate metabolism and accumulation of substances (eg, serum bilirubin) that can displace drugs from protein-binding sites. With decreased protein binding, the serum concentration of active drug is increased and the drug is distributed to sites of action and elimination more rapidly. Thus, onset of drug action may be faster, peak blood levels may be higher and cause adverse effects, and the duration of action may be shorter because the drug is metabolized and excreted more quickly.

(continued)

TABLE 2-1	Effects of Pathologic Conditions on Drug Pharmacokinetics (*continued*)
Pathologic Conditions	**Pharmacokinetic Consequences**
	With cirrhosis, oral drugs are distributed directly into the systemic circulation rather than going through the portal circulation and the liver first. This shunting of blood around the liver means that oral drugs that are normally extensively metabolized during their first pass through the liver (eg, propranolol) must be given in reduced doses to prevent high blood levels and toxicity. *Metabolism* may be impaired by hepatic and nonhepatic disorders that reduce hepatic blood flow. In addition, an impaired liver may not be able to synthesize adequate amounts of drug-metabolizing enzymes. *Excretion* may be increased when protein binding is impaired because larger amounts of free drug are circulating in the bloodstream and being delivered more rapidly to sites of metabolism and excretion. The result is a shorter drug half-life and duration of action. Excretion is decreased when the liver is unable to metabolize lipid-soluble drugs into water-soluble metabolites that can be excreted by the kidneys.
Renal impairment—acute renal failure (ARF) and chronic renal failure (CRF)	ARF and CRF can interfere with all pharmacokinetic processes. *Absorption* of oral drugs may be decreased indirectly by changes that often occur with renal failure (eg, delayed gastric emptying, changes in gastric pH, GI symptoms such as vomiting and diarrhea). Also, in the presence of generalized edema, edema of the GI tract may impair absorption. In CRF, gastric pH may be increased by administration of oral alkalinizing agents (eg, sodium bicarbonate, citrate) and the use of antacids for phosphate-binding effects. This may decrease absorption of oral drugs that require an acidic environment for dissolution and absorption and increase absorption of drugs that are absorbed from a more alkaline environment. *Distribution* of many drugs may be altered by changes in extracellular fluid volume (ECF), plasma protein binding, and tissue binding. Water-soluble drugs are distributed throughout the ECF, including edema fluid, which is usually increased in renal impairment because the kidney's ability to eliminate water and sodium is impaired. Drug binding with albumin, the main drug-binding plasma protein for acidic drugs, is usually decreased with renal impairment. Protein binding may be decreased because of less albumin or decreased binding capacity of albumin for a drug. Reasons for decreased albumin include hypermetabolic states (*eg*, stress, trauma, sepsis) in which protein breakdown exceeds protein synthesis, nephrotic states in which albumin is lost in the urine, and liver disease that decreases hepatic synthesis of albumin. Reasons for reduced binding capacity include structural changes in the albumin molecule or uremic toxins that compete with drugs for binding sites. When less drug is bound to albumin, the higher serum drug levels of unbound or active drug can result in drug toxicity. In addition, more unbound drug is available for distribution into tissues and sites of metabolism and excretion so that faster elimination can decrease drug half-life and therapeutic effects. For basic drugs (eg, clindamycin, propafenone), alpha$_1$-acid glycoprotein (AAG) is the main binding protein. The amount of AAG increases in some patients, including those with renal transplants and those receiving hemodialysis. If these patients are given a basic drug, a larger amount is bound and a smaller amount is free to exert a pharmacologic effect. Finally, some conditions that often occur in renal impairment (eg, metabolic acidosis, respiratory alkalosis, others) may alter tissue distribution of some drugs. For example, digoxin can be displaced from tissue-binding sites by metabolic products that cannot be adequately excreted by impaired kidneys. *Metabolism* can be increased, decreased, or unaffected by renal impairment. One factor is alteration of drug metabolism in the liver. In uremia, reduction and hydrolysis reactions may be slower, but oxidation by cytochrome P450 enzymes and conjugation with glucuronide or sulfate usually proceed at normal rates. Another factor is the inability of impaired kidneys to eliminate drugs and pharmacologically active metabolites, which may lead to accumulation and adverse drug reactions with long-term drug therapy. Metabolites may have pharmacologic activity similar to or different from that of the parent drug. A third factor may be impaired renal metabolism of drugs. Although the role of the kidneys in excretion of drugs and drug metabolites is well known, their role in drug metabolism has received little attention. The kidney itself contains

TABLE 2-1	Effects of Pathologic Conditions on Drug Pharmacokinetics (*continued*)
Pathologic Conditions	**Pharmacokinetic Consequences**
	many of the same metabolizing enzymes found in the liver, including renal cytochrome P450 enzymes, which metabolize a variety of chemicals and drugs. *Excretion* of many drugs and metabolites is reduced by renal impairment. The kidneys normally excrete both the parent drug and metabolites produced by the liver and other tissues. Processes of renal excretion include glomerular filtration, tubular secretion, and tubular reabsorption, all of which may be affected by renal impairment. If the kidneys are unable to excrete drugs and metabolites, some of which may be pharmacologically active, these substances may accumulate and cause adverse or toxic effects.
Respiratory impairments	Respiratory impairment may indirectly affect drug metabolism. For example, hypoxemia leads to decreased enzyme production in the liver, decreased efficiency of the enzymes that are produced, and decreased oxygen available for drug biotransformation. Mechanical ventilation leads to decreased blood flow to the liver.
Sepsis-induced alterations in cardiovascular function and hepatic blood flow	Sepsis may affect all pharmacokinetic processes. Early sepsis is characterized by hyperdynamic circulation, with increased cardiac output and shunting of blood to vital organs. As a result, absorption, distribution, metabolism, and excretion may be accelerated. Late sepsis is characterized by hypodynamic circulation, with diminished cardiac output and reduced blood flow to major organs. Thus, absorption, distribution, metabolism, and excretion may be impaired.
Shock-induced alterations in cardiovascular function and blood flow	Shock may inhibit all pharmacokinetic processes. *Absorption* is impaired by decreased blood flow to sites of drug administration. *Distribution* is impaired by decreased blood flow to all body tissues. *Metabolism* is impaired by decreased blood flow to the liver. *Excretion* is impaired by decreased blood flow to the kidneys.

More serious effects include bleeding or ulceration (most often with aspirin and nonsteroidal anti-inflammatory agents) and severe diarrhea/colitis (most often with antibiotics).

3. *Hematologic effects* (blood coagulation disorders, bleeding disorders, bone marrow depression, anemias, leukopenia, agranulocytosis, thrombocytopenia) are relatively common and potentially life threatening. Excessive bleeding is most often associated with anticoagulants and thrombolytics; bone marrow depression is usually associated with antineoplastic drugs.

4. *Hepatotoxicity* (hepatitis, hepatic necrosis, biliary tract inflammation or obstruction) is relatively rare but potentially life threatening. Because most drugs are metabolized by the liver, the liver is especially susceptible to drug-induced injury. Drugs that are hepatotoxic include acetaminophen (Tylenol), chlorpromazine (Thorazine), isoniazid (INH), methotrexate (Mexate), phenelzine (Nardil), phenytoin (Dilantin), and aspirin and other salicylates. In the presence of drug- or disease-induced liver damage, the metabolism of many drugs is impaired. Consequently, drugs metabolized by the liver tend to accumulate in the body and cause adverse effects. Besides actual hepatotoxicity, many drugs produce abnormal values in liver function tests without producing clinical signs of liver dysfunction.

5. *Nephrotoxicity* (nephritis, renal insufficiency or failure) occurs with several antimicrobial agents (eg, gentamicin and other aminoglycosides), nonsteroidal anti-inflammatory agents (eg, ibuprofen and related drugs), and others. It is potentially serious because it may interfere with drug excretion, thereby causing drug accumulation and increased adverse effects.

6. *Hypersensitivity* or *allergy* may occur with almost any drug in susceptible clients. It is largely unpredictable and unrelated to dose. It occurs in those who have previously been exposed to the drug or a similar substance (antigen) and who have developed antibodies. When readministered, the drug reacts with the antibodies to cause cell damage and the release of histamine and other intracellular substances. These substances produce reactions ranging from mild skin rashes to anaphylactic shock. Anaphylactic shock is a life-threatening hypersensitivity reaction characterized by respiratory distress and cardiovascular collapse. It occurs within a few minutes after drug administration and requires emergency treatment with epinephrine. Some allergic reactions (eg, serum sickness) occur 1 to 2 weeks after the drug is given.

7. *Drug fever* is a fever associated with administration of a medication. Drugs can cause fever by several mechanisms, including allergic reactions, damaging body tissues, increasing body heat or interfering

with its dissipation, or acting on the temperature-regulating center in the brain. The most common mechanism is an allergic reaction. Fever may occur alone or with other allergic manifestations (eg, skin rash, hives, joint and muscle pain, enlarged lymph glands, eosinophilia) and its pattern may be low grade and continuous or spiking and intermittent. It may begin within hours after the first dose if the client has taken the drug before, or within approximately 10 days of continued administration if the drug is new to the client. If the causative drug is discontinued, fever usually subsides within 48 to 72 hours unless drug excretion is delayed or significant tissue damage has occurred (eg, hepatitis).

Many drugs have been implicated as causes of drug fever, including most antimicrobials, several cardiovascular agents (eg, beta blockers, hydralazine, methyldopa, procainamide, quinidine), drugs with anticholinergic properties (eg, atropine, some antihistamines, phenothiazine antipsychotic agents, and tricyclic antidepressants), and some anticonvulsants.

8. *Idiosyncrasy* refers to an unexpected reaction to a drug that occurs the first time it is given. These reactions are usually attributed to genetic characteristics that alter the person's drug-metabolizing enzymes.

9. *Drug dependence* may occur with mind-altering drugs, such as opioid analgesics, sedative-hypnotic agents, antianxiety agents, and CNS stimulants. Dependence may be physiologic or psychological. Physiologic dependence produces unpleasant physical symptoms when the dose is reduced or the drug is withdrawn. Psychological dependence leads to excessive preoccupation with drugs and drug-seeking behavior. Drug dependence is discussed further in Chapter 15.

10. *Carcinogenicity* is the ability of a substance to cause cancer. Several drugs are carcinogens, including some hormones and anticancer drugs. Carcinogenicity apparently results from drug-induced alterations in cellular DNA.

11. *Teratogenicity* is the ability of a substance to cause abnormal fetal development when given to pregnant women. Drug groups considered teratogenic include analgesics, diuretics, antihistamines, antibiotics, antiemetics, and others.

TOLERANCE AND CROSS-TOLERANCE

Drug *tolerance* occurs when the body becomes accustomed to a particular drug over time so that larger doses must be given to produce the same effects. Tolerance may be acquired to the pharmacologic action of many drugs, especially narcotic analgesics, alcohol, and other CNS

depressants. Tolerance to pharmacologically related drugs is called *cross-tolerance*. For example, a person who regularly drinks large amounts of alcohol becomes able to ingest even larger amounts before becoming intoxicated—this is tolerance to alcohol. If the person is then given sedative-type drugs or a general anesthetic, larger-than-usual doses are required to produce a pharmacologic effect—this is cross-tolerance.

Tolerance and cross-tolerance are usually attributed to activation of drug-metabolizing enzymes in the liver, which accelerates drug metabolism and excretion. They also are attributed to decreased sensitivity or numbers of receptor sites.

Nursing Notes: Apply Your Knowledge

Answer: Half-life is the time required for the serum concentration of a drug to decrease by 50%. After 1 hour, the serum concentration would be 50 units/mL (100/2). After 2 hours, the serum concentration would be 25 units/mL (50/2) and reach the nontoxic range.

How Can You Avoid This Medication Error?

Answer: More complete client teaching could have prevented this adverse effect for Mr. Jones. Although few OTC cold remedies still contain aspirin, some contain ibuprofen, a close relative of aspirin (see Chap. 7). The combination of warfarin and ibuprofen could have caused Mr. Jones' bruising. Clients taking warfarin should be instructed to consult their physician or read the labels very carefully before taking any OTC medications.

 REVIEW AND APPLICATION EXERCISES

1. What are some factors that decrease absorption of an oral drug?

2. Drug dosage is a major determinant of both therapeutic and adverse drug effects. How can you use this knowledge in monitoring a client's response to drug therapy?

3. Does protein binding speed or slow drug distribution to sites of action?

4. Are drugs equally distributed throughout the body? Why or why not?

5. What are the implications of hepatic enzyme induction and inhibition in terms of drug metabolism and elimination from the body?

6. For a drug in which biotransformation produces active metabolites, is drug action shortened or lengthened? What difference does this make in client care?

7. Which pharmacokinetic processes are likely to be impaired with severe cardiovascular disease and with severe renal disease?

8. What are the main elements of the receptor theory of drug action?

9. When drug–drug interactions occur, are drug actions increased or decreased?

10. Giving the same drug and dosage to different clients often results in differences in blood levels and other client responses. What are some reasons for individual differences in responses to drugs?

SELECTED REFERENCES

Benet, L.Z., Kroetz, D.L., & Sheiner, L.B. (1996). Pharmacokinetics: The dynamics of drug absorption, distribution, and elimination. In J.G. Hardman, L.E. Limbird, P.B. Molinoff, & R.W. Ruddon (Eds.), *Goodman & Gilman's The pharmacological basis of therapeutics*, 9th ed., pp. 3–27. New York: McGraw-Hill.

DiPiro, J.T. & Stafford, C.T. (1997). Allergic and pseudoallergic drug reactions. In J.T. DiPiro, R.L. Talbert, G.C. Yee, G.R. Matzke, B.G. Wells, & L.M. Posey (Eds.), *Pharmacotherapy: A pathophysiologic approach*, 3rd ed., pp. 1675–1688. Stamford, CT: Appleton & Lange.

Edwards, J. (1997). Guarding against adverse drug events. *American Journal of Nursing, 97*(5), 26–31.

Haken, V. (1996). Interactions between drugs and nutrients. In L.K. Mahan & S. Escott-Stump, *Krause's food, nutrition, and diet therapy*, 9th ed., pp. 387–402. Philadelphia: W.B. Saunders.

Lawson, W.B. (1996). Clinical issues in the pharmacotherapy of African-Americans. *Psychopharmacology Bulletin, 32*(2), 275–281.

Mackowiak, P.A. (1997). Approach to the febrile patient. In W.N. Kelley (Ed.), *Textbook of internal medicine*, 3rd ed, pp. 1565–1570. Philadelphia: Lippincott-Raven.

Nies, A.S. & Spielberg, S.P. (1996). Principles of therapeutics. In J.G. Hardman, L.E. Limbird, P.B. Molinoff, & R.W. Ruddon (Eds.), *Goodman & Gilman's The pharmacological basis of therapeutics*, 9th ed., pp. 43–62. New York: McGraw-Hill.

Rock, A. (1998). A dose of trouble. *Money, 27*(12), 122–128.

Ross, E.M. (1996). Pharmacodynamics: Mechanisms of drug action and the relationship between drug concentration and effect. In J.G. Hardman, L.E. Limbird, P.B. Molinoff, & R.W. Ruddon (Eds.), *Goodman & Gilman's The pharmacological basis of therapeutics*, 9th ed., pp. 29–41. New York: McGraw-Hill.

Administering Medications

Objectives

After studying this chapter, the student will be able to:

1. List the five rights of drug administration.

2. Discuss knowledge and skills needed to implement the five rights.

3. List requirements of a complete drug order or prescription.

4. Accurately interpret drug orders containing common abbreviations.

5. Discuss advantages and disadvantages of oral, parenteral, and topical routes of drug administration.

6. Identify supplies, techniques, and observations needed for safe and accurate administration by different routes.

Ms. Mabel Zack is transferred to your rehabilitation facility after a cerebral vascular accident (stroke) 2 weeks ago. When you review her chart, it indicates she has right-sided hemiparesis, memory deficits, and dysphagia (difficulty swallowing).

Reflect on:

▶ Outline appropriate assessments to determine if it is safe to give Ms. Zack oral medications.

▶ If a swallowing evaluation indicates that Ms. Zack can take medications orally, what precautions can you take to help ensure her safety?

▶ How might you individualize your teaching plan, considering Ms. Zack's memory deficits?

Drugs given for therapeutic purposes are called *medications*. Giving medications to clients is an important nursing responsibility in many health care settings, including ambulatory care, hospitals, long-term care facilities, and clients' homes. The basic requirements for accurate drug administration are often called the "five rights": giving the right *drug*, in the right *dose*, to the right *client*, by the right *route*, at the right *time*. Each "right" requires knowledge, skills, and specific nursing interventions:

1. Right drug
   a. Interpret the physician's order accurately (ie, name of drug).
   b. Question the prescriber if the name of the drug is unclear or if the drug seems inappropriate for the client's condition.
   c. If the drug is unfamiliar, seek information from an authoritative source.
   d. Read labels of drug containers accurately.
2. Right dose
   a. Interpret abbreviations and measurements accurately.
   b. Calculate and measure doses accurately.
   c. Question the prescriber if the dose is unclear or seems inappropriate for the client's age and condition.
3. Right client
   a. Check identification bands on institutionalized clients.
   b. Verify identity of ambulatory clients.
4. Right route
   a. Use correct techniques for all routes of administration.
   b. Always use appropriate anatomic landmarks to identify sites for intramuscular (IM) injections.
   c. For intravenous (IV) medications, follow manufacturers' instructions for preparation and administration.
5. Right time
   a. Schedule to maximize therapeutic effects and minimize adverse effects.
   b. Omit or delay doses as indicated by the client's condition.

Drug administration in children is potentially more problematic than in most other clients. One reason is that many drugs are prepared in dosage forms and concentrations suitable for adults. This often requires dilution (which may change the drug's stability and compatibility), calculation, preparation, and administration of minute doses (which are more likely to be inaccurate and possibly toxic than standard doses). In addition, children have limited sites for administration of IV drugs, and several may be given through the same site. In many cases, the need for small volumes of fluid precludes extensive flushing between drugs (which may produce undesirable interactions with other drugs and IV solutions).

How Can You Avoid This Medication Error?

You are administering 6 AM medications to a client on a medical unit. You enter Mr. Gonzales' room, gently shake him awake, and call him by name. He slowly awakens and appears groggy. You explain that you have his medications, which he takes and quickly falls back to sleep. On exiting the room, you look at the room number and realize that you just gave medications to Mr. Sanchez.

PREVENTING MEDICATION ERRORS

There are several steps and numerous people involved in getting each dose of a medication to the intended client. Each step or person has a potential for contributing to a medication error.

Physicians are usually very knowledgeable about disease processes. However, in relation to drug therapy, they may write orders illegibly; order a drug that is not indicated by the client's condition; fail to order a drug that is indicated; fail to consider the client's age, size, kidney function, liver function, and disease process when selecting a drug or dosage; fail to consider other medications the client is taking, including prescription and over-the-counter drugs; lack sufficient knowledge about the drug; fail to monitor for, or instruct others to monitor for, effects of administered drugs; and fail to discontinue drugs appropriately.

Pharmacists are usually very knowledgeable about drugs and their uses in various situations. However, in many instances, they do not have access to information about individual clients or they are not consulted and involved in client care. As a result, they may not recognize an inappropriate or erroneous physician's order. They may dispense incorrect medications, mislabel containers, or fail to ask outpatients about other drugs being taken.

Nurses may have inadequate knowledge about a drug or about the client receiving the drug; not follow the "five rights"; not read drug labels sufficiently; give unfamiliar drugs; fail to question the physician's order when indicated; and assume that the physician has ordered and the pharmacist has dispensed the correct medication. In addition, nurses must be able to distinguish among drugs with similar names or similar packaging.

Clients/consumers may take drugs from several physicians; fail to inform one physician about drugs prescribed by another; get prescriptions filled at more than one pharmacy; fail to get prescriptions filled or refilled; underuse or overuse an appropriately prescribed drug; take drugs left over from a previous illness or prescribed for someone else; fail to follow instructions for drug administration or storage; fail to keep appointments for follow-up care; and fail to ask for information about prescribed and unprescribed drugs when needed.

All health care providers involved in drug therapy must be extremely vigilant in all phases of medication administration. The rest of this chapter emphasizes general information needed to fulfill nursing responsibilities related to drug administration.

MEDICATION SYSTEMS

Each agency has a system for dispensing drugs. The unit-dose system, in which most drugs are dispensed in single-dose containers, is widely used. Drug orders are checked by a pharmacist or pharmacy technician, who then places the indicated number of doses in the client's medication drawer at scheduled intervals. When a dose is due, the nurse removes the medication and takes it to the client. Unit-dose wrappings of oral drugs should be left in place until the medication is given at the client's bedside. Each dose of a drug must be recorded on a medication administration record (MAR), which becomes part of the client's permanent medical record.

Advantages of the unit-dose system include spending less time preparing drugs for administration, being able to identify most drugs until they are administered to the client, and having to calculate fewer doses. The major disadvantage is having to reorder or otherwise obtain a needed dose when it is not in the client's medication drawer. This may lead to delayed or omitted doses.

Controlled drugs, such as opioid analgesics, are usually kept as a stock supply in a locked drawer or cabinet and replaced as needed. Each dose is signed out on a special narcotic sheet and recorded on the client's MAR. Each nurse must comply with legal regulations and agency policies for dispensing and recording controlled drugs.

MEDICATION ORDERS

Nurses administer medications from orders by licensed physicians, dentists, or nurse practitioners. Drug orders should include the full name of the client; the generic or trade name of the drug; the dose, route, and frequency of administration; and the date, time, and signature of the prescriber.

For clients in a hospital or other health care agency, written orders are safer and much preferred, but occasionally verbal or telephone orders are acceptable. These are written on the client's order sheet, signed by the person taking the order, and later countersigned by the physician. Once the order is written, a copy is sent to the pharmacy, where the order is recorded and the drug is dispensed to the appropriate client care unit. In many institutions, pharmacy staff prepare a computer-generated MAR for each 24-hour period.

For clients in ambulatory care settings, the procedure is essentially the same for drugs to be given immediately. For drugs to be taken at home, written prescriptions are given. In addition to the previous information, a prescription should include instructions for taking the drug (eg, dose and frequency) and whether the prescription can be refilled. Prescriptions for Schedule II controlled drugs cannot be refilled; a new prescription is required.

To interpret medication orders accurately, the nurse must know commonly used abbreviations for routes, dosages, and times of drug administration (Table 3-1). If the nurse cannot read the physician's order or if the order seems erroneous, he or she must question the order before giving the drug.

DRUG PREPARATIONS AND DOSAGE FORMS

Drug preparations and dosage forms vary according to the drug's chemical characteristics, purpose, and route of

TABLE 3-1	Common Abbreviations

Routes of Drug Administration

IM	intramuscular
IV	intravenous
OD	right eye
OS	left eye
OU	both eyes
PO	by mouth, oral
SC	subcutaneous
SL	sublingual

Drug Dosages

cc	cubic centimeter
g	gram
gr	grain
gt	drop*
mg	milligram
mL	milliliter
oz	ounce
tbsp	tablespoon
tsp	teaspoon

Times of Drug Administration

ac	before meals
ad lib	as desired
bid	twice daily
hs	bedtime
pc	after meals
PRN	when needed
qd	every day, daily
q4h	every four hours
qid	four times daily
qod	every other day
stat	Immediately
tid	three times daily

*drops = gtt.

administration. Some drugs are available in only one dosage form; others are available in several forms.

Dosage forms of systemic drugs include liquids, tablets, capsules, suppositories, and transdermal and pump delivery systems. Systemic liquids are given orally (PO) or parenterally. Those given by injection must be sterile.

Tablets and capsules are given PO. Tablets contain active drug plus binders, colorants, preservatives, and other substances. Capsules contain active drug enclosed in a gelatin capsule. Most tablets and capsules dissolve in the acid fluids of the stomach and are absorbed in the alkaline fluids of the upper small intestine. Enteric-coated tablets and capsules are coated with a substance that is insoluble in stomach acids. This delays dissolution until the medication reaches the intestine, usually to avoid gastric irritation or to keep the drug from being destroyed by gastric acid. Tablets for sublingual or buccal administration must be specifically formulated for such use.

Several controlled-release dosage forms or drug delivery systems have been developed to allow less frequent administration and more consistent serum drug levels. Newer formulations and mechanisms of release continue to be developed. Transdermal (skin patch) formulations include systemically absorbed clonidine, estrogen, fentanyl, nitroglycerin, and scopolamine. Pump delivery systems may be external or implanted under the skin and refillable or long acting without refills. Pumps are used to administer insulin, narcotic analgesics, antineoplastics, and other drugs.

Ointments, creams, and suppositories are applied topically to skin or mucous membranes. They are formulated for the intended route of administration.

CALCULATING DRUG DOSAGES

Nurses in most practice settings are infrequently required to calculate drug doses because pharmacists usually perform the necessary calculations before dispensing drugs. Still, when calculations are needed, the importance of accuracy cannot be overemphasized. Accuracy requires basic skills in mathematics, knowledge of common units of measurement, and methods of using data in performing calculations.

Commonly Used Systems of Measurement

The most commonly used system of measurement is the *metric system*, in which the meter is used for linear measure, the gram for weight, and the liter for volume. One milliliter (mL) equals 1 cubic centimeter (cc), and both equal 1 gram (g) of water. The *apothecary system*, now obsolete and rarely used, has units called grains, minims, drams, ounces, pounds, pints, and quarts. The *household system*, with units of drops, teaspoons, tablespoons, and cups, is infrequently used in health care agencies but may be used at home. Table 3-2 lists equivalent measurements within and among these systems. Equivalents are approximate.

A few drugs are ordered and measured in terms of units or milliequivalents (mEq). Units express biologic activity in animal tests (ie, the amount of drug required to produce a particular response). Units are unique for each drug. For example, concentrations of insulin and heparin are both expressed in units, but there is no relation between a unit of insulin and a unit of heparin. These drugs are usually ordered in the number of units per dose (eg, NPH insulin 30 units subcutaneously [SC] every morning, or heparin 5000 units SC q12h) and labeled in number of units per milliliter (U 100 insulin contains 100 units/mL; heparin may have 1000, 5000, or 10,000 units/mL). Milliequivalents express the ionic activity of a drug. Drugs such as potassium chloride are ordered and labeled in the number of milliequivalents per dose, tablet, or milliliter.

Mathematical Calculations

Most drug orders and labels are expressed in metric units of measurement. If the amount specified in the order is the same as that on the drug label, no calculations are required, and preparing the right dose is a simple matter. For example, if the order reads "acetaminophen 325 mg PO" and the drug label reads "acetaminophen 325-mg tablets," it is clear that one tablet is to be given.

What happens if the order calls for a 650-mg dose and 325-mg tablets are available? The question is, "How many 325-mg tablets are needed to give a dose of 650 mg?"

TABLE 3-2	Equivalents		
Metric		**Apothecary**	**Household**
1 mL = 1 cc		= 15 or 16 minims	= 15 or 16 drops
4 or 5 mL		= 1 fluid dram	= 1 tsp
60 or 65 mg		= 1 gr	
30 or 32 mg		= ½ gr	
30 g = 30 mL		= 1 oz	= 2 tbsp
250 mL		= 8 oz	= 1 cup
454 g		= 1 lb	
500 mL = 500 cc		= 16 oz = 1 pint	= 1 pint
1 L = 1000 mL		= 32 oz = 1 quart	= 1 quart
1000 μg* = 1 mg			
1000 mg = 1 g			
1000 g = 1 kg		= 2.2 lb	= 2.2 lb
0.6 g = 600 mg or 650 mg		= 10 gr	

*μg = microgram.

In this case, the answer can be readily calculated mentally to indicate two tablets. This is a simple example that also can be used to illustrate mathematical calculations. This problem can be solved by several acceptable methods; the following formula is presented because of its relative simplicity for students lacking a more familiar method.

$$\frac{D}{H} = \frac{X}{V}$$

D = desired dose (dose ordered, often in milligrams)
H = on-hand or available dose (dose on the drug label, often in mg/tablet, capsule, or milliliter)
X = unknown (number of tablets, in this example)
V = unit (one tablet, here)

$$\frac{650 \text{ mg}}{325 \text{ mg}} = \frac{X \text{ tablets}}{1 \text{ tablet}}$$

Cross multiply:

$$325X = 650$$

$$X = \frac{650}{325} = 2 \text{ tablets}$$

What happens if the order and the label are written in different units? For example, the order may read "amoxicillin 0.5 g" and the label may read "amoxicillin 500 mg/capsule." To calculate the number of capsules needed for the dose, the first step is to convert 0.5 g to the equivalent number of milligrams, or convert 500 mg to the equivalent number of grams. The desired or ordered dose and the available or label dose *must* be in the same units of measurement. Using the equivalents (ie, 1 g = 1000 mg) listed in Table 3-2, an equation can be set up as follows:

$$\frac{1 \text{ g}}{1000 \text{ mg}} = \frac{0.5 \text{ g}}{X \text{ mg}}$$

$$X = 0.5 \times 1000 = 500 \text{ mg}$$

The next step is to use the new information in the formula, which then becomes:

$$\frac{D}{H} = \frac{X}{V}$$

$$\frac{500 \text{ mg}}{500 \text{ mg}} = \frac{X \text{ capsules}}{1 \text{ capsule}}$$

$$500X = 500$$

$$X = \frac{500}{500} = 1 \text{ capsule}$$

The same procedure and formula can be used to calculate portions of tablets or dosages of liquids. These are illustrated in the following problems:

1. Order: 25 mg PO
   Label: 50-mg tablet

$$\frac{25 \text{ mg}}{50 \text{ mg}} = \frac{X \text{ tablet}}{1 \text{ tablet}}$$

$$50X = 25$$

$$X = \frac{25}{50} = 0.5 \text{ tablet}$$

2. Order: 25 mg IM
   Label: 50 mg in 1 cc

$$\frac{25 \text{ mg}}{50 \text{ mg}} = \frac{X \text{ cc}}{1 \text{ cc}}$$

$$50X = 25$$

$$X = \frac{25}{50} = 0.5 \text{ cc}$$

3. Order: 50 mg PO
   Label: 10 mg/cc

$$\frac{50 \text{ mg}}{10 \text{ mg}} = \frac{X \text{ cc}}{1 \text{ cc}}$$

$$10X = 50$$

$$X = \frac{50}{10} = 5 \text{ cc}$$

4. Order: Heparin 5000 units
   Label: Heparin 10,000 units/mL

$$\frac{5000 \text{ units}}{10,000 \text{ units}} = \frac{X \text{ mL}}{1 \text{ mL}}$$

$$10,000X = 5000$$

$$X = \frac{5000}{10,000} = 0.5 \text{ mL}$$

5. Order: KCl 20 mEq
   Label: KCl 10 mEq/5 mL

$$\frac{20 \text{ mEq}}{10 \text{ mEq}} = \frac{X \text{ mL}}{5 \text{ mL}}$$

$$10X = 100$$

$$X = \frac{100}{10} = 10 \text{ mL}$$

ROUTES OF ADMINISTRATION

Routes of administration depend on drug characteristics, client characteristics, and desired responses. The major routes are oral, parenteral, and topical. Each has advantages, disadvantages, indications for use, and specific techniques of administration.

Oral Route

The oral route is most often used. It is simple, convenient, and relatively inexpensive, and it can be used by most people. The main disadvantages are slower drug action and irritation of gastrointestinal mucosa, which may produce adverse effects such as anorexia, nausea, vomiting, diarrhea, and ulceration.

Drugs also may be given through tubes placed into the gastrointestinal tract, such as nasogastric or gastrostomy tubes. In people who cannot take drugs orally for prolonged periods, this route is preferable to injections.

Parenteral Routes

The term *parenteral* refers to any route other than gastrointestinal (enteral), but is commonly used to indicate SC, IM, and IV injections. Injections require special drug preparations, equipment, and techniques.

Drugs for Injection

Parenteral drugs must be prepared, packaged, and administered in ways to maintain sterility. Vials are closed glass or plastic containers with rubber stoppers through which a sterile needle can be inserted for withdrawing medication. Single-dose vials usually do not contain a preservative and must be discarded after a dose is withdrawn; multiple-dose vials contain a preservative and may be reused if aseptic technique is maintained.

Ampules are sealed glass containers, the tops of which must be broken off to allow insertion of a needle and withdrawal of the medication. Broken ampules and any remaining medication are discarded; they are no longer sterile and cannot be reused. When vials or ampules contain a powder form of the drug, a sterile solution of water or 0.9% sodium chloride must be added and the drug dissolved before withdrawal. Use a filter needle to withdraw the medication from an ampule because broken glass may need to be removed from the drug solution.

Many injectable drugs, including various concentrations of commonly used parenteral opioid analgesics, are available in ready-to-use plastic or glass syringes with attached needles. These units are inserted into specially designed holders and used like other needle/syringe units.

Equipment for Injections

Sterile needles and syringes are used to contain, measure, and administer parenteral medications. They may be packaged together or separately. Needles are available in various gauges and lengths. The term *gauge* refers to lumen size, with larger numbers indicating smaller lumen sizes. For example, a 25-gauge needle is smaller than an 18-gauge needle. Choice of needle gauge and length depends on the route of administration, the viscosity of the solution to

be given, and the size of the client. Usually, a 25-gauge, ⅝-inch needle is used for SC injections and a 22- or 20-gauge, 1½-inch needle for IM injections. Other needle sizes are available for special uses, such as intradermal injections.

In many settings, needleless systems are being used. These involve a plastic cannula on the syringe instead of a needle and vials that can be entered with the cannula and then reseal themselves. They were developed because of the risk of injury and spread of blood-borne pathogens, such as the viruses that cause acquired immunodeficiency syndrome and hepatitis B. When needles are used, avoid recapping them, and dispose of them appropriately.

Syringes also are available in various sizes. The 3-mL size is probably used most often. It is usually plastic and is available with or without an attached needle. Syringes are calibrated so that drug doses can be measured accurately. However, the calibrations vary according to the size and type of syringe.

Insulin and tuberculin syringes are used for specific purposes. Insulin syringes are calibrated to measure up to 100 units of insulin. Safe practice requires that *only* insulin syringes be used to measure insulin and that they be used for no other drugs. Tuberculin syringes have a capacity of 1 mL. They should be used for small doses of any drug because measurements are more accurate than with larger syringes.

Subcutaneous Route

The SC route involves the injection of drugs under the skin. This route is used for a small volume (approximately 1 mL or less) of drug. Absorption is slower and drug action is usually longer with SC injections than with IV or IM injections. The SC route is commonly used for only a few drugs (eg, insulin). Many drugs cannot be given SC because they are irritating to tissues and may cause tissue necrosis and abscess formation. Common sites for SC injections are the upper arms, abdomen, back, and thighs (Fig. 3-1).

Intramuscular Route

The IM route involves the injection of drugs into certain muscles. This route is used for several drugs, usually in doses of 3 mL or less. Absorption is more rapid than from SC injections because muscle tissue has a greater blood supply. Site selection is especially important with IM injections because incorrect needle placement may damage blood vessels or nerves. Commonly used sites are the deltoid, dorsogluteal, ventrogluteal, and vastus lateralis. These sites must be selected by first identifying anatomic landmarks (Figs. 3-2 through 3-5).

Intravenous Route

The IV route involves the injection of a drug into the bloodstream. Drugs given IV act rapidly, and larger amounts can

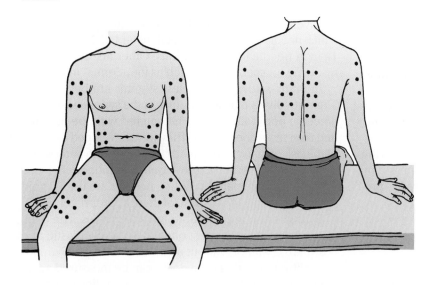

FIGURE 3-1 Subcutaneous injection sites.

be given than by SC or IM injection. One way of giving drugs IV is to prepare the drug with a needle and syringe, insert the needle into a vein, and inject the drug. More often, however, drugs are given through an established IV line, intermittently or continuously. Direct injection is useful for emergency drugs, intermittent infusion is often used for antibiotics, and continuous infusion is used for potassium chloride and a few other drugs. The nurse should wear latex gloves to start IV infusions for protection against exposure to blood-borne pathogens.

Drug administration is usually more comfortable and convenient for the client through an IV line. Disadvantages of this route include the time and skill required for venipuncture, the difficulty of maintaining an IV line, the greater potential for adverse reactions from rapid drug action, and possible complications of IV therapy (ie, bleeding, infection, fluid overload).

Other Parenteral Routes

Other parenteral routes include injection into layers of the skin (intradermal), arteries (intra-arterial), joints (intra-articular), and cerebrospinal fluid (intrathecal). Nurses may administer drugs intradermally or intra-arterially (if

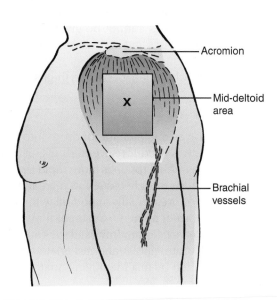

FIGURE 3-2 Placement of the needle for insertion into the deltoid muscle. The area of injection is bounded by the lower edge of the acromion on the top to a point on the side of the arm opposite the axilla on the bottom. The side boundaries of the rectangular site are parallel to the arm and one third and two thirds of the way around the side of the arm.

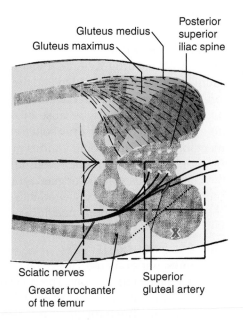

FIGURE 3-3 Proper placement of the needle for an intramuscular injection into the dorsogluteal site. It is above and outside a diagonal line drawn from the greater trochanter of the femur to the posterior superior iliac spine. Notice how this site allows the nurse to avoid entering an area near the sciatic nerve and the superior gluteal artery.

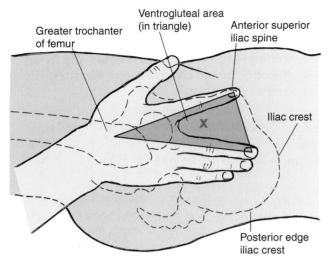

FIGURE 3–4 Placement of the needle for insertion into the ventrogluteal area. Notice how the nurse's palm is placed on the greater trochanter and the index finger on the anterior superior iliac spine. The middle finger is spread posteriorly as far as possible along the iliac crest. The injection is made in the middle of the triangle formed by the nurse's fingers and the iliac crest.

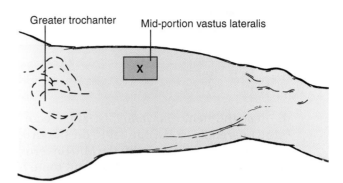

FIGURE 3–5 Placement of the needle for insertion into the vastus lateralis. It is usually easier to have the client lying on his or her back. However, the client may be sitting when using this site for intramuscular injections. It is a suitable site for children when the nurse grasps the muscle in her hand to concentrate the muscle mass for injection.

an established arterial line is present); physicians administer intra-articular and intrathecal medications.

Topical Routes

Topical administration involves the application of drugs to the skin or mucous membranes. Application to mucous membranes includes drugs given by nasal or oral inhalation; by instillation into the lungs, eyes, or nose; and by insertion under the tongue (sublingual), into the cheek (buccal), and into the vagina or rectum.

An advantage of topical administration is that many of the drugs act locally where applied; therefore, the likelihood of systemic adverse reactions is decreased. (How-

ever, several drugs are given topically for systemic effects.) A disadvantage is that specific drug preparations must be used for the various routes. Thus, only dermatologic preparations are safe to use on the skin, only ophthalmic drugs are used in the eyes, only a few drugs are given sublingually or buccally, and only vaginal or rectal preparations are given by those respective routes.

(*text continues on page 40*)

Nursing Notes: Apply Your Knowledge

Your client has a nasogastric feeding tube in place. You will be administering morning medications, including 4 tablets, 1 capsule, and 10 cc of an elixir. Describe how you will safely administer medications through a feeding tube to this client.

NURSING ACTIONS	Drug Administration

NURSING ACTIONS	**RATIONALE/EXPLANATION**
1. **Follow general rules for administering medications safety and effectively.**	
a. Prepare and give drugs in well-lighted areas, as free of interruptions and distractions as possible.	To prevent errors in selecting ordered drugs, calculating dosages, and identifying clients
b. Wash hands before preparing medications and, if needed, during administration.	To prevent infection and cross-contamination
c. Use sterile technique in preparing and administering injections.	To prevent infection. Sterile technique involves using sterile needles and syringes, using sterile *(continued)*

NURSING ACTIONS	**RATIONALE/EXPLANATION**
	drug solutions, not touching sterile objects to any unsterile objects, and cleansing injection sites with an antiseptic.
d. Read the medication administration record (MAR) carefully. Read the label on the drug container, and compare with the MAR in terms of drug, dosage or concentration, and route of administration.	For accurate drug administration. Most nursing texts instruct the nurse to read a drug label three times: when removing the container, while measuring the dose, and before returning the container.
e. Do not leave medications unattended.	To prevent accidental or deliberate ingestion by anyone other than the intended person. Also, to prevent contamination or spilling of medications.
f. Identify the client, preferably by comparing the identification wristband to the medication sheet.	This is the best way to verify identity. Calling by name, relying on the name on a door or bed, and asking someone else are unreliable methods, although they must be used occasionally when the client lacks a name band.
g. Identify yourself, if indicated, and state your reason for approaching the client. For example, "I'm . . . I have your medication for you."	Explaining actions helps to decrease client anxiety and increase cooperation in taking prescribed medication.
h. Position the client appropriately for the intended route of administration.	To prevent complications, such as aspiration of oral drugs into the lungs
i. Provide water or other supplies as needed.	To promote comfort of the client and to ensure drug administration
j. Do not leave medications at the bedside as a general rule. Common exceptions are antacids, nitroglycerin, and eye medications.	To prevent omitting or losing the drug or hoarding of the drug by the client
k. Do not give a drug when signs and symptoms of toxicity are present. Notify the physician, and record that the drug was omitted and why.	Additional doses of a drug increase toxicity. However, drugs are not omitted without a careful assessment of the client's condition and a valid reason.
l. Record drug administration (or omission) as soon as possible and according to agency policies.	To maintain an accurate record of drugs received by the client
m. If it is necessary to omit a scheduled dose for some reason, the decision to give the dose later or omit it depends largely on the drug and frequency of administration. Generally, give drugs ordered once or twice daily at a later time. For others, omit the one dose, and give the drug at the next scheduled time.	Clients may be unable to take the drug at the scheduled time because of diagnostic tests or many other reasons. A temporary change in the time of administration—usually for one dose only—may be necessary to maintain therapeutic effects.
n. For medications ordered as needed (PRN), assess the client's condition; check the physician's orders or MAR for the name, dose, and frequency of administration; and determine the time of the most recently administered dose.	Administration of PRN medications requires nursing assessment and decision making. Analgesics, antiemetics, and antipyretics are often ordered PRN.
o. For narcotics and other controlled substances, sign drugs out on separate narcotic records according to agency policies.	To meet legal requirements for dispensing controlled substances

(continued)

NURSING ACTIONS	RATIONALE/EXPLANATION
p. If, at any time during drug preparation or administration, any question arises regarding the drug, the dose, or whether the client is supposed to receive it, check the original physician's order. If the order is not clear, call the physician for clarification before giving the drug.	To promote safety and prevent errors. The same procedure applies when the client questions drug orders at the bedside. For example, the client may state he has been receiving different drugs or different doses.
2. For oral medications:	
a. With adults	
(1) To give tablets or capsules, open the unit-dose wrapper, place medication in a medicine cup, and give the cup to the client. For solutions, hold the cup at eye level, and measure the dosage at the bottom of the meniscus. For suspensions, shake or invert containers to mix the medication before measuring the dose.	To maintain clean technique and measure doses accurately. Suspensions settle on standing, and if not mixed, diluent may be given rather than the active drug.
(2) Have the client in a sitting position when not contraindicated.	To decrease risks of aspirating medication into lungs. Aspiration may lead to difficulty in breathing and aspiration pneumonia.
(3) Give before, with, or after meals as indicated by the specific drug.	Food in the stomach usually delays drug absorption and action. It also decreases gastric irritation, a common side effect of oral drugs. Giving drugs at appropriate times in relation to food intake can increase therapeutic effects and decrease adverse effects.
(4) Give most oral drugs with a full glass (8 oz) of water or other fluid.	To promote dissolution and absorption of tablets and capsules. Also, to decrease gastric irritation by diluting drug concentration.
b. With children, liquids or chewable tablets are usually given.	Children under 5 years of age are often unable to swallow tablets or capsules.
(1) Measure and give liquids to infants with a dropper or syringe, placing medication on the tongue or buccal mucosa and giving slowly.	For accurate measurement and administration. Giving slowly decreases risks of aspiration.
(2) Medications are often mixed with juice, applesauce, or other vehicle.	To increase the child's ability and willingness to take the medication. If this is done, use a small amount, and be sure the child takes all of it; otherwise, less than the ordered dose is given.
c. Do not give oral drugs if the client is:	
(1) NPO (receiving nothing by mouth)	Oral drugs and fluids may interfere with diagnostic tests or be otherwise contraindicated. Most drugs can be given after diagnostic tests are completed. If the client is having surgery, preoperative drug orders are cancelled. New orders are written postoperatively.
(2) Vomiting	Oral drugs and fluids increase vomiting. Thus, no benefit results from the drug. Also, fluid and electrolyte problems may result from loss of gastric acid.

(continued)

NURSING ACTIONS	RATIONALE/EXPLANATION
(3) Excessively sedated or unconscious	To avoid aspiration of drugs into the lungs owing to impaired ability to swallow
3. For medications given by nasogastric tube:	
a. Use a liquid preparation when possible. If necessary, crush a tablet or empty a capsule into about 30 mL of water and mix well. **Do not crush enteric-coated or sustained-release products, and do not empty sustained-release capsules.**	Particles of tablets or powders from capsules may obstruct the tube lumen. Altering sustained-release products increases risks of overdosage and adverse effects.
b. Use a clean bulb syringe or other catheter-tipped syringe.	The syringe allows aspiration and serves as a funnel for instillation of medication and fluids into the stomach.
c. Before instilling medication, aspirate gastric fluid or use another method to check tube placement.	To be sure the tube is in the stomach
d. Instill medication by gravity flow, and follow it with at least 50 mL of water. Do not allow the syringe to empty completely between additions.	Gravity flow is safer than applying pressure. Water "pushes" the drug into the stomach and rinses the tube, thereby maintaining tube patency. Additional water or other fluids may be given according to fluid needs of the client. Add fluids to avoid instilling air into the stomach unnecessarily, with possible client discomfort.
e. Clamp off the tube from suction or drainage for at least 30 minutes.	To avoid removing the medication from the stomach
4. For subcutaneous (SC) injections:	
a. Use only sterile drug preparations labeled or commonly used for SC injections.	Many parenteral drugs are too irritating to subcutaneous tissue for use by this route.
b. Use a 25-gauge, ⅝-inch needle for most SC injections.	This size needle is effective for most clients and drugs.
c. Select an appropriate injection site, based on client preferences, drug characteristics, and visual inspection of possible sites. In long-term therapy, such as with insulin, rotate injection sites. Avoid areas with lumps, bruises, or other lesions.	These techniques allow the client to participate in his or her care; avoid tissue damage and unpredictable absorption, which occur with repeated injections in the same location; and increase client comfort and cooperation.
d. Cleanse the site with an alcohol sponge.	To prevent infection
e. Tighten the skin or pinch a fold of skin and tissue between thumb and fingers.	Either is acceptable for most clients. If the client is obese, tightening the skin may be easier. If the client is very thin, the tissue fold may keep the needle from hitting bone.
f. Hold the syringe like a pencil, and insert the needle quickly at a 45-degree angle. Use enough force to penetrate the skin and subcutaneous tissue in one smooth movement.	To give the drug correctly with minimal client discomfort.
g. Release the skin so that both hands are free to manipulate the syringe. Pull back gently on the plunger (aspirate). If no blood enters the	To prevent accidental injection into the bloodstream. Blood return in the syringe is an uncommon occurrence.

(continued)

NURSING ACTIONS	RATIONALE/EXPLANATION
syringe, inject the drug. If blood is aspirated into the syringe, remove the needle, and reprepare the medication.	
h. Remove the needle quickly and apply gentle pressure for a few seconds.	To prevent bleeding
5. For intramuscular (IM) injections:	
a. Use only drug preparations labeled or commonly used for IM injections. Check label instructions for mixing drugs in powder form.	Some parenteral drug preparations cannot be given safely by the IM route.
b. Use a 1½-inch needle for most adults and a ⅝- to 1½-inch needle for children, depending on the size of the client.	A long needle is necessary to reach muscle tissue, which underlies subcutaneous fat.
c. Use the smallest-gauge needle that will accommodate the medication. A 22-gauge is satisfactory for most drugs; a 20-gauge may be used for viscous medications.	To decrease tissue damage and client discomfort
d. Select an appropriate injection site, based on client preferences, drug characteristics, anatomic landmarks, and visual inspection of possible sites. Rotate sites if frequent injections are being given, and avoid areas with lumps, bruises, or other lesions.	To increase client comfort and participation and to avoid tissue damage. Identification of anatomic landmarks is mandatory for safe administration of IM drugs.
e. Cleanse the site with an alcohol sponge.	To prevent infection
f. Tighten the skin, hold the syringe like a pencil, and insert the needle quickly at a 90-degree angle. Use enough force to penetrate the skin and subcutaneous tissue into the muscle in one smooth motion.	To give the drug correctly with minimal client discomfort
g. Aspirate (see 4g, SC injections).	
h. Remove the needle quickly and apply pressure for several seconds.	To prevent bleeding
6. For intravenous (IV) injections:	
a. Use only drug preparations that are labeled for IV use.	Others are not pure enough for safe injection into the bloodstream or are not compatible with the blood pH (7.35–7.45).
b. Check label instructions for the type and amount of fluid to use for dissolving or diluting the drug.	Some drugs require special preparation techniques to maintain solubility or pharmacologic activity. Most drugs in powder form can be dissolved in sterile water or sodium chloride for injection. Most drug solutions can be given with dextrose or dextrose and sodium chloride IV solutions.
c. Prepare drugs just before use, as a general rule. Also, add drugs to IV fluids just before use.	Some drugs are unstable in solution. In some agencies, drugs are mixed and added to IV fluids in the pharmacy. This is the preferred method because sterility can be better maintained.
d. For venipuncture and direct injection into a vein, apply a tourniquet, select a site in the	For safe and accurate drug administration with minimal risk to the client. The length of time required to

(continued)

NURSING ACTIONS	RATIONALE/EXPLANATION
arm, cleanse the skin with an antiseptic (eg, povidone-iodine or alcohol), insert the needle, and aspirate a small amount of blood into the syringe to be sure that the needle is in the vein. Remove the tourniquet, and inject the drug slowly. Remove the needle and apply pressure until there is no evidence of bleeding.	give the drug depends on the specific drug and the amount. Slow administration, over several minutes, allows immediate discontinuation if adverse effects occur.
e. For administration by an established IV line:	
(1) Check the infusion for patency and flow rate. Check the venipuncture site for signs of infiltration and phlebitis before each drug dose.	The solution must be flowing freely for accurate drug administration. If infiltration or phlebitis is present, do not give the drug until a new IV line is begun.
(2) For direct injection, cleanse an injection site on the IV tubing, insert the needle, and inject the drug slowly.	Most tubings have injection sites to facilitate drug administration.
(3) To use a volume-control set, fill it with 50 to 100 mL of IV fluid, and clamp it so that no further fluid enters the chamber and dilutes the drug. Inject the drug into an injection site after cleansing the site with an alcohol sponge and infuse, usually in 1 hour or less. Once the drug is infused, add solution to maintain the infusion.	This method is used for administration of antibiotics on an intermittent schedule. Dilution of the drug decreases adverse effects.
(4) To use a "piggyback" method, add the drug to 50 to 100 mL of IV solution in a separate container. Attach the IV tubing and a needle. Insert the needle in an injection site on the main IV tubing after cleansing the site. Infuse the drug over 15 to 60 minutes, depending on the drug.	This method is also used for intermittent administration of antibiotics and other drugs. Whether a volume-control or piggyback apparatus is used depends on agency policy and equipment available.
f. When more than one drug is to be given, flush the line between drugs. Do not mix drugs in syringes or in IV fluids unless the drug literature states that the drugs are compatible.	Physical and chemical interactions between the drugs may occur and cause precipitation, inactivation, or increased toxicity. Most nursing units have charts depicting drug compatibility, or information may be obtained from the pharmacy.
7. For application to skin:	
a. Use drug preparations labeled for dermatologic use. Cleanse the skin, remove any previously applied medication, and apply the drug in a thin layer. For broken skin or open lesions, use sterile gloves, tongue blade, or cotton-tipped applicator to apply the drug.	To promote therapeutic effects and minimize adverse effects
8. For instillation of eye drops:	
a. Use drug preparations labeled for ophthalmic use. Wash your hands, open the eye to expose the conjunctival sac, and drop the medication into the sac, not on the eyeball, without touching the dropper tip to anything. Provide a tissue for blotting any excess drug. If two or more eye drops are scheduled at the same time, wait 1 to 5 minutes between instillations.	Ophthalmic preparations must be sterile to avoid infection. Blot any excess drug from the inner canthus near the nose to decrease systemic absorption of the drug.

(continued)

NURSING ACTIONS	RATIONALE/EXPLANATION
With children, prepare the medication, place the child in a head-lowered position, steady the hand holding the medication on the child's head, gently retract the lower lid, and instill the medication into the conjunctival sac.	Careful positioning and restraint to avoid sudden movements are necessary to decrease risks of injury to the eye.
9. For instillation of nose drops and nasal sprays:	
a. Have the client hold his or her head back, and drop the medication into the nostrils. Give only as ordered With children, place in a supine position with the head lowered, instill the medication, and maintain the position for 2 to 3 minutes. Then, place the child in a prone position.	When nose drops are used for rhinitis and nasal congestion accompanying the common cold, overuse results in a rebound congestion that may be worse than the original symptom.
10. For instillation of ear medications:	
a. Open the ear canal by pulling the ear up and back for adults, down and back for children, and drop the medication on the side of the canal.	To straighten the canal and promote maximal contact between medication and tissue
11. For rectal suppositories:	
a. Lubricate the end with a water-soluble lubricant, wear a glove or finger cot, and insert into the rectum the length of the finger. Place the suppository next to the mucosal wall. If the client prefers and is able, provide supplies for self-administration.	To promote absorption. Allowing self-administration may prevent embarrassment to the client. Be sure the client knows the correct procedure.
12. For vaginal medications:	
a. Use gloves or an applicator for insertion. If an applicator is used, wash thoroughly with soap and water after each use. If the client prefers and is able, provide supplies for self-administration.	Some women may be embarrassed and prefer self-administration. Be sure the client knows the correct procedure.

How Can You Avoid This Medication Error?

Answer: This medication error occurred because the medication was given to the wrong client. The nurse did not check the client's name band and relied on the client to respond to her calling his name. In this situation, the client had been asleep and may have been responding simply to being awakened. Also, language and culture may have been a factor. Accurate identification of the client is imperative, especially when the client may be confused or unable to respond appropriately.

Nursing Notes: Apply Your Knowledge

Answer: First check tube placement by aspirating gastric content or instilling air into the stomach (listen with a stethoscope for a swishing sound over the gastric area). Use liquid preparations when possible. When a liquid formulation is not available, crush a tablet or empty a capsule into 15 to 30 mL of warm water and mix well. Note: Do **not** crush enteric-coated or sustained-release products because this alters their rate of absorption and could be dangerous to the client.

To administer, flush the feeding tube with tap water, draw medication into a syringe, and slowly instill the medication into the tube, then flush the tube again. Preferably, give each medication separately and rinse the tube between medications. When all medications are given, flush the tube with 50 mL of water unless the client is on a fluid restriction. Small feeding tubes occlude very easily and must be rinsed well to prevent clogging.

REVIEW AND APPLICATION EXERCISES

1. When giving an oral medication, what are some interventions to aid absorption and hasten therapeutic effects?

2. What are the advantages and disadvantages of the oral route and the IV route of drug administration?

3. For a client who receives all medications through a nasogastric feeding tube, which dosage forms are acceptable? Which are unacceptable, and why?

4. Which dosage forms must be kept sterile during administration?

5. What are some legal factors that influence a nurse's administration of medications?

6. When administering medications, what safety precautions are needed with various routes?

7. What safety precautions must the nurse practice consistently to avoid self-injury and exposure to blood-borne pathogens?

8. With a client who refuses an important medication, what approaches or interventions might persuade the client to take the medication? Would the same approach be indicated if the medication were a vitamin supplement or a laxative?

SELECTED REFERENCES

Beyea, S.C. & Nicoll, L.H. (1996). Administering IM injections the right way. *American Journal of Nursing, 96*(1), 34–35.

Drug facts and comparisons. (Updated monthly). St. Louis: Facts and Comparisons.

Konick-McMahan, J. (1996). Full speed ahead with caution: Pushing intravenous medications. *Nursing, 26*(6), 26–31.

Kokotis, K. (1998). Preventing chemical phlebitis. *Nursing, 28*(11), 41–46.

McConnell, E.A. (1997). Clinical do's and don't's: Using transdermal medication patches. *Nursing, 27*(7), 18.

Mitchell, J.F. (1998). Oral dosage forms that should not be crushed: 1998 update. *Hospital Pharmacy, 33*, 399–415.

Nursing Process in Drug Therapy

Objectives

After studying this chapter, the student will be able to:

1. Develop personal techniques for learning about drugs and using drug knowledge in client care.

2. Assess clients' conditions in relation to age, weight, health–illness status, and lifestyle habits likely to influence drug effects.

3. Obtain a medication history about the client's use of prescription, over-the-counter, and social drugs.

4. Identify nondrug interventions to prevent or decrease the need for drug therapy.

5. Discuss interventions to increase benefits and decrease hazards of drug therapy.

6. Discuss guidelines for rational choices of drugs, dosages, routes, and times of administration.

7. Observe clients for therapeutic and adverse responses to drug therapy.

8. Teach clients and family members how to use prescription and over-the-counter drugs safely and effectively.

9. Discuss application of the nursing process in home care settings.

10. Discuss legal implications of drug therapy.

11. Describe major differences in drug therapy for clients with impaired renal or hepatic function or critical illness.

You are making the first home visit for an elderly client with arthritis and hypertension who is taking the following medications:

Ibuprofen 800 mg every 4 hours
Prednisone 5 mg daily
Lasix 20 mg twice a day
Captopril 25 mg twice a day
Pepcid 20 mg at bedtime

Look up each of these medications. Note the drug class and why you think this client is taking them. Are these acceptable doses for elderly clients? What criteria will you use to determine therapeutic effects for each drug? Note any side effects that are likely for each drug and what assessment data will be important to collect.

41

Drug therapy involves the use of drugs to prevent or treat disease processes and manifestations. It may save lives, improve the quality of life, and otherwise benefit recipients. It also may cause adverse effects. Adverse effects and failure to achieve therapeutic effects may occur with correct use, but they are more likely to occur with incorrect use. Physicians, pharmacists, clients, and nurses all have important roles to play in the safe and effective use of drugs.

For the nurse, drug therapy is one of many responsibilities in client care. To fulfill this responsibility, the nurse must be knowledgeable about pharmacology (drugs and their effects on the body), physiology (normal body functions), and pathophysiology (alterations in mental and physical functions due to disease processes), and must be adept at using all steps of the nursing process.

Chapter 1 included general information about drugs and cellular physiology. Chapter 2 described concepts and processes essential to understanding drug effects in humans. Chapter 3 emphasized techniques of preparing and administering drugs safely and effectively. Although the importance of safe and accurate administration cannot be overemphasized, this is only one aspect of the nursing process in drug therapy. The nurse also must monitor responses to drug therapy, both therapeutic and adverse, and teach clients about drugs, both prescribed and over-the-counter. To help the nurse acquire knowledge and skills related to drug therapy, this chapter includes suggestions for studying pharmacology, legal responsibilities, nursing process guidelines, general principles of drug therapy, and general nursing actions.

USING THE PROTOTYPE APPROACH TO STUDY PHARMACOLOGY

The beginning student of pharmacology is faced with bewildering numbers and types of drugs. These can be greatly reduced by concentrating initial study on therapeutic classifications or groups of drugs and prototypes of those groups. For example, narcotic analgesics is one group, and morphine is the prototype of that group. Morphine and other opioid analgesics have many common characteristics, including the following:

1. They are used primarily to relieve pain.
2. They produce central nervous system (CNS) depression ranging from slight drowsiness to unconsciousness, depending on dose and tolerance.
3. A major adverse reaction is respiratory depression (depression of the respiratory center in the brain as part of the CNS depression). Thus, the nurse must check rate and depth of respiration.
4. They have a high potential for abuse and dependence; therefore, their use is regulated by narcotic laws and requires special records and procedures.
5. They must be used with caution in people who already have respiratory depression or an impaired level of consciousness.

Understanding these characteristics makes studying all other opioid analgesics easier because other drugs are compared with morphine, especially in their ability to relieve pain and their likelihood of causing respiratory depression.

Once you know the characteristics of the major drug groups, you must continue to build your drug knowledge. Most new or unfamiliar drugs fit into an established classification. For example, you may know that the unfamiliar drug is a thiazide diuretic. By recalling your knowledge of this drug classification, you have a base of general information to which you can add specific information about the unfamiliar drug.

Guidelines for Effective Study

Because there is a great deal of information available about individual drugs, you need to be selective about the drugs and the information you try to learn. Some guidelines for effective study include the following:

1. *Try to understand how the drug acts in the body.* This allows you to predict therapeutic effects and to predict, prevent, or minimize adverse effects by early detection and treatment.
2. *Concentrate your study efforts on major characteristics.* These include the main indications for use, common and potentially serious adverse effects, conditions in which the drug is contraindicated or must be used cautiously, usual dosage ranges, and related nursing care needs.
3. *Compare the drug with a prototype when possible.* Relating the unknown to the known aids learning and retention of knowledge.
4. *Keep an authoritative, up-to-date drug reference readily available, preferably at work and home.* This is a much more reliable source of drug information than memory. Use the reference freely whenever you encounter an unfamiliar drug or when a question arises about a familiar one.
5. *Use your own words when taking notes or writing drug information cards.* The mental processing required to put information in your own words aids learning and retention.
6. *Mentally practice applying drug knowledge in nursing care* by asking yourself, "What if I have a client who is receiving this drug? What must I do? For what must I observe? What if my client is an elderly person or a child?"

LEGAL RESPONSIBILITIES OF THE NURSE

Registered and licensed practical nurses are legally empowered, under state nurse practice acts, to give medications ordered by licensed physicians and dentists. In some states, nurse practitioners may prescribe medications.

When giving medications, the nurse is legally responsible for safe and accurate administration (right drug, right dose, right client, right route, and right time). This means the nurse may be held liable for *not* giving a drug or for giving a wrong drug or a wrong dose. Also, *the nurse is expected to have sufficient drug knowledge to recognize and question erroneous orders*. If, after questioning the prescribing physician and seeking information from other authoritative sources, the nurse considers that giving the drug is unsafe, the nurse must refuse to give the drug. The fact that a physician wrote an erroneous order does not excuse the nurse from legal liability if he or she carries out that order. The nurse also is legally responsible for actions delegated to people who are inadequately prepared for or legally barred from administering medications (such as nursing assistants). However, certified medical assistants (CMAs) administer medications in physicians' offices and certified medication aides (nursing assistants with a short course of training, also called CMAs) often administer medications in long-term care facilities.

The nurse is responsible for storing narcotics and other controlled substances in locked containers, administering them only to people for whom they are prescribed, recording each dose given on appropriate narcotic sheets and on the client's medication administration record, counting the amount of each drug at regular intervals, and reporting any discrepancies to the proper authorities.

The nurse who follows safe practices in giving medications does not need to be excessively concerned about legal liability. The basic techniques and guidelines listed in Chapter 3 are aimed at safe and accurate preparation and administration; most errors result when these practices are not followed consistently.

Legal responsibilities in other aspects of drug therapy are less tangible and clear-cut. However, nurses are in general expected to observe clients for therapeutic and adverse effects and to teach clients safe and effective self-administration of drugs when indicated.

APPLYING THE NURSING PROCESS IN DRUG THERAPY

The nursing process is a systematic way of gathering and using information to plan and provide client care and to evaluate the outcomes of care. Knowledge and skill in the nursing process are required for drug therapy, as in other aspects of client care. Each of the five steps of the nursing process is described and illustrated below.

Assessment

The first step involves collecting data about client characteristics known to affect drug therapy. This can be done by observing and interviewing the client, interviewing family members or others involved in client care, completing a physical assessment, reviewing medical records for pertinent laboratory and diagnostic test reports, and other methods. Information is also sought about the ordered drugs, if needed. Data from all sources are then analyzed.

Nursing Diagnoses

These statements, as developed by the North American Nursing Diagnosis Association, describe client problems or needs and are based on assessment data. They should be individualized according to the client's condition and the drugs prescribed. Thus, the nursing diagnoses needed to adequately reflect the client's condition vary considerably. Because almost any nursing diagnosis may apply in specific circumstances, this text emphasizes those diagnoses that generally apply to any course of drug therapy.

Planning/Goals

This step involves stating the expected outcomes of the prescribed drug therapy. As a general rule, goals should be stated in terms of client behavior, not nurse behavior.

Interventions

This step involves implementing the planned activities. Areas of nursing intervention may include drug administration, teaching about medications, problem solving, promoting compliance, identifying barriers to compliance, identifying resources (eg, financial assistance for obtaining medications), and others.

General interventions include preventing the need for drug therapy and using nondrug measures to increase safety and effectiveness. Specific interventions include actions needed once a drug is ordered (ie, accurate administration, observing for therapeutic and adverse effects).

Teaching clients, family members, or other caregivers is one of the most important nursing interventions because it makes the client/caregiver an active participant and partner in health care. In relation to drug therapy, client teaching is important because most medications are self-administered and clients need information and assistance to use the drugs safely and effectively. When medications are given by another caregiver, rather than self-administered, the caregiver needs to understand about the medication. *Client*, as used in this text, includes family/friend caregivers. Some factors to consider in preparing to teach a client or caregiver include the following:

- Assess learning needs and ability to manage a drug therapy regimen (ie, read printed instructions and drug labels, remember dosage schedules, self-administer medications by ordered routes). A medication history (Box 4-1) helps to assess the client's knowledge and attitudes about drug therapy.

BOX 4–1   **MEDICATION HISTORY**

Name_____ Age_____

Health problems, acute and chronic

Are you allergic to any medications?

If yes, describe specific effects or symptoms.

Part 1: Prescription Medications

1. Do you take any prescription medications on a regular basis?
2. If yes, ask the following about each medication.

Name	Dose
Frequency	Specific times
How long taken	Reason for use

3. Are you able to take this medicine as prescribed?
4. Does anyone else help you take your medications?
5. What information or instructions were you given when the medications were first prescribed?
6. Do you think the medication is doing what it was prescribed to do?
7. Have you had any problems that you attribute to the medication?
8. Do you take any prescription medications on an irregular basis? If yes, ask the following about each medication.

Name	Dose
Frequency	Reason
How long taken	

Part 2: Nonprescription Medications

Do you take over-the-counter medications?

		Medication		
Problem	*Yes/No*	*Name*	*Amount*	*Frequency*
Pain				
Headache				
Sleep				
Cold				
Indigestion				
Heartburn				
Diarrhea				
Constipation				
Other				

Part 3: Social Drugs

	Yes/No	*Amount*
Coffee		
Tea		
Cola drinks		
Alcohol		
Tobacco		

- From assessment data, develop an individualized teaching plan. This saves time for both nurse and client by avoiding repetition of known material and promotes compliance with the prescribed drug therapy regimen.
- Reassess learning needs when medication orders are changed (eg, with a new illness). Clients are more likely to make medication errors with large numbers of medications or changes in the medication regimen.
- Clients and caregivers may feel overwhelmed by complicated medication regimens. Try to decrease their anxiety and provide positive reinforcement for effort.
- Choose an appropriate time (eg, when the client is mentally alert and not in acute distress from pain, dif-

ficulty in breathing, or other symptoms) and a place with minimal noise and distractions.

- Proceed slowly, in small steps; emphasize essential information; and provide ample opportunities to express concerns or ask questions.

- Usually, a combination of verbal and written instructions is more effective than either alone. Minimize medical jargon and be aware that clients may have difficulty understanding and retaining the material being taught because of the stress of the illness.

- When explaining a drug therapy regimen to a hospitalized client, describe the name, purpose, expected effects, and so on. In many instances, the drug is familiar and can be described from personal knowledge. If the drug is unfamiliar, use available resources (eg, drug reference books, pharmacists, pharmacy information sheets) to learn about the drug and provide accurate information to the client.

  The client should know the name, preferably both the generic and a trade name, of any drugs being taken. Such knowledge is a safety measure, especially if an allergic or other potentially serious adverse reaction or overdose occurs. It also decreases the risk of mistaking one drug for another and promotes a greater sense of control and responsibility regarding drug therapy.

  The client should also know the purpose of prescribed drugs. Although people vary in the amount of drug information they want and need, the purpose can usually be simply stated in terms of symptoms to be relieved or other expected benefits.

- When teaching a client about medications to be taken at home, provide specific instructions about taking the medications. Also teach the client and caregiver to observe for beneficial and adverse effects. If side effects occur, teach them how to manage minor ones and which ones to report to a health care provider. In addition, discuss specific ways to take medications so that usual activities of daily living are minimally disrupted. Planning with a client to develop a convenient routine, within the limitations imposed by individual drugs, may help increase compliance with the prescribed regimen. Allow time for questions and try to ensure that the client understands how, when, and why to take the medications.

- When teaching a client about potential adverse drug effects, the goal is to provide needed information without causing unnecessary anxiety. Most drugs produce undesirable effects; some of these are minor, and others are potentially serious. Many people stop taking a drug rather than report adverse reactions. If reactions are reported, it may be possible to continue drug therapy by reducing dosage or by implementing other measures. The occurrence of severe reactions indicates that the drug should be stopped and the prescribing physician should be notified.

- Throughout the teaching session and perhaps at other contacts, emphasize the importance of taking medications as prescribed. Common client errors include taking incorrect doses, taking doses at the wrong times, forgetting to take doses, and stopping a medication too soon. Treatment failure can often be directly traced to these errors. For example, missed doses of glaucoma medication can lead to optic nerve damage and blindness.

There are several areas that may need to be included in teaching, depending on the client's learning needs. General information and instructions for prescription drugs are included in *Client teaching guidelines: Safe and effective use of prescription medications*; more specific guidelines for particular drug groups and selected individual drugs are included in the appropriate chapters. General information and instructions for using nonprescription drugs are included in *Client teaching guidelines: Safe and effective use of over-the-counter (OTC) medications*.

Evaluation

This step involves evaluating the client's status in relation to stated goals and expected outcomes. Some outcomes can be evaluated within a few minutes of drug administration (eg, relief of acute pain after administration of an analgesic). Most, however, require much longer periods of time, often extending from hospitalization and direct observation by the nurse to self-care at home and occasional contact with a health care provider.

With the current emphasis on outpatient treatment and short hospitalizations, the client is likely to experience brief contacts with many health care providers rather than extensive contacts with a few health care providers. These factors, plus a client's usual reluctance to admit noncompliance, contribute to difficulties in evaluating outcomes of drug therapy. These difficulties can be managed by using appropriate techniques and criteria of evaluation.

Techniques include directly observing the client's status; interviewing the client, family members, or other health care providers; and checking medication records and laboratory and diagnostic test reports. With outpatients, "pill counts" may be done to compare doses remaining with the number prescribed during a designated time. These techniques may be used at every contact with a client, if appropriate.

General criteria include progress toward stated outcomes, such as relief of symptoms, accurate administration, avoidance of preventable adverse effects, compliance with instructions, and others. Specific criteria indicate the parameters that must be measured to evaluate responses to particular drugs (eg, blood sugar with antidiabetic drugs, blood pressure with antihypertensive drugs).

Each step of the nursing process is more specifically illustrated in the following sections.

CLIENT TEACHING GUIDELINES
Safe and Effective Use of Prescription Medications

General Considerations

✔ Use drugs cautiously and only when necessary because all drugs affect body functions and may cause adverse effects.

✔ Use nondrug measures, when possible, to prevent the need for drug therapy or to enhance beneficial effects and decrease adverse effects of drugs.

✔ Do not take drugs left over from a previous illness or prescribed for someone else and do not share prescription drugs with anyone else. The likelihood of having the right drug in the right dose is remote and the risk of adverse effects is high in such circumstances.

✔ Keep all health care providers informed about all the drugs being taken, including over-the-counter (OTC) products. One way to do this is to keep a written record of all current medicines, including their names and doses and how they are taken. It is a good idea to carry a copy of this list at all times. This information can help avoid new prescriptions or OTC drugs that have similar effects or cancel each other's effects.

✔ Take drugs as prescribed and for the length of time prescribed; notify a health care provider if unable to obtain or take a medication. Therapeutic effects greatly depend on taking medications correctly. Altering the dose or time may cause underdosage or overdosage. Stopping a medication may cause a recurrence of the problem for which it was given or withdrawal symptoms. Some medications need to be tapered in dosage and gradually discontinued. If problems occur with taking the drug, report them to the prescribing physician rather than stopping the drug. Often, an adjustment in dosage or other aspect of administration may solve the problem.

✔ Follow instructions for follow-up care (eg, office visits, laboratory or other diagnostic tests that monitor therapeutic or adverse effects of drugs). Some drugs require more frequent monitoring than others. However, safety requires periodic checks with essentially all medications. With long-term use of a medication, responses may change over time with aging, changes in kidney function, and so on.

✔ Take drugs in current use when seeing a physician for any health-related problem. It may be helpful to remind the physician periodically of the medications being taken and ask if any can be discontinued or reduced in dosage.

✔ Get all prescriptions filled at the same pharmacy, when possible. This is an important safety factor in helping to avoid several prescriptions of the same or similar drugs and to minimize undesirable interactions of newly prescribed drugs with those already in use.

✔ Report any drug allergies to all health care providers and wear a medical identification emblem that lists allergens.

✔ Ask questions (and write down the answers) about newly prescribed medications, such as:

What is the medicine's name?

What is it supposed to do (ie, what symptoms or problems will it relieve)?

How and when do I take it, and for how long?

Should it be taken with food or on an empty stomach?

While taking this medicine, should I avoid certain foods, beverages, other medications, certain activities? (For example, alcoholic beverages and driving a car should be avoided with medications that cause drowsiness or decrease alertness.)

Will this medication work safely with the others I'm already taking?

What side effects are likely and what do I do if they occur?

Will the medication affect my ability to sleep or work?

What should I do if I miss a dose?

Is there a drug information sheet I can have?

✔ Store medications out of reach of children and never refer to medications as "candy" to prevent accidental ingestion.

✔ Develop a plan for renewing or refilling prescriptions so that the medication supply does not run out when the prescribing physician is unavailable or the pharmacy is closed.

✔ When taking prescription medications, talk to a doctor, pharmacist, or nurse before starting an OTC medication. This is a safety factor to avoid undesirable drug interactions.

✔ Inform health care providers if you have diabetes or kidney or liver disease. These conditions require special precautions with drug therapy.

✔ If pregnant, consult your obstetrician before taking any medications prescribed by another physician.

✔ If breastfeeding, consult your obstetrician or pediatrician before taking any medications prescribed by another physician.

Self-administration

✔ Develop a routine for taking medications (eg, at the same time and place each day). A schedule that minimally disrupts usual household activities is more convenient and more likely to be followed accurately.

✔ Take medications in a well-lighted area and read labels of containers to ensure taking the intended drug. Do not take medications if you are not alert or cannot see clearly.

✔ Most tablets and capsules should be taken whole. If unable to take them whole, ask a health care provider before splitting, chewing, or crushing tablets or taking the medication out of capsules. Some long-acting preparations are dangerous if altered so that the entire dose is absorbed at the same time.

(continued)

CLIENT TEACHING GUIDELINES
Safe and Effective Use of Prescription Medications *(continued)*

✔ As a general rule, take oral medications with 6 to 8 oz of water, in a sitting or standing position. The water helps tablets and capsules dissolve in the stomach, "dilutes" the drug so that it is less likely to upset the stomach, and promotes absorption of the drug into the bloodstream. The upright positions helps the drug reach the stomach rather than getting stuck in the throat or esophagus.

✔ Take most oral drugs at evenly spaced intervals around the clock. For example, if ordered once daily, take about the same time every day. If ordered twice daily or morning and evening, take about 12 hours apart.

✔ Follow instructions about taking a medication with food or on an empty stomach, about taking with other medications, or taking with fluids other than water. Prescription medications often include instructions to take on an empty stomach or with food. If taking several medications, ask a health care provider whether they may be taken together or at different times. For example, an antacid usually should not be taken at the same time as other oral medications because the antacid decreases absorption of many other drugs.

✔ If a dose is missed, most authorities recommend taking the dose if remembered soon after the scheduled time and omitting the dose if it is not remembered for several hours. If a dose is omitted, the next dose should be taken at the next scheduled time. **Do not double the dose.**

✔ If taking a liquid medication (or giving one to a child), measure with a calibrated medication cup or measuring spoon. A dose cannot be measured accurately with household teaspoons or tablespoons because they are different sizes and deliver varying amounts of medication. If the liquid medication is packaged with a measuring cup that shows teaspoons or tablespoons, that should be used to measure doses, for adults or children. This is especially important for young children because most of their medications are given in liquid form.

✔ Use other types of medications according to instructions. If not clear how a medication is to be used, be sure to ask a health care provider. Correct use of oral or nasal inhalers, eye drops, and skin medications is essential for therapeutic effects.

✔ Report problems or new symptoms to a health care provider.

✔ Store medications safely, in a cool, dry place. Do not store them in a bathroom; heat, light, and moisture may cause them to decompose. Do not store them near a dangerous substance, which could be taken by mistake. Keep medications in the container in which they were dispensed by the pharmacy, where the label identifies it and gives directions. Do not put several different tablets or capsules in one container. Although this may be more convenient, especially when away from home for work or travel, it is never a safe practice because it increases the likelihood of taking the wrong drug.

✔ Discard outdated medications; do not keep drugs for long periods. Drugs are chemicals that may deteriorate over time, especially if exposed to heat and moisture. In addition, having many containers increases the risks of medication errors and adverse drug interactions.

CLIENT TEACHING GUIDELINES
Safe and Effective Use of Over-the-Counter (OTC) Medications

✔ Read product labels carefully. The labels contain essential information about the name, ingredients, indications for use, usual dosage, when to stop using the medication or when to see a doctor, possible side effects, and expiration dates.

✔ Use a magnifying glass, if necessary, to read the fine print.

✔ If you do not understand the information on labels, ask a physician, pharmacist, or nurse.

✔ Do not take OTC medications longer or in higher doses than recommended.

✔ Note that all OTC medications are not safe for everyone. Many OTC medications warn against use with certain illnesses (eg, hypertension, thyroid disorders). Consult a health care provider before taking the product if you have one of the contraindicated conditions.

✔ If taking any prescription medications, consult a health care provider before taking any nonprescription drugs to avoid undesirable drug interactions and adverse effects. Some specific precautions include the following:

Avoid alcohol if taking antihistamines, cough or cold remedies containing dextromethorphan, or sleeping pills. Because all these drugs cause drowsiness, combining any of them with alcohol may result in excessive, potentially dangerous, sedation.

Avoid OTC sleeping aids if you are taking a prescription sedative-type drug (eg, for nervousness or depression).

(continued)

CLIENT TEACHING GUIDELINES
Safe and Effective Use of OTC Medications (continued)

Ask a health care provider before taking products containing aspirin if you are taking an anticoagulant (eg, Coumadin).

Ask a health care provider before taking other products containing aspirin if you are already taking a regular dose of aspirin to prevent blood clots, heart attack, or stroke. Aspirin is commonly used for this purpose, often in doses of 81 mg (a child's dose) or 325 mg.

Do not take a laxative if you have stomach pain, nausea, or vomiting to avoid worsening the problem.

Do not take multisymptom cold remedies (eg, Comtrex, Dimetapp, many others) or weight-control medicines (eg, Dexatrim) that contain phenylpropanolamine (PPA) if you are taking medications for high blood pressure or depression; if you have heart disease, diabetes, or thyroid disease; or if you are taking other medications containing PPA.

Do not take a nasal decongestant (eg, Sudafed) or multisymptom cold remedy containing pseudoephedrine (eg, Actifed, Sinutab) with any product that contains PPA. Pseudoephedrine and PPA are similar drugs that, among other things, raise blood pressure; taking them concurrently could cause severe hypertension and stroke.

Do not take a nasal decongestant if you are taking a prescription medication for high blood pressure or depression, or if you have thyroid disease, diabetes, or prostate enlargement.

✔ Store OTC drugs in a cool, dry place, in their original containers; check expiration dates periodically and discard those that have expired.

✔ If pregnant, consult your obstetrician before taking any OTC medications.

✔ If breastfeeding, consult your pediatrician or family doctor before taking any OTC medications.

✔ For children, follow any age limits on the label.

✔ Measure liquid OTC medications with the measuring device that comes with the product (some have a dropper or plastic cup calibrated in milliliters, teaspoons, or tablespoons). If such a device is not available, use a measuring spoon. It is not safe to use household teaspoons or tablespoons because they are different sizes and deliver varying amounts of medication. Accurate measurement of doses is especially important for young children because most of their medications are given in liquid form.

✔ Do not assume continued safety of an OTC medication you have taken for years. Older people are more likely to have adverse drug reactions and interactions because of changes in heart, kidneys, and other organs that occur with aging and various disease processes.

✔ Note tamper-resistant features and do not buy products with damaged packages.

NURSING PROCESS

Assessment

Initially (before drug therapy is started or on first contact), assess the client regarding age, weight, health status, pathologic conditions, and ability to function in usual activities of daily living. The effects of these client-related factors on drug therapy are discussed in Chapter 2.

Assess for previous and current use of prescription, nonprescription, and nontherapeutic (eg, alcohol, caffeine, nicotine, cocaine, marijuana) drugs. A medication history (see Box 4-1) is useful, or the information can be incorporated into any data collection tool. Some specific questions and areas of assessment include:

- What are current drug orders?
- What does the client know about current drugs? Is teaching needed?
- What drugs has the client taken before? Include any drugs taken regularly, such as those taken for chronic illnesses (eg, hypertension, diabetes mellitus, arthritis). It also may be helpful to ask about nonprescription drugs for headache, colds, indigestion, or constipation, because some people do not think of these preparations as drugs.

- Has the client ever had an allergic reaction to a drug? If so, what signs and symptoms occurred? This information is necessary because many people describe minor nausea and other symptoms as allergic reactions. Unless the reaction is further explored, the client may have therapy withheld inappropriately.

- What are the client's attitudes about drugs? Try to obtain information to help assess whether the client takes drugs freely or reluctantly, is likely to comply with a prescribed drug regimen, and is likely to abuse drugs.

- If long-term drug therapy is likely, can the client afford to buy medications? Is transportation available for obtaining medications or seeing a health care provider for monitoring and follow-up care?

- Can the client communicate his or her needs, such as requesting medication? Can he or she swallow oral medications?

- Are any other conditions present that influence drug therapy? For example, all seriously ill clients should be assessed for risk factors and manifestations of impaired function of vital organs. Early recognition and treatment may prevent or decrease organ impairment.

In addition to nursing assessment data, use progress notes, laboratory reports, and other sources as available and relevant. As part of the initial assessment, obtain baseline data on measurements to be used in monitoring therapeutic or adverse effects. Specific data to be acquired depend on the medication and the client's condition. Laboratory tests of liver, kidney, and bone marrow function are often helpful because some drugs may damage these organs. Also, if liver or kidney damage exists, drug metabolism or excretion may be altered. Some specific laboratory tests include serum potassium levels before diuretic therapy, culture and susceptibility studies before antimicrobial therapy, and blood clotting tests before anticoagulant therapy. Other data that may be relevant include vital signs, weight, and urine output.

After drug therapy is begun, continue to assess the client's response in relation to therapeutic and adverse effects, ability and willingness to take the drugs as prescribed, and other aspects of safe and effective drug therapy.

Nursing Diagnoses

- Knowledge Deficit: Drug therapy regimen (eg, drug ordered, reason for use, expected effects, and monitoring of response by health care providers, including diagnostic tests and office visits)
- Knowledge Deficit: Safe and effective self-administration (when appropriate)
- Risk for Injury related to adverse drug effects
- Noncompliance: Overuse
- Noncompliance: Underuse

Planning/Goals

The client will:

- Receive or take drugs as prescribed
- Experience relief of signs and symptoms
- Avoid preventable adverse drug effects
- Avoid unnecessary drug ingestion
- Self-administer drugs safely and accurately
- Verbalize essential drug information
- Keep appointments for monitoring and follow-up

Interventions

Use nondrug measures when appropriate to decrease the need for drugs, to enhance therapeutic effects, or to decrease adverse effects. General interventions include:

- Promoting healthful lifestyles in terms of nutrition, fluids, exercise, rest, and sleep
- Hand washing and other measures to prevent infection
- Positioning
- Assisting to cough and deep breathe
- Ambulating
- Applying heat or cold
- Increasing or decreasing sensory stimulation
- Scheduling activities to allow periods of rest or sleep
- Recording vital signs, fluid intake, urine output, and other assessment data
- Implementing specific interventions indicated by a particular drug or the client's condition
  - Weighing seriously ill clients early in treatment when possible, then periodically throughout the illness. Accurate weights help in calculating dosages of several drugs and in assessing changes in clients' fluid balance or nutritional status.
  - When serum drug levels are being used to guide drug therapy, be sure that blood samples are drawn at correct times in relation to administered doses.
  - In clients at risk for development of acute renal failure (ARF), try to prevent ARF by ensuring adequate fluid intake and adequate blood pressure and avoiding or following safety precautions with nephrotoxic drugs (eg, aminoglycoside antibiotics).

Evaluation

Observe and interview clients and check appropriate medical records about drug usage, compliance with prescribed therapy, relief of symptoms, adverse effects, and drug knowledge.

INTEGRATING NURSING PROCESS, DRUG THERAPY, AND CLINICAL PATHWAYS

In an increasing number of circumstances, nursing responsibilities related to drug therapy are designated in clinical pathways (also called *critical pathways* or *care maps*). Clinical pathways are guidelines for the care of clients with particular conditions. Additional characteristics include the following:

- Major components include a medical diagnosis, aspects of care related to the medical diagnosis, desired client outcomes, and time frames (usually days) for achieving the desired outcomes during the expected length of stay.
- Medical diagnoses for which clinical pathways are usually developed are those often encountered in

an agency and those that often result in complications or prolonged lengths of stay. In many agencies, clinical pathways have been developed for clients having coronary artery bypass grafts, myocardial infarction, and hip or knee replacement.

- Development and implementation of the clinical pathways should be an interdisciplinary, collaborative effort. Thus, all health care professionals usually involved in the care of a client with a particular medical diagnosis should be represented.
- In hospital settings, case managers, who may be non-nurses, usually assess clients' conditions daily to evaluate progress toward the desired outcomes.
- Although clinical pathways are used mainly in hospitals, they are likely to be developed in ambulatory settings as well. Eventually, comprehensive client pathways may be developed that extend from illness onset and initial contact with a health care provider through treatment and recovery. Such pathways could promote continuity of care among agencies, departments of agencies, and health care providers.

Depending on the medical diagnoses, many clinical pathways have specific guidelines related to drug therapy. These guidelines may affect any step of the nursing process. With assessment, for example, the clinical pathway may state, "Assess for bleeding if on anticoagulant."

GENERAL PRINCIPLES OF DRUG THERAPY

General Guidelines

1. *The goal of drug therapy should be to maximize beneficial effects and minimize adverse effects.*
2. *Expected benefits should outweigh potential adverse effects.* Thus, drugs usually should not be prescribed for trivial problems or problems for which nondrug measures are effective.
3. *Drug therapy should be individualized.* Many variables influence a drug's effects on the human body. Failure to consider these variables may decrease therapeutic effects or increase risks of adverse effects to an unacceptable level.
4. *Drug costs and effects on quality of life should be considered.* Pharmacoeconomic data that compare costs of pharmaceutical products are increasingly being considered a major factor in choosing medications. More specifically, for drugs of equal efficacy and toxicity, there is considerable pressure on prescribers to prescribe the less costly drug. There is also more emphasis on quality-of-life issues in current research, with greater expectations of measurable improvement as a result of drug therapy.

General Drug Selection and Dosage Considerations

Numerous factors must be considered when choosing a drug and dosage range for a particular client, including the following:

1. For the most part, use as few drugs in as few doses as possible. Minimizing the number of drugs and the frequency of administration increases client compliance with the prescribed drug regimen and decreases risks of serious adverse effects, including hazardous drug–drug interactions. There are notable exceptions to this basic rule. For example, multiple drugs are commonly used to treat severe hypertension or serious infections.
2. Although individual drugs allow greater flexibility of dosage than fixed-dose combinations, fixed-dose combinations are increasingly available and commonly used, mainly because clients are more likely to take them. Also, many of the combination products are formulated to be long acting, which also promotes compliance.
3. The least amount of the least potent drug that yields therapeutic benefit should be given to decrease adverse reactions. For example, if a mild non-narcotic and a strong narcotic analgesic are both ordered, give the non-narcotic drug if it is effective in relieving pain.
4. Recommended dosages are listed in amounts likely to be effective for most people, but they are only guidelines to be interpreted according to the client characteristics discussed previously. For example, clients with serious illnesses may require larger doses of some drugs than clients with milder illnesses; clients with severe kidney disease often need much smaller doses of renally excreted drugs.
5. A drug can be started rapidly or slowly. If it has a long half-life and optimal therapeutic effects do not usually occur for several days or weeks, the physician may order a limited number of relatively large (loading) doses followed by a regular schedule of smaller (maintenance) doses. When drug actions are not urgent, therapy may be initiated with a maintenance dose.
6. Different salts of the same drug rarely differ pharmacologically. Hydrochloride, sulfate, and sodium salts are often used. Pharmacists and chemists choose salts on the basis of cost, convenience, solubility, and stability. For example, solubility is especially important with parenteral drugs; taste is a factor with oral drugs.

Drug Therapy in Children

Drug therapy during infancy (1 month to 1 year) and childhood (approximately 1 to 12 years) requires special consideration because of the child's changing size, developmental level, and organ function. Physiologic differences alter drug pharmacokinetics (Table 4-1), and drug therapy is less predictable than in adults. Most drug use in children is empiric in nature because few studies have been done in that population. For many drugs, manufacturers' literature states that "safety and effectiveness for use in children have not been established." Neonates (birth to 1 month) are especially vulnerable to adverse drug effects because of their immature liver and kidney function (see Table 4-1). Neonatal therapeutics are discussed further in Chapter 67.

Most drugs given to adults also are given to children and general principles, techniques of drug administration, and nursing process guidelines apply. Additional principles and guidelines include the following:

1. All aspects of pediatric drug therapy must be guided by the child's age, weight, and level of growth and development.
2. Choice of drug is often restricted because many drugs commonly used in adult drug therapy have not been sufficiently investigated to ensure safety and effectiveness in children.
3. Safe therapeutic dosage ranges are less well defined for children than for adults. Some drugs are not recommended for use in children, and therefore dosages have not been established. For many drugs, doses for children are extrapolated from those established for adults. When pediatric dosage ranges are listed in drug literature, these should be used. Often, however, they are expressed in the amount of drug to be given per kilogram of body weight or square meter of body surface area, and the amount needed for a specific dose must be calculated as a fraction of the adult dose. The following methods are used for these calculations:

   a. Clark's rule is based on weight and is used for children at least 2 years of age:

   $$\frac{\text{Weight (in pounds)}}{150} \times \text{adult dose} = \text{child's dose}$$

   b. Calculating dosage based on body surface area is considered a more accurate method than those based on other characteristics. Body surface area, based on height and weight, is estimated using a nomogram (Fig. 4-1). Use the estimated body surface area in the following formula to calculate the child's dose:

   $$\frac{\text{Body surface area (in square meters)}}{1.73 \text{ square meters (m}^2\text{)}}$$
   $$\times \text{ adult dose } = \text{ child's dose}$$

   c. Dosages obtained from these calculations are approximate and must be individualized. These doses can be used initially and then increased or decreased according to the child's response.

TABLE 4-1   Children: Physiologic Characteristics and Pharmacokinetic Consequences

Physiologic Characteristics	Pharmacokinetic Consequences
Increased thinness and permeability of skin in neonates and infants	Increased absorption of topical drugs (eg, corticosteroids may be absorbed sufficiently to suppress adrenocortical function)
Immature blood–brain barrier in neonates and infants	Increased distribution of drugs into the central nervous system because myelinization (which creates the blood–brain barrier to the passage of drugs) is not mature until approximately 2 years of age
Increased percentage of body water (70% to 80% in neonates and infants, compared with 50% to 60% in children older than 2 years of age and adults)	Usually increased volume of distribution in infants and young children, compared to adults. This would seem to indicate a need for larger doses. However, prolonged drug half-life and decreased rate of drug clearance may offset. The net effect is often a need for decreased dosage.
Altered protein binding until approximately 1 year of age, when it reaches adult levels	The amount and binding capacity of plasma proteins may be reduced. This may result in a greater proportion of unbound or pharmacologically active drug and greater risks of adverse drug effects. Dosage requirements may be decreased or modified by other factors. Drugs with decreased protein binding in neonates, compared with older children and adults, include ampicillin (Omnipen, others), diazepam (Valium), digoxin (Lanoxin), lidocaine (Xylocaine), nafcillin (Unipen), phenobarbital, phenytoin (Dilantin), salicylates (eg, aspirin), and theophylline (Theolair).
Decreased glomerular filtration rate in neonates and infants, compared with older children and adults. Kidney function develops progressively during the first few months of life and is fairly mature by 1 year of age.	In neonates and infants, slowed excretion of drugs eliminated by the kidneys. Dosage of these drugs may need to be decreased, depending on the infant's age and level of growth and development.
Decreased activity of liver drug-metabolizing enzyme systems in neonates and infants	Decreased capacity for biotransformation of drugs. This results in slowed metabolism and elimination, with increased risks of drug accumulation and adverse effects.
Increased activity of liver drug-metabolizing enzyme systems in children	Increased capacity for biotransformation of some drugs. This results in a rapid rate of metabolism and elimination. For example, theophylline is cleared about 30% faster in a 7-year-old child than in an adult and approximately four times faster than in a neonate.

Nomogram for estimating the surface area of infants and young children

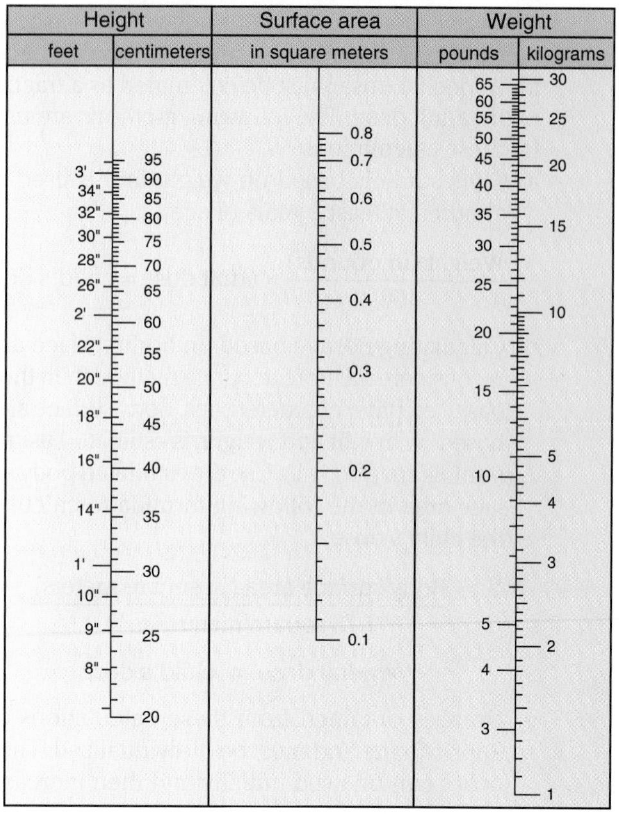

Height		Surface area	Weight	
feet	centimeters	in square meters	pounds	kilograms

Nomogram for estimating the surface area of older children and adults

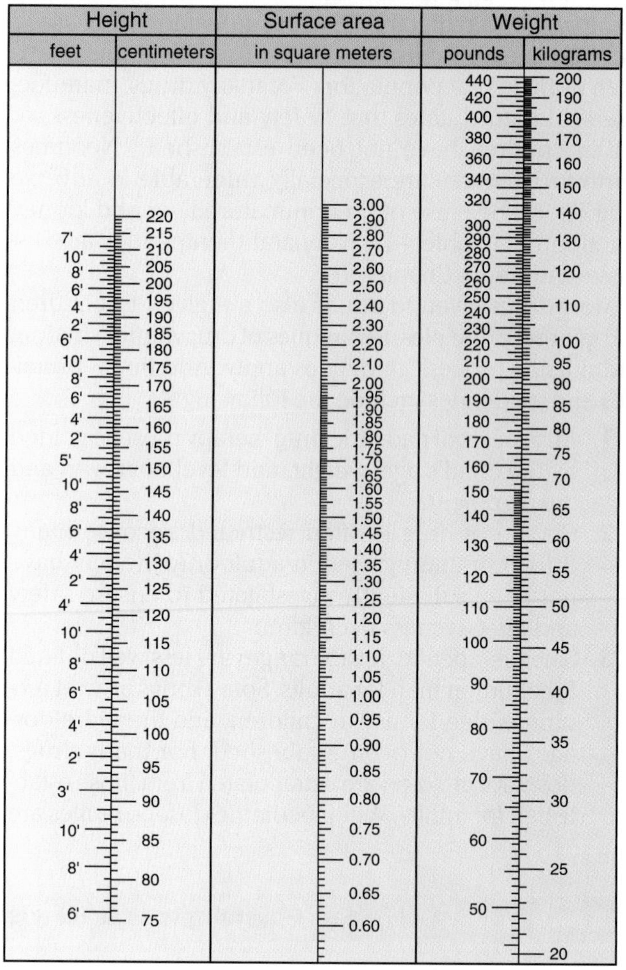

Height		Surface area	Weight	
feet	centimeters	in square meters	pounds	kilograms

FIGURE 4–1 Body surface nomograms. To determine the surface area of the client, draw a straight line between the point representing his or her height on the left vertical scale to the point representing weight on the right vertical scale. The point at which this line intersects the middle vertical scale represents the client's surface area in square meters. (Courtesy of Abbott Laboratories)

4. Use the oral route of drug administration when possible. Try to obtain the child's cooperation; never force oral medications because forcing may lead to aspiration.
5. If intramuscular injections are required in infants, use the thigh muscles because the deltoid muscles are quite small and the gluteal muscles do not develop until the child is walking.
6. For safety, keep all medications in childproof containers, out of reach of children, and do not refer to medications as "candy."

Drug Therapy in Older Adults

Aging is a continuum; precisely when a person becomes an "older adult" is not clearly established, but in this book

---

Nursing Notes: Apply Your Knowledge

Calculate the correct pediatric dosage, using the nomogram (see Fig. 4-1) and given the following information:

• Height: 55 cm
• Weight: 7 kg
• Normal adult daily dose: 2 g

How Can You Avoid This Medication Error?

Amoxicillin is prescribed for Jamie for an ear infection. The order is for 300 mg daily, to be administered q8h in equally divided doses. Jamie weighs 10 kg and the recommendations for infants are 20 to 40 mg/kg/day. The amoxicillin is supplied in syrup containing 100 mg/10 cc. The nurse gives Jamie 30 cc of amoxicillin for his morning dose.

people 65 years of age and older are so categorized. In this population, general nursing process guidelines and principles of drug therapy apply. In addition, adverse effects are likely because of physiologic changes associated with aging (Table 4-2), pathologic changes due to disease processes, multiple drug therapy for acute and chronic disorders, impaired memory and cognition, and difficulty in complying with drug orders. Overall, the goal of drug therapy may be "care" rather than "cure," with efforts to prevent or control symptoms and maintain the client's ability to function in usual activities of daily living. Additional principles include the following:

1. Although age in years is an important factor, older adults are quite heterogeneous in their responses to drug therapy. Thus, responses differ widely within the same age group. Responses also differ in the same person over time. Physiologic age (ie, organ function) is more important than chronologic age.

2. It may be difficult to separate the effects of aging from the effects of disease processes or drug therapy, particularly long-term drug therapy. Symptoms attributed to aging or disease may be caused by medications. This occurs because older adults in general metabolize and excrete drugs less efficiently, and thus drugs are more likely to accumulate.

3. Medications—both prescription and nonprescription drugs—should be taken only when necessary.

4. Review current medications, including nonprescription drugs, before prescribing new drugs; discontinue unnecessary drugs.

5. When drug therapy is required, the choice of drug should be based on available drug information regarding effects in older adults.

6. The basic principle of giving the smallest effective number of drugs applies especially to older adults. A regimen of several drugs increases the incidence of adverse reactions and potentially hazardous drug interactions. In addition, many older adults are unable or unwilling to self-administer more than three or four drugs correctly.

7. All drugs should be given for the shortest effective time. This interval is not established for most drugs, and many drugs are continued for years, regardless of whether they are needed. Health care providers must reassess drug regimens periodically to see whether drugs, dosages, or other aspects need to be revised. This is especially important when significant changes in health status have occurred.

8. The smallest number of effective doses should be prescribed. This allows less disruption of usual activities and promotes compliance with the prescribed regimen.

9. When any drug is started, the dosage in general should be smaller than for younger adults. The dosage can then be increased or decreased according to response. If an increased dosage is indicated, increments should be smaller and made at longer intervals in older adults. This conservative, safe approach is sometimes called "start low, go slow."

10. Use nondrug measures to decrease the need for drugs and to increase their effectiveness or de-

---

TABLE 4-2 **Older Adults: Physiologic Characteristics and Pharmacokinetic Consequences**

Physiologic Characteristics	Pharmacokinetic Consequences
Decreased gastrointestinal secretions and motility	Slower absorption of oral drugs and delayed onset of action. However, total absorption may be increased because drug molecules have more contact with sites of absorption in the small intestine.
Decreased cardiac output	Slower absorption from sites of administration (eg, gastrointestinal tract, subcutaneous or muscle tissue). Decreased distribution to sites of action in tissues, with potential for delaying the onset and reducing the extent of therapeutic effects.
Decreased blood flow to the liver and kidneys	The resultant delays in metabolism and excretion may lead to drug accumulation and increased risks of adverse or toxic effects.
Decreased total body water and lean body mass per kg of weight; increased body fat	Water-soluble drugs (eg, ethanol, lithium) are distributed into a smaller area, with resultant higher plasma concentrations and higher risks of toxicity with a given dose. Fat-soluble drugs (eg, diazepam) are distributed to a larger area, accumulate in fat, and have a longer duration of action in the body.
Decreased serum albumin	Decreased availability of protein for binding and transporting drug molecules. This increases serum concentration of free, pharmacologically active drug, especially for those that are normally highly protein bound (eg, aspirin, warfarin). This may increase risks of adverse effects. However, the drug also may be metabolized and excreted more rapidly, thereby offsetting at least some of the risks.
Decreased blood flow to the liver; decreased number and activity of drug-metabolizing enzymes	Slowed metabolism and detoxification, with increased risks of drug accumulation and toxic effects
Decreased blood flow to the kidneys, decreased number of functioning nephrons, decreased glomerular filtration rate, and decreased tubular secretion	Impaired drug excretion, prolonged half-life, and increased risks of toxicity

crease their adverse effects. For example, insomnia is a common complaint among older adults. Preventing it (eg, by avoiding caffeine-containing beverages and excessive napping) is much safer than taking sedative-hypnotic drugs.

11. For people receiving long-term drug therapy at home, use measures to help them take drugs safely and effectively.
    a. If vision is impaired, label drug containers with large lettering for easier readability. A magnifying glass also may be useful.
    b. Be sure the client can open drug containers. For example, avoid childproof containers for an older adult with arthritic hands.
    c. Several devices may be used to schedule drug doses and decrease risks of omitting or repeating doses. These include written schedules, calendars, and charts. Also available are drug containers with doses prepared and clearly labeled as to the day and time each dose is to be taken. With the latter system, the client can tell at a glance whether a dose has been taken.
    d. Enlist family members or friends when necessary.
12. When a client acquires new symptoms or becomes less capable of functioning in usual activities of daily living, consider the possibility of adverse drug effects. Often, new signs and symptoms are attributed to aging or disease. They may then be ignored or treated by prescribing a new drug, when stopping or reducing the dose of an old drug is the indicated intervention.

Drug Therapy in Renal Impairment

Many clients have or are at risk for impaired renal function. Clients with disease processes such as diabetes, hypertension, or heart failure may have renal insufficiency on first contact, and this may be worsened by illness, major surgery or trauma, or administration of nephrotoxic drugs. In clients with normal renal function, renal failure may develop from depletion of intravascular fluid volume, shock due to sepsis or blood loss, seriously impaired cardiovascular function, major surgery, nephrotoxic drugs, or other conditions. Acute renal failure (ARF) may occur in any illness in which renal blood flow or function is impaired. Chronic renal failure (CRF) usually results from disease processes that destroy renal tissue.

With ARF, renal function may recover if the impairment is recognized promptly, contributing factors are eliminated or treated effectively, and medication dosages are adjusted according to the extent of renal impairment. With CRF, effective treatment can help to conserve functioning nephrons and delay progression to end-stage renal disease (ESRD). If ESRD develops, some type of dialysis or transplantation is required.

In relation to drug therapy, the major concern with renal impairment is the high risk of drug accumulation and adverse effects because the kidneys are unable to excrete drugs and drug metabolites. Guidelines have been established for the use of many drugs; health care providers need to know and use these recommendations to maximize the safety and effectiveness of drug therapy. Some general guidelines are listed here; specific guidelines for particular drug groups are included in appropriate chapters.

1. Drug therapy must be especially cautious in clients with renal impairment because of the risks of drug accumulation and adverse effects. When possible, nephrologists should design drug therapy regimens. However, all health care providers need to be knowledgeable about risk factors for development of renal impairment, illnesses and their physiologic changes (eg, hemodynamic, renal, hepatic, and metabolic alterations) that affect renal function, and the effects of various drugs on renal function.
2. Renal status should be monitored in any client with renal insufficiency or risk factors for development of renal insufficiency. Signs and symptoms of ARF include decreased urine output (<600 mL/24 hours), increased blood urea nitrogen or increased serum creatinine (>2 mg/dL or an increase of ≥0.5 mg/dL over a baseline value of <3.0 mg/dL). In addition, an adequate fluid intake is required to excrete drugs by the kidneys. Any factors that deplete extracellular fluid volume (eg, inadequate fluid intake, diuretic drugs, loss of body fluids with blood loss, vomiting or diarrhea) increase the risk of worsening renal impairment in clients who already have impairment or of causing impairment in those who previously had normal function.
3. Clients with renal impairment may respond to a drug dose or serum concentration differently than clients with normal renal function because of the physiologic and biochemical changes. Thus, drug therapy must be individualized according to the extent of renal impairment. This is usually determined by measuring serum creatinine, which is then used to calculate creatinine clearance as a measure of the glomerular filtration rate (GFR). Because serum creatinine is determined by muscle mass as well as the GFR, the serum creatinine measurement cannot be used as the sole indicator of renal function unless the client is a young, relatively healthy, well-nourished person with a sudden acute illness. Estimations of creatinine clearance are more accurate for clients with stable renal function (ie, stable serum creatinine) and average muscle mass (for their age, weight, and height). Estimations are less accurate for emaciated and obese clients and for those with changing renal function, as often occurs in acute illness. If a fluctuating serum creatinine is used to calculate the GFR, an erroneous value will be obtained. If a client is oliguric (<400 mL urine/24 hours), for example, the creatinine clearance should be estimated to be less than 10 mL/minute, regardless of the serum creatinine concentration.

Serum creatinine is also a relatively unreliable indicator of renal function in elderly or malnourished clients. Because these clients usually have diminished muscle mass, they may have a normal serum level of creatinine even if their renal function and GFR are markedly reduced.

Some medications can increase serum creatinine levels and create a false impression of renal failure. These drugs, which include cimetidine and trimethoprim, interfere with secretion of creatinine into kidney tubules. As a result, serum creatinine levels are increased without an associated decrease in renal function.

4. **Drug selection** should be guided by baseline renal function and the known effects of drugs on renal function, when possible. Many commonly used drugs may adversely affect renal function, including nonsteroidal anti-inflammatory drugs such as prescription or over-the-counter ibuprofen (Motrin, Advil). Some drugs are excreted exclusively (eg, aminoglycoside antibiotics, lithium) and most are excreted primarily or to some extent by the kidneys. Some drugs are contraindicated in renal impairment (eg, tetracyclines except doxycycline); others can be used if safety guidelines are followed (eg, reducing dosage, monitoring serum drug levels and renal function tests, avoiding dehydration). Drugs known to be nephrotoxic should be avoided when possible. However, in some instances, there are no effective substitutes and nephrotoxic drugs must be given. Some commonly used nephrotoxic drugs include aminoglycoside antibiotics, amphotericin B, and cisplatin.

5. **Dosage** of many drugs needs to be decreased in renal failure, including aminoglycoside antibiotics, most cephalosporin antibiotics, fluoroquinolones, and digoxin. For some drugs, a smaller dose or a longer interval between doses is recommended for clients with moderate (creatinine clearance 10 to 50 mL/minute) or severe renal insufficiency (creatinine clearance <10 mL/minute). However, for many commonly used drugs, the most effective dosage adjustments are based on the client's clinical responses and serum drug levels.

For clients receiving renal replacement therapy (eg, hemodialysis or some type of filtration), the treatment removes variable amounts of drugs that are usually excreted through the kidneys. With some drugs, such as many antimicrobials, additional loading doses may be needed to maintain therapeutic blood levels of drug.

Drug Therapy in Hepatic Impairment

Most drugs are eliminated from the body by hepatic metabolism, renal excretion, or both. Hepatic metabolism depends mainly on blood flow and enzyme activity in the liver and protein binding in the plasma. Clients at

risk for impaired liver function include those with primary liver disease (eg, hepatitis, cirrhosis) and those with disease processes that impair blood flow to the liver (eg, heart failure, shock, major surgery or trauma) or hepatic enzyme production. An additional factor is hepatotoxic drugs. Fortunately, although the liver is often damaged, it has a great capacity for cell repair and may be able to function with as little as 10% of undamaged hepatic cells.

In relation to drug therapy, acute liver impairment may interfere with drug metabolism and elimination, whereas chronic cirrhosis or severe liver impairment may affect all pharmacokinetic processes. It is difficult to predict the effects of drug therapy because of wide variations in liver function and few helpful diagnostic tests. In addition, with severe hepatic impairment, extrahepatic sites of drug metabolism (eg, intestine, kidneys, lungs) may become more important in eliminating drugs from the body. Thus, guidelines for drug selection, dosage, and duration of use are not well established. Some general guidelines for increasing drug safety and effectiveness are listed here; known guidelines for particular drug groups are included in appropriate chapters.

1. During drug therapy, clients with impaired liver function require close monitoring for signs and symptoms (eg, nausea, vomiting, jaundice, liver enlargement) and abnormal results of laboratory tests of liver function (see 4, below).

2. **Drug selection** should be based on knowledge of drug effects on hepatic function. Hepatotoxic drugs should be avoided when possible. If they cannot be avoided, they should be used in the smallest effective doses, for the shortest effective time. Commonly used hepatotoxic drugs include acetaminophen, isoniazid, and cholesterol-lowering statins. Alcohol is toxic to the liver by itself and increases the risks of hepatotoxicity with other drugs.

In addition to hepatotoxic drugs, many other drugs can cause or aggravate liver impairment by decreasing hepatic blood flow and drug-metabolizing capacity. For example, epinephrine and related drugs may cause vasoconstriction in the hepatic artery and portal vein, the two main sources of the liver's blood supply. Beta-adrenergic blocking agents decrease hepatic blood flow by decreasing cardiac output. Several drugs (eg, cimetidine, fluoxetine, ketoconazole) inhibit hepatic metabolism of many coadministered drugs. The consequence may be toxicity from the inhibited drugs if the dose is not decreased.

3. **Dosage** should be reduced for drugs that are extensively metabolized in the liver because, if doses are not reduced, serum drug levels are higher, elimination is slower, and toxicity is more likely to occur in a client with hepatic disease. For example, lidocaine is normally rapidly deactivated by hepatic metabolism. If blood flow is impaired so that lidocaine molecules in the blood are unable to reach drug-metabolizing liver cells, more drug stays in the

bloodstream longer. Also, some oral drugs are normally extensively metabolized during their "first pass" through the liver, so that a relatively small portion of an oral dose reaches the systemic circulation. With cirrhosis, the blood carrying the drug molecules is shunted around the liver so that oral drugs go directly into the systemic circulation. Some drugs whose dosages should be decreased in hepatic failure include cefoperazone, cimetidine, clindamycin, diazepam, labetalol, lorazepam, meperidine, morphine, phenytoin, propranolol, quinidine, ranitidine, theophylline, and verapamil.

4. Liver function tests should be monitored in clients with or at risk for liver impairment, especially when clients are receiving potentially hepatotoxic drugs. Indicators of hepatic impairment include serum bilirubin levels above 4 to 5 mg/dL, a prothrombin time greater than 1.5 times control, a serum albumin below 2.0 g/dL, and elevated serum alanine (ALT) and aspartate (AST) aminotransferases. In some clients, abnormal liver function test results may occur without indicating severe liver damage and are often reversible.

Drug Therapy in Critical Illness

The term *critical illness*, as used here, denotes the care of clients who are experiencing acute, serious, or life-threatening illness. Critically ill clients are at risk for multiple organ damage, including cardiovascular, renal, and hepatic impairments that influence all aspects of drug therapy. Overall, critically ill clients exhibit varying degrees of organ dysfunction and their conditions tend to change rapidly, so that drug pharmacokinetics and pharmacodynamics vary widely. Although blood volume is often decreased, drug distribution is usually increased because of less protein binding and increased extracellular fluid. Drug elimination is usually impaired because of decreased blood flow and decreased function of the liver and kidneys.

Although critical care nursing is a specialty area of practice and much of critical care is performed in an intensive care unit (ICU), nurses in numerous other settings also care for these clients. For example, nurses in emergency departments often initiate and maintain treatment for several hours; nurses on other hospital units care for clients who are transferred to or from ICUs; and, increasingly, clients formerly cared for in an ICU are on medical-surgical hospital units, in long-term care facilities, or even at home. Moreover, increasing numbers of nursing students are introduced to critical care during their educational programs, many new graduates seek employment in critical care settings, and experienced nurses may transfer to an ICU. Thus, all nurses need to know about drug therapy in critically ill clients. Some general guidelines to increase safety and effectiveness of drug therapy in critical illness are listed here; more specific guidelines related to particular drugs are included in the appropriate chapters.

1. Drug therapy in clients who are critically ill is often more complex, more problematic, and less predictable than in most other populations. One reason is that clients often have multiple organ impairments that alter drug effects and increase the risks of adverse drug reactions. Another reason is that critically ill clients often require aggressive treatment with large numbers, large doses, and combinations of highly potent medications. Overall, therapeutic effects may be decreased and risks of adverse reactions and interactions may be increased because the client's body may be unable to process or respond to drugs effectively.

   In this at-risk population, safe and effective drug therapy requires that all involved health care providers be knowledgeable about common critical illnesses, the physiologic changes (eg, hemodynamic, renal, hepatic, and metabolic alterations) that can be caused by the illnesses, and the drugs used to treat the illnesses. Nurses need to be especially diligent in administering drugs and vigilant in observing client responses.

2. Drugs used in critical illness represent most drug classifications and are also discussed in other chapters. Commonly used drugs include analgesics, antimicrobials, cardiovascular agents, gastric acid suppressants, neuromuscular blocking agents, and sedatives.

3. In many instances, the goal of drug therapy is to support vital functions and relieve life-threatening symptoms until healing can occur or definitive treatment can be instituted.

4. **Drug selection** should be guided by the client's clinical status (eg, symptoms, severity of illness) and organ function, especially cardiovascular, renal, and hepatic functions.

5. **Route of administration** should also be guided by the client's clinical status. Most drugs are given intravenously (IV) because critically ill clients are often unable to take oral medications and require many drugs, rapid drug action, and relatively large doses. In addition, the IV route achieves more reliable and measurable blood levels.

   When a drug is given IV, it reaches the heart and brain quickly because the sympathetic nervous system and other homeostatic mechanisms attempt to maintain blood flow to the heart and brain at the expense of blood flow to other organs such as the kidneys, gastrointestinal (GI) tract, liver, and skin. As a result, cardiovascular and CNS effects may be faster, more pronounced, and longer lasting than usual. If the drug is a sedative, effects may include excessive sedation and cardiac depression.

   If the client is able to take oral medications, this is probably the preferred route. However, many factors may interfere with drug effects (eg, impaired function of the GI tract, heart, kidneys, or liver) and drug–drug and drug–diet interactions may occur if precautions are not taken. For example, anti-ulcer drugs, which are often given to prevent stress ulcers and GI bleeding, may decrease absorption of other drugs.

For clients who receive oral medications or nutritional solutions through a nasogastric, gastrostomy, or jejunostomy tube, there may be drug–food interactions that impair drug absorption. In addition, crushing tablets or opening capsules to give a drug by a GI tube may alter the absorption and chemical stability of the drug.

Sublingual, oral inhalation, and transdermal medications may be used effectively in some critically ill clients. However, few drugs are available in these formulations.

For clients in shock, drugs usually should not be given orally, subcutaneously, intramuscularly, or by skin patch because shock impairs absorption from their sites of administration, distribution to body cells is unpredictable, the liver cannot metabolize drugs effectively, and the kidneys cannot excrete drugs effectively.

6. **Dosage** requirements may vary considerably among clients and within the same client at different times during an illness. A standard dose may be effective, subtherapeutic, or toxic. Thus, it is especially important that initial dosages are individualized according to the severity of the condition being treated and client characteristics such as age and organ function, and that maintenance dosages are titrated according to client responses and changes in organ function (eg, as indicated by symptoms or laboratory tests).

7. With many drugs, the timing of administration may be important in increasing therapeutic effects and decreasing adverse effects. Once-daily drug doses should be given at approximately the same time each day; multiple-daily doses should be given at approximately even intervals around the clock.

8. Weigh clients when possible, initially and periodically, because dosage of many drugs is based on weight. In addition, periodic weights help to assess clients for loss of body mass or gain in body water, both of which affect the pharmacokinetics of the drugs administered.

9. Laboratory tests are often needed before and during drug therapy of critical illnesses to assess the client's condition (eg, cardiovascular, renal and hepatic functions, fluid and electrolyte balance) and response to treatment. Other tests may include measurement of serum drug levels. The results of these tests may indicate that changes are needed in drug therapy.

10. Serum protein levels should be monitored in critically ill clients because drug binding may be significantly altered. Serum albumin, which binds acidic drugs such as phenytoin and diazepam, is usually decreased during critical illness for a variety of reasons, including inadequate production by the liver. If there is not enough albumin to bind a drug, blood levels are higher and may cause adverse effects. Also, unbound molecules are metabolized and excreted more readily so that therapeutic effects may be decreased.

Alpha$_1$-acid glycoprotein binds basic drugs and its synthesis may increase during critical illness. As a result, the bound portion of a dose increases for some drugs (eg, meperidine, propranolol, imipramine, lidocaine) and therapeutic blood levels may not be achieved unless higher doses are given. In addition, these drugs are eliminated more slowly than usual.

 Home Care

Home care is an expanding area of health care. This trend evolved from efforts to reduce health care costs, especially the costs of hospitalization. The consequences of this trend include increased outpatient care and brief hospitalizations for severe illness or major surgery. In both instances, clients of all age groups are often discharged to their homes for follow-up care and recovery. Skilled nursing care, such as managing medication regimens, is often required during follow-up. Most general principles and nursing responsibilities related to drug therapy apply in home care as in other health care settings. Some additional principles and factors include the following:

1. Clients may require short- or long-term drug therapy. In most instances, the role of the nurse is to teach the client or caregiver to administer medications and monitor their effects.

2. In a client's home, the nurse is a guest and must work within the environment to establish rapport, elicit cooperation, and provide nursing care. The initial contact is usually by telephone, and one purpose is to schedule a home visit, preferably at a convenient time for the client and caregiver. In addition, state the main purpose of the visit and approximately how long the visit will be. Establish a method for contact in case the appointment must be canceled by either party.

3. Assess the client's attitude toward the prescribed medication regimen and his or her ability to provide self-care. If the client is unable, who will be the primary caregiver for medication administration and observing for medication effects? What are the learning needs of the client or caregiver in relation to the medication regimen?

4. Ask to see all prescribed and over-the-counter medications the client takes, and ask how and when the client takes each one. With this information, the nurse may be able to reinforce the client's compliance or identify potential problem areas (eg, differences between instructions and client usage

of medications, drugs with opposing or duplicate effects, continued use of medications that were supposed to be discontinued, drugs discontinued because of adverse effects).

5. Assess the environment for potential safety hazards (eg, risk of infection with corticosteroids and other immunosuppressants, risk of falls and other injuries with narcotic analgesics and other drugs with sedating effects). In addition, assess the client's ability to obtain medications and keep appointments for follow-up visits to health care providers.

6. Provide whatever information and assistance is needed for home management of the drug therapy regimen. Most people are accustomed to taking oral drugs, but they may need information about timing in relation to food intake, whether a tablet can be crushed, when to omit the drug, and other aspects. With other routes, the nurse may initially need to demonstrate administration or coach the client or caregiver through each step. Demonstrating and having the client or caregiver do a return demonstration is a good way to teach psychomotor skills such as giving a medication through a GI tube, preparing and administering an injection, or manipulating an intravenous infusion pump.

7. In addition to safe and accurate administration, teach the client and caregiver to observe for beneficial and adverse effects. If side effects occur, teach them how to manage minor ones and which ones to report to a health care provider.

8. Between home visits, the home care nurse can maintain telephone contact with clients and caregivers to monitor progress, answer questions, identify problems, and provide reassurance. Clients and caregivers should be given a telephone number to call with questions about medications, side effects, and so forth. The nurse may wish to schedule a daily time for receiving and making nonemergency calls.

NURSING ACTIONS | **Monitoring Drug Therapy**

NURSING ACTIONS	RATIONALE/EXPLANATION
1. Prepare and administer drugs accurately (see Chap. 3).	
a. Practice the five rights of drug administration (right *drug*, right *client*, right *dose*, right *route*, and right *time*).	These rights are ensured if the techniques described in Chapter 3 are consistently followed. The time may vary by approximately 30 minutes. For example, a drug ordered for 9 AM can be given between 8:30 AM and 9:30 AM. No variation is allowed in the other rights.
b. Use correct techniques for different routes of administration.	For example, sterile equipment and techniques are required for injection of any drug.
c. Follow label instructions regarding mixing or other aspects of giving specific drugs.	Some drugs require specific techniques of preparation and administration.
2. Observe for therapeutic effects	In general, the nurse should know the expected effects and when they are likely to occur. Specific observations depend on the specific drug or drugs being given.
3. Observe for adverse effects	All drugs are potentially harmful, although the incidence and severity of adverse reactions vary among drugs and clients. People most likely to have adverse reactions are those with severe liver or kidney disease, those who are very young or very old, those receiving several drugs, and those receiving large doses of any drug. Specific adverse effects for which to observe depend on the drugs being given.
4. Observe for drug interactions	The nurse must be knowledgeable about common and potentially significant drug interactions. Also, because interactions may occur whenever the client is receiving two or more drugs concurrently, they should be considered as a possible cause of unexpected responses to drug therapy.

Nursing Notes: Apply Your Knowledge

Answer: First calculate the body surface area (BSA) of the infant using the nomogram. Drawing a line between 55 cm and 7 kg will result in a body surface area of 0.3 meters squared. Divide 0.3 by 1.73, which equals 0.173. The adult dose is 2 g, which equals 2000 mg. Multiply 2000 mg by 0.173 to get 346 mg, which is the correct pediatric dosage.

How Can You Avoid This Medication Error?

Answer: The nurse administered the wrong dose of medication to Jamie. Thirty cc would provide the entire daily dose of amoxicillin, rather than 100 mg, which should be administered every 8 hours. Carefully reread the order and recalculate the dosage ordered. Unit dosing can help double-check calculations and avoid errors.

REVIEW AND APPLICATION EXERCISES

1. Why must nurses know the adverse effects of the drugs they give?

2. Given a newly assigned client, what information is needed about present and previous medications?

3. Anticipate the questions a client might ask about a drug and rehearse possible answers, including drugs that are well known to you and those that are not.

4. With children, what are some potential difficulties with drug administration, and how can they be prevented or minimized?

5. With older adults, what are some potential difficulties with drug administration, and how can they be prevented or minimized?

6. For older adults, explain what is meant by "start low, go slow" and why it is a good approach to drug therapy.

7. Why is client teaching about drug therapy needed, and what information should usually be included?

8. Describe at least three important nursing considerations for clients who have renal or hepatic impairment or critical illness.

9. For the home care nurse assisting with a medication regimen, what are some likely differences between the nursing care needed by a child and an adult?

SELECTED REFERENCES

Broussard, M.C. & Pitre, S. (1996). Medication problems in the elderly: A home healthcare nurse's perspective. *Home Healthcare Nurse, 14,* 441–443.

Ghalib, R. (1998). Hepatic diseases. In C.F. Carey, H.H. Lee, & K.F. Woeltje (Eds.), *The Washington manual of medical therapeutics,* 29th ed., pp. 329–342. Philadelphia: Lippincott Williams & Wilkins.

Lee, M. (1996). Drugs and the elderly: Do you know the risks? *American Journal of Nursing, 96*(7), 25–32.

Morrison, G. (1996). Drug dosing in the intensive care unit: The patient with renal failure. In J.M. Rippe, R.S. Irwin, M.P. Fink, & F.B. Cerra (Eds.), *Intensive Care Medicine,* 3rd ed., pp. 1023–1057. Boston: Little, Brown and Company.

Nies, A.S. & Spielberg, S.P. (1996). Principles of therapeutics. In J.G. Hardman, L.E. Limbird, P.B. Molinoff, & R.W. Ruddon (Eds.), *Goodman & Gilman's The pharmacological basis of therapeutics,* 9th ed., pp. 43–62. New York: McGraw-Hill.

Todi, S.K. & Hartmann, R.A. (1997). Pharmacologic principles. In J.M. Civetta, R.W. Taylor, & R.R. Kirby (Eds.), *Critical care,* 3rd ed., pp. 475–488. Philadelphia: Lippincott-Raven.

Drugs Affecting the Central Nervous System

5

Physiology of the Central Nervous System

Objectives

After studying this chapter, the student will be able to:

1. Describe the process of neurotransmission.

2. Describe major neurotransmitters and their roles in nervous system functioning.

3. Discuss signs and symptoms of central nervous system (CNS) depression.

4. Discuss general types and characteristics of CNS depressant drugs.

The central nervous system (CNS), composed of the brain and spinal cord, acts as the control center for regulating physical and mental body processes. Afferent or sensory neurons carry messages to the CNS; efferent or motor neurons carry messages away from the CNS. More specifically, the CNS constantly receives information about blood levels of oxygen and carbon dioxide, body temperature, and sensory stimuli and sends messages to effector organs to adjust the environment toward homeostasis. It is also concerned with higher intellectual functions (eg, thought, learning, reasoning, problem solving, memory) and with muscle function, both skeletal and smooth.

The CNS has complex interactions with other parts of the body, and components of the CNS have complex interactions with each other. Although various components of brain function are often studied individually, it is the overall coordination of the "mind/body" connections that produces mental and physical health. A lack of coordination or imbalances among the components may lead to mental or physical disorders. Thus, emotions can strongly influence neural control of body function, and alterations in neural functions can strongly influence psychological behavior.

More specific characteristics are reviewed in the following sections to aid understanding of drugs that act by altering CNS functions.

CHARACTERISTICS AND FUNCTIONS OF THE CENTRAL NERVOUS SYSTEM

Neurons

The CNS is composed mainly of two types of cells: the *glia* protect, support, and nourish the neuron; the *neuron* is the basic functional unit. Most neurons are composed of a cell body, a dendrite, and an axon. Nerve cell bodies usually occur in groups or clusters, called ganglia or nuclei. A cluster of cell bodies or nuclei with the same function is called a center (eg, the vasomotor and respiratory centers in the medulla oblongata). A dendrite has a branching structure with many synapses or sites for receiving stimuli or messages, which are then conducted toward the cell body. An axon is a finger-like projection that carries impulses away from the cell body. The end of the axon branches into presynaptic fibers that end with small, knob-like structures called vesicles. These structures project into the synapse and contain the granules where neurotransmitters are stored. Many axons are covered by a fatty substance called myelin. The myelin cover or sheath protects and insulates the axon. An axon together with its myelin sheath is called a nerve fiber. Nerve fibers involved in the transmission of the same type of impulses (eg, pain signals) are found together in a common pathway or tract.

Neurons must be able to communicate with other neurons and body tissues. This communication involves a complex network of electrical and chemical signals that receive, interpret or modify, and send messages. Characteristics that allow neurons to communicate with other cells include excitability (the ability to produce an action potential or be stimulated) and conductivity (the ability to convey electrical impulses). More specific components of the communication network include neurotransmitters, synapses, and receptors (described below).

Neurotransmitters

Neurotransmitters are chemical substances that carry messages from one neuron to another, or from a neuron to other body tissues, such as cardiac or skeletal muscle. They are synthesized and stored in presynaptic nerve terminals and released in response to an electrical impulse (action potential) arriving at the end of the first neuron (presynaptic fiber). The basis for the action potential is the transient opening of ion channels. The entry of calcium ions is required for neurotransmitter release from storage sites in small sacs called synaptic vesicles. Storage of neurotransmitters allows them to be available quickly when needed and to avoid degradation by enzymes in the nerve terminal.

When released from the synaptic vesicles, molecules of neurotransmitter cross the synapse, bind to receptors in the cell membrane of the postsynaptic neuron (Fig. 5-1), and excite or inhibit postsynaptic neurons. Free neurotransmitter molecules (ie, those not bound to receptors) are rapidly removed from the synapse by three mechanisms: transportation back into the presynaptic nerve terminal (re-uptake) for reuse, diffusion into surrounding body fluids, or destruction by enzymes (eg, acetylcholine is degraded by cholinesterase; norepinephrine is metabolized by monoamine oxidase and catecholomethyl transferase).

The three types of neurotransmitters thus far identified are amines, amino acids, and peptides, all of which are

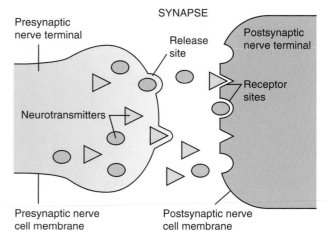

FIGURE 5–1 Neurotransmission in the central nervous system. Neurotransmitter molecules (eg, norepinephrine and acetylcholine), released by the presynaptic nerve, cross the synapse and bind with receptor proteins in the cell membrane of the postsynaptic nerve.

derived from body proteins. Most acute CNS responses are caused by small-molecule, rapidly acting neurotransmitters, such as acetylcholine, the amines (dopamine, norepinephrine, serotonin), and amino acids (aspartate, gamma-aminobutyric acid [GABA], glutamate, and glycine). Most prolonged CNS responses are caused by large-molecule, slowly acting neurotransmitters, such as the neuropeptide hormones (eg, adrenocorticotropic hormone [ACTH or corticotropin] and antidiuretic hormone [ADH]). Prolonged effects are thought to involve closure of calcium channels, changes in cellular metabolism, changes in activation or deactivation of specific genes in the cell nucleus, and alterations in the numbers of excitatory or inhibitory postsynaptic membrane receptors. Some peptides (eg, ADH) serve as chemical messengers in both the nervous system and the endocrine system.

Several factors affect the availability and function of neurotransmitters. One factor is the availability of precursor proteins and enzymes required to synthesize particular neurotransmitters. Another factor is the number and binding capacity of *receptors* in the cell membranes of presynaptic and postsynaptic nerve endings. A particular neurotransmitter may interact with many different receptors. Other important factors include *acid–base imbalances* (acidosis decreases synaptic transmission; alkalosis increases synaptic transmission); *hypoxia*, which causes CNS depression (coma occurs within seconds without oxygen); and *drugs*, which may alter neurotransmitter synthesis, release, degradation, or binding to receptors to cause either CNS stimulation or depression.

Synapses

Neurons in a chain are separated by a microscopic gap called a *synapse* or synaptic cleft. Synapses may be *electrical*, in which sodium and potassium ions can rapidly conduct an electrical impulse from one neuron to another, or *chemical*, in which a neurotransmitter conducts the message to the next neuron. The chemical synapse is more commonly used to communicate with other neurons or target cells. Neurotransmitter release and removal occur in the synapses.

Receptors

Receptors are proteins embedded in the cell membranes of neurons. In the CNS, most receptors are on postsynaptic neurons, but some are on presynaptic nerve terminals. For most receptors, several subtypes have been identified, for which specific characteristics and functions have not yet been delineated. A neurotransmitter must bind to receptors to exert an effect on the next neuron in the chain. Some receptors act rapidly to open ion channels; others interact with a variety of intracellular proteins to initiate a second messenger system. For example, when

norepinephrine binds with alpha- or beta-adrenergic receptors, intracellular events include activation of the enzyme adenyl cyclase and the production of cyclic adenosine monophosphate (cAMP). In this case, the cAMP is a second messenger that activates cellular functions and the physiologic responses controlled by the alpha- and beta-adrenergic receptors. A neurotransmitter–receptor complex may have an excitatory or inhibitory effect on the postsynaptic neuron.

Receptors increase in number and activity (up-regulation) when there is underactivity at the synapse. They decrease in number and activity (down-regulation) when there is overactivity. Like other protein molecules in the body, receptors are constantly being synthesized and degraded. More specifically, it is believed that receptor proteins are constantly being formed by the endoplasmic reticulum–Golgi apparatus and inserted into presynaptic and postsynaptic membranes. If the synapses are overused and excessive amounts of neurotransmitter combine with receptor proteins, it is then postulated that many of the receptor proteins are inactivated and removed from the synaptic membrane. Thus, synaptic fatigue and downgrading or upgrading of receptors work with other control mechanisms of the nervous system to readjust abnormally stimulated or depressed nerve function toward normal.

Neurotransmission Systems

Neurons function through communication networks that may be called neurotransmission systems, the major elements of which are neurotransmitters, synapses, and receptors. Although neurotransmitters, synapses, and receptors are discussed separately here, it is the interaction among these elements that promotes order or disorder in the body's physical and mental processes. Although many details of neuronal function remain elusive, a great deal of knowledge has been gained. For example, numerous neurotransmitters and subtypes of receptors have been identified and characterized. Major neurotransmission systems are the cholinergic, dopaminergic, GABA-ergic, noradrenergic, and serotonergic networks.

The **cholinergic system** uses *acetylcholine* as its neurotransmitter. Acetylcholine, the first substance to be designated as a neurotransmitter in the CNS, is located in many areas of the brain, with especially high concentrations in the motor cortex and basal ganglia. It is also a neurotransmitter in the autonomic nervous system and at peripheral neuromuscular junctions. Acetylcholine exerts excitatory effects at synapses and nerve–muscle junctions and inhibitory effects at some peripheral sites, such as organs supplied by the vagus nerves. In the CNS, acetylcholine is associated with level of arousal, memory, motor conditioning, and speech.

The **dopaminergic system** uses *dopamine* as its neurotransmitter. Dopamine is derived from tyrosine, an amino acid, and is a precursor substance in the synthesis of norepinephrine and epinephrine. Dopamine makes up more than half the catecholamine content in the brain and is found in the substantia nigra, the midbrain, and the hypothalamus, with high concentrations in the substantia nigra and basal ganglia. Much of the information about dopamine is derived from studies of antipsychotic drugs (see Chap. 9) and Parkinson's disease, a disorder caused by destruction of dopamine-producing neurons in the substantia nigra. Dopamine also occurs outside the brain, in renal and mesenteric blood vessels.

In the CNS, dopamine is thought to be inhibitory in the basal ganglia but may be excitatory in other areas. Repeated stimulation of dopamine receptors decreases their numbers (down-regulation) and their sensitivity to dopamine (desensitization). Prolonged blockade of dopamine receptors increases their numbers and sensitivity to dopamine. Some receptors (called autoreceptors) occur on the presynaptic nerve terminal. When released, dopamine stimulates these receptors and a negative feedback system is initiated that inhibits further dopamine synthesis and release.

Two groups of dopamine receptors have been identified. They are differentiated by the intracellular events that follow dopamine–receptor binding. One group includes D_1 and D_5 receptors, which activate adenyl cyclase to produce cAMP. The other group includes D_2, D_3, and D_4 receptors. D_2 receptors have been described most thoroughly; they are thought to inhibit activation of adenyl cyclase and subsequent production of cAMP, suppress calcium ion currents, and activate potassium ion currents. D_3 and D_4 receptor functions have not been delineated. Overall, dopamine actions at the cellular level depend on the subtype of receptor to which it binds and the simultaneous effects of other neurotransmitters at the same target neurons.

The **GABA-ergic system** uses *GABA* as its neurotransmitter. GABA is synthesized in the brain (cerebellum, basal ganglia, and cerebral cortex) and spinal cord in abundant amounts. It is the major inhibitory neurotransmitter in the CNS, with a role in many neuronal circuits (estimated at nearly one third of CNS synapses). GABA receptors have been divided into two main types, A and B. The $GABA_A$ receptor is a chloride ion channel that opens when GABA is released from presynaptic neurons. $GABA_B$ has not been delineated, but it is thought to function in the regulation of ion channels and biochemical pathways. There is evidence of multiple subtypes of GABA receptors and important functional differences among them.

The **noradrenergic** (norepinephrine) **system** uses *norepinephrine* as its neurotransmitter and extends to virtually every area of the brain. Like dopamine, norepinephrine is a catecholamine synthesized from tyrosine. It is found in relatively large amounts in the hypothalamus and the limbic system and in smaller amounts in most areas of the brain, including the reticular formation. Norepinephrine is mainly an excitatory neurotransmitter that stimulates the brain to generalized increased activity. However, it is inhibitory in a few areas because of inhibitory receptors at some nerve synapses.

Norepinephrine receptors in the CNS, as in the sympathetic nervous system, are divided into alpha- and beta-adrenergic receptors and their subtypes. Activation of $alpha_1$, $beta_1$, and $beta_2$ receptors is thought to stimulate activity of intracellular adenyl cyclase and the production of cAMP. Activation of $alpha_2$ receptors is associated with inhibition of adenyl cyclase activity and decreased production of cAMP. However, the effects of norepinephrine–$alpha_2$ receptor coupling are thought to stem mainly from activation of receptor-operated potassium ion channels and suppression of voltage-operated calcium ion channels. These effects on ion channels may increase membrane resistance to stimuli and inhibit the firing of CNS neurons. In addition, $alpha_2$ receptors on the presynaptic nerve ending are believed to regulate norepinephrine release. In other words, when high levels of extracellular norepinephrine act on presynaptic $alpha_2$ receptors, the effect is similar to that of a negative feedback system that inhibits the release of norepinephrine. Overall, the noradrenergic system is associated with mood, motor activity, regulation of arousal, and reward. It is thought to play an important role in producing rapid-eye-movement (REM) sleep, during which dreaming occurs.

The **serotonergic system** uses *serotonin* (also called 5-hydroxytryptamine or 5-HT) as its neurotransmitter. Serotonin-synthesizing neurons are widely distributed in the CNS, beginning in the midbrain and projecting into the thalamus, hypothalamus, cerebral cortex, and spinal cord. Because serotonin is synthesized from the amino acid tryptophan, the amount of tryptophan intake in the diet and the enzyme tryptophan hydroxylase control the rate of serotonin production. CNS serotonin is usually an inhibitory neurotransmitter and is associated with mood, the sleep–wake cycle, habituation, and sensory perceptions, including inhibition of pain pathways in the spinal cord. Serotonin is thought to produce sleep by inhibiting CNS activity and arousal.

Serotonin receptors are found in regions of the CNS that are associated with mood and anxiety and are also thought to be involved in temperature regulation. Activation of some receptors leads to hyperpolarization and neuronal inhibition. Several subtypes of serotonin receptors have been identified, some of which are linked to inhibition of adenyl cyclase activity or to regulation of potassium or calcium ion channels.

Serotonin is also found outside the CNS, mainly in mast cells of the lungs and platelets. It plays a major role in the blood coagulation process, during which it is released from platelets and causes vasoconstriction. It may also be involved in the vascular spasm associated with some pulmonary allergic reactions (during which it is released from mast cells) and migraine headaches. However, peripheral serotonin cannot cross the blood–brain barrier.

Other systems of neurotransmission include several amino acids that may serve as both structural components for protein synthesis and neurotransmitters. Amino acids were recognized as neurotransmitters relatively recently, and their roles and functions in this regard have not been completely elucidated. A summary of their characteristics follows.

Aspartate is an excitatory neurotransmitter found in high concentrations in the brain. Aspartate and glutamate are considered the major fast-acting, excitatory neurotransmitters in the brain.

Glycine is an inhibitory neurotransmitter found in the brain stem and spinal cord. Glycine receptors have many of the features described for GABA$_A$ receptors; subtypes have been identified but their functions are unknown.

Glutamate is considered the most important excitatory neurotransmitter in the CNS. It occurs in high concentrations in virtually every area of the CNS, including the cerebral cortex, basal ganglia, limbic structures, and hippocampus. Several subtypes of glutamate receptors have been identified, each with a unique distribution in the CNS. The functions of these receptor subtypes have not been established, but research suggests that the *N*-methyl D-aspartate (NMDA) glutamate receptor subtype plays a role in memory.

Although some glutamate is apparently necessary for normal neurotransmission, brief exposure of neurons to high concentrations can lead to neuronal cell death. Events leading to neuronal death are triggered by excessive activation of NMDA receptors and movement of calcium ions into the neurons. This process may be similar to the neurotoxicity that occurs after ischemia or hypoglycemia in the brain, where increased release and impaired reuptake of glutamate lead to excessive stimulation of glutamate receptors and subsequent cell death.

Neurotransmission Systems in Selected Central Nervous System Disorders

Abnormalities in neurotransmission systems (eg, dysfunction or destruction of the neurons that normally produce neurotransmitters or altered receptor response to neurotransmitters) are implicated in many CNS disorders. For example, decreased acetylcholine is a characteristic of Alzheimer's disease; dopamine abnormalities occur in psychosis and Parkinson's disease; GABA abnormalities occur in anxiety, hyperarousal states, and seizure disorders; glutamate has been implicated in the pathogenesis of epilepsy, stroke, and Huntington's disease; and serotonin abnormalities are thought to be involved in mental depression and sleep disorders.

Although most research has focused on single neurotransmitters and their respective receptors, CNS function in both health and disease is probably determined by interactions among neurotransmission systems. In health, for example, complex mechanisms regulate the amounts and binding capacities of neurotransmitters and receptors,

as well as the balance between excitatory and inhibitory forces. When abnormalities occur in any of these elements, the resulting dysregulation and imbalances lead to signs and symptoms of CNS disorders. Overall, then, neurotransmission systems function interdependently; one system may increase, decrease, or otherwise modify the effects of another system.

Except for mental depression, most psychiatric symptoms result from CNS stimulation and usually involve physical and mental hyperactivity. Such hyperactivity reflects a wide range of observable behaviors and nonobservable thoughts and feelings. In most people, manifestations may include pleasant feelings of mild euphoria and high levels of enthusiasm, energy, and productivity. In people with psychiatric illnesses, such as severe anxiety or psychosis, manifestations include unpleasant feelings of tension, psychomotor agitation, nervousness, and decreased ability to rest and sleep, even when very tired. Many psychiatric disorders, therapeutic drugs, and drugs of abuse may cause varying degrees of CNS stimulation. In general, the pathogenesis of excessive CNS stimulation may involve one or more of the following mechanisms:

1. Excessive amounts of excitatory neurotransmitters (eg, norepinephrine)
2. Increased numbers or sensitivity of excitatory receptors
3. Insufficient amounts of inhibitory neurotransmitters (eg, GABA)
4. Decreased numbers or sensitivity of inhibitory receptors

Cerebral Cortex

The cerebral cortex is involved in all conscious processes, such as learning, memory, reasoning, verbalization, and voluntary body movements. Some parts of the cortex receive incoming nerve impulses and are called *sensory areas*; other parts send impulses to peripheral structures and are called *motor areas*. Around the sensory and motor areas are the "association" areas, which occupy the greater portion of the cortex. These areas analyze the information received by the sensory areas and decide on the appropriate response. In some instances, the response may be to store the perception in memory; in others, it may involve stimulation of motor centers to produce movement or speech.

Thalamus

The thalamus receives impulses carrying sensations such as heat, cold, pain, and muscle position sense. These sensations produce only a crude awareness at the thalamic level. They are relayed to the cerebral cortex, where they are interpreted regarding location, quality, intensity, and significance. The thalamus also relays motor impulses from the cortex to the spinal cord.

Hypothalamus

The hypothalamus has extensive neurologic and endocrine functions. In the CNS, it is connected with the thalamus, medulla oblongata, spinal cord, reticular activating system, and limbic system. In the autonomic nervous system, it is the center for motor control. In the endocrine system, the hypothalamus controls the secretion of all pituitary hormones. It is anatomically connected to the posterior pituitary gland, and it regulates the activity of the anterior pituitary. It constantly collects information about the internal environment of the body and helps maintain homeostasis by making continuous adjustments in water balance, body temperature, hormone levels, arterial blood pressure, heart rate, gastrointestinal motility, and other body functions. The hypothalamus is stimulated or inhibited by nerve impulses from different portions of the nervous system and by concentrations of nutrients, electrolytes, water, and hormones in the blood. Specific neuroendocrine functions include:

1. Producing oxytocin and ADH, which are stored in the posterior pituitary gland and released in response to nerve impulses from the hypothalamus. Oxytocin initiates uterine contractions to begin labor and delivery and helps to release milk from breast glands during breastfeeding. ADH helps maintain fluid balance by controlling water excretion. ADH secretion is controlled by the osmolarity of the extracellular fluid. When osmolarity is high, more ADH is secreted. This means that water is retained in the body to dilute the extracellular fluid and return it toward normal or homeostatic levels. When osmolarity is low, less ADH is secreted, and more water is excreted in the urine.
2. Regulating body temperature. When body temperature is elevated, sweating and dilation of blood vessels in the skin lower the temperature. When body temperature is low, sweating ceases and vasoconstriction occurs. When heat loss is decreased, the temperature is raised.
3. Assisting in regulation of arterial blood pressure by its effects on the vasomotor center. The vasomotor center in the medulla oblongata and pons maintains a state of partial contraction in blood vessels (vasomotor tone). The hypothalamus can exert excitatory or inhibitory effects on the vasomotor center, depending on which portions of the hypothalamus are stimulated. When nerve impulses from the hypothalamus excite the vasomotor center, vasomotor tone or vasoconstriction is increased, and blood pressure is raised. When the impulses from the hypothalamus inhibit the vasomotor center, vasomotor tone or vasoconstriction is decreased, with the overall effect of relative vasodilation and lowering of arterial blood pressure.
4. Regulating anterior pituitary hormones, including thyroid-stimulating hormone, ACTH, and growth hormone. The hypothalamus secretes "releasing factors," which cause the anterior pituitary to secrete these hormones. There is a hypothalamic releasing factor for each hormone. The hypothalamic factor called prolactin-inhibiting factor inhibits secretion of prolactin, another anterior pituitary hormone.
5. Regulating food and water intake by the hypothalamic thirst, appetite, hunger, and satiety centers.
6. Regulating the physical changes associated with emotions (eg, increased blood pressure and heart rate). The hypothalamus, thalamus, and cerebral cortex interact to produce the feelings associated with emotions.

Medulla Oblongata

The medulla oblongata contains groups of neurons that form the vital cardiac, respiratory, and vasomotor centers. For example, if the respiratory center is stimulated, respiratory rate and depth are increased. If the respiratory center is depressed, respiratory rate and depth are decreased. The medulla also contains reflex centers for coughing, vomiting, sneezing, swallowing, and salivating.

The medulla and pons varolii also contain groups of neurons from which originate cranial nerves 5 through 12. Together with the midbrain, these structures form the brain stem.

Reticular Activating System

The reticular activating system is a network of neurons that extends from the spinal cord through the medulla and pons to the thalamus and hypothalamus. It receives impulses from all parts of the body, evaluates the significance of the impulses, and decides which impulses to transmit to the cerebral cortex. It also excites or inhibits motor nerves that control both reflex and voluntary movement. Stimulation of these neurons produces wakefulness and mental alertness; depression causes sedation and loss of consciousness.

Limbic System

The limbic system borders and interconnects with the thalamus, hypothalamus, basal ganglia, hippocampus, amygdala, and septum. It participates in regulation of feeding behavior, the sleep–wake cycle, emotions (eg, pleasure, fear, anger, sadness), and behavior (eg, aggression, laughing, crying). Many nerve impulses from the limbic system are transmitted through the hypothalamus; thus, physiologic changes in blood pressure, heart rate, respiration, and hormone secretion occur in response to the emotions.

Cerebellum

The cerebellum, which is connected with motor centers in the cerebral cortex and basal ganglia, coordinates muscular activity. When several skeletal muscles are involved, some are contracted and some are relaxed for smooth, purposeful movements. It also helps to maintain balance and posture by receiving nerve impulses from the inner ear that produce appropriate reflex responses.

Basal Ganglia

The basal ganglia are concerned with skeletal muscle tone and orderly activity. Normal function is influenced by dopamine, a neurotransmitter produced in several areas of the brain. Degenerative changes in one of these areas, the substantia nigra, cause dopamine to be released in decreased amounts. This process is a factor in the development of Parkinson's disease, which is characterized by rigidity and increased muscle tone.

Pyramidal and Extrapyramidal Systems

The pyramidal and extrapyramidal systems are pathways out of the cerebral cortex. In the pyramidal or corticospinal tract, nerve fibers originate in the cerebral cortex, go down the brain stem to the medulla, where the fibers cross, and continue down the spinal cord, where they end at various levels. Impulses are then carried from the spinal cord to skeletal muscle. Because the fibers cross in the medulla, impulses from the right side of the cerebral cortex control skeletal muscle movements of the left side of the body, and impulses from the left control muscle movements of the right side.

In the extrapyramidal system, fibers originate mainly in the premotor area of the cerebral cortex and travel to the basal ganglia and brain stem. The fibers are called extrapyramidal because they do not enter the medullary pyramids and cross over.

Pyramidal and extrapyramidal systems intermingle in the spinal cord; disease processes affecting higher levels of the CNS involve both tracts.

Brain Metabolism

To function correctly, the brain must have an adequate and continuous supply of nutrients, especially oxygen, glucose, and thiamine.

Oxygen is carried to the brain by the carotid and vertebral arteries. The brain requires more oxygen than any other organ. Cerebral cortex cells are very sensitive to lack of oxygen (hypoxia), and interruption of blood supply causes immediate loss of consciousness. Brain stem cells are less sensitive to hypoxia. People in whom hypoxia is relatively prolonged may survive, although they may have irreversible brain damage.

Glucose is required as an energy source for brain cell metabolism. Hypoglycemia (low blood sugar) may cause mental confusion, dizziness, convulsions, loss of consciousness, and permanent damage to the cerebral cortex.

Thiamine is required for production and use of glucose. Thiamine deficiency can reduce glucose use by approximately half and can cause degeneration of the myelin sheaths of nerve cells. Such degeneration in central neurons leads to a form of encephalopathy known as Wernicke-Korsakoff syndrome. Degeneration in peripheral nerves leads to polyneuritis and muscle atrophy, weakness, and paralysis.

Spinal Cord

The spinal cord is continuous with the medulla oblongata and extends down through the vertebral column to the sacral area. It consists of 31 segments, each of which is the point of origin for a pair of spinal nerves. The cord is a pathway between the brain and the peripheral nervous system. It carries impulses to and from the brain, along sensory and motor nerve fibers, and is a center for reflex actions. Reflexes are involuntary responses to certain nerve impulses received by the spinal cord (eg, the knee-jerk and pupillary reflexes).

DRUGS AFFECTING THE CENTRAL NERVOUS SYSTEM

Drugs affecting the CNS, sometimes called centrally active drugs, are broadly classified as depressants or stimulants. CNS depressant drugs (eg, antipsychotics, narcotic analgesics, sedative-hypnotics) produce a general depression of the CNS when given in sufficient dosages. Mild CNS depression is characterized by lack of interest in surroundings and inability to focus on a topic (short attention span). As depression progresses, there is drowsiness or sleep, decreased muscle tone, decreased ability to move, and decreased perception of sensations such as pain, heat, and cold. Severe CNS depression produces unconsciousness or coma, loss of reflexes, respiratory failure, and death.

Central nervous system stimulants produce a variety of effects. Mild stimulation is characterized by wakefulness, mental alertness, and decreased fatigue. Increasing stimulation produces hyperactivity, excessive talking, nervousness, and insomnia. Excessive stimulation can cause convulsive seizures, cardiac arrhythmias, and death. Because it is difficult to avoid excessive, harmful CNS stimulation by these drugs, CNS stimulants are less useful for therapeutic purposes than are CNS depressants.

REVIEW AND APPLICATION EXERCISES

1. Where are neurotransmitters synthesized and stored?

2. What events occur at the synapse between two neurons?

3. Once a neurotransmitter is released and acts on receptors, how are the remaining molecules inactivated?

4. What are the main functions of acetylcholine, dopamine, GABA, norepinephrine, and serotonin?

5. What part of the brain is concerned mainly with thoughts, reasoning, and learning?

6. What part of the brain contains vital respiratory and cardiovascular centers?

7. How would you expect a person with CNS depression to look and behave?

8. How would you expect a person with excessive CNS stimulation to look and behave?

SELECTED REFERENCES

Bloom, F.E. (1996). Neurotransmission and the central nervous system. In J.G. Hardman, L.E. Limbird, P.B. Molinoff, & R.W. Ruddon (Eds.), *Goodman and Gilman's The pharmacological basic of therapeutics*, 9th ed., pp. 267–293. New York: McGraw-Hill.

Guyton, A.C. & Hall, J.E. (1996). *Textbook of medical physiology*, 9th ed. Philadelphia: W.B. Saunders.

McCrone, S.H. (1996). Physical dimensions of the journey: Neurobiological influences. In V.B. Carson & E.N. Arnold (Eds.), *Mental health nursing: The nurse-patient journey*, pp. 127–149. Philadelphia: W.B. Saunders.

6

Opioid Analgesics and Opioid Antagonists

Objectives

After studying this chapter, the student will be able to:

1. Discuss characteristics of pain.

2. Discuss the nurse's role in assessing and managing clients' pain.

3. List characteristics of opioid analgesics in terms of mechanism of action, indications for use, and major adverse effects.

4. Describe morphine as the prototype of opioid analgesics.

5. Discuss morphine dosage forms and dosage ranges for various clinical uses.

6. Explain why higher doses of opioid analgesics are needed when the drugs are given orally.

7. Contrast the use of opioid analgesics in opiate-naive and opiate-tolerant clients.

8. Assess level of consciousness and respiratory status before and after administering opioids.

9. Discuss principles of therapy and nursing process for using opioid analgesics in special populations.

10. Describe signs and symptoms of opioid overdose and withdrawal and the treatment of each.

11. Teach clients about safe, effective use of opioid analgesics.

12. Discuss the clinical use of opioid antagonists.

John Shone, 65 years of age, has terminal cancer that was diagnosed 9 months ago. One month ago, he was prescribed morphine (MS Contin 30 mg bid) for pain. When you assess him, you note that he is very quiet and seems reluctant to move. His vital signs are BP 152/88, p 88, r 20. He rates his pain as 9 on a 1-to-10 scale, saying that during the last week his pain seems to be getting much worse. Previously, John and his wife expressed their concern regarding "having to take so much medication and not wanting to become addicted to pain medication."

Reflect on:

▶ Your assessment of John's pain based on the data collected.

▶ Teaching that John and his wife may need regarding chronic pain and its treatment. What suggestions do you have for John's pain management plan?

Pain, the most common symptom prompting people to seek health care, is an unpleasant sensation that usually indicates tissue damage and impels the person to remove the cause of the damage. Opioid (narcotic) analgesics are drugs that relieve moderate to severe pain. To aid understanding of drug actions, selected characteristics of pain and endogenous pain-relieving substances are described.

PAIN

Pain occurs when tissue damage activates the free nerve endings (pain receptors or nociceptors) of peripheral nerves. Nociceptors are abundant in the skin and underlying soft tissue, joint surfaces, arterial walls, and periosteum; most internal organs, such as lung and uterine tissue, contain few nociceptors. Causes of tissue damage may be physical (eg, heat, cold, pressure) or chemical (eg, pain related to substances released from damaged cells and products of inflammation, including bradykinin, histamine, and prostaglandins). Bradykinin, one of the strongest pain-producing substances, is quickly metabolized and therefore may be involved mainly in acute pain. Prostaglandins increase bradykinin's pain-provoking effects by increasing the sensitivity of pain receptors. Several other substances are also thought to produce pain, including acetylcholine, adenosine triphosphate, histamine, leukotrienes, potassium, serotonin, and substance P. Overall, these chemical mediators produce pain by activating and sensitizing peripheral nociceptors or stimulating the release of pain-producing substances.

When pain receptors are activated, the message of tissue damage is transmitted to the dorsal horn of the spinal cord by two groups of afferent nerve fibers. One group is the small, myelinated, A-delta fibers, which are activated by thermal and mechanical stimuli and transmit fast, sharp, well-localized pain signals. These fibers release glutamate and aspartate (neurotransmitter amino acids) at synapses in the spinal cord. The other group is unmyelinated C fibers that respond to thermal, mechanical, and chemical stimulation and mediate slow, burning, poorly localized pain signals. C fibers release somatostatin and substance P at synapses in the spinal cord. Substance P is a peptide neurotransmitter that is thought to play an important role in transmitting pain signals from peripheral tissues to the central nervous system (CNS).

The dorsal horn of the spinal cord is the control center or relay station for information from the A-delta and C nociceptive fibers, for local modulation of the pain impulse, and for descending influences from higher centers in the CNS (eg, attention, emotion, memory). Here, nociceptive nerve fibers synapse with non-nociceptive nerve fibers (neurons that carry information other than pain signals). The brain also contains powerful descending pathways that modify nociceptive input. Some brain nuclei are serotonergic and project to the dorsal horn of the spinal cord, where they suppress nociceptive transmission. Another major inhibitory pathway is noradrenergic and originates in the pons. Thus, increasing the concentration of norepinephrine and serotonin in the synapse interrupts or inhibits transmission of nerve impulses that carry pain signals to the brain and spinal cord. (This is thought to account for the pain-relieving effects of the tricyclic antidepressants, drugs that increase the amounts of serotonin and norepinephrine in the synapse by inhibiting their reuptake by presynaptic nerve endings.)

In the brain, the thalamus is a relay station for incoming sensory stimuli, including pain. Perception of pain is a primitive awareness in the thalamus, and sensation is not well localized or specific. From the thalamus, pain messages are relayed to the cerebral cortex, where they are perceived more specifically and analyzed to determine actions needed.

Pain is often described as acute or chronic and superficial or deep.

Acute pain is usually caused by tissue-damaging stimuli, and the duration is usually less than 6 months. It serves as a protective or warning system by demanding the sufferer's attention and compelling behavior to seek relief. It is often accompanied by anxiety and objective signs of discomfort (eg, facial expressions of distress; moaning or crying; positioning to protect the affected part; tenderness, edema, and skin color or temperature changes in the affected part; and either restlessness and excessive movement or limited movement, if movement increases pain).

Chronic pain, usually defined as pain of 6 months or longer, demands attention less urgently, may not be characterized by visible signs, and is often accompanied by depression and changes in personality, lifestyle, and functional ability. It may occur with or without evidence of tissue damage. It may include acute pain that persists beyond the normal healing time, pain related to a chronic disease, pain without an identifiable cause, and pain associated with cancer. It is important to differentiate between chronic pain and acute pain because they are managed quite differently.

Superficial pain originates in the skin or underlying structures and produces sharp pain with a burning quality that is readily localized by the sufferer. Superficial pain or pain of low to moderate intensity usually stimulates the sympathetic nervous system and produces increased blood pressure, pulse, and respiration; dilated pupils; and increased skeletal muscle tension, such as rigid posture or clenched fists.

Deep pain originates in bones and abdominal or thoracic organs and produces a dull, aching sensation that is hard to localize. Deep or severe pain stimulates the parasympathetic nervous system and produces decreased blood pressure and pulse, nausea and vomiting, weakness, syncope, and possibly loss of consciousness.

ENDOGENOUS ANALGESIA SYSTEM

The CNS has its own system for suppressing the transmission of pain signals from peripheral nerves. The system can be activated by nervous signals entering the periaqueductal gray area of the brain or by morphine-like drugs. Important elements include opiate receptors and endogenous peptides with actions similar to those of morphine. Opiate receptors are highly concentrated in some regions of the CNS, including the ascending and descending pain pathways and portions of the brain essential to the endogenous analgesia system. The opioid peptides (ie, the enkephalins, dynorphins, and beta-endorphins) interact with opiate receptors to inhibit pain transmission. All are important in the endogenous opiate system, but the three types of peptides differ in precursors and anatomic locations. Enkephalins are believed to interrupt the transmission of pain signals at the spinal cord level by inhibiting the release of substance P from C nerve fibers. The endogenous analgesia system may also inhibit pain signals at other points in the pain pathway.

OPIOID ANALGESICS

Opioid analgesics are drugs that relieve moderate to severe pain by reducing the perception of pain sensation, producing sedation, and decreasing the emotional upsets often associated with pain. Most of these analgesics are Schedule II drugs under federal narcotic laws and may lead to drug abuse and dependence. **Morphine** is the prototype of these analgesics and the standard by which others are measured. These drugs are called *opioids* because they act like morphine in the body.

Opioid analgesics are well absorbed with oral, intramuscular, or subcutaneous administration. Oral preparations undergo significant first-pass metabolism in the liver, so that oral doses must be larger than parenteral doses for equivalent therapeutic effects. The drugs are extensively metabolized in the liver and metabolites are excreted in urine. Morphine and meperidine form pharmacologically active metabolites. Thus, liver impairment can interfere with metabolism and kidney impairment can interfere with excretion. Drug accumulation and increased adverse effects may occur if dosage is not reduced.

Morphine and other opioids exert widespread pharmacologic effects, especially in the CNS and the gastrointestinal (GI) system. These effects occur with usual doses and may be therapeutic or adverse, depending on the reason for use. CNS effects include analgesia, CNS depression ranging from drowsiness to sleep to unconsciousness, decreased mental and physical activity, respiratory

depression, nausea and vomiting, and pupil constriction. Sedation and respiratory depression are major adverse effects and are potentially life threatening. Most newer opioid analgesics have been developed in an effort to find drugs as effective as morphine in relieving pain while causing less sedation, respiratory depression, and dependence. However, this effort has not been successful: *equianalgesic doses of these drugs produce sedative and respiratory depressant effects comparable with those of morphine.* In the GI system, opioid analgesics slow motility and may cause smooth muscle spasms in the bowel and biliary tract.

Mechanism of Action

Opioids relieve pain by binding to opioid receptors in the brain and spinal cord and activating the endogenous analgesia system. Six major types of receptors have been identified (Table 6-1). Opioid analgesics and opioid antagonists bind to different receptors to varying degrees, and their pharmacologic actions can be differentiated and classified on this basis.

Indications for Use

The main indication for the use of opioids is to prevent or relieve acute or chronic pain. Specific conditions in which opioid drugs are used for analgesic effects include acute myocardial infarction, biliary colic, renal colic, burns and other traumatic injuries, postoperative states, and cancer. These drugs are usually given for chronic pain only when

TABLE 6-1 Opioid Receptors and their Effects		
Drug Group	**Receptor**	**Effects**
Agonists (eg, morphine)	Mu-1	Analgesia
	Mu-2	Constipation
		Euphoria
		Physical dependence
		Respiratory depression
	Kappa	Analgesia
		Miosis
		Sedation
	Delta?	Analgesia
	Epsilon	Analgesia
Agonist/antagonists (eg, pentazocine)	Kappa	Analgesia
		Miosis
		Sedation
	Sigma	Dysphoria
		Hallucinations
		Respiratory stimulation
		Vasomotor stimulation

other measures and milder drugs are ineffective, as in terminal malignancy. Other clinical uses include:

1. Before and during surgery to promote sedation, decrease anxiety, facilitate induction of anesthesia, and decrease the amount of anesthesia required
2. Before and during invasive diagnostic procedures, such as angiograms and endoscopic examinations
3. During labor and delivery (obstetric analgesia)
4. Treating GI disorders, such as abdominal cramping and diarrhea
5. Treating acute pulmonary edema (morphine is used)
6. Treating severe, unproductive cough (codeine is usually used)

Contraindications to Use

These drugs are contraindicated or must be used very cautiously in people with respiratory depression, chronic lung disease, liver or kidney disease, prostatic hypertrophy, increased intracranial pressure, or hypersensitivity reactions to opiates and related drugs.

CLASSIFICATIONS AND INDIVIDUAL DRUGS

Agonists

Opioid agonists include morphine and morphine-like drugs. These agents have activity at mu, kappa, and possibly delta opioid receptors and thus produce prototypical opioid effects.

Morphine is a naturally occurring opium alkaloid used mainly to relieve severe acute or chronic pain. It is a Schedule II narcotic that is given orally and parenterally. Client response depends on route and dosage. After intravenous (IV) injection, maximal analgesia and respiratory depression usually occur within 10 to 20 minutes. After intramuscular (IM) injection, these effects occur in about 30 minutes. With subcutaneous (SC) injection, effects may be delayed up to 60 to 90 minutes.

Oral administration of morphine is common for chronic pain associated with cancer. When given orally, relatively high doses are required because part of each dose is metabolized in the liver and never reaches the systemic circulation. Concentrated solutions (eg, Roxanol, which contains 20 mg morphine/mL) and controlled-release tablets (eg, MS Contin, which contains 30 mg/tablet) have been developed for oral administration of these high doses. In some cases of severe pain that cannot be controlled by other methods, morphine is administered as a continuous IV infusion. Other routes of administration include epidural, in which the drug is instilled through a catheter placed in the epidural space and slowly diffuses into the spinal cord, and intrathecal, in which the drug is injected directly into the spinal cord. Epidural and intrathecal morphine provide pain relief with very small doses, once or twice daily. When clients cannot take oral medication and injections are undesirable, rectal suppositories are often given.

Morphine is primarily metabolized in the liver and excreted by the kidneys. Consequently, impaired liver and kidney function may cause prolonged drug action and accumulation, with a subsequent increase in the incidence and severity of adverse effects.

ROUTES AND DOSAGE RANGES

Adults: PO 10–30 mg q4h PRN or as ordered by physician

PO controlled-release tablets, 30 mg q8–12h or as ordered by physician

IM, SC 5–20 mg/70 kg q4h PRN

IV injection, 2.5–15 mg/70 kg, diluted in 5 mL water for injection and injected slowly, for approximately 5 min, PRN

IV continuous infusion, 0.1–1 mg/mL in 5% dextrose in water, by controlled infusion pump

Epidural injection, 5 mg/24 h; continuous infusion, 2–4 mg/24 h

Intrathecal injection, 0.2–1 mg/24 h

Rectal, 10–20 mg q4h or as ordered by physician

Infants and children: IM, SC 0.1–0.2 mg/kg (up to 15 mg) q4h

Alfentanil (Alfenta), **fentanyl** (Sublimaze), and **sufentanil** (Sufenta) are potent drugs with a short duration of action. They are most often used in anesthesia (see Chap. 14) as analgesic adjuncts or primary anesthetic agents in open heart surgery or complicated neurologic and orthopedic procedures. Fentanyl also is used for preanesthetic medication, postoperative analgesia, and chronic pain that requires an opioid analgesic. A transmucosal formulation (Fentanyl Oralet, also called a lozenge or "lollipop") is available for conscious sedation or anesthesia premedication in children and adults. Because of a high risk of respiratory depression, recommended dosages must not be exceeded, and the drug should be given only in an area with staff and equipment for emergency care (eg, intensive care unit, operating room, emergency room). As with other routes of administration, dosage of the oral lozenge should be individualized according to age, weight, illness, other medications, type of procedure and anesthesia, and other factors. A transdermal formulation (Duragesic) is used in the treatment of chronic pain. The active drug is deposited in the skin and slowly absorbed systemically. Thus, the skin patches have a slow onset of action (approximately 12 to 24 hours), but they last approximately 3 days. When a patch is removed, the drug continues to be absorbed from the skin deposits for 24 hours or longer.

Alfentanil

ROUTES AND DOSAGE RANGES

Adults: Analgesic adjunct in general anesthesia, IV initial dose 8–50 µg/kg; maintenance injection, 3–5 µg/kg; maintenance infusion, 0.5–1 µg/kg/min

Anesthesia induction, IV injection 130–245 µg/kg over 3 min or IV infusion 50–75 µg/kg

Anesthesia maintenance, IV infusion 0.5–3 µg/kg/min

Fentanyl

ROUTES AND DOSAGE RANGES

Adults: Preanesthetic, IM 0.05–0.1 mg 30–60 min before surgery; oral lozenge, 200–400 µg, 20 to 40 min before a procedure, with instructions to suck, not chew, the medication. Maximum dose of oral lozenge, 400 µg.

Analgesic adjunct to general anesthesia, IV total dose of 0.002–0.05 mg/kg, depending on type and length of surgical procedure

Adjunct to regional anesthesia, IM or slow IV (over 1–2 min) 0.05–0.1 mg PRN

Postoperative analgesia, IM 0.05–0.1 mg, repeat in 1–2 h if needed

General anesthesia, IV 0.05–0.1 mg/kg with oxygen and a muscle relaxant (maximum dose 0.15 mg/kg with open heart surgery, other major surgeries, and complicated neurologic or orthopedic procedures)

Chronic pain, transdermal system 2.5–10 mg every 72 h

Children <12 y: General anesthesia induction and maintenance, IV 1.7–3.3 mg/kg (20–30 µg/20–25 lb)

Children weighing at least 15 kg: Conscious sedation or preanesthetic sedation, 5–15 µg/kg of body weight (200–400 µg), depending on weight, type of procedure, and other factors. Maximum dose, 400 µg, regardless of age and weight

Sufentanil

ROUTES AND DOSAGE RANGES

Adults: Analgesic adjunct to general anesthesia, IV initial dose 1–8 µg/kg; maintenance, 10–25 µg PRN

General anesthesia, IV induction, 8–30 µg/kg; maintenance, 25–50 µg PRN

Children <12 y: General anesthesia, IV induction 10–25 µg with 100% oxygen; maintenance 25–50 µg PRN

Codeine is a naturally occurring opium alkaloid used for analgesic and antitussive effects. Codeine produces weaker analgesic and antitussive effects and milder adverse effects than morphine. Compared with other opioid analgesics, codeine is more effective when given orally and is less likely to lead to abuse and dependence. Parenteral administration is more effective in relieving pain than oral administration, but onset (15 to 30 minutes) and duration of action (4 to 6 hours) are approximately the same. Larger doses are required for analgesic than for antitussive effects. Codeine is often given with acetaminophen for additive analgesic effects.

ROUTES AND DOSAGE RANGES

Adults: PO, SC, IM 15–60 mg q4–6h PRN
Cough, PO 10–20 mg q4h PRN
Children: PO, SC, IM 0.5 mg/kg q4–6h PRN

Cough, children 6–12 y, PO 5–10 mg q4–6h
Cough, children 2–6 y, PO 2.5–5 mg q4–6h

Hydrocodone, which is similar to codeine in its analgesic and antitussive effects, is a Schedule III drug. It is available only in combination products for cough (eg, Hycodan) and with acetaminophen for pain. Most products (eg, Hydrocet, Lortab, Vicodin) are analgesic combinations containing hydrocodone and acetaminophen.

ROUTE AND DOSAGE RANGES

Adults: PO 5–10 mg q6–8h
Children: PO 0.6 mg/kg/day in three or four divided doses

Hydromorphone (Dilaudid) is a semisynthetic derivative of morphine that has the same actions, uses, contraindications, and adverse effects as morphine. Hydromorphone is more potent on a milligram basis and is relatively more effective orally than morphine. Effects occur in 15 to 30 minutes, peak in 30 to 90 minutes, and last 4 to 5 hours.

ROUTES AND DOSAGE RANGES

Adults: PO 2–4 mg q4–6h PRN
IM, SC, IV 1–1.5 mg q4–6h PRN (may be increased to 4 mg for severe pain)
Rectal suppository 3 mg q6–8h

Levorphanol (Levo-Dromoran) is a synthetic drug that is chemically and pharmacologically related to morphine. It has the same uses and produces the same adverse effects, although some reports indicate less nausea and vomiting. The average dose is probably equianalgesic with 10 mg of morphine. Maximal analgesia occurs 60 to 90 minutes after SC injection. Effects last 4 to 8 hours.

ROUTES AND DOSAGE RANGE

Adults: PO, SC 2–3 mg q4–6h PRN

Meperidine (Demerol) is a frequently prescribed synthetic drug that is similar to morphine in pharmacologic actions. A parenteral dose of 80 to 100 mg is equivalent to 10 mg of morphine. Oral meperidine is only half as effective as a parenteral dose because approximately half is metabolized in the liver and never reaches the systemic circulation. Meperidine produces sedation and respiratory depression comparable to morphine. Meperidine differs from morphine as follows:

1. It has a shorter duration of action and requires more frequent administration. After parenteral administration, analgesia occurs in approximately 10 to 20 minutes, peaks in approximately 1 hour, and lasts approximately 2 to 4 hours.
2. It has little antitussive effect. However, excessive sedation with meperidine reduces the ability to cough effectively.
3. It causes less respiratory depression in the newborn when used for obstetric analgesia.
4. It causes less smooth muscle spasm and is preferred in renal and biliary colic.

5. With chronic use, toxic doses, or renal failure, meperidine may cause CNS stimulation characterized by tremors, hallucinations, and seizures. These effects are attributed to accumulation of a metabolite, normeperidine.

ROUTES AND DOSAGE RANGES

Adults: IM, IV, SC, PO 50–100 mg q2–4h
  Obstetric analgesia, IM, SC 50–100 mg q2–4h for three or four doses

Methadone (Dolophine) is a synthetic drug with the same pharmacologic actions as morphine. Compared with morphine, methadone has a longer duration of action and is relatively more effective when given orally. Analgesia occurs within 10 to 20 minutes after injection and 30 to 60 minutes after oral administration. Methadone is used for severe pain and in the detoxification and maintenance treatment of opiate addicts.

ROUTES AND DOSAGE RANGES

Adults: IM, SC 2.5–10 mg q3–4h PRN
  PO 5–20 mg q6–8h PRN

Oxycodone is a semisynthetic derivative of codeine used to relieve moderate pain. It is reportedly less potent and less likely to produce dependence than morphine but is more potent and more likely to produce dependence than codeine. It is a drug of abuse. Pharmacologic actions are similar to those of other opioid analgesics. Oxycodone is available alone (Roxicodone) and in combination with aspirin (Percodan) or acetaminophen (Percocet, Tylox).

ROUTE AND DOSAGE RANGE

Adults: PO 5 mg q6h PRN
Children: Not recommended for children <12 y

Oxymorphone (Numorphan) is a semisynthetic derivative of morphine. Its actions, uses, and adverse effects are similar to those of morphine, except that it has little antitussive effect.

ROUTES AND DOSAGE RANGES

Adults: IM, SC 1–1.5 mg q4–6h PRN
  IV 0.5 mg q4–6h PRN
  Rectal suppository, 5 mg q4–6h PRN
  Obstetric analgesia, IM 0.5–1 mg

Propoxyphene (Darvon) is a synthetic drug chemically related to methadone. It is used for mild to moderate pain but is considered no more effective than 650 mg of aspirin or acetaminophen, with which it is usually given. It is not recommended for use in children or in clients at risk for suicide or addiction. Propoxyphene is abused (alone and with alcohol or other CNS depressant drugs), and deaths have occurred from overdoses. An overdose causes respiratory depression, excessive sedation, and circulatory failure. Despite these characteristics and dangers, the drug continues to be prescribed. Propoxyphene is a Schedule IV drug.

Propoxyphene Hydrochloride

ROUTE AND DOSAGE RANGE

Adults: PO 65 mg q4h PRN (maximal daily dose, 390 mg)
Children: Not recommended

Propoxyphene Napsylate

ROUTE AND DOSAGE RANGE

Adults: PO 100 mg q4h PRN (maximal daily dose, 600 mg)
Children: Not recommended

Tramadol (Ultram) is an oral, synthetic, centrally active analgesic for moderate to severe pain. It is not chemically related to opioids. Its mechanism of action is unclear but includes binding to mu opioid receptors and inhibiting reuptake of norepinephrine and serotonin in the brain. Analgesia occurs within 1 hour after administration and peaks in approximately 2 to 3 hours. Tramadol causes significantly less respiratory depression than morphine but may cause other morphine-like adverse effects (eg, drowsiness, nausea, constipation, pruritus, orthostatic hypotension).

Tramadol is well absorbed after oral administration, even if taken with food. It is minimally bound (approximately 20%) to plasma proteins. It is extensively metabolized; approximately 30% of a dose is excreted unchanged in the urine and approximately 60% is excreted as metabolites. Dosage should be reduced in people with severe renal impairment.

ROUTE AND DOSAGE RANGE

Adults: PO 50–100 mg q4–6h PRN (maximal daily dose, 400 mg)
  Adults with renal impairment (ie, creatinine clearance <30 mL/min): PO 50–100 mg q12h (maximal daily dose, 200 mg)
  Adults with hepatic impairment (cirrhosis): PO 50 mg q12h
  Elderly adults (65–75 y): Same as above, unless they also have renal or hepatic impairment
  Elderly adults (>75 y): <300 mg daily, in divided doses
Children: Dosage not established

Agonists/Antagonists

These agents have agonist activity at some receptors and antagonist activity at others. Because of their agonist activity, they are potent analgesics with a lower abuse potential than pure agonists; because of their antagonist activity, they may produce withdrawal symptoms in people with opiate dependence.

Buprenorphine (Buprenex) is a semisynthetic opioid with a long duration of action and a low incidence of causing physical dependence. These characteristics are attributed to its high affinity for and slow dissociation from mu receptors. With IM administration, analgesia onset occurs in 15 minutes, peaks in 60 minutes, and lasts approximately

6 hours. It is highly protein bound (approximately 96%) and has an elimination half-life of 2 to 3 hours. It is metabolized in the liver, and clearance is related to hepatic blood flow. It is excreted mainly in feces.

ROUTES AND DOSAGE RANGE

Adults: IM or slow IV (over 2 min) 0.3 mg q6h PRN

Butorphanol (Stadol) is a synthetic agonist analgesic similar to morphine and meperidine in analgesic effects and ability to cause respiratory depression. It is used in moderate to severe pain and is given parenterally or topically to nasal mucosa by a metered spray (Stadol NS). After IM or IV administration, analgesia peaks in approximately 30 to 60 minutes. After nasal application, analgesia peaks within 1 to 2 hours. Butorphanol also has antagonist activity and therefore should not be given to people who have been receiving opioid analgesics or who have opioid dependence. Other adverse effects include drowsiness and nausea and vomiting. Butorphanol is not recommended for use in children younger than 18 years of age.

ROUTES AND DOSAGE RANGES

Adults: IM, IV 1–4 mg q3–4h PRN
   Nasal spray 1 mg (one spray in one nostril) q3–4h PRN
Children: Not recommended

Dezocine (Dalgan) is a synthetic analgesic used for moderate to severe pain. It is given parenterally. It is similar to morphine in its effects. Onset of analgesia occurs within 15 minutes after IV administration and within 30 minutes after IM injection. Like other drugs in this group, dezocine may cause respiratory depression, sedation, nausea and vomiting, and other adverse effects. It also may cause allergic reactions, especially in people with asthma or allergy to sulfites because it contains metabisulfite.

ROUTES AND DOSAGE RANGES

Adults: IM 5–20 mg q3–6h PRN
   IV 2.5–10 mg q2–4h PRN
Children: Not recommended

Nalbuphine (Nubain) is a synthetic analgesic used for moderate to severe pain. It is given parenterally. Onset, duration, and extent of analgesia and respiratory depression are comparable with those produced by morphine. Other adverse effects include sedation, sweating, headache, and psychotic symptoms, but these are reportedly minimal at doses of 10 mg or less.

ROUTES AND DOSAGE RANGE

Adults: IM, IV, SC 10 mg/70 kg q3–6h PRN

Pentazocine (Talwin) is a synthetic analgesic drug of abuse and may produce physical and psychological dependence. It is a Schedule IV drug. Pentazocine usually is used for the same clinical indications as other strong analgesics and causes similar adverse effects. Recommended doses for analgesia are less effective than usual doses of morphine or meperidine, but some people may tolerate pentazocine better than morphine or meperidine. Parenteral pentazocine usually produces analgesia within 10 to 30 minutes and lasts 2 to 3 hours. Adverse effects include hallucinations, bizarre dreams or nightmares, depression, nervousness, feelings of depersonalization, extreme euphoria, tissue damage with ulceration and necrosis or fibrosis at injection sites with long-term use, and respiratory depression.

Oral pentazocine tablets contain naloxone 0.5 mg, a narcotic antagonist that prevents the effects of pentazocine if the oral tablet is injected. It has no pharmacologic action if taken orally. Naloxone was added to prevent a method of abuse in which oral tablets of pentazocine and tripelennamine, an antihistamine, were dissolved and injected IV. The mixture caused such adverse effects as pulmonary emboli and stroke (from obstruction of blood vessels by talc and other insoluble ingredients in the tablets).

ROUTES AND DOSAGE RANGES

Adults: PO 50–100 mg q3–4h (maximal daily dose, 600 mg)
   IM, SC, IV 30–60 mg q3–4h (maximal daily dose, 360 mg)
Children: Not recommended for children <12 y

Opioid Antagonists

Opioid antagonists reverse or block analgesia, CNS and respiratory depression, and other physiologic effects of opioid agonists. They compete with opioids for opioid receptor sites in the brain and thereby prevent opioid binding with receptors or displace opioids already occupying receptor sites. When an opioid cannot bind to receptor sites, it is "neutralized" and cannot exert its effects on body cells. Opioid antagonists do not relieve the depressant effects of other drugs, such as sedative-hypnotic, antianxiety, and antipsychotic agents. The chief clinical use of these drugs is to relieve CNS and respiratory depression induced by therapeutic doses or overdoses of opioids. The drugs are also used to reverse postoperative opioid depression, and naltrexone is approved for the treatment of opioid and alcohol dependence. These drugs produce withdrawal symptoms when given to opiate-dependent people.

Naloxone (Narcan), **nalmefene** (Revex), and **naltrexone** (ReVia) are structurally and pharmacologically similar. Naloxone is the oldest of the three drugs and has long been the drug of choice in respiratory depression known or thought to be caused by a narcotic. Therapeutic effects occur within minutes after parenteral injection and last 1 to 2 hours. Naloxone has a shorter duration of action than opioids, and repeated injections are usually needed. For a long-acting drug such as methadone, injections may be needed for 2 to 3 days. Naloxone produces few adverse effects, and repeated injections can be given safely. This drug should be readily available in all health care settings where opioids are given. Nalmefene is a newer agent whose main difference from naloxone is a longer duration of action. It may be preferred when opioid depression results from long-acting drugs such as methadone, pentazocine, or propoxyphene. Nalmefene is available in two concentrations: one for postoperative use and one for treatment of clients with opiate overdoses. Health care personnel must use the appropriate concentration for the intended purpose. Naltrexone is used in the maintenance of opiate-free states in opiate addicts. It is apparently effective in highly motivated, detoxified people. If given before the client is detoxified, acute withdrawal symptoms occur. Clients receiving naltrexone do not respond to analgesics if pain control is needed. The drug is recommended for use in conjunction with psychological and social counseling.

Naloxone

ROUTES AND DOSAGE RANGES

Adults: IV, IM, SC 0.1–0.4 mg, repeated IV q2–3 min PRN
Children: IV, IM, SC 0.01 mg/kg initially, repeated IV q2–3 min PRN

Nalmefene

ROUTE AND DOSAGE RANGES

Adults, reversal of postoperative opioid depression: (Blue label, 1-mL ampules containing 100 µg) IV according to body weight (50 kg, 0.125 mL; 60 kg, 0.15 mL; 70 kg, 0.175 mL; 80 kg, 0.2 mL; 90 kg, 0.225 mL; 100 kg, 0.25 mL)
Adults, treatment of opioid overdose: (Green label, 2-mL ampules containing 1 mg) IV 0.5 mg/70 kg as initial dose for clients who are not opioid dependent, followed by 1 mg/70 kg in 2–5 min if necessary. For known or suspected opioid-dependent people, give a test dose of 0.1 mg/70 kg. If no signs of opiate withdrawal occur within 2 min, proceed with the above dosage.

Naltrexone

ROUTE AND DOSAGE RANGE

Adults: PO 50 mg/day

NURSING PROCESS

Assessment

Pain is a subjective experience (whatever the person says it is), and humans display a wide variety of responses. Although pain thresholds (the point at which a tissue-damaging stimulus produces a sensation of pain) are similar, people differ in their perceptions, behaviors, and tolerance of pain. Differences in pain perception may result from psychological components. Stressors such as anxiety, depression, fatigue, anger, and fear tend to increase pain; rest, mood elevation, and diversionary activities tend to decrease pain. Differences in behaviors may or may not indicate pain to observers, and overt signs and symptoms are not reliable indicators of the presence or extent of pain. Especially with chronic pain, overt signs and symptoms may be absent. Differences in tolerance of pain (the amount or duration of pain a person is willing to suffer before seeking relief) often reflect the person's concern about the meaning of the pain and the type or intensity of the painful stimulus. Thus, pain is a complex physiologic, psychological, and sociocultural phenomenon that must be thoroughly assessed if it is to be managed effectively.

The nurse must assess every client in relation to pain, initially to determine appropriate interventions and later to determine whether the interventions were effective in preventing or relieving pain. Although the client is usually the best source of data, other people may be questioned about the client's words and behaviors that indicate pain. This is especially important with young children. During assessment, keep in mind that acute pain may coexist with or be superimposed on chronic pain. Specific assessment data usually include:

- **Location.** Determining the location may assist in relieving the pain or identifying its underlying cause. Ask the client to show you where it hurts, if possible, and whether the pain stays in one place or radiates to other parts of the body. The term *referred pain* is used when pain arising from tissue damage in one area of the body is felt in another area. Patterns of referred pain may be helpful in diagnosis. For example, pain of cardiac origin may radiate to the neck, shoulders, chest muscles, and down the arms, often on the left side. This form of pain usually results from myocardial ischemia due to atherosclerosis of coronary arteries. Stomach pain is usually referred to the epigastrium and may indicate gastritis or peptic ulcer. Gallbladder and bile duct pain is often localized in the right upper quadrant of the abdomen. Uterine pain is usually felt as abdominal cramping or low back pain. Deep or chronic pain is usually more difficult to localize than superficial or acute pain.

- **Intensity or severity.** Because pain is a subjective experience and cannot be objectively measured, assessment of severity is based on the client's description and the nurse's observations. Various scales have been developed to measure and quantify pain. These include verbal descriptor scales in which the client is asked to rate pain as mild, moderate, or severe; numeric scales, with 0 representing no pain and 10 representing severe, intense pain; and visual analog scales, in which the client chooses the location indicating the level of pain on a continuum.

- **Relation to time, activities, and other signs and symptoms.** Specific questions include:
  - When did the pain start?
  - What activities were occurring when the pain started?
  - Does the pain occur with exercise or when at rest?
  - Do other signs and symptoms occur before, during, or after the pain?
  - Is this the first episode or a recurrent pain?
  - How long does the pain last?
  - What, if anything, decreases or relieves the pain?
  - What, if anything, aggravates the pain?
- **Other data.** For example, do not assume that postoperative pain is incisional and requires narcotic analgesics for relief. A person who has had abdominal surgery may have headache, musculoskeletal discomfort, or "gas pains." Also, restlessness may be caused by hypoxia or anxiety rather than pain.

Nursing Diagnoses

- Pain
- Impaired Gas Exchange related to sedation and decreased mobility
- Risk for Injury related to sedation and decreased mobility
- Constipation related to slowed peristalsis
- Altered Tissue Perfusion related to drug-induced decrease in cardiac output and blood pressure
- Urinary Retention related to decreased bladder contractility

How Can You Avoid This Medication Error?

Mr. Segel, a postoperative patient with a history of congestive heart failure and renal insufficiency, has the following orders for pain: morphine sulfate 4–6 mg IV q2–4h.

His wife asks you if her husband can have something for pain because she has seen him twitch and she thinks he is having pain. When you enter his room, he is dozing, so you administer the IV pain medication without waking him up. One hour later, the nursing assistant tells you he obtained the following vital signs: BP 112/64, pulse 66, respirations 6/minute and shallow.

- Knowledge Deficit: Effects and appropriate use of opioid analgesics
- Noncompliance: Drug dependence related to overuse

Planning/Goals

The client will:

- Avoid or be relieved of pain
- Use opioid analgesics appropriately
- Avoid preventable adverse effects
- Be closely monitored for excessive sedation and respiratory depression
- Be able to communicate and perform other activities of daily living when feasible

Interventions

Use measures to prevent, relieve, or decrease pain when possible. General measures include those that promote optimal body functioning and those that prevent trauma, inflammation, infection, and other sources of painful stimuli. Specific measures include:

- Encourage pulmonary hygiene techniques (eg, coughing, deep breathing, ambulation) to promote respiration and prevent pulmonary complications, such as pneumonia and atelectasis.
- Use sterile technique when caring for wounds, urinary catheters, or IV lines.
- Use exercises, ambulation, and position changes to promote circulation and musculoskeletal function.
- Handle any injured tissue very gently to avoid further trauma.
- Prevent bowel or bladder distention.
- Apply heat or cold.
- Use relaxation or distraction techniques.
- If a client is in pain on initial contact, try to relieve the pain as soon as possible. Once pain is controlled, plan with the client to avoid or manage future episodes.
- If a client is not in pain initially but anticipates surgery or an uncomfortable diagnostic procedure, plan with the client ways to minimize and manage discomfort.

Evaluation

- Ask clients about their levels of comfort or relief from pain.
- Observe behaviors that indicate the presence or absence of pain.
- Observe participation and ability to function in usual activities of daily living.
- Observe for presence or absence of sedation and respiratory depression.
- Observe for drug-seeking behavior (possibly indicating dependence).

CLIENT TEACHING GUIDELINES
Opioid (Narcotic) Analgesics

General Considerations

✔ Use nonpharmacologic treatments of pain (eg, exercise, heat and cold applications) instead of or along with analgesics, when effective.

✔ Use of a narcotic analgesic for acute pain is acceptable and unlikely to lead to addiction.

✔ For pain that is not relieved by a non-narcotic analgesic, a combination product containing a narcotic and non-narcotic (eg, Percocet, Vicodin, Tylenol No. 3) may be effective. Also, a narcotic may be alternated with a non-narcotic analgesic (eg, acetaminophen or ibuprofen).

✔ For acute episodes of pain, most opioids may be taken as needed; for chronic pain, the drugs should be taken on a regular schedule, around the clock.

✔ When a choice of analgesics is available, use the least amount of the mildest drug that is likely to be effective in a particular situation.

✔ Take only as prescribed. If desired effects are not achieved, report to the physician. Do not increase the dose and do not take medication more often than prescribed. Although these principles apply to all medications, they are especially important with opioid analgesics because of potentially serious adverse reactions, including drug dependence, and because analgesics may mask pain for which medical attention is needed.

✔ Do not drink alcohol or take other drugs that cause drowsiness (eg, some antihistamines, sedative-type drugs for nervousness or anxiety, sleeping pills) while taking opioid analgesics. Combining drugs with similar effects may lead to excessive sedation, even coma, and difficulty in breathing.

✔ Do not smoke, cook, drive a car, or operate machinery when drowsy or dizzy or when vision is blurred from medication.

✔ Stay in bed at least 30 to 60 minutes after receiving an opioid analgesic by injection. Injected drugs may cause dizziness, drowsiness, and falls when walking around. If it is necessary to get out of bed, ask someone for assistance.

✔ When hospitalized, ask the physician or nurse about potential methods of pain management. For example, if anticipating surgery, ask how postoperative pain will be handled, how you need to report pain and request pain medication, and so on. It is better to take adequate medication and be able to cough, deep breathe, and ambulate than to avoid or minimize pain medication and be unable to perform activities that promote recovery and healing. Do not object to having bedrails up and asking for assistance to ambulate when receiving a strong narcotic analgesic. These are safety measures to prevent falls or other injuries because these analgesics may cause drowsiness, weakness, unsteady gait, and blurred vision.

✔ Constipation is a common adverse effect of opioid analgesics. It may be prevented or managed by eating high-fiber foods, such as whole-grain cereals, fruits, and vegetables; drinking 2 to 3 quarts of fluid daily; and being as active as tolerated. For someone unable to take these preventive measures, Metamucil daily or a mild laxative every other day may be needed.

Self-administration

✔ Take oral narcotics with 6 to 8 oz of water, with or after food to reduce nausea.

✔ Do not crush or chew long-acting tablets (eg, MS Contin, MSIR). The tablets are formulated to release the active drug slowly, over several hours. Crushing or chewing causes immediate release of the drug, with a high risk of overdose and adverse effects, and shortens the duration of action.

✔ Omit one or more doses if severe adverse effects occur (eg, excessive drowsiness, difficulty in breathing, severe nausea, vomiting, or constipation) and report to a health care provider.

PRINCIPLES OF THERAPY

Need for Effective Pain Management

Numerous studies have indicated ineffective management of clients' pain, especially moderate to severe pain associated with surgery or cancer. Much of the difficulty has been attributed to inadequate or improper use of opioid analgesics, including administering the wrong drug, prescribing inadequate dosage, or leaving long intervals between doses. Even when ordered appropriately, nurses or clients and family members may not administer the drugs effectively. Traditionally, concerns about respiratory depression, excessive sedation, drug dependence, and other adverse effects have contributed to reluctance and delay in administering narcotic analgesics. Inadequate management of pain often leads to anxiety, depression, and other emotional upsets from anticipation of pain recurrence.

In recent years, a more humane approach to pain management has evolved. Basic assumptions of this approach are that no one should suffer pain needlessly; that pain occurs when the client says it does and should be relieved by whatever means required, including pharmacologic and nonpharmacologic treatments; that doses of opioids should be titrated to achieve maximal effectiveness and minimal toxicity; and that dependence rarely results from drugs taken for physical pain. Proponents of this view emphasize the need to assess and monitor all clients receiving opioid analgesics.

Drug Selection

1. Morphine is often the drug of first choice for severe pain. It is effective, available in various dosage strengths and forms, useful on a short- or long-term basis, and its adverse effects are well known. In addition, it is a "nonceiling" drug because there is no upper limit to the dosage that can be given to clients who have developed tolerance to previous dosages. This characteristic is especially valuable in clients with severe cancer-related pain because the drug dosage can be increased and titrated to relieve pain when pain increases or tolerance develops. Thus, some clients have safely received extremely large doses. Hydromorphone, levorphanol, and methadone are other nonceiling drugs.

    In contrast, meperidine and pentazocine are "ceiling" drugs: doses cannot be increased sufficiently or titrated to relieve increasing pain without greatly increasing the incidence and severity of adverse effects. These drugs are not recommended for the treatment of chronic cancer pain.

2. When more than one analgesic drug is ordered, use the least potent drug that is effective in relieving pain. For example, use a non-opioid analgesic, such as acetaminophen, rather than an opioid analgesic when feasible.

3. Non-opioid analgesics may be alternated or given concurrently with opioid analgesics, especially in chronic pain. This increases client comfort, reduces the likelihood of drug abuse and dependence, and decreases tolerance to the pain-relieving effects of the opioid analgesics.

4. In many instances, the drug preparation of choice may be one that combines an opioid and a non-opioid. The drugs act by different mechanisms and therefore produce greater analgesic effects. Commonly used examples are Tylenol No. 3 (acetaminophen 325 mg and codeine 30 mg/tablet) and Percocet (acetaminophen 325 mg and oxycodone 5 mg/tablet).

Route Selection

Opioid analgesics can be given by several routes, either noninvasively (orally, rectally, or transdermally) or invasively (SC, IV, or by spinal infusion). *When the route is changed (eg, from oral to injection or vice versa), the dose must also be changed to prevent overdosage or underdosage.*

1. Oral drugs are preferred when feasible, and most clients achieve relief with a short-acting or sustained-release oral preparation.

2. IV injection is usually preferred for rapid relief of acute, severe pain. Small, frequent IV doses are often effective in relieving pain with minimal risk of serious adverse effects. This is especially advantageous during a serious illness or after surgery.

    A technique called *patient-controlled analgesia* allows self-administration. One device consists of a syringe of diluted drug connected to an IV line and infusion pump; another device uses a specially designed IV bag and special tubing. These devices deliver a dose when the client pushes a button. The amount of drug delivered with each dose and the intervals between doses are preset and limited. Studies indicate that analgesia is more effective, client satisfaction is high, and smaller amounts of drug are used than with conventional PRN administration.

3. Continuous IV infusion may be used to treat severe pain.

4. Two other routes of administration are used to manage acute pain. One route involves injection of opioid analgesics directly into the CNS through a catheter placed into the epidural or intrathecal space by an anesthesiologist or other physician. This method provides effective analgesia while minimizing depressant effects. This type of pain control was developed after opioid receptors were found on neurons in the spinal cord. The other route involves the injection of local anesthetics to provide local or regional analgesia. Both of these methods interrupt the transmission of pain signals and are effective in

relieving pain, but they also require special techniques and monitoring procedures for safe use.

5. For clients with chronic pain and contraindications to oral or injected medications, some opioids are available in rectal suppositories or skin patches. Morphine, oxymorphone, and hydromorphone can be given rectally with similar potencies and half-lives as when given orally. For clients who cannot take oral medications and whose opioid requirement is too large for rectal administration, the transdermal route is preferred to IV or SC routes. A fentanyl skin patch (Duragesic) is effective and commonly used. When first applied, pain relief is delayed approximately 12 hours (as the drug is gradually absorbed). A steady-state plasma concentration is reached in approximately 14 to 20 hours and lasts approximately 72 hours. Because of the delayed effects, doses of a short-acting opioid should be ordered and given as needed during the first 48 hours after the patch is applied. With continued use, the old patch is removed and a new one applied approximately every 72 hours. Opioid overdose can occur with fentanyl patches if the client has fever (hastens drug absorption) or liver impairment (slows drug metabolism).

Dosage

Dosages of opioid analgesics should be sufficient to relieve pain without causing unacceptable adverse effects. Thus, dosages should be individualized according to the type and severity of pain; the client's age, size, and health status; whether the client is opiate naive (has not received sufficient opioids for development of tolerance) or opiate tolerant (has previously taken opioids and drug tolerance has developed, so that larger-than-usual doses are needed to relieve pain); whether the client has progressive or worsening disease; and other characteristics that influence responses to pain. Guidelines include:

1. Small to moderate doses relieve constant, dull pain; moderate to large doses relieve intermittent, sharp pain caused by trauma or conditions affecting the viscera.
2. When a narcotic analgesic is ordered in variable amounts (eg, 8 to 10 mg of morphine), give the smaller amount as long as it is effective in relieving pain.
3. Dosages of narcotic analgesics should be reduced for clients who also are receiving other CNS depressants, such as sedating antianxiety, antidepressant, antihistaminic, antipsychotic, or other sedative-type drugs.
4. Dosages often differ according to the route of administration. Oral doses undergo extensive metabolism on their first pass through the liver so that oral doses are usually much larger than IV doses.

Scheduling

Opioid analgesics may be given as needed, within designated time limits, or on a regular schedule. Traditionally, the drugs have often been scheduled every 4 to 6 hours PRN. Numerous studies have indicated that such a schedule is often ineffective in managing clients' pain. Because these analgesics are used for moderate to severe pain, they should in general be scheduled to provide effective and consistent pain relief. Some guidelines for scheduling drugs include:

1. When analgesics are ordered PRN, have a clear-cut system by which the client reports pain or requests medication. The client should know that analgesic drugs have been ordered and will be given promptly when needed. If a drug cannot be given or if administration must be delayed, explain this to the client. In addition, offer or give the drug when indicated by the client's condition rather than waiting for the client to request medication.
2. In acute pain, opioid analgesics are most effective when given parenterally and at the onset of pain. In chronic, severe pain, opioid analgesics are most effective when given on a regular schedule, around the clock. To prevent pain recurrence, sleeping clients should be awakened to take their medication.
3. When needed, analgesics should be given before coughing and deep-breathing exercises, dressing changes, and other therapeutic and diagnostic procedures.
4. Opioids are not recommended for prolonged periods except for advanced malignant disease. Health care agencies usually have an automatic "stop order" for opioids after 48 to 72 hours; this means that the drug is discontinued when the time limit expires if the physician does not reorder it.

Drug Use in Specific Situations

Cancer

Pain associated with cancer is caused mainly by tumor spread into pain-sensitive tissues (eg, bone, nerves, soft tissues, viscera) and the resulting tissue destruction. Pain may also accompany treatment of cancer by surgery, chemotherapy, or radiation therapy. When opioid analgesics are required in chronic pain associated with malignancy, the main consideration is client comfort, not preventing drug addiction. Effective treatment requires that pain be relieved and prevented from recurring. With disease progression and the development of drug tolerance, extremely large doses and frequent administration may be required. Additional guidelines include the following:

1. Analgesics should be given on a regular schedule, around the clock. Clients should be awakened, if necessary, to prevent pain recurrence.

2. Oral, rectal, and transdermal routes of administration are generally preferred over injections.
3. A non-narcotic analgesic (see Chap. 7) may be used alone for mild pain.
4. Oxycodone or codeine can be used for moderate pain, often with a non-narcotic analgesic. A combination of the two types of drugs produces additive analgesic effects and may allow smaller doses of the opioid.
5. Morphine or another strong opioid is given for severe pain. Although the dose of morphine can be titrated upward for adequate analgesia, unacceptable adverse effects (eg, excessive sedation, respiratory depression, nausea and vomiting) may limit the dose. The oral route of administration is preferred; the initial oral dosage of morphine is usually 10 to 20 mg every 3 to 4 hours.
6. When long-acting forms of opioid analgesics are being given on a regular schedule (eg, sustained-release forms of morphine or fentanyl skin patches), fast-acting forms also need to be ordered and available for "breakthrough" pain. If additional doses are needed frequently, the baseline dose of long-acting medication may need to be increased.
7. In addition to opioid analgesics, other drugs may be used to increase client comfort. For example, tricyclic antidepressants (TCAs) have analgesic effects, especially in neuropathic pain. Lower doses of TCAs are required for analgesia than for depression, but analgesic effects may not occur for 2 to 3 weeks. Antiemetics may be given for nausea and vomiting, and laxatives are usually needed to prevent or relieve constipation.

Biliary, Renal, or Ureteral Colic

When opioid analgesics are used to relieve the acute, severe pain associated with various types of colic, an antispasmodic drug such as atropine may be needed as well. Opioid analgesics may increase smooth muscle tone and cause spasm. Atropine does not have strong antispasmodic properties of its own in usual doses, but it reduces the spasm-producing effects of opioid analgesics.

Postoperative Use

When analgesics are used postoperatively, the goal is to relieve pain without excessive sedation so that clients can do deep-breathing exercises, cough, ambulate, and implement other measures to promote recovery.

Burns

In severely burned clients, opioid analgesics should be used cautiously. A common cause of respiratory arrest in burned clients is excessive administration of analgesics. Agitation in a burned person usually should be interpreted as hypoxia or hypovolemia rather than pain, until proved

otherwise. When opioid analgesics are necessary, they are usually given IV in small doses. Drugs given by other routes are absorbed erratically in the presence of shock and hypovolemia and may not relieve pain. In addition, unabsorbed drugs may be rapidly absorbed when circulation is improved, with the potential for excessive dosage and toxic effects.

Management of Toxicity or Overdose

Acute toxicity or opioid overdose can occur from therapeutic use or from abuse by drug-dependent people. Overdose may produce severe respiratory depression and coma. The main goal of treatment is to restore and maintain adequate respiratory function. This can be accomplished by inserting an endotracheal tube and starting mechanical ventilation, or by giving an opioid antagonist, such as naloxone or nalmefene. Thus, emergency supplies should be readily available in any setting where opioid analgesics are used, including ambulatory settings and clients' homes.

Prevention and Management of Withdrawal Symptoms

Abstinence from opiates after chronic use produces a withdrawal syndrome characterized by anxiety; aggressiveness; restlessness; generalized body aches; insomnia; lacrimation; rhinorrhea; perspiration; pupil dilation; piloerection (goose flesh); anorexia, nausea, and vomiting; diarrhea; elevation of body temperature, respiratory rate, and systolic blood pressure; abdominal and other muscle cramps; dehydration; and weight loss. Although all opioids produce similar withdrawal syndromes, the onset, severity, and duration vary. With morphine, symptoms begin within a few hours of the last dose, reach peak intensity in 36 to 72 hours, and subside over approximately 10 days. With methadone, symptoms begin in 1 to 2 days, peak in approximately 3 days, and subside over several weeks. Heroin, meperidine, methadone, morphine, oxycodone, and oxymorphone are associated with more severe withdrawal symptoms than other opioids. If an opioid antagonist, such as naloxone (Narcan), is given, withdrawal symptoms occur rapidly and are more intense but of shorter duration. Despite the discomfort that occurs, withdrawal from opioids is rarely life threatening unless other problems are present. An exception is opioid withdrawal in neonates, which has a high mortality rate if not treated effectively. Signs and symptoms in neonates include tremor, jitteriness, increased muscle tone, screaming, fever, sweating, tachycardia, vomiting, diarrhea, respiratory distress, and possibly seizures.

Recognition and treatment of early, mild symptoms of withdrawal can prevent progression to severe symptoms. Both opioids and nonopioids are used for treatment. Opioids may be used in two ways to provide a safe, comfortable, and therapeutic withdrawal. One technique is to give the opioid from which the person is withdrawing, which immediately reverses the signs and symptoms of withdrawal. Then, dosage is gradually reduced over several days. Another technique is to substitute a long-acting opioid (eg, methadone) for a short-acting opioid of abuse. Methadone is usually given in an adequate dose to control symptoms, once or twice daily, then gradually tapered over 5 to 10 days. In neonates undergoing opioid withdrawal, methadone or paregoric may be used.

Clonidine, an antihypertensive drug, is a nonopioid that may be used to treat opioid withdrawal. Clonidine reduces the release of norepinephrine in the brain and thus reduces symptoms associated with excessive stimulation of the sympathetic nervous system (eg, anxiety, restlessness, insomnia). Blood pressure must be closely monitored during clonidine therapy. Other medications (non-opioid analgesics, antiemetics, antidiarrheals) are often required to treat other symptoms.

Use in Opiate-Tolerant People

Whether opiate tolerance results from the use of prescribed, therapeutic drugs or the abuse of street drugs, there are two main considerations in using opioid analgesics in this population. First, larger-than-usual doses are required to treat pain. Second, signs and symptoms of withdrawal occur if adequate dosage is not maintained or if opioid antagonists are given.

Use in Children

In general, there is little understanding of the physiology, pathology, assessment, and management of pain in children. Many authorities indicate that children's pain is often ignored or undertreated, including children having surgical and other painful procedures for which adults routinely receive an anesthetic, a strong analgesic, or both. This is especially true in preterm and full-term neonates. One reason for inadequate prevention and management of pain in newborns has been a common belief that they did not experience pain because of immature nervous systems. However, research indicates that neonates have abundant C fibers and that A-delta fibers are developing during the first few months of life. These are the nerve fibers that carry pain signals from peripheral tissues to the spinal cord. In addition, brain pain centers and the endogenous analgesia system seem to be developed and functional. Endogenous opioids are released at birth and in response to fetal and neonatal distress such as asphyxia or other difficulty associated with the birth process.

Older infants and children may experience pain even when analgesics have been ordered and are readily available. For example, children may fear injections or may be unable to communicate their discomfort. Health care providers or parents may fear adverse effects of narcotic analgesics, including excessive sedation, respiratory depression, and addiction.

Other than reduced dosage, there have been few guidelines about the use of opioid analgesics in children. With increased knowledge about pain mechanisms and the recommendations prepared by the Acute Pain Management Guideline Panel in 1992, every nurse who works with children should be able to manage pain effectively. Some specific considerations include the following:

1. Opioid analgesics administered during labor and delivery may depress fetal and neonatal respiration. The drugs cross the blood–brain barrier of the infant more readily than that of the mother. Therefore, doses that do not depress maternal respiration may profoundly depress the infant's respiration. Respiration should be monitored closely in neonates, and the opioid antagonist naloxone should be readily available.

2. Expressions of pain may differ according to age and developmental level. Infants may cry and have muscular rigidity and thrashing behavior. Preschoolers may behave aggressively or complain verbally of discomfort. Young school-aged children may express pain verbally or behaviorally, often with regression to behaviors used at younger ages. Adolescents may be reluctant to admit they are uncomfortable or need help. With chronic pain, children of all ages tend to withdraw and regress to an earlier stage of development.

3. The Acute Pain Management Guideline Panel recommends that opioid analgesics be given by routes (eg, PO, IV, epidurally) other than IM injections, because IM injections are painful and frightening for children. For any child receiving parenteral opioids, vital signs and level of consciousness must be assessed regularly.

4. Opioid formulations specifically for children are not generally available. When children's doses are calculated from adult doses, the fractions and decimals that often result greatly increase the risk of a dosage error.

5. Opioid rectal suppositories may be used more often in children than in adults. Although they may be useful when oral or parenteral routes are not indicated, the dose of medication actually received by the child is unknown because drug absorption is erratic and because adult suppositories are sometimes cut in half or otherwise altered.

6. Opioid effects in children may differ from those expected in adults because of physiologic and pharmacokinetic differences. Assess regularly and be alert for unusual signs and symptoms.

7. Hydromorphone, methadone, oxycodone, oxymorphone, and propoxyphene are not recommended

for use in children because safety, efficacy, or dosages have not been established.

8. Like adults, children seem more able to cope with pain when they are informed about what is happening to them and are assisted in developing coping strategies. Age-appropriate doll play, a favorite videotape, diversionary activities, and other techniques can be used effectively. However, such techniques should be used in conjunction with adequate analgesia, not as a substitute for pain medication.

Use in Older Adults

Opioid analgesics should be used cautiously in older adults, especially if they are debilitated; have hepatic, renal, or respiratory impairment; or are receiving other drugs that depress the CNS. Older adults are especially sensitive to respiratory depression, excessive sedation, confusion, and other adverse effects. However, they are entitled to and should receive adequate analgesia, along with vigilant monitoring. Specific recommendations include the following:

1. Use nondrug measures (eg, heat applications, exercise) and non-opioid analgesics to relieve pain, when effective.
2. When opioid analgesics are needed, use those with short half-lives (eg, oxycodone or hydromorphone) because they are less likely to accumulate.
3. Start with low doses and increase doses gradually, if necessary.
4. Give the drugs less often than for younger adults because the duration of action may be longer.
5. Monitor carefully for sedation or confusion. Also, monitor voiding and urine output because acute urinary retention is more likely to occur in older adults.
6. Assess older adults for ability to self-administer opioid analgesics safely. Those with short-term memory loss (common in this population) may require assistance and supervision.

Use in Renal Impairment

Most opioid analgesics and related drugs are extensively metabolized in the liver to metabolites that are then excreted in urine. In clients with renal impairment, the drugs should be given in minimal doses, for the shortest effective time, because usual doses may produce profound sedation and a prolonged duration of action. Morphine, for example, produces an active metabolite that may accumulate in renal impairment. Meperidine (Demerol) should not be used in clients with renal impairment because a toxic metabolite, normeperidine, may accumulate. Normeperidine is pharmacologically active and a CNS stimulant that may cause muscle spasms, seizures, and psychosis.

These effects are not reversed by opioid antagonists such as naloxone (Narcan).

Use in Hepatic Impairment

Because opioid analgesics and related drugs are extensively metabolized by the liver, they may accumulate and cause increased adverse effects in the presence of hepatic impairment. Dosages may need to be reduced, especially with chronic use.

Use in Critical Illness

Opioid analgesics are commonly used to manage pain associated with disease processes and invasive diagnostic and therapeutic procedures. In intensive care units, they are also used for synergistic effects with sedatives and neuromuscular blocking agents, which increases the risks of adverse drug reactions and interactions. In critical illness, opioid analgesics are usually given by IV bolus or continuous infusion. Guidelines include the following:

1. Assume that all critically ill clients are in pain or at high risk for development of pain.
2. Assess for pain on a regular schedule around the clock (eg, every 1 to 2 hours in critical care units). Use a consistent method for assessing severity, such as a visual analog or numeric scale. If the client is able to communicate, ask about the location, severity, and so forth. If the client is unable to communicate needs for pain relief, as is often the case with critically ill clients, the nurse must evaluate posture, body language, risk factors, and other possible indicators of pain.
3. Prevent pain when possible. Interventions include being very gentle when performing nursing care, to avoid tissue trauma, and positioning clients to prevent ischemia, edema, and misalignment. In addition, give analgesics before painful procedures, when indicated.
4. When pain occurs, manage it appropriately to provide relief and prevent its recurrence. Some helpful techniques include obtaining orders for adequate initial or renewal analgesics; giving analgesics on a regular schedule, with additional PRN doses for breakthrough pain; and treating pain as soon as possible.
5. Opioid analgesics are often given by IV infusion over a prolonged period in trauma and other critical illnesses. They may also be given orally, by transdermal patch, or epidural infusion, depending on the client's condition.
6. Consult specialists in pain management (eg, anesthesiologists, clinical pharmacists, or nurses) when pain is inadequately controlled with usual measures.

Home Care

Opioid analgesics are widely used in the home for both acute and chronic pain. With acute pain, such as post-operative recovery, the use of a opioid analgesic is often limited to a short period and clients self-administer their medications. The need for strong pain medication recedes as healing occurs. The home care nurse may teach clients and caregivers safe usage of the drugs (eg, that the drugs decrease mental alertness and physical agility, so potentially hazardous activities should be avoided), nonpharmacologic methods of managing pain, and ways to prevent adverse effects of opioids (eg, excessive sedation, constipation). Physical dependence is uncommon with short-term use of opioid analgesics for acute pain.

With some types of chronic pain, such as that occurring with low back pain or osteoarthritis, opioid analgesics are not indicated for long-term use. Treatment involves non-opioid medications, physical therapy, and other measures. The home care nurse may need to explain the reasons for not using opioids on a long-term basis and to help clients and caregivers learn alternative methods of relieving discomfort.

With cancer pain, as previously discussed, the goal of treatment is to prevent or relieve pain and keep clients comfortable, without concern about addiction. Consequently, the home care nurse must assist clients and caregivers in understanding the appropriate use of opioid analgesics in cancer care, including administration on a regular schedule. The nurse also must be proficient in using and teaching various routes of drug administration and in arranging regimens with potentially very large doses and various combinations of drugs. In addition, an active effort is needed to prevent or manage adverse effects, such as a bowel program to prevent constipation.

(*text continues on page 89*)

NURSING ACTIONS Opioid Analgesics

NURSING ACTIONS	RATIONALE/EXPLANATION
1. Administer accurately	
a. Check the rate, depth, and rhythm of respirations before each dose. If the rate is below 12 per minute, delay or omit the dose and report to the physician.	Respiratory depression is a major adverse reaction to strong analgesics. Assessing respirations before each dose can help prevent or minimize potentially life-threatening respiratory depression.
b. Have the client lie down to receive injections of opioid analgesics and for at least a few minutes afterward.	To prevent or minimize hypotension, nausea, and vomiting. These side effects are more likely to occur in the ambulatory client. Also, the client may be sedated enough to make ambulation hazardous without help.
c. When injecting opioid analgesics intravenously, give small doses; inject slowly over several minutes; and have opioid antagonist drugs, artificial airways, and equipment for artificial ventilation readily available.	Large doses or rapid intravenous injection may cause severe respiratory depression and hypotension.
d. Give meperidine and pentazocine intramuscularly rather than subcutaneously.	Subcutaneous injections of these drugs may cause pain, tissue irritation, and possible abscess. This reaction is more likely with long-term use.
e. Put siderails up; instruct the client not to smoke or try to ambulate without help. Keep the call light within reach.	To prevent falls or other injuries.
f. When giving controlled-release tablets of morphine, do NOT crush them, and instruct the client not to chew them.	Crushing or chewing causes immediate release of drug, with a high risk of overdose and toxicity.
g. To apply transdermal fentanyl: (1) Clip (do not shave) hair, if needed, on a flat surface of the upper trunk.	Correct preparation of the site and application of the medicated adhesive patch are necessary for drug absorption and effectiveness.

(*continued*)

NURSING ACTIONS	RATIONALE/EXPLANATION
(2) If it is necessary to cleanse the site, use plain water; do not use soaps, oils, lotions, alcohol, or other substances. Let the skin dry.	
(3) Apply the skin patch and press it in place for a few seconds.	
(4) Leave in place for 72 hours.	
(5) When a new patch is to be applied, remove the old one, fold it so that the medication is on the inside, and flush the patch down the toilet. Apply the new patch to a different skin site.	
2. **Observe for therapeutic effects**	Therapeutic effects depend on the reason for use, usually for analgesic effects, sometimes for antitussive or antidiarrheal effects.
a. A verbal statement of pain relief	
b. Decreased behavioral manifestations of pain or discomfort	
c. Sleeping	
d. Increased participation in usual activities of daily living, including interactions with other people in the environment	
e. Fewer and shorter episodes of nonproductive coughing when used for antitussive effects	Opioid analgesics relieve cough by depressing the cough center in the medulla oblongata.
f. Lowered blood pressure, decreased pulse rate, slower and deeper respirations, and less dyspnea when morphine is given for pulmonary edema	Morphine may relieve pulmonary edema by causing vasodilation, which in turn decreases venous return to the heart and decreases cardiac work.
g. Decreased diarrhea when given for constipating effects	These drugs slow secretions and motility of the gastrointestinal tract. Constipation is usually an adverse effect. However, in severe diarrhea or with ileostomy, the drugs decrease the number of bowel movements and make the consistency more paste-like than liquid.
3. **Observe for adverse effects**	
a. Respiratory depression—hypoxemia, restlessness, dyspnea, slow, shallow breathing, changes in blood pressure and pulse, decreased ability to cough	Respiratory depression is a major adverse effect of opioid analgesics and results from depression of the respiratory center in the medulla oblongata. Respiratory depression occurs with usual therapeutic doses and increases in incidence and severity with large doses or frequent administration.
b. Hypotension	Hypotension stems from drug effects on the vasomotor center in the medulla oblongata that cause peripheral vasodilation and lowering of blood pressure. This is a therapeutic effect with pulmonary edema.
c. Excessive sedation—drowsiness, slurred speech, impaired mobility and coordination, stupor, coma	This is caused by depression of the central nervous system (CNS) and is potentially life threatening.
d. Nausea and vomiting	Opioid analgesics stimulate the chemoreceptor trigger zone in the brain. Consequently, nausea and

(continued)

NURSING ACTIONS	RATIONALE/EXPLANATION
	vomiting may occur with oral or parenteral routes of administration. They are more likely to occur with ambulation than with recumbency.
e. Constipation	This is caused by the drug's slowing effects on the gastrointestinal tract. Constipation may be alleviated by activity, adequate food and fluid intake, and regular administration of mild laxatives.
4. Observe for drug interactions	
a. Drugs that *increase* effects of opioid analgesics:	
(1) CNS depressants—alcohol, general anesthetics, antianxiety agents, tricyclic antidepressants, antihistamines, antipsychotic agents, barbiturates, and other sedative-hypnotic drugs	All these drugs alone, as well as the opioid analgesics, produce CNS depression. When combined, additive CNS depression results. If dosage of one or more interacting drugs is high, severe respiratory depression, coma, and death may ensue.
(2) Diuretics	Orthostatic hypotension, an adverse effect of strong analgesics and diuretics, may be increased if the two drug groups are given concurrently.
(3) Monoamine oxidase (MAO) inhibitors	These drugs interfere with detoxification of some opioid analgesics, especially meperidine. They may cause additive CNS depression with hypotension and respiratory depression or CNS stimulation with hyperexcitability and convulsions. If an MAO inhibitor is necessary, dosage should be reduced because the combination is potentially life threatening.
b. Drugs that *decrease* effects of opioid analgesics:	
(1) Opioid antagonists	These drugs reverse respiratory depression produced by opioid analgesics. This is their only clinical use, and they should not be given unless severe respiratory depression is present. They do not reverse respiratory depression caused by other CNS depressants.
(2) Butorphanol, nalbuphine, and pentazocine	These analgesics are weak antagonists of opioid analgesics, and they may cause withdrawal symptoms in people who have been receiving opiates or who are physically dependent on opioid analgesics.

How Can You Avoid This Medication Error?

Answer: Mr. Segel has received too much morphine which has caused his respiration rate to fall to a dangerously slow rate. Before giving any patient a PRN narcotic, it is important to check vital signs and when the last dose of the narcotic was administered. This situation does not indicate that those assessments were completed. Also, the medication was administered when the patient was sleeping. Before administering pain medications, a pain assessment should be completed, rather than depending on the impressions of a relative or visitor. The nurse should have been more cautious in administering pain medication to a postoperative patient with renal impairment because he will be less able to excrete the drug.

REVIEW AND APPLICATION EXERCISES

1. When assessing a client for pain, what are the major guidelines?

2. What kinds of behaviors may indicate acute pain? Are similar behaviors associated with chronic pain?

3. What are some nonpharmacologic interventions for pain, and why should they be used instead of or along with analgesics?

4. What are the major adverse effects of opioid analgesics? How do opioid antagonists counteract adverse effects?

5. For a client who has had major surgery during the previous 24 to 72 hours, what type of analgesic is indicated? Why?

6. What are the potential differences in dosage between short-term (a few days) and long-term (weeks or months) administration of morphine?

7. Explain the rationale for using both opioid analgesics and non-opioid analgesics in the treatment of pain.

8. For a client with chronic cancer pain, what are the advantages and disadvantages of using opioid analgesics?

9. Why is meperidine (Demerol) not recommended for the management of chronic cancer pain?

10. For a client with chronic cancer pain, should opioid analgesics be given as needed or on a regular schedule? Why?

11. For a client who is receiving large doses of an opioid analgesic, what signs and symptoms would make you suspect drug toxicity or overdose? What interventions are needed for suspected toxicity?

12. For a client who has been taking an opioid analgesic for a long time, what signs and symptoms would make you suspect opioid withdrawal? What interventions are needed for suspected withdrawal?

13. On a initial visit to a client with cancer who is receiving an opioid analgesic, how would you assess the effectiveness of pain management?

SELECTED REFERENCES

Abrahm, J.L. (1997). Cancer pain management. In W.N. Kelley (Ed.), *Textbook of internal medicine*, 3rd ed., pp. 1538–1543. Philadelphia: Lippincott-Raven.

Acute Pain Management Guideline Panel. (1992). *Acute pain management: Operative or medical procedures and trauma. Clinical practice guideline*. AHCPR Pub. No. 92-0032. Rockville, MD: Agency for Health Care Policy and Research, Public Health Service, U.S. Department of Health and Human Services for Health Care Policy and Research.

Baumann, T.J. (1997). Pain management. In J.T. DiPiro, R.L. Talbert, P.E. Hayes, G.C. Yee, G.R. Matzke, B.G. Wells, & L.M. Posey (Eds.), *Pharmacotherapy: A pathophysiologic approach*, 3rd ed., pp. 1259–1278. Stamford, CT: Appleton & Lange.

Curtis, S.M., Kolytolo, C., & Broome, M.E. (1998). Somatosensory function and pain. In C.M. Porth (Ed.), *Pathophysiology: Concepts of altered health states*, 5th ed., pp. 959–992. Philadelphia: Lippincott Williams & Wilkins.

Drug facts and comparisons. (Updated monthly). St. Louis: Facts and Comparisons.

Guyton, A.C. & Hall, J.E. (1996). *Textbook of medical physiology*, 9th ed. Philadelphia: W.B. Saunders.

Haack, M.R. (1998). Treating acute withdrawal from alcohol and other drugs. *Nursing Clinics of North America, 33*(1), 75–92.

Hoyt, D.B., Winchell, R.J., & Ferris, N. (1996). Analgesia and sedation. In J.A. Weigelt & F.R. Lewis, Jr. (Eds.), *Surgical critical care*. Philadelphia: W.B. Saunders.

Moulin, D. (1997). Approach to the patient with chronic pain. In W.N. Kelley (Ed.), *Textbook of internal medicine*, 3rd ed., pp. 212–215. Philadelphia: Lippincott-Raven.

Reisine, T. & Pasternak, G. (1996). Opioid analgesics and antagonists. In J.G. Hardman, L.E. Limbird, P.B. Molinoff, & R.W. Ruddon (Eds.), *Goodman & Gilman's The pharmacological basis of therapeutics*, 9th ed., pp. 521–555. New York: McGraw-Hill.

7

Analgesic–Antipyretic–Anti-inflammatory and Related Drugs

Objectives

After studying this chapter, the student will be able to:

1. Discuss the role of prostaglandins in the etiology of pain, fever, and inflammation.

2. Discuss aspirin and other nonsteroidal anti-inflammatory drugs (NSAIDs) in terms of mechanism of action, indications for use, contraindications to use, nursing process, and principles of therapy.

3. Compare and contrast aspirin, other NSAIDs, and acetaminophen in terms of indications for use and adverse effects.

4. Differentiate among antiplatelet, analgesic, and anti-inflammatory doses of aspirin.

5. Differentiate between traditional NSAIDs and the newer cyclooxygenase-2 inhibitors.

6. Teach clients interventions to prevent or decrease adverse effects of aspirin, other NSAIDs, and acetaminophen.

7. Identify factors influencing the use of aspirin, NSAIDs, and acetaminophen in special populations.

8. Discuss the use of acetylcysteine (Mucomyst) as an antidote for acetaminophen overdose.

9. Discuss the use of NSAIDs and antigout drugs.

10. Discuss the use of NSAIDs, triptans, and ergot antimigraine drugs.

You are working in an emergency room when parents bring in their 2-year-old son who has just ingested half a bottle of acetaminophen (Tylenol). His parents have recently come to this country from Mexico and speak very little English. The child does not appear acutely ill and the parents become very upset when the physician wants to admit the child.

Reflect on:

▶ Why is Tylenol overdose potentially so serious for this young child?

▶ What would emergency and follow-up treatment for Tylenol overdose be?

▶ How has this child's developmental stage increased the likelihood for accidental poisoning?

▶ Develop a teaching plan for this family to prevent recurrence.

DESCRIPTION

The analgesic–antipyretic–anti-inflammatory drugs relieve symptoms (ie, pain, fever, and inflammation) that may be associated with many different illnesses. **Acetylsalicylic acid** (ASA, aspirin) is the prototype of the group. Except for acetaminophen, the drugs in this group also are called nonsteroidal anti-inflammatory drugs (NSAIDs). (Adrenal corticosteroids, the "steroidal" anti-inflammatory drugs, are discussed in Chap. 24.) Several NSAIDs are used primarily for their analgesic and anti-inflammatory effects in musculoskeletal disorders, such as arthritis. Acetaminophen (Tylenol, others) is not an NSAID because it does not have anti-inflammatory effects. It is included in this chapter because of its extensive use as an analgesic and antipyretic. With gout and migraine, these drugs and others are used for prevention and treatment of acute attacks.

Aspirin and related drugs inhibit the synthesis of prostaglandins, and both therapeutic and adverse effects are attributed primarily to this action. Found in most body tissues, prostaglandins are chemical mediators that help regulate many cell functions and participate in the inflammatory response to tissue injury (see Chap. 1). To aid understanding of prostaglandins, their physiologic effects are listed in Table 7-1 and their roles in pain, fever, and inflammation are described in the following section.

PAIN, FEVER, AND INFLAMMATION

Pain is the sensation of discomfort, hurt, or distress. It is a common human ailment and may occur with tissue injury and inflammation. Prostaglandins sensitize pain receptors and increase the pain associated with other chemical mediators, such as bradykinin and histamine.

Fever is an elevation of body temperature above the normal range. Body temperature is controlled by a regulating center in the hypothalamus. Normally, there is a balance between heat production and heat loss so that a constant body temperature is maintained. When there is excessive heat production, mechanisms to increase heat loss are activated. As a result, blood vessels dilate, more blood flows through the skin, sweating occurs, and body temperature usually stays within normal range. When fever occurs, the heat-regulating center in the hypothalamus is reset so that it tolerates a higher body temperature. Fever may be produced by dehydration, inflammatory and infectious processes, some drugs, brain injury, or diseases involving the hypothalamus. Prostaglandin formation is stimulated by such circumstances and, along with bacterial toxins and other substances, prostaglandins act as pyrogens (fever-producing agents).

Inflammation is the normal body response to tissue damage from any source, and it may occur in any tissue or organ. It is an attempt by the body to remove the damaging agent and repair the damaged tissue. The local manifestations of inflammation are redness, heat, edema, and pain. Redness and heat result from vasodilation and increased blood supply; edema results from leakage of blood plasma into the area; and pain is produced by the pressure of edema and secretions on nerve endings and by chemical irritation of bradykinin, histamine, and other substances released by the damaged cells. Prostaglandins also are released and increase the pain and edema caused by other substances. Systemic manifestations of inflammation include leukocytosis, increased erythrocyte sedimentation rate, fever, headache, loss of appetite, lethargy or malaise, and weakness. Both local and systemic manifestations vary according to the cause and extent of tissue damage.

GOUT

Gout is a disorder characterized by an inability to metabolize uric acid, a waste product of protein metabolism. The resulting hyperuricemia may be asymptomatic or may lead to urate deposits in various tissues. In the musculoskeletal system, often in the feet, urate deposits produce periodic episodes of severe pain, edema, and inflammation (gouty arthritis). In the kidneys, urate deposits may form renal calculi or cause other damage.

MIGRAINE

Migraine is a type of headache characterized by periodic attacks of pain, nausea, and increased sensitivity to light and sound. The pain is often worse on one side of the head, throbbing or pulsating in nature, moderate or severe in intensity, and disruptive of usual activities of daily living. The etiology is unknown, but one theory is that certain

TABLE 7-1	Prostaglandins and Their Effects
Prostaglandin	**Effects**
D_2	Bronchoconstriction
E_2	Vasodilation
	Bronchodilation
	Increased activity of GI smooth muscle
	Gastroprotective effects
	Increased sensitivity to pain
	Increased body temperature
F_2	Bronchoconstriction
	Increased uterine contraction
	Increased activity of GI smooth muscle
I_2 (Prostacyclin)	Vasodilation
	Decreased platelet aggregation
	Gastroprotective effects
Thromboxane A_2	Vasoconstriction
	Increased platelet aggregation

GI, gastrointestinal.

circumstances cause an imbalance of chemicals (eg, serotonin, prostaglandins) in the brain. This imbalance results in vasodilation, release of inflammatory mediators, and irritation of nerve endings. Numerous circumstances have been implicated as "triggers" for the chemical imbalance and migraine, including alcohol (especially red wine), some foods (eg, chocolate, aged cheeses), some medications (eg, antihypertensives, oral contraceptives), irregular patterns of eating and sleeping, and physical and emotional stress. Migraine occurs more often in women than men and may be associated with menses.

MECHANISM OF ACTION

Aspirin, acetaminophen, and NSAIDs inactivate cyclooxygenases (COX), the enzymes required for formation of prostaglandins. This action inhibits formation of prosta-

glandins and thereby inhibits their effects on body tissues. This antiprostaglandin effect is considered the primary mechanism by which these drugs produce both therapeutic and adverse effects (Fig. 7-1).

Aspirin and traditional NSAIDs are nonselective COX inhibitors because they inhibit both COX enzymes, called COX-1 and COX-2. COX-1 is normally present in the blood vessels, kidneys, and stomach. Prostaglandins produced by COX-1 help to regulate cellular functions in these tissues and are associated with protective effects on the stomach and kidneys. In the stomach, prostaglandins decrease gastric acid secretion, increase mucus secretion, and regulate blood circulation. In the kidneys, prostaglandins are produced mainly when renal blood flow is impaired and they help to maintain adequate renal blood flow and function.

Cyclooxygenase-2 is found in inflamed tissues; its presence is induced by inflammatory mediators, white blood cells, and cytokines. Prostaglandins produced by COX-2 are associated with pain and all the signs of inflammation.

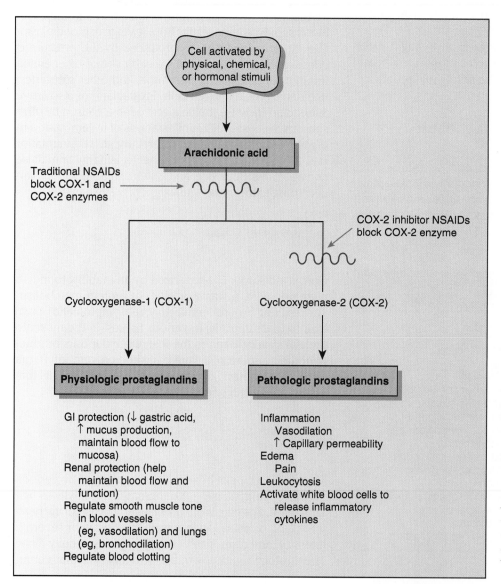

FIGURE 7–1 Physiologic and pathologic (ie, inflammatory) prostaglandins: Actions of antiprostaglandin drugs. Prostaglandins play important roles in normal body functions as well as inflammatory processes. Inhibition of both COX-1 and COX-2 by traditional NSAIDs produces adverse effects on the stomach (eg, irritation, ulceration, bleeding) and possibly on the kidneys (eg, decreased blood flow and function) as well as anti-inflammatory effects. Selective inhibition of COX-2 produces anti-inflammatory effects while maintaining protective effects on the stomach and perhaps the kidneys.

Newer types of NSAID, celecoxib (Celebrex) and rofe-coxib (Vioxx), are selective COX-2 inhibitor drugs. They were designed to relieve pain, fever, and inflammation as effectively as older NSAIDs, but with fewer adverse effects, especially stomach damage.

To relieve pain, aspirin acts both centrally and periph-erally to block the transmission of pain impulses. Related analgesic–antipyretic–anti-inflammatory drugs act periph-erally to prevent sensitization of pain receptors to various chemical substances released by damaged cells. To relieve fever, the drugs act on the hypothalamus to decrease its response to pyrogens and reset the "thermostat" at a lower level. For inflammation, they prevent prostaglandins from increasing the pain and edema produced by bradykinin and other substances released by damaged cells. Although these drugs relieve symptoms and contribute greatly to the client's comfort and quality of life, they do not cure the underlying disorders that cause the symptoms.

Antiplatelet effects of aspirin and other NSAIDs differ in mechanism and extent. When aspirin (also called ASA) is absorbed into the bloodstream, the acetyl portion disso-ciates, then binds irreversibly to platelet COX. This action prevents synthesis of thromboxane A_2 and thereby inhibits platelet aggregation. A small single dose ($\leq$325 mg) irre-versibly acetylates circulating platelets within a few min-utes, and effects last for the lifespan of the platelets (7 to 10 days). Other NSAIDs bind reversibly with platelet COX so that antiplatelet effects occur only while the drug is pres-ent in the blood. Thus, aspirin has greater effects, but all the drugs except acetaminophen and the COX-2 inhibitors inhibit platelet aggregation, cause hypoprothrombinemia, interfere with blood coagulation, and increase the risk of bleeding.

In migraine, aspirin, acetaminophen, and NSAIDs may alleviate symptoms by inhibiting prostaglandin synthesis and reducing serotonin.

INDICATIONS FOR USE

Despite many similarities, aspirin and other NSAIDs dif-fer in their approved indications for use. Aspirin can be used in many disorders characterized by pain, fever, or inflammation. It also is often prescribed for clients at high risk of myocardial infarction or stroke from thrombosis. This indication stems from its antiplatelet activity and resultant effects on blood coagulation (ie, decreased clot formation).

Acetaminophen, which differs chemically from aspirin and other NSAIDs, is commonly used as an aspirin sub-stitute for pain and fever, but it lacks anti-inflammatory and antiplatelet effects. It is also used to relieve pain asso-ciated with osteoarthritis because the disease process is degenerative rather than inflammatory. Ibuprofen (Motrin, others) and other propionic acid derivatives are widely used as anti-inflammatory agents and analgesics. Ibupro-fen, ketoprofen, and naproxen are available in prescrip-

tion and over-the-counter (OTC) formulations. Ketorolac (Toradol), which can be given orally and parenterally, is used only as an analgesic. Most of the other NSAIDs are too toxic to use as analgesics and antipyretics. They are used primarily in rheumatoid arthritis and other musculo-skeletal disorders that do not respond to safer drugs. Celecoxib is indicated for rheumatoid arthritis and osteoarthritis; rofecoxib is used for osteoarthritis, acute pain, and dysmenorrhea. Some drugs and their indica-tions for use are summarized in Table 7-2.

CONTRAINDICATIONS TO USE

Contraindications to clinical use of aspirin and nonselec-tive NSAIDs include peptic ulcer disease, gastrointestinal (GI) or other bleeding disorders, history of hypersensitiv-ity reactions, and impaired renal function. In people who are allergic to aspirin, nonaspirin NSAIDs also are contra-indicated because hypersensitivity reactions may occur with any drugs that inhibit prostaglandin synthesis. In chil-dren and adolescents, aspirin is contraindicated in the presence of viral infections such as influenza or chicken-pox because of its association with Reye's syndrome. Selective COX-2 inhibitors are contraindicated for clients with a history of ulcers, GI bleeding, asthma, an allergic reaction to other NSAIDs, or severe renal impairment.

Over-the-counter products containing these drugs are contraindicated for chronic alcohol abusers because of possible liver damage (with acetaminophen) or stomach bleeding (with aspirin and other salicylates, ibuprofen, ketoprofen, or naproxen). The Food and Drug Adminis-tration (FDA) requires an alcohol warning on the labels of all OTC pain relievers and fever reducers stating that people who drink three or more alcoholic drinks every day ask their doctor about taking the products.

INDIVIDUAL DRUGS

Nonselective Cyclooxygenase Inhibitor Drugs

Aspirin is the prototype of the analgesic–antipyretic–anti-inflammatory drugs and the most commonly used sa-licylate. Aspirin is effective in pain of low to moderate intensity, especially that involving the skin, muscles, joints, and other connective tissue. It is useful in inflam-matory disorders, such as rheumatoid arthritis, but many people prefer drugs that cause less gastric irritation.

Because aspirin is a nonprescription drug, it is a home remedy for headaches, colds, influenza and other res-piratory infections, muscular aches, and fever. It can be purchased in plain, chewable, enteric-coated, and effer-vescent tablets and rectal suppositories. It is not marketed in liquid form because it is unstable in solution.

TABLE 7-2 Clinical Indications for Commonly Used Analgesic–Antipyretic–Anti-inflammatory Drugs

Generic/Trade Name	Pain	Fever	Osteoarthritis	Rheumatoid Arthritis	Juvenile Rheumatoid Arthritis	Dysmenorrhea	Acute Painful Shoulder	Ankylosing Spondylitis	Bursitis	Gout	Tendinitis
Acetaminophen (Tylenol, others)	✔	✔									
Acetylsalicylic acid (Aspirin)	✔	✔	✔	✔	✔	✔	✔	✔	✔	✔	✔
Diclofenac (Voltaren)			✔	✔				✔			
Diflunisal (Dolobid)	✔		✔	✔							
Etodolac (Lodine)	✔		✔								
Fenoprofen (Nalfon)	✔		✔	✔							
Flurbiprofen (Ansaid)			✔	✔							
Ibuprofen (Motrin, others)	✔	✔	✔	✔		✔				✔	✔
Indomethacin (Indocin)			✔	✔			✔	✔	✔	✔	✔
Ketoprofen (Orudis)	✔		✔	✔		✔			✔	✔	✔
Ketorolac (Toradol)	✔										
Nabumetone (Relafen)			✔	✔							
Naproxen (Naprosyn)	✔		✔	✔	✔	✔		✔	✔	✔	✔
Oxaprozin (Daypro)			✔	✔							
Piroxicam (Feldene)			✔	✔							
Sulindac (Clinoril)			✔	✔			✔	✔	✔	✔	✔
Tolmetin (Tolectin)			✔	✔	✔						

ROUTE AND DOSAGE RANGES

Adults: Analgesia and antipyresis, orally (PO) 325–650 mg q4h PRN; usual single dose, 650 mg

Arthritis and other rheumatic conditions, PO 3.2–6 g/d in divided doses

Myocardial infarction prophylaxis, PO 81–325 mg/d

Acute rheumatic fever, PO 5–8 g/d, initially, in divided doses

Transient ischemic attacks in men, PO 1300 mg/d in divided doses (650 mg twice a day or 325 mg four times a day)

Children: Analgesia and antipyresis, PO 10–15 mg/kg q4h, up to 60–80 mg/kg/d. Recommended doses for specific weight ranges: 24–35 lb (10.6–15.9 kg), 162 mg; 36–47 lb (16–21.4 kg), 243 mg; 48–59 lb (21.5–26.8 kg), 324 mg; 60–71 lb (26.9–32.3 kg), 405 mg; 72–95 lb (32.4–43.2 kg), 486 mg; 96 lb or above (43.3 kg or above), 648 mg

Juvenile rheumatoid arthritis, PO 60–110 mg/kg/d in divided doses q6–8h. Reduce amount for long-term use.

Acute rheumatic fever, PO 100 mg/kg/d, in divided doses, for 2 wk, then 75 mg/kg/d for 4–6 wk

Diflunisal (Dolobid) is a salicylic acid derivative that differs chemically from aspirin. It is reportedly equal or superior to aspirin in mild to moderate pain, rheumatoid arthritis, and osteoarthritis. Compared with aspirin, it has less antipyretic effect and causes less gastric irritation; its longer duration of action allows for twice-daily administration.

ROUTE AND DOSAGE RANGES

Adults: Mild to moderate pain, PO 500–1000 mg initially, then 250–500 mg q8–12h

Rheumatoid arthritis, osteoarthritis PO 500–1000 mg/d, in two divided doses, increased to a maximum of 1500 mg/d if necessary

Acetaminophen USP (Tylenol, others) is a nonprescription drug commonly used as an aspirin substitute because it does not cause nausea, vomiting, or GI bleeding, and it does not interfere with blood clotting. It is equal to aspirin in analgesic and antipyretic effects, but it lacks anti-inflammatory activity.

Acetaminophen is well absorbed from oral administration and peak plasma concentrations are reached within 30 to 120 minutes. It is metabolized in the liver; approximately 94% is excreted in the urine as inactive glucuronate and sulfate conjugates. Approximately 4% is metabolized to a toxic metabolite, which is normally inactivated by conjugation with glutathione and excreted in urine. Glutathione is important in liver detoxification of acetaminophen and an adequate supply is usually available in liver cells. In acute or chronic overdose situations, however, the supply of glutathione may become depleted. In the absence of glutathione, the toxic metabolite combines with liver cells and causes damage or fatal liver necrosis. In alcoholics, usual therapeutic doses may cause or increase liver damage. The probable mechanism for increased risk of hepatotoxicity in this population is that ethanol induces drug-metabolizing enzymes in the liver. The resulting rapid metabolism of acetaminophen produces enough toxic metabolite to exceed the available glutathione.

Acetaminophen is available in tablet, liquid, and rectal suppository forms and is in numerous combination products marketed as analgesics and cold remedies. It is often prescribed with codeine or oxycodone for added analgesic effects.

ROUTES AND DOSAGE RANGES

Adults: PO 325–650 mg q4–6h, or 1000 mg three or four times per day; maximum 4 g/d
Rectal suppository 650 mg q4–6h, maximum of 6 in 24 h

Children: PO 10 mg/kg or according to age as follows: 0–3 mo, 40 mg; 4–11 mo, 80 mg; 1–2 y, 120 mg; 2–3 y, 160 mg; 4–5 y, 240 mg; 6–8 y, 320 mg; 9–10 y, 400 mg; 11 y, 480 mg. Doses may be given q4–6h to a maximum of 5 doses in 24 h.
Rectal suppository: age under 3 y, consult physician; age 3–6 y, 120 mg q4–6h, maximum 720 mg in 24 h; age 6–12 y, 325 mg q4–6h, maximum 2.6 g in 24 h

Fenoprofen (Nalfon), **flurbiprofen** (Ansaid), **ibuprofen** (Motrin, others), **ketoprofen** (Orudis), **naproxen** (Naprosyn, Anaprox), and **oxaprozin** (Daypro) are propionic acid derivatives that are chemically and pharmacologically similar. In addition to their use as anti-inflammatory agents in rheumatoid arthritis, gout, tendinitis, and bursitis, they are used as analgesics in conditions not necessarily related to inflammation (eg, dysmenorrhea, episiotomy, minor trauma) and as antipyretics.

Ibuprofen, ketoprofen, and naproxen are available OTC, with recommended doses usually smaller than those for prescription formulations. Although these drugs are usually better tolerated than aspirin, they are much more expensive and may cause all the adverse effects associated with aspirin and other prostaglandin inhibitors.

Fenoprofen

ROUTE AND DOSAGE RANGES

Adults: Rheumatoid arthritis, osteoarthritis, PO 300–600 mg three or four times per day; maximum 3200 mg/d
Mild to moderate pain, PO 200 mg q4–6h PRN

Flurbiprofen

ROUTE AND DOSAGE RANGE

Adults: Rheumatoid arthritis, osteoarthritis, PO 200–300 mg/d in two, three, or four divided doses

Ibuprofen

ROUTE AND DOSAGE RANGES

Adults: Rheumatoid arthritis, osteoarthritis, PO 300–600 mg 3 or 4 times per day; maximum 2400 mg/d
Mild to moderate pain, PO 200–400 mg q4–6h PRN
Primary dysmenorrhea, PO 400 mg q4h PRN

Children: Fever, age 1–12 y, initial temperature 39.2°C (102.5°F) or less, PO 5 mg/kg q6–8 h; initial temperature above 39.2°C (102.5°F), PO 10 mg/kg q6–8h; maximum 40 mg/kg/d
Juvenile arthritis, PO 20–40 mg/kg/d, in three or four divided doses

Ketoprofen

ROUTE AND DOSAGE RANGES

Adults: Rheumatoid arthritis, osteoarthritis, PO 150–300 mg/d in three or four divided doses; maximum 300 mg/d. Sustained-release (Oruvail SR), 200 mg once daily
Mild to moderate pain, primary dysmenorrhea, PO 25–50 mg q6–8h PRN; maximum 300 mg/d

Naproxen

ROUTE AND DOSAGE RANGES

Adults: Rheumatoid arthritis, osteoarthritis, ankylosing spondylitis, PO 250–375 mg twice a day
Acute gout, PO 750 mg initially, then 250 mg q8h until the attack subsides
Mild to moderate pain, primary dysmenorrhea, acute tendinitis and bursitis, PO 500 mg initially, then 250 mg q6–8h

Children: Juvenile arthritis, PO 10 mg/kg/d in two divided doses; OTC preparation not recommended for children under 12 y

Naproxen Sodium

ROUTE AND DOSAGE RANGES

Adults: Rheumatoid arthritis, osteoarthritis, ankylosing spondylitis, PO 275 mg twice a day
Acute gout, PO 825 mg initially, then 275 mg q8h until the attack subsides
Mild to moderate pain, primary dysmenorrhea, acute tendinitis and bursitis, PO 550 mg initially, then 275 mg q6–8h

Oxaprozin

ROUTE AND DOSAGE RANGE

Adults: Rheumatoid arthritis, osteoarthritis, PO 600–1200 mg once daily; maximum, 1800 mg/d in divided doses

Indomethacin (Indocin), **sulindac** (Clinoril), and **tolmetin** (Tolectin) are acetic acid derivatives used for moderate to severe rheumatoid arthritis, osteoarthritis, ankylosing spondylitis, acute gouty arthritis, and acute painful shoulder (bursitis, tendinitis). These drugs have potent anti-inflammatory effects but are associated with a greater incidence and severity of adverse effects than aspirin and the propionic acid derivatives. Thus, they are not recommended for general use as analgesics or antipyretics. Uncommon but potentially serious adverse effects include GI ulceration, bone marrow depression, hemolytic anemia, mental confusion, depression, and psychosis. These adverse effects are especially associated with indomethacin; the other drugs were developed in an effort to find equally effective but less toxic derivatives of indomethacin. Although adverse reactions occur less often with sulindac and tolmetin, they are still common.

In addition to the aforementioned uses, tolmetin is approved for treatment of juvenile rheumatoid arthritis, and intravenous (IV) indomethacin is approved for treatment of patent ductus arteriosus in premature infants. (The ductus arteriosus joins the pulmonary artery to the aorta in the fetal circulation. When it fails to close, blood is shunted from the aorta to the pulmonary artery, causing severe cardiopulmonary problems.)

Newer drugs related to this group are **etodolac** (Lodine), **ketorolac** (Toradol), and **nabumetone** (Relafen). Etodolac is used for pain and osteoarthritis and reportedly causes less gastric irritation, especially in older adults at high risk for GI bleeding. Ketorolac is used only for pain, and although it can be given orally, its unique characteristic is that it can be given by injection. Parenteral ketorolac is reportedly comparable with morphine and other opiates in analgesic effectiveness for moderate or severe pain. However, hematomas and wound bleeding have been reported with postoperative use, and its use is limited to 5 days. Nabumetone is approved for treatment of rheumatoid arthritis and osteoarthritis.

Etodolac

ROUTE AND DOSAGE RANGES

Adults: Osteoarthritis, PO 600–1200 mg/d in two to four divided doses; maximum dose, 1200 mg/d
Pain, PO 200–400 mg q6–8h PRN; maximum dose, 1200 mg/d

Indomethacin

ROUTES AND DOSAGE RANGES

Adults: PO, rectal suppository, 75 mg/d initially, increased by 25 mg/d at weekly intervals to a maximum of 150–200 mg/d, if necessary
Acute gouty arthritis, acute painful shoulder, PO 75–150 mg/d in three or four divided doses until pain and inflammation are controlled (approximately 3–5 d for gout, 7–14 d for painful shoulder), then discontinued
Children: Premature infants with patent ductus arteriosus, IV 0.2–0.3 mg/kg q12h for a total of three doses

Ketorolac

ROUTES AND DOSAGE RANGES

Adults: PO 10 mg q4–6h for limited duration; maximum dose, 40 mg/d
Intramuscularly (IM) 30–60 mg initially, then 15–30 mg q6h on a regular schedule or as needed to control pain, up to 5 d

Nabumetone

ROUTE AND DOSAGE RANGE

Adults: Osteoarthritis, rheumatoid arthritis, PO 1000–2000 mg/d in one or two doses. For long-term treatment, use the lowest effective dose.

Sulindac

ROUTE AND DOSAGE RANGES

Adults: PO 150–200 mg twice a day; maximum 400 mg/d
Acute gouty arthritis, acute painful shoulder, PO 200 mg twice a day until pain and inflammation are controlled (approximately 7–14 d), then discontinued

Tolmetin

ROUTE AND DOSAGE RANGES

Adults: PO 400 mg three times per day initially, increased to 1600 mg/d for osteoarthritis or 2000 mg/d for rheumatoid arthritis, if necessary
Children: Rheumatoid arthritis, PO 20 mg/kg/d in three or four divided doses

Diclofenac sodium (Voltaren) is chemically different but pharmacologically similar to other NSAIDs. It is indicated for use in rheumatoid arthritis, osteoarthritis, and ankylosing spondylitis. **Diclofenac potassium** (Cataflam) may be given for pain and primary dysmenorrhea when rapid pain relief is desired.

ROUTE AND DOSAGE RANGES

Adults: Rheumatoid arthritis, PO 150–200 mg/d in three or four divided doses
Osteoarthritis, PO 100–150 mg/d in three or four divided doses
Ankylosing spondylitis, PO 100–125 mg/d in three or four divided doses
Pain and primary dysmenorrhea (diclofenac potassium only), PO 150 mg/d, in three divided doses

Piroxicam (Feldene) is an oxicam NSAID that differs chemically from other agents but has similar pharmacologic properties. Approved for treatment of rheumatoid arthritis and osteoarthritis, it reportedly causes less GI irritation than aspirin. Its long half-life allows for once-daily dosing, but optimal efficacy may not occur for 1 to 2 weeks.

ROUTE AND DOSAGE RANGE

Adults: PO 20 mg/d

Selective Cyclooxygenase-2 Inhibitor Drugs

Celecoxib (Celebrex) and **rofecoxib** (Vioxx) are newer prescription NSAIDs that block production of prostaglandins associated with pain and inflammation without blocking production of prostaglandins associated with protective effects on gastric mucosa. Thus, they produce less gastric irritation than aspirin and the older NSAIDs.

Celecoxib is indicated for use in rheumatoid arthritis and osteoarthritis. Celecoxib is well absorbed with oral administration, highly bound to plasma proteins, and metabolized by the cytochrome P450 enzymes in the liver to inactive metabolites that are then excreted in the urine. A small amount is excreted unchanged in the urine. Peak plasma levels occur approximately 3 hours after an oral dose.

Rofecoxib is approved for treatment of osteoarthritis, acute pain, and dysmenorrhea. Its similarities and differences in relation to celecoxib and older NSAIDs are being delineated.

Celecoxib

ROUTE AND DOSAGE RANGES

Adults: Osteoarthritis, PO 100 mg bid or 200 mg once daily
Rheumatoid arthritis, PO 100–200 mg bid

Rofecoxib

ROUTE AND DOSAGE RANGES

Adults: Osteoarthritis, PO 12.5–25 mg once daily
Acute pain, PO 50 mg once daily
Dysmenorrhea, PO 50 mg once daily

Drugs Used in Gout and Hyperuricemia

Allopurinol (Zyloprim) is used to prevent or treat hyperuricemia, which occurs with gout and with antineoplastic drug therapy. Uric acid is formed by purine metabolism and an enzyme called xanthine oxidase. Allopurinol prevents formation of uric acid by inhibiting xanthine oxidase. It is especially useful in chronic gout characterized by tophi (deposits of uric acid crystals in the joints, kidneys, and soft tissues) and impaired renal function.

The drug promotes resorption of urate deposits and prevents their further development. Acute attacks of gout may result when urate deposits are mobilized. These may be prevented by concomitant administration of colchicine until serum uric acid levels are lowered.

ROUTE AND DOSAGE RANGES

Adults: Mild gout, PO 200–400 mg/d
Severe gout, PO 400–600 mg/d
Hyperuricemia in clients with renal insufficiency, PO 100–200 mg/d
Secondary hyperuricemia from anticancer drugs, PO 100–200 mg/d; maximum 800 mg/d
Children: Secondary hyperuricemia from anticancer drugs: <6 y, PO 150 mg/d; 6–10 y, PO 300 mg/d

Colchicine is an anti-inflammatory drug used to prevent or treat acute attacks of gout. In acute attacks, it is the drug of choice for relieving joint pain and edema. Colchicine decreases inflammation by decreasing the movement of leukocytes into body tissues containing urate crystals. It has no analgesic or antipyretic effects.

ROUTES AND DOSAGE RANGES

Adults: Acute attacks, PO 0.5 mg q1h until pain is relieved or toxicity (nausea, vomiting, diarrhea) occurs; 3-d interval between courses of therapy
IV 1–2 mg initially, then 0.5 mg q3–6h until response is obtained; maximum total dose 4 mg
Prophylaxis, PO 0.5–1 mg/d

Probenecid (Benemid) increases the urinary excretion of uric acid. This uricosuric action is used therapeutically to treat hyperuricemia and gout. It is not effective in acute attacks of gouty arthritis but prevents hyperuricemia and tophi associated with chronic gout. Probenecid may precipitate acute gout until serum uric acid levels are within the normal range; concomitant administration of colchicine prevents this effect. (Probenecid also is used with penicillin, most often in treating sexually transmitted diseases. It increases blood levels and prolongs the action of penicillin by decreasing the rate of urinary excretion.)

ROUTE AND DOSAGE RANGES

Adults: PO 250 mg twice a day for 1 wk, then 500 mg twice a day
Children over 2 years: PO 40 mg/kg/d in divided doses

Sulfinpyrazone (Anturane) is a uricosuric agent similar to probenecid. It is not effective in acute gout but prevents or decreases tissue changes of chronic gout. Colchicine is usually given during initial sulfinpyrazone therapy to prevent acute gout.

ROUTE AND DOSAGE RANGE

Adults: PO 100–200 mg twice a day, gradually increased over 1 wk to a maximum of 400–800 mg/d

Drugs Used to Treat Acute Migraine Attacks

Naratriptan (Amerge), **rizatriptan** (Maxalt), **sumatriptan** (Imitrex), and **zolmitriptan** (Zomig) are newer drugs developed specifically for the treatment of moderate or severe migraines. They are called selective serotonin 5-HT$_1$ receptor agonists because they act on a specific subtype of serotonin receptor to increase serotonin (5-hydroxytryptamine) in the brain. They relieve migraine by constricting blood vessels in the brain. Because of their vasoconstrictive properties, the drugs are contraindicated in clients with a history of angina pectoris, myocardial infarction, or uncontrolled hypertension. The drugs produce fewer adverse effects than ergot alkaloids, and those that occur (anxiety, dizziness, and drowsiness) are usually mild and of short duration.

Naratriptan

ROUTE AND DOSAGE RANGE

Adults: PO 1–2.5 mg as a single dose; may repeat in 4 h, if necessary; maximum dose, 5 mg/d

Rizatriptan

ROUTE AND DOSAGE RANGE

Adults: PO 5–10 mg as a single dose; may repeat after 2 h, if necessary; maximum dose, 30 mg/d

Sumatriptan

ROUTE AND DOSAGE RANGE

Adults: PO 25–100 mg as a single dose; maximum dose, 300 mg/d

Subcutaneously (SC) 6 mg as a single dose; maximum dose, 12 mg/d

Nasal spray 5, 10, or 20 mg by unit-dose spray device; maximum dose, 40 mg/d

Zolmitriptan

ROUTE AND DOSAGE RANGE

Adults: PO 1.25–2.5 mg as a single dose; may repeat after 2 h, if necessary; maximum dose, 10 mg/d

Ergotamine tartrate (Ergomar) is an ergot alkaloid used only in the treatment of migraine. Ergot preparations relieve migraine by constricting blood vessels in the brain. Ergotamine is most effective when given sublingually or by inhalation at the onset of headache. When given orally, ergotamine is erratically absorbed, and therapeutic effects may be delayed for 20 to 30 minutes.

Ergotamine is contraindicated during pregnancy and in the presence of severe hypertension, peripheral vascular disease, coronary artery disease, renal or hepatic disease, and severe infections.

ROUTES AND DOSAGE RANGES

Adults: PO, sublingually 1–2 mg at onset of acute migraine attack, then 2 mg q30 min, if necessary, to a maximum of 6 mg/24 h or 10 mg/wk

Inhalation, 0.36 mg (one inhalation) at onset of acute migraine, repeated in 5 min, if necessary, to a maximum of 6 inhalations/24 h

Ergotamine tartrate and caffeine (Cafergot) is a commonly used antimigraine preparation. Caffeine reportedly increases the absorption and vasoconstrictive effects of ergotamine. The combination product is available in oral tablets containing ergotamine 1 mg and caffeine 100 mg and in rectal suppositories containing ergotamine 2 mg and caffeine 100 mg.

ROUTES AND DOSAGE RANGES

Adults: PO 2 tablets at the onset of acute migraine, then 1 tablet every 30 min, if necessary, up to 6 tablets per attack or 10 tablets/wk

Rectal suppository 0.5–1 suppository at the onset of acute migraine, repeated in 1 h, if necessary, up to two suppositories per attack or five suppositories/wk

Children: PO 0.5–1 tablet initially, then 0.5 tablet every 30 min, if necessary, to a maximum of three tablets

Dihydroergotamine mesylate (DHE 45) is a semi-synthetic derivative of ergotamine that is less toxic and less effective than the parent drug.

ROUTES AND DOSAGE RANGES

Adults: IM 1 mg at onset of acute migraine, repeated hourly, if necessary, to a total of 3 mg

IV 1 mg, repeated, if necessary, after 1 h; maximum dose 2 mg. Do not exceed 6 mg/wk.

NURSING PROCESS

Assessment

- Assess for signs and symptoms of pain, such as location, severity, duration, and factors that cause or relieve the pain (see Chap. 6).
- Assess for fever (thermometer readings above 99.6°F [37.3°C] are usually considered fever). Hot, dry skin; flushed face; reduced urine output; and concentrated urine may accompany fever if the person also is dehydrated.
- Assess for inflammation. Local signs are redness, heat, edema, and pain or tenderness; systemic signs include fever, elevated white blood cell count (leukocytosis), and weakness.
- With arthritis or other musculoskeletal disorders, assess for pain and limitations in activity and mobility.
- Ask about use of OTC analgesic, antipyretic, or anti-inflammatory drugs.
- Ask about allergic reactions to aspirin or NSAIDs.
- Assess for history of peptic ulcer disease, GI bleeding, or kidney disorders.
- With migraine, assess severity and patterns of occurrences.

Nursing Diagnoses

- Pain
- Chronic Pain
- Activity Intolerance related to pain and impaired physical mobility
- Impaired Physical Mobility related to pain and inflammation
- Risk for Injury related to adverse drug effects (GI bleeding, renal insufficiency)
- Knowledge Deficit: Comparative characteristics of OTC and prescription drugs for pain, fever, and inflammation
- Knowledge Deficit: Therapeutic and adverse effects of commonly used drugs
- Knowledge Deficit: Correct use of OTC drugs for pain, fever, and inflammation

Planning/Goals

The client will:

- Experience relief of discomfort with minimal adverse drug effects
- Experience increased mobility and activity tolerance
- Inform health care providers if taking aspirin or an NSAID regularly
- Self-administer the drugs safely
- Verbalize signs and symptoms of adverse drug effects to be reported to health care providers
- Avoid overuse of the drugs
- Use measures to prevent accidental ingestion or overdose, especially in children
- Experience fewer and less severe attacks of migraine

Interventions

Implement measures to prevent or minimize pain, fever, and inflammation:

- Treat the disease processes (eg, infection, arthritis) or circumstances (eg, impaired blood supply, lack of physical activity, poor positioning or body alignment) thought to be causing pain, fever, or inflammation
- Treat pain as soon as possible; early treatment may prevent severe pain and anxiety and allow the use of milder analgesic drugs. Use distraction, relaxation techniques, other nonpharmaco-

logic techniques along with drug therapy, when appropriate.

- With acute musculoskeletal injuries (eg, sprains), cold applications can decrease pain, swelling, and inflammation. Apply for approximately 20 minutes, then remove.
- Assist clients with migraine to identify and avoid "triggers."

Assist clients to drink approximately 3 L of fluid daily when taking an NSAID regularly. This decreases gastric irritation and helps to maintain good kidney function. With long-term use of aspirin, fluids help to prevent precipitation of salicylate crystals in the urinary tract. With antigout drugs, fluids help to prevent precipitation of urate crystals and formation of urate kidney stones. Fluid intake is especially important initially when serum uric acid levels are high and large amounts of uric acid are being excreted.

Evaluation

- Interview and observe regarding relief of symptoms.
- Interview and observe regarding mobility and activity levels.
- Interview and observe regarding safe, effective use of the drugs.
- Select drugs appropriately.

CLIENT TEACHING GUIDELINES
Acetaminophen, Aspirin, and Other NSAIDs

General Considerations

✔ Aspirin and other nonsteroidal anti-inflammatory drugs (commonly called NSAIDs) are used to relieve pain, fever, and inflammation. Aspirin is the oldest of these drugs and is as effective as the more costly prescription and nonprescription NSAIDs. Although all the drugs can cause similar adverse effects, the NSAIDs are somewhat less likely to cause stomach irritation and bleeding problems. This distinction is probably lost with high doses of NSAIDs.

Because these drugs are so widely used and available, the risk of overdosing on different products containing the same drug or products containing similar drugs is high. Knowing drug names, carefully reading product labels, and using the following precautions can increase safety in using these drugs:

1. If you are taking aspirin or an NSAID regularly, avoid over-the-counter (OTC) aspirin or products containing

aspirin (eg, Alka-Seltzer, Anacin, Arthritis Pain Formula, Ascriptin, Bufferin, Doan's Pills/Caplets, Ecotrin, Excedrin, Midol, Vanquish). However, it is probably safe to take additional aspirin or an NSAID for pain or fever if taking a small dose of aspirin (usually 81–325 mg/day) to prevent heart attack or stroke.

2. If you are taking any prescription NSAID regularly, avoid OTC products containing ibuprofen (eg, Advil, Dristan Sinus, Midol IB, Motrin IB, Sine-Aid IB), ketoprofen (Actron, Orudis KT), or naproxen (Aleve). Also, do not combine the OTC products with each other or with aspirin. These drugs are available as both prescription and OTC products. OTC ibuprofen is the same medication as prescription Motrin; OTC naproxen is the same as prescription Naprosyn; OTC ketoprofen is the same as prescription Orudis. Recommended doses are smaller for OTC products than for prescription drugs. However, any combination of these drugs could constitute an overdose.

(continued)

CLIENT TEACHING GUIDELINES
Acetaminophen, Aspirin, and Other NSAIDs (continued)

3. Acetaminophen is available in its generic form and with many brand names (eg, Tylenol). Most preparations contain 500 mg of drug per tablet or capsule. In addition, many OTC pain relievers (usually labeled "nonaspirin") and cold remedies contain acetaminophen. Thus, all consumers should read product labels carefully to avoid duplicate sources and potential overdoses. Overuse may cause life-threatening liver damage.

✔ With NSAIDs, if one is not effective, another one may work because people vary in responses to the drugs. Improvement of symptoms depends on the reason for use. When taken for pain, the drugs act within approximately 30 to 60 minutes; when taken for inflammatory disorders, such as arthritis, improvement may occur within 24 to 48 hours with aspirin and 1 to 2 weeks with other NSAIDs.

✔ Taking a medication for fever is not usually recommended unless the fever is high or is accompanied by other uncomfortable signs and symptoms. Fever is one way the body fights infection.

✔ Do not take OTC ibuprofen more than 3 days for fever or 10 days for pain. If these symptoms persist or worsen, or if new symptoms develop, contact a health care provider.

✔ Avoid aspirin for approximately 2 weeks before and after major surgery or dental work to decrease the risk of excessive bleeding. If pregnant, do not take aspirin for approximately 2 weeks before the estimated delivery date.

✔ Inform any health care provider if taking aspirin, ibuprofen, or any other NSAID regularly.

✔ Inform health care providers if you have ever had an allergic reaction (eg, asthma, difficulty in breathing, hives) or severe GI symptoms (eg, ulcer, bleeding) after taking aspirin, ibuprofen, or similar drugs.

✔ Avoid or minimize alcoholic beverages. With aspirin and other NSAIDs, alcohol increases gastric irritation and risks of bleeding; with acetaminophen, alcohol increases risk of liver damage. The Food and Drug Administration requires an alcohol warning on the labels of OTC pain and fever relievers and urges people who drink three or more alcoholic drinks every day to ask their doctors about using the products.

✔ Acetaminophen is an effective aspirin substitute for pain or fever but not for inflammation or preventing heart attack or stroke.

✔ Store aspirin in a closed childproof container and keep out of children's reach. Never call aspirin "candy." A closed container reduces exposure of the drug to moisture and air, which cause chemical breakdown. Aspirin that is deteriorating smells like vinegar. Special precautions are needed with children because aspirin ingestion is a common cause of drug poisoning in children.

✔ When colchicine is taken for acute gout, pain is usually relieved in 4 to 12 hours with IV administration and 24 to 48 hours with oral administration. Inflammation and edema may not decrease for several days.

✔ When allopurinol is taken, blood levels of uric acid usually decrease to normal range within 1 to 3 weeks.

Self-administration

✔ Take aspirin, ibuprofen, and other NSAIDs with a full glass of liquid and food to decrease stomach irritation. Acetaminophen may be taken on an empty stomach.

✔ Swallow enteric-coated aspirin (eg, Ecotrin) whole; do not chew or crush. The coating is applied to decrease stomach irritation by making the tablet dissolve in the intestine. Also, do not take with an antacid, which can cause the table to dissolve in the stomach.

✔ Drink 2½ to 3 quarts of fluid daily when taking an NSAID regularly. This decreases gastric irritation and helps to maintain good kidney function. In addition, with long-term use of aspirin, adequate fluid intake is needed to prevent precipitation of salicylate crystals in the urinary tract.

✔ Report signs of bleeding (eg, nose bleed, vomiting blood, bruising, blood in urine or stools), difficulty breathing, skin rash or hives, ringing in ears, dizziness, severe stomach upset, or swelling and weight gain.

✔ With colchicine for chronic gout, carry the drug and start taking it as directed (usually one pill every hour for several hours until relief is obtained or nausea, vomiting, and diarrhea occur) when joint pain starts. This prevents or minimizes an attack of gouty arthritis.

✔ Drink 2½ to 3 quarts of fluid daily with antigout drugs. An adequate fluid intake helps prevent precipitation of urate crystals and formation of urate kidney stones. Fluid intake is especially important initially when serum uric acid levels are high and large amounts of uric acid are being excreted in the urine.

PRINCIPLES OF THERAPY

Guidelines for Therapy With Aspirin

When pain, fever, or inflammation is present, aspirin is effective across a wide range of clinical conditions. Because it is a nonprescription drug and is widely available, people tend to underestimate its usefulness. Like any other drug, aspirin must be used appropriately to maximize therapeutic benefits and minimize adverse reactions. Some guidelines for correct usage include the following:

CLIENT TEACHING GUIDELINES
Drugs for Migraine

General Considerations

✔ Try to identify and avoid situations known to precipitate acute attacks of migraine.

✔ For mild or infrequent migraine attacks, acetaminophen, aspirin, or another nonsteroidal anti-inflammatory drug may be effective.

✔ For moderate to severe migraine attacks, the drug of first choice is probably sumatriptan (Imitrex) or a related drug, if not contraindicated (eg, by heart disease or hypertension). However, one of these drugs should not be taken if an ergot preparation has been taken within the previous 24 hours.

✔ If you have frequent or severe migraine attacks, consult a physician about medications to prevent or reduce the frequency of acute attacks.

✔ Never take an antimigraine medication prescribed for someone else or allow someone else to take yours. The medications used to relieve acute migraines can constrict blood vessels, raise blood pressure, and cause serious adverse effects.

Self-administration

✔ Take medication at onset of pain, when possible, to prevent development of more severe symptoms.

✔ With triptans, take oral drugs (except for rizatriptan orally disintegrating tablets) with fluids. If symptoms recur, a second dose may be taken. However, do not take a second dose of sumatriptan or zolmitriptan sooner than 2 hours after the first dose, or a second dose of naratriptan sooner than 4 hours after the first dose. **Do not**

take more than 300 mg of sumatriptan, 5 mg of naratriptan, or 10 mg of zolmitriptan in any 24-hour period.

✔ Rizatriptan is available in a regular tablet, which can be taken with fluids, and in an orally disintegrating tablet, which can be dissolved on the tongue and swallowed without fluids. The tablet should be removed from its package with dry hands and placed on the tongue immediately.

✔ Sumatriptan can be taken by mouth, injection, or nasal spray. Instructions should be strictly followed for the prescribed method of administration. For the nasal spray, the usual dose is one spray into one nostril. If symptoms return, a second spray may be taken 2 hours or longer after the first spray. **Do not take more than 40 mg of nasal spray in any 24-hour period.** If self-administering injectable sumatriptan, be sure to give in fatty tissue under the skin. This drug must not be taken intravenously; serious, potentially fatal reactions may occur.

✔ If symptoms of an allergic reaction (eg, shortness of breath, wheezing, heart pounding, swelling of eyelids, face or lips, skin rash, or hives) occur after taking a triptan drug, tell your prescribing physician immediately and do not take any additional doses without specific instructions to do so.

✔ With ergot preparations, report signs of vascular insufficiency, such as tingling sensation or coldness, numbness, or weakness of the extremities. These are symptoms of ergot toxicity. To avoid potentially serious adverse effects, do not exceed recommended doses.

---

1. For *pain*, aspirin is useful alone when the discomfort is of low to moderate intensity. For more severe pain, aspirin may be combined with an opioid or given between opioid doses for better analgesia or to allow lower doses of the opioid. Aspirin and opioid analgesics act by different mechanisms, so such use is rational. Aspirin may be used with codeine or other opioids in clients who can take oral medications. For acute pain, aspirin is taken when the pain occurs and is often effective within a few minutes. For chronic pain, a regular schedule of administration, such as every 4 to 6 hours, is more effective.

2. For *fever*, aspirin is effective if drug therapy is indicated. In children, however, aspirin is contraindicated because of its association with Reye's syndrome.

3. For *inflammation*, aspirin is useful in both short- and long-term therapy of conditions characterized by pain and inflammation, such as rheumatoid arthritis. Although effective, the high doses and frequent

administration required for anti-inflammatory effects increase the risks of GI upset and ulceration.

4. For acute pain or fever, plain aspirin tablets are preferred. For chronic pain, long-term use in rheumatoid arthritis, and daily use for antiplatelet effects, enteric-coated tablets may be better tolerated. Rectal suppositories are sometimes used when oral administration is contraindicated.

5. Aspirin dosage depends mainly on the condition being treated. Low doses are used for antiplatelet effects in preventing arterial thrombotic disorders such as myocardial infarction or stroke. Lower-than-average doses are needed for clients with low serum albumin levels because a larger proportion of each dose is free to exert pharmacologic activity. Larger doses are needed for anti-inflammatory effects than for analgesic and antipyretic effects.

6. To decrease risks of toxicity, plasma salicylate levels should be measured periodically when large doses of aspirin are taken for anti-inflammatory effects. Therapeutic levels are 150 to 300 µg/mL. Chronic

administration of large doses saturates a major metabolic pathway, thereby slowing drug elimination, prolonging the serum half-life, and causing drug accumulation.

7. Salicylate intoxication may occur with an acute overdose or chronic use of therapeutic doses. Manifestations of salicylism include nausea, vomiting, fever, fluid and electrolyte deficiencies, tinnitus, decreased hearing, visual changes, drowsiness, confusion, hyperventilation, and others. Severe central nervous system dysfunction (eg, delirium, stupor, coma, seizures) indicates life-threatening toxicity.

8. In mild salicylism, stopping the drug or reducing the dose is usually sufficient. In severe salicylate overdose, treatment is symptomatic and aimed at preventing further absorption from the GI tract; increasing urinary excretion; and correcting fluid, electrolyte, and acid–base imbalances. When the drug may still be in the GI tract, gastric lavage and activated charcoal help reduce absorption. IV sodium bicarbonate produces an alkaline urine in which salicylates are more rapidly excreted, and hemodialysis effectively removes salicylates from the blood. IV fluids are indicated when high fever or dehydration is present. The specific content of IV fluids depends on the serum electrolyte and acid–base status.

Guidelines for Therapy With Acetaminophen

Acetaminophen is effective and widely used for the treatment of pain and fever. A major advantage over aspirin is that acetaminophen does not cause gastric irritation and upset. It is the drug of choice for children with febrile illness (because of the association of aspirin with Reye's syndrome), elderly adults with impaired renal function (because aspirin and NSAIDs may cause further impairment), and pregnant women (because aspirin is associated with several maternal and fetal disorders, including bleeding).

The major drawback to acetaminophen is potential liver damage. Factors related to identification and treatment of hepatotoxicity include the following:

1. Acute hepatic failure may occur with a single large dose, usually approximately 10 to 15 g, but it has been reported with 6 g. Acute acetaminophen poisoning may be characterized by jaundice, vomiting, and central nervous system stimulation with excitement and delirium followed by vascular collapse, coma, and death. Early symptoms (within 24 hours after ingestion) are nonspecific (eg, anorexia, nausea, vomiting). Peak hepatotoxicity occurs in 3 to 4 days, and recovery occurs in 7 to 8 days.

2. If overdose is detected soon after ingestion, activated charcoal can be given to inhibit absorption. However, the specific antidote is acetylcysteine (Mucomyst), a mucolytic agent given by inhalation in respiratory disorders (see Chap. 49). For acetaminophen poisoning, it is given orally. The drug provides cysteine, a precursor substance required for the synthesis of glutathione. Glutathione combines with a toxic metabolite and decreases hepatotoxicity if acetylcysteine is given. Acetylcysteine is most beneficial if given within 8 to 10 hours of acetaminophen ingestion, but may be helpful up to 36 hours. It does not reverse damage that has already occurred.

3. Hepatotoxicity also occurs with chronic ingestion of acetaminophen (5 to 8 g/day for several weeks or 3 to 4 g/day for 1 year) and short-term ingestion of usual therapeutic doses in alcoholics. Although no safe dosage range has been established for chronic alcohol abusers, it is recommended that they ingest no more than 2 g daily. If they ingest three or more alcoholic drinks daily, they should avoid acetaminophen or consult their physician before taking even small doses.

Guidelines for Therapy With NSAIDs

Nonaspirin NSAIDs are widely used and preferred by many people because of less gastric irritation and GI upset, compared with aspirin. Many NSAIDs are prescription drugs used primarily for analgesic and anti-inflammatory effects in arthritis and other musculoskeletal disorders. However, several are approved for more general use as an analgesic or antipyretic. Ibuprofen, ketoprofen, and naproxen are available by prescription and OTC. Clients must be instructed to avoid combined use of prescription and nonprescription NSAIDs because of the high risk of adverse effects. NSAIDs commonly cause gastric mucosal damage and prolonged use may lead to gastric ulceration and bleeding. Because NSAIDs lead to renal impairment in some clients, blood urea nitrogen and serum creatinine should be checked approximately 2 weeks after starting any of these agents.

Nonsteroidal anti-inflammatory drugs inhibit platelet activity only while drug molecules are in the bloodstream, not for the life of the platelet (approximately 1 week), as aspirin does. Thus, they are *not* prescribed therapeutically for antiplatelet effects.

Guidelines for Treating Rheumatoid Arthritis and Related Disorders

The primary goals of treatment are to control pain and inflammation and to minimize immobilization and disability. Rest, exercise, physical therapy, and drugs are used to attain these goals. None of these measures prevents joint destruction.

Aspirin relieves pain and inflammation, and it is inexpensive, an important factor in the long-term treatment of chronic musculoskeletal disorders. Dosage should be individualized to relieve symptoms, maintain therapeutic salicylate blood levels, and minimize adverse effects. Regular administration of aspirin every 4 to 6 hours usually produces a therapeutic serum salicylate level of 150 to 300 µg/mL.

For people who cannot take aspirin because of gastric irritation, peptic ulcer disease, bleeding disorders, and other contraindications, another NSAID is usually ordered. The choice of a specific drug is largely empiric; one person may respond better to one NSAID than another. A drug may be given for 2 or 3 weeks on a trial basis. If therapeutic benefits occur, the drug may be continued; if no benefits seem evident or toxicity occurs, another drug may be tried. Ibuprofen and other propionic acid derivatives are often used because they are associated with fewer GI adverse effects than most other NSAIDs.

Several other drugs also may be used to treat rheumatoid arthritis. These include adrenal corticosteroids and the disease-modifying antirheumatic drugs, such as gold, hydroxychloroquine (Plaquenil), penicillamine (Cuprimine, Depen), azathioprine (Imuran), cyclophosphamide (Cytoxan), and methotrexate. These drugs have anti-inflammatory and immunosuppressant effects and may cause significant toxicity. The disease-modifying drugs are used to slow tissue damage, which aspirin and other NSAIDs cannot do. Leflunomide (Arava) is a newer drug approved only for treatment of rheumatoid arthritis; it reportedly relieves symptoms and slows structural damage.

Guidelines for Perioperative Use of Aspirin and Other NSAIDs

Aspirin should in general be avoided for 1 to 2 weeks before and after surgery because it increases the risk of bleeding. Most other NSAIDs should be discontinued approximately 3 days before surgery; nabumetone and piroxicam have long half-lives and must be discontinued approximately 1 week before surgery. After surgery, especially after relatively minor procedures, such as dental extractions and episiotomies, several of the drugs are used

Nursing Notes: Apply Your Knowledge

Mrs. Whynn, a 73-year-old widow, has severe osteoarthritis. To control the pain, she takes ibuprofen 400 mg every 4 hours while awake and prednisone 5 mg daily. Also, she swims and uses moist heat to decrease stiffness and discomfort. Lately, she has been feeling weak and tired. She has also experienced dizziness when getting up from bed, and today she fainted. She asks you if this could be related to the medications she is taking and what she should do.

to relieve pain. Caution is needed because of increased risks of bleeding, and the drugs should not be given if there are other risk factors for bleeding. In addition, ketorolac, the only injectable NSAID, has been used in more extensive surgeries. Although the drug has several advantages over opioid analgesics, bleeding and hematomas may occur.

Use of Acetaminophen, Aspirin, and Other NSAIDs in Cancer Pain

Cancer often produces chronic pain from tumor invasion of tissues or complications of treatment (chemotherapy, surgery, or radiation). As with acute pain, these drugs prevent sensitization of peripheral pain receptors by inhibiting prostaglandin formation. They are especially effective for pain associated with bone metastases. For mild pain, acetaminophen, aspirin, or another NSAID may be used alone; for moderate to severe pain, these drugs may be continued and a opioid analgesic added. Non-opioid and opioid analgesics can be given together or alternated; a combination of analgesics is often needed to provide optimal pain relief.

Use of Acetaminophen, Aspirin, and Other NSAIDs in Children

Acetaminophen is usually the drug of choice for pain or fever in children. Children seem less susceptible to liver toxicity than adults, apparently because they form less of the toxic metabolite during metabolism of acetaminophen. Ibuprofen also may be given for fever. Aspirin is not recommended because of its association with Reye's syndrome, a life-threatening illness characterized by encephalopathy, hepatic damage, and other serious problems. Reye's syndrome usually occurs after a viral infection, such as influenza B or chickenpox, during which aspirin was given for fever. For children with juvenile rheumatoid arthritis, aspirin, ibuprofen, naproxen, or tolmetin may be given. Pediatric indications for use and dosages have not been established for most of the other drugs. Ibuprofen (Children's Advil, Children's Motrin) is available in a liquid suspension containing 100 mg/5 mL.

When an NSAID is given during late pregnancy to prevent premature labor, the fetus' kidneys may be adversely affected. When one is given shortly after birth to close a patent ductus arteriosus, the neonate's kidneys may be adversely affected.

Use of Acetaminophen, Aspirin, and Other NSAIDs in Older Adults

Acetaminophen is usually safe in recommended doses unless liver damage is present or the person is a chronic alcohol abuser. Aspirin is usually safe in the small doses prescribed for prevention of myocardial infarction and stroke (antiplatelet effects). Aspirin and NSAIDs are probably safe in therapeutic doses for occasional use as an analgesic or antipyretic. However, older adults have a high incidence of musculoskeletal disorders (eg, osteoarthritis), and an NSAID is often prescribed. Long-term use of the relatively high doses required for anti-inflammatory effects increases the risk of serious GI bleeding. Small doses, gradual increments, and taking the drug with food or a full glass of water may decrease GI effects. In addition, misoprostol (Cytotec) may be given. Misoprostol can be used to prevent gastric ulcers in older adults, although its adverse effects of abdominal cramping and diarrhea may not be tolerated very well. The newer COX-2 inhibitor NSAIDs may be especially beneficial in older adults because they are less likely to cause gastric ulceration and bleeding. Older adults also are more likely than younger adults to acquire nephrotoxicity with NSAIDs, especially with high doses or long-term use, because the drugs may reduce blood flow to the kidneys.

Guidelines for Treating Hyperuricemia and Gout

Opinions differ regarding treatment of asymptomatic hyperuricemia. Some authorities do not think drug therapy is indicated; others think that lowering serum uric acid levels may prevent joint inflammation and renal calculi. Allopurinol, probenecid, or sulfinpyrazone may be given for this purpose. Colchicine also should be given for several weeks to prevent acute attacks of gout while serum uric acid levels are being lowered. During initial administration of these drugs, a high fluid intake (to produce approximately 2000 mL of urine per day) and alkaline urine are recommended to prevent renal calculi. Urate crystals are more likely to precipitate in acid urine.

Guidelines for Treating Migraine

For infrequent or mild migraine attacks, acetaminophen, aspirin, or other NSAIDs may be effective. For example, NSAIDs are often effective in migraines associated with menstruation. For moderate to severe migraine attacks, sumatriptan and related drugs are effective and they cause fewer adverse effects than ergot preparations. They are usually well tolerated; adverse effects are relatively minor and usually brief. However, because they are strong vasoconstrictors, they should not be taken by people with coronary artery disease or hypertension. They are also expensive compared with other antimigraine drugs. If an ergot preparation is used, it should be given at the onset of headache, and the client should lie down in a quiet, darkened room.

For frequent (two or more per month) or severe migraine attacks, prophylactic therapy is needed. Those for whom the triptans and ergot preparations are contraindicated for acute attacks and those whose attacks are predictable (eg, perimenstrual) may also need drug therapy to reduce the incidence and severity of acute attacks. Numerous medications have been used for prophylaxis, including aspirin (650 mg bid) and NSAIDs (ibuprofen 300 to 600 mg tid; ketoprofen 50 to 75 mg bid or tid; naproxen 250 to 750 mg daily or 250 mg tid). When used to prevent migraine associated with menses, they should be started approximately 1 week before and continued through the menstrual period. Although these drugs are usually well tolerated, long-term use is not recommended because of GI and renal toxicity associated with chronic inhibition of prostaglandin production. Other prophylactic drugs include propranolol and other beta-adrenergic blocking agents (see Chap. 19).

Use in Renal Impairment

Acetaminophen, aspirin, and other NSAIDs can cause or aggravate renal impairment even though they are eliminated mainly by hepatic metabolism. Acetaminophen is normally metabolized mainly in the liver to metabolites that are excreted through the kidneys; these metabolites may accumulate in renal failure. In addition, acetaminophen is nephrotoxic in overdose because it forms a metabolite that attacks kidney cells and may cause necrosis. Aspirin is nephrotoxic in high doses, and protein binding of aspirin is reduced in renal failure so that blood levels of active drug are higher. In addition, aspirin and other NSAIDs can decrease blood flow in the kidneys by inhibiting synthesis of prostaglandins that dilate renal blood vessels. When renal blood flow is normal, these prostaglandins have limited activity. When renal blood flow is decreased, however, their synthesis is increased and they protect the kidneys from ischemia and hypoxia by antagonizing the vasoconstrictive effects of angiotensin II, norepinephrine, and other substances. Thus, in clients who depend on prostaglandins to maintain an adequate renal blood flow, the prostaglandin-blocking effects of aspirin and NSAIDS result in constriction of renal arteries and arterioles, decreased renal blood flow, decreased glomerular filtration rate, and retention of salt and water. NSAIDs can also cause kidney damage by other mechanisms, including a hypersensitivity reaction that leads to acute renal failure, manifested by proteinuria, hematuria, or pyuria. Biopsy reports usually indicate inflammatory reactions such as glomerulonephritis or interstitial nephritis.

People at highest risk from the use of these drugs are those with pre-existing renal impairment; those older than 50 years of age; those taking diuretics; and those with hypertension, diabetes, or heart failure. Measures to prevent or minimize renal damage include avoiding nephrotoxic drugs when possible, treating the disorders that increase risk of renal damage, stopping the NSAID if renal impairment occurs, monitoring renal function, reducing dosage, and maintaining hydration.

The role of COX-2 inhibitor NSAIDs in renal impairment is not clear. Although it was hoped that these drugs would have protective effects on the kidneys as they do on the stomach, studies indicate that their effects on the kidneys are similar to those of the older NSAIDs.

Use in Hepatic Impairment

Except for acetaminophen, the effects of NSAIDs on liver function and the effects of hepatic impairment on most NSAIDs are largely unknown. Because the drugs are metabolized in the liver, they should be used with caution and perhaps in lower doses in people with impaired hepatic function or a history of liver disease.

Acetaminophen can cause fatal liver necrosis in overdose because it forms a metabolite that can destroy liver cells. The hepatotoxic metabolite is formed more rapidly when drug-metabolizing enzymes in the liver have been stimulated by ingestion of alcohol, cigarette smoking, and drugs such as anticonvulsants and others. Thus, alcoholics are at high risk of hepatotoxicity with usual therapeutic doses.

In cirrhotic liver disease, naproxen and sulindac may be metabolized more slowly and aggravate hepatic impairment if dosage is not reduced. In liver impairment, blood levels of oral sumatriptan and related antimigraine drugs may be high because less drug is metabolized on its first pass through the liver and a higher proportion of a dose reaches the systemic circulation. Thus, the drugs should be used cautiously, possibly in reduced dosage.

Use in Critical Illness

Acetaminophen, aspirin, and other NSAIDs are infrequently used during critical illness, partly because they are usually given orally and many clients are unable to take oral medications. Pain is more likely to be treated with injectable opioid analgesics in this population. Acetaminophen may be given by rectal suppository for pain or fever in clients who are unable to take oral drugs.

These drugs may be risk factors for renal or hepatic impairment or bleeding disorders. For example, if a client has a history of taking aspirin, including the low doses prescribed for antithrombotic effects, there is a risk of bleeding from common therapeutic (eg, IM injections, starting IV lines, inserting urinary catheters or GI tubes) or diagnostic procedures (eg, drawing blood, angiography). If a client has been taking an NSAID regularly, he or she may be more likely to experience renal failure if the critical illness causes dehydration or requires treatment with one or more nephrotoxic drugs. If a client presents with acute renal failure, NSAID ingestion must be considered as a possible cause. If a client is known to drink alcoholic beverages and take acetaminophen, he or she may be more likely to experience impaired liver function.

Home Care

Home use of acetaminophen and NSAIDs is extremely widespread. Many people are aware of the drugs' beneficial effects in relieving pain, but many may not be adequately informed about potential problems associated with use of the drugs. Thus, the home care nurse may need to assist clients in perceiving a need for additional information and provide that information. Specific suggestions include reading and following instructions on labels of OTC analgesics, not exceeding recommended dosages without consulting a health care provider, and avoiding combinations of NSAIDs (eg, multiple OTC NSAIDs or an OTC and a prescription NSAID). In addition, adverse drug effects should be reviewed with clients, and clients should be assessed for characteristics (eg, older age group, renal impairment, overuse of the drugs) that increase the risks of adverse effects.

(*text continues on page 109*)

NURSING ACTIONS	Analgesic–Antipyretic–Anti-inflammatory and Related Drugs

NURSING ACTIONS	RATIONALE/EXPLANATION
1. Administer accurately **a.** Give aspirin and other nonsteroidal anti-inflammatory drugs (NSAIDs) with a full glass of water or other fluid and with or just after food.	To decrease gastric irritation. Even though food delays absorption and decreases peak plasma levels of some of the drugs, it is probably safer to give them with food. (*continued*)

NURSING ACTIONS	RATIONALE/EXPLANATION
b. Give antimigraine preparations at the onset of headache.	To prevent development of more severe symptoms
2. Observe for therapeutic effects	
a. When drugs are given for pain, observe for decreased or absent manifestations of pain.	Pain relief is usually evident within 30 to 60 minutes.
b. When drugs are given for fever, record temperature every 2 to 4 hours, and observe for a decrease.	
c. When drugs are given for arthritis and other inflammatory disorders, observe for decreased pain, edema, redness, heat, and stiffness of joints. Also observe for increased joint mobility and exercise tolerance.	With aspirin, improvement is usually noted within 24 to 48 hours. With most of the NSAIDs, 1 to 2 weeks may be required before beneficial effects become evident.
d. When colchicine is given for acute gouty arthritis, observe for decreased pain and inflammation in involved joints.	Therapeutic effects occur within 4 to 12 hours after intravenous colchicine administration and 24 to 48 hours after oral administration. Edema may not decrease for several days.
e. When allopurinol, probenecid, or sulfinpyrazone is given for hyperuricemia, observe for normal serum uric acid level (approximately 2–8 mg/100 mL).	Serum uric acid levels usually decrease to normal range within 1 to 3 weeks.
f. When the above drugs are given for chronic gout, observe for decreased size of tophi, absence of new tophi, decreased joint pain and increased joint mobility, and normal serum uric acid levels.	
g. When triptans or ergot preparations are given in migraine headache, observe for relief of symptoms.	Therapeutic effects are usually evident within 15 to 30 minutes.
3. Observe for adverse effects	
a. With analgesic–antipyretic–anti-inflammatory and antigout agents, observe for:	
(1) Gastrointestinal problems—anorexia, nausea, vomiting, diarrhea, bleeding, ulceration	These are common reactions, more likely with aspirin, indomethacin, piroxicam, sulindac, tolmetin, colchicine, and sulfinpyrazone and less likely with acetaminophen, diflunisal, etodolac, fenoprofen, ibuprofen, and naproxen. A prostaglandin called misoprostol (Cytotec) may be given concurrently with aspirin and other NSAIDs to prevent gastric ulcers (see Chap. 60).
(2) Hematologic problems—petechiae, bruises, hematuria, melena, epistaxis, and bone marrow depression (leukopenia, thrombocytopenia, anemia)	Bone marrow depression is more likely to occur with colchicine.
(3) Central nervous system effects—headache, dizziness, fainting, ataxia, insomnia, confusion, drowsiness	These effects are relatively common with indomethacin and may occur with most of the other drugs, especially with high dosages.
(4) Skin rashes, dermatitis	

(continued)

NURSING ACTIONS	RATIONALE/EXPLANATION
(5) Hypersensitivity reactions with dyspnea, bronchospasm, skin rashes	These effects may simulate asthma in people who are allergic to aspirin and aspirin-like drugs.
(6) Tinnitus, blurred vision	Tinnitus (ringing or roaring in the ears) is a classic sign of aspirin overdose (salicylate intoxication). It occurs with NSAIDs as well, especially with over-dosage.
(7) Nephrotoxicity—decreased urine output, increased blood urea nitrogen (BUN), increased serum creatinine, hyperkalemia, retention of sodium and water with resultant edema	More likely to occur in people with preexisting renal impairment, especially when fluid intake is decreased or fluid loss is increased. Elderly adults are at greater risk because of decreased renal blood flow and increased incidence of congestive heart failure and diuretic therapy. Renal damage is usually reversible when the drug is discontinued.
(8) Cardiovascular and hepatic effects	These are not common with usual therapeutic doses, but all vital organs may be adversely affected with overdoses.
b. With triptan antimigraine drugs, observe for:	Most adverse effects are mild and transient. However, because of their vasoconstrictive effects, they may cause or aggravate angina pectoris and hypertension.
(1) Chest tightness or pain, hypertension, drowsiness, dizziness, nausea, fatigue, paresthesias	
c. With ergot antimigraine drugs, observe for:	
(1) Nausea, vomiting, diarrhea	These drugs have a direct effect on the vomiting center of the brain and stimulate contraction of gastrointestinal smooth muscle.
(2) Symptoms of ergot poisoning (ergotism)—coolness, numbness, and tingling of the extremities, headache, vomiting, dizziness, thirst, convulsions, weak pulse, confusion, angina-like chest pain, transient tachycardia or bradycardia, muscle weakness and pain, cyanosis, gangrene of the extremities	The ergot alkaloids are highly toxic; poisoning may be acute or chronic. Acute poisoning is rare; chronic poisoning is usually a result of overdosage. Circulatory impairments may result from vasoconstriction and vascular insufficiency. Large doses also damage capillary endothelium and may cause thrombosis and occlusion. Gangrene of extremities rarely occurs with usual doses unless peripheral vascular disease or other contraindications are also present.
(3) Hypertension	Blood pressure may rise as a result of generalized vasoconstriction induced by the ergot preparation.
(4) Hypersensitivity reactions—local edema and pruritus, anaphylactic shock	Allergic reactions are relatively uncommon.
4. Observe for drug interactions	
a. Drugs that *increase* effects of aspirin and other NSAIDs:	
(1) Acidifying agents (eg, ascorbic acid)	Acidify urine and thereby decrease the urinary excretion rate of salicylates
(2) Alcohol	Increases gastric irritation and occult blood loss
(3) Anticoagulants, oral	Increase risk of bleeding substantially. People taking anticoagulants should not take aspirin or aspirin-containing products.
(4) Codeine, other opioid analgesics, and some related analgesics such as methotri-	Additive analgesic effects because of different mechanisms of action. Aspirin can be used with these

(continued)

NURSING ACTIONS	RATIONALE/EXPLANATION
meprazine (Levoprome) and pentazocine (Talwin)	drugs to provide adequate pain relief without excessive doses and sedation, in many cases.
(5) Corticosteroids (eg, prednisone)	Additive gastric irritation and ulcerogenic effects
b. Drugs that *decrease* effects of aspirin and other NSAIDs:	
(1) Alkalinizing agents (eg, sodium bicarbonate)	Increase rate of renal excretion
(2) Misoprostol (Cytotec)	This drug, a prostaglandin, was developed specifically to prevent aspirin and NSAID-induced gastric ulcers.
c. Drugs that *increase* effects of indomethacin:	
(1) Anticoagulants, oral	Increase risk of gastrointestinal bleeding. Indomethacin causes gastric irritation and is considered an ulcerogenic drug.
(2) Corticosteroids	Increase ulcerogenic effect
(3) Salicylates	Increase ulcerogenic effect
(4) Heparin	Increases risk of bleeding. These drugs should not be used concurrently.
d. Drugs that *decrease* effects of indomethacin:	Delay absorption from the gastrointestinal tract
(1) Antacids	
e. Drugs that *decrease* effects of allopurinol, probenecid, and sulfinpyrazone:	
(1) Alkalinizing agents (eg, sodium bicarbonate)	Decrease risks of renal calculi from precipitation of uric acid crystals. Alkalinizing agents are recommended until serum uric acid levels return to normal.
(2) Colchicine	Decreases attacks of acute gout. Recommended for concurrent use until serum uric acid levels return to normal.
(3) Diuretics	Decrease uricosuric effects
(4) Salicylates	Mainly at salicylate doses less than 2 g/day, decrease uricosuric effects of probenecid and sulfinpyrazone but do not interfere with the action of allopurinol. Salicylates are uricosuric at doses greater than 5 g/day
f. Drugs that *increase* effects of ergot preparations:	
(1) Vasoconstrictors (eg, ephedrine, epinephrine, phenylephrine)	Additive vasoconstriction with risks of severe, persistent hypertension and intracranial hemorrhage
g. Drugs that *increase* the effects of triptan antimigraine drugs:	
(1) Monoamine oxidase inhibitors (MAOIs)	Increase serum levels of triptans and may cause serious adverse effects, including cardiac arrhythmias and myocardial infarction. **Triptans and MAOIs must not be taken concurrently; a triptan should not be taken for at least 2 weeks after an MAOI is discontinued.**
(2) Ergot preparations	**Triptans and ergot preparations should not be taken concurrently or within 24 hours of each other, because severe hypertension and stroke may occur.**

Nursing Notes: Apply Your Knowledge

Answer: The symptoms may be related to her medications, but you need to collect more information before you can be sure. A very common side effect of aspirin (and all nonsteroidal anti-inflammatory drugs) is gastric irritation that can cause gastrointestinal ulceration and bleeding. Blood loss is often gradual, so patients get used to the fatigue. When patients become volume depleted secondary to the blood loss, they can exhibit signs of dizziness and syncope. Take Mrs. Whynn's postural blood pressure. Refer her to her physician, who will test her stool for blood, and if blood is present, will do some diagnostic tests. Most important, to prevent falls and accidental injury, make sure Mrs. Whynn seeks care promptly.

 ## REVIEW AND APPLICATION EXERCISES

1. How do aspirin and other NSAIDs produce analgesic, antipyretic, anti-inflammatory, and antiplatelet effects?

2. What adverse effects occur with aspirin and other NSAIDs, especially with daily ingestion?

3. Compare and contrast the uses and effects of aspirin and acetaminophen.

4. For a 6-year-old child with fever, would aspirin or acetaminophen be preferred? Why?

5. For a 50-year-old adult with rheumatoid arthritis, would aspirin, another NSAID, or acetaminophen be preferred? Why?

6. For a 75-year-old adult with osteoarthritis and a long history of "stomach trouble," would aspirin, another NSAID, or acetaminophen be preferred? Why?

7. What are some nursing interventions to decrease the adverse effects of aspirin, other NSAIDs, and acetaminophen?

8. When teaching a client about home use of aspirin, other NSAIDs, and acetaminophen, what information must be included?

9. What is the rationale for using acetylcysteine in the treatment of acetaminophen toxicity?

10. What is the rationale for combining opioid and nonopioid analgesics in the treatment of moderate pain?

11. If you were a client, what information do you think would be most helpful in home management of migraine headaches?

SELECTED REFERENCES

Becket, B.E. (1997). Headache disorders. In J.T. DiPiro, R.L. Talbert, P.E. Hayes, G.C. Yee, G.R. Matzke, B.G. Wells, & L.M. Posey (Eds.), *Pharmacotherapy: A pathophysiologic approach*, 3rd ed., pp. 1279–1291. Stamford, CT: Appleton & Lange.

Boh, L.E. (1997). Osteoarthritis. In J.T. DiPiro, R.L. Talbert, P.E. Hayes, G.C. Yee, G.R. Matzke, B.G. Wells, & L.M. Posey (Eds.), *Pharmacotherapy: A pathophysiologic approach*, 3rd ed., pp. 1735–1753. Stamford, CT: Appleton & Lange.

Courts, N.F. (1996). Salicylism in the elderly: "A little aspirin never hurt anybody." *Geriatric Nursing, 17*(2), 55–59.

Davis, W.M. (1998). New perspectives on headache. *Drug Topics, 42*(12), 76–83.

Drug facts and comparisons. (Updated monthly). St. Louis: Facts and Comparisons.

Hawkins, D.W. (1997). Gout and hyperuricemia. In J.T. DiPiro, R.L. Talbert, P.E. Hayes, G.C. Yee, G.R. Matzke, B.G. Wells, & L.M. Posey (Eds.), *Pharmacotherapy: A pathophysiologic approach*, 3rd ed., pp. 1755–1761. Stamford, CT: Appleton & Lange.

Insel, P.A. (1996). Analgesic-antipyretic and antiinflammatory agents and drugs employed in the treatment of gout. In J.G. Hardman, L.E. Limbird, P.B. Molinoff, & R.W. Ruddon (Eds.), *Goodman & Gilman's The pharmacological basis of therapeutics*, 9th ed., pp. 617–657. New York: McGraw-Hill.

Lance, J.W. (1997). Approach to the patient with headache. In W.N. Kelley (Ed.), *Textbook of internal medicine*, 3rd ed., pp. 206–212. Philadelphia: Lippincott-Raven.

McCaffery, M. (1998). How to make the most of nonopioid analgesics. *Nursing 28*(8), 54–55.

Porth, C.M. (1998). *Pathophysiology: Concepts of altered health states*, 5th ed. Philadelphia: Lippincott Williams & Wilkins.

Samuels, M.A. (1998). Update in neurology. *Annals of Internal Medicine, 129*, 878–885.

8

Antianxiety and Sedative-Hypnotic Drugs

Objectives

After studying this chapter, the student will be able to:

1. Discuss characteristics, sources, and signs and symptoms of anxiety.

2. Discuss functions of sleep and consequences of sleep deprivation.

3. Describe nondrug interventions to decrease anxiety and insomnia.

4. List characteristics of benzodiazepine antianxiety and hypnotic drugs in terms of mechanism of action, indications for use, nursing process implications, and potential for abuse and dependence.

5. Describe strategies for preventing, recognizing, or treating benzodiazepine withdrawal reactions.

6. Contrast characteristics of selected nonbenzodiazepines and benzodiazepines.

7. Teach clients guidelines for rational, safe use of antianxiety and sedative-hypnotic drugs.

8. Discuss the use of flumazenil (Romazicon) and other treatment measures for overdose of benzodiazepines.

Jane Morgan, 37 years of age and recently divorced, goes to her primary care provider complaining of anxiety and inability to sleep at night. A prescription is written for diazepam (Valium) 5 mg tid and triazolam (Halcion) 0.25 mg hs PRN. You are the nurse responsible for developing a teaching plan for Ms. Morgan.

Reflect on:

▶ How to establish a therapeutic rapport while obtaining additional important information.

▶ How to include nonpharmacologic methods to reduce anxiety and improve sleep.

▶ Identify essential information about these new medications that can be taught in 5 minutes.

▶ Discuss teaching and evaluation strategies that might be helpful in this situation.

Antianxiety and sedative-hypnotic agents are central nervous system (CNS) depressants with similar effects. Antianxiety drugs and sedatives promote relaxation; hypnotics produce sleep. The difference between the effects depends largely on dosage: large doses of antianxiety and sedative agents produce sleep, and small doses of hypnotics produce antianxiety or sedative effects. In addition, therapeutic doses of hypnotics given at bedtime may have residual sedative effects ("morning hangover") the following day. Because these drugs produce varying degrees of CNS depression, some are also used as anticonvulsant and anesthetic agents.

The drugs most often used to treat both anxiety and insomnia belong to a chemical group called *benzodiazepines*. Although chlordiazepoxide (Librium) was the first benzodiazepine, diazepam (Valium) quickly became more commonly used and for a wider range of clinical indications. Thus, **diazepam** is the prototypical benzodiazepine, although alprazolam (Xanax) and lorazepam (Ativan) may be more commonly prescribed.

To aid understanding of the uses and effects of these drugs, anxiety and insomnia are described in the following sections. The clinical manifestations of these disorders are similar and overlapping—that is, daytime anxiety may be manifested as nighttime difficulty in sleeping because the person cannot "turn off" worries, and difficulty in sleeping may be manifested as anxiety, fatigue, and decreased ability to function during usual waking hours.

ANXIETY

Anxiety is a common disorder that may be referred to as apprehension, fear, nervousness, tension, worry, or other terms that denote an unpleasant feeling state. It occurs when a person perceives a situation as threatening to physical, emotional, social, or economic well-being. Many causes occur with everyday events associated with home, work, school, social activities, and chronic illness. Others occur episodically, such as an acute illness, death, divorce, loss of a job, starting a new job, or taking a test. Situational anxiety is a normal response to a stressful situation. It may be beneficial when it motivates the person toward constructive, problem-solving, coping activities. Symptoms may be quite severe, but they usually last only 2 to 3 weeks.

Anxiety is called an *anxiety disorder* when it is severe or prolonged and impairs the ability to function in usual activities of daily living. The American Psychiatric Association delineates anxiety disorders as medical diagnoses in the *Diagnostic and Statistical Manual of Mental Disorders*, 4th Edition (Revised). This classification includes phobias and panic, obsessive-compulsive, post-traumatic stress, and atypical anxiety disorders, as well as generalized anxiety disorder. Although the pathophysiology of anxiety

disorders is unknown, there is evidence of a biologic basis and possible imbalances among several neurotransmission systems. A simplistic view involves an excess of excitatory neurotransmitters (eg, norepinephrine) or a deficiency of inhibitory neurotransmitters (eg, gamma-aminobutyric acid [GABA]).

Generalized anxiety disorder is emphasized in this chapter. Major diagnostic criteria include worry about two or more circumstances and multiple symptoms for 6 months or longer, and elimination of disease processes or drugs as possible causes. Symptoms are related to motor tension (eg, muscle tension, restlessness, trembling, fatigue), overactivity of the autonomic nervous system (eg, dyspnea, palpitations, tachycardia, sweating, dry mouth, dizziness, nausea, diarrhea), and increased vigilance (feeling fearful, nervous, or keyed up; difficulty concentrating, irritability, insomnia). Numerous disease processes may be accompanied by symptoms of anxiety, including hyperthyroidism, cardiovascular disease, cancer, and others.

When the symptoms are secondary to medical illness, they may decrease as the illness improves. Symptoms also occur with several psychiatric illnesses (eg, mood disorders, schizophrenia, substance use disorders). Drugs that affect the CNS are often associated with anxiety. With CNS stimulants (eg, nasal decongestants, antiasthma drugs, nicotine, caffeine, diet aids), symptoms of anxiety occur with administration; with CNS depressants (eg, alcohol, sedative-type drugs), symptoms are more likely to occur when the drug is stopped, especially if stopped abruptly.

SLEEP AND INSOMNIA

Sleep is a recurrent period of decreased mental and physical activity during which the person is relatively unresponsive to sensory and environmental stimuli. Normal sleep allows rest, renewal of energy for performing activities of daily living, and alertness on awakening. When a person retires for sleep, there is an initial period of drowsiness or sleep latency, which lasts approximately 30 minutes. Once the person is asleep, cycles occur approximately every 90 minutes during the sleep period. During each cycle, the sleeper progresses from drowsiness (stage I) to deep sleep (stage IV). These stages are characterized by depressed body functions, non-rapid eye movements (non-REM), and nondreaming, and are thought to be physically restorative. Stage IV is followed by a period of 5 to 20 minutes of REM, dreaming, and increased physiologic activity. REM sleep is thought to be mentally and emotionally restorative; REM deprivation can lead to serious psychological problems, including psychosis.

Insomnia, prolonged difficulty in going to sleep or staying asleep long enough to feel rested, is the most common sleep disorder. Insomnia has many causes, including such stressors as pain, anxiety, illness, changes in lifestyle or environment, and various drugs. Occasional sleeplessness is a normal response to many stimuli and is not usually harmful.

DRUGS USED TO TREAT ANXIETY AND INSOMNIA

Drugs used to treat anxiety and insomnia include barbiturates, benzodiazepines, and others.

Barbiturates

Barbiturates are the prototype sedative-hypnotic drugs, although they are rarely used (Table 8-1). They have similar pharmacologic actions but differ in onset and duration of action. They are usually described as ultrashort, short, intermediate, and long acting. The ultrashort-acting drugs are used mainly for anesthesia and are discussed in Chapter 14. Barbiturates are metabolized into water-soluble, inactive metabolites in the liver; the metabolites are excreted by the kidneys.

Before the benzodiazepines were introduced in the early 1960s, the barbiturates were widely used. Four major problems associated with their use were suppression of REM sleep, induction of drug-metabolizing enzymes in the liver, development of tolerance and cross-tolerance, and development of dependence and abuse.

Suppression of REM sleep occurs when barbiturates are given in hypnotic doses for insomnia. Decreased REM sleep is followed by a compensatory increase in REM sleep when the drug is discontinued, as though the mind must make up the lost dreaming time. This REM rebound effect can occur when barbiturates are used for only 3 or 4 days. With longer drug use, REM rebound may be severe and accompanied by vivid dreams, nightmares, restlessness, and frequent awakening. This may promote dependence and abuse because people continue taking the drugs to avoid REM rebound. Normal sleep patterns may not return for several weeks after a barbiturate is discontinued, especially if it is stopped abruptly.

Enzyme induction means that barbiturates stimulate liver cells to produce larger amounts of drug-metabolizing enzymes. This allows larger amounts of a drug or other substance to be metabolized during a given period of time. Thus, barbiturates increase the liver's ability to metabolize themselves, several other drugs (eg, phenytoin, alcohol), and numerous substances that may be endogenous or administered as drugs (eg, adrenal corticosteroids, bile salts, sex hormones, vitamin K). Enzyme induction leads to tolerance, in which barbiturates lose their effectiveness as sedative-hypnotics in approximately 2 weeks of daily use, and cross-tolerance with other CNS depressants and other drugs metabolized by the same enzyme system in the liver. Barbiturate-induced enzyme induction disappears a few weeks after the drug is discontinued. Barbiturates have a high potential for dependence and abuse (see Chap. 15).

Benzodiazepines

Benzodiazepines are widely used for anxiety and insomnia and are also used for several other indications (Table 8-2). They have several advantages over the barbiturates. They have a wider margin of safety between therapeutic and toxic doses and are rarely fatal, even in overdose, unless combined with other CNS depressant drugs, such as alcohol. They do not induce drug-metabolizing enzymes or suppress REM sleep. They also cause less physical and psychological dependence than the barbiturates. Because they are drugs of abuse and may cause physiologic dependence, withdrawal symptoms (see Chap. 15) occur if the drugs are stopped abruptly. To avoid withdrawal symptoms, the drugs should be gradually tapered and discontinued.

In addition to abuse and dependence, benzodiazepines may cause characteristic effects of CNS depression, including excessive sedation, impairment of physical and mental activities, and respiratory depression. These drugs are Schedule IV under the Controlled Substances Act, and none is recommended for long-term use. They are well absorbed with oral administration, and most are given orally; a few (eg, diazepam, lorazepam) are given both orally and parenterally.

These drugs are highly lipid soluble, widely distributed in body tissues, and highly bound to plasma proteins. They are metabolized in the liver by the cytochrome P450 (microsomal) enzymes and glucuronide conjugation. Most benzodiazepines are oxidized by the enzymes to metabolites that are then conjugated and excreted through the kidneys. For example, diazepam and halazepam are converted to N-desmethyldiazepam (N-DMDZ), an active metabolite with a long elimination half-life of 36 to 200 hours. N-DMDZ is further oxidized to oxazepam, then conjugated and excreted. With repeated drug doses, N-DMDZ accumulates and may contribute to both long-lasting antianxiety effects and to adverse effects. If oxidation is impaired (eg, in the elderly, in liver disease, or with concurrent use of drugs that inhibit oxidation), higher blood levels of both the parent drug and metabolites increase the risks of adverse drug effects. In contrast, lorazepam, oxazepam, and temazepam are conjugated only, so their elimination is not impaired by the above factors.

Pharmacologically, all the benzodiazepines have similar characteristics and effects. However, they differ in clinical uses because the manufacturers developed and promoted them for particular purposes. The drugs also differ in serum half-lives, production of active metabolites, and duration of action. Several (eg, diazepam, flurazepam) have long half-lives and produce pharmacologically active metabolites that also have long half-lives. As a result, these drugs require approximately 5 to 7 days to reach steady-state serum levels. Therapeutic effects (eg, decreased anxiety or insomnia) and adverse effects (eg, sedation, ataxia) are more likely to occur after 2 or
(*text continues on page 115*)

TABLE 8-1 **Barbiturate Sedative-Hypnotics**

Generic/Trade Name	Major Clinical Use	Routes and Dosage Ranges		Remarks
		Adults	Children	
Short-acting				
Pentobarbital sodium (Nembutal)	Hypnotic, preoperative sedation	*Sedative:* PO 30 mg 3–4 times daily; rectal 120–200 mg *Hypnotic:* PO 100 mg; rectal 120–200 mg; IM 150–200 mg; IV 100 mg	*Sedative:* PO, rectal 2 mg/kg per day in 4 divided doses *Hypnotic:* IM 25–80 mg; rectal under 1 y, 30 mg; 1–4 y, 30 or 60 mg; 5–12 y, 60 mg; 12–14 y, 60 or 120 mg	Pentobarbital and seco-barbital are Schedule II controlled substances. They lose effectiveness as hypnotics in approximately 2 weeks of continuous administration. Do not divide rectal suppositories.
Secobarbital sodium (Seconal)	Hypnotic, preoperative sedation	*Sedative:* PO, rectal 120–200 mg *Hypnotic:* PO 100 mg; rectal 120–200 mg; IV 50–250 mg; IM 100–200 mg	*Sedative:* PO, rectal 6 mg/kg per day in 3 divided doses *Hypnotic:* IM 3–5 mg/kg; maximum dose, 100 mg	See pentobarbital
Intermediate-acting				
Amobarbital sodium (Amytal)	Hypnotic	*Sedative:* PO 50–300 mg daily in divided doses *Hypnotic:* PO 65–200 mg: IM, IV 65–500 mg	*Sedative:* over 12 y, same as adult dosage; under 12 y, PO 2 mg/kg per day in 4 divided doses *Hypnotic:* over 12 years, same as adult dosage	Schedule II drug
Aprobarbital (Alurate)	Sedative, hypnotic	*Sedative:* PO 40 mg 3 times daily *Hypnotic:* PO 40–160 mg		Schedule III drug
Butabarbital sodium (Butisol)	Sedative	*Sedative:* PO 50–120 mg daily in 3–4 divided doses *Hypnotic:* PO 50–100 mg	*Sedative:* PO 2 mg/kg per day in 3 divided doses	Schedule IV drug
Long-acting				
Mephobarbital (Mebaral)	Anticonvulsant	PO 200 mg at bedtime, up to 600 mg daily in divided doses	*Over 5 years:* PO 32–64 mg 3–4 times daily *Under 5 years:* PO 16–32 mg 3–4 times daily	Serum levels of pheno-barbital can be used as guidelines for adjusting dosage because mephobarbital is metabolized to phenobarbital.
Phenobarbital (Luminal, others)	Sedative, anticonvulsant	*Sedative:* PO, IM, IV 30–120 mg daily in 2–3 divided doses *Hypnotic:* PO, IM, IV 100–300 mg *Anticonvulsant:* PO 100–300 mg daily in 2–3 divided doses	*Sedative:* PO, rectal 1–2 mg/kg per day in 2–3 divided doses *Hypnotic:* PO 2–4 mg/kg *Anticonvulsant:* PO 5 mg/kg per day in 2–3 divided doses	Schedule IV drug. Not likely to produce abuse or dependence with chronic administration of anticonvulsant doses. Therapeutic plasma levels in seizure disorders are usually 10–25 μg/mL.

IM, intramuscular; IV, intravenous; PO, oral.

TABLE 8-2	Benzodiazepines			
Generic/Trade Name	**Clinical Indications**	**Half-life (h)**	**Metabolite(s)**	**Routes and Dosage Ranges**
Antianxiety Agents				
Alprazolam (Xanax)	Anxiety Panic attacks	Short (7–15)	Active	*Adults:* PO 0.25–0.5 mg 3 times daily; maximal dose, 4 mg daily in divided doses *Elderly or debilitated adults:* 0.25 mg 2–3 times daily, increased gradually if necessary
Chlordiazepoxide (Librium)	Anxiety Acute alcohol withdrawal	Long (5–30)	Active	*Adults:* PO 15–100 mg daily, once at bedtime or in 3–4 divided doses. IM, IV 50–100 mg, maximal daily dose 300 mg; for short-term use *Elderly or debilitated adults:* PO 5–10 mg 2–4 times daily *Children over 6 y:* PO, IM 0.5 mg/kg per day in 3–4 divided doses *Children under 6 y:* Not recommended
Clonazepam (Klonopin)	Seizure disorders	Long (20–40)	Inactive	*Adults:* PO 0.5 mg 3 times daily, increased by 0.5–1 mg every 3 days until seizures are controlled or adverse effects occur. Maximal daily dose, 20 mg
Clorazepate (Tranxene)	Anxiety Seizure disorders	Long (30–100)	Active	*Adults:* PO 7.5 mg 3 times daily, increased by no more than 7.5 mg/wk. Maximal daily dose, 90 mg *Children 9–12 y:* PO 7.5 mg 2 times daily, increased by no more than 7.5 mg/wk. Maximal daily dose, 60 mg *Children under 9 y:* Not recommended
Diazepam (Valium)	Anxiety Seizure disorders Acute alcohol withdrawal Muscle spasm Preoperative sedation Hypnotic	Long (20–50)	Active	*Adults:* PO 2–10 mg 2–4 times daily; sustained release, PO 15–30 mg once daily; IM, IV 5–10 mg, repeated in 3–4 hours if necessary *Elderly or debilitated adults:* PO 2–5 mg once or twice daily, increased gradually if needed and tolerated. *Children:* PO 1–2.5 mg 3–4 times daily, increased gradually if needed and tolerated *Children over 30 days and under 5 y of age:* Seizures IM, IV 0.2–0.5 mg/2–5 min to a maximum of 5 mg *Children 5 y or older:* Seizures, IM, IV 1 mg/2–5 min to a maximum of 10 mg
Lorazepam (Ativan)	Anxiety Preoperative sedation	Short (8–15)	Inactive	*Adults:* PO 2–6 mg/d in 2–3 divided doses. IM 0.05 mg/kg to a maximum of 4 mg. IV 2 mg, diluted with 2 ml of sterile water, sodium chloride, or 5% dextrose injection, injected over 1 min or longer *Elderly or debilitated adults:* PO 1–2 mg/d in divided doses

(continued)

TABLE 8-2	Benzodiazepines (*continued*)			
Generic/Trade Name	**Clinical Indications**	**Half-life (h)**	**Metabolite(s)**	**Routes and Dosage Ranges**
Midazolam (Versed)	Preoperative sedation Sedation before short diagnostic tests and endoscopic examinations Induction of general anesthesia Supplementation of nitrous oxide/oxygen anesthesia for short surgical procedures	Short (1–12)	Active	*Adults:* Preoperative sedation, IM 0.05–0.08 mg/kg approximately 1 hour before surgery *Prediagnostic test sedation.* IV 0.1–0.15 mg/kg or up to 0.2 mg/kg initially; maintenance dose, approximately 25% of initial dose. Reduce dose by 25% to 30% if a narcotic is also given. *Induction of anesthesia.* IV 0.3–0.35 mg/kg initially, then reduce dose as above for maintenance. Reduce initial dose to 0.15–0.3 mg/kg if a narcotic is also given. *Children:* Preoperative or preprocedure sedation, induction of anesthesia. PO syrup 0.25–1 mg/kg (maximum dose, 20 mg) as a single dose
Oxazepam (Serax)	Anxiety Acute alcohol withdrawal	Short (5–15)	Inactive	*Adults:* PO 30–120 mg daily in 3–4 divided doses *Elderly or debilitated adults:* PO 30 mg daily in 3 divided doses, gradually increased to 45–60 mg daily if necessary
Prazepam (Centrax)	Anxiety	Long (30–100)	Active	*Adults:* PO 20–40 mg daily in divided doses *Elderly or debilitated adults:* PO 10–15 mg daily in divided doses
Estazolam (ProSom)	Hypnotic	Intermediate (10–24)	Inactive	*Adults:* PO 1–2 mg
Flurazepam (Dalmane)	Hypnotic	Long (47–100)	Active	*Adults:* PO 15–30 mg
Quazepam (Doral)	Hypnotic	Long (39)	Active	*Adults:* PO 7.5–15 mg
Temazepam (Restoril)	Hypnotic	Short (9–12)	Inactive	*Adults:* PO 15–30 mg
Triazolam (Halcion)	Hypnotic	Ultrashort (1.5–5.5)	Inactive	*Adults:* PO 0.125–0.25 mg

IM, intramuscular; IV, intravenous; PO, oral.

3 days of therapy than initially. Such effects accumulate with chronic usage and persist for several days after the drugs are discontinued. Other drugs have short half-lives and produce inactive metabolites (eg, lorazepam, oxazepam); thus, their durations of action are much shorter, and they do not accumulate.

Miscellaneous Drugs

Several nonbarbiturate, nonbenzodiazepine drugs of varied characteristics are also used as antianxiety and sedative-hypnotic agents. These include buspirone, clomipramine, and hydroxyzine as antianxiety agents and chloral hydrate and zolpidem as hypnotics. Selected characteristics of the drugs are described here; dosages are listed in Table 8-3.

Buspirone differs chemically and pharmacologically from other antianxiety drugs. Its mechanism of action is unclear, but it apparently interacts with serotonin and dopamine receptors in the brain. Compared with the benzodiazepines, buspirone lacks muscle relaxant and anti-

convulsant effects, does not cause sedation or physical or psychological dependence, does not increase the CNS depression of alcohol and other drugs, and is not a controlled substance. Adverse effects include nervousness and excitement. Thus, clients wanting and accustomed to sedative effects may not like the drug or comply with instructions for its use. Its only clinical indication for use is the short-term treatment of anxiety. Although some beneficial effects may occur within 7 to 10 days, optimal effects may require 3 to 4 weeks. Because therapeutic effects may be delayed, buspirone is not considered beneficial for immediate effects or occasional (PRN) use. Buspirone is rapidly absorbed after oral administration. Peak plasma levels occur within 45 to 90 minutes. It is metabolized by the liver to inactive metabolites, which are then excreted in the urine and feces. Its elimination half-life is 2 to 3 hours.

Clomipramine is a tricyclic antidepressant (see Chap. 10) used for the treatment of obsessive-compulsive disorder.

Hydroxyzine is an antihistamine with sedative and antiemetic properties. Clinical indications for use include

TABLE 8-3   Miscellaneous Antianxiety and Sedative-Hypnotic Agents

Generic/Trade Name	Major Clinical Use	Routes and Dosage Ranges	
		Adults	Children
Antianxiety Agents			
Buspirone (BuSpar)	Anxiety	PO 5 mg 3 times daily, increased by 5 mg/d at 2- to 3-day intervals if necessary. Usual maintenance dose 20–30 mg/d in divided doses; maximum dose 60 mg/d	Not recommended
Clomipramine (Anafranil)	Obsessive–compulsive disorder	PO 25 mg/d initially; increase to 100 mg/d during the first 2 wk and to a maximum dose of 250 mg/d over several weeks if necessary	PO 25 mg/d initially; increase to 3 mg/kg or 100 mg, whichever is smaller, during the first 2 wk and to 3 mg/kg or 200 mg, whichever is smaller, over several weeks if necessary
Hydroxyzine (Vistaril)	Anxiety, sedative, pruritus	PO 75–400 mg/d in 3 or 4 divided doses. Pre- and postoperative and pre and postpartum sedation, IM 25–100 mg in a single dose	PO 2 mg/kg per day in 4 divided doses. Pre- and postoperative sedation, IM 1 mg/kg in a single dose
Sedative-hypnotic Agents			
Chloral hydrate	Sedative, hypnotic	*Sedative:* PO, rectal suppository 250 mg 3 times per day, after meals *Hypnotic:* PO, rectal suppository 500–1000 mg at bedtime; maximum dose, 2 g/d	*Sedative:* PO, rectal suppository 25 mg/kg per day, in 3 or 4 divided doses. *Hypnotic:* PO, rectal suppository 50 mg/kg at bedtime; maximum single dose, 1 g
Zolpidem (Ambien)	Hypnotic	PO 10 mg at bedtime. Elderly, hepatic impairment, PO 5 mg	Not recommended

IM, intramuscular; PO, oral.

anxiety, preoperative sedation, nausea and vomiting associated with surgery or motion sickness, and pruritus and urticaria associated with allergic dermatoses.

Chloral hydrate, the oldest sedative-hypnotic drug, is relatively safe, effective, and inexpensive in usual therapeutic doses. It reportedly does not suppress REM sleep. Tolerance develops after approximately 2 weeks of continual use. It is a drug of abuse and may cause physical dependence.

Zolpidem is a hypnotic that differs structurally from the benzodiazepines, but produces similar effects. It is a Schedule IV drug approved for short-term treatment (≤10 days) of insomnia and does not adversely affect sleep patterns. It is well absorbed with oral administration and has a rapid onset of action. Its half-life is approximately 2.5 hours and its hypnotic effects last approximately 6 to 8 hours. Adverse effects are usually few and mild (eg, daytime drowsiness, dizziness, nausea, diarrhea), but rebound insomnia may occur for a night or two after stopping the drug, and withdrawal symptoms may occur if it is stopped abruptly after approximately a week of regular use. Zolpidem is metabolized to inactive metabolites that are then eliminated mainly by renal excretion. Dosage should be reduced for clients of advanced age or those with liver disease.

In addition, several antihistamines cause drowsiness and are used as hypnotics, although they are not approved by the Food and Drug Administration (FDA) for this purpose. **Diphenhydramine** (Benadryl) is used in hospital-ized clients and is available over the counter. An antihistamine is the active ingredient in nonprescription sleep aids (eg, diphenhydramine in Compoz, Nytol, Sominex, Sleep-Eze; doxylamine in Unisom).

Mechanisms of Action

Barbiturates produce CNS depression by inhibiting functions of nerve cells, such as electrical stimulation, depolarization, impulse transmission, and neurotransmitter release. Neurons in the reticular formation, which control cerebral cortex activity and level of arousal or wakefulness, are especially sensitive to the depressant effects of barbiturates.

Benzodiazepines bind with a receptor complex in the nerve cells of the brain; this receptor complex also has binding sites for GABA, an inhibitory neurotransmitter (see Chap. 5). This GABA–benzodiazepine receptor complex regulates the entry of chloride ions into the cell. When GABA binds to the receptor complex, chloride ions enter the cell and stabilize (hyperpolarize) the cell membrane so that it is less responsive to excitatory neurotransmitters, such as norepinephrine. Benzodiazepines bind at a different site on the receptor complex and enhance the inhibitory effect of GABA to relieve anxiety, tension, and nervousness and to produce sleep. Other antianxiety and sedative-hypnotic drugs have varied mechanisms of action.

Indications for Use

Major clinical uses of the benzodiazepines are as antianxiety, hypnotic, and anticonvulsant agents. They also are given for preoperative sedation, prevention of agitation and delirium tremens in acute alcohol withdrawal, and treatment of anxiety symptoms associated with depression, acute psychosis, or mania. Thus, they are often given concurrently with antidepressants, antipsychotics, and mood stabilizers. Not all benzodiazepines are approved for all uses; Table 8-2 lists indications for the use of individual benzodiazepines. Diazepam has been extensively studied and has more approved uses than others.

Clinical indications for the use of sedative-hypnotics include short-term treatment of insomnia and sedation before surgery or invasive diagnostic tests (eg, angiograms, endoscopies). Barbiturates also are used for their general anesthetic and anticonvulsant effects.

Contraindications to Use

Contraindications to benzodiazepines include severe respiratory disorders, severe liver or kidney disease, hypersensitivity reactions, and a history of alcohol or other drug abuse. The drugs must be used very cautiously when taken concurrently with any other CNS depressant drugs.

NURSING PROCESS

Assessment

Assess the client's need for antianxiety or sedative-hypnotic drugs, including intensity and duration of symptoms. Manifestations are more obvious with moderate to severe anxiety or insomnia. Some guidelines for assessment include the following:

- What is the client's statement of the problem? Does the problem interfere with usual activities of daily living? If so, how much and for how long?
- Try to identify factors that precipitate anxiety or insomnia in the client. Some common ones are physical symptoms; feeling worried, tense, or nervous; factors such as illness, death of a friend or family member, divorce, or job stress; and excessive CNS stimulation from caffeine-containing beverages or drugs such as bronchodilators and nasal decongestants. In addition, excessive daytime sleep and too little exercise and activity may cause insomnia, especially in older clients.
- Observe for behavioral manifestations of anxiety, such as psychomotor agitation, facial grimaces, tense posture, and others.
- Observe for physiologic manifestations of anxiety. These may include increased blood pressure and pulse rate, increased rate and depth of respiration, increased muscle tension, and pale, cool skin.
- If behavioral or physiologic manifestations seem to indicate anxiety, try to determine whether this is actually the case. Because similar manifestations may indicate pain or other problems rather than anxiety, the observer's perceptions must be validated by the client before appropriate action can be taken.
- If insomnia is reported, observe for signs of sleep deprivation such as drowsiness, slow movements or speech, and difficulty concentrating or focusing attention.
- Obtain a careful drug history, including the use of alcohol and sedative-hypnotic drugs, and assess the likelihood of drug abuse and dependence. People who abuse other drugs, including alcohol, are likely to abuse antianxiety and sedative-hypnotic drugs. Also assess for use of prescription and nonprescription CNS stimulants (eg, appetite suppressants, bronchodilators, nasal decongestants, excessive caffeine, cocaine).
- Identify coping mechanisms used in managing previous situations of stress, anxiety, and insomnia. These are very individualized. Reading, watching television, listening to music, or talking to a friend are examples. Some people are quiet and inactive; others participate in strenuous activity. Some prefer to be alone; others prefer being with a friend or family member or a group.
- Once drug therapy for anxiety or insomnia is begun, assess the client's level of consciousness and functional ability before each dose so that excessive sedation can be avoided.

Nursing Diagnoses

- Ineffective Individual Coping related to need for antianxiety or sedative-hypnotic drug
- Knowledge Deficit: Appropriate uses and effects of antianxiety or sedative-hypnotic drugs
- Knowledge Deficit: Nondrug measures for relieving anxiety and insomnia
- Noncompliance: Overuse
- Risk for Injury related to sedation, respiratory depression, impaired mobility, and other adverse effects
- Altered Thought Processes related to confusion (especially in older adults)
- Sleep Pattern Disturbance: Insomnia related to one or more causes (eg, anxiety, daytime sleep)

Planning/Goals

The client will:

- Feel more calm, relaxed, and comfortable with anxiety; experience improved quantity and quality of sleep with insomnia

- Be monitored for excessive sedation and impaired mobility to prevent falls or other injuries (in health care settings)
- Verbalize and demonstrate nondrug activities to reduce or manage anxiety or insomnia
- Demonstrate safe, accurate drug usage
- Notify a health care provider if he or she wants to stop taking a benzodiazepine; will not stop taking a benzodiazepine abruptly
- Avoid preventable adverse effects, including abuse and dependence

Interventions

Use nondrug measures to relieve anxiety or to enhance the effectiveness of antianxiety drugs.

- Assist clients to identify and avoid or decrease situations that cause anxiety and insomnia, when possible. In addition, help them to understand that medications do not solve underlying problems.
- Support the client's usual coping mechanisms when feasible. Provide the opportunity for reading, exercising, listening to music, or watching television; promote contact with significant others, or simply allow the client to be alone and uninterrupted for a while.
- Use interpersonal and communication techniques to help the client manage anxiety. The degree of anxiety and the clinical situation largely determine which techniques are appropriate. For example, staying with the client, showing interest, listening, and allowing him or her to verbalize concerns may be beneficial.
- Providing information may be a therapeutic technique when anxiety is related to medical conditions. People vary in the amount and kind of information they want, but usually the following topics should be included:
  - The overall treatment plan, including medical or surgical treatment, choice of outpatient care or hospitalization, expected length of treatment, and expected outcomes in terms of health and ability to function in activities of daily living
  - Specific diagnostic tests, including preparation, after-effects if any, and how the client will be informed of results
  - Specific medication and treatment measures, including expected therapeutic results
  - What the client must do to carry out the plan of treatment
- When offering information and explanations, keep in mind that anxiety interferes with intellectual functioning. Thus, communication should be brief, clear, and repeated as necessary because clients may misunderstand or forget what is said.
- Modify the environment to decrease anxiety-provoking stimuli. Modifications may involve altering temperature, light, and noise levels.
- Use measures to increase physical comfort. These may include a wide variety of activities, such as positioning, helping the client bathe or ambulate, giving back rubs, or providing fluids of the client's choice.
- Consult with other services and departments on the client's behalf. For example, if financial problems were identified as a cause of anxiety, social services may be able to help.
- When a benzodiazepine is used with diagnostic tests or minor surgery, provide instructions for postprocedure care to the client or to family members, preferably in written form.

Implement measures to decrease the need for or increase the effectiveness of sedative-hypnotic drugs, such as the following:

- Modify the environment to promote rest and sleep (eg, reduce noise and light).
- Plan care to allow uninterrupted periods of rest and sleep when possible.
- Relieve symptoms that interfere with rest and sleep. Drugs such as analgesics for pain or antitussives for cough are usually safer and more effective than sedative-hypnotic drugs. Nondrug measures, such as positioning, exercise, and back rubs, may be helpful in relieving muscle tension and other discomforts. Allowing the client to verbalize concerns, providing information so that he or she knows what to expect, or consulting other personnel (eg, social worker, chaplain) may be useful in decreasing anxiety.
- Help the client modify lifestyle habits to promote rest and sleep (eg, limiting intake of caffeine-containing beverages, limiting intake of fluids during evening hours if nocturia interferes with sleep, avoiding daytime naps, having a regular schedule of rest and sleep periods, increasing physical activity, and not trying to sleep unless tired or drowsy).

Evaluation

- Decreased symptoms of anxiety or insomnia and increased rest and sleep are reported or observed.
- Excessive sedation and motor impairment are not observed.
- The client reports no serious adverse effects.
- Monitoring of prescriptions (eg, "pill counts") does not indicate excessive use.

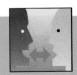

CLIENT TEACHING GUIDELINES
Antianxiety and Sedative-Hypnotic Drugs

General Considerations

✔ "Nerve pills" and "sleeping pills" can relieve symptoms temporarily but do not cure or solve the underlying problems. With rare exceptions, these drugs are recommended only for short-term use. For long-term relief, counseling or psychotherapy may be more beneficial than drug therapy.

✔ Use nondrug measures to promote relaxation, rest, and sleep when possible. Physical exercise, reading, craft work, stress management, and relaxation techniques are safer than any drug.

✔ Try to identify and avoid factors that cause nervousness or insomnia, such as caffeine-containing beverages and stimulant drugs. This may prevent or decrease the severity of nervousness or insomnia so that sedative-type drugs are not needed. If the drugs are used, these factors can cancel or decrease the drugs' effects. Stimulant drugs include asthma and cold remedies and appetite suppressants.

✔ Most "nerve pills" and "sleeping pills" belong to a chemical group called benzodiazepines. All benzodiazepines have similar characteristics and effects, including the potential to cause dependence. Thus, there is no logical reason to take a combination of the drugs for anxiety, or to take one drug for daytime sedation and another for sleep.

✔ Inform all health care providers when taking a sedative-type medication, preferably by the generic and trade names. This helps avoid multiple prescriptions of drugs with similar effects and reduces the risk of serious adverse effects from overdose.

✔ Do not perform tasks that require alertness if drowsy from medication. The drugs often impair mental and physical functioning, especially during the first several days of use, and thereby make routine activities potentially hazardous. Avoid smoking, ambulating without help, driving a car, operating machinery, and other potentially hazardous tasks. These activities may lead to falls or other injuries if undertaken while alertness is impaired.

✔ Avoid alcohol and other depressant drugs (eg, over-the-counter [OTC] antihistamines and sleeping pills, narcotic analgesics) while taking any antianxiety or sedative-hypnotic drugs (except buspirone). An antihistamine that causes drowsiness is the active ingredient in OTC sleep aids (eg, Compoz, Nytol, Sominex, Unisom) and many pain reliever products with "PM" as part of their names (eg, Tylenol PM). Because these drugs depress brain functioning when taken alone, combining them produces additive depression and may lead to excessive drowsiness, difficulty breathing, traumatic injuries, and other potentially serious adverse drug effects.

✔ Store drugs safely, out of reach of children and adults who are confused or less than alert. Accidental or intentional ingestion may lead to serious adverse effects. Also, do not keep the drug container at the bedside, because a person sedated by a previous dose may take additional doses.

✔ Do not share these drugs with anyone else. These mind-altering, brain-depressant drugs should be taken only by those people for whom they are prescribed.

✔ Do not increase dosage, do not increase frequency of administration, and do not take for prolonged periods.

✔ Do not stop taking a benzodiazepine drug abruptly. Withdrawal symptoms can occur. When being discontinued, dosage should be gradually reduced, as directed and with the supervision of a health care provider.

✔ Do not take "sleeping pills" every night. These drugs lose their effectiveness in 2 to 4 weeks if taken nightly, and cause sleep disturbances when stopped.

✔ Alprazolam (Xanax), a commonly prescribed benzodiazepine, is sometimes confused with ranitidine (Zantac), a drug for heartburn and peptic ulcers.

Self-administration

✔ Follow instructions carefully about how much, how often, and how long to take the drugs. These drugs produce more beneficial effects and fewer adverse reactions when used in the smallest effective doses and for the shortest duration feasible in particular circumstances. All of the benzodiazepines and zolpidem can produce psychological and physiologic dependence, which may eventually cause worse problems than the original anxiety or insomnia.

✔ Take sleeping pills just before going to bed so that you are lying down when the expected drowsiness occurs.

✔ Omit one or more doses if excessive drowsiness occurs to avoid difficulty breathing, falls, and other adverse drug effects.

✔ Take oral benzodiazepines with a glass of water; they may be taken with food if stomach upset occurs.

✔ Take buspirone on a daily schedule. It is not fully effective until after 3 to 4 weeks of regular use; it is ineffective for occasional use.

✔ Take zolpidem on an empty stomach, at bedtime, because the drug acts quickly to cause drowsiness.

Nursing Notes: Apply Your Knowledge

Georgia Summers is admitted to your unit for elective surgery. During your admission assessment, she states she has been taking alprazolam (Xanax) 1 mg tid and hs for the last 3 years. She claims to be a social drinker, consuming two to three drinks per evening. During the interview she appears nervous and asks you at least five times whether the doctor will order her Xanax while she is in the hospital. Discuss your interpretation of these assessment data and how it will affect your plan of care for Ms. Summers.

PRINCIPLES OF THERAPY

Use in Anxiety

Antianxiety drugs are not recommended for treating everyday stress and anxiety. Some authorities believe such use promotes reliance on drugs and decreases development of healthier coping mechanisms. For severe anxiety associated with a temporary stressful situation, an anxiolytic drug may be beneficial for short-term, "as-needed" use; prolonged drug therapy is not recommended. These drugs are most clearly indicated when anxiety causes disability and interferes with job performance, interpersonal relationships, and other activities of daily living. The drugs are not recommended for long-term use and chronic anxiety states are probably more effectively treated with psychotherapy. Because anxiety often accompanies pain, antianxiety agents are sometimes used to manage pain. In the management of chronic pain, however, antianxiety drugs have not demonstrated a definite benefit. Anxiety about recurrence of pain is probably better controlled by adequate analgesia than by antianxiety drugs.

The antianxiety benzodiazepines are often the drugs of choice for treating anxiety. Because they are equally effective in relieving anxiety, other factors may assist the prescriber in choosing a particular drug for a particular client. For example, alprazolam, clorazepate, and diazepam decrease anxiety within 30 to 60 minutes. Thus, one of these drugs may be preferred when rapid onset of drug action is desired. Lorazepam, oxazepam, and prazepam have a slower onset of action and thus are not recommended for acute symptoms of anxiety. Because they have short half-lives and their elimination does not depend on the cytochrome P450 oxidizing enzymes in the liver, lorazepam and oxazepam are the drugs of choice for clients who are elderly, have liver disease, or are taking drugs that interfere with hepatic drug-metabolizing enzymes.

Buspirone is also an effective antianxiety agent, especially for clients with conditions that may be aggravated by the sedative and respiratory depressant effects of benzodiazepines (eg, chronic obstructive lung disease). However, anxiety-relieving effects may be delayed for 3 to 4 weeks. Thus, buspirone is not useful for acute episodes of anxiety and it may be difficult to persuade some clients to take the drug long enough to be effective.

Use in Insomnia

In general, sedative-hypnotic drugs should be used only when insomnia causes significant distress and resists management by nonpharmacologic means; they should not be used for occasional sleeplessness. When drug therapy is required, the goal of treatment is to relieve anxiety or sleeplessness without permitting sensory perception, responsiveness to the environment, or alertness to drop below safe levels. Additional guidelines include the following:

1. Do not give sedative-hypnotic drugs every night unless necessary. Intermittent administration helps maintain drug effectiveness and decreases the risks of drug abuse and dependence. It also decreases disturbances of normal sleep patterns.
2. When sedative-hypnotic drugs are prescribed for outpatients, the prescription should limit the number of doses dispensed and the number of refills. This is one way of decreasing the risk of abuse and suicide.
3. In chronic insomnia, no hypnotic drug is recommended for long-term treatment. Most benzodiazepine hypnotics lose their effectiveness in producing sleep after approximately 4 weeks of daily use; triazolam loses effectiveness in approximately 2 weeks. It is not helpful to switch from one drug to another because cross-tolerance develops. To restore the sleep-producing effect, administration of the hypnotic drug must be interrupted for 1 to 2 weeks.
4. As with the antianxiety benzodiazepines, most hypnotic benzodiazepines are oxidized in the liver by the cytochrome P450 (microsomal) enzymes to metabolites that are then conjugated and excreted through the kidneys. An exception is temazepam, which is eliminated only by conjugation with glucuronide. Thus, temazepam is the drug of choice for clients who are elderly, have liver disease, or are taking drugs that interfere with hepatic drug-metabolizing enzymes.
5. Zolpidem is an acceptable alternative to a benzodiazepine for short-term treatment of insomnia. It is metabolized in the liver to inactive metabolites, and its use is not associated with tolerance. Lower doses are recommended for clients who are elderly or have impaired liver function.

Duration of Therapy

Benzodiazepines should be given for the shortest effective period to decrease the likelihood of drug abuse and physiologic and psychological dependence. Few problems develop with short-term use unless an overdose is taken or other CNS depressant drugs (eg, alcohol) are taken concurrently. Most problems occur with long-term use, especially of larger-than-usual doses. In general, an antianxiety benzodiazepine should not be taken for longer than 4 months and a hypnotic benzodiazepine should not be taken more than 3 or 4 nights a week for approximately 3 weeks.

For buspirone, recommendations for duration of therapy have not been established. For zolpidem, the recommended duration is no longer than 10 days.

Dosage

With benzodiazepines, dosage must be individualized and carefully titrated because requirements vary widely among clients. With antianxiety agents, the goal is to find the lowest effective dose that does not cause excessive daytime drowsiness or impaired mobility. In general, start with the smallest dose likely to be effective (eg, diazepam 2 mg three times daily or equivalent doses of others). Then, according to client response, doses can be titrated upward to relieve symptoms of anxiety and avoid adverse drug effects. The maximum daily dose is diazepam 40 mg/day or equivalent doses of others. With hypnotics, the lowest effective doses should be taken on an intermittent basis, not every night. Additional guidelines include the following:

1. Smaller-than-usual doses may be indicated in clients receiving cimetidine or several other drugs that decrease the hepatic metabolism of most benzodiazepines and in elderly or debilitated clients. With alprazolam (Xanax), the most commonly prescribed benzodiazepine, the dose should be reduced by 50% if given concurrently with nefazodone (Serzone) or fluvoxamine (Luvox).

   In the elderly, most benzodiazepines are metabolized more slowly, and half-lives are longer than in younger adults. Exceptions are lorazepam and oxazepam, whose half-lives and dosages are the same for elderly adults as for younger ones. The recommended initial dose of zolpidem is 5 mg, one-half of that recommended for younger adults.

2. Larger-than-usual doses may be needed for clients who are severely anxious or agitated. Also, large doses are usually required to relax skeletal muscle, control muscle spasm, control seizures, and provide sedation before surgery, cardioversion, endoscopy, and angiography.

3. When benzodiazepines are used with opioid analgesics, the analgesic dose should be reduced initially and increased gradually to avoid excessive CNS depression.

Scheduling

The antianxiety benzodiazepines are often given in three or four daily doses. This is necessary for the short-acting agents, but there is no pharmacologic basis for multiple daily doses of the long-acting drugs. Because of their prolonged actions, all or most of the daily dose can be given at bedtime. This schedule promotes sleep, and there is usually enough residual sedation to maintain antianxiety effects throughout the next day. If necessary, one or two small supplemental doses may be given during the day. Although the hypnotic benzodiazepines vary in their onset of action, they should be taken at bedtime because it is safer for clients to be recumbent when drowsiness occurs. Zolpidem also should be taken at bedtime because it has a rapid onset of action.

Prevention and Management of Benzodiazepine Withdrawal

Physical dependence on benzodiazepines is indicated by withdrawal symptoms when the drugs are stopped. Mild symptoms occur in approximately half the clients taking therapeutic doses for 6 to 12 weeks; severe symptoms are most likely to occur when high doses are taken regularly for more than 4 months and then abruptly discontinued. Although the drugs have not been proven effective for more than 4 months of regular use, this period is probably exceeded quite often in clinical practice.

Withdrawal symptoms may be caused by the abrupt separation of benzodiazepine molecules from their receptor sites and the acute decrease in GABA neurotransmission that results. Because GABA is an inhibitory neurotransmitter, less GABA may produce a less inhibited CNS and symptoms of hyperarousal or CNS stimulation.

Thus, common manifestations include increased anxiety, psychomotor agitation, insomnia, irritability, headache, tremor, and palpitations. Less common but more serious manifestations include confusion, abnormal perception of movement, depersonalization, psychosis, and seizures.

Severe symptoms are most likely to occur with short-acting drugs such as alprazolam, lorazepam, and triazolam unless they are discontinued very gradually. Symptoms may occur within 24 hours of stopping a short-acting drug, but usually occur 4 to 5 days after stopping a long-acting drug such as diazepam. Symptoms can be relieved by administration of a benzodiazepine.

To prevent withdrawal symptoms, the drug should be tapered in dose and gradually discontinued. Reducing the dose by 10% to 25% every 1 or 2 weeks over 4 to 16 weeks usually is effective. However, the rate may need to be even slower with high doses or long-term use. Once the drug is discontinued, the client should be monitored for a few weeks for symptoms of withdrawal or recurrence of symptoms for which the drug was originally prescribed.

Management of Benzodiazepine Toxicity

Flumazenil is a specific antidote that competes with benzodiazepines for benzodiazepine receptors and reverses sedation, coma, and respiratory depression. Clinical indications for use include benzodiazepine overdose and reversal of sedation after diagnostic or therapeutic procedures. The degree of sedation reversal depends on the plasma concentration of the ingested benzodiazepine and the flumazenil dose and frequency of administration. The drug acts rapidly, with onset within 2 minutes and peak effects within 6 to 10 minutes. However, the duration of action is short (serum half-life of 60 to 90 minutes) compared with that of most benzodiazepines, so repeated doses are usually required. Adverse effects include precipitation of acute benzodiazepine withdrawal symptoms, agitation, confusion, and seizures. Resedation and hypoventilation may occur if flumazenil is not given long enough to coincide with the duration of action of the benzodiazepine.

The drug should be injected into a freely flowing intravenous (IV) line in a large vein. Dosage recommendations vary with use. For reversal of conscious sedation or general anesthesia, the initial dose is 0.2 mg over 15 seconds, then 0.2 mg every 60 seconds, if necessary, to a maximum of 1.0 mg (total of five doses). For overdose, the initial dose is 0.2 mg over 30 seconds, wait 30 seconds, then 0.3 mg over 30 seconds, then 0.5 mg every 60 seconds up to a total dose of 3 mg, if necessary, for the client to reach the desired level of consciousness. Slow administration and repeated doses are recommended to awaken the client gradually and decrease the risks of causing acute withdrawal symptoms. A client who does not respond within 5 minutes of administering the total recommended dose should be reassessed for other causes of sedation.

Use in Children

Anxiety is a common disorder among children and adolescents. When given antianxiety and sedative-hypnotic drugs, they may have unanticipated or variable responses, including paradoxical CNS stimulation and excitement rather than CNS depression and calming. Few studies have been done in children. Thus, much clinical usage of these drugs is empiric, not approved by the FDA, and not supported by data. Some considerations include the following:

1. Drug pharmacodynamics and pharmacokinetics are likely to be different in children than in adults. Pharmacodynamic differences may stem from changes in neurotransmission systems in the brain as the child grows. Pharmacokinetic differences may stem from changes in distribution or metabolism of drugs; absorption seems similar to that of adults. In relation to distribution, children usually have a lesser percentage of body fat than adults. Thus, antianxiety and sedative-hypnotic drugs, which are usually highly lipid soluble, cannot be as readily stored in fat as they are in adults. This often leads to shorter half-

lives and the need for more frequent administration. In relation to metabolism, young children (eg, preschoolers) usually have a faster rate than adults and may therefore require relatively high doses for their size and weight. In relation to excretion, renal function is usually similar to that of adults and most of the drugs are largely inactive. Thus, with normal renal function, excretion probably has little effect on blood levels of active drug or the child's response to the drug.

2. Oral and parenteral diazepam has been used extensively in children, in all age groups older than 6 months. Other benzodiazepines are not recommended for particular age groups (eg, oral chlordiazepoxide under 6 years of age; parenteral chlordiazepoxide under 12 years of age; clorazepate under 9 years of age; oral lorazepam under 12 years of age; alprazolam, halazepam, prazepam, and injectable lorazepam under 18 years of age).

3. As with other populations, benzodiazepines should be given to children only when clearly indicated, in the lowest effective dose, for the shortest effective time.

4. Effects of buspirone and zolpidem in children are unknown.

Use in Older Adults

Most antianxiety and sedative-hypnotic drugs are metabolized and excreted more slowly in older adults, so the effects of a given dose last longer. Also, several of the benzodiazepines produce pharmacologically active metabolites, which prolong drug actions. Thus, the drugs may accumulate and increase adverse effects if dosages are not reduced. The initial dose of any antianxiety or sedative-hypnotic drug should be small and any increments should be made gradually to decrease the risks of adverse effects. Adverse effects include oversedation, dizziness, confusion, hypotension, and impaired mobility, which may contribute to falls and other injuries unless clients are carefully monitored and safeguarded.

Benzodiazepines should be tapered rather than discontinued abruptly in older adults, as in other populations. Withdrawal symptoms may occur within 24 hours after abruptly stopping a short-acting drug but may not occur for several days after stopping a long-acting agent.

For anxiety, short-acting benzodiazepines, such as alprazolam or lorazepam, are preferred over long-acting agents, such as diazepam. Buspirone may be preferred over a benzodiazepine because it does not cause sedation, psychomotor impairment, or increased risk of falls. However, it must be taken on a regular schedule and is not effective for PRN use.

For insomnia, sedative-hypnotic drugs should usually be avoided or their use minimized in older adults. Finding and treating the causes and using nondrug measures to aid sleep are much safer. If a sedative-hypnotic is used, shorter-acting benzodiazepines are preferred because they are eliminated more rapidly and are therefore less likely to accumulate and cause adverse effects. In addition, dosages should be smaller than for younger adults, the drugs should not be used every night or for longer than a few days, and older adults should be monitored closely for adverse effects. If zolpidem is used, the recommended dose for older adults is half that of younger adults (5 mg).

Use in Hypoalbuminemia

Clients with hypoalbuminemia (eg, from malnutrition or liver disease) are at risk of adverse effects with drugs that are highly bound to plasma proteins, such as the benzodiazepines, buspirone, and zolpidem. If a benzodiazepine is given to clients with low serum albumin levels, alprazolam or lorazepam is preferred because these drugs are less extensively bound to plasma proteins and less likely to cause adverse effects. If buspirone or zolpidem is given, dosage may need to be reduced.

Use in Renal Impairment

Clients with renal impairment are often given sedatives to relieve anxiety and depression, and excessive sedation is the major adverse effect. It may be difficult to assess the client for excessive sedation because drowsiness, lethargy, and mental status changes are also common symptoms of uremia.

All benzodiazepines undergo hepatic metabolism and then elimination in urine. Several of the drugs produce active metabolites that are normally excreted by the kidney. If renal excretion is impaired, the active metabolites may accumulate and cause excessive sedation and respiratory depression.

Buspirone is contraindicated in clients with severe renal impairment. Zolpidem may be used in renal impairment and does not require dosage reduction.

Use in Hepatic Impairment

Benzodiazepines undergo hepatic metabolism and then elimination in urine. In the presence of liver disease (eg, cirrhosis, hepatitis), the metabolism of most benzodiazepines is slowed, with resultant accumulation and increased risk of adverse effects. If a benzodiazepine is needed, lorazepam and oxazepam are preferred antianxiety agents and temazepam is the preferred hypnotic. These drugs require only conjugation with glucuronide for elimination and liver disease does not significantly affect this process. If other benzodiazepines are given to clients with

advanced liver disease, small initial doses and slow, gradual increases are indicated. Buspirone is metabolized in the liver and should not be used in clients with severe hepatic impairment. Zolpidem is metabolized more slowly in clients with liver impairment; if used, dosage should be reduced to 5 mg.

Use in Critical Illness

Antianxiety and sedative-hypnotic drugs are often used in critically ill clients to relieve stress, anxiety, and agitation. By their calming effects, they may also decrease cardiac workload (eg, heart rate, blood pressure, force of myocardial contraction, myocardial oxygen consumption) and respiratory effort. Additional benefits include improving tolerance of treatment measures (eg, mechanical ventilation); keeping confused clients from harming themselves by pulling out IV catheters, feeding or drainage tubes, wound drains, and other treatment devices; and allowing clients to rest or sleep more. In addition to sedation, the drugs often induce amnesia, which may be a desirable effect in the critically ill.

Commonly used drugs are injectable benzodiazepines, often in conjunction with opioid analgesics. When psychoactive drugs are combined, the risk of adverse effects and adverse drug interactions is increased. The drugs are often given by IV infusion, sometimes by intermittent bolus injection. The infusions may be given on a short-term (eg, a few days) or long-term (eg, weeks) basis. Most pharmacokinetic and pharmacodynamic data were derived from short-term administration of the drugs to non-critically ill adults and may differ significantly with long-term infusions and administration to the critically ill. For example, the drugs may have a longer duration of action in critically ill clients and may require dosage reduction.

Lorazepam is probably the benzodiazepine of first choice for treating anxiety in intensive care units. It has a slow onset of action because of delayed brain penetration, but an intermediate to prolonged duration. Midazolam is also used in critically ill clients, but its effects are less predictable than in other groups because of changes in protein binding, hepatic metabolism, and other factors. As a result of these changes, drug disposition and duration of action vary widely among recipients. In critically ill clients, midazolam has prolonged sedation in those being mechanically ventilated, those who have had cardiac surgery, and those with septic shock or acute renal failure. In renal failure, active metabolites may accumulate to high levels.

 Home Care

Although antianxiety and sedative-hypnotic drugs are not recommended for long-term use, they are often used at home. Previously described precautions and teaching needs related to safe use of the drugs apply in home care as in other settings. The home care nurse should encourage the client to use nondrug methods of reducing anxiety and insomnia and should review the risks of injuries if mental and physical responses are slowed by the drugs. In addition, assess the client for signs and symptoms of

overuse, withdrawal, and use of other sedating drugs, including alcohol, sedating antihistamines, and other prescription drugs. Although the home care nurse is more likely to encounter these drugs as legal prescriptions, they are also commonly abused street drugs.

(*text continues on page 128*)

NURSING ACTIONS: Antianxiety and Sedative-Hypnotic Drugs

NURSING ACTIONS	RATIONALE/EXPLANATION
1. Administer accurately	
a. If a client appears excessively sedated when a dose of an antianxiety or sedative-hypnotic drug is due, omit the dose and record the reason.	To avoid excessive sedation and other adverse effects
b. For oral sedative-hypnotics:	
(1) Prepare the client for sleep before giving hypnotic doses of any drug.	Most of the drugs cause drowsiness within 15 to 30 minutes. The client should be in bed when he or she becomes drowsy to increase the therapeutic effectiveness of the drug and to decrease the likelihood of falls or other injuries.
(2) Give with a glass of water or other fluid.	The fluid enhances dissolution and absorption of the drug for a quicker onset of action.
(3) Raise bedrails and instruct the client to stay in bed or ask for help if necessary to get out of bed.	To avoid falls and other injuries related to sedation and impaired mobility
c. For benzodiazepines:	
(1) Give orally, when feasible.	These drugs are well absorbed from the gastrointestinal (GI) tract, and onset of action occurs within a few minutes. Diazepam is better absorbed orally than IM. When given IM, the drug crystallizes in tissue and is absorbed very slowly.
(2) Do not mix injectable diazepam with any other drug in a syringe or add to intravenous (IV) fluids.	Diazepam is physically incompatible with other drugs and solutions.
(3) Give intramuscular (IM) benzodiazepines undiluted, deeply, into large muscle masses, such as the gluteus muscle of the hip.	These drugs are irritating to tissues and may cause pain at injection sites.
(4) With IV benzodiazepines, be very careful to avoid intra-arterial injection or extravasation into surrounding tissues. Have equipment available for respiratory assistance.	These drugs are very irritating to tissues and may cause venous thrombosis, phlebitis, local irritation, edema, and vascular impairment. They may also cause respiratory depression and apnea.
(5) Give IV **diazepam** slowly, over at least 1 minute for 5 mg (1 mL); into large veins (not hand or wrist veins); by direct injection into the vein or into IV infusion tubing as close as possible to the venipuncture site.	To avoid apnea and tissue irritation
(6) Give IV **lorazepam** slowly, over at least 1 minute for 2 mg, by direct injection into the	To avoid apnea and tissue irritation

(continued)

NURSING ACTIONS	RATIONALE/EXPLANATION
vein or into IV infusion tubing. Immediately before injection, dilute with an equal volume of sterile water for injection, sodium chloride injection, or 5% dextrose injection.	
(7) Give IV **midazolam** slowly, over approximately 2 minutes, after diluting the dose with 0.9% sodium chloride injection or 5% dextrose in water.	Rapid IV injection may cause severe respiratory depression and apnea; dilution facilitates slow injection.
(8) Midazolam may be mixed in the same syringe with morphine sulfate, meperidine, and atropine sulfate.	No apparent chemical or physical incompatibilities occur with these substances.
d. When giving **barbiturates** parenterally, do not give solutions that are cloudy or contain a precipitate. Do not mix with any other drugs in the same syringe. Give IM injections deeply into a large muscle mass. Give IV injections slowly and have equipment available for artificial ventilation. Be very careful to avoid extravasation of the drug into surrounding tissues and accidental intra-arterial injection.	Parenteral barbiturate solutions are highly alkaline and irritating to tissues. These precautions are needed to ensure safe administration and minimize tissue irritation.
e. Give **hydroxyzine** orally or deep IM only. When given IM for preoperative sedation, it can be mixed in the same syringe with atropine, meperidine, and most other opioid analgesics likely to be ordered at the same time.	IM hydroxyzine is very irritating to tissues.
f. Give **clomipramine** in divided doses, with meals, initially; after titration to a stable dose, give the total daily dose at bedtime.	Giving with meals decreases adverse effects on the GI tract; giving the total dose once daily at bedtime decreases daytime sedation.
2. Observe for therapeutic effects	Therapeutic effects depend largely on the reason for use. With benzodiazepines, decreased anxiety and drowsiness may appear within a few minutes.
a. When a drug is given for antianxiety effects, observe for:	
(1) An appearance of being relaxed, perhaps drowsy, but easily aroused	With buspirone, antianxiety effects may occur within 7 to 10 days of regular use, with optimal effects in 3 to 4 weeks.
(2) Verbal statements such as "less worried," "more relaxed," "resting better"	
(3) Decrease in or absence of manifestations of anxiety, such as rigid posture, facial grimaces, crying, elevated blood pressure and heart rate	
b. When a drug is given for hypnotic effects, drowsiness should be evident within approximately 30 minutes, and the client usually sleeps for several hours.	
c. When diazepam or lorazepam is given IV for control of acute convulsive disorders, seizure activity should decrease or stop almost immediately. When a drug is given for chronic anticonvulsant effects, lack of seizure activity is a therapeutic effect.	

(*continued*)

NURSING ACTIONS	RATIONALE/EXPLANATION
d. When hydroxyzine is given for nausea and vomiting, absence of vomiting and verbal statements of relief indicate therapeutic effects.	
e. When hydroxyzine is given for antihistaminic effects in skin disorders, observe for decreased itching and fewer statements of discomfort.	
3. Observe for adverse effects	Most adverse effects are caused by central nervous system (CNS) depression.
a. Excessive sedation—drowsiness, stupor, difficult to arouse, impaired mental processes, impaired mobility, respiratory depression, confusion	These effects are more likely to occur with large doses or if the recipient is elderly, debilitated, or has liver disease that slows drug metabolism. Respiratory depression and apnea stem from depression of the respiratory center in the medulla oblongata; they are most likely to occur with large doses or rapid IV administration of diazepam, lorazepam, or midazolam. Excessive drowsiness is more likely to occur when drug therapy is begun, and it usually decreases within a week.
b. Hypotension	Hypotension probably results from depression of the vasomotor center in the brain and is more likely to occur with large doses or rapid IV administration of diazepam, lorazepam, or midazolam.
c. Pain and induration at injection sites	Parenteral solutions are irritating to tissues.
d. Paradoxical excitement, anger, aggression, and hallucinations	
e. Chronic intoxication—sedation, confusion, emotional lability, muscular incoordination, impaired mental processes, mental depression, GI problems, weight loss	These signs and symptoms may occur with benzodiazepines or barbiturates and are similar to those occurring with chronic alcohol abuse (see Chap. 15).
f. Withdrawal or abstinence syndrome—anxiety, insomnia, restlessness, irritability, tremors, postural hypotension, seizures	These signs and symptoms may occur when benzodiazepines or barbiturates are discontinued abruptly, especially after high doses or long-term use.
g. With buspirone, the most common adverse effects are headache, dizziness, nausea, nervousness, fatigue, and excitement. Less frequent effects include dry mouth, chest pain, tachycardia, palpitations, drowsiness, confusion, and depression	
h. With zolpidem, common adverse effects include daytime drowsiness, dizziness, headache, nausea and diarrhea. Less frequent effects include ataxia, confusion, paradoxical excitation, allergic reactions.	
4. Observe for drug interactions	
a. Drugs that *increase* effects of antianxiety and sedative-hypnotic drugs:	
(1) CNS depressants—alcohol, opioid analgesics, tricyclic antidepressants, antihistamines, phenothiazine and other antipsychotic agents	All these drugs produce CNS depression when given alone. Any combination increases CNS depression, sedation, and respiratory depression. Combinations of these drugs are hazardous and *(continued)*

NURSING ACTIONS	RATIONALE/EXPLANATION
	should be avoided. Ingesting alcohol with antianxiety or sedative-hypnotic drugs may cause respiratory depression, coma, and convulsions. Although buspirone does not appear to cause additive CNS depression, concurrent use with other CNS depressants is best avoided.
(2) Cimetidine, disulfiram, fluoxetine, fluvoxamine, isoniazid, ketoconazole, metoprolol, nefazodone, omeprazole, oral contraceptives, propranolol, ritonavir, valproic acid	These drugs interfere with the hepatic metabolism of diazepam and other benzodiazepines. They do not affect elimination of lorazepam or oxazepam.
b. Drugs that *decrease* effects of antianxiety and sedative-hypnotic agents:	
(1) CNS stimulants—appetite suppressants (eg, phenylpropanolamine), bronchodilators (eg, albuterol, theophylline), nasal decongestants (eg, phenylephrine, phenylpropanolamine, pseudoephedrine), and social drugs (eg, caffeine, nicotine)	Phenylpropanolamine is the active ingredient in over-the-counter (OTC) diet aids such as Dexatrim and a component of multisymptom cold remedies. Phenylephrine and pseudoephedrine are available alone or in multisymptom cold remedies. OTC asthma remedies are also CNS stimulants.
(2) Enzyme inducers (eg, barbiturates)	With chronic use, these drugs antagonize their own actions and the actions of other drugs metabolized in the liver. They increase the rate of drug metabolism and elimination from the body.
c. Drugs that *increase* effects of barbiturates (in addition to those that increase effects of antianxiety and sedative-hypnotic agents in general):	
(1) Acidifying agents (eg, ascorbic acid)	These agents increase absorption of barbiturates in the GI tract and increase drug reabsorption in renal tubules (except for phenobarbital).
(2) Benzodiazepines (eg, diazepam)	May potentiate sedative and respiratory effects of barbiturates
d. Drugs that *decrease* effects of barbiturates:	
(1) Alkalinizing agents (eg, sodium bicarbonate)	Increase renal excretion of phenobarbital; have been used in treating phenobarbital overdose
e. Drug that increases effects of zolpidem:	
(1) Ritonavir	Inhibits hepatic metabolism of zolpidem and may cause severe sedation and respiratory depression. **These drugs should not be given concurrently.**

Nursing Notes: Apply Your Knowledge

Answer: Xanax, a benzodiazepine, is used for short-term treatment of anxiety. The length of time and high dose of Xanax indicates that Ms. Summers has developed tolerance to this drug. Alcohol works synergistically with benzodiazepines to increase effects such as central nervous system depression and sedation. The nurse should consult with the surgeon and anesthesiologist concerning Ms. Summers' use of Xanax and alcohol. Abruptly stopping these medications before surgery could result in withdrawal. A long-term plan that avoids dependence on benzodiazepines should be developed to assist Ms. Summers with her anxiety.

REVIEW AND APPLICATION EXERCISES

1. What is anxiety, and how may it be manifested?
2. How do benzodiazepines act to relieve anxiety?
3. What are some nonpharmacologic interventions to decrease anxiety?
4. When assessing a client before giving an antianxiety benzodiazepine, what assessment data would cause the nurse to omit the dose?
5. Why is sleep necessary? What functions does sleep fulfill?
6. Why are nonpharmacologic interventions to promote relaxation and sleep usually preferred over the use of sedative-hypnotic drugs?
7. What is the main difference between sedatives and hypnotics?
8. In terms of nursing care, what difference does it make whether a benzodiazepine is metabolized to active or inactive metabolites?
9. What are drug dependence, tolerance, and withdrawal symptoms in relation to the benzodiazepines?
10. What are some special precautions for using sedatives and hypnotics in older adults and those with renal or hepatic impairment or critical illness?
11. For an ambulatory client beginning a prescription for a benzodiazepine antianxiety or hypnotic agent, what instructions must be emphasized for safe, effective, and rational drug use?
12. When assisting in home care of a client taking a benzodiazepine, what kinds of data would the nurse collect to evaluate whether the client is using the drug appropriately or abusing it?

SELECTED REFERENCES

Baldessarini, R.J. (1996). Drugs and the treatment of psychiatric disorders: Psychosis and anxiety. In J.G. Hardman, L.E. Limbird, P.B. Molinoff, & R.W. Ruddon (Eds.), *Goodman & Gilman's The pharmacological basis of therapeutics*, 9th ed., pp. 399–430. New York: McGraw-Hill.

Birmaker, B., Yelovich, K., & Renaud, J. (1998). Pharmacologic treatment for children and adolescents with anxiety disorders. *Pediatric Clinics of North America, 45*, 1187–1204.

Drug facts and comparisons. (Updated monthly). St. Louis: Facts and Comparisons.

Flaherty, J.H. (1998). Psychotherapeutic agents in older adults. Commonly prescribed and over-the-counter remedies: Causes of confusion. *Clinics in Geriatric Medicine 14*, 101–127.

Hobbs, W.R., Rall, T.W., & Verdoorn, T.A. (1996). Hypnotics and sedatives; ethanol. In J.G. Hardman, L.E. Limbird, P.B. Molinoff, & R.W. Ruddon (Eds.), *Goodman & Gilman's The pharmacological basis of therapeutics*, 9th ed., pp. 361–396. New York: McGraw-Hill.

Kirkwood, C.K. & Hayes, P.E. (1997). Anxiety disorders. In J.T. DiPiro, R.L. Talbert, P.E. Hayes, G.C. Yee, G.R. Matzke, B.G. Wells, & L.M. Posey (Eds.), *Pharmacotherapy: A pathophysiologic approach*, 3rd ed., pp. 1443–1462. Stamford, CT: Appleton & Lange.

Kirkwood, C.K. & Sood, R.K. (1997). Sleep disorders. In J.T. DiPiro, R.L. Talbert, P.E. Hayes, G.C. Yee, G.R. Matzke, B.G. Wells, & L.M. Posey (Eds.), *Pharmacotherapy: A pathophysiologic approach*, 3rd ed., pp. 1477–1488. Stamford, CT: Appleton & Lange.

Pies, R.W. (1998). *Handbook of essential psychopharmacology.* Washington, DC: American Psychiatric Press, Inc.

Tosyali, M.C. & Greenhill, L.L. (1998). Child and adolescent psychopharmacology. *Pediatric Clinics of North America 45*, 1021–1035.

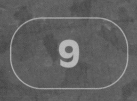

9

Antipsychotic Drugs

Objectives

After studying this chapter, the student will be able to:

1. Discuss common manifestations of psychotic disorders, including schizophrenia.

2. Discuss characteristics of phenothiazines and related antipsychotics in terms of mechanism of action, indications for use, adverse effects, nursing process implications, and principles of therapy.

3. Compare characteristics of "atypical" antipsychotic drugs with those of "typical" phenothiazines and related antipsychotic drugs.

4. Describe the main elements of acute and long-term treatment of psychotic disorders.

5. List interventions to decrease adverse effects of antipsychotic drugs.

6. State interventions to promote compliance with outpatient use of antipsychotic drugs.

As a nurse in an acute psychiatric facility, you attend the family conference for a young man who has recently been diagnosed as schizophrenic and started on antipsychotic medications. It is apparent that the family members are in shock, still not believing that a member of their family could be mentally ill. They also have just experienced a very stressful week in which the young man was psychotic, experiencing delusions and severe agitation and threatening the family.

Reflect on:

▶ How would you feel if someone you love is diagnosed with a serious, chronic mental health condition? How are these feelings similar to or different from when a loved one is diagnosed with a chronic physical condition?

▶ What questions do you think these family members might ask about schizophrenia or the medications prescribed to control it?

▶ What factors might influence compliance with antipsychotic medications?

PSYCHOSIS

Antipsychotic drugs are used mainly for the treatment of *psychosis*, a severe mental disorder characterized by disordered thought processes (disorganized and often bizarre thinking); blunted or inappropriate emotional responses; bizarre behavior ranging from hypoactivity to hyperactivity with agitation, aggressiveness, hostility, and combativeness; autism (self-absorption in which the person pays no attention to the environment or to other people); deterioration from previous levels of occupational and social functioning (poor self-care and interpersonal skills); hallucinations; and paranoid delusions. *Hallucinations* are sensory perceptions of people or objects that are not present in the external environment. More specifically, people see, hear, or feel stimuli that are not visible to external observers and cannot distinguish between these false perceptions and reality. Hallucinations occur with delirium, dementias, schizophrenia, and other psychotic states. Those occurring in schizophrenia or bipolar affective disorder are usually auditory, those in delirium are usually visual or tactile, and those in dementias are usually visual. *Delusions* are false beliefs that persist in the absence of reason or evidence. Deluded people often believe that other people control their thoughts, feelings, and behaviors or seek to harm them (paranoia). Delusions indicate severe mental illness. Although they are commonly associated with schizophrenia, delusions also occur with delirium, dementias, and other psychotic disorders.

Psychosis may be acute or chronic. Acute episodes, also called confusion or delirium, have a sudden onset over hours to days and may be precipitated by physical disorders (eg, brain damage related to cerebrovascular disease or head injury, metabolic disorders, infections); drug intoxication with adrenergics, antidepressants, some anticonvulsants, amphetamine, cocaine, and others; and drug withdrawal after chronic use (eg, alcohol, benzodiazepine antianxiety or sedative-hypnotic agents). In addition, acute psychotic episodes may be superimposed on chronic dementias and psychoses, such as schizophrenia. This chapter focuses primarily on schizophrenia as a chronic psychosis.

SCHIZOPHRENIA

Although schizophrenia is often referred to as a single disease, it includes a variety of related disorders. Risk factors include a genetic predisposition and environmental stresses. Symptoms may begin gradually or suddenly, usually during adolescence or early adulthood. According to the American Psychiatric Association's *Diagnostic and Statistical Manual of Mental Disorders*, 4th Edition (Revised), overt psychotic symptoms must be present for 6 months before schizophrenia can be diagnosed.

Behavioral manifestations of schizophrenia are categorized as positive and negative symptoms. Positive symptoms are characterized by central nervous system (CNS) stimulation and include agitation, delusions, hallucinations, insomnia, and paranoia. Negative symptoms are characterized by a lack of pleasure (anhedonia), a lack of motivation, a blunted affect, poor grooming and hygiene, poor social skills, and poverty of speech. However, all of these symptoms may occur with other disorders.

Etiology

Although the etiology is unclear, there is evidence that schizophrenia results from dysfunction of the dopaminergic and other neurotransmission systems in the brain (see Chap. 5). The dopaminergic system has been more extensively studied than other systems because schizophrenia has long been attributed to increased dopamine activity in the brain. This etiology is supported by the findings that antipsychotic drugs exert their therapeutic effects by decreasing dopamine activity (ie, blocking dopamine receptors) and that drugs that increase dopamine levels in the brain (eg, bromocriptine, levodopa) can cause signs and symptoms of psychosis.

In addition to the increased amount of dopamine, dopamine receptors are also involved. Two groups of dopamine receptors have been differentiated, mainly by the effects of the dopamine–receptor complex on intracellular functions. One group consists of D_1 and D_5 receptors, which stimulate cellular functions. The other group consists of D_2, D_3, and D_4 receptors, which decrease cellular functions and alter the movement of calcium and potassium ions across neuronal cell membranes. The D_2 group of dopamine receptors is considered important in the pathophysiology of schizophrenia; antipsychotic drugs bind to these receptors and block the action of dopamine (Fig. 9-1).

Thus, at the cellular level, dopamine activity is determined by its interaction with various receptors and the simultaneous actions of other neurotransmitters at the same target neurons.

In addition to dopamine, other neurotransmitters and receptors may be involved in producing psychosis. One indication of such involvement is the wide variety of drugs that may cause psychosis, including adrenergics (increase norepinephrine), antidepressants (increase norepinephrine, serotonin, or both), some anticonvulsants (increase the effects of gamma-aminobutyric acid), and others with unknown effects on neurotransmitters and receptors. Amino acid neurotransmitters, especially glutamate, are also receiving attention as possible etiologic factors.

Schizophrenia is a complex disorder and probably has multiple etiologies. Current emphasis is on abnormal neurotransmission systems in the brain. In addition to the dopaminergic system, there is evidence of abnormalities in the

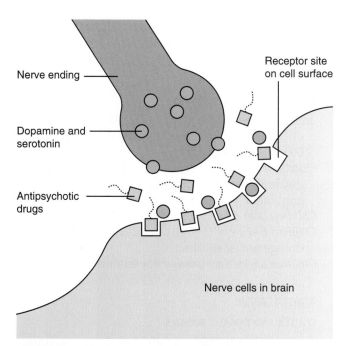

FIGURE 9–1 Antipsychotic drugs prevent dopamine and serotonin from occupying receptor sites on neuronal cell membranes and exerting their effects on cellular functions. This action leads to changes in receptors and cell functions that account for therapeutic effects (ie, relief of psychotic symptoms).

Nerve ending

Dopamine and serotonin

Antipsychotic drugs

Receptor site on cell surface

Nerve cells in brain

glutamate and serotonin systems. There is also evidence of extensive interactions among neurotransmission systems, whereby other systems can alter dopaminergic activity. The disease probably results from imbalances and abnormal integration among neurotransmission systems.

ANTIPSYCHOTIC DRUGS

Antipsychotic drugs are derived from several chemical groups and broadly categorized as "typical" or traditional (phenothiazines and nonphenothiazines with similar pharmacologic actions) and the "atypical" agents. The term *atypical* is used for newer drugs that differ from older ones by producing few, if any, movement disorders (extrapyramidal symptoms) and possibly being more effective in relieving negative symptoms of schizophrenia. **Chlorpromazine** (Thorazine) is the prototype of the phenothiazines; **clozapine** (Clozaril) is the prototype of the atypical agents.

The phenothiazines, the largest group of antipsychotic drugs, have been used since the 1950s. They are well absorbed after oral and parenteral administration. With oral drugs, peak plasma levels occur in approximately 2 to 3 hours; with intramuscular (IM) administration, peak levels occur in approximately 20 to 30 minutes. Phenothiazines are distributed to most body tissues and reach high concentrations in the brain. They are metabolized in the liver by the cytochrome P450 enzyme system; several produce pharmacologically active metabolites. Metabolites

are excreted in urine. These drugs do not cause psychological dependence, but they may cause physical dependence manifested by withdrawal symptoms (eg, lethargy and difficulty sleeping) if abruptly discontinued.

Phenothiazines exert many effects in the body, including CNS depression, autonomic nervous system depression (antiadrenergic and anticholinergic effects), antiemetic effects, lowering of body temperature, hypersensitivity reactions, and others. They differ mainly in potency and adverse effects. Differences in potency are demonstrated by the fact that some phenothiazines (piperazine subgroup) are as effective in doses of a few milligrams as others (aliphatic and piperadine subgroups) are in doses of several hundred milligrams. All phenothiazines produce the same kinds of adverse effects, but the subgroups differ in the incidence and severity of particular adverse effects.

Some nonphenothiazines, such as thiothixene (Navane) and haloperidol (Haldol), differ chemically from the phenothiazines, but their pharmacologic actions, clinical uses, and adverse effects are similar to those of the phenothiazines.

The atypical agents, such as clozapine (Clozaril), have both similarities and differences compared with other antipsychotic drugs and with each other. The main similarity is their effectiveness in treating the positive symptoms of psychosis; the main differences are fewer extrapyramidal effects and perhaps greater effectiveness in relieving negative symptoms of schizophrenia. The drugs' ability to decrease adverse effects is seen as a significant advantage because clients are more likely to take the drugs. Better compliance with drug therapy helps to prevent acute episodes of psychosis and repeated hospitalizations. A disadvantage is that these drugs are much more expensive than the older ones.

Mechanism of Action

Most antipsychotic drugs occupy or block dopamine receptors in the brain, thereby decreasing the effects of dopamine. However, drug binding to the receptors does not explain antipsychotic effects because binding occurs within a few hours after a drug dose and antipsychotic effects may not occur until the drugs have been given for a few weeks. Manifestations of hyperarousal (eg, anxiety, agitation, hyperactivity, insomnia, aggressive or combative behavior) are relieved more quickly than hallucinations, delusions, and thought disorders. One view of the delayed effects is that the blockade of dopamine receptors leads to changes in the receptors and postreceptor effects on cell metabolism and function. With chronic drug administration (ie, chronic blockade of dopamine receptors), there is an increased number of dopamine receptors on postsynaptic and possibly presynaptic nerve cell membranes (up-regulation). Clozapine and other atypical agents block both dopamine and serotonin receptors.

Overall, the drugs apparently reregulate the abnormal neurotransmission systems associated with psychosis.

Indications for Use

The major clinical indication for use of antipsychotic drugs is schizophrenia. The drugs also are used to treat psychotic symptoms associated with brain impairment induced by head injury, tumor, stroke, alcohol withdrawal, overdoses of CNS stimulant drugs, and other disorders. They may be useful in the manic phase of bipolar affective disorder to control manic behavior until lithium, the drug of choice, becomes effective.

The phenothiazines are also used for clinical indications not associated with psychiatric illness. These include treatment of nausea, vomiting, and intractable hiccups. The drugs relieve nausea and vomiting by blocking dopamine receptors in the chemoreceptor trigger zone, a group of neurons in the medulla oblongata that causes nausea and vomiting when activated by physical or psychological stimuli. The mechanism by which the drugs relieve hiccups is unclear.

Contraindications to Use

Because of their wide-ranging adverse effects, antipsychotic drugs may cause or aggravate a number of conditions. Thus, they are contraindicated in clients with liver damage, coronary artery disease, cerebrovascular disease, parkinsonism, bone marrow depression, severe hypotension or hypertension, coma, or severely depressed states. They should be used cautiously in seizure disorders, diabetes mellitus, glaucoma, prostatic hypertrophy, peptic ulcer disease, and chronic respiratory disorders.

INDIVIDUAL ANTIPSYCHOTIC DRUGS

Phenothiazines

Commonly used phenothiazine antipsychotic drugs are listed in Table 9-1. **Promethazine** (Phenergan) is a phenothiazine that is not used clinically for antipsychotic effects but is often used for sedative, antiemetic, and antihistaminic effects.

Phenothiazine-Similar Drugs

Chlorprothixene (Taractan) and **thiothixene** (Navane) are thioxanthenes. They are used clinically only for their antipsychotic effects, although they produce other effects similar to those of the phenothiazines. A 100-mg dose of chlorprothixene is therapeutically equivalent to 100 mg

of chlorpromazine; a 4-mg dose of thiothixene is equivalent to 100 mg of chlorpromazine.

Chlorprothixene

ROUTES AND DOSAGE RANGES

Adults: Acute psychosis, oral (PO), IM 75–200 mg/d in divided doses, increased to a maximal oral dose of 600 mg/d, if necessary
Elderly or debilitated adults: PO, IM 30–100 mg/d in divided doses, reduced when symptoms have been controlled
Children over 12 y: IM, same as adults
Children 6–12 y: PO 30–100 mg/d in divided doses; IM dosage not established
Children under 6 y: Dosage not established

Thiothixene

ROUTES AND DOSAGE RANGES

Adults: PO 6–10 mg/d in divided doses; maximum 60 mg/d
Acute psychosis, IM 8–16 mg/d in divided doses; maximum 30 mg/d
Elderly or debilitated adults: PO, IM one third to one half the usual adult dosage
Children 12 y and older: Same as adults
Children under 12 y: Dosage not established

Haloperidol (Haldol) is a butyrophenone and the only drug of this group available for use in psychiatric disorders; a related drug, droperidol (Inapsine), is used in anesthesia and as an antiemetic. Haloperidol is a frequently used antipsychotic agent that is chemically different but pharmacologically similar to the phenothiazines. A potent, long-acting drug, it is readily absorbed after oral or intramuscular administration, metabolized in the liver, and excreted in urine and bile. Haloperidol may cause adverse effects similar to those of the phenothiazines and thioxanthenes. Usually, it produces a relatively low incidence of hypotension and sedation and a high incidence of extrapyramidal effects.

Haloperidol is used as the initial drug for treating psychotic disorders or as a substitute in clients who are hypersensitive or refractory to the phenothiazines. It also is used for some conditions in which other antipsychotic drugs are not used, including mental retardation with hyperkinesia (abnormally increased motor activity), Tourette syndrome (a rare disorder characterized by involuntary movements and vocalizations), and Huntington's disease (a rare genetic disorder that involves progressive psychiatric symptoms and involuntary movements). A 2-mg dose is therapeutically equivalent to 100 mg of chlorpromazine. For clients who are unable or unwilling to take the oral drug as prescribed, a slowly absorbed, long-acting formulation (haloperidol decanoate) may be given intramuscularly, once monthly.

(*text continues on page 135*)

TABLE 9-1 Phenothiazine Antipsychotic Drugs

Generic/Trade Name	Routes of Administration and Dosage Ranges	Major Side Effects (Incidence)			Remarks
		Sedation	Extrapyramidal Reactions	Hypotension	
Acetophenazine (Tindal)	*Adults:* PO 60 mg daily in divided doses, may be gradually increased by 20 mg daily until therapeutic or adverse effects occur. Usual optimal dosage is 80–120 mg daily. *Elderly or debilitated adults:* one third to one half usual adult dose *Children:* 0.8–1.6 mg/kg per day in 3 divided doses (maximum, 80 mg daily)	Moderate	High	Low	20 mg is equivalent to 100 mg of chlorpromazine.
Chlorpromazine (Thorazine)	*Adults:* PO 200–600 mg daily in divided doses. Dose may be increased by 100 mg daily q2–3 days until symptoms are controlled, adverse effects occur, or a maximum daily dose of 2 g is reached. IM 25–100 mg initially for acute psychotic symptoms, repeated in 1–4 hours PRN until control is achieved. *Elderly or debilitated adults:* PO one third to one half usual adult dose, increased by 25 mg daily q2–3 days if necessary. IM 10 mg q6–8h until acute symptoms are controlled *Children:* PO, IM 0.5 mg/kg q4–8h. Maximum IM dose, 40 mg daily in children under 5 y of age and 75 mg for older children	High	Moderate	Moderate to high	Sustained-release capsules and liquid concentrates are available.
Fluphenazine decanoate and enanthate (Prolixin Decanoate; Prolixin Enanthate)	*Adults under 50 y:* IM; SC 12.5 mg initially followed by 25 mg every 2 weeks. Dosage requirements rarely exceed 100 mg q2–6 wk. *Adults over 50 y, debilitated clients, or clients with a history of extrapyramidal reactions:* 2.5 mg initially followed by 2.5–5 mg q10–14 days *Children:* No dosage established	Low to moderate	High	Low	
Fluphenazine hydrochloride (Prolixin, Permitil)	*Adults:* PO 2.5–10 mg initially, gradually reduced to maintenance dose of 1–5 mg (doses above 3 mg are rarely necessary). Acute psychosis: 1.25 mg initially, increased gradually to 2.5–10 mg daily in 3–4 divided doses *Elderly or debilitated adults:* PO 1–2.5 mg daily; IM one third to one half the usual adult dose *Children:* PO 0.75–10 mg daily in children 5 to 12 y. IM no dosage established	Low to moderate	High	Low	2 mg of the oral hydrochloride salt is equivalent to 100 mg of chlorpromazine.

(continued)

TABLE 9-1 **Phenothiazine Antipsychotic Drugs** (*continued*)

Generic/Trade Name	Routes of Administration and Dosage Ranges	Major Side Effects (Incidence)			Remarks
		Sedation	Extrapyramidal Reactions	Hypotension	
Mesoridazine (Serentil)	*Adults and children over 12 y:* PO 150 mg daily in divided doses initially, increased gradually in 50-mg increments until symptoms are controlled. Usual dose range, 100–400 mg. IM 25–175 mg daily in divided doses *Elderly and debilitated adults:* one third to one half usual adult dose *Children under 12 y:* no dosage established	High	Low	Moderate	50 mg is equivalent to 100 mg of chlorpromazine.
Perphenazine (Trilafon)	*Adults:* PO 16–64 mg daily in divided doses. Acute psychoses: IM 5–10 mg initially, then 5 mg q6h if necessary. Maximum daily dose, 15 mg for ambulatory clients and 30 mg for hospitalized clients *Elderly or debilitated adults:* PO, IM one-third to one-half usual adult dose *Children:* PO dosages not established, but the following amounts have been given in divided doses: ages 1–6 y, 4–6 mg daily; 6–12 y, 6 mg daily; over 12 y, 6–12 mg daily	Low to moderate	High	Low	8 mg is equivalent to 100 mg of chlorpromazine.
Prochlorperazine (Compazine)	*Adults:* PO 10 mg 3–4 times daily, increased gradually (usual daily dose, 100–150 mg). IM 10–20 mg; may be repeated in 2–4 h. Switch to oral form as soon as possible. *Children over 2 y:* PO, rectal 2.5 mg 2–3 times daily, IM 0.06 mg/lb	Moderate	High	Low	10 mg is equivalent to 100 mg of chlorpromazine.
Promazine (Sparine)	*Adults:* Initially, 50–150 mg IM; maintenance, PO, IM 10–200 mg q4–6h *Children over 12 y:* 10–25 mg q4–6h	Moderate	Moderate	Moderate	200 mg is equivalent to 100 mg of chlorpromazine.
Thioridazine (Mellaril)	*Adults:* PO 150–300 mg daily in divided doses, gradually increased if necessary to a maximum daily dose of 800 mg *Elderly or debilitated adults:* PO one third to one half the usual adult dose *Children 2 y and over:* 1 mg/kg per day in divided doses. Maximum dose, 3 mg/kg per day *Children under 2 y:* no dosage established	High	Low	Moderate	Thioridazine lacks antiemetic effects and has little, if any, effect on seizure threshold; 100 mg is equivalent to 100 mg of chlorpromazine.

(*continued*)

TABLE 9-1 **Phenothiazine Antipsychotic Drugs** (*continued*)

Generic/Trade Name	Routes of Administration and Dosage Ranges	Major Side Effects (Incidence)			Remarks
		Sedation	Extrapyramidal Reactions	Hypotension	
Trifluoperazine (Stelazine)	*Adults:* Outpatients PO 2–4 mg daily in divided doses. Hospitalized clients, PO 4–10 mg daily in divided doses. Acute psychoses: IM 1–2 mg q4–5h, maximum of 10 mg daily *Elderly or debilitated adults:* PO, IM one third to one half usual adult dose. If given IM, give at less frequent intervals than above. *Children 6 y and over:* PO, IM 1–2 mg daily, maximum daily dose 15 mg *Children under 6 y:* no dosage established	Moderate	High	Low	5 mg is equivalent to 100 mg of chlorpromazine.

IM, intramuscular; PO, oral.

ROUTES AND DOSAGE RANGES

Adults: Acute psychosis, PO 1–15 mg/d initially in divided doses, gradually increased to 100 mg/d, if necessary; usual maintenance dose, 2–8 mg daily; IM 2–10 mg q1–8h until symptoms are controlled (usually within 72 h)

Chronic schizophrenia, PO 6–15 mg/d; maximum 100 mg/d; dosage is reduced for maintenance, usually 15–20 mg/d. Haloperidol decanoate IM, initial dose up to 100 mg, depending on the previous dose of oral drug, then titrated according to response. Usually given every 4 weeks

Tourette syndrome, PO 6–15 mg/d; maximum 100 mg/d; usual maintenance dose, 9 mg/d

Mental retardation with hyperkinesia, PO 80–120 mg/d, gradually reduced to a maintenance dose of approximately 60 mg/d; IM 20 mg/d in divided doses, gradually increased to 60 mg/d if necessary. Oral administration should be substituted after symptoms are controlled.

Elderly or debilitated adults: Same as for children <12 y

Children 12 y and older: Acute psychosis, chronic refractory schizophrenia, Tourette syndrome, mental retardation with hyperkinesia: same as for adults

Children under 12 y: Acute psychosis, PO 0.5–1.5 mg/d initially, gradually increased in increments of 0.5 mg; usual maintenance dose, 2–4 mg/d. IM dosage not established.

Chronic refractory schizophrenia, dosage not established

Tourette syndrome, PO 1.5–6 mg/d initially in divided doses; usual maintenance dose, approximately 1.5 mg/d

Mental retardation with hyperkinesia, PO 1.5 mg/d initially in divided doses, gradually increased to a maximum of 15 mg/d, if necessary. When symptoms are controlled, dosage is gradually reduced to the minimum effective level. IM dosage not established.

Loxapine (Loxitane) is pharmacologically similar to phenothiazines and related drugs. It is recommended for use only in the treatment of schizophrenia.

ROUTE AND DOSAGE RANGES

Adults and adolescents 16 y and older: PO 10 mg twice a day to a total of 50 mg/d in severe psychoses; usual maintenance dose 60–100 mg/d; maximum dose, 250 mg/d

Elderly or debilitated adults: One third to one half the usual adult dosage

Children under 6 y: Dosage not established

Molindone (Moban) differs chemically from other agents but has similar pharmacologic actions. A 20-mg dose is equivalent to 100 mg of chlorpromazine.

ROUTE AND DOSAGE RANGES

Adults: PO 50–75 mg/d, increased gradually if necessary up to 225 mg/d, then reduced for maintenance; usual maintenance dose, 15–40 mg/d

Elderly or debilitated adults: One third to one half the usual adult dosage

Children under 12 y: Dosage not established

Pimozide (Orap) is an antipsychotic drug approved only for the treatment of Tourette syndrome in clients who fail to respond to haloperidol. Potentially serious adverse effects include tardive dyskinesia, major motor seizures, and sudden death.

ROUTE AND DOSAGE RANGE

Adults: PO 1–2 mg/d in divided doses initially, increased if necessary; usual maintenance dose, approximately 10 mg/d; maximum dose, 20 mg/d

Atypical Drugs

Clozapine (Clozaril), the prototype of the atypical agents, is chemically different from the older antipsychotic drugs. It blocks both dopamine and serotonin receptors in the brain. It is recommended only for clients with schizophrenia, for whom it may improve negative symptoms and does not cause the extrapyramidal effects (eg, acute dystonia, parkinsonism, akathisia, tardive dyskinesia) associated with most antipsychotic agents. Despite these advantages, however, it is considered a second-line drug, recommended only for clients who have not responded to treatment with at least two other antipsychotic drugs or who have disabling tardive dyskinesia. The reason for clozapine's second-line status is its association with agranulocytosis, a life-threatening decrease in white blood cells (WBCs), which usually occurs during the first 3 months of therapy. Weekly WBC counts are required. In addition, clozapine is reportedly more likely to cause constipation, dizziness, drowsiness, hypotension, seizures, and weight gain than other atypical agents (ie, olanzapine, quetiapine, risperidone).

ROUTE AND DOSAGE RANGE

Adults: PO 50–900 mg/d
Children: Dosage not established

Olanzapine (Zyprexa) is an atypical antipsychotic with therapeutic effects similar to those of clozapine, but its adverse effects may differ. Compared with clozapine, olanzapine may be more likely to cause extrapyramidal effects (eg, acute dystonia, parkinsonism, akathisia, tardive dyskinesia), but is less likely to cause agranulocytosis. Compared with typical antipsychotics, olanzapine reportedly causes less sedation, extrapyramidal symptoms, anticholinergic effects, and orthostatic hypotension.

The drug is well absorbed after oral administration; its absorption is not affected by food. A steady-state concentration is reached in approximately 1 week of once-daily administration. It is highly metabolized and excreted in urine and feces.

ROUTE AND DOSAGE RANGE

Adults: PO 5–10 mg/d initially; given once daily at bedtime; increased over several weeks to 20 mg/d, if necessary
Children: Dosage not established

Quetiapine (Seroquel), like the other atypical agents, blocks both dopamine and serotonin receptors and relieves both positive and negative symptoms of psychosis. After oral administration, quetiapine is well absorbed and may be taken without regard for meals. Peak plasma levels

are reached in 2 to 4 hours and last 8 to 10 hours. It is extensively metabolized in the liver by the cytochrome P450 enzyme system. Clinically significant drug interactions may occur with drugs that induce or inhibit the liver enzymes; dosage of quetiapine may need to be increased with enzyme inducers (eg, phenytoin) or decreased with enzyme inhibitors (eg, cimetidine, erythromycin). Common adverse effects include drowsiness, headache, orthostatic hypotension, and weight gain.

ROUTE AND DOSAGE RANGE

Adults: PO 25 mg bid initially; increased by 25–50 mg two or three times daily on second and third days, as tolerated, to a dosage range of 300–400 mg in two or three divided doses on the fourth day. Additional increments or decrements can be made at 2-day intervals; maximum dosage 800 mg/d.
Elderly or debilitated adults: Use lower initial doses and increase more gradually, to a lower target dose than for other adults
Hepatic impairment: PO, same as for elderly or debilitated adults
Children: Dosage not established

Risperidone (Risperdal), like other atypical antipsychotic agents, blocks both dopamine and serotonin receptors and relieves both positive and negative symptoms of psychosis. It was marketed in 1993 for the treatment of schizophrenia in people who did not respond to other antipsychotic drugs. Since then, however, it has become a frequently prescribed, first-choice agent. It is usually well tolerated, and client compliance is better than with older antipsychotic drugs.

Risperidone is well absorbed with oral administration, is metabolized mainly in the liver by the cytochrome P450 enzyme system, and produces an active metabolite. Effects are attributed approximately equally to risperidone and the metabolite. Elimination half-life is 20 to 30 hours; 70% is excreted in urine and 14% in feces. Peak blood levels occur in 1 to 2 hours, but therapeutic effects are delayed for 1 to 2 weeks. Adverse effects include agitation, anxiety, headache, insomnia, dizziness, and hypotension. It may also cause parkinsonism and other movement disorders, especially at higher doses, but is less likely to do so than phenothiazines and other typical drugs.

ROUTE AND DOSAGE RANGES

Adults: PO, initially 1 mg twice daily (2 mg/d); increase to 2 mg twice daily on the second day (4 mg/d); increase to 3 mg twice daily on the third day (6 mg/d), if necessary. Usual maintenance dose, 4 to 8 mg/d. After initial titration, dosage increases or decreases should be made at a rate of 1 mg/wk.
Elderly or debilitated adults: PO, initially 0.5 mg twice daily (1 mg/d); increase in 0.5-mg increments to 1.5 mg twice daily (3 mg/d)
Renal or hepatic impairment: PO, same as for elderly or debilitated adults
Children under 12 y: Dosage not established

You are assigned to care for John Chou, hospitalized 2 weeks ago and started on fluphenazine hydrochloride (Prolixin) to treat acute psychotic symptoms. During your assessment, John appears restless, unable to sit still, and uncoordinated. He also has a fine hand tremor. How would you interpret these data?

NURSING PROCESS

Assessment

Assess the client's mental health status, need for antipsychotic drugs, and response to drug therapy. There is a wide variation in response to drug therapy. Close observation of physical and behavioral reactions is necessary to evaluate effectiveness and to individualize dosage schedules. Accurate assessment is especially important when starting drug therapy and when increasing or decreasing dosage. Some assessment factors include the following:

- Interview the client and family members. Attempts to interview an acutely psychotic person yield little useful information because of the client's distorted perception of reality. The nurse may be able to assess the client's level of orientation and delusional and hallucinatory activity. If possible, try to determine from family members or others what the client was doing or experiencing when the acute episode began (ie, predisposing factors, such as increased environmental stress or alcohol or drug ingestion); whether this is a first or a repeated episode of psychotic behavior; whether the person has physical illnesses, takes any drugs, or uses alcohol; whether the client seems to be a hazard to self or others; and some description of pre-illness personality traits, level of social interaction, and ability to function in usual activities of daily living.
- Observe the client for the presence or absence of psychotic symptoms such as agitation, hyperactivity, combativeness, and bizarre behavior.
- Obtain baseline data to help monitor the client's response to drug therapy. Some authorities advocate initial and periodic laboratory tests of liver, kidney, and blood functions, as well as electrocardiograms. Although such tests do not help greatly in preventing adverse reactions, they may assist in earlier detection and treatment of adverse reactions. Baseline blood pressure readings also may be helpful.

- Continue assessing the client's response to drug therapy and his or her ability to function in activities of daily living, whether the client is hospitalized or receiving outpatient treatment.

Nursing Diagnoses

- Altered Thought Processes related to the disease, especially during the first few weeks of antipsychotic drug therapy
- Self-Care Deficit related to the disease process or drug-induced sedation
- Impaired Physical Mobility related to sedation
- Decreased Cardiac Output related to hypotension
- Altered Tissue Perfusion related to hypotension
- Risk for Injury related to excessive sedation and movement disorders (extrapyramidal effects)
- Risk for Violence: Self-Directed or Directed at Others
- Noncompliance related to underuse of prescribed drugs
- Knowledge Deficit: Expected recurrence of symptoms and hospitalization if drug therapy is not continued in chronic schizophrenia

Planning/Goals
The client will:

- Become less agitated within a few hours after drug therapy is started and less psychotic within a few days
- Be kept safe while sedated during early drug therapy
- Be cared for by staff in areas of nutrition, hygiene, exercise, and social interactions when unable to provide self-care
- Improve in ability to participate in self-care activities
- Avoid preventable adverse drug effects, especially those that impair safety
- Be helped to take medications as prescribed and return for follow-up appointments with health care providers

Interventions

Use nondrug measures when appropriate to increase the effectiveness of drug therapy and to decrease adverse reactions.

- Obviously, drug therapy will be ineffective if the client does not receive sufficient medication. For numerous reasons, many people are unable or unwilling to take medications as prescribed. Any nursing action aimed toward more accurate drug administration increases the effectiveness of drug therapy.

CLIENT TEACHING GUIDELINES
Antipsychotic Drugs

Antipsychotic drugs are given to clients with schizophrenia, a chronic mental illness. Because of the nature of the disease, a responsible adult caregiver is needed to prompt a client about taking particular doses and to manage other aspects of the drug therapy regimen, as follows.

General Considerations

✔ Ask about the planned drug therapy regimen, including the desired results, when results can be expected, and the tentative length of drug therapy.

✔ Maintain an adequate supply of medication to ensure regular administration. Consistent blood levels are necessary to control symptoms and prevent recurring episodes of acute illness and hospitalization.

✔ Do not allow the client to drive a car, operate machinery, or perform activities that require alertness when drowsy from medication. Drowsiness, slowed thinking, and impaired muscle coordination are especially likely during the first 2 weeks of drug therapy but tend to decrease with time.

✔ Report unusual side effects and all physical illnesses, because changes in drug therapy may be indicated.

✔ Try to prevent the client from taking unprescribed medications, including those available without prescription or those prescribed for another person, to prevent undesirable drug interactions. Alcohol and sleeping pills should be avoided because they may cause excessive drowsiness and decreased awareness of safety hazards in the environment.

✔ Keep all physicians informed about all the medications being taken by the client, to decrease risks of undesirable drug interactions.

✔ These drugs should be tapered in dosage and discontinued gradually; they should not be stopped abruptly.

Medication Administration

Assist or prompt the client to:

✔ Take medications in the correct doses and at the correct times, to maintain blood levels and beneficial effects.

✔ Avoid taking these medications with antacids. If an antacid is needed (eg, for heartburn), it should be taken 1 hour before or 2 hours after the antipsychotic drug. Antacids decrease absorption of these drugs from the intestine.

✔ Lie down for approximately an hour after receiving medication, if dizziness and faintness occur.

✔ Take the medication at bedtime, if able, so that drowsiness aids sleep and is minimized during waking hours.

✔ Practice good oral hygiene, including dental checkups, thorough and frequent toothbrushing, drinking fluids, and frequent mouth rinsing. Mouth dryness is a common side effect of the drugs. Although it is usually not serious, dry mouth can lead to mouth infections and dental cavities.

✔ Minimize exposure to sunlight, wear protective clothing, and use sunscreen lotions. Sensitivity to sunlight occurs with some of the drugs and may produce a sunburn-type of skin reaction.

✔ Avoid exposure to excessive heat. Some of these medications may cause fever and heat prostration with high environmental temperatures. In hot weather or climates, keep the client indoors and use air conditioning or fans during the hours of highest heat levels.

Specific nursing actions must be individualized to the client. Some general nursing actions that may be helpful include emphasizing the therapeutic benefits expected from drug therapy, answering questions or providing information about drug therapy and other aspects of the treatment plan, devising a schedule of administration times that is as convenient as possible for the client, giving the drug in the form (eg, syrup, capsule) most acceptable to the client, and assisting the client or caregiver in preventing or managing adverse drug effects. Most adverse effects are less likely to occur or be severe with the newer atypical drugs than with phenothiazines and other older drugs.

• Supervise ambulation to prevent falls or other injuries if the client is drowsy or elderly or has postural hypotension.

• Several measures can help prevent or minimize hypotension, such as having the client lie down for approximately an hour after a large oral dose or an injection of antipsychotic medication; applying elastic stockings; and instructing the client to change positions gradually, elevate legs when sitting, avoid standing for prolonged periods, and avoid hot baths (hot baths cause vasodilation and increase the incidence of hypotension). In addition, the daily dose can be decreased or divided into smaller amounts.

• Dry mouth and oral infections can be decreased by frequent brushing of the teeth, rinsing the mouth with water, chewing sugarless gum or candy, and ensuring an adequate fluid intake. Excessive water intake should be discouraged because it may lead to serum electrolyte deficiencies.

- The usual measures of increasing fluid intake, dietary fiber, and exercise can help prevent constipation.
- Support caregivers in efforts to maintain contact with inpatients and provide care for outpatients. One way is to provide caregivers with telephone numbers of health care providers and to make periodic telephone calls to caregivers.

Evaluation

- Interview the client to determine the presence and extent of hallucinations and delusions.
- Observe the client for decreased signs and symptoms. Document abilities and limitations in self-care.
- Note whether any injuries have occurred during drug therapy.
- Interview the caregiver about the client's behavior and medication response (ie, during a home visit or telephone call).

PRINCIPLES OF THERAPY

Goals of Treatment

For acute psychosis, the goal of treatment during the first week is to decrease symptoms (eg, aggression, agitation, combativeness, hostility) and normalize patterns of sleeping and eating. The next goal may be increased ability for self-care and increased socialization. Therapeutic effects usually occur gradually, over 1 to 2 months. Long-term goals include increasing the client's ability to cope with the environment, promoting optimal functioning in self-

Nursing Notes: Ethical/Legal Dilemma

Mr. Seager, 37 years of age and homeless, has been diagnosed and treated for schizophrenia and alcohol abuse for the last 15 years. He is admitted to the hospital for pneumonia. When you enter his room to administer his prescribed antipsychotic medication and his antibiotic, he swears at you and tells you to leave the room because he has no plans to take that poison.

Reflect on:

- Does Mr. Seager have the right to refuse to take his medication?
- Does his psychiatric history alter his rights?
- Role play how you would respond to Mr. Seager if you were the nurse in this situation.

care and activities of daily living, and preventing acute episodes and hospitalizations. With drug therapy, clients often can participate in psychotherapy, group therapy, or other treatment modalities; return to community settings; and return to their pre-illness level of functioning.

Drug Selection

The physician caring for a client with psychosis has a greater choice of drugs than ever before. Some general factors to consider include the client's age and physical condition, the severity and duration of illness, the frequency and severity of adverse effects produced by each drug, the response to antipsychotic drugs in the past, the subjective response to the drugs, the supervision available, and the physician's experience with a particular drug. Some specific factors include the following:

1. The atypical drugs (eg, olanzapine, risperidone) are probably the drugs of choice, especially for newly diagnosed schizophrenics, because they may be more effective in relieving some symptoms, they usually produce milder adverse effects, and clients seem to take them more consistently. A major drawback is their high cost.
2. The traditional or typical antipsychotic drugs are apparently equally effective, but some clients who do not respond well to one may respond to another. Because the drugs are similarly effective, some physicians base their choice on a drug's adverse effects. In addition, some physicians use a phenothiazine first and prescribe a nonphenothiazine as a second-line agent for clients with chronic schizophrenia whose symptoms have not been controlled by the phenothiazines and for clients with hypersensitivity reactions to the phenothiazines.
3. Unless the choice of drug is dictated by the client's previous favorable response to a particular drug, the preferred drug should be available in both parenteral and oral forms for flexibility of administration.
4. Clients who are unable or unwilling to take daily doses of a maintenance antipsychotic drug may be given periodic injections of a long-acting form of fluphenazine or haloperidol.
5. Any person who has had an allergic or hypersensitivity reaction to an antipsychotic drug usually should not be given that drug again or any drug in the same chemical subgroup. Cross-sensitivity occurs, and the likelihood of another allergic reaction is high.
6. There is no logical basis for giving more than one antipsychotic agent at a time. There is no therapeutic advantage, and the risk of serious adverse reactions is increased.
7. If therapeutic ineffectiveness or unacceptable adverse effects require that another antipsychotic drug be substituted for the one a client is currently

receiving, this substitution must be done gradually; abrupt substitution may cause reappearance of symptoms. This can be avoided by gradually decreasing doses of the old drug while substituting equivalent doses of the new one.

Dosage and Administration

Dosage and route of administration must be individualized according to the client's condition and response. Oral drugs undergo extensive first-pass metabolism in the liver so that a significant portion of a dose does not reach the systemic circulation and low serum drug levels are produced. In contrast, IM doses avoid first-pass metabolism and produce serum drug levels approximately double those of oral doses. Thus, usual IM doses are approximately half the oral doses.

Initial drug therapy for acute psychotic episodes usually requires high dosage, IM administration, divided doses, and hospitalization. Symptoms are usually controlled within 48 to 72 hours, after which oral drugs can be given and dosage gradually reduced to the lowest effective amount. For maintenance therapy, drug dosages are usually much smaller, oral drugs are preferred, and a single bedtime dose is effective for most clients. This schedule increases compliance with prescribed drug therapy, allows better nighttime sleep, and decreases hypotension and daytime sedation. Effective maintenance therapy requires close supervision and contact with the client and family members.

Duration of Therapy

In schizophrenia, antipsychotic drugs are usually given for years because there is a high rate of relapse (acute psychotic reactions) when drug therapy is discontinued, most often by clients who become unwilling or unable to continue their medication regimen. Drug therapy usually is indicated for at least 1 year after an initial psychotic episode and for at least 5 years, perhaps for life, after multiple episodes. Several studies indicate that low-dose, continuous maintenance therapy is effective in long-term prevention of recurrent psychosis. With wider use of maintenance therapy and the newer, better-tolerated antipsychotic drugs, clients may experience fewer psychotic episodes and hospitalizations.

Management of Drug Withdrawal

Antipsychotic drugs can cause symptoms of withdrawal when suddenly or rapidly discontinued. Specific symptoms are related to a drug's potency, extent of dopaminergic blockade, and its anticholinergic effects. Low-potency drugs (eg, chlorpromazine), for example, have strong anticholinergic effects and sudden withdrawal can cause cholinergic effects such as diarrhea, drooling, and insomnia. To prevent withdrawal symptoms, drugs should be tapered in dosage and gradually discontinued over several weeks.

Management of Extrapyramidal Symptoms

Extrapyramidal effects (eg, abnormal movements) are more likely to occur with older antipsychotic drugs than with the newer atypical agents. If they do occur, an anticholinergic antiparkinson drug (see Chap. 12) can be given. Such neuromuscular symptoms appear in fewer than half the clients taking traditional antipsychotic drugs and are better handled by reducing dosage, if this does not cause recurrence of psychotic symptoms. If antiparkinson drugs are given, they should be gradually discontinued in approximately 3 months. Extrapyramidal symptoms do not usually recur despite continued administration of the same antipsychotic drug at the same dosage.

Ethnic or Genetic Considerations

Antipsychotic drug therapy for nonwhite populations in the United States is based primarily on dosage recommendations, pharmacokinetic data, adverse effects, and other characteristics of antipsychotic drugs derived from white recipients. Most of the differences are attributed to variations in hepatic drug metabolizing enzymes. Those with strong enzyme activity are known as extensive or fast metabolizers, whereas those with slower rates of enzyme activity are poor or slow metabolizers. Fast metabolizers eliminate drugs rapidly and may need a larger-than-usual dose to achieve therapeutic effects; poor metabolizers eliminate drugs slowly and therefore are at risk of drug accumulation and adverse effects. Although little research has been done and other factors may be involved, several studies document differences in antipsychotic drug effects in nonwhite populations, including the following:

1. *African Americans* tend to respond more rapidly, experience a higher incidence of adverse effects, including tardive dyskinesia, and metabolize antipsychotic drugs more slowly than whites.

   In addition, compared with whites with psychotic disorders, African Americans may be given higher doses and more frequent injections of long-acting antipsychotic drugs, both of which may increase the incidence and severity of adverse effects.

2. *Asians* in general metabolize antipsychotic drugs slowly and therefore have higher plasma drug levels for a given dose than whites. Most studies have been done with haloperidol and in a limited number of Asian subgroups. Thus, it cannot be assumed that all antipsychotic drugs and all people of Asian

heritage respond in the same way. To avoid drug toxicity, initial doses should be approximately half the usual doses given to whites and later doses should be titrated according to clinical response and serum drug levels.

3. *Hispanics'* responses to antipsychotic drugs are largely unknown. Some are extremely fast metabolizers who may have low plasma drug levels in relation to a given dose.

Use in Perioperative Periods

A major concern about giving traditional antipsychotic drugs perioperatively is their potential for adverse interactions with other drugs. For example, the drugs potentiate the effects of general anesthetics and other CNS depressants that are often used before, during, and after surgery. As a result, risks of hypotension and excessive sedation are increased unless doses of other agents are reduced. If hypotension occurs and requires vasopressor drugs, phenylephrine (Neo-Synephrine) or norepinephrine (Levophed) should be used rather than epinephrine (Adrenalin) because antipsychotic drugs inhibit the vasoconstrictive (blood pressure–raising) effects of epinephrine. Guidelines for perioperative use of the newer atypical agents have not been developed. Cautious use is indicated because they may also cause hypotension, sedation, and other adverse effects.

Use in Children

Antipsychotic drugs are used mainly for childhood schizophrenia, which is often characterized by more severe symptoms and a more chronic course than adult schizophrenia. Drug therapy is largely empiric because few studies have been done in children and adolescents and few guidelines have been developed. A child's age, weight, and severity of symptoms are not usually helpful. Some considerations include the following:

1. Drug pharmacodynamics and pharmacokinetics are likely to be different in children, compared with adults. Pharmacodynamic differences may stem from changes in neurotransmission systems in the brain as the child grows. Pharmacokinetic differences may stem from changes in distribution or metabolism of drugs; absorption seems similar to that of adults. In relation to distribution, children usually have a lesser percentage of body fat than adults. Thus, antipsychotic drugs, which are highly lipid soluble, cannot be as readily stored in fat as they are in adults. This often leads to shorter half-lives and the need for more frequent administration. In relation to metabolism, children usually have a faster rate than adults and may therefore require relatively high doses for their size and weight. In relation to excretion, renal function is usually similar to that of adults and most of the drugs are largely inactivated by liver metabolism. Thus, with normal renal function, excretion probably has little effect on blood levels of active drug or the child's response to the drug.

2. It is not clear which types of antipsychotics are safest and most effective in children and adolescents. Traditional drugs are not usually recommended for children younger than 12 years of age. However, thioridazine, prochlorperazine, trifluoperazine, and haloperidol may be used in children aged 2 to 12 years. Some authors recommend the newer atypical drugs (eg, olanzapine, quetiapine, risperidone) because they are less likely to cause extrapyramidal effects than older agents. However, children's dosages have not been established for olanzapine or quetiapine.

3. Dosage regulation is difficult because children may require lower plasma levels for therapeutic effects, but they also metabolize antipsychotic drugs more rapidly than adults. A conservative approach is to begin with a low dose and increase it gradually (no more than once or twice a week), if necessary. Divided doses may be useful initially, with later conversion to once daily at bedtime. Older adolescents may require doses comparable with those of adults.

4. Adverse effects may be different in children. For example, extrapyramidal symptoms with conventional drugs are more likely to occur in children than adults. If they do occur, dosage reduction is more effective in alleviating them than the anticholinergic antiparkinson drugs commonly used in adults. In addition, hypotension is more likely to develop in children. Blood pressure should be closely monitored during initial dosage titration.

5. A treatment plan should include nonpharmacologic interventions, as for other populations.

Use in Older Adults

Antipsychotic drugs should be used cautiously in older adults. Before they are started, a thorough assessment is needed because psychiatric symptoms are often caused by organic disease or other drugs. If this is the case, treating the disease or stopping the offending drug may cancel the need for an antipsychotic drug. In addition, older adults are more likely to have problems in which the drugs are contraindicated (eg, severe cardiovascular disease, liver damage, Parkinson's disease) or must be used very cautiously (diabetes mellitus, glaucoma, prostatic hypertrophy, peptic ulcer disease, chronic respiratory disorders).

For older adults in long-term care facilities, there is concern that antipsychotic drugs may be overused to control agitated or disruptive behavior that is caused by non-psychotic disorders and for which other treatments are preferable. For example, clients with dementias may become agitated from environmental or medical problems. Alleviating such causes, when possible, is safer and more effective than administering antipsychotic drugs. Inappropriate use of the drugs exposes clients to adverse drug effects and does not resolve underlying problems. Because of the many implications for client safety and welfare, federal regulations were established for the use of antipsychotics in facilities receiving Medicare and Medicaid funds. These regulations include appropriate (eg, psychotic disorders, delusions, schizophrenia, and dementia and delirium that meet certain criteria) and inappropriate (eg, agitation not thought to indicate potential harm to the resident or others, anxiety, depression, uncooperativeness, wandering) indications. When the drugs are required for psychosis or dementia in older adults, considerations include the following:

1. *Drug selection.* With traditional antipsychotic drugs, chlorpromazine and thioridazine are not recommended because of their strong anticholinergic effects. Haloperidol and fluphenazine may be better tolerated but cause a high incidence of extrapyramidal symptoms. With atypical drugs, clozapine is a second-line agent because it produces many adverse effects. Olanzapine, quetiapine, and risperidone may be useful, but little information is available about their use in older adults.

2. *Dosage.* When the drugs are required, dosage should be reduced by 30% to 50% and increased gradually, if necessary, according to clinical response. The basic principle of "start low, go slow" is especially applicable. Once symptoms are controlled, dosage should be reduced to the lowest effective level. Some specific drugs and dosage ranges include haloperidol 0.25 to 1.5 mg qd to qid; clozapine 6.25 mg qd, initially; risperidone 0.5 mg qd, initially; quetiapine, a lower initial dose, slower dose titration, and a lower target dose in older adults.

   As in other populations, antipsychotic drugs should be tapered in dosage and discontinued gradually rather than discontinued abruptly.

3. *Adverse effects.* Older adults are at high risk of adverse effects because metabolism and excretion are usually slower or more likely to be impaired than in younger adults. With traditional antipsychotic drugs, anticholinergic effects (eg, confusion, memory impairment, hallucinations, urinary retention, constipation, heat stroke) may be especially problematic. In addition, cardiovascular (hypotension, arrhythmias) effects may be especially dangerous in older adults, who often have underlying cardiovascular diseases. Tardive dyskinesia, which may occur with long-term use of antipsychotic drugs, may develop more rapidly and at lower drug doses in older adults than in younger clients. There is also a risk of neuroleptic malignant syndrome, a rare but serious disorder characterized by confusion, dizziness, fever, and rigidity. Other adverse effects include oversedation, dizziness, confusion, and impaired mobility, which may contribute to falls and other injuries unless clients are carefully monitored and safeguarded. With atypical drugs, many of these adverse effects are less likely to occur, especially at the reduced doses recommended for older adults.

Use in Renal Impairment

Because most antipsychotic drugs are extensively metabolized in the liver and the metabolites are excreted through the kidneys, the drugs should be used cautiously in clients with impaired renal function. Renal function should be monitored periodically during long-term therapy. If renal function test results (eg, blood urea nitrogen) become abnormal, the drug may need to be lowered in dosage or discontinued. Because risperidone is metabolized to an active metabolite, recommended dosage reductions and titrations for clients with renal impairment are the same as those for older adults.

With highly sedating antipsychotic drugs, it may be difficult to assess the client for excessive sedation because drowsiness, lethargy, and mental status changes may also occur with renal impairment.

Use in Hepatic Impairment

Antipsychotic drugs undergo extensive hepatic metabolism and then elimination in urine. In the presence of liver disease (eg, cirrhosis, hepatitis), metabolism may be slowed and drug elimination half-lives prolonged, with resultant accumulation and increased risk of adverse effects. Thus, the drugs should be used cautiously in clients with hepatic impairment.

Jaundice has been associated with phenothiazines, usually after 2 to 4 weeks of therapy. It is considered a hypersensitivity reaction and clients should not be reexposed to a phenothiazine. If antipsychotic drug therapy is required in these clients, a drug from a different chemical group should be given. Overall, there is no conclusive evidence that preexisting liver impairment increases a client's risk for development of jaundice, and clients with alcoholic cirrhosis have been treated without complications. With risperidone, recommended dosage reductions and titrations for clients with hepatic impairment are the same as those for older adults. With quetiapine, higher plasma levels occur in clients with hepatic impairment and a slower rate of dose titration and a lower target dose are recommended.

Periodic liver function tests (eg, gamma-glutamyl transpeptidase, alkaline phosphatase, bilirubin) are probably indicated, especially with long-term therapy or the use of clozapine, haloperidol, phenothiazines, or thiothixenes.

Use in Critical Illness

Antipsychotic drugs are infrequently used in clients who are critically ill. Haloperidol is sometimes given to calm clients with acute agitation and delirium. Some physicians prefer to use a benzodiazepine-type of sedative because of the adverse effects associated with haloperidol.

For clients with chronic schizophrenia who are stabilized on an antipsychotic drug when they experience a critical illness, either continuing or stopping the drug may cause difficulties. Continuing the drug may worsen signs and symptoms of the critical illness (eg, hypotension); stopping it may cause symptoms of withdrawal.

Little information is available about the newer drugs. If quetiapine is used, very low doses are recommended in older adults, clients with hepatic impairment, debilitated

clients, and those predisposed to hypotension. A critically ill client could have all of these conditions.

 Home Care

Chronically mentally ill clients, such as those with schizophrenia, are among the most challenging in a home care nurse's caseload. Major recurring problems include failure to take antipsychotic medications as prescribed and the concurrent use of alcohol and other drugs of abuse. Either problem is likely to lead to acute psychotic episodes and hospitalizations. The home care nurse must assist and support caregivers' efforts to maintain medications and manage adverse drug effects, other aspects of daily care, and follow-up psychiatric care. In addition, the home care nurse may need to coordinate the efforts of several health and social service agencies or providers.

(*text continues on page 148*)

NURSING ACTIONS Antipsychotic Drugs

NURSING ACTIONS	RATIONALE/EXPLANATION
1. Administer accurately	
a. When feasible, give oral antipsychotic drugs once daily, within 1 to 2 hours of bedtime.	Peak sedation occurs approximately 2 hours after administration and aids sleep. Hypotension, dry mouth, and other adverse reactions are less bothersome with this schedule. Although antipsychotic drugs are probably more often prescribed in two or three daily doses, their long duration of action usually allows once-daily dosage.
b. When preparing oral concentrated solutions or parenteral solutions, try to avoid contact with the solution. If contact is made, wash the area immediately.	These solutions are irritating to the skin and many cause contact dermatitis.
c. Mix liquid concentrates with at least 60 mL of fruit juice or water just before administration.	To mask the taste. If the client does not like juice or water, check the package insert for other diluents. Some of the drugs may be mixed with coffee, tea, milk, or carbonated beverages.
d. Mix oral solution of risperidone with 3 to 4 oz of water, coffee, orange juice, or low-fat milk; do not mix with cola drinks or tea.	Manufacturer's recommendation
e. For intramuscular injections.	
(1) Give only those preparations labeled for intramuscular use.	
(2) Do not mix any other drugs in the same syringe with antipsychotic drugs.	These drugs are physically incompatible with many other drugs, and a precipitate may occur.
(3) Change the needle after filling the syringe for injection.	Parenteral solutions of these drugs are highly irritating to body tissues. Changing needles helps pro-

(continued)

NURSING ACTIONS	RATIONALE/EXPLANATION
	tect the tissues of the injection tract from unnecessary contact with the drug.
(4) Inject slowly and deeply into gluteal muscles.	Using a large muscle mass for the injection site decreases tissue irritation.
(5) Have the client lie down for 30 to 60 minutes after the injection.	To observe for adverse reactions. Orthostatic hypotension is likely if the client tries to ambulate.
f. Do not give antipsychotic drugs subcutaneously, except for fluphenazine decanoate and fluphenazine enanthate.	More tissue irritation occurs with subcutaneous administration than with intramuscular administration.
g. When parenteral fluphenazine is ordered, check the drug preparations very closely.	The hydrochloride solution of fluphenazine is given intramuscularly only. The decanoate and enanthate preparations (long-acting, sesame oil preparations) can be given intramuscularly or subcutaneously.
2. Observe for therapeutic effects	
a. When the drug is given for acute psychotic episodes, observe for decreased agitation, combativeness, and psychomotor activity.	The sedative effects of antipsychotic drugs are exerted within 48 to 72 hours. Sedation that occurs with treatment of acute psychotic episodes is a therapeutic effect. Sedation that occurs with treatment of nonacute psychotic disorders, or excessive sedation at any time, is an adverse reaction.
b. When the drug is given for acute or chronic psychosis, observe for decreased psychotic behavior, such as:	These therapeutic effects may not be evident for 3 to 6 weeks after drug therapy is begun.
(1) Decreased auditory and visual hallucinations	
(2) Decreased delusions	
(3) Continued decrease in or absence of agitation, hostility, hyperactivity, and other behavior associated with acute psychosis	
(4) Increased socialization	
(5) Increased ability in self-care activities	
(6) Increased ability to participate in other therapeutic modalities along with drug therapy.	
c. When the drug is given for antiemetic effects, observe for decreased or absent nausea or vomiting.	
3. Observe for adverse effects	
a. With phenothiazines and related drugs, observe for:	
(1) Excessive sedation—drowsiness, lethargy, fatigue, slurred speech, impaired mobility, and impaired mental processes	Excessive sedation is most likely to occur during the first few days of treatment of an acute psychotic episode, when large doses are usually given. Psychotic clients also seem sedated because the drug lets them catch up on psychosis-induced sleep deprivation. Sedation is more likely to occur in elderly or debilitated people. Tolerance to the drugs' sedative effects develops, and sedation tends to decrease with continued drug therapy.

(continued)

NURSING ACTIONS	RATIONALE/EXPLANATION
(2) Extrapyramidal reactions *Akathisia*—compulsive, involuntary restlessness and body movements	Akathisia is the most common extrapyramidal reaction, and it may occur about 5 to 60 days after the start of antipsychotic drug therapy. The motor restlessness may be erroneously interpreted as psychotic agitation necessitating increased drug dosage. This condition can sometimes be controlled by substituting an antipsychotic drug that is less likely to cause extrapyramidal effects or by giving an anticholinergic antiparkinson drug.
Parkinsonism—loss of muscle movement (akinesia), muscular rigidity and tremors, shuffling gait, postural abnormalities, mask-like facial expression, hypersalivation, and drooling	These symptoms are the same as those occurring with idiopathic Parkinson's disease. They can be controlled with anticholinergic antiparkinson drugs, given along with the antipsychotic drug for about 3 months, then discontinued. This reaction may occur about 5 to 30 days after antipsychotic drug therapy is begun.
Dyskinesias (involuntary, rhythmic body movements) and *dystonias* (uncoordinated, bizarre movements of the neck, face, eyes, tongue, trunk, or extremities)	These are less common extrapyramidal reactions, but they may occur suddenly, approximately 1 to 5 days after drug therapy is started, and be very frightening to the client and health care personnel. The movements are caused by muscle spasms and result in exaggerated posture and facial distortions. These symptoms are sometimes misinterpreted as seizures, hysteria, or other disorders. Antiparkinson drugs are given parenterally during acute dystonic reactions, but continued administration is not usually required. These reactions occur most often in younger people.
Tardive dyskinesia—hyperkinetic movements of the face (sucking and smacking of lips, tongue protrusion, and facial grimaces) and choreiform movements of the trunk and limbs	This syndrome occurs after months or years of high-dose antipsychotic drug therapy. The drugs may mask the symptoms so that the syndrome is more likely to be diagnosed when dosage is decreased or the drug is discontinued for a few days. It occurs gradually and at any age but is more common in older people, women, and people with organic brain disorders. The condition is usually irreversible, and there is no effective treatment. Symptoms are not controlled and may be worsened by antiparkinson drugs. Low dosage and short-term use of antipsychotic drugs help prevent tardive dyskinesia; drug-free periods may aid early detection.
(3) Antiadrenergic effects—hypotension, tachycardia, dizziness, faintness, and fatigue.	Hypotension is potentially one of the most serious adverse reactions to the antipsychotic drugs. It is most likely to occur when the client assumes an upright position after sitting or lying down (orthostatic or postural hypotension) but it does occur in the recumbent position. It is caused by peripheral vasodilation. Orthostatic hypotension can be assessed by comparing blood pressure readings taken with the client in supine and standing positions.

(continued)

NURSING ACTIONS	RATIONALE/EXPLANATION
	Tachycardia occurs as a compensatory mechanism in response to hypotension and as an anticholinergic effect in which the normal vagus nerve action of slowing the heart rate is blocked.
(4) Anticholinergic effects—dry mouth, dental caries, blurred vision, constipation, paralytic ileus, urinary retention	These atropine-like effects are common with therapeutic doses and are increased with large doses of phenothiazines.
(5) Respiratory depression—slow, shallow breathing and decreased ability to breathe deeply, cough, and remove secretions from the respiratory tract	This stems from general central nervous system (CNS) depression, which causes drowsiness and decreased movement. It may cause pneumonia or other respiratory problems, especially in people with hypercarbia and chronic lung disease.
(6) Endocrine effects—menstrual irregularities, possibly impotence and decreased libido in the male client, weight gain	These apparently result from drug-induced changes in pituitary and hypothalamic functions.
(7) Hypothermia or hyperthermia	Antipsychotic drugs may impair the temperature-regulating center in the hypothalamus. Hypothermia is more likely to occur. Hyperthemia occurs with high doses and warm environmental temperatures.
(8) Hypersensitivity reactions:	
Cholestatic hepatitis—may begin with fever and influenza-like symptoms followed in approximately 1 week by jaundice	Cholestatic hepatitis results from drug-induced edema of the bile ducts and obstruction of the bile flow. It occurs most often in women and after 2 to 4 weeks of receiving the drug. It is usually reversible if the drug is discontinued.
Blood dyscrasias—leukopenia, agranulocytosis (fever, sore throat, weakness)	Some degree of leukopenia occurs rather often and does not seem to be serious. Agranulocytosis, on the other hand, occurs rarely but is life threatening. Agranulocytosis is most likely to occur during the first 4 to 10 weeks of drug therapy, in women, and in older people.
Skin reactions—photosensitivity, dermatoses	Skin pigmentation and discoloration may occur with exposure to sunlight.
(9) Electrocardiogram (ECG) changes	The mechanism and clinical significance of ECG changes are not completely clear. However, some antipsychotic drugs, especially thioridazine, alter normal impulse conduction through the ventricles. There is probably increased risk of cardiac arrhythmias, which may be serious in a person with cardiovascular disease.
(10) Neuroleptic malignant syndrome—fever (may be confused with heat stroke), muscle rigidity, agitation, confusion, delirium, dyspnea, tachycardia, respiratory failure, acute renal failure	A rare but potentially fatal reaction that may occur hours to months after initial drug use. Symptoms usually develop rapidly over 24 to 72 hours. Treatment includes stopping the antipsychotic drug, giving supportive care related to fever and other symptoms, and drug therapy (dantrolene, a skeletal muscle relaxant, and amantadine or bromocriptine, dopamine-stimulating drugs).

(continued)

NURSING ACTIONS	RATIONALE/EXPLANATION
b. With clozapine, observe for:	
(1) CNS effects—drowsiness, dizziness, headache, seizures	
(2) Gastrointestinal (GI) effects—nausea, vomiting, constipation	
(3) Cardiovascular effects—hypotension, tachycardia	
(4) Hematologic effects—agranulocytosis	This is the most life-threatening adverse effect of clozapine. Clients' white blood cell counts must be checked before starting clozapine, every week during therapy, and for 4 weeks after the drug is discontinued.
c. With olanzapine, observe for:	
(1) CNS effects—drowsiness, dizziness, akathisia, tardive dyskinesia, neuroleptic malignant syndrome	
(2) GI effects—constipation	
(3) Cardiovascular effects—hypotension, tachycardia	
d. With quetiapine, observe for:	
(1) CNS effects—drowsiness, dizziness, headache, tardive dyskinesia, neuroleptic malignant syndrome	
(2) GI effects—anorexia, nausea, vomiting	
(3) Cardiovascular effects—orthostatic hypotension, tachycardia	
e. With risperidone, observe for:	
(1) CNS effects—agitation, anxiety, drowsiness, dizziness, headache, insomnia, tardive dyskinesia, neuroleptic malignant syndrome	
(2) GI effects—nausea, vomiting, constipation	
(3) Cardiovascular effects—orthostatic hypotension, arrhythmias	
(4) Other—photosensitivity	
4. Observe for drug interactions	
a. Drugs that *increase* effects of antipsychotic drugs:	
(1) Anticholinergic drugs (eg, atropine)	Additive anticholinergic effects, especially with thioridazine
(2) Antidepressants, tricyclic	Potentiation of sedative and anticholinergic effects. Additive CNS depression, sedation, orthostatic hypotension, urinary retention, and glaucoma may occur unless dosages are decreased. Apparently these two drug groups inhibit the metabolism of each other, thus prolonging the actions of both groups if they are given concomitantly.

(continued)

NURSING ACTIONS	RATIONALE/EXPLANATION
(3) Antihistamines	Additive CNS depression and sedation
(4) CNS depressants—alcohol, opioid analgesics, antianxiety agents, barbiturates and other sedative-hypnotics	Additive CNS depression. Also, severe hypotension, urinary retention, seizures, severe atropine-like reactions, and others may occur, depending on which group of CNS depressant drugs is given.
(5) Propranolol (Inderal)	Additive hypotensive and ECG effects
(6) Thiazide diuretics, such as hydrochlorothiazide (HydroDIURIL)	Additive hypotension
(7) Lithium	Acute encephalopathy, including irreversible brain damage and dyskinesias, has been reported.
b. Drugs that *decrease* effects of antipsychotic drugs:	
(1) Antacids	Oral antacids, especially aluminum hydroxide and magnesium trisilicate, may inhibit gastrointestinal absorption of antipsychotic drugs.
(2) Barbiturates, carbamazepine, phenytoin	By induction of drug-metabolizing enzymes in the liver
(3) Norepinephrine (Levophed), phenylephrine (Neo-Synephrine)	Antagonize the hypotensive effects of antipsychotic drugs

Nursing Notes: Apply Your Knowledge

Answer: Although these symptoms may accompany some psychiatric disorders, it is important to consider that John may be experiencing extrapyramidal side effects from the antipsychotic medication (Prolixin) he is taking. Notify the physician of the new symptoms. The dose of Prolixin may be lowered or an antiparkinson agent may be ordered to treat the extrapyramidal symptoms.

REVIEW AND APPLICATION EXERCISES

1. How do antipsychotic drugs act to relieve psychotic symptoms?

2. What are some uses of antipsychotic drugs other than the treatment of schizophrenia?

3. Do the phenothiazine, butyrophenone, and thioxanthene antipsychotic drugs differ significantly in therapeutic effects?

4. What are major adverse effects of antipsychotic drugs?

5. When instructing a client to rise slowly from a sitting or lying position, which adverse effect of an antipsychotic drug is the nurse trying to prevent?

6. In a client receiving an antipsychotic drug, what appearances or behaviors would lead the nurse to suspect an extrapyramidal reaction?

7. Describe potential difficulties in getting psychotic clients to take their drugs as prescribed and interventions to overcome these difficulties.

8. Are antipsychotic drugs likely to be overused and abused? Why or why not?

9. In an older client taking an antipsychotic drug, what special safety measures are needed? Why?

10. How do clozapine, olanzapine, quetiapine, and risperidone compare with older antipsychotic drugs in terms of therapeutic and adverse effects?

11. What can the home care nurse do to prevent acute psychotic episodes and hospitalization of chronically mentally ill clients?

SELECTED REFERENCES

American Psychiatric Association. (1994). *Diagnostic and statistical manual of mental disorders*, 4th ed (Revised). Washington, D.C.: American Psychiatric Association.

Bendik, M.F. (1996). The schizophrenias. In K.M. Fortinash & P.A. Holoday-Worret (Eds.), *Psychiatric-mental health nursing*, pp. 284–316. St. Louis: Mosby.

Cardinale, V. (1997). Mental health and pharmacy. *Drug Topics 4* (Suppl), 1s–47s.

Crismon, M.L. & Dorson, P.G. (1997). Schizophrenia. In J.T. DiPiro, R.L. Talbert, P.E. Hayes, G.C. Yee, G.R. Matzke, B.G. Wells, & L.M. Posey (Eds.), *Pharmacotherapy: A pathophysiologic approach*, 3rd ed., pp. 1367–1394. Stamford, CT: Appleton & Lange.

Drug facts and comparisons. (Updated monthly). St. Louis: Facts and Comparisons.

Findling, R.L., Schulz, S.C., Reed, M.D., & Blumer, J.L. (1998). The antipsychotics: A pediatric perspective. *Pediatric Clinics of North America, 45,* 1205–1232.

Jessen, L.M. (1998). New treatment options for schizophrenia. *US Pharmacist 23*(5), 117–128.

Jones, P. & Cannon, M. (1998). The new epidemiology of schizophrenia. *Psychiatric Clinics of North America 21,* 1–25.

Lasley, S.M. (1997). Antipsychotic drugs. In C.R. Craig & R.E. Stitzel (Eds.), *Modern pharmacology with clinical applications,* 5th ed., pp. 421–428. Boston: Little, Brown & Co.

McBride, A.B. & Austin, J.K. (1996). *Psychiatric-mental health nursing.* Philadelphia: W.B. Saunders.

McCrone, S.H. (1996). Physical dimensions of the journey: Neurobiological influences. In V.B. Carson & E.L. Arnold (Eds.), *Mental health nursing: The nurse-patient journey,* pp. 127–149. Philadelphia: W.B. Saunders.

Mohr, W. (1998). Cross-ethnic variations in the care of psychiatric patients. *Journal of Psychosocial Nursing, 36*(5), 16–21.

Smith, T.E. & Docherty, J.P. (1998). Standards of care and clinical algorithms for treating schizophrenia. *Psychiatric Clinics of North America 21,* 203–220.

Tosyali, M.C. & Greenhill, L.L. (1998). Child and adolescent psychopharmacology. *Pediatric Clinics of North America 45,* 1021–1035.

10

Antidepressants

Objectives

After studying this chapter, the student will be able to:

1. Define types and characteristics of depression.

2. Differentiate between mental depression and general central nervous system depression.

3. Discuss characteristics of antidepressants in terms of mechanism of action, indications for use, adverse effects, principles of therapy, and nursing process implications.

4. Compare and contrast selective serotonin reuptake inhibitors with tricyclic antidepressants.

5. Discuss selected characteristics of bupropion, nefazodone, and venlafaxine.

6. Describe the use of lithium in bipolar disorder.

7. Discuss interventions to increase safety of lithium therapy.

8. Describe the nursing role in preventing, recognizing, and treating overdoses of antidepressant drugs and lithium.

9. Analyze important factors in using antidepressant drugs and lithium in special populations.

Betty McGrath, 73 years of age, was recently widowed. She depended on her husband to handle their finances, maintain their home, and make major decisions. She enjoyed the role of homemaker and never worked outside the home. Her children live out of state, but they write and call often. Betty's daughter calls you because she is concerned about her mother. Mrs. McGrath seems to be losing weight, stays home most of the time, complains she feels very tired, and sleeps much more than usual. She is also reluctant to go out with friends or visit her children.

▶ List factors that might increase Mrs. McGrath's risk for depression.

▶ What symptoms does Mrs. McGrath have that may indicate she is depressed?

▶ What additional data would support a diagnosis of depression?

▶ At this point, what suggestions would you have for Mrs. McGrath and her daughter?

DEPRESSION

Depression is an affective disorder often described as the most common mental illness. It is characterized by depressed mood, feelings of sadness, or emotional upset, and it occurs in all age groups. Numerous terms have been used to describe depression. Mild depression occurs in everyone as a normal response to life stresses and losses and usually does not require treatment; severe or major depression is a psychiatric illness and requires treatment. Depression also is categorized as unipolar, in which people of usually normal moods experience recurrent episodes of depression, and bipolar disorder, in which episodes of depression alternate with episodes of mania.

Major Depression

The American Psychiatric Association's *Diagnostic and Statistical Manual of Mental Disorders*, 4th Edition (Revised), lists two major categories of depression. One category is *major depression*, which consists of a depressed mood plus at least five of the following symptoms:

Loss of energy
Fatigue
Indecisiveness
Difficulty thinking and concentrating
Loss of interest in appearance, work, and leisure and sexual activities
Inappropriate feelings of guilt and worthlessness
Loss of appetite and weight loss, or excessive eating and weight gain
Sleep disorders (hypersomnia or insomnia)
Somatic symptoms (eg, constipation, headache, atypical pain)
Obsession with death, thoughts of suicide
Psychotic symptoms, such as hallucinations and delusions

Dysthymia

The other category is *dysthymia*, a chronically depressed mood or loss of interest in usual activities that is not severe enough or does not last long enough to meet the criteria for major depression. Dysthymia is further described as primary or secondary. Primary depression cannot be related to an identifiable cause; secondary depression may be precipitated by the following:

Environmental stress (eg, job loss or dissatisfaction, financial worries)
Adverse life events (eg, divorce, death of a family member or friend)
Drugs (alcohol; antiarrhythmics, such as lidocaine, procainamide, and tocainide; antihypertensive drugs, such as clonidine, methyldopa, and prazosin; beta blockers; corticosteroids; opiates; and oral contraceptives)
Concurrent disease states, including endocrine disorders (hypothyroidism and hyperthyroidism, diabetes mellitus, adrenal insufficiency or excess), central nervous system (CNS) disorders (stroke, tumors, or other brain lesions; Parkinson's disease), cardiovascular disorders (myocardial infarction, congestive heart failure, hypertension), and miscellaneous disorders (rheumatoid arthritis, infectious disease, malnutrition)

Differentiating between major depression and dysthymia is difficult because the symptoms are similar; the main differences are the severity and duration of symptoms.

Seasonal affective disorder, a type of depression that occurs during the winter, also has been described. Its classification and differentiation from major depression and dysthymia are unclear.

Etiology

Despite extensive study, the etiology of depression has not been clearly delineated. Depression usually is attributed to neurotransmitter or receptor abnormalities in the brain, with much of the available information derived from studies about the actions of antidepressant drugs. Some possible etiologic factors are described in the following sections.

Neurotransmitters

An early hypothesis was that depression results from a deficiency of norepinephrine, serotonin, or both. This theory was supported by studies demonstrating that antidepressant drugs increased the amounts of one or both of these neurotransmitters in the CNS synapse by inhibiting their reuptake into the presynaptic neuron. Since the advent of the selective serotonin reuptake inhibitor (SSRI) antidepressants, much research has been focused on the role of serotonin. Serotonin helps regulate several behaviors that are disturbed in depression and other psychiatric disorders, such as mood, sleep, appetite, energy level, and cognitive and psychomotor functions. Thus, a disturbance in the serotonin system may play a primary or secondary role in the etiology of depression. Other neurotransmitters, such as dopamine and acetylcholine, probably also play a role.

Receptors

Emphasis shifted toward receptors because the neurotransmitter hypothesis did not explain why the amounts of neurotransmitter were increased within minutes to hours after single doses of a drug, but relief of depression occurred only after several weeks of drug therapy.

Researchers identified changes in norepinephrine and serotonin receptors with chronic antidepressant drug therapy. Studies demonstrated that chronic drug administration (ie, increased neurotransmitter in the synapse for several weeks) results in fewer receptors on the postsynaptic membrane. This down-regulation of receptors, first noted with beta-adrenergic receptors, corresponds with therapeutic drug effects. All known treatments for depression (including electroconvulsive shock) lead to the down-regulation of beta receptors and occur in the same period as the behavioral changes associated with antidepressant drug therapy.

Alpha$_2$-adrenergic receptors (called autoreceptors), located on presynaptic nerve terminals, may also play a role in depression. When these receptors are stimulated, they inhibit the release of norepinephrine. There is evidence that alpha$_2$ receptors are also down-regulated by antidepressant drugs, thus allowing increased norepinephrine release. With serotonin receptors, available antidepressants may increase the sensitivity of postsynaptic receptors and decrease the sensitivity of presynaptic receptors.

Physiologically, presynaptic receptors regulate the release and reuptake of neurotransmitters; postsynaptic receptors participate in the transmission of nerve impulses to target tissues. It seems apparent that long-term administration of antidepressant drugs produces complex changes in the sensitivities of both presynaptic and postsynaptic receptor sites.

Neurotransmission Systems

There is an increasing awareness that depression is a complex disorder and probably has multiple causes. Moreover, the balance, integration, and interactions among neurotransmission systems are probably more important etiologic factors than single neurotransmitter or receptor alterations. For example, disturbances in the norepinephrine or serotonin neurotransmission system (see Chap. 5) are often implicated in depression. One current view is that the serotonin and norepinephrine systems are related and in balance in the CNS and that depression may result from an imbalance or an alteration in their relationship.

Genetic and Endocrine Factors

Genetic factors are considered important in depression, with close relatives of a depressed person more likely to experience depression. In addition, endocrine abnormalities are often present in people who are depressed. These include disturbances in the hypothalamic–pituitary–adrenal axis, excessive secretion of cortisol, and altered thyroid function.

In bipolar disorder, periods of depression alternate with periods of mania, an excited state characterized by excessive CNS stimulation with physical and mental hyperactivity (eg, energetic and constant movement, decreased sleep, talkativeness, racing thoughts, short attention span, grandiose ideation). *Hypomania* is the term used to indicate less CNS stimulation and hyperactivity than mania. Like depression, mania and hypomania may result from abnormal functioning of neurotransmitters or receptors, such as a relative excess of excitatory neurotransmitters (eg, norepinephrine) or a relative deficiency of inhibitory neurotransmitters (eg, gamma-aminobutyric acid [GABA]). Drugs that stimulate the CNS can cause manic and hypomanic behaviors that are easily confused with schizophreniform psychoses.

ANTIDEPRESSANT DRUGS

Antidepressant drugs are used in the pharmacologic management of depressive disorders (also called mood or affective disorders). They are derived from several chemical groups. Older or first-generation antidepressants include the tricyclic antidepressants (TCAs) and the monoamine oxidase inhibitors (MAOIs). Newer or second-generation drugs include serotonin enhancers and several other drugs, some of which differ chemically from the tricyclics but are similar in pharmacologic actions and antidepressant effectiveness.

With oral administration, the drugs are absorbed from the small bowel, enter the portal circulation, and circulate through the liver, where they undergo extensive first-pass metabolism before reaching the systemic circulation. Like most psychotropic drugs, antidepressants are metabolized by the cytochrome P450 enzymes in the liver. Many antidepressants and other drugs are metabolized by a subgroup of the enzymes, 2D6 or 3A4. Thus, antidepressants may interact with each other, with other mind-altering drugs (eg, antianxiety or antipsychotic agents), and a wide variety of nonpsychotropic drugs that are normally metabolized by the same subgroups of enzymes. The drugs are also highly protein bound.

Additional characteristics of these drugs and lithium, an antimanic agent used for bipolar affective disorder, are described in the following sections.

Tricyclic Antidepressants

Tricyclic antidepressants are chemically and pharmacologically similar drugs. They contain a triple-ring nucleus from which their name is derived. The drugs are structurally similar to phenothiazine antipsychotic agents (see Chap. 9) and have similar antiadrenergic and anticholinergic adverse effects. They produce a relatively high incidence of sedation, orthostatic hypotension, cardiac dysrhythmias, and other adverse effects. TCAs are well absorbed after oral administration. However, first-pass metabolism by the liver results in blood level variations of 10- to 30-fold among people given identical doses. Once absorbed, these drugs are widely distributed throughout body tissues and metabolized by the liver to active and inactive metabolites. Because of adverse effects on the heart, especially in overdose, baseline and follow-up electrocardiograms (ECGs) are recommended for all clients. **Amitriptyline** (Elavil) is a commonly used TCA.

Selective Serotonin Reuptake Inhibitors

Selective serotonin reuptake inhibitors, of which **fluoxetine** (Prozac) is the prototype, are as effective as TCAs and have a similar onset of action. Although the drugs share some characteristics, they also differ in structure and pharmacodynamic effect. They are well absorbed with oral administration, undergo extensive first-pass metabolism in the liver, are highly protein bound (approximately 95%), and have a half-life of 24 to 72 hours, which may lead to accumulation with chronic administration. Fluoxetine also forms an active metabolite with a half-life of 7 to 9 days. Thus, steady-state blood levels are achieved slowly, over several weeks, and drug effects decrease slowly (over 2 to 3 months) when fluoxetine is discontinued. Sertraline and citalopram also have active metabolites, but fluoxetine and paroxetine are more likely to accumulate than other SSRIs. Paroxetine, sertraline, and fluvoxamine reach steady-state concentrations in 1 to 2 weeks.

Because SSRIs are highly bound to plasma proteins, the drugs compete with endogenous compounds and other medications for binding sites. Because they are highly lipid soluble, they accumulate in the CNS and other adipose-rich tissue.

Selective serotonin reuptake inhibitors do not produce the sedation, anticholinergic effects, orthostatic hypotension, cardiac arrhythmias, and weight gain associated with TCAs. Their adverse effects include CNS stimulation (eg, anxiety, nervousness, insomnia), gastrointestinal (GI) effects (nausea, diarrhea, weight loss), and a skin rash that sometimes requires stopping the drug. The available drugs in this group are usually given once daily.

Serious, sometimes fatal, reactions have occurred from combined therapy with an SSRI and an MAOI, and the drugs should not be given concurrently or within 2 weeks of each other. If a client on an SSRI is to be transferred to an MAOI, most SSRIs should be discontinued at least 14 days before starting the MAOI; fluoxetine should be discontinued at least 5 weeks before starting an MAOI.

Monoamine Oxidase Inhibitors

Monoamine oxidase inhibitors are well absorbed after oral administration and produce maximal inhibition of MAO within 5 to 10 days. However, clinical improvement in depression may require 2 to 3 weeks.

Monoamine oxidase inhibitors may interact with numerous foods and drugs to produce hypertensive crisis (ie, severe hypertension, severe headache, fever, possible myocardial infarction, or intracranial hemorrhage). Foods that interact with MAOIs are those containing tyramine, a monoamine precursor of norepinephrine. Normally, tyramine is deactivated in the gastrointestinal tract and liver so that large amounts do not reach the systemic circulation. However, when deactivation of tyramine is blocked by MAOIs, tyramine is absorbed systemically and transported to adrenergic nerve terminals, where it causes a sudden release of large amounts of norepinephrine. Hypertensive crisis may result. Several drugs also may interact with MAOIs to cause hypertensive crisis. Foods and drugs to be avoided during (and 2 to 3 weeks after) drug therapy with MAOIs are listed in Table 10-1.

Miscellaneous Antidepressants

Bupropion (Wellbutrin, Zyban) inhibits the reuptake of dopamine, norepinephrine, and serotonin. It was marketed with warnings related to seizure activity. Seizures are most likely to occur with doses above 450 mg/day and in clients known to have a seizure disorder.

After an oral dose, peak plasma levels are reached in approximately 2 hours. The average drug half-life is approximately 14 hours. The drug is metabolized in the liver and excreted primarily in the urine. Several metabolites are pharmacologically active. Dosage should be reduced with impaired hepatic or renal function. Acute episodes of depression usually require several months of drug therapy.

TABLE 10-1	Foods and Drugs to be Avoided During Therapy With Monoamine Oxidase Inhibitor Drugs
Foods to Avoid	**Drugs to Avoid**
Aged cheese (eg, cheddar, Camembert, Stilton, Gruyere)	Amphetamines
Alcoholic beverages (beer, Chianti and other red wines)	Antiallergy and antiasthmatic drugs (eg, ephedrine, epinephrine, phenylpropanolamine, pseudoephedrine)
Avocados and guacamole dip	Antidepressants (tricyclic antidepressants, serotonin reuptake inhibitors)
Bananas	
Caffeine-containing beverages (coffee, tea, cola drinks)	Antihistamines (including over-the-counter cough and cold remedies)
Chicken livers	
Chocolate (in large amounts)	Antihypertensive drugs (ie, methyldopa)
Fava bean pods	Levodopa
Figs (canned)	Meperidine
Meat tenderizers	
Pickled herring	
Raisins	
Sour cream	
Soy sauce	
Yogurt	

Bupropion may also be used up to 12 weeks as a smoking cessation aid, if progress is being made.

In addition to seizures, the drug has CNS stimulant effects (agitation, anxiety, excitement, increased motor activity, insomnia, restlessness) that may require a sedative during the first few days of administration. These effects may increase the risk of abuse. Other common adverse effects include dry mouth, headache, nausea and vomiting, and constipation.

Maprotiline (Ludiomil) is a tetracyclic antidepressant that also has anxiolytic properties. It causes adverse effects similar to those with the TCAs and seems to have few, if any, advantages over the TCAs.

Mirtazapine (Remeron) is a newer antidepressant that blocks presynaptic alpha$_2$-adrenergic receptors, which increases the release of norepinephrine and serotonin. The drug is well absorbed after oral administration, and peak plasma levels occur in approximately 2 hours after an oral dose. It is metabolized in the liver, mainly to inactive metabolites. Common adverse effects include drowsiness (with accompanying cognitive and motor impairment), increased appetite, weight gain, dizziness, dry mouth, and constipation. Mirtazapine should not be taken concurrently with other CNS depressants (eg, alcohol or benzodiazepine antianxiety or hypnotic agents) because of additive sedation. In addition, it should not be taken concurrently with an MAOI or for 14 days after stopping an MAOI. An MAOI should not be started until at least 14 days after stopping mirtazapine.

Nefazodone (Serzone) inhibits the neuronal reuptake of serotonin and norepinephrine, thereby increasing the amount of these neurotransmitters in the brain. It is contraindicated in pregnancy and should be used with caution in people with cardiovascular or cerebrovascular disorders, dehydration, hypovolemia, mania, hypomania, suicidal ideation, hepatic cirrhosis, electroconvulsive therapy, debilitation, and lactation. It has a long half-life (2 to 3 days) and crosses the placenta. It is metabolized in the liver and excreted in breast milk, urine, and feces.

Adverse effects resemble those of SSRIs and TCAs, including agitation, confusion, dizziness, GI symptoms (nausea, vomiting, diarrhea), headache, insomnia, orthostatic hypotension, sedation, and skin rash. Potentially significant drug–drug interactions include the risk of severe toxic effects if taken with MAOIs. This combination should be avoided. If a client on nefazodone is to be transferred to an MAOI, the nefazodone should be discontinued at least 7 days before starting the MAOI; if a client on an MAOI is to be transferred to nefazodone, the MAOI should be discontinued at least 14 days before starting nefazodone. There is also a risk of increased CNS depression with general anesthetics.

Trazodone (Desyrel) represents a different chemical class of antidepressants. Oral trazodone is well absorbed, and peak plasma concentrations are obtained within 30 minutes to 2 hours. Trazodone is metabolized by the liver and excreted primarily by the kidneys. Although trazodone reportedly produces less anticholinergic activity than the TCAs, it causes a number of other adverse effects, including sedation, dizziness, edema, cardiac arrhythmias, and priapism (prolonged and painful penile erection). It is used more often for sedation and sleep than for depression because high doses (>300 mg/day) are required for antidepressant effects and these amounts cause excessive sedation for many clients. Trazodone is often given concurrently with a stimulating antidepressant, such as an SSRI.

Venlafaxine (Effexor), which is chemically related to bupropion, inhibits the reuptake of norepinephrine, serotonin, and dopamine, thereby increasing the activity of these neurotransmitters in the brain. The drug crosses the placenta and may enter breast milk. It is metabolized in the liver and excreted in urine. It is contraindicated during pregnancy, and women should use effective birth control methods while taking this drug. Adverse effects include CNS (anxiety, dizziness, dreams, insomnia, nervousness, somnolence, tremors), GI (anorexia, nausea, vomiting, constipation, diarrhea), cardiovascular (hypertension, tachycardia, vasodilation), genitourinary (abnormal ejaculation, impotence, urinary frequency), and dermatologic (sweating, rash, pruritus) symptoms. Venlafaxine should not be taken concurrently with MAOIs because of increased serum levels and risks of toxicity. If a client on venlafaxine is to be transferred to an MAOI, the venlafaxine should be discontinued at least 7 days before starting the MAOI; if a client on an MAOI is to be transferred to venlafaxine, the MAOI should be discontinued at least 14 days before starting venlafaxine.

Mood-Stabilizing Agent

Lithium carbonate (Eskalith) is a naturally occurring metallic salt used in the management of bipolar affective disorder. Lithium is more effective in the treatment and prevention of mania than in preventing depression. It is sometimes described as an "antimanic" drug.

Lithium is well absorbed after oral administration, with peak serum levels in 1 to 3 hours after a dose and steady-state concentrations in 5 to 7 days. Because serum concentrations of lithium vary widely among clients taking comparable doses, frequent monitoring of the serum lithium concentration is required.

Lithium is not metabolized by the body; it is entirely excreted by the kidneys, so adequate renal function is a prerequisite for lithium therapy. Approximately 80% of a lithium dose is reabsorbed in the proximal renal tubules. The amount of reabsorption depends on the concentration of sodium in the proximal renal tubules. A deficiency of sodium causes more lithium to be reabsorbed and increases the risk of lithium toxicity; excessive sodium intake causes more lithium to be excreted (ie, lithium diuresis) and may lower serum lithium levels to nontherapeutic ranges.

Before lithium therapy is begun, baseline studies of renal, cardiac, and thyroid status should be obtained because adverse drug effects involve these organ systems. Baseline electrolyte studies are also necessary.

Mechanisms of Action

Antidepressant drugs apparently normalize abnormal neurotransmission systems in the brain by increasing the amounts of neurotransmitters and altering the number or sensitivity of receptors. After neurotransmitters are released from presynaptic nerve endings, the molecules that are not bound to receptors are normally inactivated by reuptake into the presynaptic nerve fibers that released them or metabolized by MAO. Most antidepressants prevent the reuptake of multiple neurotransmitters; SSRIs selectively inhibit the reuptake of serotonin. MAOIs prevent the metabolism of neurotransmitter molecules. These mechanisms thereby increase the amount of neurotransmitter available to bind to receptors.

With chronic drug administration, receptors adapt to the presence of increased neurotransmitter by decreasing their number or sensitivity to the neurotransmitter. More specifically, norepinephrine receptors, especially postsynaptic beta receptors and presynaptic $alpha_2$ receptors, are down-regulated. The $serotonin_2$ receptor, a postsynaptic receptor, may also be down-regulated.

Thus, antidepressant effects are attributed to changes in receptors rather than changes in neurotransmitters. Although some of the drugs act more selectively on one neurotransmission system than another initially, this selectivity seems to be lost with chronic administration.

With lithium, the exact mechanism of action is unknown. However, it is known to affect the synthesis, release, and reuptake of several neurotransmitters in the brain, including acetylcholine, dopamine, GABA, and norepinephrine. For example, the drug may increase the activity of GABA, an inhibitory neurotransmitter. It also stabilizes postsynaptic receptor sensitivity to neurotransmitters, probably by competing with calcium, magnesium, potassium, and sodium ions for binding sites.

Indications for Use

Antidepressant drug therapy may be indicated if depressive symptoms persist at least 2 weeks, impair social relationships or work performance, and occur independently of life events. In addition, some SSRIs are used for the treatment of obsessive–compulsive disorder and are being studied for possible use in numerous other disorders such as panic disorder, obesity, eating disorders, substance abuse, and chronic pain. TCAs may be used in children and adolescents in the management of enuresis (bedwetting), involuntary urination resulting from a physical or psychological disorder. In this setting, a TCA may be given after physical causes (eg, urethral irritation, excessive intake of fluids) have been ruled out. MAOIs are considered third-line drugs, largely because of their potential for serious and fatal interactions with certain foods and other drugs.

Contraindications to Use

Antidepressant drugs are contraindicated or must be used with caution in clients with acute schizophrenia; mixed mania and depression; suicidal tendencies; severe renal, hepatic, or cardiovascular disease; narrow-angle glaucoma; and seizure disorders.

INDIVIDUAL ANTIDEPRESSANTS

Table 10-2 lists the names, routes, and dosage ranges of individual antidepressants.

TABLE 10-2 **Antidepressant Agents**

Generic/Trade Name	Routes and Dosage Ranges	
	Adults	Children
Tricyclic Antidepressants		
Amitriptyline (Elavil, Endep, others)	PO 75–100 mg daily in divided doses, gradually increased to 150–300 mg daily if necessary. Maintenance dose, 50–100 mg once daily at bedtime. IM 80–120 mg daily in 4 divided doses *Older adults:* PO 10 mg 3 times daily and 20 mg at bedtime	Adolescents, PO 10 mg 3 times daily and 20 mg at bedtime Enuresis in children 5–14 years: PO 25 mg once daily at bedtime
Amoxapine (Asendin)	PO 50 mg 3 times daily, increased to 100 mg 3 times daily on the third day. Maintenance dose may be given in a single dose at bedtime.	Not recommended for children younger than 16 years of age
Desipramine (Pertofrane, Norpramin)	PO 75 mg daily in divided doses, gradually increased to a maximum of 200–300 mg daily if necessary *Older adults:* PO 25–50 mg daily in divided doses, gradually increased to 100 mg daily if necessary	Not recommended

(continued)

TABLE 10-2 **Antidepressant Agents** (*continued*)

Generic/Trade Name	Routes and Dosage Ranges	
	Adults	Children
Doxepin (Sinequan, Adapin)	PO 75–150 mg daily, gradually increased to a maximum of 300 mg daily if necessary	Not recommended
Imipramine (Tofranil)	PO 75 mg daily in 3 divided doses, gradually increased to a maximum of 300 mg daily if necessary. Maintenance dose, 75–150 mg daily *Older adults:* PO 30–40 mg daily in divided doses, increased to 100 mg daily if necessary	Enuresis: PO 25–50 mg 1 hour before bedtime
Nortriptyline (Aventyl, Pamelor)	PO 40 mg daily in divided doses, gradually increased to 100–150 mg daily if necessary	Enuresis: PO 25 mg once daily at bedtime
Protriptyline (Vivactil)	PO 15 mg daily in divided doses, increased to 60 mg daily if necessary	
Trimipramine maleate (Surmontil)	PO 75–100 mg daily, gradually increased to 300 mg daily if necessary	
Monoamine Oxidase Inhibitor Antidepressants		
Isocarboxazid (Marplan)	PO 10 mg twice daily, increased by 10 mg every 2–4 days to 40 mg daily in 1 week, in 2 to 4 doses.	Dosage not established
Phenelzine (Nardil)	PO 60 mg daily in 3 divided doses, increased to 90 mg daily if necessary	Dosage not established
Tranylcypromine (Parnate)	PO 20 mg daily in 2 divided doses in the morning and afternoon for 2 weeks, then adjusted according to client's response. Maximal daily dose, 30 mg	Dosage not established
Selective Serotonin Reuptake Inhibitor Antidepressants		
Citalopram (Celexa)	PO 20 mg once daily in the morning or evening, increased to 40 mg daily in 1 week, if necessary *Elderly/hepatic impairment:* PO 20 mg daily	Dosage not established
Fluoxetine (Prozac)	PO 20 mg once daily in the morning, increased after several weeks if necessary. Divide doses larger than 20 mg, and give morning and noon; maximum daily dose, 80 mg.	Dosage not established
Fluvoxamine (Luvox)	PO 50 mg once daily at bedtime, increased in 50-mg increments every 4–7 days if necessary. For daily amounts above 100 mg, give in 2 divided doses. Maximum daily dose, 300 mg	Dosage not established
Paroxetine (Paxil)	PO 20 mg once daily in the morning, increased after 3–4 weeks if necessary; maximum dose, 50 mg daily (40 mg for older adults)	Dosage not established
Sertraline (Zoloft)	PO 50 mg once daily morning or evening, increased at 1-week or longer intervals to a maximum daily dose of 200 mg	Dosage not established
Miscellaneous Antidepressants		
Bupropion (Wellbutrin)	PO 100 mg twice daily, increased to 100 mg 3 times daily if necessary. Maximal single dose, 150 mg	Dosage not established
Maprotiline (Ludiomil)	PO 75 mg daily in single or divided doses, increased to a maximum of 300 mg daily if necessary	Not recommended for children younger than 18 years of age
Mirtazapine (Remeron)	PO 15 mg/d, in a single dose, at bedtime	Dosage not established
Nefazodone (Serzone)	PO 200 mg daily in 2 divided doses; increase at 1-week intervals in increments of 100–200 mg/d; usual range, 300–600 mg/d. *Elderly or debilitated adults:* PO initially 100 mg/d in 2 divided doses	Not recommended in children younger than 18 years of age
Trazodone (Desyrel)	PO 100–300 mg daily, increased to a maximum dose of 600 mg daily if necessary	
Venlafaxine (Effexor)	PO initially 75 mg/d in 2 or 3 divided doses, with food. May be increased slowly up to 225 mg/d if necessary. In hepatic or renal impairment, reduce dose by 50% and increase very slowly.	Not recommended in children younger than 18 years of age
Mood-Stabilizing Agent		
Lithium carbonate (Eskalith)	Bipolar disorder (formerly called manic–depressive disorder), PO 900–1200 mg daily in divided doses, gradually increased in 300-mg increments if necessary, according to serum lithium levels and client's response	Not Food and Drug Administration approved for use in children younger than 12 years of age but sometimes given PO 300–900 mg or 30 mg/kg per day, in divided doses

PO, oral.

NURSING PROCESS

Assessment

Assess the client's condition in relation to depressive disorders.

- Identify clients at risk for current or potential depression. Areas to assess include health status, family and social relationships, and work status. Severe or prolonged illness, impaired interpersonal relationships, inability to work, and job dissatisfaction may precipitate depression. Depression also occurs without an identifiable cause.
- Observe for the signs and symptoms of depression listed previously. Manifestations may occur in any client, not just those who have or are suspected of having psychiatric illness. Clinical manifestations are nonspecific and vary in severity. For example, fatigue and insomnia may be caused by a variety of disorders and range from mild to severe. When symptoms are present, try to determine their frequency, duration, and severity.
- When a client appears depressed or has a history of depression, assess for suicidal thoughts and behaviors. Statements indicating a detailed plan, accompanied by the intent, ability, and method for carrying out the plan, place the client at high risk for suicide.
- Identify the client's usual coping mechanisms for stressful situations. Coping mechanisms vary widely, and behavior that may be helpful to one client may not be helpful to another. For example, one person may prefer being alone or having decreased contact with family and friends, whereas another may find increased contact desirable.

Nursing Diagnoses

- Dysfunctional Grieving related to loss (of health, ability to perform usual tasks, job, significant other, and so forth)
- Self Care Deficit related to fatigue and self-esteem disturbance with depression or sedation with antidepressant drugs
- Sleep Pattern Disturbance related to depression or insomnia with SSRIs
- Impaired Physical Mobility related to sedation with TCAs and related antidepressants
- Altered Thought Processes related to confusion (especially in older adults)
- Knowledge Deficit: Effects and appropriate use of antidepressant drugs
- Decreased Cardiac Output related to cardiac arrhythmias and hypotension with TCAs and related antidepressants

- Altered Tissue Perfusion related to hypotension with TCAs and related antidepressants
- Risk for Injury related to sedation with TCAs and related antidepressants
- Risk for Violence: Self-Directed or Directed at Others

Planning/Goals

The client will:

- Experience improvement of mood and depressive state
- Receive or self-administer the drugs correctly
- Be kept safe while sedated during therapy with the TCAs and related drugs
- Be assessed regularly for suicidal tendencies. If present, caretakers will implement safety measures.
- Be cared for by staff in areas of nutrition, hygiene, exercise, and social interactions when unable to provide self-care
- Resume self-care and other usual activities
- Avoid preventable adverse drug effects

Interventions

Use measures to prevent or decrease the severity of depression. General measures include supportive psychotherapy and reduction of environmental stress. Specific measures include the following:

- Support the client's usual mechanisms for handling stressful situations, when feasible. Helpful actions may involve relieving pain or insomnia, scheduling rest periods, and increasing or decreasing socialization.
- Call the client by name, encourage self-care activities, allow him or her to participate in setting goals and making decisions, and praise efforts to accomplish tasks. These actions promote a positive self-image.
- When signs and symptoms of depression are observed, initiate treatment before depression becomes severe. Institute suicide precautions for clients at risk. These usually involve close observation, often on a one-to-one basis, and removal of potential weapons from the environment. For clients hospitalized on medical-surgical units, transfer to a psychiatric unit may be needed.

Evaluation

- Observe for behaviors indicating lessened depression.
- Interview regarding feelings and mood.
- Observe and interview regarding adverse drug effects.
- Observe and interview regarding suicidal thoughts and behaviors.

CLIENT TEACHING GUIDELINES
Antidepressants and Lithium

General Considerations

✔ Take antidepressants as directed to maximize therapeutic benefits and minimize adverse effects. Do not alter doses when symptoms subside. Antidepressants are usually given for several months, perhaps years; lithium therapy may be lifelong.

✔ Therapeutic effects (relief of symptoms) may not occur for 2 to 4 weeks after drug therapy is started. As a result, it is very important not to think the drug is ineffective and stop taking it prematurely.

✔ Do not take other prescription or over-the-counter drugs without consulting a health care provider, including over-the-counter cold remedies. Potentially serious drug interactions may occur.

✔ Inform any physician, surgeon, or dentist about the antidepressant drugs being taken. Potentially serious adverse effects or drug interactions may occur if certain other drugs are prescribed.

✔ Avoid activities that require alertness and physical coordination (eg, driving a car, operating other machinery) until reasonably sure the medication does not impair ability to perform the activities safely.

✔ Avoid alcohol and other central nervous system depressants (eg, any drugs that cause drowsiness). Excessive drowsiness, dizziness, difficulty breathing, and low blood pressure may occur, with potentially serious consequences.

✔ Learn the name and type of a prescribed antidepressant drug to help avoid undesirable interactions with other drugs or a physician prescribing other drugs with similar effects. There are several different types of antidepressant drugs, with different characteristics and precautions for safe and effective usage.

✔ Bupropion is a unique drug prescribed for depression (brand name, Wellbutrin) and for smoking cessation (brand name, Zyban). It is extremely important not to increase the dose or take the two brand names at the same time (as might happen with different physicians or filling prescriptions at different pharmacies). Overdoses may cause seizures, as well as other adverse effects. When used for smoking cessation, Zyban is recommended for up to 12 weeks if progress is being made. If significant progress is not made by approximately 7 weeks, it is considered unlikely that longer drug use will be helpful.

✔ Do not stop taking any antidepressant drug without discussing it with a health care provider. If a problem occurs, the type of drug, the dose, or other aspects may be changed to solve the problem and continue taking the medication.

✔ Counseling, support groups, relaxation techniques, and other nonmedication treatments are recommended along with drug therapy.

Self-administration

✔ With a selective serotonin reuptake inhibitor (eg, Celexa, Paxil, Prozac, Zoloft), take in the morning because the drug may interfere with sleep if taken at bedtime. In addition, notify a health care provider if a skin rash or other allergic reaction occurs. Allergic reactions are uncommon but may require that the drug be discontinued.

✔ With a tricyclic antidepressant (eg, amitriptyline), take at bedtime. These drugs cause drowsiness and may aid sleep as well as decrease other side effects. Also, report urinary retention, fainting, irregular heartbeat, seizures, restlessness, and mental confusion. These are potentially serious adverse drug effects.

✔ With nefazodone (Serzone) and venlafaxine (Effexor), take as directed or ask for instructions. These drugs are often taken twice daily. Notify a health care provider if a skin rash or other allergic reaction occurs. An allergic reaction may require that the drug be discontinued.

✔ With bupropion, take two or three times daily, as prescribed.

✔ With lithium, several precautions are needed for safe use:
1. Take with food or milk or soon after a meal to decrease stomach upset.
2. Do not alter dietary salt intake. Decreased salt intake (eg, low-salt diet) increases risk of adverse effects from lithium. Increased intake may decrease therapeutic effects.
3. Drink 8 to 12 glasses of fluids daily; avoid excessive intake of caffeine-containing beverages. Caffeine has a diuretic effect and dehydration increases lithium toxicity.
4. Minimize activities that cause excessive perspiration. Loss of salt in sweat increases the risk of adverse effects from lithium.
5. Report for measurements of lithium blood levels as instructed, and do not take the morning dose of lithium until the blood sample has been obtained. Regular measurements of blood lithium levels are necessary for safe and effective lithium therapy. Accurate measurement of serum drug levels requires that blood be drawn approximately 12 hours after the previous dose of lithium.
6. If signs of overdose occur (eg, vomiting, diarrhea, unsteady walking, tremor, drowsiness, muscle weakness), stop taking lithium and contact the prescribing physician or other health care provider.

PRINCIPLES OF THERAPY

Drug Selection

Because the available drugs seem similarly effective, the choice of an antidepressant depends on the client's age, medical conditions, previous history of drug response, if any, and the specific drug's adverse effects. Cost also needs to be considered. The newer drugs are much more expensive than the TCAs. However, they may be more cost effective overall because TCAs are more likely to cause serious adverse effects, they require monitoring of plasma drug levels and ECGs, and clients are more likely to stop taking them. Additional guidelines for choosing a drug include the following:

1. The SSRIs are the drugs of first choice. These drugs are effective and usually produce fewer and milder adverse effects than other drugs. Guidelines for choosing one SSRI over another have not been established.
2. With TCAs, initial selection may be based on the client's previous response or susceptibility to adverse effects. For example, if a client (or a close family member) responded well to a particular drug in the past, that is probably the drug of choice for repeated episodes of depression. The response of family members to individual drugs may be significant because there is a strong genetic component to depression and drug response. If therapeutic effects do not occur within 4 weeks, the TCA proba-

bly should be discontinued or changed, because some clients tolerate or respond better to one TCA than to another. For a potentially suicidal client, an SSRI or another newer drug is preferred over a TCA because the TCAs are much more toxic in overdoses.
3. MAOIs are third-line drugs for the treatment of depression because of their potential interactions with other drugs and certain foods. An MAOI is most likely to be prescribed when the client does not respond to other antidepressant drugs or when electroconvulsive therapy is refused or contraindicated.
4. Criteria for choosing bupropion, mirtazapine, nefazodone, and venlafaxine are not clearly defined. Nefazodone has sedating and anxiolytic properties that may be useful for clients with severe insomnia, anxiety, and agitation.
5. For clients with cardiovascular disorders, most antidepressants can cause hypotension, but the SSRIs, bupropion, nefazodone, and venlafaxine are rarely associated with cardiac arrhythmias. Venlafaxine and MAOIs can increase blood pressure.
6. For clients with seizure disorders, bupropion, clomipramine, and maprotiline should be avoided; SSRIs, MAOIs, and desipramine are less likely to cause seizures.
7. For clients with diabetes mellitus, SSRIs may have a hypoglycemic effect and bupropion and venlafaxine have little effect on blood sugar levels.
8. Lithium is the drug of choice for clients with bipolar disorder. When used therapeutically, lithium is effective in controlling mania in approximately 65% to 80% of clients. When used prophylactically, the drug decreases the frequency and intensity of manic cycles. Carbamazepine (Tegretol), an anticonvulsant, may be as effective as lithium as a mood-stabilizing agent. It is often used in clients who do not respond to lithium, although it is not approved by the Food and Drug Administration for that purpose.

Dosage and Administration

Dosage of antidepressant drugs should be individualized according to clinical response. Antidepressant drug therapy is usually initiated with small, divided doses that are gradually increased until therapeutic or adverse effects occur. Specific guidelines for dosage include the following:

1. With SSRIs, nefazodone, and venlafaxine, therapy is begun with once-daily oral administration of the manufacturer's recommended dosage. Dosage may be increased after 3 or 4 weeks if depression is not relieved. With nefazodone, an optimal response may require 300 mg to 500 mg daily. As with most other drugs, smaller doses may be indicated in older adults and clients taking multiple medications.

2. With TCAs, therapy is begun with small doses, which are increased to the desired dose over 1 to 2 weeks. Minimal effective doses are approximately 150 mg/day of imipramine or its equivalent. TCAs can be administered once or twice daily because they have long elimination half-lives. Once dosage is established, TCAs are often given once daily at bedtime. This regimen is effective and well tolerated by most clients. Elderly clients may experience fewer adverse reactions if divided doses are continued. With TCAs, plasma levels are helpful in adjusting dosages.

3. With bupropion, seizures are more likely to occur with large single doses, large total doses, and large or abrupt increases in dosage. Recommendations to avoid these risk factors are:
   a. Give the drug in equally divided doses, preferably at least 6 hours apart.
   b. Single doses are usually 100 mg; the maximal single dose is 150 mg.
   c. The recommended initial dose is 200 mg, gradually increased to 300 mg. If no clinical improvement occurs after several weeks of 300 mg/day, dosage may be increased to 450 mg, the maximal daily dose.
   d. The recommended maintenance dose is the lowest amount that maintains remission.

4. With lithium therapy, dosage should be based on serum lithium levels, control of symptoms, and occurrence of adverse effects. Serum levels are required because therapeutic doses are only slightly lower than toxic doses and because clients vary widely in rates of lithium absorption and excretion. Thus, a dose that is therapeutic in one client may be toxic in another. Lower doses are indicated for older adults and for clients with conditions that impair lithium excretion (eg, diuretic drug therapy, dehydration, low-salt diet, renal impairment, decreased cardiac output).

When lithium therapy is being initiated, the serum drug concentration should be measured two or three times weekly in the morning, 12 hours after the last dose of lithium. For most clients, the therapeutic range of serum levels is 0.5 to 1.2 mEq/L (SI units, 0.5 to 1.2 mmol/L). Serum lithium levels should not exceed 1.5 mEq/L because the risk of serious toxicity is increased at higher levels.

Once symptoms of mania are controlled, lithium doses should be lowered. Serum lithium levels should be measured at least every 3 months during long-term maintenance therapy.

Duration of Drug Therapy

Guidelines for the duration of antidepressant drug therapy are not well established, and there are differences of opinion. However, evidence is accumulating that 6 to 12 months of treatment are needed for an acute episode of depression and that long-term maintenance therapy may be desirable. One argument for long-term maintenance therapy is that depression tends to relapse or recur, and successive episodes often are more severe and more difficult to treat. Thus, some authorities recommend indefinite drug therapy for clients who have had three or more episodes of major depression.

Maintenance therapy for depression requires close supervision and periodic reassessment of the client's condition and response. With the use of TCAs for acute depression, maintenance therapy usually consists of low doses for several months after recovery, followed by gradual tapering of the dose and drug discontinuation. However, recent studies indicate that full therapeutic doses (if clients can tolerate the adverse effects) for up to 5 years are effective in preventing recurrent episodes. The long-term effects (beyond 2 to 4 months) of SSRIs and newer agents have not been studied.

With lithium, long-term therapy is the usual practice because of a high recurrence rate if the drug is discontinued. When lithium is discontinued, most often because of adverse effects or the client's lack of adherence to the prescribed regimen, gradually tapering the dose over 2 to 4 weeks delays recurrence of symptoms.

Effects of Antidepressants on Nonpsychotropic Drugs

The SSRIs are strong inhibitors of the cytochrome P450 enzyme system that metabolizes many drugs, including adrenal corticosteroids, antiarrhythmics (eg, propafenone), beta-adrenergic blocking agents, benzodiazepine antianxiety and hypnotic agents, calcium channel blockers, carbamazepine, erythromycin, lidocaine, quinidine, and opiate analgesics. Inhibiting the enzymes that normally metabolize or inactivate a drug produces the same effect as an excessive dose of the inhibited drug. As a result, serum drug levels and risks of adverse effects are greatly increased.

Nefazodone also inhibits these enzymes. If nefazodone is given with alprazolam or triazolam (benzodiazepines), dosage of the benzodiazepine should be reduced by 50% or more.

Recognition and Management of Toxicity

Some antidepressant drugs are highly toxic and potentially lethal when taken in large doses. Toxicity is most likely to occur in depressed clients who intentionally ingest large amounts of drug in suicide attempts and in young children who accidentally gain access to improperly stored medication containers. Measures to prevent acute poisoning from drug overdose include dispensing only a few days' supply (ie, 5 to 7 days) to clients with suicidal tendencies and storing the drugs in places inaccessible to young children. General measures to treat acute poisoning include early detection of signs and symptoms, stopping the drug, and instituting treatment if indicated. Specific measures include the following:

SSRI overdose: Symptoms include nausea, vomiting, agitation, restlessness, hypomania, and other signs of CNS stimulation. Management includes symptomatic and supportive treatment, such as maintaining an adequate airway and ventilation and administering activated charcoal.

TCA overdose: Symptoms occur approximately 1 to 4 hours after drug ingestion and consist primarily of CNS depression and cardiovascular effects (eg, nystagmus, tremor, restlessness, seizures, hypotension, arrhythmias, myocardial depression). Death usually results from cardiac, respiratory, and circulatory failure. Management of TCA toxicity consists of performing gastric lavage and giving activated charcoal to reduce drug absorption, establishing and maintaining a patent airway, performing continuous ECG monitoring of comatose clients or those with respiratory insufficiency or wide QRS intervals, giving intravenous fluids and vasopressors for severe hypotension, and giving intravenous phenytoin or a parenteral benzodiazepine (eg, lorazepam) if seizures occur.

MAOI overdose: Symptoms occur 12 hours or more after drug ingestion and consist primarily of adrenergic effects (eg, tachycardia, increased rate of respiration, agitation, tremors, convulsive seizures, sweating, heart block, hypotension, delirium, coma). Management consists of diuresis, acidification of urine, or hemodialysis to remove the drug from the body.

Bupropion overdose: Symptoms include agitation and other mental status changes, nausea and vomiting, and seizures. General treatment measures include hospitalization, decreasing absorption (eg, giving activated charcoal to conscious clients), and supporting vital functions. If seizures occur, an intravenous benzodiazepine (eg, lorazepam) is the drug of first choice.

Nefazodone or venlafaxine overdose: Symptoms include increased incidence or severity of adverse effects, with nausea, vomiting, and drowsiness most often reported. Hypotension and excessive sedation may occur with nefazodone, seizures and diastolic hypertension with venlafaxine. There are no specific antidotes; treatment is symptomatic and supportive.

Lithium overdose: Toxic manifestations occur with serum lithium levels above 2.5 mEq/L and include nystagmus, tremors, oliguria, confusion, impaired consciousness, visual or tactile hallucinations, choreiform movements, convulsions, coma, and death.

Treatment involves supportive care to maintain vital functions, including correction of fluid and electrolyte imbalances. With severe overdoses, hemodialysis is preferred because it removes lithium from the body.

Prevention and Management of Withdrawal Symptoms

Withdrawal symptoms have been reported with sudden discontinuation of most antidepressant drugs. In general, symptoms occur more rapidly and may be more intense with drugs having a short half-life. As with other psychotropic drugs, these drugs should be tapered in dosage and discontinued gradually unless severe drug toxicity, anaphylactic reactions, or other life-threatening conditions are present. Most antidepressants may be tapered and discontinued over approximately a week without serious withdrawal symptoms. For a client on maintenance drug therapy, the occurrence of withdrawal symptoms may indicate omitted doses or noncompliance.

The most clearly delineated withdrawal syndromes are associated with SSRIs and TCAs. With SSRIs, withdrawal symptoms include dizziness, nausea, and headache and last from several days to several weeks. More serious symptoms may include aggression, hypomania, mood disturbances, and suicidal tendencies. Fluoxetine has a long half-life and has not been associated with withdrawal symptoms. Other SSRIs have short half-lives and may cause withdrawal reactions if stopped abruptly. Paroxetine, which has a half-life of approximately 24 hours and does not produce active metabolites, is associated with rather severe withdrawal symptoms even when discontinued gradually, over 7 to 10 days. Symptoms may include a flu-like syndrome with nausea, vomiting, fatigue, muscle aches, dizziness, headache, and insomnia. The short-acting SSRIs should be tapered in dosage and gradually discontinued to prevent or minimize withdrawal reactions.

With TCAs, the main concern is over those with strong anticholinergic effects. When stopped abruptly, especially with high doses, these drugs can cause symptoms of excessive cholinergic activity (ie, hypersalivation, diarrhea, urinary urgency, abdominal cramping, and sweating). A recommended rate for tapering TCAs is approximately 25 to 50 mg every 2 to 3 days.

Ethnic or Genetic Considerations

Antidepressant drug therapy for nonwhite populations in the United States is based primarily on dosage recommendations, pharmacokinetic data, and adverse effects derived from white recipients. However, several studies document differences in drug effects in nonwhite populations. The differences are mainly attributed to ethnic or genetic variations in drug-metabolizing enzymes in the liver. Although all ethnic groups are genetically heterogeneous and individual members may respond differently, health care providers need to consider potential differences in responses to drug therapy.

1. *African Americans* tend to have higher plasma levels for a given dose, respond more rapidly, experience a higher incidence of adverse effects, and metabolize tricyclic antidepressants (TCAs) more slowly than whites. To decrease adverse effects, initial doses may need to be lower than those given to whites and later doses should be titrated according to clinical response and serum drug levels. In addition, baseline and periodic ECGs are recommended to detect adverse drug effects on the heart. Studies have not been done with newer antidepressants. With lithium, African Americans report more adverse reactions than whites and may need smaller doses.

2. *Asians* tend to metabolize antidepressant drugs slowly and therefore have higher plasma drug levels for a given dose than whites. Most studies have been done with TCAs and a limited number of Asian subgroups. Thus, it cannot be assumed that all antidepressant drugs and all people of Asian heritage respond the same. To avoid drug toxicity, initial doses should be approximately half the usual doses given to whites and later doses should be titrated according to clinical response and serum drug levels. This recommendation is supported by a survey from several Asian countries that reported the use of much smaller doses of TCAs than in the United States. In addition, in Asians as in African Americans, baseline and periodic ECGs are recommended to detect adverse drug effects on the heart. Studies have not been done with newer antidepressants. With lithium, there are no apparent differences between effects in Asians and whites.

3. *Hispanics'* responses to antidepressant drugs are largely unknown. Few studies have been done, with some reporting a need for lower doses of TCAs and greater susceptibility to anticholinergic effects, whereas others report no differences between Hispanics and whites.

Use in Perioperative Periods

Antidepressants must be used very cautiously, if at all, perioperatively because of the risk of serious adverse effects and adverse interactions with anesthetics and other commonly used drugs. MAOIs are contraindicated and should be discontinued at least 10 days before elective surgery. TCAs should be discontinued several days before elective surgery and resumed several days after surgery. SSRIs and miscellaneous antidepressants have not been studied in relation to perioperative use; however, it seems reason-

able to discontinue the drugs when feasible because of potential adverse effects, especially on the cardiovascular system and CNS. It is usually recommended that antidepressants be tapered in dosage and gradually discontinued. Lithium should be stopped 1 to 2 days before surgery and resumed when full oral intake of food and fluids is allowed. Lithium may prolong the effects of anesthetics and neuromuscular blockers.

Use in Children

Depression is considered common in children and adolescents and antidepressant drugs are widely prescribed. However, drug therapy is largely empiric and of unproven effectiveness. Although some antidepressants are approved for other uses in children (eg, two SSRIs, fluvoxamine and sertraline, are approved for treatment of obsessive–compulsive disorder, and some TCAs are approved for treatment of enuresis), none is approved for treatment of depression. Moreover, the long-term effects of antidepressant drugs on the developing brain are unknown. Overall, there are few reliable data or guidelines for the use of antidepressants in children and adolescents. Considerations include the following:

1. For most children and adolescents, it is probably best to reserve drug therapy for those who do not respond to nonpharmacologic treatment and those whose depression is persistent or severe enough to impair function in usual activities of daily living.

2. For adolescents, it may be important to discuss sexual effects because most antidepressants can cause sexual dysfunction (eg, anorgasmia, decreased libido, erectile dysfunction).

3. SSRIs are not approved in children (<18 years of age) and their safety and effectiveness have not been established. However, for children, as for other groups, these drugs are considered first-line antidepressants and safer than TCAs and MAOIs. Common adverse effects include sedation and activation; it is often difficult to distinguish therapeutic effects (improvement of mood, increased energy and motivation) from the adverse effects of behavioral activation (agitation, hypomania, restlessness).

4. TCAs are not recommended for use in children younger than 12 years of age except for short-term treatment of enuresis in children older than 6 years of age. However, they are used to treat depression. Commonly used TCAs include imipramine, amitriptyline, nortriptyline, desipramine, and clomipramine. Because of potentially serious adverse effects, blood pressure, ECGs, and plasma drug levels should be monitored. There is evidence that children metabolize TCAs faster than adults, and withdrawal symptoms (eg, increased GI motility, malaise, headache) are more common in children than in adults.

Divided doses may be better tolerated and minimize withdrawal symptoms. When a TCA is used for enuresis, effectiveness may decrease over time, and no residual benefits continue once the drug is stopped. Common adverse effects include sedation, fatigue, nervousness, and sleep disorders. A TCA probably is not a drug of first choice for adolescents because TCAs are more toxic in overdose than other antidepressants and suicide is a leading cause of death in adolescents.

5. Safety and effectiveness have not been established for amoxapine and MAOIs in children younger than 16 years of age or for bupropion, maprotiline, nefazodone, and venlafaxine in children younger than 18 years of age.

6. Lithium is not approved for use in children younger than 12 years of age, but it has been used to treat bipolar disorder and aggressiveness. Children normally excrete lithium more rapidly than adults. As with adults, initial doses should be relatively low and gradually increased according to regular measurements of serum drug levels.

Use in Older Adults

Selective serotonin reuptake inhibitors are probably the drugs of choice in older adults as in younger ones because they cause fewer sedative, anticholinergic, cardiotoxic, and psychomotor adverse effects than the TCAs and related antidepressants. These drugs produce similar adverse effects in older adults as in younger adults. Although their effects in older adults are not well delineated, SSRIs may be eliminated more slowly, and smaller or less frequent doses may be prudent. The weight loss often associated with SSRIs may be undesirable in older adults. Nefazodone and venlafaxine may also be used in older adults, with smaller initial doses and increments recommended.

Tricyclic antidepressants may cause or aggravate conditions that are common in older adults (eg, cardiac conduction abnormalities, urinary retention, narrow-angle glaucoma). In addition, impaired compensatory mechanisms make older adults more likely to experience anticholinergic effects, confusion, hypotension, and sedation. If a TCA is chosen for an older adult, nortriptyline or desipramine is preferred. In addition, any TCA should be given in small doses initially and gradually increased over several weeks, if necessary, to achieve therapeutic effects. Initial and maintenance doses should be small because the drugs are metabolized and excreted more slowly than in younger adults. Initial dosage should be decreased by 30% to 50% to avoid serious adverse reactions; increments should be small. Vital signs, serum drug levels, and ECGs should be monitored regularly.

Monoamine oxidase inhibitors may be more likely to cause hypertensive crises in older adults because cardiovascular, renal, and hepatic functions are often diminished. With lithium, initial doses should be low and increased gradually, according to regular measurements of serum drug levels.

Use in Renal Impairment

Antidepressants should be used cautiously in the presence of severe renal impairment. Mild or moderate impairment has few effects, but severe impairment may increase plasma levels and adverse effects of virtually all antidepressants. Thus, small initial doses, slow increases, and less frequent dosing are indicated.

Lithium is eliminated only by the kidneys and it has a very narrow therapeutic range. If given to a client with renal impairment or unstable renal function, the dose must be markedly reduced and plasma lithium levels must be closely monitored.

Use in Hepatic Impairment

Hepatic impairment leads to reduced first-pass metabolism of most antidepressant drugs, with resultant higher plasma levels after oral administration. The drugs should be used cautiously in clients with severe liver impairment. Cautious use means lower doses, longer intervals between doses, and slower dose increases than usual.

Fluoxetine and sertraline are less readily metabolized to their active metabolites with hepatic impairment, including cirrhosis. In clients with cirrhosis, for example, the average half-life of fluoxetine may increase from 2 to 3 days to more than 7 days, and that of norfluoxetine, the active metabolite, from 7 to 9 days to 12 days. Clearance of sertraline is also decreased in clients with cirrhosis. Paroxetine has a short half-life and no active metabolites, but increased plasma levels can occur with severe hepatic impairment.

Tricyclic antidepressants are also less readily metabolized with severe hepatic impairment such as in severe cirrhosis. This increases the risk of adverse effects such as sedation or hypotension.

Use in Critical Illness

Critically ill clients may be receiving an antidepressant drug when the critical illness develops or may need a drug to combat the depression that often develops with major illness. The decision to continue or start an antidepressant drug should be based on a thorough assessment of the client's condition, other drugs being given, potential adverse drug effects, and other factors. If an antidepressant is given, its use must be cautious and slow and the client's responses carefully monitored because critically ill clients are often frail and unstable, with multiple organ dysfunctions.

 Home Care

Whatever the primary problem for which a home care nurse is visiting a client, he or she must be vigilant for signs and symptoms of major depression. Depression often accompanies any serious physical illness and may occur in many other circumstances as well. The main role of the nurse may be in recognizing depressive states and referring clients for treatment. If antidepressant medications were recently started, the nurse may need to remind the client that it takes 2 or 3 weeks to feel better; the nurse should encourage the client to continue taking the medication. Also, the nurse needs to observe the client's response and assess for suicidal thoughts or plans.

(*text continues on page 167*)

NURSING ACTIONS	Antidepressants

NURSING ACTIONS	**RATIONALE/EXPLANATION**
1. Administer accurately	
a. Give most selective serotonin reuptake inhibitors (SSRIs) in the morning; sertraline may be given morning or evening.	To prevent insomnia
b. Give tricyclic antidepressants (TCAs) and mirtazapine at bedtime.	To aid sleep and decrease daytime sedation
c. Give venlafaxine and lithium with food.	To decrease gastrointestinal (GI) effects (eg, nausea and vomiting)
2. Observe for therapeutic effects	
a. With antidepressants, observe for statements of feeling better or being less depressed; increased appetite, physical activity, and interest in surroundings; improved sleep patterns; improved appearance; decreased anxiety; decreased somatic complaints.	Therapeutic effects usually do not occur for 2 to 3 weeks after drug therapy is started.
b. With lithium, observe for decreases in manic behavior and mood swings.	Therapeutic effects do not occur until approximately 7 to 10 days after therapeutic serum drug levels are attained. In mania, a benzodiazepine or an antipsychotic drug is usually given to reduce agitation and control behavior until the lithium takes effect.
3. Observe for adverse effects	
a. With SSRIs, nefazodone, and venlafaxine, observe for headache, nervousness, insomnia, nausea, diarrhea, dizziness, dry mouth, constipation, sedation, skin rash, sexual dysfunction.	GI upset and diarrhea are common with SSRIs; GI upset, diarrhea, and orthostatic hypotension are common with nefazodone; GI upset, diarrhea, agitation, and insomnia are common with venlafaxine. Although numerous adverse effects may occur, they are usually less serious than those occurring with most other antidepressants. Compared with the TCAs, SSRIs and other newer drugs are less likely to cause significant sedation, hypotension, and cardiac arrhythmias but are more likely to cause nausea, nervousness, and insomnia.
b. With TCAs, observe for:	Most adverse effects result from anticholinergic or antiadrenergic activity. Cardiovascular effects are most serious in overdose.
(1) Central nervous system (CNS) effects—drowsiness, dizziness, confusion	

(*continued*)

NURSING ACTIONS	**RATIONALE/EXPLANATION**
(2) Cardiovascular effects—cardiac arrhythmias, tachycardia, orthostatic hypotension	
(3) GI effects—nausea, dry mouth, constipation	
(4) Other effects—blurred vision, urinary retention, sexual dysfunction, weight gain	
c. With monoamine oxidase inhibitors (MAOIs), observe for blurred vision, constipation, dizziness, dry mouth, hypotension, urinary retention, hypoglycemia.	Anticholinergic effects are common. Hypoglycemia results from a drug-induced reduction in blood sugar.
d. With bupropion, observe for seizure activity, CNS stimulation (agitation, insomnia, hyperactivity, hallucinations, delusions), headache, nausea and vomiting, and weight loss.	Adverse effects are most likely to occur if recommended doses are exceeded.
e. With mirtazapine, observe for sedation, confusion, dry mouth, constipation, nausea and vomiting, hypotension, tachycardia, urinary retention, photosensitivity, skin rash, weight gain.	Common effects are drowsiness, dizziness, and weight gain. Has CNS depressant and anticholinergic effects.
f. With lithium, observe for:	Most clients who take lithium experience adverse effects. Symptoms listed in (1) are common, occur at therapeutic serum drug levels (0.8–1.2 mEq/L), and usually subside during the first few weeks of drug therapy. Symptoms listed in (2) occur at higher serum drug levels (1.5–2.5 mEq/L). Nausea may be decreased by giving lithium with meals. Propranolol (Inderal), 20–120 mg daily, may be given to control tremors. Severe adverse effects may be managed by decreasing lithium dosage, omitting a few doses, or discontinuing the drug temporarily. Toxic symptoms occur at serum drug levels above 2.5 mEq/L.
(1) Metallic taste, hand tremors, nausea, polyuria, polydipsia, diarrhea, muscular weakness, fatigue, edema, and weight gain	
(2) More severe nausea and diarrhea, vomiting, ataxia, incoordination, dizziness, slurred speech, blurred vision, tinnitus, muscle twitching and tremors, increased muscle tone	
(3) Leukocytosis	Lithium mobilizes white blood cells (WBCs) from bone marrow to the bloodstream. Maximum increase in WBCs occurs in 7 to 10 days.
4. Observe for drug interactions	
a. Drugs that *increase* effects of SSRIs:	Drug interactions with the SSRIs vary with individual drugs.
(1) Cimetidine	May increase serum drug levels of SSRIs by slowing their metabolism
(2) MAOIs	**SSRIs and MAOIs should not be given concurrently or close together because serious and fatal reactions have occurred.** The reaction, attributed to excess serotonin and called the *serotonin syndrome*, may cause hyperthermia, muscle spasm, agitation, delirium, and coma. To avoid this reaction, an SSRI should not be started for at least 2 weeks after an MAOI is discontinued, and an MAOI should not be started for at least 2 weeks after an SSRI has been

(continued)

NURSING ACTIONS	RATIONALE/EXPLANATION
	discontinued (5 weeks with fluoxetine, because of its long half-life).
b. Drugs that *decrease* effects of SSRIs:	
(1) Anticonvulsants (phenobarbital, phenytoin)	These drugs induce liver enzymes that accelerate the metabolism of the SSRIs.
(2) Cyproheptadine	This is an antihistamine with antiserotonin effects.
c. Drugs that *increase* the effects of nefazodone and venlafaxine:	
(1) MAOIs	See SSRIs, above. **These drugs and MAOIs should not be given concurrently or close together because serious and fatal reactions have occurred.** Nefazodone or venlafaxine should be discontinued at least 7 days before starting an MAOI, and an MAOI should be stopped at least 14 days before starting nefazodone or venlafaxine.
d. Drugs that increase effects of TCAs:	
(1) Antiarrhythmics (eg, quinidine, disopyramide, procainamide)	Additive effects on cardiac conduction, increasing risk of heart block
(2) Antihistamines, atropine, and other drugs with anticholinergic effects	Additive anticholinergic effects (eg, dry mouth, blurred vision, urinary retention, constipation)
(3) Antihypertensives	Additive hypotension
(4) Cimetidine	Increases risks of toxicity by decreasing hepatic metabolism and increasing blood levels of TCAs.
(5) CNS depressants (eg, alcohol, benzodiazepine antianxiety and hypnotic agents, opioid analgesics)	Additive sedation and CNS depression
(6) MAOIs	**TCAs should not be given with MAOIs or within 2 weeks after an MAOI drug;** hyperpyrexia, convulsions, and death have occurred with concurrent use.
(7) SSRIs	Inhibit metabolism of TCAs
e. Drugs that *decrease* effects of TCAs:	
(1) Barbiturates, nicotine (cigarette smoking)	These drugs decrease blood levels of TCAs by increasing the rate of hepatic metabolism of the antidepressant agent.
f. Drugs that *increase* effects of MAOIs:	
(1) Anticholinergic drugs (eg, atropine, antipsychotic agents, TCAs)	Additive anticholinergic effects
(2) Adrenergic agents (eg, epinephrine, phenylephrine), alcohol (some beers and wines), levodopa, meperidine	Hypertensive crisis and stroke may occur.
g. Drugs that *increase* effects of lithium:	
(1) Angiotensin-converting enzyme inhibitors (eg, captopril)	Decrease renal clearance of lithium and thus increase serum lithium levels and risks of toxicity.
(2) Diuretics (eg, furosemide, hydrochlorothiazide)	Increase neurotoxicity and cardiotoxicity of lithium by increasing excretion of sodium and potassium and thereby decreasing excretion of lithium.

(continued)

NURSING ACTIONS	RATIONALE/EXPLANATION
(3) Nonsteroidal anti-inflammatory drugs	Decrease renal clearance of lithium and thus increase serum levels and risks of lithium toxicity.
(4) Phenothiazines	Increased risk of hyperglycemia
(5) TCAs	May increase antidepressant effects of lithium and are sometimes combined with lithium for this purpose. These drugs also may precipitate a manic episode and increase risks of hypothyroidism.
h. Drugs that *decrease* effects of lithium: (1) Acetazolamide, sodium chloride (in excessive amounts), drugs with a high sodium content (eg, ticarcillin), theophylline	Increase excretion of lithium

How Can You Avoid This Medication Error?

Answer: Do not leave medications at the bedside of a client. Often they can be forgotten or taken away with the food tray. Missing a dose of a medication can affect therapeutic blood levels. In this situation, special care should be taken to supervise all medications. Depressed clients could save up medication to commit suicide by overdosing. The risk for this increases as the antidepressant drugs start to work, giving the client more energy to carry out suicidal actions. Wake Jane up and firmly encourage her to take her medications as you watch.

Nursing Notes: Apply Your Knowledge

Answer: Prozac has a long half-life (24 to 72 hours), so it takes longer than a week to reach steady state. The dosage is usually not increased for 3 to 4 weeks. It is important to teach all clients beginning therapy with antidepressants that they may not see significant improvement in their depression for a number of weeks. Ms. Jordan's sleeping difficulty could be a symptom of her depression or a side effect of the Prozac. If it is a drug side effect, it might help to take the drug in the morning.

REVIEW AND APPLICATION EXERCISES

1. During the initial assessment of any client, what kinds of appearances or behaviors may indicate depression?

2. Is antidepressant drug therapy indicated for most episodes of temporary sadness? Why or why not?

3. What are the major groups of antidepressant drugs?

4. How do the drugs act to relieve depression?

5. When a client begins antidepressant drug therapy, why is it important to explain that relief of depression may not occur for a few weeks?

6. What are common adverse effects of TCAs, and how may they be minimized?

7. What is the advantage of giving a TCA at bedtime rather than in the morning?

8. For a client taking an MAOI, what information would you provide for preventing a hypertensive crisis?

9. How do the SSRIs differ from TCAs?

10. How do the newer drugs, mirtazapine, nefazodone, and venlafaxine, compare with the SSRIs in terms of adverse effects and adverse drug–drug interactions?

11. List the main elements of treatment for antidepressant overdoses.

12. What are common adverse effects of lithium, and how may they be minimized?

13. What is the nurse's role in assessing and managing depression in special populations? In the home setting?

SELECTED REFERENCES

American Psychiatric Association. (1994). *Diagnostic and statistical manual of mental disorders*, 4th ed (Revised). Washington, D.C.: American Psychiatric Association.

Daly, J.M. & Wilens, T. (1998). The use of tricyclic antidepressants in children and adolescents. *Pediatric Clinics of North America, 45,* 1123–1135.

Depression Guideline Panel. (1993). *Clinical practice guideline: Depression in primary care, 2: Treatment of major depression.* Rockville, MD: U.S. Department of Health and Human Services, Public Health Service, Agency for Health Care Policy and Research; AHCPR publication No. 93-0551.

Drug facts and comparisons. (Updated monthly). St. Louis: Facts and Comparisons.

Fankhauser, M.P. & Benefield, W.H. (1997). Bipolar disorder. In J.T. DiPiro, R.L. Talbert, P.E. Hayes, G.C. Yee, G.R. Matzke, B.G. Wells, & L.M. Posey (Eds.), *Pharmacotherapy: A pathophysiologic approach,* 3rd ed., pp. 1419–1441. Stamford, CT: Appleton & Lange.

Isaacs, A. (1998). Depression and your patient. *American Journal of Nursing, 98*(7), 26–31.

Knies, R.C. (1998). Discontinuation of some depression, migraine, and anxiety drugs can cause reactions. *Journal of Emergency Nursing, 24,* 424–426.

Labellarte, M.J., Walkup, J.T., & Riddle, M.A. (1998). The new antidepressants: Selective serotonin reuptake inhibitors. *Pediatric Clinics of North America, 45,* 1137–1155.

Mohr, W.K. (1998). Cross-ethnic variations in the care of psychiatric patients: A review of contributing factors and practice considerations. *Journal of Psychosocial Nursing, 36*(5), 16–21.

Mohr, W.K. (1998). Updating what we know about depression in adolescents. *Journal of Psychosocial Nursing, 36*(9), 12–19.

O'Toole, S.M. & Johnson, D.A. (1997). Psychobiology and psychopharmacotherapy of unipolar major depression: A review. *Archives of Psychiatric Nursing, 11,* 304–313.

Pies, R.W. (1998). *Handbook of essential psychopharmacology.* Washington, D.C.: American Psychiatric Press, Inc.

Risby, E.D. (1996). Ethnic considerations in the pharmacotherapy of mood disorders. *Psychopharmacology Bulletin, 32,* 231–234.

Sherr, J. (1996). Psychopharmacology and other biologic therapies. In K.M. Fortinash & P.A. Holoday-Worret (Eds.), *Psychiatric-mental health nursing,* pp. 531–564. St. Louis: C.V. Mosby.

Tosyali, M.C. & Greenhill, L.L. (1998). Child and adolescent psychopharmacology. *Pediatric Clinics of North America, 45,* 1021–1035.

Wells, B.G., Mandos, L.A., & Hayes, P.E. (1997). Depressive disorders. In J.T. DiPiro, R.L. Talbert, P.E. Hayes, G.C. Yee, G.R. Matzke, B.G. Wells, & L.M. Posey (Eds.), *Pharmacotherapy: A pathophysiologic approach,* 3rd ed., pp. 1395–1417. Stamford, CT: Appleton & Lange.

Zimmerman, P.G. (1997). Tricyclic antidepressant overdose. *American Journal of Nursing, 97*(10), 39.

11

Antiseizure Drugs

Objectives

After studying this chapter, the student will be able to:

1. Define terms commonly used to describe seizure disorders.

2. Discuss major factors that influence choice of an antiseizure drug for a client with a seizure disorder.

3. Differentiate uses and effects of commonly used antiseizure drugs.

4. Differentiate characteristics of older and newer antiseizure drugs.

5. Apply the nursing process with clients experiencing selected seizure disorders.

You are caring for 6-month-old Jamie, who was just diagnosed with tonic-clonic seizures. He was started on valproic acid (Depakene) 30 mg qid and has only had one seizure during his 4-day hospitalization. He will be discharged today to his single, teenaged mother, who will be the primary caregiver.

Reflect on:

▶ How you would feel as a new parent if your infant were diagnosed with a seizure disorder. What would be your most significant fears?

▶ Given 15 minutes for discharge teaching, prioritize your teaching plan, considering the following: safe administration of an anticonvulsant medication to a 6-month-old; methods to avoid skipping doses, which could increase risk of seizures; management of Jamie during a seizure to ensure safety.

SEIZURE DISORDERS

Antiseizure drugs are also called antiepileptic drugs (AEDs) or anticonvulsants. The terms *seizure* and *convulsion* are often used interchangeably, although they are not the same. A seizure involves a brief episode of abnormal electrical activity in nerve cells of the brain that may or may not be accompanied by visible changes in appearance or behavior. A convulsion is a common, tonic-clonic type of seizure characterized by spasmodic contractions of involuntary muscles.

Seizures may occur as single events in response to hypoglycemia, fever, electrolyte imbalances, overdoses of numerous drugs (eg, cocaine, isoniazid, lidocaine, lithium, phenothiazine antipsychotic drugs, theophylline), and withdrawal of alcohol or sedative-hypnotic drugs. In these instances, treatment of the underlying problem or temporary use of an AED may relieve the seizures.

Epilepsy

When seizures occur in a chronic, recurrent pattern, the disorder is called *epilepsy*, and drug therapy is usually required. Epilepsy is characterized by abnormal and excessive electrical discharges of nerve cells. It is diagnosed by clinical signs and symptoms of seizure activity and by the presence of abnormal brain wave patterns on the electroencephalogram. The cause of most cases of epilepsy is unknown. When epilepsy begins in infancy, causes include developmental defects, metabolic disease, or birth injury. When it begins in adulthood, it is usually caused by an acquired brain disorder, such as head injury, disease or infection of the brain and spinal cord, cerebrovascular accident (stroke), metabolic disorder, primary or metastatic brain tumor, or other recognizable neurologic disease.

Epilepsy is classified as partial and generalized seizures. *Partial or focal seizures* begin in a specific area of the brain and produce symptoms ranging from simple motor and sensory manifestations to more complex abnormal movements and bizarre behavior. Movements are usually automatic, repetitive, and inappropriate to the situation, such as chewing, swallowing, or aversive movements. Behavior is sometimes so bizarre that the person is diagnosed as psychotic or schizophrenic.

Generalized seizures are bilateral and symmetric and have no discernible point of origin in the brain. The most common type is the tonic-clonic or major motor seizure, formerly called grand mal seizures. The tonic phase involves sustained contraction of skeletal muscles; abnormal postures, such as opisthotonos; and absence of respiration, during which the person becomes cyanotic. The clonic phase is characterized by rapid rhythmic and symmetric jerking movements of the body. Tonic-clonic sei-

zures are sometimes preceded by an aura, a brief warning, such as a flash of light or a specific sound.

Another type of generalized seizure is the absence seizure, characterized by abrupt alterations in consciousness that last only a few seconds. The person may have a blank, staring expression with or without blinking of the eyelids, twitching of the head or arms, and other motor movements. Other types of generalized seizures include the myoclonic type (contraction of a muscle or group of muscles) and the akinetic type (absence of movement). Some people are subject to mixed seizures.

Status epilepticus is a life-threatening emergency characterized by generalized tonic-clonic convulsions occurring at close intervals. The client does not regain consciousness between seizures, and hypotension, hypoxia, and cardiac arrhythmias may occur. There is a high risk of permanent brain damage and death unless prompt, appropriate treatment is instituted. In a person taking medications for a diagnosed seizure disorder, the most common cause of status epilepticus is abruptly stopping AEDs. In other clients, regardless of whether they have a diagnosed seizure disorder, causes of status epilepticus include brain trauma or tumors, systemic or central nervous system (CNS) infections, alcohol withdrawal, and overdoses of drugs (eg, cocaine, theophylline).

ANTISEIZURE DRUGS

Antiseizure drugs, which belong to several different chemical groups, can control seizure activity but do not cure the underlying disorder. Long-term administration is usually required. Most AEDs can be taken orally and are absorbed through the intestinal mucosa. After absorption, the drugs pass through the liver and undergo transformation by liver enzymes, during which some of the drug is inactivated. Most AEDs are metabolized in the liver.

Mechanism of Action

Antiepileptic drugs are thought to act in two main ways to control seizure activity. One way is to block the movement of sodium ions into nerve cells. Because movement of sodium and other ions is required for normal conduction of nerve impulses, blocking sodium ions decreases responsiveness to stimuli and results in stabilized, less excitable cell membranes. A second way is to enhance the activity of gamma-aminobutyric acid (GABA), the major inhibitory neurotransmitter in the brain. Benzodiazepines and most of the newer AEDs increase the effects of GABA. The actions of both sodium channel blockers and GABA enhancers raise the amount of stimulation required to produce a seizure (called the *seizure threshold*). Some of the drugs may also inhibit glutamate, the major excitatory neurotransmitter in the brain.

Indications for Use

The major clinical indication for AEDs is the prevention or treatment of seizures, especially the chronic recurring seizures of epilepsy. Indications for particular drugs depend on the types of seizures involved. In addition to maintenance treatment of epilepsy, AEDs also are used to stop acute, tonic-clonic convulsions and status epilepticus. The drug of choice for this purpose is an intravenous (IV) benzodiazepine, usually lorazepam (Ativan). Once acute seizure activity is controlled, a longer-acting drug, such as phenytoin, is given to prevent recurrence. AEDs also are used prophylactically in clients with brain trauma from injury or surgery.

Contraindications to Use

Antiepileptic drugs are contraindicated or must be used with caution in clients with CNS depression. Phenytoin, carbamazepine, gabapentin, lamotrigine, tiagabine, topiramate, and valproate are contraindicated in clients who have experienced a hypersensitivity reaction to the particular drug (usually manifested by a skin rash, arthralgia, and other symptoms). Phenytoin, carbamazepine, ethosuximide, lamotrigine, and topiramate are contraindicated or must be used cautiously in clients with hepatic or renal impairment. Additional contraindications include phenytoin with sinus bradycardia or heart block; carbamazepine with bone marrow depression (eg, leukopenia, agranulocytosis); and tiagabine and valproic acid with liver disease.

INDIVIDUAL ANTISEIZURE DRUGS

Individual drugs are described in this section; the types of seizures for which each drug is used and routes and dosage ranges are listed in Table 11-1.

Phenytoin (Dilantin), the prototype, is one of the oldest and most widely used AEDs. It is often the initial drug of choice, especially in adults. In addition to treatment of seizure disorders, it is also used to prevent seizures in people who have had brain surgery or brain injury. The drug also is used occasionally to treat cardiac arrhythmias.

Oral phenytoin is slowly absorbed from the small intestine. The rate and extent of absorption vary with the drug formulation. Prompt-acting forms reach peak plasma levels in approximately 2 to 3 hours, and long-acting forms in approximately 12 hours. Intramuscular (IM) phenytoin is poorly absorbed and this route is not recommended. Phenytoin is highly bound to plasma proteins (approximately 90%). It is metabolized in the liver to inactive metabolites that are excreted in the urine. The rate of metabolism varies, but the average half-life is approximately 18 to 24 hours. The clinical significance of this relatively long

half-life is that phenytoin can be given once or twice daily and that, when it is started at usual maintenance doses, a steady-state concentration in plasma is not reached for approximately 1 to 3 weeks.

The most common adverse effects of phenytoin affect the CNS (eg, ataxia, drowsiness, lethargy) and gastrointestinal (GI) tract (nausea, vomiting). Gingival hyperplasia is also common, especially in children. Serious reactions are uncommon but may include allergic reactions, hepatitis, nephritis, bone marrow depression, and mental confusion.

Phenytoin may have clinically important interactions with many other drugs. It is a strong inducer of drug-metabolizing enzymes in the liver. Thus, it can increase the metabolism of itself and many other drugs, both AEDs and non-AEDs. Also, many other drugs can affect phenytoin metabolism and protein binding. For any client receiving phenytoin and one or more other drugs, precautions should be taken to reduce the risk of serious adverse drug interactions.

Phenytoin is available in generic and brand name (Dilantin) capsules, a chewable tablet, an oral suspension, and an injectable solution. The injectable solution is highly irritating to tissues and special techniques are required when the drug is given IV.

Fosphenytoin (Cerebyx) is a prodrug formulation that is rapidly hydrolyzed to phenytoin after IV or IM injection. It is approved for treatment of status epilepticus and for short-term use in clients who cannot take oral phenytoin. In contrast to other preparations of injectable phenytoin, fosphenytoin causes minimal tissue irritation, can be diluted with 5% dextrose or 0.9% sodium chloride solution, and can be given IV more rapidly. The disadvantages of fosphenytoin include higher costs and potential confusion with dosage and administration. The manufacturer recommends that all dosages be expressed in phenytoin equivalents (PE). Fosphenytoin is available in 2-mL and 10-mL vials with 50 mg PE/mL (fosphenytoin 75 mg/mL). For IV administration, fosphenytoin can be diluted to a concentration of 1.5 to 25 mg PE/mL, and infused at a maximal rate of 150 mg PE/minute.

Carbamazepine (Tegretol) is related chemically to the tricyclic antidepressants and pharmacologically to phenytoin. In addition to seizure disorders, carbamazepine also is used to treat facial pain associated with trigeminal neuralgia and some psychiatric disorders, including unipolar and bipolar depression.

Carbamazepine is given orally and peak blood levels are reached in approximately 1.5 hours with the liquid suspension, 4 to 5 hours with conventional tablets, and 3 to 12 hours with extended-release forms (tablets and capsules). It is metabolized in the liver to an active metabolite. Because it induces its own metabolism, its half-life is approximately 12 to 17 hours with chronic administration. Carbamazepine is contraindicated in clients with previous bone marrow depression or hypersensitivity to carbamaze-

(*text continues on page 175*)

TABLE 11-1   Antiseizure Drugs

Generic/Trade Name	Types of Seizures Used to Treat	Routes and Dosage Ranges		Remarks
		Adults	**Children**	
Phenytoin (Dilantin)	Generalized tonic-clonic and some partial seizures, such as psychomotor seizures	PO 100 mg three times daily initially; 300 mg (long-acting) once daily as maintenance IV 100 mg q6–8h; maximum 50 mg/min	PO 4–7 mg/kg/d in divided doses; maximum dose, 300 mg/d	The therapeutic serum level is 5 to 20 µg/mL (SI units 40–80 µmol/L). Concentrations at or above the upper therapeutic level may be associated with toxicity.
Fosphenytoin (Cerebyx)	Status epilepticus and short-term use in clients who cannot take oral phenytoin	Nonemergent seizures, IV, IM loading dose 1–20 mg PE/kg; maintenance dose 4–6 mg PE/kg/d; status epilepticus, IV 15–20 mg PE/kg, at a rate of 100–150 mg PE/min	Dosage not established	Much easier to give IV than phenytoin; can also be given IM
Carbamazepine (Tegretol)	Psychomotor, generalized tonic-clonic, and mixed seizures	Epilepsy, PO 200 mg twice daily, increased gradually to 600–1200 mg if needed, in 3 or 4 divided doses Trigeminal neuralgia, PO 200 mg/d, increased gradually to 1200 mg if necessary	>12 y: PO 200 mg twice daily, gradually increased to 20–30 mg/kg/d if necessary 6–12 y: PO 100 mg twice daily, gradually increased to 20–30 mg/kg/d, in 3 or 4 divided doses, if necessary	Therapeutic range of serum drug levels is approximately 4 to 12 µg/mL (SI units, 17–51 µmol/L).
Clonazepam (Klonopin)	Myoclonic or akinetic seizures, alone or with other AEDs; possibly effective in generalized tonic-clonic and psychomotor seizures	PO 1.5 mg/d, increased by 0.5 mg/d every 3–7 days if necessary; maximum dose, 20 mg/d	PO 0.01–0.03 mg/kg/d, increased by 0.25–0.5 mg/d every 3–7 days if necessary; maximum dose, 0.2 mg/kg/d	Schedule IV drug
Clorazepate (Tranxene)	Partial seizures, with other AEDs	PO maximal initial dose 7.5 mg 3 times daily; increased by 7.5 mg every week, if necessary; maximum dose, 90 mg/d	>12 y: PO same as adults 9–12 y: PO maximal initial dose 7.5 mg two times daily; increased by 7.5 mg every week, if necessary; maximum dose, 60 mg/d	Schedule IV drug
Diazepam (Valium)	Acute convulsive seizures, status epilepticus	IV 5–10 mg at no more than 2 mg/min; repeat every 5–10 min if needed; maximum dose, 30 mg. Repeat in 2–4 hours if necessary; maximum dose, 100 mg/24 h.	>30 d and <5 y: IV 0.2–0.5 mg over 2–3 min, every 2–5 min up to a maximum of 5 mg. ≥5 y: IV 1 mg every 2–5 min up to a maximum of 10 mg. Repeat in 2–4 hours if necessary.	Schedule IV drug
Ethosuximide (Zarontin)	Absence seizures; also may be effective in myoclonic and akinetic epilepsy	PO initially 500 mg/d, increased by 250 mg at weekly intervals until seizures are controlled or toxicity occurs; maximum dose, approximately 1500 mg/d	PO initially 250 mg/d, increased at weekly intervals until seizures are controlled or toxicity occurs; maximum dose, approximately 750–1000 mg/d	The therapeutic range of serum drug levels is approximately 40 to 80 µg/mL.
Gabapentin (Neurontin)	Partial seizures that do not respond adequately to a single drug; given with other AEDs	PO Day 1, 300 mg once; day 2, 300 mg twice (600 mg); day 3, 300 mg three times (900 mg); increase by 250 mg each week until	>12 y: Same as adults <12 y: Safety and dosage not established	Reportedly does not cause significant drug–drug interactions

Drug	Indications for Use	Routes and Dosage Ranges (Adults)	Routes and Dosage Ranges (Children)	Comments
		seizures are controlled or toxicity occurs, up to 1800 mg/d. Usual maintenance dose, 900–1800 mg/d, in 3 divided doses. Renal impairment: Creatinine clearance (Crcl) >60 mL/min, 400 mg 3 times daily (1200 mg/d); Crcl 30–60 mL/min, 300 mg 2 times daily (600 mg/d); Crcl 15–30 mL/min, 300 mg 2 times daily, 300 mg once daily; Crcl <15 mL/min, 300 mg every other day. For patients on hemodialysis, 200–300 mg after each 4 h of hemodialysis.		
Lamotrigine (Lamictal)	Partial seizures, in combination with other AEDs	With AEDs other than valproic acid: PO 50 mg once daily for 2 wk, then 50 mg twice daily (100 mg/d) for 2 wk, then increase by 100 mg/d at weekly intervals to a maintenance dose. Usual maintenance dose, 300–500 mg/d in 2 divided doses. Adults receiving AEDs plus valproic acid: PO 25 mg every other day for 2 wk, then 25 mg once daily for 2 wk, then increase by 25 to 50 mg/d every 1 to 2 wk to a maintenance dose. Usual maintenance dose, 100–150 mg/d in 2 divided doses.	<16 y: Safety and dosage not established	Valproic acid slows lamotrigine's metabolism by approximately 50%. If lamotrigine is combined with other AEDs plus valproic acid, dosage must be substantially reduced.
Lorazepam (Ativan)	Acute convulsive seizures, status epilepticus	IV 2–10 mg, diluted in an equal amount of sterile water for injection, 0.9% sodium chloride injection, or 5% dextrose in water, and injected over 2 min	Dosage not established	Schedule IV drug
Phenobarbital	Generalized tonic-clonic epilepsy and temporal lobe and other partial seizures. It also may be used to treat status epilepticus.	PO 100–300 mg daily in 2 to 3 divided doses	PO 5 mg/kg per day in 2 to 3 divided doses	Serum drug levels of 10 to 25 µg/mL are in the therapeutic range.
Primidone (Mysoline)	Generalized tonic-clonic, psychomotor, or partial seizures, alone or with other AEDs	PO 500–1500 mg/d in divided doses	PO 5–20 mg/kg/d	The therapeutic ranges are phenobarbital 10 to 20 µg/mL; primidone, 5 to 10 µg/mL; and phenylethylmalonamide, 7 to 15 µg/mL.
Tiagabine (Gabitril)	Partial seizures, with other AEDs	PO 4 mg daily for 1 wk, increased by 4–8 mg/wk until desired effect; maximum dose 56 mg/d in 2 to 4 divided doses	12–18 y: PO 4 mg daily for 1 wk, increased to 8 mg/d in 2 divided doses for 1 wk; then increased by 4–8 mg/wk up to a maximum of 32 mg/d in 2 to 4 divided doses <12 y: not recommended	Most experience obtained in patients receiving at least one concomitant enzyme-inducing AED. Use in noninduced patients (eg, those receiving valproate monotherapy) may require lower doses or a slower dose titration.

(continued)

TABLE 11-1   **Antiseizure Drugs** *(continued)*

Generic/Trade Name	Types of Seizures Used to Treat	Routes and Dosage Ranges		Remarks
		Adults	Children	
Topiramate (Topamax)	Partial seizures, with other AEDs	PO wk 1, 50 mg every PM; wk 2, 50 mg AM and PM; wk 3, 50 mg AM and 100 mg PM; wk 4, 100 mg AM and PM; wk 5, 100 mg AM and 150 mg PM; wk 6, 150 mg AM and PM; wk 7, 150 mg AM and 200 mg PM; wk 8 and maintenance, 200 mg AM and PM	Safety and effectiveness not established	
Valproic acid (Depakene capsules)	Absence, mixed, and complex partial seizures	PO 10–15 mg/kg/d, increasing each wk by 5–10 mg/kg/d, until seizures controlled, adverse effects occur, or the maximum recommended dose (60 mg/kg/d) is reached. Give amounts >250 mg/d in divided doses. Usual daily dose, 1000–1600 mg, in divided doses	PO 15–30 mg/kg/d	Therapeutic plasma levels are approximately 50 to 100 μg/mL (SI units 350–700 μmol/L) *Note:* Dosage ranges are the same for the different formulations; doses are in valproic acid equivalents.
Sodium valproate (Depakene syrup; Depacon injection)				
Divalproex sodium (Depakote enteric-coated tablets)		IV client's usual dose, diluted in 5% dextrose or 0.9% sodium chloride injection, infused over 60 min, not more than 20 mg/min		Do not give IV >14 days; switch to oral product when possible.

AED, antiepileptic drug; IM, intramuscular; IV, intravenous; PE, phenytoin equivalent; PO, oral.

pine or tricyclic antidepressants and in clients receiving monoamine oxidase inhibitors (MAOIs). MAOIs should be discontinued at least 14 days before carbamazepine is started.

Clonazepam (Klonopin), **clorazepate** (Tranxene), **diazepam** (Valium), and **lorazepam** (Ativan) are benzodiazepines (see Chap. 8) used in seizure disorders. Clonazepam and clorazepate are used in long-term treatment of seizure disorders, alone or with other AEDs. Tolerance to antiseizure effects develops with long-term use. Clonazepam has a long half-life and may require weeks of continued administration to achieve therapeutic serum levels. As with other benzodiazepines, clonazepam produces physical dependence and withdrawal symptoms. Because of clonazepam's long half-life, withdrawal symptoms may appear several days after administration is stopped. Abrupt withdrawal may precipitate seizure activity or status epilepticus.

Diazepam and lorazepam are used to terminate acute convulsive seizures, especially the life-threatening seizures of status epilepticus. Diazepam has a short duration of action and must be given in repeated doses. In status epilepticus, it is followed with a long-acting anticonvulsant, such as phenytoin. Lorazepam has become the drug of choice for status epilepticus because its effects last longer than those of diazepam.

Ethosuximide (Zarontin) is the AED of choice for absence seizures. It is well absorbed with oral administration and reaches peak serum levels in 3 to 7 hours; a steady-state serum concentration is reached in approximately 5 days. It is eliminated mainly by hepatic metabolism to inactive metabolites; approximately 20% is excreted unchanged through the kidneys. The elimination half-life is approximately 30 hours in children and 60 hours in adults. Ethosuximide may be used with other AEDs for treatment of mixed types of seizures.

Gabapentin (Neurontin) is used with other AEDs for treatment of partial seizures that do not respond adequately to a single drug. Its mechanism of action is unknown. Gabapentin is approximately 60% absorbed from usual therapeutic doses, circulates largely in a free state because it does not bind significantly to plasma proteins, is not appreciably metabolized, and is eliminated by the kidneys as unchanged drug. The elimination half-life is approximately 5 to 7 hours with normal renal function and up to 50 hours with impaired renal function, depending on creatinine clearance.

Adverse effects include dizziness, drowsiness, fatigue, loss of muscle coordination, tremor, nausea, vomiting, constipation, abnormal vision, gingivitis, and pruritus. Most adverse effects subside spontaneously or with dosage reduction. Gabapentin is not metabolized in the liver and reportedly does not cause significant drug–drug interactions. Because gabapentin is eliminated only by the kidneys, dosage must be reduced in clients with renal impairment.

Lamotrigine (Lamictal) is used with other AEDs for treatment of adults with partial seizures. It is thought to reduce the release of glutamate, an excitatory neurotransmitter, in the brain. It is well absorbed after oral administration, with peak plasma levels reached in approximately 1.5 to 4.5 hours. Lamotrigine is approximately 55% bound to plasma proteins. It is metabolized in the liver to an inactive metabolite and eliminated mainly in the urine.

Adverse effects include dizziness, drowsiness, headache, ataxia, blurred or double vision, nausea and vomiting, and weakness. Because a serious skin rash may occur, especially in children, lamotrigine should not be given to children younger than 16 years of age. If a skin rash develops in an adult, lamotrigine should be discontinued.

Lamotrigine does not significantly affect the metabolism of other AEDs, but other AEDs affect lamotrigine's metabolism. Phenytoin, carbamazepine, and phenobarbital induce drug-metabolizing enzymes in the liver and accelerate lamotrigine's metabolism. Valproic acid inhibits those enzymes and thereby slows lamotrigine's metabolism by approximately 50%. If lamotrigine is combined with other AEDs plus valproic acid, dosage must be substantially reduced. To discontinue, dosage should be tapered over at least 2 weeks.

Phenobarbital is a long-acting barbiturate that has been widely used alone or with another AED (most often phenytoin). Its use has declined with the advent of other AEDs that cause less sedation and cognitive impairment. CNS depression and other adverse effects associated with barbiturates may occur, but drug dependence and barbiturate intoxication are unlikely with usual antiepileptic doses. Because phenobarbital has a long half-life, it takes approximately 2 to 3 weeks to reach therapeutic serum levels and 3 to 4 weeks to reach a steady-state concentration.

Primidone (Mysoline) is used alone or with other AEDs. Because it produces marked sedation, primidone is an alternative rather than a primary drug. Excessive sedation is minimized by increasing dosage gradually. Sedation decreases with continued administration of the drug. Primidone is converted to two metabolites, phenobarbital and phenylethylmalonamide. The parent drug and both metabolites exert antiseizure effects. Therefore, measurements of plasma drug levels should include all three chemicals.

Tiagabine (Gabitril) is a newer AED believed to increase GABA levels in the brain. It is used with other AEDs in clients with partial seizures. After oral administration, tiagabine is rapidly and well absorbed. Peak plasma levels occur in approximately 45 minutes if taken on an empty stomach and approximately 2.5 hours if taken with food. It is metabolized in the liver and the metabolites are excreted in urine and feces. Only a small amount, approximately 2%, is excreted unchanged in the urine. The elimination half-life is approximately 4 to 7 hours in clients receiving enzyme-inducing AEDs (eg, phenytoin, carbamazepine, phenobarbital, primidone). Clients with impaired liver function may need smaller doses because the drug is cleared more slowly. CNS effects (eg, confusion, drowsiness, impaired concentration or speech) are the most common adverse effects. GI upset and a serious skin rash may also occur.

Topiramate (Topamax) is a newer AED with a broad spectrum of antiseizure activity. It may act by increasing the effects of GABA and other mechanisms. It is rapidly absorbed and produces peak plasma levels in approximately 2 hours after oral administration. The average elimination half-life is approximately 21 hours, and steady-state concentrations are reached in approximately 4 days with normal renal function. It is approximately 20% bound to plasma proteins. It is not extensively metabolized and is primarily eliminated unchanged through the kidneys. For clients with a creatinine clearance below 70 mL/minute, dosage should be reduced by half.

The most common adverse effects are ataxia, drowsiness, dizziness, and nausea. Additive CNS depression may occur with alcohol and other CNS depressant drugs.

Valproic acid preparations are chemically unrelated to other AEDs. They are thought to act by enhancing the effects of GABA in the brain, and perhaps by other mechanisms. They are also used to treat manic reactions in bipolar disorder and to prevent migraine headaches.

Valproic acid preparations are well absorbed after oral administration and produce peak plasma levels in approximately 1 to 4 hours (15 minutes to 2 hours with the syrup). They are highly bound (90%) to plasma proteins. They are primarily metabolized in the liver and metabolites are excreted through the kidneys.

These preparations produce less sedation and cognitive impairment than phenytoin and phenobarbital. Although they are uncommon, potentially serious adverse effects include hepatotoxicity and pancreatitis. The drugs are contraindicated in people who have had hypersensitivity reactions to any of the preparations and people with hepatic disease or impaired hepatic function.

Valproic acid (Depakene) is available in capsules; sodium valproate is a syrup formulation. Divalproex sodium (Depakote) contains equal parts of valproic acid and sodium valproate and is available as delayed-release tablets and sprinkle capsules. Depacon is an injectable formulation of valproate. Dosages of all formulations are expressed in valproic acid equivalents.

NURSING PROCESS

Assessment

Assess client status in relation to seizure activity and other factors:

- If the client has a known seizure disorder and is taking antiseizure drugs, helpful assessment data can be obtained by interviewing the client. Some questions and guidelines include the following:
  - How long has the client had the seizure disorder?
  - How long has it been since seizure activity occurred, or what is the frequency of seizures?
  - Does any particular situation or activity precipitate a seizure?
  - How does the seizure affect the client? For example, what parts of the body are involved? Does he or she lose consciousness? Is he or she drowsy and tired afterward?
  - Which antiseizure drugs are taken? How do they affect the client? How long has the client taken the drugs? Is the currently ordered dosage the same as what the client has been taking? Does the client usually take the drugs as prescribed, or does he or she find it difficult to do so?
  - What other drugs are taken? This includes both prescription and nonprescription drugs, as well as those taken regularly or periodically. This information is necessary because many drugs interact with antiseizure drugs to decrease seizure control or increase drug toxicity.
  - What is the client's attitude toward the seizure disorder? Clues to attitude may include terminology, willingness or reluctance to discuss the seizure disorder, compliance or rejection of drug therapy, and others.
- Check reports of serum drug levels for abnormal values.
- Identify risk factors for seizure disorders. In people without previous seizure activity, seizure disorders may develop with brain surgery, head injury, hypoxia, hypoglycemia, drug overdosage (CNS stimulants, such as amphetamines, or local anesthetics, such as lidocaine), and withdrawal from CNS depressants, such as alcohol and barbiturates.
- To observe and record seizure activity accurately, note the location (localized or generalized); specific characteristics of abnormal movements or behavior; duration; concomitant events, such as loss of consciousness and loss of bowel or bladder control; and postseizure behavior.
- Assess for risk of status epilepticus. Risk factors include recent changes in antiseizure drug therapy, chronic alcohol ingestion, use of drugs known to cause seizures, and infection.

Nursing Diagnoses

- Ineffective Individual Coping related to anger or denial of the disease process and need for long-term drug therapy
- Self-Esteem Disturbance related to having a seizure disorder
- Impaired Social Interaction related to perceived stigma of epilepsy
- Knowledge Deficit: Disease process
- Knowledge Deficit: Drug effects

- Risk for Injury: Trauma related to ataxia, drowsiness, confusion
- Risk for Injury: Seizure activity
- Noncompliance: Underuse of medications

Planning/Goals

The client will:

- Take medications as prescribed
- Experience control of seizures
- Avoid adverse drug effects
- Verbalize knowledge of the disease process and treatment regimen
- Avoid discontinuing antiseizure medications abruptly
- Keep follow-up appointments with health care providers

Interventions

Use measures to minimize seizure activity. Guidelines include the following:

- Help the client identify conditions under which seizures are likely to occur. These precipitating factors, to be avoided or decreased when possible, may include ingestion of alcoholic beverages or stimulant drugs, such as amphetamines; fever; severe physical or emotional stress; and sensory stimuli, such as flashing lights and loud noises.
- Assist the client in planning how to get enough rest and exercise and eat a balanced diet, if needed.
- Discuss the seizure disorder, the plan for treatment, and the importance of complying with prescribed drug therapy with the client and family members.
- Involve the client in decision making when possible.
- Inform the client and family that seizure control is not gained immediately when drug therapy is started. The goal is to avoid unrealistic expectations and excessive frustration while drugs and dosages are being changed in an effort to determine the best combination for the client.
- Discuss social and economic factors that promote or prevent compliance.
- Protect a client experiencing a generalized tonic-clonic seizure by:
  - Placing a pillow or piece of clothing under the head if injury could be sustained from the ground or floor.
  - Not restraining the client's movements; fractures may result.
  - Loosening tight clothing, especially around the neck and chest, to promote respiration.
  - Turning the client to one side so that accumulated secretions can drain from the mouth and throat when convulsive movements stop. The cyanosis, abnormal movements, and loss of consciousness that characterize a generalized tonic-clonic seizure can be quite alarming to witnesses. Most of these seizures, however, subside within 3 or 4 minutes, and the person starts responding and regaining normal skin color. If the person has one seizure after another (status epilepticus), has trouble breathing or continued cyanosis, or has sustained an injury, further care is needed, and a physician should be notified immediately.
- When risk factors for seizures, especially status epilepticus, are identified, try to prevent or minimize their occurrence.

Evaluation

- Interview and observe for decrease in or absence of seizure activity.
- Interview and observe for avoidance of adverse drug effects, especially those that impair safety.
- When available, check laboratory reports of serum drug levels for therapeutic ranges or evidence of underdosing or overdosing.

How Can You Avoid This Medication Error?

Ms. Hammerly is admitted to your unit for neurosurgery in the morning. She is NPO after midnight. The nurse holds all medications, including her antiseizure medication, which is usually taken at midnight and 6 AM. In the morning, Ms. Hammerly's surgery is delayed so you decide to help her with her shower. While showering, Ms. Hammerly experiences a generalized seizure.

PRINCIPLES OF THERAPY

Drug Selection

The goal of drug therapy for epilepsy is to control seizure activity without severe adverse drug effects. To meet this goal, therapy must be individualized.

1. The choice of drugs is determined largely by the type of seizure. Therefore, an accurate diagnosis is essential before drug therapy is started. For generalized convulsive and focal seizures, phenytoin, carbamazepine, phenobarbital, and valproic acid are effective. For absence seizures, ethosuximide is the drug of choice; clonazepam and valproic acid also are effective. For mixed seizures, a combination of drugs is usually necessary. Guidelines for optimal usage of the newer drugs (gabapentin, lamotrigine,

CLIENT TEACHING GUIDELINES
Antiseizure Medications

General Considerations

✔ Take the medications as prescribed. This is extremely important. These drugs must be taken regularly to maintain blood levels adequate to control seizure activity. At the same time, additional doses must not be taken because of increased risks of serious adverse reactions.

✔ Do not suddenly stop taking any antiseizure medication. Severe, even life-threatening, seizures may occur if the drugs are stopped abruptly.

✔ Discuss any problems (eg, seizure activity, excessive drowsiness, other adverse effects) associated with an antiseizure medication with the prescribing physician or other health care professional. Adjusting dosage or time of administration may relieve the problems.

✔ Do not drive a car, operate machinery, or perform other activities requiring physical and mental alertness when drowsy from antiseizure medications. Excessive drowsiness, decreased physical coordination, and decreased mental alertness increase the likelihood of injury.

✔ Do not take other drugs without the physician's knowledge and inform any other physician or dentist about taking antiseizure medications. There are many potential drug interactions in which the effects of the antiseizure drug or other drugs may be altered when drugs are given concomitantly.

✔ Do not take any other drugs that cause drowsiness, including over-the-counter antihistamines and sleeping aids.

✔ Carry identification, such as a MedicAlert device, with the name and dose of the medication being taken. This is necessary for rapid and appropriate treatment in the event of a seizure, accidental injury, or other emergency situation.

✔ Notify your physician if you become pregnant or intend to become pregnant during therapy.

✔ Notify your physician if you are breastfeeding or intend to breastfeed during therapy.

Self-administration

✔ Take antiseizure medications with food or a full glass of fluid. This will prevent or decrease nausea, vomiting, and gastric distress, which are adverse reactions to most of these drugs.

✔ When taking generic phenytoin or the Dilantin brand of phenytoin:

1. Ask for the same formulation of the drug when renewing prescriptions. There may be differences in formulations from different manufacturers. These differences, such as how fast and how completely the drug is absorbed into the bloodstream, influence seizure control and the likelihood of adverse reactions.
2. Ask your physician if you should take (or give a child) supplements of folic acid, calcium, vitamin D, or vitamin K. These supplements may help to prevent some adverse effects of phenytoin.
3. Brush and floss your teeth and have regular dental care to prevent or delay a gum disorder called gingival hyperplasia.
4. If you have diabetes, you may need to check your blood sugar more often or take a higher dose of your antidiabetic medication. Phenytoin may inhibit the release of insulin and increase blood sugar.
5. Notify your physician or another health care professional if you develop a skin rash, severe nausea and vomiting, swollen glands, bleeding, swollen or tender gums, yellowish skin or eyes, joint pain, unexplained fever, sore throat, unusual bleeding or bruising, persistent headache, or any indication of infection or bleeding, and if you become pregnant.
6. If you are taking phenytoin liquid suspension or giving it to a child, mix it thoroughly immediately before use and measure it with a calibrated medicine cup or a measuring teaspoon. Do not use regular teaspoons because they hold varying amounts of medication.

✔ With valproic acid, the regular capsule should not be opened and the tablet should not be crushed for administration. The sprinkle capsule may be opened and the contents sprinkled on soft food for administration. The syrup formulation may be diluted in water or milk but should not be mixed in carbonated beverages.

✔ Swallow tablets or capsules of valproic acid (Depakene or Depakote) whole; chewing or crushing may cause irritation of the mouth and throat.

✔ Taking valproic acid at bedtime may reduce dizziness and drowsiness.

✔ Lamotrigine may cause photosensitivity. When outdoors, wear protective clothing and sunscreen.

✔ If taking lamotrigine, notify the physician immediately if a skin rash or decreased seizure control develops.

---

tiagabine, and topiramate) have not been established. These agents are approved for combination therapy with other AEDs in clients whose seizures are not adequately controlled with a single drug.

Because most types of seizures can be treated effectively by a variety of drugs, adverse effects of drugs are an important factor in drug selection. Numerous studies have documented cognitive and psychomotor impairment with the sedating antiseizure drugs (eg, phenobarbital, phenytoin), so carbamazepine and valproic acid are increasingly used. However, carbamazepine and valproic acid may cause other potentially serious adverse effects. Other factors influencing drug choice include drug cost and client willingness to comply with the prescribed regimen.

2. A single drug (monotherapy) is recommended when possible. If effective in controlling seizures, monotherapy has the advantages of fewer adverse drug effects, fewer drug–drug interactions, lower costs, and usually greater client compliance. If adequate doses of a single drug do not control seizures, alternative interventions include reassessing the client for type of seizure or compliance with the prescribed drug therapy, adding a second drug, or substituting another antiseizure drug. When substituting, the second drug should be added and allowed to reach therapeutic blood levels before the first drug is gradually decreased in dosage and discontinued.

3. It is likely that the newer AEDs (eg, gabapentin, lamotrigine, tiagabine, and topiramate) will be increasingly used because they are less likely to have significant interactions with other drugs than the older agents.

Drug Dosage

1. Usually, larger doses are needed for a single drug than for multiple drugs; for people with a large body mass (assuming normal liver and kidney function); and in cases involving trauma, surgery, and emotional stress.

2. Smaller doses are usually required when liver disease is present and when multiple drugs are being given. Smaller doses of gabapentin must be given in the presence of renal impairment, and smaller doses of lamotrigine must be given when combined with valproic acid and another AED.

3. For most drugs, initial doses are relatively low; doses are gradually increased until seizures are controlled or adverse effects occur.

4. When fosphenytoin is substituted for oral phenytoin, the same total daily dosage (in PE) may be given IV or IM.

Monitoring Antiepileptic Drug Therapy

1. The effectiveness of drug therapy is evaluated primarily by client response in terms of therapeutic or adverse effects. Measuring serum drug levels may be helpful in validating drug dosages, assessing client compliance with the prescribed drug regimen, and documenting toxicity or adverse drug effects. Serum drug levels must be interpreted in relation to clinical responses because there are wide variations among clients receiving similar doses, probably owing to differences in hepatic metabolism. In other words, doses should not be increased or decreased solely to maintain a certain serum drug level.

2. Most antiseizure drugs have the potential for causing blood, liver, and kidney disorders. For this reason, it is usually recommended that baseline blood studies (complete blood count, platelet count) and liver function tests (eg, bilirubin, serum protein, aspartate aminotransferase) be performed before drug therapy starts and periodically thereafter.

3. When drug therapy fails to control seizures, there are several possible causes. A common one is the client's failure to take the antiseizure drug as prescribed. Other causes include incorrect diagnosis of the type of seizure, use of the wrong drug for the type of seizure, inadequate drug dosage, and too-frequent changes or premature withdrawal of drugs. Additional causes may include drug overdoses (eg, theophylline) and severe electrolyte imbalances (eg, hyponatremia).

Duration and Discontinuation of Therapy

Antiseizure drug therapy may be discontinued for some clients, usually after a seizure-free period of at least 2 years. Although opinions differ about whether, when, and how the drugs should be discontinued, studies indicate that medications can be stopped in approximately two thirds of clients whose epilepsy is completely controlled with drug therapy. Advantages of discontinuation include avoiding adverse drug effects and decreasing costs; disadvantages include recurrence of seizures, with possible status epilepticus. Even if drugs cannot be stopped completely, periodic attempts to decrease the number or dosage of drugs are probably desirable to minimize adverse reactions. Discontinuing drugs, changing drugs, or changing dosage must be done gradually over 2 to 3 months for each drug and with close medical supervision because sudden withdrawal or dosage decreases may cause status epilepticus. Only one drug should be reduced in dosage or gradually discontinued at a time.

Drug Therapy for Status Epilepticus

An IV benzodiazepine (eg, lorazepam) is the drug of choice for rapid control of tonic-clonic seizures. However, seizures often recur within 15 to 20 minutes unless the benzodiazepine is repeated or another, longer-acting drug is given (eg, IV phenytoin or fosphenytoin). Because there is a risk of significant respiratory depression with IV benzodiazepines, personnel and supplies for emergency resuscitation must be readily available.

Effects of Antiepileptic Drugs on Non-Antiepileptic Drugs

Antiepileptic drugs may have clinically significant interactions with many non-AEDs. Because the drugs depress the CNS and cause drowsiness, their combination with any other CNS depressant drugs may cause excessive sedation and other adverse CNS effects. They may also decrease the effects of numerous other drugs, mainly by inducing drug-metabolizing enzymes in the liver. Enzyme induction means the affected drugs are metabolized and eliminated more quickly. In some cases, larger doses of the affected drugs are needed to achieve therapeutic effects.

Phenytoin reduces the effects of cardiovascular drugs (eg, amiodarone, digoxin, disopyramide, dopamine, mexilitene, quinidine), female sex hormones (estrogens, oral contraceptives, levonorgestrel), adrenal corticosteroids, antipsychotic drugs (eg, phenothiazines, haloperidol), oral antidiabetic agents (eg, sulfonylureas), doxycycline, furosemide, levodopa, methadone, and theophylline. It also decreases the therapeutic effects of acetaminophen, but may increase the risk of hepatotoxicity by accelerating production of the metabolite that damages the liver. The consequence of increasing metabolism of oral contraceptives may be unintended pregnancy; the consequence of decreasing the effects of sulfonylureas may be greater difficulty in controlling blood sugar levels in diabetic clients who require both drugs.

Carbamazepine reduces the effects of tricyclic antidepressants, oral anticoagulants, oral contraceptives, bupropion, cyclosporine, doxycycline, felodipine, and haloperidol. The effects on acetaminophen are the same as those of phenytoin (see above).

Topiramate decreases effects of digoxin and oral contraceptives.

Use in Children

Oral drugs are absorbed slowly and inefficiently in newborns. If an antiseizure drug is necessary during the first 7 to 10 days of life, IM phenobarbital is effective. Metabolism and excretion also are delayed during the first 2 weeks of life, but rates become more rapid than those of adults by 2 to 3 months of age. In infants and children, oral drugs are rapidly absorbed and have short half-lives. This produces therapeutic serum drug levels earlier in children than in adults. Rates of metabolism and excretion also are increased. Consequently, children require higher doses per kilogram of body weight than adults.

The rapid rate of drug elimination persists until approximately 6 years of age, then decreases until it stabilizes around the adult rate by age 10 to 14 years. These drugs must be used cautiously to avoid excessive sedation and interference with learning and social development. There is little information about the effects of newer AEDs in children.

Use in Older Adults

Antiseizure drugs should be used cautiously in older adults because their liver and kidney functions may not be sufficient to metabolize and excrete the drugs. With impaired elimination, the drugs are more likely to accumulate and cause toxic effects unless dosage is reduced. In addition, older adults often have reduced levels of serum albumin, which may increase the active portion of a highly protein-bound AED (eg, phenytoin).

Use in Renal Impairment

Phenytoin is often used to prevent or treat seizure disorders in seriously ill clients. With renal impairment, protein binding is decreased and the volume of distribution is increased. Thus, the amount of free, active drug is higher in clients with renal impairment than in those with normal renal function. The use of long-acting *barbiturates* in clients with severe renal impairment requires markedly reduced dosage, close monitoring of plasma drug levels, and frequent observations for toxic effects. Smaller doses of *gabapentin* must be given in the presence of renal impairment. With *topiramate*, half the usual dose is recommended for clients with moderate or severe renal impairment because unchanged topiramate and its metabolites are eliminated primarily through the kidneys.

Use in Hepatic Impairment

Most AEDs are metabolized in the liver and may accumulate in the presence of liver disease or impaired function. The drugs should be used cautiously. *Tiagabine* is cleared more slowly in clients with liver impairment. Doses may need to be reduced or given at less frequent intervals. *Topiramate* may also be cleared more slowly even though it is eliminated mainly through the kidneys and does not undergo significant hepatic metabolism. It should be used with caution in the presence of hepatic impairment. *Valproic acid* is a hepatotoxic drug and contraindicated for use in hepatic impairment.

Use in Critical Illness

Phenytoin is often used to prevent or treat seizure disorders in critically ill clients, including those with head injuries. Phenytoin therapy can best be monitored by measuring free serum phenytoin concentrations, but laboratories usually report the total serum drug concentration. In some clients, a low total phenytoin level may still be therapeutic and a dosage increase is not indicated. The occurrence of nystagmus (abnormal movements of the eyeball) indicates phenytoin toxicity, and the drug should be discontinued until serum levels decrease. Because phenytoin is extensively metabolized in the liver, clients with severe illnesses may metabolize the drug more slowly and therefore experience toxicity.

For clients in critical care units for other disorders, a history of long-term AED therapy may be a risk factor for seizures, including status epilepticus, if the drug is stopped abruptly. At the same time, continuing an AED may complicate drug therapy of other conditions because of adverse effects and potential drug–drug interactions. For example, phenytoin decreases the effects of dopamine, a drug often used to treat hypotension and shock in critical care units. In addition, phenytoin decreases ventricular automaticity and should not be used in critically ill clients with sinus bradycardia or heart block.

 Home Care

The home care nurse must work with clients and family members to implement and monitor AED therapy. When an AED is started, a few weeks may be required to titrate the dosage and determine whether the chosen drug is effective in controlling seizures. The nurse can play an important role by clinical assessment of the client, interviewing the family about the occurrence of seizures (a log of date, time, duration, and characteristics of seizures can

---

Nursing Notes: *Apply Your Knowledge*

You are a nurse working in a clinic. Mr. Eng, an epileptic for the last 10 years, comes into the clinic complaining of problems with poor coordination and fatigue. His speech also seems somewhat slurred. His seizures have been well controlled on phenytoin (Dilantin) 300 mg hs. His Dilantin level is drawn and is 19 µg/mL. How should you proceed?

---

be very helpful), ensuring that the client keeps appointments for serum drug levels and follow-up care, and encouraging compliance with the prescribed regimen. With long-term use of the drugs, the nurse must monitor the client for therapeutic and adverse drug effects, especially with changes in drugs or dosages. With any evidence that the client is not taking medication as directed, the nurse may need to review the potential loss of seizure control and potential for status epilepticus.

(*text continues on page 185*)

NURSING ACTIONS   Antiseizure Drugs

NURSING ACTIONS	RATIONALE/EXPLANATION
1. Administer accurately	
a. Give on a regular schedule about the same time each day.	To maintain therapeutic blood levels of drugs
b. Give oral antiseizure drugs after meals or with a full glass of water or other fluid.	Most antiseizure drugs cause some gastric irritation, nausea, or vomiting. Taking the drugs with food or fluid helps decrease gastrointestinal side effects.
c. To give phenytoin: (1) Shake oral suspensions of the drug vigorously before pouring and always use the same measuring equipment.	When a drug preparation is called a *suspension*, it means that particles of drug are suspended or floating in water or other liquid. On standing, drug particles settle to the bottom of the container. Shaking the container is necessary to achieve a uniform distribution of drug particles in the liquid vehicle. If the contents are not mixed well every time a dose is given, the liquid vehicle will be given initially, and the concentrated drug will be given later. That is, underdosage will occur at first, and little if any therapeutic benefit will result. Overdosage will follow, and the risks of serious toxicity are greatly increased. Using the same measuring container ensures consistent dosage. Calibrated medication cups or measuring teaspoons or tablespoons are acceptable. Regular household teaspoons and tablespoons used for eating and serving are *not* acceptable because sizes vary widely.

(continued)

NURSING ACTIONS	RATIONALE/EXPLANATION
(2) Do not mix parenteral phenytoin in the same syringe with any other drug.	Phenytoin solution is highly alkaline (pH approximately 12) and physically incompatible with other drugs. A precipitate occurs if mixing is attempted.
(3) Give phenytoin as an undiluted intravenous (IV) bolus injection at a rate not exceeding 50 mg/min, then flush the IV line with normal saline or dilute in 50 to 100 mL of normal saline (0.9% NaCl) and administer over approximately 30 to 60 minutes. If "piggybacked" into a primary IV line, the primary IV solution must be normal saline or the line must be flushed with normal saline before and after administration of phenytoin. An inline filter is recommended.	Phenytoin cannot be diluted or given in IV fluids other than normal saline because it precipitates within minutes. Slow administration and dilution decrease local venous irritation from the highly alkaline drug solution. Rapid administration must be avoided because it may produce myocardial depression, hypotension, cardiac arrhythmias, and even cardiac arrest.
(4) Give intramuscular (IM) phenytoin deeply into a large muscle mass, and rotate injection sites.	Phenytoin is absorbed slowly when given IM and causes local tissue irritation. Correct administration helps increase absorption and decrease pain.
d. To give IV fosphenytoin:	
(1) Check the physician's order and the drug concentration carefully.	Because the dose is expressed in phenytoin equivalents (PE; fosphenytoin 50 mg PE = phenytoin 50 mg) there is a risk for error.
(2) Dilute the ordered dose in 5% dextrose or 0.9% sodium chloride solution to a concentration of 1.5 mg PE/mL to 25 mg PE/mL and infuse no faster than 150 mg PE/min.	The drug is preferably diluted in the pharmacy and labeled with the concentration and duration of the infusion. For a 100-mg PE dose, diluting with 4 mL yields the maximum concentration of 25 mg PE/mL; this amount could be infused in about 1 min at the maximal recommended rate. A 1-g loading dose could be added to 50 mL of 0.9% sodium chloride and infused in approximately 10 min at the maximal recommended rate.
(3) Consult a pharmacist or the manufacturer's literature if any aspect of the dose or instructions for administration are unclear.	To avoid error until becoming accustomed to using this parenteral dosage form of phenytoin
e. To give carbamazepine and phenytoin suspensions by nasogastric (NG) feeding tube, dilute with an equal amount of water, and rinse the NG tube before and after administration.	Absorption is slow and decreased, possibly because of drug adherence to the NG tube. Dilution and tube irrigation decrease such adherence.
2. Observe for therapeutic effects	
a. When the drug is given on a long-term basis to prevent seizures, observe for a decrease in or absence of seizure activity.	Therapeutic effects begin later with antiseizure drugs than with most other drug groups because the antiseizure drugs have relatively long half-lives. Optimum therapeutic benefits of phenytoin occur approximately 7 to 10 days after drug therapy is started. Those of phenobarbital occur in approximately 2 weeks; those of ethosuximide, in approximately 5 days.
b. When the drug is given to stop an acute convulsive seizure, seizure activity usually slows or stops within a few minutes.	Lorazepam is the drug of choice for controlling an acute convulsion because it acts rapidly. Even when given IV, phenytoin and phenobarbital do not act for several minutes.

(continued)

NURSING ACTIONS	RATIONALE/EXPLANATION
3. Observe for adverse effects	
a. Central nervous system (CNS) effects—drowsiness, sedation, ataxia, diplopia, nystagmus	These effects are common, especially during the first week or two of drug therapy.
b. Gastrointestinal effects—anorexia, nausea, vomiting	These common effects of oral drugs can be reduced by taking the drugs with food or a full glass of water.
c. Skin disorders—rash, urticaria, exfoliative dermatitis, Stevens-Johnson syndrome (a severe reaction accompanied by headache, arthralgia, and other symptoms in addition to skin lesions)	These may occur with almost all the antiseizure drugs. Some are mild; some are potentially serious but rare. Most skin reactions are apparently caused by hypersensitivity or idiosyncratic reactions and are usually sufficient reason to discontinue the drug.
d. Blood dyscrasias—anemia, leukopenia, thrombocytopenia, agranulocytosis	Most antiseizure drugs produce decreases in the levels of folic acid, which may progress to megaloblastic anemia. The other disorders indicate bone marrow depression and are potentially life threatening. They do not usually occur with phenytoin, phenobarbital, or primidone but may infrequently occur with most other antiseizure drugs.
e. Respiratory depression	This is not likely to be a significant adverse reaction except when a depressant drug, such as diazepam or a barbiturate, is given IV to control acute seizures, such as status epilepticus. Even then, respiratory depression can be minimized by avoiding overdosage and rapid administration.
f. Liver damage—hepatitis symptoms, jaundice, abnormal liver function test results	Hepatic damage may occur with phenytoin, and fatal hepatotoxicity has been reported with valproic acid.
g. Gingival hyperplasia	Occurs often with phenytoin, especially in children. It may be prevented or delayed by vigorous oral hygiene or treated surgically by gingivectomy.
h. Hypocalcemia	May occur when antiseizure drugs are taken in high doses and over long periods
i. Lymphadenopathy resembling malignant lymphoma	This reaction has occurred with several antiseizure drugs, most often with phenytoin.
4. Observe for drug interactions	
a. Drugs that *increase* effects of antiseizure drugs:	
(1) CNS depressants	Additive CNS depression
(2) Other antiseizure drugs	Additive or synergistic effects
b. Drugs that *decrease* effects of antiseizure drugs:	
(1) Tricyclic antidepressants, antipsychotic drugs	These drugs may lower the seizure threshold and precipitate seizures. Dosage of antiseizure drugs may need to be increased.
(2) Barbiturates and other enzyme inducers	These drugs inhibit themselves and other antiseizure drugs by activating liver enzymes and accelerating the rate of drug metabolism.

(continued)

NURSING ACTIONS	**RATIONALE/EXPLANATION**
c. Additional drugs that alter effects of phenytoin and fosphenytoin:	
(1) Alcohol (acute ingestion), allopurinol, amiodarone, benzodiazepines, chloramphenicol, chlorpheniramine, cimetidine, disulfiram, fluconazole, isoniazid, metronidazole, miconazole, omeprazole, and trimethoprim increase effects.	These drugs increase phenytoin toxicity by inhibiting hepatic metabolism of phenytoin or by displacing it from plasma protein-binding sites.
(2) Alcohol (chronic ingestion), antacids, antineoplastics, folic acid, loxapine, nitrofurantoin, pyridoxine, rifampin, sucralfate, and theophylline decrease effects.	These drugs decrease effects of phenytoin by decreasing absorption, accelerating metabolism, or by unknown mechanisms.
(3) Phenobarbital has variable interactions with phenytoin.	Phenytoin and phenobarbital have complex interactions with unpredictable effects. Interactions are considered separately because the two drugs are often used at the same time. Although phenobarbital induces drug metabolism in the liver and may increase the rate of metabolism of other anticonvulsant drugs, its interaction with phenytoin differs. Phenobarbital apparently decreases serum levels of phenytoin and perhaps its half-life. Still, the anticonvulsant effects of the two drugs together are greater than those of either drug given alone. The interaction apparently varies with dosage, route, time of administration, the degree of liver enzyme induction already present, and other factors. Thus, whether a significant interaction will occur in a client is unpredictable. Probably the most important clinical implication is that close observation of the client is necessary when either drug is being added or withdrawn.
d. Additional drugs that alter effects of carbamazepine:	
(1) Cimetidine, erythromycin, isoniazid, and valproic acid increase effects.	These drugs inhibit hepatic drug-metabolizing enzymes, thereby increasing blood levels of carbamazepine.
(2) Alcohol, phenytoin, phenobarbital, and primidone decrease effects.	These drugs increase activity of hepatic drug-metabolizing enzymes, thereby decreasing blood levels of carbamazepine.
e. Drugs that alter the effects of gabapentin:	
(1) Antacids	Reduce absorption of gabapentin. Gabapentin should be given at least 2 hours after a dose of an antacid to decrease interference with absorption.
f. Drugs that alter effects of lamotrigine:	
(1) Valproic acid increases effects.	Valproic acid inhibits the liver enzymes that metabolize lamotrigine, thereby increasing blood levels and slowing metabolism of lamotrigine. As a result, lamotrigine dosage must be substantially reduced when the drug is given in a multidrug regimen that includes valproic acid.
(2) Carbamazepine, phenytoin, phenobarbital decrease effects.	These drugs induce drug-metabolizing enzymes in the liver and thereby increase the rate of metabolism of themselves and of lamotrigine.

(continued)

NURSING ACTIONS	RATIONALE/EXPLANATION
g. Additional drugs that alter effects of valproate: (1) Chlorpromazine, cimetidine, and salicylates increase effects.	These drugs decrease clearance and increase blood levels of valproic acid.
h. Interactions with phenobarbital: (1) Valproic acid	May increase plasma levels of phenobarbital as much as 40%, probably by inhibiting liver metabolizing enzymes.
(2) Other drugs	Many drugs interact with the barbiturates, the drug group of which phenobarbital is a member. These drug interactions are listed in Chapter 8.
i. Interactions with clonazepam, lorazepam, and diazepam	These drugs are benzodiazepines, discussed in Chapter 8.

How Can You Avoid This Medication Error?

Answer: Blood levels need to remain within a therapeutic range to prevent seizures. Even missing two doses could affect this level. Frequently, surgery patients are permitted to take medications with a sip of water, even when they are NPO. Good judgment requires a nurse to check with the physician when significant medications are withheld.

Nursing Notes: Apply Your Knowledge

Answer: Although Mr. Eng's Dilantin level falls within the high end of normal (10–20 µg/mL), his symptoms indicate phenytoin toxicity. Laboratory values are guides for appropriate dosing, but it is important that treatment be based on clinical data. Mr. Eng should be referred to his physician for evaluation of Dilantin toxicity and adjustment of Dilantin dosage.

REVIEW AND APPLICATION EXERCISES

1. For a client with a newly developed seizure disorder, why is it important to verify the type of seizure by electroencephalogram before starting antiseizure drug therapy?

2. What are the indications for use of the major AEDs?

3. What are the major adverse effects of commonly used AEDs, and how can they be minimized?

4. What are the advantages and disadvantages of treatment with a single drug and of treatment with multiple drugs?

5. Which of the benzodiazepines (antianxiety agents and hypnotics) are used as antiseizure agents?

6. What are the advantages of carbamazepine and valproic acid compared with the benzodiazepines, phenytoin, and phenobarbital?

7. How are the newer drugs, tiagabine and topiramate, similar to or different from phenytoin?

8. What is the treatment of choice for an acute convulsion or status epilepticus?

9. Why is it important when teaching clients to emphasize that none of the AEDs should be stopped abruptly?

10. How can a home care nurse monitor AED therapy during a home visit?

SELECTED REFERENCES

Craig, C.R. (1997). Anticonvulsant drugs. In C.R. Craig & R.E. Stitzel (Eds.), *Modern pharmacology with clinical applications*, 5th ed., pp. 391–405. Boston: Little, Brown.

Delgado-Escueta, A.V. & Serratosa, J.M. (1997). Approach to the patient with seizures. In W.N. Kelley (Ed.), *Textbook of internal medicine*, 3rd ed., pp. 2347–2354. Philadelphia: Lippincott-Raven.

Drug facts and comparisons. (Updated monthly). St. Louis: Facts and Comparisons.

Garnett, W.R. (1997). Epilepsy. In J.T. DiPiro, R.L. Talbert, P.E. Hayes, G.C. Yee, G.R. Matzke, B.G. Wells, & L.M. Posey (Eds.), *Pharmacotherapy: A pathophysiologic approach*, 3rd ed., pp. 1179–1209. Stamford, CT: Appleton & Lange.

McNamara, J.O. (1996). Drugs effective in the therapy of the epilepsies. In J.G. Hardman, L.E. Limbird, P.B. Molinoff, & R.W. Ruddon (Eds.), *Goodman & Gilman's The pharmacological basis of therapeutics*, 9th ed., pp. 461–486. New York: McGraw-Hill.

Wallace, S.J., Binnie, C.D., Brown, S.W., Duncan, J.S., McKee, P., & Ridsdale, L. (1998). Epilepsy—a guide to medical treatment 1: Antiepileptic drugs. *Hospital Medicine*, 59, 380–387.

Willmore, L.J. (1998). Antiepileptic drug therapy in the elderly. *Pharmacology and Therapeutics*, 78(1), 9–16.

12

Antiparkinson Drugs

Objectives

After studying this chapter, the student will be able to:

1. Describe major characteristics of Parkinson's disease.

2. Differentiate the types of commonly used antiparkinson drugs.

3. Discuss therapeutic and adverse effects of dopaminergic and anticholinergic drugs.

4. Apply the nursing process with clients experiencing parkinsonism.

Mr. Rod was diagnosed with Parkinson's disease 1 week ago. His symptoms included slow, shuffling gait; stooped posture; fine tremor at rest; and mask-like facial expression. His physician started him on levodopa 500 mg tid and benztropine (Cogentin) 1 mg hs. You are a home health nurse visiting Mr. Rod.

Reflect on:

▶ How can Parkinson's disease affect Mr. Rod's ability to function normally?

▶ How does each medication work to restore the balance of neurotransmitters?

▶ What assessment data will you collect to evaluate whether the antiparkinson medications are effective?

▶ What assessment data should be collected to detect adverse effects of antiparkinson drugs?

PARKINSON'S DISEASE

Parkinson's disease is a chronic, progressive, degenerative disorder of the central nervous system (CNS) characterized by abnormalities in movement and posture (tremor, brady-kinesia, joint and muscular rigidity). It occurs equally in men and women, usually between 50 and 80 years of age. Classic parkinsonism probably results from destruction or degenerative changes in dopamine-producing nerve cells. Signs and symptoms of the disease also may occur with other CNS diseases or trauma and with the use of anti-psychotic drugs.

The basal ganglia in the brain normally contain sub-stantial amounts of the neurotransmitters dopamine and acetylcholine. The correct balance of dopamine and acetyl-choline is important in regulating posture, muscle tone, and voluntary movement. People with Parkinson's disease have an imbalance in these neurotransmitters, resulting in a decrease in brain dopamine and a relative increase in acetylcholine. Other neurotransmitters (eg, norepineph-rine, serotonin) may be involved as well, but their roles have not been elucidated.

ANTIPARKINSON DRUGS

Drugs used in Parkinson's disease act to increase levels of dopamine (levodopa, dopamine agonists, monoamine oxidase [MAO] inhibitors, catechol-*O*-methyltransferase [COMT] inhibitors) or inhibit the actions of acetylcholine (anticholinergic agents) in the brain. Thus, the drugs help adjust the balance of neurotransmitters.

Dopaminergic Drugs

Levodopa, carbidopa, amantadine, bromocriptine, per-golide, pramipexole, ropinirole, selegiline, and tolcapone increase dopamine concentrations in the brain and exert dopaminergic activity, directly or indirectly. Levodopa is the mainstay of drug therapy for classic or idiopathic parkin-sonism. Carbidopa is used only in conjunction with levo-dopa. The other drugs are used as adjunctive agents, usually with levodopa.

Anticholinergic Drugs

Anticholinergic drugs are discussed in Chapter 21 and are described here only in relation to their use in the treatment of Parkinson's disease. Only anticholinergic drugs that are centrally active (ie, those that penetrate the blood–brain barrier) are useful in treating parkinsonism. Atropine and scopolamine are centrally active but are not used because of a high incidence of adverse reactions. In addition to the primary anticholinergic drugs, an antihistamine (diphen-hydramine) is used for parkinsonism because of its strong anticholinergic effects.

Mechanisms of Action

Dopaminergic drugs increase the amount of dopamine in the brain by various mechanisms. Amantadine increases dopamine release and decreases dopamine reuptake by presynaptic nerve fibers. Bromocriptine, pergolide, pra-mipexole, and ropinirole are dopamine agonists that directly stimulate postsynaptic dopamine receptors. Levo-dopa is a precursor substance that enters the brain rapidly and is converted to dopamine. Selegiline blocks one of the enzymes (MAO-B) that normally inactivates dopamine. Tolcapone blocks another enzyme (COMT) that normally inactivates dopamine and levodopa. Anticholinergic drugs decrease the effects of acetylcholine. This decreases the apparent excess of acetylcholine in relation to the amount of dopamine.

Indications for Use

Levodopa, pergolide, pramipexole, ropinirole, selegiline, and tolcapone are indicated for the treatment of idio-pathic or acquired parkinsonism; carbidopa is used only to decrease peripheral breakdown of levodopa. Some of the other drugs have additional uses. For example, aman-tadine is also used to prevent and treat influenza A viral infections. Bromocriptine is also used in the treatment of amenorrhea and galactorrhea associated with hyper-prolactinemia.

Anticholinergic drugs are used in idiopathic parkinson-ism to decrease salivation, spasticity, and tremors. They are used primarily for people who have minimal symptoms or who cannot tolerate levodopa, or in combination with other antiparkinson drugs. Anticholinergic agents also are used to relieve symptoms of parkinsonism that can occur with the use of antipsychotic drugs. If used for this purpose, a course of therapy of approximately 3 months is recom-mended because symptoms usually subside by then even if the antipsychotic drug is continued.

Contraindications to Use

Levodopa is contraindicated in clients with narrow-angle glaucoma, hemolytic anemia, severe angina pectoris, tran-sient ischemic attacks, or a history of melanoma or un-diagnosed skin disorders, and in clients taking MAO in-hibitor drugs. In addition, levodopa must be used with caution in clients with severe cardiovascular, pulmonary, renal, hepatic, or endocrine disorders. Bromocriptine and pergolide are ergot derivatives and therefore are contraindicated in people hypersensitive to ergot alkaloids or those with uncontrolled hypertension. Selegiline and tolcapone are contraindicated in people with hypersensitivity reactions to the drugs.

Anticholinergic drugs are contraindicated in clients with glaucoma, gastrointestinal obstruction, prostatic hypertrophy, urinary bladder neck obstruction, and myasthenia gravis. The drugs must be used cautiously in clients with cardiovascular disorders (eg, tachycardia, arrhythmias, hypertension) and liver or kidney disease.

INDIVIDUAL ANTIPARKINSON DRUGS

Dopaminergic antiparkinson drugs are described in this section; generic and trade names, routes, and dosage ranges are listed in Table 12-1.

Levodopa is the most effective drug available for the treatment of Parkinson's disease. It relieves all major symptoms, especially bradykinesia and rigidity. Although levodopa does not alter the underlying disease process, it may improve a client's quality of life.

TABLE 12–1	Antiparkinson Drugs
Generic/Trade Name	**Routes and Dosage Ranges**
Dopaminergic Agents	
Levodopa (Larodopa)	PO 0.5–1 g/d initially in 3 or 4 divided doses, increase gradually by no more than 0.75 g/d, every 3–7 d. The rate of dosage increase depends mainly on the client's tolerance of adverse effects, especially nausea and vomiting. Average maintenance dose, 3–6 g/d; maximum dose, 8 g/d. Dosage must be reduced when carbidopa is also given (see carbidopa, below).
Carbidopa (Lodosyn)	PO 70–100 mg/d, depending on dosage of levodopa; maximum dose, 200 mg/d
Levodopa/carbidopa (Sinemet)	*Clients not receiving levodopa:* PO 1 tab. of 25 mg carbidopa/100 mg levodopa 3 times daily or 1 tab. of 10 mg carbidopa/100 mg levodopa 3 or 4 times daily, increased by 1 tablet every day or every other day until a dosage of 8 tablets daily is reached.
	Sinemet CR PO 1 tab. twice daily at least 6 h apart initially, increased up to 8 tablets daily and q4h intervals if necessary
	Clients receiving levodopa: Discontinue levodopa at least 8 h before starting Sinemet. PO 1 tab. of 25 mg carbidopa/250 mg levodopa 3 or 4 times daily for clients taking >1500 mg levodopa or 1 tab. of 25 mg carbidopa/100 mg levodopa for clients taking <1500 mg levodopa.
Amantadine (Symmetrel)	PO 100 mg twice a day
Bromocriptine (Parlodel)	PO 1.25 mg twice a day with meals, increased by 2.5 mg/d every 2–4 wk if necessary for therapeutic benefit. Reduce dose gradually if severe adverse effects occur.
Pergolide (Permax)	PO 0.05–0.1 mg/d at bedtime, increased by 0.05–0.15 mg every 3 d to a maximum dose of 6 mg/d if necessary
Pramipexole (Mirapex)	PO wk 1, 0.125 mg 3 times daily; wk 2, 0.25 mg 3 times daily; wk 3, 0.5 mg 3 times daily; wk 4, 0.75 mg 3 times daily; wk 5, 1 mg 3 times daily; wk 6, 1.25 mg 3 times daily; wk 7, 1.5 mg 3 times daily
	Renal impairment: Creatinine clearance (Crcl) >60 mL/min, 0.125 mg 3 times daily initially, up to a maximum of 1.5 mg 3 times daily; Crcl 35–59 mL/min, 0.125 mg 2 times daily initially, up to a maximum of 1.5 mg 2 times daily; Crcl 15–34 mL/min, 0.125 mg once daily, up to a maximum of 1.5 mg once daily
Ropinirole (Requip)	PO wk 1, 0.25 mg 3 times daily; wk 2, 0.5 mg 3 times daily; wk 3, 0.75 mg 3 times daily; wk 4, 1 mg 3 times daily
Selegiline (Eldepryl)	PO 5 mg twice daily, morning and noon
Tolcapone (Tasmar)	PO 100–200 mg 3 times daily; maximum dose, 600 mg daily
Anticholinergic Agents	
Benztropine (Cogentin)	PO 0.5–1 mg at bedtime initially, gradually increased to 4–6 mg daily if necessary
Biperiden (Akineton)	Parkinsonism, PO 2 mg 3–4 times daily
	Drug-induced extrapyramidal reactions, PO 2 mg 1–3 times daily, IM 2 mg repeated q30min if necessary to a maximum of 8 mg in 24 h
Diphenhydramine (Benadryl)	PO 25 mg 3 times daily, gradually increased to 50 mg 4 times daily if necessary
	Adults: Drug-induced extrapyramidal reactions, IM, IV 10–50 mg; maximal single dose, 100 mg; maximal daily dose, 400 mg
	Children: Drug-induced extrapyramidal reactions, IM 5 mg/kg per day; maximal daily dose, 300 mg
Procyclidine (Kemadrin)	PO 5 mg twice daily initially, gradually increased to 5 mg 3–4 times daily if necessary
Trihexyphenidyl (Artane)	PO 1–2 mg daily initially, gradually increased to 12–15 mg daily, until therapeutic or adverse effects occur
	Adults: Drug-induced extrapyramidal reactions, PO 1 mg initially, gradually increased to 5–15 mg daily if necessary

IM, intramuscular; IV, intravenous; PO, oral.

Levodopa acts to replace dopamine in the basal ganglia of the brain. Dopamine cannot be used for replacement therapy because it does not enter the brain in sufficient amounts. Levodopa readily penetrates the CNS and is converted to dopamine by the enzyme amino acid decarboxylase (AADC). The dopamine is stored in presynaptic dopaminergic neurons and functions like endogenous dopamine. In advanced stages of Parkinson's disease, there are fewer dopaminergic neurons and thus less storage capacity for dopamine derived from levodopa. As a result, levodopa has a shorter duration of action and drug effects "wear off" between doses.

In peripheral tissues (eg, liver, kidney, gastrointestinal tract), levodopa is extensively metabolized by decarboxylase, whose concentration is greater in peripheral tissues than in the brain. It is metabolized to a lesser extent by the enzyme COMT. Consequently, most levodopa is metabolized in peripheral tissues and large amounts are required to obtain therapeutic levels of dopamine in the brain. Peripheral metabolism of levodopa can be reduced (and the amounts reaching the brain can be increased) by giving the AADC inhibitor, carbidopa. The combination of levodopa and carbidopa greatly increases the amount of available levodopa, so that the levodopa dosage can be reduced by approximately 70%. The two drugs are usually given together in a fixed-dose formulation called Sinemet. When carbidopa inhibits the decarboxylase pathway of levodopa metabolism, the COMT pathway becomes more important (see tolcapone, a COMT inhibitor, below).

Levodopa is well absorbed from the small intestine after oral administration and has a short serum half-life (1 to 3 hours). Absorption is decreased by delayed gastric emptying, hyperacidity of gastric juice, and competition with amino acids (from digestion of protein foods) for sites of absorption in the small intestine. Levodopa is metabolized to 30 or more metabolites, some of which are pharmacologically active and probably contribute to drug toxicity; the metabolites are excreted primarily in the urine, usually within 24 hours.

Because of side effects and recurrence of parkinsonian symptoms after a few years of levodopa therapy, levodopa is often reserved for clients with significant symptoms and functional disabilities. In addition to treating Parkinson's disease, levodopa also may be useful in other CNS disorders in which symptoms of parkinsonism occur (eg, juvenile Huntington's chorea, chronic manganese poisoning). Levodopa relieves only parkinsonian symptoms in these conditions.

Carbidopa (Lodosyn) inhibits the enzyme AADC. As a result, less levodopa is decarboxylated in peripheral tissues; more levodopa reaches the brain, where it is decarboxylated to dopamine; and much smaller doses of levodopa can be given. Carbidopa does not penetrate the blood–brain barrier. Although carbidopa is available alone, it is most often given in a levodopa/carbidopa fixed-dose combination product called Sinemet.

How Can You Avoid This Medication Error?

Mr. Evans, a patient with Parkinson's disease, has carbidopa/levodopa (Sinemet) 25/100 ordered tid. Your pharmacy supplies you with Sinemet 25/250. You administer 1 tablet to Mr. Evans for his morning dose.

Amantadine (Symmetrel) is a synthetic antiviral agent initially used to prevent infection from influenza A virus. Amantadine increases the release and inhibits the reuptake of dopamine in the brain, thereby increasing dopamine levels. The drug relieves symptoms rapidly, within 1 to 5 days, but it loses efficacy with approximately 6 to 8 weeks of continuous administration. Consequently, it is usually given for 2- to 3-week periods during initiation of drug therapy with longer-acting agents (eg, levodopa), or when symptoms worsen. Amantadine is often given in conjunction with levodopa. Compared with other antiparkinson drugs, amantadine is considered less effective than levodopa but more effective than anticholinergic agents.

Amantadine is well absorbed from the gastrointestinal tract and has a relatively long duration of action. It is excreted unchanged in the urine. Dosage must be reduced with impaired renal function to avoid drug accumulation.

Bromocriptine (Parlodel) and **pergolide** (Permax) are ergot derivatives that directly stimulate dopamine receptors in the brain. They are used in the treatment of idiopathic Parkinson's disease, with levodopa/carbidopa, to prolong effectiveness and allow reduced dosage of levodopa. Pergolide has a longer duration of action than bromocriptine and may be effective in some clients unresponsive to bromocriptine. Adverse effects are similar for the two drugs.

Pramipexole (Mirapex) and **ropinirole** (Requip) are newer drugs that directly stimulate dopamine receptors in the brain. They are approved for both beginning and advanced stages of Parkinson's disease. In early stages, one of the drugs can be used alone to improve motor performance, improve ability to participate in usual activities of daily living, and to delay levodopa therapy. In advanced stages, one of the drugs can be used with levodopa and perhaps other antiparkinson drugs to provide more consistent relief of symptoms between doses of levodopa and allow reduced dosage of levodopa. These drugs are not ergot derivatives and may not cause some adverse effects associated with bromocriptine and pergolide (eg, pulmonary and peritoneal fibrosis and constriction of coronary arteries).

Pramipexole is rapidly absorbed with oral administration. Peak serum levels are reached in 1 to 3 hours after a dose and steady-state concentrations in approximately 2 days. It is less than 20% bound to plasma proteins and has an elimination half-life of 8 to 12 hours. Most of the drug is excreted unchanged in the urine; only 10% of the drug is metabolized. As a result, renal failure may cause higher-than-usual plasma levels and possible toxicity, but hepatic disease is unlikely to alter drug effects.

Ropinirole is also well absorbed with oral administration. It reaches peak serum levels in 1 to 2 hours and steady-state concentrations within 2 days. It is approximately 40% bound to plasma proteins and has an elimination half-life of approximately 6 hours. It is metabolized by the cytochrome P450 enzymes in the liver to inactive metabolites, which are excreted through the kidneys. Less than 10% of ropinirole is excreted unchanged in the urine. Thus, liver failure may decrease metabolism, allow drug accumulation, and increase adverse effects. Renal failure does not appear to alter drug effects.

Selegiline (Eldepryl) increases dopamine in the brain by inhibiting its metabolism by MAO. MAO exists in two types, MAO-A and MAO-B, both of which are found in the CNS and peripheral tissues. They are differentiated by their relative specificities for individual catecholamines. MAO-A acts more specifically on tyramine, norepinephrine, epinephrine, and serotonin. It is the main subtype in gastrointestinal mucosa and the liver and is responsible for metabolizing dietary tyramine. If MAO-A is inhibited in the intestine, tyramine in various foods is absorbed systemically rather than deactivated. As a result, there is excessive stimulation of the sympathetic nervous system and severe hypertension and stroke can occur. This life-threatening reaction can also occur with medications that are normally metabolized by MAO.

MAO-B metabolizes dopamine; in the brain, most MAO activity is due to type B. At oral doses of 10 mg/day or less, selegiline inhibits MAO-B selectively and is unlikely to cause severe hypertension and stroke. At doses higher than 10 mg/day, however, selectivity is lost and metabolism of both MAO-A and MAO-B is inhibited. Doses above 10 mg/day should be avoided in Parkinson's disease. Selegiline inhibition of MAO-B is irreversible and drug effects persist until more MAO is synthesized in the brain, which may take several months.

In early Parkinson's disease, selegiline may be effective as monotherapy. In advanced disease, it is given to enhance the effects of levodopa. Its addition aids symptom control and allows the dosage of levodopa/carbidopa to be reduced.

Tolcapone (Tasmar) is the first of a new class of antiparkinson drugs called COMT inhibitors. COMT plays a role in brain metabolism of dopamine and metabolizes approximately 10% of peripheral levodopa. By inhibiting COMT, tolcapone increases levels of dopamine in the brain and relieves symptoms more effectively and consistently. Although the main mechanism of action seems to be inhibiting the metabolism of levodopa in the bloodstream, tolcapone may also inhibit COMT in the brain and prolong the activity of dopamine at the synapse. The drug is used only in conjunction with levodopa/carbidopa, and dosage of levodopa must be reduced.

Tolcapone is well absorbed with oral administration. Its elimination half-life is 2 to 3 hours and it is metabolized in the liver. Diarrhea was a common adverse effect during clinical trials. In addition, elevation of liver aminotransferase enzymes (serum alanine aminotransferase and aspartate aminotransferase) occurred during clinical trials and a few deaths from liver failure have been reported. As a result, liver aminotransferase enzymes should be monitored every month for 3 months, then every 6 weeks for 3 months.

Nursing Notes: Apply Your Knowledge

Mr. Simmons has had Parkinson's disease for 4 years and, despite treatment with Sinemet, his functional abilities continue to decline. His physician prescribes a tricyclic antidepressant. He comes to the clinic 3 weeks later complaining of constipation and difficulty voiding. Are these symptoms related to his medications?

NURSING PROCESS

Assessment

Assess for signs and symptoms of Parkinson's disease and drug-induced extrapyramidal reactions. These may include the following, depending on the severity and stage of progression:

- Slow movements (bradykinesia) and difficulty in changing positions, assuming an upright position, eating, dressing, and other self-care activities
- Stooped posture
- Accelerating gait with short steps
- Tremor at rest (eg, "pill rolling" movements of fingers)
- Rigidity of arms, legs, and neck
- Mask-like, immobile facial expression
- Speech problems (eg, low volume, monotonous tone, rapid, difficult to understand)
- Excessive salivation and drooling
- Dysphagia
- Excessive sweating
- Constipation from decreased intestinal motility
- Mental depression from self-consciousness and embarrassment over physical appearance and activity limitations. The intellect is usually intact until the late stages of the disease process.

Nursing Diagnoses

- Self Care Deficit: Total related to tremors and impaired motor function

- Impaired Physical Mobility related to alterations in balance and coordination
- Body Image Disturbance related to disease and disability
- Knowledge Deficit: Safe usage and effects of antiparkinson drugs
- Altered Thought Processes related to impaired mentation
- Altered Nutrition: Less Than Body Requirements related to difficulty in chewing and swallowing food
- Risk for Injury: Dizziness, hypotension related to adverse drug effects

Planning/Goals

The client will:

- Experience relief of excessive salivation, muscle rigidity, spasticity, and tremors
- Experience improved motor function, mobility, and self-care abilities
- Experience improvement of self-concept and body image
- Increase knowledge of the disease process and drug therapy
- Take medications as instructed
- Avoid falls and other injuries from the disease process or drug therapy.

Interventions

Use measures to assist the client and family in coping with symptoms and maintaining function. These include the following:

- Provide physical therapy for heel-to-toe gait training, widening stance to increase balance and base of support, other exercises.
- Encourage ambulation and frequent changes of position, assisted if necessary.
- Help with active and passive range-of-motion exercises.
- Encourage self-care as much as possible. Cutting meat; opening cartons; giving frequent, small meals; and allowing privacy during mealtime may be helpful. If the client has difficulty chewing or swallowing, chopped or soft foods may be necessary. Velcro-type fasteners or zippers are easier to handle than buttons. Slip-on shoes are easier to manage than laced ones.
- Spend time with the client and encourage socialization with other people. Victims of Parkinson's disease tend to become withdrawn, isolated, and depressed.
- Schedule rest periods. Tremor and rigidity are aggravated by fatigue and emotional stress.
- Provide facial tissues if drooling is a problem.

CLIENT TEACHING GUIDELINES
Antiparkinson Drugs

General Considerations

✔ Beneficial effects of antiparkinson drugs may not occur for a few weeks or months; do not stop taking them before they have had a chance to work.

✔ Do not take other drugs without the physician's knowledge and consent. This is necessary to avoid adverse drug interactions. Prescription and nonprescription drugs may interact with antiparkinson drugs to increase or decrease effects.

✔ Avoid driving an automobile or operating other potentially hazardous machinery if vision is blurred or drowsiness occurs with levodopa.

✔ Change positions slowly, especially when assuming an upright position, and wear elastic stockings, if needed, to prevent dizziness from a drop in blood pressure.

Self- or Caregiver Administration

✔ With levodopa, take on an empty stomach, if possible, because drug absorption is better. If nausea occurs, take it with a small amount of food. Limit intake of alcohol and high-protein foods (eg, meat, poultry, fish, milk, eggs, cheese) and do not take multivitamin preparations that contain vitamin B_6. Alcohol, protein, and vitamin B_6 may decrease therapeutic effects of levodopa.

✔ Take most antiparkinson drugs (except levodopa) with or just after food intake to prevent or reduce anorexia, nausea, and vomiting.

✔ Take or give selegiline in the morning and at noon. This schedule decreases central nervous system stimulating effects that may interfere with sleep if the drug is taken in the evening.

✔ Decrease excessive mouth dryness by maintaining an adequate fluid intake (2000 to 3000 mL daily if not contraindicated) and using sugarless chewing gum and hard candies. Both anticholinergics and levodopa may cause mouth dryness. This is usually a therapeutic effect in Parkinson's disease. However, excessive mouth dryness causes discomfort and dental caries.

✔ Report adverse effects. Adverse effects can often be reduced by changing drugs or dosages. However, some adverse effects usually must be tolerated for control of disease symptoms.

Evaluation

- Interview and observe for relief of symptoms.
- Interview and observe for increased mobility and participation in activities of daily living.
- Interview and observe regarding correct usage of medications.

PRINCIPLES OF THERAPY

Goals of Treatment

The goals of antiparkinson drug therapy are to control symptoms, maintain functional ability in activities of daily living, minimize adverse drug effects, and slow disease progression.

Drug Selection

Choices of antiparkinson drugs depend largely on the type of parkinsonism (idiopathic or drug induced) and the severity of symptoms. In addition, because of difficulties with levodopa therapy (eg, adverse effects, loss of effectiveness in a few years, possible acceleration of the loss of dopaminergic neurons in the brain), several drug therapy strategies and combinations are used to delay the start of levodopa therapy and, once started, to reduce levodopa dosage.

1. For drug-induced parkinsonism or extrapyramidal symptoms, an anticholinergic agent is the drug of choice.

2. For early idiopathic parkinsonism, when symptoms and functional disability are relatively mild, several drugs may be used as monotherapy.

   An anticholinergic agent may be the initial drug of choice in clients younger than 60 years of age, especially when tremor is the major symptom. An anticholinergic relieves tremor in approximately 50% of clients.

   Amantadine may be useful in relieving bradykinesia or tremor.

   A dopamine agonist may improve functional disability related to bradykinesia, rigidity, impaired physical dexterity, impaired speech, shuffling gait, and tremor.

3. For advanced idiopathic parkinsonism, a combination of medications is used. Two advantages of combination therapy are better control of symptoms and reduced dosage of individual drugs.

   An anticholinergic agent may be given with levodopa alone or with a levodopa/carbidopa combination.

   Amantadine may be given in combination with levodopa or other antiparkinson agents.

A dopamine agonist is usually given with levodopa/carbidopa. The combination provides more effective relief of symptoms and allows lower dosage of levodopa. Although all four of the available dopamine agonists are similarly effective, the newer agents (pramipexole and ropinirole) may cause fewer or less severe adverse effects than bromocriptine and pergolide.

The levodopa/carbidopa combination is probably the most effective drug when bradykinesia and rigidity become prominent. However, because levodopa becomes less effective after approximately 5 to 7 years, many clinicians use other drugs first and reserve levodopa for use when symptoms become more severe.

Selegiline may be given with levodopa/carbidopa. Although evidence is limited, it is thought that selegiline may have a neuroprotective effect and slow the loss of dopaminergic neurons in the brain.

Tolcapone is used only with levodopa/carbidopa. However, in contrast to AADC inhibitors, which increase the bioavailability of levodopa without increasing its plasma half-life, simultaneous administration of COMT and AADC inhibitors significantly increases the plasma half-life of levodopa.

Selegiline and tolcapone may both be used with levodopa/carbidopa because tolcapone acts peripherally and selegiline acts in the brain. Inhibition of levodopa/dopamine metabolism is a valuable addition to levodopa as an exogenous source of dopamine.

4. When changes are made in a drug therapy regimen, one change at a time is recommended so that effects of the change are clear.

Drug Dosage

The dosage of antiparkinson drugs is highly individualized. The general rule is to start with a low initial dose and gradually increase the dosage until therapeutic effects, adverse effects, or maximum drug dosage is achieved. Additional guidelines include the following.

1. The optimal dose is the lowest one that allows the client to function adequately. Optimal dosage may not be established for 6 to 8 weeks with levodopa.

2. Doses need to be adjusted as parkinsonism progresses.

3. Dosage must be individualized for levodopa and carbidopa. Only 5% to 10% of a dose of levodopa reaches the CNS, even with the addition of carbidopa. When carbidopa is given with levodopa, the dosage of levodopa must be reduced by approximately 75%. A daily dose of approximately 70 to 100 mg of carbidopa is required to saturate peripheral amino acid decarboxylase.

A levodopa/carbidopa combination is available in three dosage formulations (10 mg carbidopa/100 mg levodopa, 25 mg carbidopa/100 mg levodopa, and 25 mg carbidopa/250 mg levodopa) of immediate-release tablets (Sinemet) and two dosage formulations (25 mg carbidopa/100 mg levodopa, 50 mg carbidopa/200 mg levodopa) of sustained-release tablets (Sinemet CR). Various preparations can be mixed to administer optimal amounts of each ingredient. Sinemet CR is not as well absorbed as the short-acting form, and a client being transferred to Sinemet CR needs a dosage increase of approximately one third.

4. With levodopa, therapeutic effects may be increased and adverse effects decreased by frequent administration of small doses.
5. With pramipexole and ropinirole, dosage is started at low levels and gradually increased over several weeks. When the drugs are discontinued, they should be tapered in dosage over 1 week. With pramipexole, lower doses are indicated in older adults and those with renal impairment; with ropinirole, lower doses may be needed with hepatic impairment.
6. When combinations of drugs are used, dosage adjustments of individual components are often necessary. When levodopa is added to a regimen of anticholinergic drug therapy, for example, the anticholinergic drug need not be discontinued or reduced in dosage. However, when a dopaminergic drug is added to a regimen containing levodopa/carbidopa, dosage of levodopa/carbidopa must be reduced.

Use in Children

Safety and effectiveness for use in children have not been established for most antiparkinson drugs, including the centrally acting anticholinergics (all ages), levodopa (<12 years), and bromocriptine (<15 years). However, anticholinergics are sometimes given to children who have drug-induced extrapyramidal reactions.

Because parkinsonism is a degenerative disorder of adults, antiparkinson drugs are most likely to be used for other purposes in children. Amantadine for influenza A prevention or treatment is not recommended for neonates or infants younger than 1 year of age but may be given to children 9 to 12 years of age.

Use in Older Adults

Dosage of amantadine may need to be reduced because the drug is excreted mainly through the kidneys and renal function is usually decreased in older adults. Dosage of levodopa/carbidopa may need to be reduced because of an age-related decrease in peripheral AADC, the enzyme that carbidopa inhibits.

Anticholinergic drugs may cause blurred vision, dry mouth, tachycardia, and urinary retention. They also decrease sweating and may cause fever or heatstroke. Fever may occur in any age group, but heatstroke is more likely to occur in older adults, especially with cardiovascular disease, strenuous activity, and high environmental temperatures. When centrally active anticholinergics are given for Parkinson's disease, agitation, mental confusion, hallucinations, and psychosis may occur. In addition to the primary anticholinergics, many other drugs have significant anticholinergic activity. These include many antihistamines, including those in over-the-counter cold remedies and sleep aids; tricyclic antidepressants; and phenothiazine antipsychotic drugs. When an anticholinergic is needed by an older adult, dosage should be minimized, combinations of drugs with anticholinergic effects should be avoided, and clients should be closely monitored for adverse drug effects.

Older clients are at increased risk of having hallucinations with dopamine agonist drugs. In addition, pramipexole dosage may need to be reduced in older adults with impaired renal function.

Use in Renal Impairment

Amantadine is excreted primarily by the kidneys and should be used with caution in clients with renal failure. With pramipexole, clearance is reduced in clients with moderate or severe renal impairment and lower initial and maintenance doses are recommended. With ropinirole and tolcapone, no dosage adjustments are recommended for moderate renal impairment. The drugs have not been studied in severe renal impairment, but should be used with caution.

Use in Hepatic Impairment

Ropinirole should be used cautiously in hepatic impairment and dosage may need to be reduced. With tolcapone, elevated liver enzymes and a few deaths from liver failure have been reported. In clients with noncirrhotic liver disease, dosage reductions are not needed. In clients with hepatic cirrhosis, however, tolcapone metabolism is impaired and plasma drug levels are high. Dosage should be reduced and maintenance dosage should be less than the 600 mg daily recommended for noncirrhotic clients. In addition, liver transaminase enzymes should be monitored every month for 3 months, then every 6 weeks for 3 months.

 Home Care

The home care nurse must help clients and caregivers understand that the purpose of drug therapy is to control symptoms and that noticeable improvement may not occur for several weeks. In addition, teaching may be needed about preventing or managing adverse drug effects.

(*text continues on page 197*)

NURSING ACTIONS Antiparkinson Drugs

NURSING ACTIONS	RATIONALE/EXPLANATION
1. Administer accurately	
a. Give levodopa on an empty stomach, if tolerated. Give with food if nausea occurs.	Food slows the rate and extent of absorption, especially high-protein foods such as meats and dairy products.
b. Give other antiparkinson drugs with or just after food.	To prevent or reduce anorexia, nausea, and vomiting
c. Give selegiline in the morning and at noon.	To decrease central nervous system (CNS) stimulating effects that may interfere with sleep if the drug is taken in the evening
2. Observe for therapeutic effects	
a. With anticholinergic agents, observe for decreased tremor, salivation, drooling, and sweating.	Decreased salivation and sweating are therapeutic effects when these drugs are used in Parkinson's disease, but they are adverse effects when the drugs are used in other disorders.
b. With levodopa and dopaminergic agents, observe for improvement in mobility, balance, posture, gait, speech, handwriting, and self-care ability. Drooling and seborrhea may be abolished, and mood may be elevated.	Therapeutic effects are usually evident within 2 to 3 weeks, as levodopa dosage approaches 2 to 3 g/d, but may not reach optimum levels for 6 months.
3. Observe for adverse effects	
a. With anticholinergic drugs, observe for atropine-like effects, such as:	
(1) Tachycardia and palpitations	These effects may occur with usual therapeutic doses but are not likely to be serious except in people with underlying heart disease.
(2) Excessive CNS stimulation (tremor, restlessness, confusion, hallucinations, delirium)	This effect is most likely to occur with large doses of trihexyphenidyl (Artane) or benztropine (Cogentin). It may occur with levodopa.
(3) Sedation and drowsiness	These are most likely to occur with benztropine. The drug has antihistaminic and anticholinergic properties, and sedation is attributed to the antihistamine effect.
(4) Constipation, impaction, paralytic ileus	These effects result from decreased gastrointestinal motility and muscle tone. They may be severe because decreased intestinal motility and constipation also are characteristics of Parkinson's disease; thus, additive effects may occur.
(5) Urinary retention	This reaction is caused by loss of muscle tone in the bladder and is most likely to occur in elderly men who have enlarged prostate glands.
(6) Dilated pupils (mydriasis), blurred vision, photophobia	Ocular effects are due to paralysis of accommodation and relaxation of the ciliary muscle and the sphincter muscle of the iris.
b. With levodopa, observe for:	
(1) Anorexia, nausea, and vomiting	These symptoms usually disappear after a few months of drug therapy. They may be minimized by

(continued)

NURSING ACTIONS	RATIONALE/EXPLANATION
	giving levodopa with food, gradually increasing dosage, administering smaller doses more frequently, or adding carbidopa so that dosage of levodopa can be reduced.
(2) Orthostatic hypotension—check blood pressure in both sitting and standing positions q4h while the client is awake.	This effect is common during the first few weeks but usually subsides eventually. It can be minimized by arising slowly from supine or sitting positions and by wearing elastic stockings.
(3) Cardiac arrhythmias (tachycardia, premature ventricular contractions) and increased myocardial contractility	Levodopa and its metabolites stimulate beta-adrenergic receptors in the heart. People with pre-existing coronary artery disease may need a beta-adrenergic blocking agent (eg, propranolol) to counteract these effects.
(4) Dyskinesia—involuntary movements that may involve only the tongue, mouth, and face or the whole body	Dyskinesia eventually develops in most people who take levodopa. It is related to duration of levodopa therapy rather than dosage. Carbidopa may heighten this adverse effect, and there is no way to prevent it except by decreasing levodopa dosage. Many people prefer dyskinesia to lowering drug dosage and subsequent return of the parkinsonism symptoms.
(5) CNS stimulation—restlessness, agitation, confusion, delirium	This is more likely to occur with levodopa/carbidopa combination drug therapy.
(6) Abrupt swings in motor function (on–off phenomenon)	This fluctuation may indicate progression of the disease process. It often occurs after long-term levodopa use.
c. With amantadine, observe for:	
(1) CNS stimulation—insomnia, hyperexcitability, ataxia, dizziness, slurred speech, mental confusion, hallucinations	Compared with other antiparkinson drugs, amantadine produces few adverse effects. The ones that occur are mild, transient, and reversible. However, adverse effects increase if daily dosage exceeds 200 mg.
(2) Livedo reticularis—patchy, bluish discoloration of skin on the legs	This is a benign but cosmetically unappealing condition. It usually occurs with long-term use of amantadine and disappears when the drug is discontinued.
d. With bromocriptine and pergolide, observe for:	
(1) Nausea	These symptoms are usually mild and can be minimized by starting with low doses and increasing the dose gradually until the desired effect is achieved. If adverse effects do occur, they usually disappear with a decrease in dosage.
(2) Confusion and hallucinations	
(3) Hypotension	
e. With pramipexole and ropinirole, observe for:	These effects occurred more commonly than others during clinical trials.
(1) Nausea	
(2) Confusion, hallucinations	
(3) Dizziness, drowsiness	
(4) Dyskinesias	
(5) Orthostatic hypotension	

(continued)

NURSING ACTIONS	RATIONALE/EXPLANATION
f. With selegiline, observe for: (1) CNS effects—agitation, ataxia, bradykinesia, confusion, dizziness, dyskinesias, hallucinations, insomnia (2) Nausea, abdominal pain	
g. With tolcapone, observe for: (1) Anorexia, nausea, vomiting, diarrhea, constipation (2) Dizziness, drowsiness (3) Dyskinesias and dystonias (4) Hallucinations (5) Orthostatic hypotension	These effects occurred more commonly than others during clinical trials.
4. Observe for drug interactions	
a. Drugs that *increase* effects of anticholinergic drugs: (1) Antihistamines, disopyramide (Norpace, an antiarrhythmic agent), phenothiazines, thioxanthene agents, and tricyclic antidepressants	These drugs have anticholinergic properties and produce additive anticholinergic effects.
b. Drugs that *decrease* effects of anticholinergic drugs: (1) Cholinergic agents	These drugs counteract the inhibition of gastrointestinal motility and tone, which is a side effect of anticholinergic drug therapy.
c. Drugs that *increase* effects of levodopa: (1) Amantadine, anticholinergic agents, bromocriptine, carbidopa, pergolide, pramipexole, ropinirole, selegiline, tolcapone	These drugs are often used in combination for treatment of Parkinson's disease.
(2) Tricyclic antidepressants	These drugs potentiate levodopa effects and increase the risk of cardiac arrhythmias in people with heart disease.
(3) Monoamine oxidase type A (MAO-A) inhibitors, including isocarboxazid (Marplan), phenelzine (Nardil), and tranylcypromine (Parnate)	The combination of a catecholamine precursor (levodopa) and MAO-A inhibitors that decrease metabolism of catecholamines can result in excessive amounts of dopamine, epinephrine, and norepinephrine. Heart palpitations, headache, hypertensive crisis, and stroke may occur. Levodopa and MAO-A inhibitors should not be given concurrently. Also, levodopa should not be started within 3 weeks after an MAO-A inhibitor is discontinued. Effects of MAO-A inhibitors persist for 1 to 3 weeks after their discontinuation.
	These effects are unlikely to occur with selegiline, an MAO-B inhibitor, which more selectively inhibits the metabolism of dopamine. However, selectivity may be lost at doses higher than the recommended 10 mg/d. Selegiline is used with levodopa.

(continued)

NURSING ACTIONS	RATIONALE/EXPLANATION
d. Drugs that *decrease* effects of levodopa:	
(1) Anticholinergics	Although anticholinergics are often given with levodopa for increased antiparkinson effects, they also may decrease effects of levodopa by delaying gastric emptying. This causes more levodopa to be metabolized in the stomach and decreases the amount available for absorption from the intestine.
(2) Alcohol, antianxiety agents (eg, diazepam [Valium] and probably other benzodiazepines), antiemetics, antipsychotic agents (phenothiazines, butyrophenones, thioxanthenes)	The mechanisms by which most of these drugs decrease effects of levodopa are not clear. Phenothiazines block dopamine receptors in the basal ganglia.
(3) Oral iron preparations	Iron binds with levodopa and reduces levodopa absorption, possibly by as much as 50%.
(4) Pyridoxine (vitamin B$_6$)	Pyridoxine stimulates decarboxylase, the enzyme that converts levodopa to dopamine. As a result, more levodopa is metabolized in peripheral tissues, and less reaches the CNS, where antiparkinson effects occur. This interaction does not occur when carbidopa is given with levodopa.
e. Drugs that *decrease* effects of dopaminergic antiparkinson drugs:	
(1) Antipsychotic drugs	These drugs are dopamine antagonists and therefore inhibit the effects of dopamine agonists.
(2) Metoclopramide	

How Can You Avoid This Medication Error?

Answer: This medication error occurred because the wrong dose of levodopa was given to Mr. Evans. When administering a combination product, it is important that the dosage be correct for each medication. In this situation, the Sinemet provided contained 25 mg of carbidopa and 250 mg of levodopa. When administering Sinemet 25/250, you give the patient 250 mg of levodopa rather than the 100 mg that was ordered. Call the pharmacy and request that Sinemet 25/100 be provided.

Nursing Notes: Apply Your Knowledge

Answer: Yes. Both Sinemet and tricyclic antidepressants have anticholinergic side effects, including urinary retention and constipation. When these medications are given together, enhanced anticholinergic effects are seen. Tachycardia and palpitations can also occur. Refer Mr. Simmons to his physician to see if another antidepressant with fewer anticholinergic side effects could be used.

REVIEW AND APPLICATION EXERCISES

1. Which neurotransmitter is deficient in idiopathic and drug-induced parkinsonism?

2. How do the antiparkinson drugs act to alter the level of the deficient neurotransmitter?

3. What are the advantages and disadvantages of the various drugs used to treat parkinsonism?

4. Why is it desirable to delay the start of levodopa therapy and, once started, reduce dosage as much as possible?

5. What is the rationale for various combinations of antiparkinson drugs?

6. What are the major adverse effects of antiparkinson drugs, and how can they be minimized?

SELECTED REFERENCES

Anonymous. (1998). New drug class for Parkinson's disease. *American Journal of Nursing, 98*(7), 16MM.

Curtis, R. & McDonald, S. (1998). Alterations in motor function. In C.M. Porth (Ed.), *Pathophysiology: Concepts of altered health states*, 5th ed., pp. 921–958. Philadelphia: Lippincott Williams & Wilkins.

Drug facts and comparisons. (Updated monthly). St. Louis: Facts and Comparisons.

Factor, S.A. (1999). Dopamine agonists. *Medical Clinics of North America, 83*, 415–443.

Hauser, R.A. & Zesiewicz, T.A. (1999). Management of early Parkinson's disease. *Medical Clinics of North America, 83*, 393–414.

Kuzel, M.D. (1999). Ropinirole: A dopamine agonist for the treatment of Parkinson's disease. *American Journal of Health-System Pharmacy, 56*, 217–224.

Nelson, M.V., Berchou, R.C., & LeWitt, P.A. (1997). Parkinson's disease. In J.T. DiPiro, R.L. Talbert, P.E. Hayes, G.C. Yee, G.R. Matzke, B.G. Wells, & L.M. Posey (Eds.), *Pharmacotherapy: A pathophysiologic approach*, 3rd ed., pp. 1243–1257. Stamford, CT: Appleton & Lange.

Pittman, J.R. & Rogers, C.M. (1998). Advances in Parkinson's disease treatment. *Drug Topics, 42*(15), 52–60.

Siderowf, A., & Kurlan, R. (1999). Monoamine oxidase and catechol-*O*-methyltransferase inhibitors. *Medical Clinics of North America, 83*, 445–467.

13

Skeletal Muscle Relaxants

Objectives

After studying this chapter, the student will be able to:

1. Discuss common symptoms/disorders for which skeletal muscle relaxants are used.

2. Differentiate uses and effects of selected drugs.

3. Describe nonpharmacologic interventions to relieve muscle spasm and spasticity.

4. Apply the nursing process with clients experiencing muscle spasm or spasticity.

John Moore was in an automobile accident 5 days ago, sustaining trauma to his back and shoulder. Although no bones were broken, he continues to have pain and muscle spasms. His physician orders Tylox PRN for the pain and cyclobenzaprine (Flexeril) tid for muscle spasms.

Reflect on:

▶ Why are two different medications ordered to manage John's discomfort?

▶ What nonpharmacologic treatments can be used to promote comfort?

▶ What teaching needs to be done before sending John home?

SKELETAL MUSCLE RELAXANTS

Skeletal muscle relaxants are used to decrease muscle spasm or spasticity that occurs in certain neurologic and musculoskeletal disorders. (Neuromuscular blocking agents used as adjuncts to general anesthesia for surgery are discussed in Chap. 14.)

Muscle spasm is sudden movement that may involve alternating contraction and relaxation (clonic) or sustained contraction (tonic). Muscle spasm may occur with musculoskeletal trauma or inflammation (eg, sprains, strains, bursitis, arthritis). It is also encountered with acute or chronic low back pain, a common condition that is primarily a disorder of posture.

Spasticity involves increased muscle tone or contraction, which produces stiff, awkward movements. Spasticity results from neurologic disorders such as cerebral palsy, stroke, paraplegia, spinal cord injury, and multiple sclerosis.

Mechanism of Action

Almost all skeletal muscle relaxants are centrally active agents. Pharmacologic action is probably caused by general depression of the central nervous system (CNS), but may result from blockage of nerve impulses that cause increased muscle tone and contraction. It is unclear whether relief of pain results from sedative effects, muscular relaxation, or a placebo effect. In addition, although parenteral administration of some drugs (eg, diazepam [Valium], methocarbamol [Robaxin]) relieves pain associated with acute musculoskeletal trauma or inflammation, it is uncertain whether oral administration of usual doses exerts a beneficial effect in acute or chronic disorders. Dantrolene (Dantrium) is the only skeletal muscle relaxant that acts peripherally on the muscle itself.

Indications for Use

Skeletal muscle relaxants are recommended for use primarily as adjuncts to other treatment measures. Occasionally, parenteral agents are given to facilitate orthopedic procedures and examinations. In spastic disorders, skeletal muscle relaxants are not usually indicated only to relieve spasticity. However, they may be indicated when spasticity causes severe pain or inability to tolerate physical therapy, sit in a wheelchair, or participate in self-care activities of daily living (eg, eating, dressing). The drugs should not be given if they cause excessive muscle weakness and impair rather than facilitate mobility and function.

Dantrolene also is indicated for prevention and treatment of malignant hyperthermia, a rare but life-threatening complication of anesthesia characterized by hypercarbia, metabolic acidosis, skeletal muscle rigidity, fever, and cyanosis. For preoperative prophylaxis in people with previous episodes of malignant hyperthermia, the drug is given orally for 1 to 2 days before surgery. For intraoperative malignant hyperthermia, the drug is given intravenously. After an occurrence during surgery, the drug is given orally for 1 to 3 days to prevent recurrence of symptoms.

Contraindications to Use

Most skeletal muscle relaxants cause CNS depression and have the same contraindications as other CNS depressants. They should be used cautiously in clients with impaired renal or hepatic function or respiratory depression, and in clients who must be alert for activities of daily living (eg, driving a car, operating potentially hazardous machinery). Orphenadrine and cyclobenzaprine have high levels of anticholinergic activity and therefore should be used cautiously with glaucoma, urinary retention, cardiac arrhythmias, or tachycardia.

Individual skeletal muscle relaxants are listed in Table 13-1.

NURSING PROCESS

Assessment
Assess for muscle spasm and spasticity.

- With muscle spasm, assess for:
  Pain. This is a prominent symptom of muscle spasm and is usually aggravated by movement. Try to determine the location as specifically as possible, as well as the intensity, duration, and precipitating factors (eg, traumatic injury, strenuous exercise).
  Accompanying signs and symptoms, such as bruises (ecchymoses), edema, or signs of inflammation (redness, heat, edema, tenderness to touch)
- With spasticity, assess for pain and impaired functional ability in self-care (eg, eating, dressing). In addition, severe spasticity interferes with physical therapy exercises to maintain joint and muscle mobility.

Nursing Diagnoses
- Pain related to muscle spasm
- Impaired Physical Mobility related to spasm and pain
- Self Care Deficit related to spasm and pain
- Knowledge Deficit: Nondrug measures to relieve muscle spasm, pain, and spasticity
- Knowledge Deficit: Safe usage and effects of skeletal muscle relaxants

TABLE 13-1	Skeletal Muscle Relaxants	
	Routes and Dosage Ranges	
Generic/Trade Name	**Adults**	**Children**
Baclofen (Lioresal)	PO 5 mg 3 times daily initially, increased to 10 mg 3 times daily after 3 days, then gradually increased further if necessary; maximal dose, 20 mg 4 times daily Dosage must be reduced in the presence of impaired renal function.	Under age 12 y, not recommended
Carisoprodol (Rela, Soma)	PO 350 mg 4 times daily	Age 5 y and over, PO 25 mg/kg per day in 4 divided doses Dosage not established
Chlorphenesin (Maolate)	PO 800 mg 3 times daily until desired effect attained, then 400 mg 4 times daily or less for maintenance as needed	
Cyclobenzaprine (Flexeril)	PO 10 mg 3 times daily. Maximal recommended duration, 3 weeks; maximal recommended dose, 60 mg daily	
Dantrolene (Dantrium)	PO 25 mg daily initially, gradually increased weekly (by increments of 50–100 mg/d) to a maximal dose of 400 mg daily in 4 divided doses Preoperative prophylaxis of malignant hyperthermia: PO 4–8 mg/kg per day in 3–4 divided doses for 1 or 2 days before surgery Intraoperative malignant hyperthermia: IV push 1 mg/kg initially, continued until symptoms are relieved or a maximum total dose of 10 mg/kg has been given Postcrisis follow-up treatment: PO 4–8 mg/kg per day in 4 divided doses for 1–3 days	PO 1 mg/kg per day initially, gradually increased to a maximal dose of 3 mg/kg 4 times daily, not to exceed 400 mg daily Same as adult
Diazepam (Valium)	PO 2–10 mg 3 or 4 times daily IM, IV 5–10 mg repeated in 3–4 hours if necessary	PO 0.12–0.8 mg/kg per day in 3 or 4 divided doses IM, IV 0.04–0.2 mg/kg in a single dose, not to exceed 0.6 mg/kg within an 8-h period
Metaxalone (Skelaxin)	PO 800 mg 3 or 4 times daily for not more than 10 consecutive days	
Methocarbamol (Robaxin)	PO 1.5–2 g 4 times daily for 48–72 hours, reduced to 1.0 g 4 times daily for maintenance IM 500 mg q8h IV 1–3 g daily at a rate not to exceed 300 mg/min (3 mL of 10% injection). Do not give IV more than 3 days.	PO, IM, IV 60–75 mg/kg per day in 4 divided doses
Orphenadrine citrate (Norflex)	PO 100 mg twice daily IM, IV 60 mg twice daily	
Tizanidine (Zanaflex)	PO 4 mg q6–8h initially, increased gradually if needed. Maximum of 3 doses and 36 mg in 24 h	Dosage not established

IM, intramuscular; IV, intravenous; PO, oral.

- Risk for Injury: Dizziness, sedation related to CNS depression

Planning/Goals

The client will:

- Experience relief of pain and spasm
- Experience improved motor function
- Increase self-care abilities in activities of daily living
- Take medications as instructed

- Use nondrug measures appropriately
- Be safeguarded when sedated from drug therapy

Interventions

Use adjunctive measures for muscle spasm and spasticity:

- Physical therapy (massage, moist heat, exercises)
- Bed rest for acute muscle spasm
- Relaxation techniques

- Correct posture and lifting techniques (eg, stooping rather than bending to lift objects, holding heavy objects close to the body, *not* lifting excessive amounts of weight)
- Regular exercise and use of warm-up exercises. Strenuous exercise performed on an occasional basis (eg, weekly or monthly) is more likely to cause acute muscle spasm.

Evaluation

- Interview and observe for relief of symptoms.
- Interview and observe regarding correct usage of medications and nondrug therapeutic measures.

Nursing Notes: Apply Your Knowledge

Sarah Johnson is experiencing severe muscle spasms. Her physician orders Valium 50 mg to be given IV stat. Your stock supply has 10 mg valium per 2 cc. Discuss how you will safely administer this medication.

PRINCIPLES OF THERAPY

Goal of Treatment

The goal of treatment is to relieve pain, muscle spasm, and muscle spasticity without impairing the ability to perform self-care activities of daily living.

Drug Selection

Choice of a skeletal muscle relaxant depends primarily on the disorder being treated:

1. For acute muscle spasm and pain, a drug that can be given parenterally (eg, diazepam, methocarbamol) is usually the drug of choice.
2. Parenteral agents are preferred for orthopedic procedures because they have greater sedative and pain-relieving effects.
3. Baclofen (Lioresal) is approved for treatment of spasticity in people with multiple sclerosis. It is variably effective, and its clinical usefulness may be limited by adverse reactions. Baclofen is not recommended for pregnant women or children younger than 12 years of age.
4. None of the skeletal muscle relaxants has been established as safe for use during pregnancy and lactation.
5. Many of the skeletal muscle relaxants have not been established as safe for use in children. Choice of drug should be limited to those with established pediatric dosages.

Use in Children

For most of the drugs, safety and effectiveness for use in children 12 years of age and younger have not been established. The drugs should be used only when clearly indicated, for short periods, when close supervision is available for monitoring drug effects (especially sedation), and when mobility and alertness are not required.

Use in Older Adults

Any CNS depressant or sedating drugs should be used cautiously in older adults. Risks of falls, mental confusion, and other adverse effects are higher in older adults because of impaired drug metabolism and excretion. In addition, tizanidine should be used with caution because drug clearance is slower and the risk of adverse effects is higher in older adults.

CLIENT TEACHING GUIDELINES
Skeletal Muscle Relaxants

General Considerations

✔ Use nondrug measures, such as exercises and applications of heat and cold, to decrease muscle spasm and spasticity.

✔ Avoid activities that require mental alertness or physical coordination (eg, driving an automobile, operating potentially dangerous machinery) if drowsy from medication.

✔ Do not take other drugs without the physician's knowledge, including nonprescription drugs. The major risk occurs with concurrent use of alcohol, antihistamines, sleeping aids, or other drugs that cause drowsiness.

Self-administration

✔ Take the drugs with milk or food, to avoid nausea and stomach irritation.

✔ Do not stop drugs abruptly. Dosage should be decreased gradually, especially with baclofen, carisoprodol, and cyclobenzaprine. Suddenly stopping baclofen may cause hallucinations; stopping the other drugs may cause fatigue, headache, and nausea.

Skeletal Muscle Relaxants

NURSING ACTIONS	RATIONALE/EXPLANATION
1. Administer accurately	
a. Give baclofen, chlorphenesin, metaxalone with milk or food.	To decrease gastrointestinal distress
b. Do not mix parenteral diazepam in a syringe with any other drugs.	Diazepam is physically incompatible with other drugs.
c. Inject intravenous (IV) diazepam directly into a vein or the injection site nearest the vein (during continuous IV infusions) at a rate of approximately 2 mg/min.	Diazepam may cause a precipitate if diluted. Avoid contact with IV solutions as much as possible. A slow rate of injection minimizes the risks of respiratory depression and apnea.
d. Avoid extravasation with IV diazepam, and inject intramuscular (IM) diazepam deeply into a gluteal muscle.	To prevent or reduce tissue irritation
e. With IV methocarbamol, inject or infuse slowly.	Rapid administration may cause bradycardia, hypotension, and dizziness.
f. With IV methocarbamol, have the client lie down during and at least 15 minutes after administration.	To minimize orthostatic hypotension and other adverse drug effects
g. Avoid extravasation with IV methocarbamol, and give IM methocarbamol deeply into a gluteal muscle. (Dividing the dose and giving two injections is preferred.)	Parenteral methocarbamol is a hypertonic solution that is very irritating to tissues. Thrombophlebitis may occur at IV injection sites, and sloughing of tissue may occur at sites of extravasation or IM injections.
2. Observe for therapeutic effects	
a. When the drug is given for acute muscle spasm, observe for:	Therapeutic effects usually occur within 30 minutes after IV injection of diazepam or methocarbamol.
(1) Decreased pain and tenderness	
(2) Increased mobility	
(3) Increased ability to participate in activities of daily living	
b. When the drug is given for spasticity in chronic neurologic disorders, observe for:	
(1) Increased ability to maintain posture and balance	
(2) Increased ability for self-care (eg, eating and dressing)	
(3) Increased tolerance for physical therapy and exercises	
3. Observe for adverse effects	
a. With centrally active agents, observe for:	
(1) Drowsiness and dizziness	These are the most common adverse effects.
(2) Blurred vision, lethargy, flushing	These effects occur more often with IV administration of drugs. They are usually transient.
(3) Nausea, vomiting, abdominal distress, constipation or diarrhea, ataxia, areflexia, flaccid paralysis, respiratory depression, tachycardia, hypotension	These effects are most likely to occur with large oral doses.

(continued)

NURSING ACTIONS	RATIONALE/EXPLANATION
(4) Hypersensitivity—skin rash, pruritus	The drug should be discontinued if hypersensitivity reactions occur. Serious allergic reactions (eg, anaphylaxis) are rare.
(5) Psychological or physical dependence with diazepam and other antianxiety agents	Most likely to occur with long-term use of large doses
b. With a peripherally active agent (dantrolene), observe for:	Adverse effects are usually transient.
(1) Drowsiness, fatigue, lethargy, weakness, nausea, vomiting	These effects are the most common.
(2) Headache, anorexia, nervousness	Less common effects
(3) Hepatotoxicity	This potentially serious adverse effect is most likely to occur in people older than 35 years of age who have taken the drug 60 days or longer. Women over age 35 years who take estrogens have the highest risk. Hepatotoxicity can be prevented or minimized by administering the lowest effective dose, monitoring liver enzymes (aspartate aminotransferase and alanine aminotransferase) during therapy, and discontinuing the drug if no beneficial effects occur within 45 days.
4. Observe for drug interactions	
a. Drugs that *increase* effects of skeletal muscle relaxants:	
(1) Central nervous system (CNS) depressants (alcohol, antianxiety agents, antidepressants, antihistamines, antipsychotic drugs, sedative-hypnotics)	Additive CNS depression with increased risks of excessive sedation and respiratory depression or apnea
(2) Monoamine oxidase inhibitors	May potentiate effects by inhibiting metabolism of muscle relaxants

Nursing Notes: Apply Your Knowledge

Answer: Check this order with the physician. Normal IV Valium dosage is 5 to 10 mg every 3 to 4 hours. A 50-mg dose is unsafe and should not be given.

REVIEW AND APPLICATION EXERCISES

1. How do skeletal muscle relaxants act to relieve spasm and pain?
2. What are the indications for the use of skeletal muscle relaxants?
3. What are the contraindications to the use of these drugs?
4. What are the major adverse effects of these drugs, and how can they be minimized?
5. What are some nonpharmacologic interventions to use instead of or along with the drugs?

SELECTED REFERENCES

Drug facts and comparisons. (Updated monthly). St. Louis: Facts and Comparisons.

Guyton, A.C. & Hall, J.E. (1996). *Textbook of medical physiology*, 9th ed. Philadelphia: W.B. Saunders.

14

Anesthetics

Objectives

After studying this chapter, the student will be able to:

1. Discuss factors considered when choosing an anesthetic agent.

2. Describe characteristics of general and regional/local anesthetic agents.

3. Compare general and local anesthetics in terms of administration, client safety, and nursing care.

4. Discuss the rationale for using adjunctive drugs before and during surgical procedures.

5. Describe the nurse's role in relation to anesthetics and adjunctive drugs.

6. Discuss the use of anesthetics and neuromuscular blocking agents in children; older adults; and clients with renal impairment, hepatic impairment, and critical illness.

You are a nurse working in the postanesthesia recovery unit of an outpatient surgery center. Patients may be given general or local anesthetics for minor surgical procedures. Your responsibilities include monitoring during the immediate recovery period as the effects of the anesthesia wear off. Patients are usually discharged on the same day.

Reflect on:

▶ What effects would you expect to see as the general anesthesia wears off?

▶ Compare and contrast how these effects might be the same or different for the patient receiving local anesthesia.

▶ Identify priorities of nursing care to maintain patient safety during this period.

Anesthesia means loss of sensation with or without loss of consciousness. Anesthetic drugs are given to prevent pain and promote relaxation during surgery, childbirth, some diagnostic tests, and some treatments. They interrupt the conduction of painful nerve impulses from a site of injury to the brain. The two basic types of anesthesia are general and regional.

GENERAL ANESTHESIA

General anesthesia is a state of profound central nervous system (CNS) depression, during which there is complete loss of sensation, consciousness, pain perception, and memory. It has three components: hypnosis, analgesia, and muscle relaxation. Several different drugs are usually combined to produce desired levels of these components without excessive CNS depression. This so-called *balanced anesthesia* also allows lower dosages of potent general anesthetics.

General anesthesia is usually induced with a fast-acting drug (eg, propofol or thiopental) given intravenously (IV) and is maintained with a gas mixture of an anesthetic agent and oxygen given by inhalation. The IV agent produces rapid loss of consciousness and provides a pleasant induction and recovery. Its rapid onset of action is attributed to rapid circulation to the brain and accumulation in the neuronal tissue of the cerebral cortex.

The drugs are short acting because they are quickly redistributed from the brain to highly perfused organs (eg, heart, liver, kidneys) and muscles, and then to fatty tissues. Because they are slowly released from fatty tissues back into the bloodstream, anesthesia, drowsiness, and cardiopulmonary depression persist into the postoperative period. Duration of action can be prolonged and accumulation is more likely to occur with repeated doses or continuous IV infusion.

An anesthetic barbiturate or propofol may be used alone for anesthesia during brief diagnostic tests or surgical procedures. Barbiturates are contraindicated in patients with acute intermittent porphyria, a rare hereditary disorder characterized by recurrent attacks of physical and mental disturbances.

Inhalation anesthetics vary in the degree of CNS depression produced and thereby vary in the rate of induction, anesthetic potency, degree of muscle relaxation, and analgesic potency. CNS depression is determined by the concentration of the drug in the CNS. Drug concentration, in turn, depends on the rate at which the drug is transported from the alveoli to the blood, transported past the blood–brain barrier to reach the CNS, redistributed by the blood to other body tissues, and eliminated by the lungs. Depth of anesthesia can be regulated readily by varying the concentration of the inhaled anesthetic gas. General inhala-tion anesthetics should be given only by specially trained people, such as anesthesiologists and nurse anesthetists, and only with appropriate equipment.

REGIONAL ANESTHESIA

Regional anesthesia involves loss of sensation and motor activity in localized areas of the body. It is induced by application or injection of local anesthetic drugs. The drugs act to decrease the permeability of nerve cell membranes to ions, especially sodium. This action stabilizes the cell membrane, prevents initiation and transmission of nerve impulses, and therefore prevents the cells from responding to pain impulses and other sensory stimuli.

Regional anesthesia is usually categorized according to the site of application. The area anesthetized may be the site of application, or it may be distal to the point of injection. Specific types of anesthesia attained with local anesthetic drugs include the following:

1. Topical or surface anesthesia involves applying local anesthetics to skin or mucous membrane. Such application makes sensory receptors unresponsive to pain, itching, and other stimuli. Local anesthetics for topical use are usually ingredients of various ointments, solutions, or lotions designed for use at particular sites. For example, preparations are available for use on eyes, ears, nose, oral mucosa, perineum, hemorrhoids, and skin.
2. Infiltration involves injecting the local anesthetic solution directly into or very close to the area to be anesthetized.
3. Peripheral nerve block involves injecting the anesthetic solution into the area of a larger nerve trunk or a nerve plexus at some access point along the course of a nerve distant from the area to be anesthetized.
4. Field block anesthesia involves injecting the anesthetic solution around the area to be anesthetized.
5. Spinal anesthesia involves injecting the anesthetic agent into the cerebrospinal fluid, usually in the lumbar spine. The anesthetic blocks sensory impulses at the root of peripheral nerves as they enter the spinal cord. Spinal anesthesia is especially useful for surgery involving the lower abdomen and legs.

   The body area anesthetized is determined by the level to which the drug solution rises in the spinal canal. This, in turn, is determined by the site of injection, the position of the client, and the specific gravity, amount, and concentration of the injected solution.

   Solutions of local anesthetics used for spinal anesthesia are either hyperbaric or hypobaric. *Hyperbaric* or heavy solutions are diluted with dextrose, have a higher specific gravity than cerebrospinal fluid, and gravitate toward the head when the client is tilted in a head-down position. *Hypobaric* or light solutions are diluted with distilled water, have a lower specific gravity than cerebrospinal fluid, and gravitate toward the lower (caudal) end of the spinal canal when the client is tilted in a head-down position.

6. Epidural anesthesia, which involves injecting the anesthetic into the epidural space, is used most often in obstetrics during labor and delivery. This route is also used to provide analgesia (often with a combination of a local anesthetic and an opioid) for clients with postoperative or other pain.

The extent and duration of anesthesia produced by injection of local anesthetics depend on several factors. In general, large amounts, high concentrations, or injections into highly vascular areas (eg, head and neck, intercostal and paracervical sites) produce rapid peak plasma levels. Duration depends on the chemical characteristics of the drug used and the rate at which it leaves nerve tissue. When a vasoconstrictor drug, such as epinephrine, has been added, onset and duration of anesthesia are prolonged because of slow absorption and elimination of the anesthetic agent. Epinephrine also controls bleeding in the affected area.

ADJUNCTS TO ANESTHESIA

Several nonanesthetic drugs are used as adjuncts or supplements to anesthetic drugs. Most are discussed elsewhere and are described here only in relation to anesthesia. Drug groups include antianxiety agents and sedative-hypnotics (see Chap. 8), anticholinergics (see Chap. 21), and opioid analgesics (see Chap. 6). The neuromuscular blocking agents are described in this chapter.

Goals of preanesthetic medication include decreased anxiety without excessive drowsiness, client amnesia for the perioperative period, reduced requirement for inhalation anesthetic, reduced adverse effects associated with some inhalation anesthetics (eg, bradycardia, coughing, salivation, postanesthetic vomiting), and reduced perioperative stress. Various regimens, usually of two or three drugs, are used.

Antianxiety Agents and Sedative-Hypnotics

Antianxiety agents and *sedative-hypnotics* are given to decrease anxiety, promote rest, and increase client safety by allowing easier induction of anesthesia and smaller doses of anesthetic agents. These drugs may be given the night before to aid sleep and 1 or 2 hours before the scheduled procedure. Hypnotic doses are usually given for greater sedative effects. A benzodiazepine such as diazepam (Valium) or midazolam (Versed) is often used. Mida-

zolam has a rapid onset and short duration of action, causes amnesia, produces minimal cardiovascular side effects, and reduces the dose of opioid analgesics required during surgery. It is often used in ambulatory surgical or invasive diagnostic procedures and regional anesthesia.

Anticholinergics

Anticholinergic drugs are given to prevent vagal effects associated with general anesthesia and surgery (eg, bradycardia, hypotension). Vagal stimulation occurs with some inhalation anesthetics; with succinylcholine, a muscle relaxant; and with surgical procedures in which there is manipulation of the pharynx, trachea, peritoneum, stomach, intestine, or other viscera and procedures in which pressure is exerted on the eyeball. Useful drugs are atropine and glycopyrrolate (Robinul).

Opioid Analgesics

Opioid analgesics induce relaxation and pain relief in the preanesthetic period. These drugs potentiate the CNS depression produced by other drugs, and less anesthetic agent is required. Morphine and fentanyl may be given in anesthetic doses in certain circumstances.

Neuromuscular Blocking Agents

Neuromuscular blocking agents cause muscle relaxation, the third component of general anesthesia, and allow the use of smaller amounts of anesthetic agent. Artificial ventilation is necessary because these drugs paralyze muscles of respiration as well as other skeletal muscles. The drugs do not cause sedation; therefore, unless the recipients are unconscious, they can see and hear environmental activities and conversations.

There are two types of neuromuscular blocking agents: depolarizing and nondepolarizing. Succinylcholine is the only commonly used depolarizing drug. Like acetylcholine, the drug combines with cholinergic receptors at the motor endplate to produce depolarization and muscle contraction initially. Repolarization and further muscle contraction are then inhibited as long as an adequate concentration of drug remains at the receptor site.

Muscle paralysis is preceded by muscle spasms, which may damage muscles. Injury to muscle cells may cause postoperative muscle pain and release potassium into the circulation. If hyperkalemia develops, it is usually mild and insignificant but may cause cardiac arrhythmias or even cardiac arrest in some situations. Succinylcholine is normally deactivated by plasma pseudocholinesterase. There is no antidote except reconstituted fresh-frozen plasma that contains pseudocholinesterase.

Nondepolarizing neuromuscular blocking agents prevent acetylcholine from acting at neuromuscular junctions. Consequently, the nerve cell membrane is not depolarized, the muscle fibers are not stimulated, and skeletal muscle contraction does not occur. The prototype drug is tubocurarine, the active ingredient of curare, a naturally occurring plant alkaloid that causes skeletal muscle relaxation or paralysis. Anticholinesterase drugs, such as neostigmine (Prostigmin; see Chap. 20), are antidotes and can be used to reverse muscle paralysis.

Several newer, synthetic nondepolarizing agents are available and are preferred over succinylcholine in most instances. (Succinylcholine remains the drug of choice when speed of onset and short duration of action are priorities.) The drugs vary in onset and duration of action. Some have short elimination half-lives (eg, mivacurium, rocuronium) that allow spontaneous recovery of neuro-

muscular function when an IV infusion is discontinued. With these agents, administration of a reversal agent may be unnecessary. The drugs also vary in routes of elimination, with most involving both hepatic and renal mechanisms. In clients with renal or hepatic impairment, the parent drug or its metabolites may accumulate and cause prolonged paralysis. As a result, neuromuscular blocking agents should be used very cautiously in clients with renal or hepatic impairment.

INDIVIDUAL ANESTHETIC AGENTS

General anesthetics are listed in Table 14-1, neuromuscular blocking agents in Table 14-2, and local anesthetics in Table 14-3.

(*text continues on page 212*)

TABLE 14-1	General Anesthetics		
Generic/Trade Name	**Characteristics**		**Remarks**
General Inhalation Anesthetics			
Desflurane (Suprane)	Similar to isoflurane		Used for induction and maintenance of general anesthesia
Enflurane (Ethrane)	Nonexplosive, nonflammable volatile liquid; similar to halothane but may produce better analgesia and muscle relaxation; sensitizes heart to catecholamines—increases risk of cardiac arrhythmias; renal or hepatic toxicity not reported		A frequently used agent
Halothane (Fluothane)	Nonexplosive, nonflammable volatile liquid Advantages: 1. Produces rapid induction with little or no excitement; rapid recovery with little excitement or nausea and vomiting 2. Does not irritate respiratory tract mucosa; therefore does not increase saliva and tracheobronchial secretions 3. Depresses pharyngeal and laryngeal reflexes, which decreases risk of laryngospasm and bronchospasm Disadvantages: 1. Depresses contractility of the heart and vascular smooth muscle, which causes decreased cardiac output, hypotension, and bradycardia 2. Circulatory failure may occur with high doses. 3. Causes cardiac arrhythmias. Bradycardia is common; ventricular arrhythmias are uncommon unless ventilation is inadequate. 4. Sensitizes heart to catecholamines; increases risk of cardiac arrhythmias 5. Depresses respiration and may produce hypoxemia and respiratory acidosis (hypercarbia) 6. Depresses functions of the kidneys, liver, and immune system 7. May cause jaundice and hepatitis 8. May cause malignant hyperthermia		Halothane has largely been replaced by newer agents with increased efficacy, decreased adverse effects, or both. It may be used in balanced anesthesia with other agents. Although quite potent, it may not produce adequate analgesia and muscle relaxation at a dosage that is not likely to produce significant adverse effects. Therefore, nitrous oxide is given to increase analgesic effects; a neuromuscular blocking agent is given to increase muscle relaxation; and an IV barbiturate is used to produce rapid, smooth induction, after which halothane is given to maintain anesthesia.

(continued)

TABLE 14-1   **General Anesthetics** (*continued*)

Generic/Trade Name	Characteristics	Remarks
Isoflurane (Forane)	Similar to halothane but less likely to cause cardiovascular depression and ventricular arrhythmias. Isoflurane may cause malignant hyperthermia but apparently does not cause hepatotoxicity.	Used for induction and maintenance of general anesthesia
Nitrous oxide	Nonexplosive gas; good analgesic, weak anesthetic; one of oldest and safest anesthetics; causes no appreciable damage to vital organs unless hypoxia is allowed to develop and persist; administered with oxygen to prevent hypoxia; rapid induction and recovery. *Note:* Nitrous oxide is an incomplete anesthetic; that is, by itself, it cannot produce surgical anesthesia.	Used in balanced anesthesia with IV barbiturates, neuromuscular blocking agents, opioid analgesics, and more potent inhalation anesthetics. It is safer for prolonged surgical procedures (see "Characteristics"). It is used alone for analgesia in dentistry, obstetrics, and brief surgical procedures.
Sevoflurane (Ultane)	Similar to isoflurane	Used for induction and maintenance of general anesthesia
General Intravenous Anesthetics		
Alfentanil (Alfenta)	Opioid analgesic-anesthetic related to fentanyl and sufentanil. Rapid acting.	May be used as a primary anesthetic or an analgesic adjunct in balanced anesthesia
Etomidate (Amidate)	A nonanalgesic hypnotic used for induction and maintenance of general anesthesia	May be used with nitrous oxide and oxygen in maintenance of general anesthesia for short operative procedures such as uterine dilation and curettage
Fentanyl and droperidol combination (Innovar)	Droperidol (Inapsine) is related to the antipsychotic agent haloperidol. It produces sedative and antiemetic effects. Fentanyl citrate (Sublimaze) is a very potent opioid analgesic whose actions are similar to those of morphine but of shorter duration. Innovar is a fixed-dose combination of the two drugs. Additional doses of fentanyl are often needed because its analgesic effect lasts approximately 30 minutes, whereas droperidol's effects last 3–6 hours.	Either drug may be used alone, but they are often used together for neuroleptanalgesia and combined with nitrous oxide for neuroleptanesthesia. Neuroleptanalgesia is a state of reduced awareness and reduced sensory perception during which a variety of diagnostic tests or minor surgical procedures can be done, such as bronchoscopy and burn dressings. Neuroleptanesthesia can be used for major surgical procedures. Consciousness returns rapidly, but respiratory depression may last 3–4 hours into the postoperative recovery period.
Ketamine (Ketalar)	Rapid-acting nonbarbiturate anesthetic; produces marked analgesia, sedation, immobility, amnesia, and a lack of awareness of surroundings (called dissociative anesthesia); may be given IV or IM; awakening may require several hours; during recovery, unpleasant psychic symptoms may occur, including dreams and hallucinations; vomiting, hypersalivation, and transient skin rashes also may occur during recovery.	Used most often for brief surgical, diagnostic, or therapeutic procedures. It also may be used to induce anesthesia. If used for major surgery, it must be supplemented by other general anesthetics. It is generally contraindicated in clients with increased intracranial pressure, severe coronary artery disease, hypertension, or psychiatric disorders. Hyperactivity and unpleasant dreams occur less often with children than adults.
Methohexital sodium (Brevital)	An ultrashort-acting barbiturate similar to thiopental	See thiopental, below.
Midazolam (Versed)	Short-acting benzodiazepine. May cause respiratory depression, apnea, death with IV administration. Smaller doses are needed if other CNS depressants (eg, opioid analgesics, general anesthetics) are given concurrently.	Given IM for preoperative sedation. Given IV for conscious sedation during short endoscopic or other diagnostic procedures; induction of general anesthesia; and maintenance of general anesthesia with nitrous oxide and oxygen for short surgical procedures
Propofol (Diprivan)	A rapid-acting hypnotic used with other agents in balanced anesthesia. May cause hypotension, apnea, and other signs of CNS depression. Recovery is rapid, occurring within minutes after the drug is stopped.	Given by IV bolus or infusion for induction or maintenance of general anesthesia or sedation in intensive care

(*continued*)

TABLE 14-1   **General Anesthetics** (*continued*)

Generic/Trade Name	Characteristics	Remarks
Remifentanil (Ultiva)	An opioid analgesic-anesthetic with a rapid onset and short duration of action	Used for induction and maintenance of general anesthesia
Sufentanil (Sufenta)	A synthetic opioid analgesic-anesthetic related to fentanyl. Compared with fentanyl, it is more potent and faster acting and may allow a more rapid recovery.	May be used as a primary anesthetic or an analgesic adjunct in balanced anesthesia
Thiopental sodium (Pentothal)	Ultrashort-acting barbiturate, used almost exclusively in general anesthesia; excellent hypnotic but does not produce significant analgesia or muscle relaxation; given IV by intermittent injection or by continuous infusion of a dilute solution.	Thiopental is commonly used. A single dose produces unconsciousness in less than 30 seconds and lasts 20–30 minutes. Usually given to induce anesthesia. It is used alone only for brief procedures. For major surgery, it is usually supplemented by inhalation anesthetics and muscle relaxants.

CNS, central nervous system; IM, intramuscular; IV, intravenous.

TABLE 14-2   **Neuromuscular Blocking Agents (Skeletal Muscle Relaxants)**

Generic/Trade Name	Characteristics	Uses
Depolarizing Type		
Succinylcholine (Anectine)	Short acting after single dose; action can be prolonged by repeated injections or continuous intravenous infusion. Malignant hyperthermia may occur.	All types of surgery and brief procedures, such as endoscopy and endotracheal intubation
Nondepolarizing Type		
Atracurium (Tracrium)	Intermediate acting*	Adjunct to general anesthesia
Cisatracurium (Nimbex)	Intermediate acting*	Same as rocuronium, below
Doxacurium (Nuromax)	Long acting*	Adjunct to general anesthesia
Metocurine (Metubine)	Long acting; more potent than tubocurarine*	Same as vecuronium, below
Mivacurium (Mivacron)	Short acting*	Adjunct to general anesthesia
Pancuronium (Pavulon)	Long acting*	Mainly during surgery after general anesthesia has been induced; occasionally to aid endotracheal intubation or mechanical ventilation
Pipecuronium (Arduan)	Long acting*	Adjunct to general anesthesia; recommended only for procedures expected to last 90 minutes or longer
Rocuronium (Zemuron)	Intermediate acting*	Adjunct to general anesthesia to aid endotracheal intubation and provide muscle relaxation during surgery or mechanical ventilation
Tubocurarine	Long acting; the prototype of nondepolarizing drugs*	Adjunct to general anesthesia; occasionally to facilitate mechanical ventilation
Vecuronium (Norcuron)	Intermediate acting*	Adjunct to general anesthesia; to facilitate endotracheal intubation and mechanical ventilation

*All the nondepolarizing agents may cause hypotension; effects of the drugs can be reversed by neostigmine (Prostigmin).

TABLE 14-3   **Local Anesthetics**

Generic/Trade Name	Characteristics	Clinical Uses
Benzocaine (Americaine)	Poorly water soluble and poorly absorbed; thus, anesthetic effects are relatively prolonged, and systemic absorption is minimal; available in many prescription and nonprescription preparations, including aerosol sprays, throat lozenges, rectal suppositories, lotions, and ointments	Topical anesthesia of skin and mucous membrane to relieve pain and itching of sunburn, other minor burns and wounds, skin abrasions, earache, hemorrhoids, sore throat, and other conditions. Caution: may cause hypersensitivity reactions.
Bupivacaine (Marcaine)	Given by injection; has a relatively long duration of action; may produce systemic toxicity	Regional anesthesia by infiltration, nerve block, and epidural anesthesia during childbirth. It is not used for spinal anesthesia.
Butamben (Butesin)	Applied topically to skin only	Used mainly in minor burns and skin irritations
Chloroprocaine (Nesacaine)	Chemically and pharmacologically related to procaine, but its potency is greater and duration of action is shorter; rapidly metabolized and less likely to cause systemic toxicity than other local anesthetics; given by injection	Regional anesthesia by infiltration, nerve block, and epidural anesthesia
Cocaine	One of the oldest local anesthetics; a naturally occurring plant alkaloid; readily absorbed through mucous membranes; a Schedule II controlled substance with high potential for abuse, largely because of euphoria and other central nervous system stimulatory effects; produces psychic dependence and tolerance with prolonged use; too toxic for systemic use	Topical anesthesia of ear, nose, and throat
Dibucaine (Nupercaine, Nupercainal)	Potent agent; onset of action slow but duration relatively long; rather high incidence of toxicity	Topical or spinal anesthesia
Dyclonine (Dyclone)	Rapid onset of action and duration comparable to procaine; absorbed through skin and mucous membranes	Topical anesthesia in otolaryngology
Etidocaine (Duranest)	A derivative of lidocaine that is more potent and more toxic than lidocaine; long duration of action	Regional nerve blocks and epidural anesthesia
Lidocaine (Xylocaine)	Given topically and by injection; more rapid in onset, intensity, and duration of action than procaine, also more toxic; acts as an antiarrhythmic drug by decreasing myocardial irritability. One of the most widely used local anesthetic drugs.	Topical anesthesia and regional anesthesia by local infiltration, nerve block, spinal, and epidural anesthesia. It also is used intravenously to prevent or treat cardiac arrhythmias (see Chap. 52). (Caution: do not use preparations containing epinephrine for arrhythmias.)
Lidocaine 2.5%/prilocaine 2.5% (EMLA)	Formulated to be absorbed through intact skin; contraindicated for use on mucous membranes or abraded skin	Topical anesthesia for vaccinations or venipuncture in children
Mepivacaine (Carbocaine)	Chemically and pharmacologically related to lidocaine; action slower in onset and longer in duration than lidocaine; effective only in large doses; not used topically	Infiltration, nerve block, and epidural anesthesia
Pramoxine (Tronothane)	Not injected or applied to nasal mucosa because it irritates tissues	Topical anesthesia for skin wounds, dermatoses, hemorrhoids, endotracheal intubation, sigmoidoscopy
Prilocaine (Citanest)	Pharmacologically similar to lidocaine with approximately the same effectiveness but slower onset, longer duration, and less toxicity because it is more rapidly metabolized and excreted	Regional anesthesia by infiltration, nerve block, and epidural anesthesia
Procaine (Novocain)	Most widely used local anesthetic for many years, but it has largely been replaced by newer drugs. It is rapidly metabolized, which increases safety but shortens duration of action.	Regional anesthesia by infiltration, nerve block, and spinal anesthesia. Not used topically.

(continued)

TABLE 14-3	Local Anesthetics (*continued*)

Generic/Trade Name	Characteristics	Clinical Uses
Proparacaine (Alcaine)	Causes minimal irritation of the eye but may cause allergic contact dermatitis of the fingers	Topical anesthesia of the eye for tonometry and for removal of sutures, foreign bodies, and cataracts
Ropivacaine (Naropin)	Given by injection or epidural infusion	Obstetric or postoperative analgesia and local or regional surgical anesthesia
Tetracaine (Pontocaine)	Applied topically or given by injection	Topical and spinal anesthesia mainly; can be used for local infiltration or nerve block

How Can You Avoid This Medication Error?

You are working in a busy postanesthesia recovery unit (PACU), caring for two patients recovering from general anesthesia. You have been asked to extend your shift because someone has called in sick. You are preparing some intravenous morphine to administer to one patient, but before you administer the morphine, you are interrupted twice. After you finally administer the drug, you realize that you administered it to the wrong patient.

NURSING PROCESS

Preoperative Assessment

- Assess nutritional status.
- Assess use of prescription and nonprescription drugs, especially those taken within the past 3 days.
- Ask about drug allergies. If use of local or regional anesthesia is anticipated, ask if the client has ever had an allergic reaction to a local anesthetic.
- Assess for risk factors for complications of anesthesia and surgery (cigarette smoking, obesity, limited exercise or activity, chronic cardiovascular, respiratory, renal, or other disease processes).
- Assess the client's understanding of the intended procedure, attitude toward anesthesia and surgery, and degree of anxiety and fear.
- Assess ability and willingness to participate in postoperative activities to promote recovery.
- Assess vital signs, laboratory data, and other data as indicated to establish baseline measurements for monitoring changes.

Postoperative Assessment

- During the immediate postoperative period, assess vital signs and respiratory and cardiovascular function every 5 to 15 minutes until reactive and stabilizing. Effects of anesthetics and adjunctive medications persist into postanesthesia recovery.

- Continue to assess vital signs, fluid balance, and laboratory and other data.
- Assess for signs of complications (eg, fluid and electrolyte imbalance, respiratory problems, thrombophlebitis, wound infection).

Nursing Diagnoses

- Risk for Injury: Trauma related to impaired sensory perception and impaired physical mobility from anesthetic or sedative drugs
- Risk for Injury: CNS depression with premedications and general anesthetics
- Pain related to operative procedure
- Decreased Cardiac Output related to effects of anesthetics, other medications, and surgery
- Impaired Gas Exchange related to effects of anesthetics, other medications, and surgery
- Risk for Ineffective Breathing Patterns related to respiratory depression
- Impaired Physical Mobility and Self Care Deficits related to sedation
- Impaired Verbal Communication related to intubation and sedation
- Anxiety or Fear related to anticipated surgery and possible outcomes

Planning/Goals

The client will:

- Receive sufficient emotional support and instruction to facilitate a smooth preoperative and postoperative course
- Be protected from injury and complications while self-care ability is impaired
- Have emergency supplies and personnel available if needed
- Have postoperative discomfort managed appropriately

Interventions

Preoperatively, assist the client to achieve optimal conditions for surgery. Some guidelines include the following:

- Provide foods and fluids to improve or maintain nutritional status (eg, those high in protein, vit-

CLIENT TEACHING GUIDELINES
Perioperative Medications

✔ If having surgery, ask how pain will be managed after surgery and what you will need to do to promote recovery. Instructions about postoperative activities vary with the type of surgery.

✔ With preanesthetic, sedative-type medications, stay in bed with the siderails up and use the call light if help is needed. You may fall or otherwise injure yourself if you get out of bed without assistance.

✔ Do not try to perform activities requiring mental alertness and physical coordination while drowsy or less than alert from general anesthesia, sedation, or pain medication.

✔ After surgery, take enough pain medication to allow ambulation, movement, coughing and deep breathing, and other exercises to promote recovery. In most instances, you will receive pain medication by injection (often intravenously) for 2 or 3 days, then by mouth.

✔ Follow instructions and try to cooperate with health care personnel in activities to prevent postoperative complications, including respiratory and wound infections.

CLIENT TEACHING GUIDELINES
Topical Anesthetics

✔ Use the drug preparation only on the part of the body for which it was prescribed. Most preparations are specifically made to apply on certain areas, and they cannot be used effectively and safely on other body parts.

✔ Use the drug only for the condition for which it was prescribed. For example, a local anesthetic prescribed to relieve itching may aggravate an open wound.

✔ Apply local anesthetics to clean areas. If needed, wash skin areas or take a sitz bath to cleanse the perineal area. For the drugs to be effective, they must have direct contact with the affected area.

✔ Do *not* apply more often than directed. Local irritation, skin rash, and hives can develop.

✔ With spray preparations, do not inhale vapors, spray near food, or store near any heat source.

✔ Use local anesthetic preparations for only a short period. If the condition for which it is being used persists, report the condition to the physician.

✔ Inform dentists or other physicians if allergic to any local anesthetic drug. Allergic reactions are rare, but if they have occurred, another type of local anesthetic can usually be substituted safely.

amin C and other vitamins, and electrolytes to promote healing).

• Help the client maintain exercise and activity, when feasible. This helps promote respiratory and cardiovascular function and decreases anxiety.

• Explain the expected course of events of the perioperative period (eg, specific preparations for surgery, close observation and monitoring during postanesthesia recovery, approximate length of stay).

• Assist clients with measures to facilitate recovery postoperatively (eg, coughing and deep-breathing exercises, leg exercises and early ambulation, maintaining fluid balance and urine output).

• Explain how postoperative pain will be managed. This is often a major source of anxiety.

Postoperatively, the major focus is on maintaining a safe environment and vital functions. Specific interventions include:

• Observe and record vital signs, level of consciousness, respiratory and cardiovascular status, wound status, and elimination frequently until sensory and motor functions return, then periodically until discharge.

• Maintain IV infusions. Monitor the site, amount, and type of fluids. If potential problems are identified (eg, hypovolemia or hypervolemia), intervene to prevent them from becoming actual problems.

• Give pain medication appropriately as indicated by the client's condition.

• Help the client to turn, cough, deep breathe, exercise legs, ambulate, and perform other self-care activities until he or she can perform them independently.

• Use sterile technique in wound care.

• Initiate discharge planning for a smooth transition to home care.

Evaluation
- Observe for absence of injury and complications (eg, no fever or other signs of infection).
- Observe for improved ability in self-care activities.
- The client states that pain has been managed satisfactorily.

PRINCIPLES OF THERAPY

Preanesthetic Medications

Principles for using preanesthetic drugs (antianxiety agents, anticholinergics, opioid analgesics) are the same when these drugs are given before surgery as at other times. They are ordered by an anesthesiologist and the choice of a particular drug depends on several factors. Some client-related factors include age; the specific procedure to be performed and its anticipated duration; the client's physical condition, including severity of illness, presence of chronic diseases, and any other drugs being given; and the client's mental status. Severe anxiety, for example, may be a contraindication to regional anesthesia, and the client may require larger doses of preanesthetic sedative-type medication.

General Anesthesia

General anesthesia can be used for almost any surgical, diagnostic, or therapeutic procedure. If a medical disorder of a vital organ system (cardiovascular, respiratory, renal) is present, it should be corrected before anesthesia, when possible. General anesthesia and major surgical procedures have profound effects on normal body functioning. When alterations due to other disorders are also involved, the risks of anesthesia and surgery are greatly increased. Because of the risks, general anesthetics and neuromuscular blocking agents should be given *only* by people with special training in correct usage and *only* in locations where staff, equipment, and drugs are available for emergency use or cardiopulmonary resuscitation.

Regional and Local Anesthesia

Regional or local anesthesia is usually safer than general anesthesia because it produces fewer systemic effects. For example, spinal anesthesia is often the anesthesia of choice for surgery involving the lower abdomen and lower extremities, especially in people who are elderly or have chronic lung disease. A major advantage of spinal anesthesia is that it causes less CNS and respiratory depression. Guidelines for injections of local anesthetic agents include the following:

1. Local anesthetics should be injected *only* by people with special training in correct usage and *only* in locations where staff, equipment, and drugs are available for emergency use or cardiopulmonary resuscitation.

2. Choice of a local anesthetic depends mainly on the reason for use or the type of regional anesthesia desired. Lidocaine, one of the most widely used, is available in topical and injectable forms.

3. Local anesthetic solutions must not be injected into blood vessels because of the high risk of serious adverse reactions involving the cardiovascular system and CNS. To prevent accidental injection into a blood vessel, needle placement must be verified by aspirating before injecting the local anesthetic solution. If blood is aspirated into the syringe, another injection site must be selected.

4. Local anesthetics given during labor cross the placenta and may depress muscle strength, muscle tone, and rooting behavior in the newborn. Apgar scores are usually normal. If excessive amounts are used (eg, in paracervical block), local anesthetics may cause fetal bradycardia, increased movement, and expulsion of meconium before birth and marked depression after birth. Dosage used for spinal anesthesia during labor is too small to depress the fetus or the newborn.

5. For spinal or epidural anesthesia, use only local anesthetic solutions that have been specifically prepared for spinal anesthesia and are in single-dose containers. Multiple-dose containers are not used because of the risk of injecting contaminated solutions.

6. Epinephrine is often added to local anesthetic solutions to prolong anesthetic effects. Such solutions require special safety precautions, such as the following:
   a. This combination of drugs should not be used for nerve blocks in areas supplied by end arteries (fingers, ears, nose, toes, penis) because it may produce ischemia and gangrene.
   b. This combination should not be given IV or in excessive dosage because the local anesthetic and epinephrine can cause serious systemic toxicity, including cardiac arrhythmias.
   c. This combination should not be used with inhalation anesthetic agents that increase myocardial sensitivity to catecholamines. Severe ventricular arrhythmias may result.
   d. These drugs should not be used in clients with severe cardiovascular disease or hyperthyroidism.
   e. If used in obstetrics, the concentration of epinephrine should be no greater than 1:200,000 because of the danger of producing vasoconstriction in uterine blood vessels. Such vasoconstriction may cause decreased placental circulation, decreased intensity of uterine contractions, and prolonged labor.

Topical Anesthesia of Mucous Membranes

When used to anesthetize nasal, oral, pharyngeal, laryngeal, tracheal, bronchial, or urethral mucosa, local anesthetics should be given in the lowest effective dosage. The drugs are well absorbed through mucous membranes and may cause systemic adverse reactions.

Use in Children

Compared with adults, children are at greater risk of complications (eg, laryngospasm, bronchospasm, aspiration) and death from anesthesia. Thus, whoever administers anesthetics to children should be knowledgeable about anesthetics and their effects in children. In addition, the nurse who cares for a child before, during, and after surgical or other procedures that require anesthesia or sedation must be skilled in using the nursing process with children.

1. Halothane has been commonly used. It causes bronchodilation and does not irritate respiratory mucosa, features that make it especially useful for children with asthma, cystic fibrosis, or other bronchospastic disorders. However, the drug dilates blood vessels in the brain and increases intracranial pressure, so it may not be indicated in clients who already have increased intracranial pressure or mass lesions. Halothane may also sensitize the myocardium to epinephrine, although children are less likely than adults to have ventricular arrhythmias.

2. Sevoflurane, a newer agent, may have some advantages over halothane in pediatric anesthesia. It allows a faster induction and emergence, does not stimulate the sympathetic nervous system or potentiate cardiac arrhythmias, and produces a minimal increase in intracranial pressure. However, it is much more expensive than halothane.

3. Propofol is approved for use in children 3 years of age and older. It has a rapid onset; a rapid metabolism rate; and a smooth emergence with little mental confusion, sedation, or nausea. It also decreases cerebral blood flow and intracranial pressure, making it useful in neurosurgery. In addition, propofol is widely used for sedation with diagnostic tests or special procedures that require children to be sedated and immobile. Propofol may be given by injection for induction or an IV infusion pump for maintenance anesthesia or sedation.

   Adverse effects include respiratory depression, hypotension, and pain with injection. Slow titration of dosage, a large-bore IV catheter, adding lidocaine, and slow drug injection into a rapidly flowing IV can minimize these effects. Propofol lacks an antimicrobial preservative and supports rapid growth of microorganisms. As a result, a dose should be prepared and administered with strict aseptic technique.

4. In general, infants and children have a higher anesthetic requirement, relative to size and weight, than healthy adults.

5. Some agencies allow parents to be present during induction of general anesthesia. This seems to reduce anxiety for both parents and children.

6. With skeletal muscle relaxants, the choice depends on the type of surgery and anesthesia, contraindications to a particular agent, the presence of client conditions that affect or preclude use of a particular drug, and the preference of the anesthetist. For short surgical procedures, intermediate-acting nondepolarizing agents (eg, atracurium, mivacurium) are commonly used. Succinylcholine, formerly a commonly used agent, is now contraindicated for routine, elective surgery in children and adolescents. This precaution stems from reports of several deaths associated with the use of succinylcholine in children with previously undiagnosed skeletal muscle myopathy. However, succinylcholine is still indicated in children who require emergency intubation or rapid securing of the airway (eg, laryngospasm, full stomach) and for intramuscular administration when a suitable vein is unavailable.

7. Children are more likely to have postoperative nausea and vomiting than adults.

8. Local anesthetics usually have the same uses, precautions, and adverse effects in children as in adults. Safety and efficacy of bupivacaine, dyclonine, and tetracaine have not been established in children younger than 12 years of age. Benzocaine should not be used in infants younger than 1 year of age. Dosages in children should be reduced according to age, body weight, and physical condition.

   With topical applications to intact skin, there is greater systemic absorption and risk of toxicity in infants. A mixture of lidocaine/prilocaine (Eutectic Mixture Local Anesthetics [EMLA]) was formulated to penetrate intact skin and provide local anesthesia and decrease pain of vaccinations and venipuncture. The cream is applied at the injection site with an occlusive dressing at least 60 minutes before vaccination or venipuncture.

   For topical application to mucous membranes, low concentrations of local anesthetics should be used. EMLA cream should not be used on mucous membranes (or abraded skin). These drugs are readily absorbed through mucous membrane and may cause systemic toxicity.

Use in Older Adults

Older adults often have physiologic changes and pathologic conditions that make them more susceptible to adverse effects of anesthetics, neuromuscular blocking agents, and adjunctive medications. Thus, lower doses of these agents are usually needed. With propofol, delayed excretion and a longer half-life lead to higher peak plasma levels. Higher plasma levels can cause hypotension, apnea, airway obstruction, and oxygen desaturation if dosage is not reduced. Long-term infusion may result in accumulation in body fat and prolonged elimination.

With injections of a local anesthetic, repeated doses may cause accumulation of the drug or its metabolites and increased risks of adverse effects. Because cardiovascular homeostatic mechanisms are often impaired, older adults may be at risk for decreased cardiac output, hypotension, heart block, and cardiac arrest.

Use in Renal Impairment

Most inhalation general anesthetic agents can be used in clients with renal impairment because they are eliminated mainly by exhalation from the lungs. However, they reduce renal blood flow, glomerular filtration, and urine volume, as do IV general anesthetics.

Most neuromuscular blocking agents are metabolized or excreted in urine to varying extents. Thus, renal effects vary among the drugs, and several may accumulate in the presence of renal impairment because of delayed elimination. With atracurium, which is mainly metabolized by the liver with a small amount excreted unchanged in urine, short-term use of bolus doses does not impair renal function. With long-term infusion, however, metabolism of atracurium produces a metabolite (laudanosine) that accumulates in renal failure and may cause neurotoxicity. With succinylcholine, liver metabolism produces active metabolites, some of which are excreted through the kidneys. These metabolites can accumulate and cause hyperkalemia in clients with renal impairment. Thus, renal impairment may lead to accumulation of neuromuscular blocking agents or their metabolites. The drugs should be used very cautiously in clients with renal impairment.

Use in Hepatic Impairment

Most inhalation general anesthetics are minimally metabolized in the liver and therefore are unlikely to accumulate with short-term usage. However, all general anesthetics reduce blood flow to the liver, and the liver's ability to metabolize other drugs may be impaired. Propofol is metabolized mainly in the liver to inactive metabolites, which are then excreted by the kidneys. Propofol clearance may be slower because of decreased hepatic blood flow.

Neuromuscular blocking agents vary in the extent to which they are metabolized in the liver. For example, atracurium, rocuronium, and vecuronium are eliminated mainly by the liver. They may accumulate with hepatic impairment because of delayed elimination. Succinylcholine is also metabolized in the liver and should be used very cautiously in clients with hepatic impairment.

With local anesthetics, injections of the amide type (eg, lidocaine), which are metabolized primarily in the liver, are more likely to reach high plasma levels and cause systemic toxicity in clients with hepatic disease. The drugs should be used cautiously, in minimally effective doses, in such clients. In addition, clients with severe hepatic impairment are more likely to acquire toxic plasma concentrations of lidocaine and prilocaine from topical use of EMLA because of impaired ability to metabolize the drug.

Use in Critical Illness

Propofol, neuromuscular blocking agents, and local anesthetics are commonly used in intensive care units. These drugs should be administered and monitored only by health care personnel who are skilled in the management of critically ill clients, including cardiopulmonary resuscitation and airway management. Critical care nurses must often care for clients receiving IV infusions of the drugs and titrate dosage and flow rate to achieve desired effects and minimize adverse effects.

Propofol is used for short-term sedation of clients who are intubated and mechanically ventilated. It has a rapid onset of action and clients awaken within a few minutes of stopping drug administration. It is given by continuous IV infusion in doses of 5 to 50 μg/kg/min. Doses can be increased in small amounts every 5 to 10 minutes to achieve sedation and decreased in small amounts every 5 to 10 minutes to allow awakening. The rate of infusion should be individualized and titrated to clinical response. As a general rule, the rate should be slower in older adults, clients receiving other CNS depressant drugs (eg, opioids or benzodiazepines), and critically ill clients. In addition, the level of sedation may be adjusted to the client's condition and needs, such as a lighter level during visiting hours or a deeper level during painful procedures.

During propofol infusion, vital functions need to be assessed and monitored at regular intervals. For neurologic assessment, dosage is decreased every 12 or 24 hours to maintain light sedation. The drug should not be stopped because rapid awakening may be accompanied by anxiety, agitation, and resistance to mechanical ventilation. After assessment, the dose is increased until the desired level of sedation occurs. For hemodynamic and respiratory assessment, vital signs, electrocardiograms, pulmonary capillary wedge pressures, arterial blood gas levels, oxygen saturation, and other measurements are needed.

Neuromuscular blocking agents are used to facilitate mechanical ventilation, control increased intracranial pressure, and treat status epilepticus. Clients requiring prolonged use of neuromuscular blocking agents usually have life-threatening illnesses such as adult respiratory distress syndrome, systemic inflammatory response syndrome, or multiple organ dysfunction syndrome.

The most commonly used are the nondepolarizing agents (eg, atracurium, vecuronium), which are given by intermittent bolus or continuous infusion. When the drugs are used for extended periods, clients are at risk for development of complications of immobility such as atelectasis, pneumonia, muscle wasting, and malnutrition. In addition, the drugs may accumulate, prolong muscle weakness, and make weaning from a ventilator more difficult. Accumulation results mainly from delayed elimination.

Local anesthetics should be used with caution in critically ill clients, especially those with impaired cardiovascular function such as dysrhythmias, heart block, hypotension, or shock. Repeated doses may cause accumulation of the drug or its metabolites or slow its metabolism. Reduced doses are indicated to decrease adverse effects. In addition to usual uses of local anesthetics, lidocaine is often given in coronary care units to decrease myocardial irritability and prevent or treat ventricular tachyarrhythmias (see Chap. 52).

(*text continues on page 222*)

NURSING ACTIONS   Anesthetic Drugs

NURSING ACTIONS	RATIONALE/EXPLANATION
1. Administer accurately	Drug administration in relation to anesthesia refers primarily to preanesthetic or postanesthetic drugs because physicians, dentists, and nurse anesthetists administer anesthetic drugs. In addition, critical care nurses may administer propofol or a neuromuscular blocking agent to patients being mechanically ventilated.
a. Schedule the administration of preanesthetic medications so that their peak effects are reached at the optimal time, if possible.	Timing is important. It is better if these medications are administered so that peak sedative effects occur before administration of anesthetics to avoid excessive central nervous system (CNS) depression. If they are given too early, the client may be sedated longer than necessary, and the risk of postanesthetic respiratory and circulatory complications is increased. Also, medication effects may wear off before induction of anesthesia. If they are given too late, the client may suffer needless anxiety and not be relaxed and drowsy when anesthesia is being initiated. Preanesthetic medications are often ordered "on call" rather than for a specific time, and the client may or may not become sedated before being transported to the surgery suite.
b. If a combination of injectable preanesthetic medications is ordered, do not mix in the same syringe and give as one injection unless the drugs are known to be compatible and the total volume is approximately 2 mL. For example, atropine and glycopyrrolate (Robinul) are compatible with morphine and meperidine. If compatibility is unknown, give two or more injections if necessary. Do not mix the drugs.	A precipitate may develop, or one of the drugs may be inactivated or altered when combined. Although larger amounts are sometimes given, probably no more than 2 to 3 mL should be given intramuscularly (IM) for both drug absorption and client comfort. Approximately 1.25 mL (20 minims) is the upper limit for subcutaneous injections.
c. With propofol intravenous (IV) infusion:	
(1) Administer through a central or large peripheral IV catheter, with an infusion pump.	The drug can irritate peripheral veins. An infusion pump is required for accurate administration and dosage titration.
(2) Do not mix with other drugs before administration.	Propofol is an emulsion that is incompatible with other drugs.
(3) Dilute with 5% dextrose injection and do not dilute to a concentration of <2 mg/mL.	Manufacturer's recommendation

(continued)

NURSING ACTIONS	RATIONALE/EXPLANATION
(4) Propofol is compatible with 5% dextrose, lactated Ringer's, lactated Ringer's and 5% dextrose, 5% dextrose and 0.45% sodium chloride, and 5% dextrose and 0.2% sodium chloride IV solutions	
(5) Change IV tubing and propofol solution every 6 hours if manufactured IV solution is not used. If manufactured solution is used and the nurse only has to access the bag of fluid, change IV tubing every 12 hours.	Strict aseptic administration and maintenance techniques are needed because of the potential for microbial contamination.
d. Have drugs and equipment for resuscitation readily available in any location where propofol, neuromuscular blocking agents, or local anesthetics are being used.	These drugs can cause cardiovascular collapse, hypotension, and respiratory failure.
e. If assisting a physician in injecting a local anesthetic solution, show the drug container to the physician and verbally verify the name of the drug, the percentage concentration, and whether the solution is plain or contains epinephrine.	Although the physician is responsible for drugs he or she administers, the nurse often assists by obtaining and perhaps holding the drug vial while the physician aspirates drug solution into a syringe. Accuracy of administration is essential so that adverse reactions can be avoided or treated appropriately if they do occur. The incidence of adverse reactions increases with the amount and concentration of local anesthetic solution injected. Also, adverse reactions to epinephrine may occur.
f. When applying local anesthetics for topical or surface anesthesia, be certain to use the appropriate preparation of the prescribed drug.	Most preparations are used in particular conditions or bodily locations. For example, lidocaine viscous is used only as an oral preparation for anesthesia of the mouth and throat. Other preparations are used only on the skin.
2. Observe for therapeutic effects	Therapeutic effects depend on the type of drug and the reason for use.
a. When adjunctive drugs are given for preanesthetic medication, observe for relaxation, drowsiness, and relief of pain.	Depending on dose and client condition, these effects are usually evident within 20 to 30 minutes after the drugs are given.
b. When local anesthetic drugs are applied for surface anesthesia, observe for relief of the symptom for which the drug was ordered, such as sore mouth or throat, pain in skin or mucous membrane, and itching of hemorrhoids.	Relief is usually obtained within a few minutes. Ask the client if the symptom has been relieved, and if not, assess the situation to determine whether further action is needed.
c. When propofol is used for sedation in an intensive care unit, observe for lack of agitation and movement, tolerance of mechanical ventilation, and arousability for neurologic assessment when drug dosage is reduced by slowing the IV infusion rate.	
d. When a neuromuscular blocking agent is used in an intensive care unit, observe for tolerance of mechanical ventilation.	

(*continued*)

NURSING ACTIONS	RATIONALE/EXPLANATION
3. Observe for adverse effects	Serious adverse effects are most likely to occur during and within a few hours after general anesthesia and major surgery. During general anesthesia, the anesthesiologist monitors the client's condition constantly to prevent, detect, or treat hypoxia, hypotension, cardiac arrhythmias, and other problems. The nurse observes for adverse effects in the preanesthetic and postanesthetic periods.
a. With preanesthetic drugs, observe for excessive sedation.	The often-used combination of an opioid analgesic and a sedative-type drug produces additive CNS depression.
b. After general anesthesia and during propofol administration in intensive care units, observe for:	
(1) Excessive sedation—delayed awakening, failure to respond to verbal or tactile stimuli	The early recovery period is normally marked by a progressive increase in alertness, responsiveness, and movement.
(2) Respiratory problems—laryngospasm, hypoxia, hypercarbia	Laryngospasm may occur after removal of the endotracheal tube used to administer general anesthesia. Hypoxia and hypercarbia indicate inadequate ventilation and may result from depression of the respiratory center in the medulla oblongata, prolonged paralysis of respiratory muscles with muscle relaxant drugs, or retention of respiratory tract secretions due to a depressed cough reflex.
(3) Cardiovascular problems—hypotension, tachycardia and other cardiac arrhythmias, fluid and electrolyte imbalances	Vital signs are often unstable during the early recovery period and therefore need to be checked frequently. Extreme changes must be reported to the surgeon or the anesthesiologist. These problems are most likely to occur while general anesthesia is being administered and progressively less likely as the patient recovers or awakens.
(4) Other problems—restlessness, nausea, and vomiting. With ketamine, unpleasant dreams or hallucinations also may occur.	Restlessness may be caused by the anesthetic, pain, or hypoxia and should be assessed carefully before action is taken. For example, if caused by hypoxia but interpreted as being caused by pain, administration of analgesics would aggravate hypoxia.
c. After regional anesthesia, observe for:	
(1) CNS stimulation at first (hyperactivity, excitement, seizure activity) followed by CNS depression	These symptoms are more likely to occur with large doses, high concentrations, injections into highly vascular areas, or accidental injection into a blood vessel.
(2) Cardiovascular depression—hypotension, arrhythmias	Local anesthetics depress myocardial contractility and the cardiac conduction system. These effects are most likely to occur with high doses. Doses used for spinal or epidural anesthesia usually have little effect on cardiovascular function.
(3) Headache and urinary retention with spinal anesthesia	Headache is more likely to occur if the person does not lie flat for 8 to 12 hours after spinal anesthesia is given. Urinary retention may occur in anyone but is more likely in older men with enlarged prostate glands.

(continued)

NURSING ACTIONS	RATIONALE/EXPLANATION
4. Observe for drug interactions	For interactions involving preanesthetic medications, see Sedative-Hypnotics and Antianxiety Drugs (Chap. 8), Anticholinergic Drugs (Chap. 21), and Opioid Analgesics (Chap. 6).
a. Drugs that *increase* effects of general anesthetic agents:	
(1) Antibiotics—aminoglycosides (gentamicin and related drugs)	These antibiotics inhibit neuromuscular transmission. When they are combined with general anesthetics, additive muscle relaxation occurs with increased likelihood of respiratory paralysis and apnea.
(2) Antihypertensives	Additive hypotension, shock, and circulatory failure may occur.
(3) Catecholamines—dopamine, epinephrine, isoproterenol, norepinephrine	Increased likelihood of cardiac arrhythmias. Halothane and a few rarely used general anesthetics sensitize the myocardium to the effects of catecholamines. If they are combined, ventricular tachycardia or ventricular fibrillation may occur. Such a combination is contraindicated.
(4) CNS depressants—alcohol, antianxiety agents, anticonvulsants, antidepressants, antihistamines, antipsychotics, barbiturates, opioid analgesics, sedative-hypnotics	CNS depressants include many different drug groups and hundreds of individual drugs. Some are used therapeutically for their CNS depressant effects; others are used mainly for other purposes, and CNS depression is a side effect. Any combination of these drugs with each other or with general anesthetic agents produces additive CNS depression. Extreme caution must be used to prevent excessive CNS depression.
(5) Corticosteroids	Additive hypotension may occur during and after surgery because of adrenocortical atrophy and reduced ability to respond to stress. For clients who have been receiving corticosteroids, most physicians recommend administration of hydrocortisone before, during, and, in decreasing doses, after surgery.
(6) Monoamine oxidase (MAO) inhibitors—isocarboxazid, isoniazid, procarbazine, tranylcypromine, others	Additive CNS depression. These drugs should be discontinued at least 10 days to 3 weeks before elective surgery. If emergency surgery is required, clients taking MAO inhibitors should not be given general anesthesia. Although they may be given spinal anesthesia, there is increased risk of hypotension. They should not be given local anesthetic solutions to which epinephrine has been added.
(7) Neuromuscular blocking agents	Additive relaxation of skeletal muscles. These drugs are given for this therapeutic effect so that smaller amounts of general anesthetics may be given.
b. Drugs that *decrease* effects of general anesthetics:	Few drugs actually decrease effects of general anesthetics. When clients are excessively depressed and hypotension, cardiac arrhythmias, respiratory depression, and other problems develop, the main *(continued)*

NURSING ACTIONS	RATIONALE/EXPLANATION
	treatment is stopping the anesthetic and supporting vital functions rather than giving additional drugs. Effects of general inhalation anesthetics decrease rapidly once administration is discontinued. Effects of IV anesthetics decrease more slowly.
(1) Alcohol	Alcohol is a CNS depressant, and acute ingestion has an additive CNS depressant effect with general anesthetic agents. With chronic ingestion, however, tolerance to the effects of alcohol and general anesthetics develops; that is, larger amounts of general anesthetic agents are required in clients who have acquired tolerance to alcohol.
(2) Atropine	Atropine is often given as preanesthetic medication to prevent reflex bradycardia, which may occur with general inhalation anesthetics.
c. Drugs that *increase* effects of local anesthetics:	
(1) Cardiovascular depressants—general anesthetics, propranolol (Inderal)	Additive depression and increased risk of hypotension and arrhythmias
(2) CNS depressants	Additive CNS depression with high doses
(3) Epinephrine	Epinephrine is often used in dental anesthesia to prolong anesthetic effects by delaying systemic absorption of the local anesthetic drug. It is contraindicated for this use, however, in clients with hyperthyroidism or severe heart disease or those receiving adrenergic blocking agents for hypertension.
(4) Succinylcholine (Anectine)	Apnea may be prolonged by the combination of a local anesthetic agent and succinylcholine.
d. Drugs that *decrease* effects of local anesthetics:	These are seldom necessary or desirable. If overdosage of local anesthetics occurs, treatment is mainly symptomatic and supportive.
(1) Succinylcholine (Anectine)	This drug may be given to treat acute convulsions resulting from toxicity of local anesthetic drugs.
e. Drugs that *increase* effects of neuromuscular blocking agents (muscle relaxants):	
(1) Aminoglycoside antibiotics (eg, gentamicin),	Additive neuromuscular blockade, apnea, and respiratory depression
(2) Diuretics, potassium-losing (eg, furosemide, hydrochlorothiazide)	Diuretics that produce hypokalemia potentiate skeletal muscle relaxants.
(3) General anesthetics	Additive muscle relaxation
(4) Local anesthetics	Prolong apnea from succinylcholine
(5) MAO inhibitors	Additive respiratory depression
(6) Opioid analgesics	Additive respiratory depression
(7) Procainamide (Pronestyl) and quinidine	Additive neuromuscular blockade
f. Drugs that *decrease* effects of neuromuscular blocking agents:	
(1) Anticholinesterase drugs (eg, neostigmine)	These drugs often are used to reverse the effects of the nondepolarizing agents. They do not reverse the effects of succinylcholine and may potentiate them instead.

How Can You Avoid This Medication Error?

Answer: The risk of administering a drug to the wrong patient is increased in the PACU because patients are unconscious and patient turnover is frequent. In these situations, it is essential that the patient is properly identified using the name band and the orders verified on the patient's chart. Other factors that could have contributed to the error include the length of time the nurse had worked (fatigue) and the interruptions that distracted her concentration.

REVIEW AND APPLICATION EXERCISES

1. When assessing a client before, during, or after general anesthesia, what are important factors to consider?
2. What are major adverse effects of general anesthetics and neuromuscular blocking agents?
3. What interventions are needed to ensure client safety during recovery from general anesthesia?
4. When assessing a client before, during, or after local or regional anesthesia, what are important factors to consider?
5. What are major adverse effects of local anesthetic agents?

6. What interventions are needed to ensure client safety during recovery from local or regional anesthesia?
7. What are the main elements of drug administration and client assessment when propofol or a neuromuscular blocking agent is used in critical care settings?

SELECTED REFERENCES

Burns, L.S. (1997). Advances in pediatric anesthesia. *Nursing Clinics of North America, 32*(1), 45–71.

Catterall, W.A. & Mackie, K. (1996). Local anesthetics. In J.G. Hardman, L.E. Limbird, P.B. Molinoff, & R.W. Ruddon (Eds.), *Goodman & Gilman's The pharmacological basis of therapeutics*, 9th ed., pp. 331–347. New York: McGraw-Hill.

Covington, H. (1998). Use of propofol for sedation in the ICU. *Critical Care Nurse, 18*(4): 3–39.

Drug facts and comparisons. (Updated monthly). St. Louis: Facts and Comparisons.

Kowalski, S.D. & Rayfield, C.A. (1999). A post hoc descriptive study of patients receiving propofol. *American Journal of Critical Care, 8*(1), 507–513.

Marshall, B.E. & Longnecker, D.E. (1996). General anesthetics. In J.G. Hardman, L.E. Limbird, P.B. Molinoff, & R.W. Ruddon (Eds.), *Goodman & Gilman's The pharmacological basis of therapeutics*, 9th ed., pp. 307–330. New York: McGraw-Hill.

Power, B.M., Forbes, A.M., Van Heerden, P.V., & Ilett, K.F. (1998). Pharmacokinetics of drugs used in critically ill adults. *Clinical Pharmacokinetics, 34*(1), 25–56.

15

Substance Abuse Disorders

Objectives

After studying this chapter, the student will be able to:

1. Identify risk factors for development of drug dependence.

2. Describe the effects of alcohol, cocaine, marijuana, and nicotine on selected body organs.

3. Compare and contrast characteristics of dependence associated with alcohol, benzodiazepines, cocaine, and opiates.

4. Describe specific antidotes for overdoses of central nervous system (CNS) depressant drugs and the circumstances indicating their use.

5. Outline major elements of treatment for overdoses of commonly abused drugs that do not have antidotes.

6. Describe interventions to prevent or manage withdrawal reactions associated with barbiturates, benzodiazepines, cocaine and other CNS stimulants, ethanol, and opiates.

You are a school nurse working in a middle school. Just after lunch, an 8th grader approaches you saying he is very worried about his friend. After lunch, on a dare, his friend drank over half a bottle of vodka. He is in the bathroom and no one has been able to wake him up.

Reflect on:

▶ Prioritize your assessment when you reach the intoxicated youth.

▶ List factors, especially during the adolescent period, that increase the likelihood that a person will experiment with or abuse alcohol.

▶ Discuss important follow-up with this adolescent and his family after the incident.

SUBSTANCE ABUSE

Abuse of alcohol and other drugs is a significant health, social, economic, and legal problem. Substance abuse is often associated with substantial damage to the individual abuser and with numerous social ills (eg, crime, child and spouse abuse, traumatic injury, death). As used in this chapter, *substance abuse* is defined as self-administration of a drug for prolonged periods or in excessive amounts to the point of producing physical or psychological dependence and reduced ability to function as a productive member of society.

Most drugs of abuse are those that affect the central nervous system (CNS) and alter the state of consciousness. These include prescription and nonprescription and legal and illegal drugs. Commonly abused drugs include CNS depressants (eg, alcohol, antianxiety/sedative-hypnotic agents, opioid analgesics), CNS stimulants (eg, amphetamines, cocaine, nicotine), and other mind-altering drugs (eg, marijuana). Although these drugs produce different effects, they are all associated with positive reinforcement, compulsive self-administration, and increased dopamine activity in the brain. Dopamine is associated with feelings of pleasure and reward.

DEPENDENCE

Drug dependence involves compulsive drug-seeking behavior. *Psychological dependence* involves feelings of satisfaction and pleasure from taking the drug. These feelings, perceived as extremely desirable by the drug-dependent person, contribute to acute intoxication, development and maintenance of drug abuse patterns, and return to drug-taking behavior after periods of abstinence.

Physical dependence involves physiologic adaptation to chronic use of a drug so that unpleasant signs and symptoms occur when the drug is stopped or its action is antagonized by another drug. The withdrawal or abstinence syndrome produces specific manifestations according to the type of drug and does not occur as long as adequate dosage is maintained. Attempts to avoid withdrawal symptoms reinforce psychological dependence and promote continuing drug use and relapses to drug-taking behavior. Tolerance is often an element of drug dependence, and increasing doses are therefore required to obtain psychological effects or avoid physical withdrawal symptoms. A person may be dependent on more than one drug.

Drug dependence is a complex phenomenon of unknown cause. One view is that drugs stimulate or inhibit neurotransmitters in the brain to produce pleasure and euphoria or to decrease unpleasant feelings such as anxiety. The specific drug and the amount, frequency, and route of administration are also important. In addition to drug effects, other influencing factors include a person's psychological and physiologic characteristics and environmental or circumstantial characteristics. Peer pressure is often an important factor in initial and continuing drug ingestion. A genetic factor seems evident in alcohol abuse: studies indicate that children of abusers are at risk of becoming abusers themselves, even if reared away from the abusing parent. Additional general characteristics of substance abuse and dependence include the following:

- Substance abuse involves all socioeconomic levels and almost all age groups, from school-aged children to elderly adults. Patterns of abuse may vary in age groups. For example, adolescents and young adults may be more likely to use illicit drugs and elderly adults are more likely to abuse alcohol and prescription drugs. Health care professionals (eg, physicians, pharmacists, nurses) are also considered at high risk for development of substance abuse disorders, at least partly because of easy access.
- A person who abuses one drug is at risk of abusing others.
- Multiple drugs are often abused concomitantly. Alcohol, for example, is often used with other drugs of abuse, probably because it is legal and readily available. In addition, alcohol, marijuana, opioids, and sedatives are often used to combat the anxiety and nervousness induced by cocaine and other CNS stimulants.
- Drug effects vary according to the type of substance being abused, the amount, route of administration, duration of use, and phase of substance abuse (eg, acute intoxication, withdrawal syndromes, organ damage, and medical illness). Thus, acute intoxication often produces profound behavioral changes and chronic abuse often leads to serious organ damage and impaired ability to function in work, family, or social settings. Withdrawal symptoms are characteristic for particular types of drugs and are usually opposite the effects originally produced. For example, withdrawal symptoms of alcohol and sedative-type drugs are mainly agitation, nervousness, and hyperactivity.
- Alcohol and other drug abusers are not reliable sources of information about the types or amounts of drugs used. Most abusers understate the amount and frequency of using abused substances; heroin addicts may overstate the amount used in attempts to obtain higher doses of methadone. In addition, those who use illegal street drugs may not know what they have taken because of varying purity, potency, additives, and names.
- Substance abusers rarely seek health care unless circumstances force the issue. Thus, most substance abuse comes to the attention of health care professionals when the abuser experiences a complication such as acute intoxication, withdrawal, or serious medical problems resulting from chronic drug overuse, misuse, or abuse.
- Smoking or inhaling drug vapors is a preferred route of administration for cocaine, marijuana, and nico-

tine because the drugs are rapidly absorbed from the large surface area of the lungs. Then, they rapidly circulate to the heart and brain without dilution by the systemic circulation or metabolism by enzymes. With crack cocaine, inhaling vapors from the heated drug produces blood levels comparable with those obtained with intravenous (IV) administration.

- Substance abusers who inject their drugs intravenously are prey to serious problems because they use impure drugs of unknown potency, contaminated needles, poor hygiene, and other dangerous practices. Specific problems include overdoses, death, and numerous infections (eg, hepatitis, human immunodeficiency virus infection, endocarditis, phlebitis, and cellulitis at injection sites).

Many drugs are abused for their mind-altering properties. Most of these have clinical usefulness and are discussed elsewhere in this text: Antianxiety and Sedative-Hypnotic Drugs (see Chap. 8), Opioid Analgesics and Opioid Antagonists (see Chap. 6), and Central Nervous System Stimulants (see Chap. 16). This chapter describes commonly abused substances, characteristics of substance-related disorders, and drugs used to treat substance-related disorders (Table 15-1).

CENTRAL NERVOUS SYSTEM DEPRESSANTS

Central nervous system depressant drugs include alcohol, antianxiety and sedative-hypnotic agents, and opiates.

Alcohol (Ethanol)

Alcohol is the most abused drug in the world. It is legal and readily available, and its use is accepted in most societies. There is no clear-cut dividing line between use and abuse, but rather a continuum of progression over several years. Alcohol exerts profound metabolic and physiologic effects on all organ systems (Box 15-1). Some of these effects are evident with acute alcohol intake, whereas others become evident with chronic intake of substantial amounts. Alcohol is thought to exert its effects on the CNS by enhancing the activity of gamma-aminobutyric acid, an inhibitory neurotransmitter, or by inhibiting the activity of glutamate, an excitatory neurotransmitter.

When alcohol is ingested orally, a portion is inactivated in the stomach (by the enzyme alcohol dehydrogenase) and not absorbed systemically. Women have less enzyme activity than men and therefore absorb approximately 30% more alcohol than men when comparable amounts are ingested according to weight and size. As a result, women are especially vulnerable to adverse effects of alcohol, including more rapid intoxication from smaller amounts of alcohol and earlier development of hepatic cirrhosis and other complications of alcohol abuse.

In men and women, alcohol is absorbed partly from the stomach but mostly from the upper small intestine. It is rapidly absorbed when the stomach and small intestine are empty. Food delays absorption by diluting the alcohol and delaying gastric emptying. Once absorbed, alcohol is quickly distributed to all body tissues, partly because it is lipid soluble and crosses cell membranes easily. The alcohol concentration in the brain rapidly approaches that in the blood, and CNS effects usually occur within a few minutes. These effects depend on the amount ingested, how rapidly it was ingested, whether the stomach was empty, and other factors. Effects with acute intoxication usually progress from a feeling of relaxation to impaired mental and motor functions to stupor and sleep. Excited behavior may occur because of depression of the cerebral cortex, which normally controls behavior. The person may seem more relaxed, talkative, and outgoing or more impulsive and aggressive because inhibitions have been lessened.

The rate of alcohol metabolism largely determines the duration of CNS effects. Most alcohol is oxidized in the liver to acetaldehyde, which can be used for energy or converted to fat and stored. When metabolized to acetaldehyde, alcohol no longer exerts depressant effects on the CNS. Although the rate of metabolism differs with acute ingestion or chronic intake and some other factors, it is approximately 120 mg/kg of body weight or approximately 10 mL/hour. This is the amount of alcohol contained in approximately 2/3 oz of whiskey, 3 to 4 oz of wine, or 8 to 12 oz of beer. *Alcohol is metabolized at the same rate regardless of the amount present in body tissues.*

In older adults, the pharmacokinetics of alcohol are essentially the same as for younger adults. However, equivalent amounts of alcohol produce higher blood levels in older adults because of changes in body composition (eg, a greater proportion of fatty tissue).

Alcohol Interactions With Other Drugs

Alcohol may cause several potentially significant interactions when used with other drugs. These interactions often differ between acute and chronic ingestion. *Acute ingestion* inhibits drug-metabolizing enzymes. This slows the metabolism of some drugs, thereby increasing their effects and the likelihood of toxicity. *Chronic ingestion* induces metabolizing enzymes. This increases the rate of metabolism and decreases drug effects. Long-term ingestion of large amounts of alcohol, however, causes liver damage and impaired ability to metabolize drugs.

Because so many variables influence alcohol's interactions with other drugs, it is difficult to predict effects of interactions in particular people. However, some important interactions include those with other CNS depressants, antihypertensive agents, antidiabetic agents, oral anticoagulants, and disulfiram. These are summarized as follows:

- With other CNS depressants (eg, sedative-hypnotics, opioid analgesics, antianxiety agents, antipsychotic

TABLE 15-1 Drugs Used to Treat Substance Abuse Disorders

Generic/Trade Name	Indications for Use	Routes and Dosage Ranges	Comments
Chlordiazepoxide (Librium)	Alcohol detoxification; benzodiazepine withdrawal	PO 50 mg q6–8h initially, then tapered over 1–2 wk	
Clonidine (Catapres)	Alcohol withdrawal; opiate withdrawal	Alcohol withdrawal PO 0.3–0.6 mg q6h Opiate withdrawal PO 2 μg/kg 3 times daily for 7–10 days	Unlabeled uses May cause hypotension
Disulfiram (Antabuse)	Chronic alcohol abuse, to prevent continued alcohol ingestion	PO 125–500 mg daily	Limited effectiveness because many alcoholics will not take the drug; should not be given until at least 12 h after alcohol ingestion
Flumazenil (Romazicon)	Acute intoxication or overdose of benzodiazepine antianxiety or sedative-hypnotic drugs	IV 0.1–0.2 mg/min up to 1 mg	May precipitate acute withdrawal symptoms
Haloperidol (Haldol)	Psychotic symptoms associated with acute intoxication with cocaine and other CNS stimulants	IM 2–5 mg every 30 min to 6 h PRN for psychotic behavior	Other antipsychotic agents may also be used
Levo-alpha-acetylmethadol (LAAM) (Orlaam)	Maintenance therapy of heroin addiction	PO 60–100 mg 3 times weekly	Reportedly as effective and well accepted by heroin addicts as methadone
Lorazepam (Ativan)	Excessive CNS stimulation associated with acute intoxication with cocaine and other CNS stimulants, hallucinogens, marijuana, inhalants, and phencyclidine; alcohol withdrawal	*Agitation*, IM q30 min–6 h PRN; *alcohol withdrawal* hallucinations or seizures, IM 2 mg, repeated if necessary; *benzodiazepine withdrawal*, PO 2 mg q6–8h initially, then tapered over 1–2 wk	1 wk of tapering usually adequate for withdrawal from short-acting benzodiazepines; 2 wk needed for long-acting benzodiazepines
Methadone	Opiate withdrawal; maintenance therapy of heroin addiction	*Withdrawal*, PO 20–80 mg daily initially, reduced by 5–10 mg daily over 7–10 days; *maintenance* PO 20–80 mg daily	Maintenance doses of 60–80 mg daily more effective than 20–30 mg daily in decreasing heroin use
Naloxone (Narcan)	Acute intoxication or overdose of opiates (heroin, morphine, others)	IV 0.4–2 mg q3min	May precipitate acute withdrawal symptoms
Naltrexone (ReVia)	Opiate dependence; alcohol dependence	PO 50 mg daily	With opiate dependence, should not be started until patient is opioid-free for at least 7 d
Nicotine (Habitrol, Nicotrol, Nicoderm, ProStep, Nicorette)	Aid smoking cessation by relieving nicotine withdrawal symptoms	*Transdermal patches, Habitrol, Nicotrol,* 21 mg/d for 6 wk; 14 mg/d for 2 wk; 7 mg/d for 2 wk *Nicoderm,* 15 mg/d for 12 wk; 10 mg/d for 2 wk; 5 mg/d for 2 wk *ProStep,* 22 mg/d for 4–8 wk; 11 mg/d for 2–4 wk *Chewing gum,* 4 mg 9–12 pieces daily (maximum of 20 pieces); 2 mg 9–12 pieces daily (maximum of 30 pieces)	Should not be used while continuing to smoke because of high risk of serious adverse effects; used patches contain enough nicotine to be toxic to children and pets; they should be discarded in a safe manner.

IM, intramuscular; IV, intravenous; PO, oral; PRN, as needed.

agents, general anesthetics, and tricyclic antidepressants), alcohol potentiates CNS depression and increases risks of excessive sedation, respiratory depression, impaired mental and physical functioning, and other effects. Combining alcohol with these drugs may be lethal and should be avoided.

- With antihypertensive agents, alcohol potentiates vasodilation and hypotensive effects.
- With oral antidiabetic drugs, alcohol potentiates hypoglycemic effects.
- With oral anticoagulants (eg, warfarin), alcohol interactions vary. Acute ingestion increases anticoagulant

BOX 15–1   EFFECTS OF ALCOHOL ABUSE

Central and Peripheral Nervous System Effects

Sedation ranging from drowsiness to coma; impaired memory, learning, and thinking processes; impaired motor coordination, with ataxia or staggering gait, altered speech patterns, poor task performance, and hypoactivity or hyperactivity; mental depression, anxiety, insomnia; impaired interpersonal relationships; brain damage, polyneuritis and Wernicke-Korsakoff syndrome.

Hepatic Effects

Induces drug-metabolizing enzymes that accelerate metabolism of alcohol and many other drugs and produces tolerance and cross-tolerance; eventually damages the liver enough to impair drug metabolism, leading to accumulation and toxic effects; decreases use and increases production of lactate, leading to lactic acidosis, decreased renal excretion of uric acid, and secondary hyperuricemia; decreases use and increases production of lipids, leading to hyperlipidemia and fatty liver. Fatty liver causes accumulation of fat and protein, leading to hepatomegaly; eventually produces severe liver injury characterized by necrosis and inflammation (alcoholic hepatitis) or by fibrous bands of scar tissue that irreversibly alter structure and function (cirrhosis).

The incidence of liver disease correlates with the amount of alcohol consumed and the progression of liver damage is attributed directly to ethanol or indirectly to the metabolic changes produced by ethanol.

Gastrointestinal Effects

Slowed gastric emptying time; increased intestinal motility, which probably contributes to the diarrhea that often occurs with alcoholism; damage to the epithelial cells of the intestinal mucosa; multiple nutritional deficiencies, including protein and water-soluble vitamins, such as thiamine, folic acid, and vitamin B_{12}; pancreatic disease, which contributes to malabsorption of fat, nitrogen, and vitamin B_{12}.

Cardiovascular Effects

Damage to myocardial cells; cardiomyopathy manifested by cardiomegaly, edema, dyspnea, abnormal heart sounds, and electrocardiographic changes indicating left ventricular hypertrophy, abnormal T waves, and conduction disturbances; possible impairment of coronary blood flow and myocardial contractility.

Hematologic Effects

Bone marrow depression due to alcohol or associated conditions, such as malnutrition, infection, and liver disease; several types of anemia including *megaloblastic anemia* from folic acid deficiency, *sideroblastic anemia* (sideroblasts are precursors of red blood cells) probably from nutritional deficiency, *hemolytic anemia* from abnormalities in the structure of red blood cells, *iron deficiency anemia* usually from gastrointestinal bleeding, and anemias from hemodilution, chronic infection, and fatty liver and bone marrow failure associated with cirrhosis; thrombocytopenia and decreased platelet aggregation from folic acid deficiency, hypersplenism, and other factors; decreased numbers and impaired function of white blood cells, which lead to decreased resistance to infection.

Endocrine Effects

Increased release of cortisol and catecholamines and decreased release of aldosterone from the adrenal glands; hypogonadism, gynecomastia, and feminization in men with cirrhosis due to decreased secretion of male sex hormones; degenerative changes in the anterior pituitary gland; decreased secretion of antidiuretic hormone from the posterior pituitary; hypoglycemia due to impaired glucose synthesis or hyperglycemia due to glycogenolysis.

Skeletal Effects

Impaired growth and development, which is most apparent in children born to alcoholic mothers. Fetal alcohol syndrome is characterized by low birth weight and length and by birth defects, such as cleft palate and cardiac septal defects. Impairment of growth and motor development persists in the postnatal period, and mental retardation becomes apparent. Other effects include decreased bone density, osteoporosis, and increased susceptibility to fractures; osteonecrosis due to obstructed blood supply; hypocalcemia, which leads to bone resorption and decreased skeletal mass; hypomagnesemia, which may further stimulate bone resorption; hypophosphatemia, probably from inadequate dietary intake of phosphorus.

Muscular Effects

Acute myopathy, which may be manifested by acute pain, tenderness, edema, and hyperkalemia; chronic myopathy, which may involve muscle weakness, atrophy, episodes of acute myopathy associated with a drinking spree, and elevated creatine phosphokinase.

effects and the risk of bleeding. Chronic ingestion decreases anticoagulant effects by inducing drug-metabolizing enzymes in the liver and increasing the rate of warfarin metabolism. However, if chronic ingestion has caused liver damage, metabolism of warfarin may be slowed. This increases the risk of excessive anticoagulant effect and bleeding.

- With disulfiram (Antabuse), alcohol produces significant distress (flushing, tachycardia, bronchospasm, sweating, nausea and vomiting). This reaction may be used to treat alcohol dependence.
- A disulfiram-like reaction also may occur with other drugs, including several cephalosporin antibiotics (cefamandole, cefonicid, cefoperazone, ceforanide, cefotetan), chlorpropamide (Diabinese), tolbutamide (Orinase), and metronidazole (Flagyl).

Alcohol Dependence

Alcohol dependence involves acute or chronic consumption of alcohol in excess of the limits accepted by the person's culture, at times considered inappropriate by that culture, and to the extent that physical health and social relationships are impaired. Psychological dependence, physical dependence, tolerance, and cross-tolerance (with other CNS depressants) are prominent characteristics.

Acute intoxication impairs thinking, judgment, and psychomotor coordination. These impairments lead to poor work performance, accidents, and disturbed relationships with other people. Conscious control of behavior is lost, and exhibitionism, aggressiveness, and assaultiveness often result. Chronic ingestion affects essentially all body systems and may cause severe organ damage and mental problems. Effects are summarized in Box 15-1.

Signs and symptoms of alcohol withdrawal include agitation, anxiety, tremors, sweating, nausea, tachycardia, fever, hyperreflexia, postural hypotension, and, if severe, convulsions and delirium. Delirium tremens, the most serious form of alcohol withdrawal, is characterized by confusion, disorientation, delusions, visual hallucinations, and other signs of acute psychosis. The intensity of the alcohol withdrawal syndrome varies with the duration and amount of alcohol ingestion. Withdrawal symptoms start within a few hours after a person's last drink and last for several days.

Treatment of Alcohol Dependence

Alcohol dependence is a progressive illness, and early recognition and treatment are desirable. The alcohol-dependent person is unlikely to seek treatment for alcohol abuse unless an acute situation forces the issue. He or she is likely, however, to seek treatment for other disorders, such as nervousness, anxiety, depression, insomnia, and gastroenteritis. Thus, health professionals may recognize alcohol abuse in its early stages if they are aware of indicative assessment data.

If the first step of treatment is recognition of alcohol abuse, the second step is probably confronting the client with evidence of alcohol abuse and trying to elicit cooperation. Unless the client admits that alcohol abuse is a problem and agrees to participate in a treatment program, success is unlikely. The client may fail to make return visits or may seek treatment elsewhere. If the client agrees to treatment, the three primary approaches are psychological counseling, referral to a self-help group such as Alcoholics Anonymous, and drug therapy.

Acute intoxication with alcohol does not usually require treatment. If the client is hyperactive and combative, a sedative-type drug may be given. The client must be closely observed because sedatives potentiate alcohol, and excessive CNS depression may occur. If the client is already sedated and stuporous, he or she can be allowed to sleep off the alcohol effects. If the client is comatose, supportive measures are indicated. For example, respiratory depression may require insertion of an artificial airway and mechanical ventilation.

Benzodiazepine antianxiety agents are the drugs of choice for treating alcohol withdrawal syndromes. They can help the client participate in rehabilitation programs and can be gradually reduced in dosage and discontinued. They provide adequate sedation and have a significant anticonvulsant effect. Seizures require treatment if they are repeated or continuous. Antiseizure drugs need not be given for more than a few days unless the person has a pre-existing seizure disorder. Clonidine may be given to reduce symptoms (eg, hyperactivity, tremors) associated with excessive stimulation of the sympathetic nervous system.

Drug therapy for maintenance of sobriety is limited, mainly because of poor compliance. The two drugs approved for this purpose are *disulfiram* (Antabuse) and *naltrexone* (ReVia). Disulfiram interferes with hepatic metabolism of alcohol and allows accumulation of acetaldehyde. If alcohol is ingested during disulfiram therapy, acetaldehyde causes nausea and vomiting, dyspnea, hypotension, tachycardia, syncope, blurred vision, headache, and confusion. Severe reactions include respiratory depression, cardiovascular collapse, cardiac arrhythmias, myocardial infarction, congestive heart failure, unconsciousness, convulsions, and death. The severity of reactions varies but is usually proportional to the amounts of alcohol and disulfiram taken. The duration of the reaction varies from a few minutes to several hours, as long as alcohol is present in the blood. Ingestion of prescription and over-the-counter medications that contain alcohol may cause a reaction in the disulfiram-treated alcoholic. Disulfiram alone may produce adverse reactions of drowsiness, fatigue, impotence, headache, and dermatitis. These are more likely to occur during the first 2 weeks of treatment, after which they usually subside. Disulfiram also interferes with the metabolism of phenytoin and warfarin, which may increase blood levels of the drugs and increase their toxicity. Because of these reactions, disulfiram must be given only with the client's full consent, cooperation, and knowledge.

Naltrexone is an opiate antagonist that reduces craving for alcohol and increases abstinence rates when combined with psychosocial treatment. A possible mechanism is blockade of the endogenous opioid system, which is thought to reinforce alcohol craving and consumption. The most common adverse effect is nausea; others include anxiety, dizziness, drowsiness, headache, insomnia, nervousness, and vomiting. Naltrexone is hepatotoxic in high doses and contraindicated in patients with acute hepatitis or liver failure.

In addition to drug therapy to treat withdrawal and maintain sobriety, alcohol abusers often need treatment of coexisting psychiatric disorders, such as depression. Antidepressant drugs seem to decrease alcohol intake as well as relieve depression.

Barbiturates and Benzodiazepines

Barbiturates are old drugs that are rarely used therapeutically but remain drugs of abuse; benzodiazepines are widely used for antianxiety and sedative-hypnotic effects (see Chap. 8) and are also widely abused.

Barbiturate and Benzodiazepine Dependence

This type of dependence resembles alcohol dependence in symptoms of intoxication and withdrawal. Other characteristics include physical dependence, psychological dependence, tolerance, and cross-tolerance. Signs and symptoms of withdrawal include anxiety, tremors and muscle twitching, weakness, dizziness, distorted visual perceptions, nausea and vomiting, insomnia, weight loss, postural hypotension, generalized tonic-clonic (grand mal) seizures, and delirium that resembles the delirium tremens of alcoholism or a major psychotic episode. Convulsions are more likely to occur during the first 48 hours of withdrawal and delirium after 48 to 72 hours. Signs and symptoms of withdrawal are less severe with the benzodiazepines than with the barbiturates.

Treatment of Barbiturate or Benzodiazepine Abuse

Treatment may involve overdose and withdrawal syndromes. Overdose produces intoxication similar to that produced by alcohol. There may be a period of excitement and emotional lability followed by progressively increasing signs of CNS depression (eg, impaired mental function, muscular incoordination, and sedation). Treatment is unnecessary for mild overdose if vital functions are adequate. The client usually sleeps off the effects of the drug. The rate of recovery depends primarily on the amount of drug ingested and its rate of metabolism. More severe overdoses cause respiratory depression and coma.

There is no antidote for barbiturate overdose; treatment is symptomatic and supportive. The goals of treatment are to maintain vital functions until the drug is metabolized and eliminated from the body. Insertion of an artificial airway and mechanical ventilation often are necessary. Gastric lavage may help if started within approximately 3 hours of drug ingestion. If the person is comatose, a cuffed endotracheal tube should be inserted and the cuff inflated before lavage to prevent aspiration. Diuresis helps to eliminate the drugs and can be induced by IV fluids or diuretic drugs. Hemodialysis also removes most of these drugs and may be used with high serum drug levels or failure to respond to other treatment measures. Hypotension and shock are usually treated with IV fluids.

These treatments were formerly used for benzodiazepine overdoses and may still be needed in some cases (eg, overdoses involving multiple drugs). However, a specific antidote is now available to reverse sedation, coma, and respiratory depression. Flumazenil (Romazicon) competes with benzodiazepines for benzodiazepine receptors. The drug has a short duration of action, and repeated IV injections are usually needed. Recipients must be closely observed because symptoms of overdose may recur when the effects of a dose of flumazenil subside and because the drug may precipitate acute withdrawal symptoms (eg, agitation, confusion, seizures) in benzodiazepine abusers.

Treatment of withdrawal may involve administration of a benzodiazepine or phenobarbital to relieve acute signs and symptoms, then tapering the dose until the drug can be discontinued. Barbiturate and benzodiazepine withdrawal syndromes can be life threatening. The person may experience cardiovascular collapse, generalized tonic-clonic seizures, and acute psychotic episodes. These can be prevented by gradually withdrawing the offending drug. If they do occur, each situation requires specific drug therapy and supportive measures. Withdrawal reactions should be supervised and managed by experienced people, such as health care professionals or staff at detoxification centers.

Opiates

Opiates are potent analgesics and extensively used in pain management (see Chap. 6). They are also commonly abused. Because therapeutic opiates are discussed elsewhere, the focus here is heroin. Heroin, a semisynthetic derivative of morphine, is a common drug of abuse. It is a Schedule I drug in the United States and is not used therapeutically.

Heroin may be taken by IV injection, smoking, or nasal application (snorting). IV injection produces intense euphoria, which occurs within seconds, lasts a few minutes, and is followed by a period of sedation. Effects diminish over approximately 4 hours, depending on the dose. Addicts may inject several times daily, cycling between desired effects and symptoms of withdrawal. Tolerance to euphoric effects develops rapidly, leading to dosage escalation and continued use to avoid withdrawal. Like other opiates, heroin causes severe respiratory depression with overdose and produces a characteristic abstinence syndrome.

Opiate Dependence

Opiates produce tolerance and high degrees of psychological and physical dependence. Most other drugs that produce dependence do so with prolonged usage of large doses, but morphine-like drugs produce dependence with repeated administration of small doses. Medical usage of these drugs produces physical dependence and tolerance but rarely leads to use or abuse for mind-altering effects. Thus, "addiction" should not be an issue when the drugs are needed for pain management in patients with cancer or other severe illnesses.

Acute effects of opiate administration vary according to dosage, route of administration, and physical and mental characteristics of the user. They may produce euphoria, sedation, analgesia, respiratory depression, postural hypotension, vasodilation, pupil constriction, and constipation.

Treatment of Opiate Dependence

Treatment may be needed for overdose or withdrawal syndromes. Overdose may produce severe respiratory depression and coma. Insertion of an endotracheal tube and mechanical ventilation may be required. Drug therapy consists of an opioid antagonist to reverse opioid effects. Giving an opioid antagonist can precipitate withdrawal symptoms. If there is no response to the opioid antagonist, the symptoms may be caused by depressant drugs other than opiates. In addition to profound respiratory depression, pulmonary edema, hypoglycemia, pneumonia, cellulitis, and other infections often accompany opiate overdose and require specific treatment measures.

Signs and symptoms of withdrawal can be reversed immediately by giving the drug producing the dependence. Therapeutic withdrawal, which is more comfortable and safer, can be managed by gradually reducing dosage over several days. Clonidine, an antihypertensive drug, is sometimes used to relieve withdrawal symptoms associated with sympathetic nervous system overactivity.

Ideally, the goal of treatment for opiate abuse is abstinence from further opiate usage. Because this goal is rarely met, long-term drug therapy may be used to treat heroin dependence. One method uses opioid substitutes to prevent withdrawal symptoms and improve a lifestyle that revolves around obtaining, using, and recovering from a drug. Methadone has long been used for this purpose, usually a single, daily, oral dose given in a methadone clinic. Proponents say that methadone blocks euphoria produced by heroin, acts longer, and reduces preoccupation with drug use. This allows a more normal lifestyle for the client

and reduces morbidity and mortality associated with the use of illegal and injected drugs. Also, because methadone is free, the heroin addict does not commit crimes to obtain drugs. Opponents say that methadone maintenance only substitutes one type of drug dependence for another. In addition, a substantial percentage of those receiving methadone maintenance therapy abuse other drugs, including cocaine.

Another drug approved for maintenance therapy is levo-alpha-acetylmethadol, also called LAAM. LAAM (Orlamm) is a synthetic opioid analgesic that is metabolized to long-acting, potent metabolites. After oral administration, effects occur within 90 minutes, peak in approximately 4 hours, and last approximately 72 hours. Its main advantage over methadone is that it can be given three times weekly rather than daily. However, if given on a Monday/Wednesday/Friday schedule, the Friday dose may need to be larger to prevent withdrawal symptoms until the Monday dose can be given. Also, initial dosage needs careful titration to prevent withdrawal symptoms but avoid overdosage when peak effects occur. Patients must be informed about the delayed effects of the drug and the risks of overdosage if they take other opiates.

A third treatment option is naltrexone (ReVia), an opioid antagonist that prevents opiates from occupying receptor sites and thereby prevents their physiologic effects. Used to maintain opiate-free states in the opiate addict, it is recommended for use in conjunction with psychological counseling to promote client motivation and compliance. If the patient taking naltrexone has mild or moderate pain, nonopioid analgesics (eg, acetaminophen or a nonsteroidal anti-inflammatory drug) should be given. If the patient has severe pain and requires an opioid, it should be given in a setting staffed and equipped for cardiopulmonary resuscitation because respiratory depression may be deeper and more prolonged than usual. In addition, patients needing elective surgery and opioid analgesics should be instructed to stop taking naltrexone at least 72 hours before the scheduled procedure.

CENTRAL NERVOUS SYSTEM STIMULANTS

Amphetamines and Related Drugs

Amphetamines and related drugs (see Chap. 16) are used for appetite suppression and other effects. However, the drugs are probably more important as drugs of abuse than therapeutic agents.

Amphetamine-Type Dependence

Amphetamines and related drugs (eg, methylphenidate, phenmetrazine) produce stimulation and euphoria, effects often sought by drug users. The user may increase the amount and frequency of administration to reach or continue the state of stimulation. One of the drugs, methamphetamine, may be chemically treated to produce potent crystals (called "ice"), which are then heated and the vapors smoked or inhaled. Psychological effects of amphetamines are similar to those produced by cocaine and are largely dose related. Small amounts produce mental alertness, wakefulness, and increased energy. Large amounts may produce psychotic behavior (eg, hallucinations and paranoid delusions). Tolerance develops to amphetamines.

Acute ingestion of these drugs masks underlying fatigue or depression; withdrawal allows these conditions to emerge in an exaggerated form. The resulting exhaustion and depression reinforce the compulsion to continue using the drugs. Users may take them alone or to counteract the effects of other drugs. In the latter case, these drugs may be part of a pattern of polydrug use in which CNS depressants, such as alcohol or sedative-type drugs ("downers"), are alternated with CNS stimulants, such as amphetamines ("uppers").

Treatment of Amphetamine-Type Abuse

Treatment of amphetamine-type abuse is mainly concerned with overdosage because these drugs do not produce physical dependence and withdrawal as alcohol, opiates, and sedative-hypnotic drugs do. Because amphetamines delay gastric emptying, gastric lavage may be helpful even if several hours have passed since drug ingestion. The client is likely to be hyperactive, agitated, and hallucinating (toxic psychosis) and may have tachycardia, fever, and other symptoms. Symptomatic treatment includes sedation, lowering of body temperature, and administration of an antipsychotic drug. Sedative-type drugs must be used with great caution, however, because depression and sleep usually follow amphetamine use, and these after-effects can be aggravated by sedative administration.

Cocaine

Cocaine is a popular drug of abuse. It produces powerful CNS stimulation by preventing reuptake of neurotransmitters (eg, dopamine, norepinephrine, serotonin), which increases and prolongs neurotransmitter effects. Cocaine is commonly inhaled (snorted) through the nose; "crack" is heated and the vapors inhaled. Acute use of cocaine or crack produces intense euphoria, increased energy and alertness, sexual arousal, tachycardia, increased blood pressure, and restlessness followed by depression, fatigue, and drowsiness as drug effects wear off. Overdosage can cause cardiac arrhythmias, convulsions, myocardial infarction, respiratory failure, stroke, and death, even in young, healthy adults and even with initial exposure. Both acute and chronic use produce numerous physiologic effects (Box 15-2).

Cocaine Dependence

Cocaine-induced euphoria is intense but brief and often leads to drug ingestion every few minutes as long as the drug is available. Cocaine is not thought to produce physical dependence, although fatigue, depression, drowsiness,

---

BOX 15–2   PHYSIOLOGIC AND BEHAVIORAL EFFECTS OF COCAINE ABUSE

Central Nervous System Effects

Cerebral infarct, subarachnoid and other hemorrhages; excessive central nervous system stimulation, manifested by anxiety, agitation, delirium, hyperactivity, irritability, insomnia, anorexia and weight loss; psychosis with paranoid delusions and hallucinations that may be indistinguishable from schizophrenia; seizures.

Cardiovascular Effects

Arrhythmias, including tachycardia, premature ventricular contractions, ventricular tachycardia and fibrillation, and asystole; cardiopathy; myocardial ischemia and acute myocardial infarction; hypertension; stroke; rupture of the aorta; constriction of coronary and peripheral arteries.

Respiratory Effects

With snorting of cocaine, rhinitis, rhinorrhea, and damage (ulceration, perforation, necrosis) of the nasal sep-

tum from vasoconstriction and ischemia. With inhalation of crack cocaine vapors, respiratory symptoms occur in up to 25% of users and may include bronchitis, bronchospasm, cough, dyspnea, pneumonia, pulmonary edema, and fatal lung hemorrhage.

Gastrointestinal Effects

Nausea; weight loss; intestinal ischemia, possible necrosis.

Genitourinary Effects

Delayed orgasm for men and women; difficulty in maintaining erection.

Effects of Intravenous Use

Hepatitis; human immunodeficiency virus infection; endocarditis; cellulitis; abscesses.

dysphoria, and intense craving occur as drug effects dissipate. Crack is a strong, inexpensive, extremely addicting, and widely used form of cocaine. It is prepared by altering cocaine hydrochloride with chemicals and heat to form rock-like formations of cocaine base. The process removes impurities and results in a very potent drug. When the drug is heated and the vapors inhaled, crack acts within a few seconds. It reportedly can cause psychological dependence with one use.

Treatment of Cocaine Abuse

Drug therapy is largely symptomatic. Thus, agitation and hyperactivity may be treated with a benzodiazepine antianxiety agent; psychosis may be treated with haloperidol or other antipsychotic agent; cardiac arrhythmias may be treated with usual antiarrhythmic drugs; myocardial infarction may be treated by standard methods; and so forth. Initial detoxification and long-term treatment are best accomplished in centers or units that specialize in substance abuse disorders.

Long-term treatment of cocaine abuse usually involves psychotherapy, behavioral therapy, and 12-step programs. In addition, many patients need treatment for coexisting psychiatric disorders.

Nicotine

Nicotine, one of many active ingredients in tobacco products, is the ingredient that promotes compulsive use, abuse, and dependence. Inhaling smoke from a cigarette produces CNS stimulation in a few seconds. The average cigarette contains approximately 8 to 9 mg of nicotine and delivers approximately 1 mg of nicotine systemically to the smoker (most is burned or dissipated as "sidestream" smoke). Nicotine obtained from chewing tobacco produces longer-lasting effects because it is more slowly absorbed than inhaled nicotine. Nicotine produces its effects by increasing levels of dopamine and other substances in the brain.

Nicotine is readily absorbed through the lungs, skin, and mucous membranes. It is extensively metabolized, mainly in the liver, and its metabolites are eliminated by the kidneys. It is also excreted in breast milk of nursing mothers. Adverse effects include nausea in new smokers at low blood levels and in experienced smokers at blood levels higher than their accustomed levels. Nicotine poisoning can occur in infants and children from ingestion of tobacco products, skin contact with used nicotine transdermal patches, or chewing nicotine gum. Poisoning may also occur with accidental ingestion of insecticide sprays containing nicotine. Oral ingestion usually causes vomiting, which limits the amount of nicotine absorbed. Toxic effects of a large dose may include hypertension, cardiac arrhythmias, convulsions, coma, respiratory arrest, and paralysis of skeletal muscle. With chronic tobacco use, nicotine is implicated in the vascular disease and sudden cardiac death associated with smoking. However, the role of nicotine in the etiology of other disorders (eg, cancer and pulmonary disease) associated with chronic use of tobacco is unknown. Effects are summarized in Box 15-3.

Nicotine Dependence

Like alcohol and opiate dependence, nicotine dependence is characterized by compulsive use and the development of tolerance and physical dependence. Mental depression is also associated with nicotine dependence. It is unknown whether depression leads to smoking or develops concomitantly with nicotine dependence. Cigarette smokers may smoke to obtain the perceived pleasure of nicotine's effects, avoid the discomfort of nicotine withdrawal, or both. Evidence indicates a compulsion to smoke when blood levels of nicotine become low. Abstinence from smoking leads to signs and symptoms of withdrawal (eg, anxiety, irritability, difficulty concentrating, restlessness, headache, increased appetite, weight gain, sleep disturbances), which usually begin within 24 hours of the last exposure to nicotine.

Treatment of Nicotine Dependence

Most tobacco users who quit do so on their own. For those who are strongly dependent and unable or unwilling to quit on their own, drug formulations of nicotine

---

BOX 15–3   EFFECTS OF NICOTINE

Central Nervous System Effects

Central nervous system stimulation with increased alertness, possibly feelings of enjoyment, decreased appetite, tremors, convulsions at high doses.

Cardiovascular Effects

Cardiac stimulation with tachycardia, vasoconstriction, increased blood pressure, increased force of myocardial contraction, and increased cardiac workload.

Gastrointestinal Effects

Increases secretion of gastric acid; increases muscle tone and motility; nausea and vomiting; aggravates gastroesophageal and peptic ulcer disease.

may be used to initiate smoking cessation. These products prevent or reduce withdrawal symptoms, but they do not produce the subjective effects or peak blood levels seen with cigarettes.

Nicotine is available in transdermal patches and chewing gum. Pieces of the gum may be chewed several times daily; the transdermal patch is applied once daily. Transdermal patches produce a steady blood level of nicotine and patients seem to use them more consistently than they use the chewing gum. These products are available over the counter. They are contraindicated in people with significant cardiovascular disease (angina pectoris, arrhythmias, or recent myocardial infarction). Adverse effects include soreness of mouth and throat (with gum), nausea, vomiting, dizziness, hypertension, arrhythmias, confusion, and skin irritation at sites of transdermal patch application.

Although nicotine products are effective in helping smokers achieve abstinence, approximately three fourths resume smoking within a year. Treatment regimens that combine counseling and behavioral therapy with drug therapy are more successful than those using nicotine replacement therapy alone.

MARIJUANA

Marijuana and other cannabis preparations are obtained from *Cannabis sativa*, the hemp plant, which grows in most parts of the world, including the entire United States. Marijuana and hashish are the two cannabis preparations used in the United States. Marijuana is obtained from leaves and stems; hashish, prepared from plant resin, is 5 to 10 times as potent as commonly available marijuana. These cannabis preparations contain several related compounds called *cannabinoids*. Delta-9-tetrahydrocannabinol (Δ-9-THC) is the main psychoactive ingredient, but metabolites and other constituents also may exert pharmacologic activity. The mechanism of action is unknown, although specific cannabinoid receptors have been identified in several regions of the brain. The endogenous substances that react with these receptors have not yet been determined.

Cannabis preparations are difficult to classify. Some people call them depressants; some call them stimulants; and others label them as mind-altering, hallucinogenic, psychotomimetic, or unique in terms of fitting into drug categories. It is also difficult to predict the effects of these drugs. Many factors apparently influence a person's response. One factor is the amount of active ingredients, which varies with the climate and soil where the plants are grown and with the method of preparation. Other factors include dose, route of administration, personality variables, and the environment in which the drug is taken.

Marijuana can be taken orally but is more often smoked and inhaled through the lungs. It is more potent and more rapid in its actions when inhaled. After smoking, subjective effects begin in minutes, peak in approximately 30 minutes, and last 2 to 3 hours. Low doses are mildly intoxicating and similar to small amounts of alcohol. Large doses can produce panic reactions and hallucinations similar to acute psychosis. Effects wear off as THC is metabolized to inactive products. Many physiologic effects (Box 15-4) and adverse reactions have been reported with marijuana use, including impaired ability to drive an automobile and perform other common tasks of everyday life.

Except for dronabinol (Marinol), marijuana and other cannabis preparations are illegal and not used therapeutically in the United States. Dronabinol, a formulation of Δ-9-THC, is used to treat nausea and vomiting associated

---

BOX 15–4 | EFFECTS OF MARIJUANA

Central Nervous System Effects

Impaired memory; perceptual and sensory distortions; disturbances in time perception; mood alteration; restlessness; depersonalization; panic reactions; paranoid ideation; impaired performance on cognitive, perceptual, and psychomotor tasks; drowsiness with high doses.

Cardiovascular Effects

Hypertension; bradycardia; peripheral vasoconstriction; orthostatic hypotension and tachycardia at high doses.

Respiratory Effects

Irritation and cellular changes in bronchial mucosa; bronchospasm; impaired gas exchange; aspergillosis in immunocompromised people; possibly increased risk of mouth, throat, and lung cancer (some known carcinogens are much higher in marijuana smoke than in tobacco smoke).

Musculoskeletal Effects

Ataxia; impaired coordination; increased reaction time.

Miscellaneous Effects

Constipation, decreased libido, thirst, decreased intraocular pressure.

with anticancer drugs and to stimulate appetite in patients with acquired immunodeficiency syndrome (AIDS). The risks of abuse are high, and the drug may cause physical and psychological dependence. It is a Schedule II controlled drug. Cannabinoids can also decrease intraocular pressure and may be useful in treating glaucoma. Some people promote legalization of marijuana for medical uses. However, clinicians state that such usage is no more effective than available legal treatments with less abuse potential.

Marijuana Dependence

Tolerance and psychological dependence do not usually develop with occasional use but may occur with chronic use; physical dependence rarely occurs. There is no specific treatment other than abstinence.

HALLUCINOGENS

Hallucinogenic drugs include a variety of substances that cause mood changes, anxiety, distorted sensory perceptions, hallucinations, delusions, depersonalization, pupil dilation, elevated body temperature, and elevated blood pressure.

LSD is a synthetic derivative of lysergic acid, a compound in ergot and some varieties of morning glory seeds. It is very potent, and small doses can alter normal brain functioning. LSD is usually distributed as a soluble powder and ingested in capsule, tablet, or liquid form. The exact mechanism of action is unknown, and effects cannot be predicted accurately. LSD alters sensory perceptions and thought processes; impairs most intellectual functions, such as memory and problem-solving ability; distorts perception of time and space; and produces sympathomimetic reactions, including increased blood pressure, heart rate, body temperature, and pupil dilation. Adverse reactions include self-injury and possibly suicide, violent behavior, psychotic episodes, "flashbacks" (a phenomenon characterized by psychological effects and hallucinations that may recur days, weeks, or months after the drug is taken), and possible chromosomal damage resulting in birth defects.

Mescaline is an alkaloid of the peyote cactus. It is the least active of the commonly used psychotomimetic agents but produces effects similar to those of LSD. It is usually ingested in the form of a soluble powder or capsule.

Phencyclidine (PCP) produces excitement, delirium, hallucinations, and other profound psychological and physiologic effects, including a state of intoxication similar to that produced by alcohol; altered sensory perceptions; impaired thought processes; impaired motor skills; psychotic reactions; sedation and analgesia; nystagmus and diplopia; and pressor effects that can cause hypertensive crisis, cerebral hemorrhage, convulsions, coma, and death. Death from overdose also has occurred as a

result of respiratory depression. Bizarre murders, suicides, and self-mutilations have been attributed to the schizophrenic reaction induced by PCP, especially in high doses. The drug also produces flashbacks.

Phencyclidine is usually distributed in liquid or crystal form and can be ingested, inhaled, or injected. It is usually sprayed or sprinkled on marijuana or herbs and smoked. Probably because it is cheap, easily synthesized, and readily available, PCP is often sold as LSD, mescaline, cocaine, or THC (the active ingredient in marijuana). It is also added to low-potency marijuana without the user's knowledge. Consequently, the drug user may experience severe and unexpected reactions, including death.

Hallucinogen Dependence

Tolerance develops, but there is no apparent physical dependence or abstinence syndrome. Psychological dependence probably occurs but is usually not intense. Users may prefer one of these drugs, but they apparently do without or substitute another drug if the one they favor is unavailable. A major danger with these drugs is their ability to impair judgment and insight, which can lead to panic reactions in which users may try to injure themselves (eg, by running into traffic).

Treatment of Hallucinogen Abuse

There is no specific treatment for hallucinogen dependence. Those who experience severe panic reactions may be kept in a safe, supportive environment until drug effects wear off or may be given a sedative-type drug.

VOLATILE SOLVENTS (INHALANTS)

These drugs include acetone, toluene, and gasoline. These solvents may be constituents of some types of glue, plastic cements, aerosol sprays, and other products. Some general inhalation anesthetics, such as nitrous oxide, have also been abused to the point of dependence. Volatile solvents are most often abused by preadolescents and adolescents who squeeze glue into a plastic bag, for example, and sniff the fumes. Suffocation sometimes occurs when the sniffer loses consciousness while the bag covers the face.

These substances produce symptoms comparable with those of acute alcohol intoxication, including initial mild euphoria followed by ataxia, confusion, and disorientation. Some substances in gasoline and toluene also may produce symptoms similar to those produced by the hallucinogens, including euphoria, hallucinations, recklessness, and loss of self-control. Large doses may cause convulsions, coma, and death. Substances containing gasoline, benzene, or carbon tetrachloride are especially likely to cause serious damage to the liver, kidneys, and bone marrow.

These substances produce psychological dependence, and some produce tolerance. There is some question about whether physical dependence occurs. If it does occur, it is considered less intense than the physical dependence associated with alcohol, barbiturates, and opiates.

Nursing Notes: Ethical/Legal Dilemma

You are working on a medical unit when Mrs. Collins is admitted for cirrhosis after an acute drinking episode. You overhear a coworker stating, in a very judgmental tone, "This is the third time she has been admitted for her drinking, and it is the taxpayers that end up paying her bill. It is very hard for me even to go in the room and take care of her."

Reflect on:

- Your feelings about caring for someone who abuses drugs or alcohol.

- How you would feel if you heard the coworker speaking judgmentally.

- Role play what you might say to the coworker.

NURSING PROCESS

Assessment

Assess clients for signs of alcohol and other drug abuse, including abuse of prescription drugs, such as antianxiety agents, opioids, and sedative-hypnotics. Some general screening-type questions are appropriate for any initial nursing assessment. The overall purpose of these questions is to determine whether a current or potential problem exists and whether additional information is needed. Some clients may refuse to answer or give answers that contradict other assessment data. Denial of excessive drinking and of problems resulting from alcohol use is a prominent characteristic of alcoholism; underreporting the extent of drug use is common in other types of drug abuse as well. Useful information includes each specific drug, the amount, the frequency of administration, and the duration of administration. If answers to general questions reveal problem areas, such as long-term use of alcohol or psychotropic drugs, more specific questions can be formulated to assess the scope and depth of the problem. It may be especially difficult to obtain needed information about illegal "street drugs," most of which have numerous, frequently changed names. For nurses who often encounter substance abusers, efforts to keep up with drug names and terminology may be helpful.

- Interview the client regarding alcohol and other drug use to help determine immediate and long-term nursing care needs. For example, information may be obtained that would indicate the likelihood of a withdrawal reaction, the risk of increased or decreased effects of a variety of drugs, and the client's susceptibility to drug abuse. People who abuse one drug are likely to abuse others, and abuse of multiple drugs is a more common pattern than abuse of a single drug. These and other factors aid effective planning of nursing care.

- Assess behavior that may indicate drug abuse, such as alcohol on the breath, altered speech patterns, staggering gait, hyperactivity or hypoactivity, and other signs of excessive CNS depression or stimulation. Impairments in work performance and in interpersonal relationships also may be behavioral clues.

- Assess for disorders that may be caused by substance abuse. These disorders may include infections, liver disease, accidental injuries, and psychiatric problems of anxiety or depression. These disorders may be caused by other factors, of course, and are nonspecific.

- Check laboratory reports, when available, for abnormal liver function test results, indications of anemia, abnormal white blood cell counts, abnormal electrolytes (hypocalcemia, hypomagnesemia, and acidosis are common in alcoholics), and alcohol and drug levels in the blood.

Nursing Diagnoses

- Ineffective Individual Coping related to reliance on alcohol or other drugs
- Risk for Injury: Adverse drug effects
- Risk for Violence related to altered thought processes, impaired judgment, and impulsive behavior
- Altered Nutrition: Less Than Body Requirements related to drug effects and drug-seeking behavior
- Altered Thought Processes related to use of psychoactive drugs
- Risk for Injury: Infection, hepatitis, AIDS related to use of contaminated needles and syringes for IV drugs

Planning/Goals

- Safety will be maintained for clients impaired by alcohol and drug abuse.
- Information will be provided regarding drug effects and treatment resources.
- The client's efforts toward stopping drug usage will be recognized and reinforced.

Interventions

- Administer prescribed drugs correctly during acute intoxication or withdrawal.

- Decrease environmental stimuli for the person undergoing drug withdrawal.
- Record vital signs; cardiovascular, respiratory, and neurologic functions; mental status; and behavior at regular intervals.
- Support use of resources for stopping drug abuse (psychotherapy, treatment programs).
- Request patient referrals to psychiatric/mental health physicians, nurse clinical specialists, or self-help programs when indicated.
- Use therapeutic communication skills to discuss alcohol or other drug-related health problems, health-related benefits of stopping substance use or abuse, and available services or treatment options.
- Teach nondrug techniques for coping with stress and anxiety.
- Provide positive reinforcement for efforts toward quitting substance abuse.
- Inform smokers with young children in the home that cigarette smoke can precipitate or aggravate asthma and upper respiratory disorders in children.
- Inform smokers with nonsmoking spouses or other members of the household that "secondhand" smoke can increase the risks of cancer and lung disease in the nonsmokers as well as the smoker.
- For smokers who are concerned about weight gain if they quit smoking, emphasize that the health benefits of quitting far outweigh the disadvantages of gaining a few pounds, and discuss ways to control weight without smoking.

Evaluation

- Observe for improved behavior (eg, less impulsiveness, improved judgment and thought processes, commits no injury to self or others).
- Observe for use or avoidance of nonprescribed drugs while hospitalized.
- Interview to determine the client's insight into personal problems stemming from drug abuse.
- Verify enrollment in a treatment program.
- Observe for appropriate use of drugs to decrease abuse of other drugs.

PRINCIPLES OF THERAPY

Prevention of Alcohol and Other Drug Abuse

Use measures to prevent substance abuse. Although there are difficulties in trying to prevent conditions for which causes are not known, some of the following communitywide and individual measures may be helpful:

1. Decrease the supply or availability of commonly abused drugs. Most efforts at prevention have tried to reduce the supply of drugs. For example, laws designate certain drugs as illegal and provide penalties for possession or use of these drugs. Other laws regulate circumstances in which legal drugs, such as opioid analgesics and barbiturates, may be used. Also, laws regulate the sale of alcoholic beverages.

2. Decrease the demand for drugs. Because this involves changing attitudes, it is very difficult but more effective in the long run. Many current attitudes seem to promote drug use, misuse, and abuse, including:

   a. The belief that a drug is available for every mental and physical discomfort and should be taken in preference to tolerating even minor discomfort. Consequently, society has a permissive attitude toward taking drugs, and this attitude is probably perpetuated by physicians who are quick to prescribe drugs and nurses who are quick to administer them. Of course, there are many appropriate uses of drugs, and clients certainly should not be denied their benefits. The difficulties emerge when there is excessive reliance on drugs as chemical solutions to problems that are not amenable to chemical solutions.

   b. The widespread acceptance and use of alcohol. In some groups, every social occasion is accompanied by alcoholic beverages of some kind.

   c. The apparently prevalent view that drug abuse refers only to the use of illegal drugs and that using alcohol or prescription drugs, however inappropriately, does not constitute drug abuse.

   d. The acceptance and use of illegal drugs in certain subgroups of the population. This is especially prevalent in high school and college students.

   Efforts to change attitudes and decrease demand for drugs can be made through education and counseling about such topics as drug effects and nondrug ways to handle the stresses and problems of daily life.

3. Each person must take personal responsibility for drinking alcoholic beverages and taking mind-altering drugs. Initially, conscious, voluntary choices are made to drink or not to drink, to take a drug or not to take it. This period varies somewhat, but drug dependence develops in most instances only after prolonged use. When mind-altering drugs are prescribed for a legitimate reason, the client must use them in prescribed doses and preferably for a short time.

4. Physicians can help prevent drug abuse by prescribing drugs appropriately, prescribing mind-altering drugs in limited amounts and for limited periods, using nondrug measures when they are likely to be

effective, educating clients about the drugs prescribed for them, participating in drug education programs, and recognizing, as early as possible, clients who are abusing or are likely to abuse drugs.

5. Nurses can help prevent drug abuse by administering drugs appropriately, using nondrug measures when possible, teaching clients about drugs prescribed for them, and participating in drug education programs.

6. Parents can help prevent drug abuse in their children by minimizing their own use of drugs and by avoiding heavy cigarette smoking. Children are more likely to use illegal drugs if their parents have a generally permissive attitude about drug taking, if either parent takes mind-altering drugs regularly, and if either parent is a heavy cigarette smoker.

7. Pregnant women should avoid alcohol, nicotine, and other drugs of abuse because of potentially harmful effects on the fetus.

Treatment Measures for Substance Abuse

Treatment measures for alcohol and other drug abuse have not been especially successful. Even people who have been institutionalized and achieved a drug-free state for prolonged periods are apt to resume their drug-taking behavior when released from the institution. So far, voluntary, self-help groups, such as Alcoholics Anonymous and Narcotics Anonymous, have been more successful than health professionals in dealing with drug abuse. Health professionals are more likely to be involved in acute situations, such as intoxication or overdose, withdrawal syndromes, or various medical-surgical conditions. As a general rule, treatment depends on the type, extent, and duration of drug-taking behavior and the particular situation for which treatment is needed. Some general management principles include the following:

1. Psychological rehabilitation efforts should be part of any treatment program for a drug-dependent person. Several approaches may be useful, including psychotherapy, voluntary groups, and other types of emotional support and counseling.

2. Drug therapy is limited in treating drug dependence for several reasons. First, specific antidotes are available only for benzodiazepines (flumazenil) and opioid narcotics (naloxone). Second, there is a high risk of substituting one abused drug for another. Third, there are significant drawbacks to giving CNS stimulants to reverse effects of CNS depressants, and vice versa. Fourth, there is often inadequate information about the types and amounts of drugs taken.

   Despite these drawbacks, however, there are some clinical indications for drug therapy, including treatment of overdose or withdrawal syndromes. Even when drug therapy is indicated, there are few guidelines for optimal use. Doses, for example, must often be estimated initially and then titrated according to response.

3. General care of clients with drug overdose is primarily symptomatic and supportive. The aim of treatment is usually to support vital functions, such as respiration and circulation, until the drug is metabolized and eliminated from the body. For example, respiratory depression from an overdose of a CNS depressant drug may be treated by inserting an artificial airway and mechanical ventilation. Removal of some drugs can be hastened by hemodialysis.

4. Treatment of substance abuse may be complicated by the presence of other disorders. For example, depression is common and may require antidepressant drug therapy.

 REVIEW AND APPLICATION EXERCISES

1. Why is it important to assess each client in relation to alcohol and other substance abuse?

2. What are signs and symptoms of overdose with alcohol, benzodiazepine antianxiety or hypnotic agents, cocaine, and opiates?

3. What are general interventions for treatment of drug overdoses?

4. What are specific antidotes for opiate and benzodiazepine overdoses, and how are they administered?

5. Which commonly abused drugs may produce life-threatening withdrawal reactions if stopped abruptly?

6. How can severe withdrawal syndromes be prevented, minimized, or safely managed?

7. What are the advantages of treating substance abuse disorders in centers established for that purpose?

SELECTED REFERENCES

Acute reactions to drugs of abuse (1996). *The Medical Letter, 38*(974), 43–46.

Adams, I.B. & Martin, B.R. (1996). Cannabis: Pharmacology and toxicology in animals and humans. *Addiction, 91*, 1585–1614.

Crabtree, B.L. & Polles, A. (1997). Substance-related disorders. In J.T. DiPiro, R.L. Talbert, G.C. Yee, G.R. Matzke, B.G. Wells, & L.M. Posey (Eds.), *Pharmacotherapy: A pathophysiologic approach*, 3rd ed., pp. 1345–1365. Stamford, CT: Appleton & Lange.

Cruz, R., Davis, M., O'Neil, H., Tamarin, F., Brandstetter, R.D., & Karetzky, M. (1998). Pulmonary manifestations of inhaled street drugs. *Heart and Lung, 27*, 297–305.

Haack, M.R. (1998). Treating acute withdrawal from alcohol and other drugs. *Nursing Clinics of North America, 33*(1), 75–92.

Kosten, T.R. (1997). Generic substance and polydrug use disorders. In A. Tasman, J. Kay, & J.A. Lieberman (Eds.), *Psychiatry*, pp. 743–754. Philadelphia: W.B. Saunders.

Munzer, A. (1997). Smoking and smoking cessation. In W.N. Kelley (Ed.), *Textbook of internal medicine*, 3rd ed., pp. 163–167. Philadelphia: Lippincott-Raven.

O'Brien, C.P. (1996). Drug addiction and drug abuse. In J.G. Hardman, L.E. Limbird, P.B. Molinoff, & R.W. Ruddon (Eds.), *Goodman & Gilman's The pharmacological basis of therapeutics*, 9th ed., pp. 557–577. New York: McGraw-Hill.

Parran, T., Jr. (1997). Prescription drug abuse: A question of balance. *Medical Clinics of North America, 81*, 967–978.

Schatzberg, A.F. & Nemeroff, C.B. (1998). (Eds.), *The American Psychiatric Press Textbook of psychopharmacology*, 2nd ed. Washington, DC: American Psychiatric Press, Inc.

Saitz, R. & O'Malley, S.S. (1997). Pharmacotherapies for alcohol abuse: Withdrawal and treatment. *Medical Clinics of North America, 81*, 881–907.

Warner, E.A., Kosten, T.R., & O'Connor, P.G. (1997). Pharmacotherapy for opioid and cocaine abuse. *Medical Clinics of North America, 81*, 909–925.

16

Central Nervous System Stimulants

Objectives

After studying this chapter, the student should be able to:

1. Describe general characteristics of central nervous system (CNS) stimulant drugs.

2. Discuss reasons for decreased use of amphetamines for therapeutic purposes.

3. Discuss the rationale for treating attention deficit-hyperactivity disorder with CNS stimulant drugs.

4. Describe characteristics and effects of xanthine drugs.

Mrs. Williams comes to your office with her 6-year-old son. She complains that he is a very active child who always seems to be getting into mischief. She likes a clean, orderly house and he likes to make messes. He seems to be doing OK in school, although she would like to see his grades improve. She was talking to a neighbor, who encouraged her to talk with a physician about prescribing Ritalin, because her son may have attention deficit-hyperactivity disorder (ADHD).

Reflect on:

- What advice you would have for Mrs. Williams.

- Possible therapeutic effects if the boy has ADHD.

- Possible negative effects if the boy does not have ADHD.

USES

Many drugs stimulate the central nervous system (CNS), but only a few are used therapeutically, and their indications for use are limited. Two disorders treated with CNS stimulants are narcolepsy and attention deficit-hyperactivity disorder (ADHD).

Narcolepsy is a rare disorder characterized by periodic "sleep attacks" in which the victim has an uncontrollable feeling of drowsiness and goes to sleep at any place or any time. In addition to excessive daytime drowsiness and fatigue, nighttime sleep patterns are disturbed. The hazards of suddenly going to sleep in unsafe environments restrict activities of daily living.

Attention deficit-hyperactivity disorder occurs in children, usually by 3 years of age and before 7 years. It is characterized by hyperactivity, a short attention span, difficulty completing assigned tasks or schoolwork, restlessness, and impulsive behavior. Formerly thought to disappear with adolescence, the disorder is now thought to continue into adolescence and adulthood in one third to two thirds of clients. In adolescents and adults, impulsiveness and inattention continue but hyperactivity is not a prominent feature. A major criterion for diagnosing later ADHD is a previous diagnosis of childhood ADHD.

TYPES OF STIMULANTS

Most CNS stimulants act by facilitating initiation and transmission of nerve impulses that excite other cells. The drugs are somewhat selective in their actions at lower doses but tend to involve the entire CNS at higher doses. The major groups of CNS stimulants are amphetamines and related drugs, analeptics, and xanthines.

Amphetamines increase the amounts of norepinephrine, dopamine, and possibly serotonin in the brain, thereby producing mood elevation or euphoria, increasing mental alertness and capacity for work, decreasing fatigue and drowsiness, and prolonging wakefulness. Larger doses, however, produce signs of excessive CNS stimulation, such as restlessness, hyperactivity, agitation, nervousness, difficulty concentrating on a task, and confusion. Overdoses can produce convulsions and psychotic behavior. Amphetamines also stimulate the sympathetic nervous system, resulting in increased heart rate and blood pressure, mydriasis, slowed gastrointestinal motility, and other symptoms. In ADHD, the drugs reduce behavioral symptoms and may improve cognitive performance.

These drugs produce tolerance and psychological dependence. They are Schedule II drugs under the Controlled Substances Act, and prescriptions for them are nonrefillable. These drugs are widely sold on the street and commonly abused (see Chap. 15).

Analeptics stimulate respiration but do not reverse the effects of CNS depressant drugs. A major drawback to their clinical use is that doses sufficient to stimulate respiration often cause convulsive seizures. Respiratory depression can be more safely and effectively treated with endotracheal intubation and mechanical ventilation than with analeptic drugs.

Xanthines stimulate the cerebral cortex, increasing mental alertness and decreasing drowsiness and fatigue. Other effects include myocardial stimulation with increased cardiac output and heart rate, diuresis, and increased secretion of pepsin and hydrochloric acid. Large doses can impair mental and physical functions by producing restlessness, nervousness, anxiety, agitation, insomnia, and cardiac arrhythmias.

Indications for Use

Amphetamines are used in the treatment of narcolepsy, ADHD, and obesity. Methylphenidate is indicated only for ADHD and narcolepsy. Analeptics are used occasionally to treat respiratory depression. Caffeine (a xanthine) is often an ingredient in nonprescription analgesics and stimulants (eg, No-Doz). A combination of caffeine and sodium benzoate is occasionally used as a respiratory stimulant in neonates.

Contraindications to Use

Central nervous system stimulants cause cardiac stimulation and thus are contraindicated in clients with cardiovascular disease (eg, angina, arrhythmias, hypertension) that is likely to be aggravated by the drugs. They also are contraindicated in clients with anxiety or agitation, glaucoma, or hyperthyroidism. They are usually contraindicated in clients with a history of drug abuse.

INDIVIDUAL CENTRAL NERVOUS SYSTEM STIMULANTS

Amphetamines and Related Drugs

Amphetamine, **dextroamphetamine** (Dexedrine), and **methamphetamine** (Desoxyn) are closely related drugs that share characteristics of the amphetamines as a group. They are more important as drugs of abuse than as therapeutic agents.

Amphetamine and Dextroamphetamine

ROUTE AND DOSAGE RANGES

Adults: Narcolepsy, oral (PO) 5–60 mg/d in divided doses

Children >6 y: Narcolepsy, PO 5 mg/d to start therapy; raise by 5 mg/wk to effective dose

ADHD, PO 5 mg once or twice daily initially, increased by 5 mg/d at weekly intervals until optimal response is obtained (usually no greater than 40 mg/d). Do not initiate dosage with a long-acting preparation.

Children 3–5 y: ADHD, PO 2.5 mg/d initially, increased by 2.5 mg/d at weekly intervals until optimal response is obtained. Do not initiate dosage with a long-acting preparation.

Methamphetamine

ROUTE AND DOSAGE RANGES

Adults: Narcolepsy, same as amphetamine
Children >6 y: Narcolepsy, no dosage established
   ADHD, same as amphetamine
Children <6 y: No dosage established

Methylphenidate (Ritalin) is chemically related to amphetamines and produces similar actions and adverse effects. It is used to treat ADHD in children and adults and narcolepsy in adults. As a CNS stimulant, methylphenidate is considered less potent than amphetamines and more potent than caffeine. Methylphenidate is a Schedule II drug because it produces psychological dependence and is a drug of abuse.

ROUTE AND DOSAGE RANGES

Adults: Narcolepsy, PO 10–60 mg/d in two or three divided doses (average dose 20–30 mg/d)
   ADHD, PO 10–15 mg q2–3h (40–90 mg/d)
Children ≥6 y: ADHD, PO 5 mg twice a day initially, increased by 5–10 mg at weekly intervals to a maximum of 60 mg/d

Analeptic Agent

Doxapram (Dopram) has limited clinical usefulness as a respiratory stimulant. Although it does increase tidal volume and respiratory rate, it also increases oxygen consumption and carbon dioxide production. Limitations include a short duration of action (5 to 10 minutes after a single intravenous [IV] dose) and therapeutic dosages near or overlapping those that produce convulsions. Mechanical ventilation is safer and more effective in relieving respiratory depression from depressant drugs or other causes. Doxapram is occasionally used by anesthesiologists and pulmonary specialists.

ROUTE AND DOSAGE RANGE

Adults: IV 0.5–1.5 mg/kg in single or divided doses; IV continuous infusion 5 mg/min initially, decreased to 2.5 mg/min or more. Dose by infusion should not exceed 3 g.

Xanthines

Caffeine is commercially prepared from tea leaves. Pharmaceutical preparations include an oral preparation and a solution for injection. Caffeine is usually prescribed as caffeine citrate for oral use and caffeine and sodium benzoate for parenteral use because these forms are more soluble than caffeine itself. Caffeine has limited therapeutic usefulness. It is an ingredient in some nonprescription analgesic preparations (Anacin, Excedrin, Vanquish) and may increase analgesia. It is also an ingredient in nonprescription stimulant (antisleep) preparations (eg, No-Doz). It is sometimes combined with an ergot alkaloid to treat migraine headaches (eg, Cafergot). A combination of caffeine and sodium benzoate is used as a respiratory stimulant in neonatal apnea unresponsive to other therapies.

Most caffeine is consumed in beverages, such as coffee, tea, cocoa, and cola drinks. One cup of coffee contains approximately 100 to 150 mg of caffeine, analgesic preparations contain 30 to 60 mg, and antisleep preparations contain 100 to 200 mg. Thus, the stimulating effects of caffeine can be obtained as readily with coffee as with a drug preparation. Caffeine produces tolerance to its stimulating effects, and psychological dependence or habituation occurs.

Theophylline preparations are xanthine derivatives used in the treatment of respiratory disorders, such as asthma and bronchitis. In these conditions, the desired effect is bronchodilation and improvement of breathing; CNS stimulation is then an adverse reaction (see Chap. 47).

NURSING PROCESS

Assessment

- Assess use of stimulant and depressant drugs (prescribed, over-the-counter, or street drugs).
- Assess for conditions that are aggravated by CNS stimulants.
- For a child with possible ADHD, assess behavior as specifically and thoroughly as possible.
- For any client receiving amphetamines or methylphenidate, assess behavior for signs of tolerance and abuse.

Nursing Diagnoses

- Sleep Pattern Disturbance related to hyperactivity, nervousness, insomnia
- Risk for Injury: Adverse drug effects (excessive cardiac and CNS stimulation, drug dependence)
- Knowledge Deficit: Drug effects on children and adults
- Noncompliance: Overuse of drug

Planning/Goals

The client will:

- Take drugs safely and accurately
- Improve attention span and task performance (children and adults with ADHD) and decrease hyperactivity (children with ADHD)

- Have fewer sleep episodes during normal waking hours (for clients with narcolepsy)

Interventions

- For a child receiving CNS stimulants, assist parents in scheduling drug administration and drug holidays (eg, weekends, summers) to increase beneficial effects and help prevent drug dependence and stunted growth.
- Record weight at least weekly.
- Promote nutrition to avoid excessive weight loss.
- Provide information about the condition for which a stimulant drug is being given and the potential consequences of overusing the drug.

Evaluation

- Reports of improved behavior and academic performance from parents and teachers of children with ADHD
- Self- or family reports of improved ability to function in work, school, or social environments for adolescents and adults with ADHD
- Reports of decreased inappropriate sleep episodes with narcolepsy

PRINCIPLES OF THERAPY

1. Stimulant drugs are often misused and abused by people who want to combat fatigue and delay sleep, such as long-distance drivers, students, and athletes. Use of amphetamines or other stimulants for this purpose is not justified. These drugs are dangerous for drivers and those involved in similar activities, and they have no legitimate use in athletics.

2. When an amphetamine or methylphenidate is prescribed, giving the smallest effective dose and limiting the number of doses obtained with one prescription decrease the likelihood of drug dependence.

3. Analeptics are not indicated for most clients with depression of the CNS or the respiratory system. Anesthesiologists, if they use analeptic drugs at all, use them only in carefully selected circumstances and with great caution. Doxapram usually should not be used to stimulate ventilation in clients with drug-induced coma or exacerbations of chronic lung disease. Respiration can be more effectively and safely controlled with mechanical ventilation than with drugs.

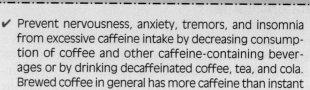

CLIENT TEACHING GUIDELINES
Methylphenidate

General Considerations

✔ This drug may mask symptoms of fatigue, impair physical coordination, and cause dizziness or drowsiness. Use caution while driving or performing other tasks requiring alertness.

✔ Notify a health care provider of nervousness, insomnia, heart palpitations, vomiting, fever, or skin rash. These are adverse drug effects and dosage may need to be reduced.

✔ Avoid other central nervous system stimulants, including caffeine.

✔ Record weight at least weekly; report excessive losses.

✔ The drug may cause weight loss; caloric intake (of nutritional foods) may need to be increased, especially in children.

✔ Take methylphenidate only as prescribed by a physician. These drugs have a high potential for abuse. The risks of drug dependence are lessened if the drugs are taken correctly.

✔ Get adequate rest and sleep. Do not take stimulant drugs to delay fatigue and sleep; these are normal, necessary resting mechanisms for the body.

✔ Prevent nervousness, anxiety, tremors, and insomnia from excessive caffeine intake by decreasing consumption of coffee and other caffeine-containing beverages or by drinking decaffeinated coffee, tea, and cola. Brewed coffee in general has more caffeine than instant coffee, tea, and other beverages.

Self-Administration and Administration to Children

✔ Take regular tablets approximately 30 to 45 minutes before meals.

✔ Take the last dose of the day in the afternoon, before 6 PM, to avoid interference with sleep.

✔ Swallow the sustained-release tablet whole, without crushing or chewing.

✔ If excessive weight loss, nervousness, or insomnia develops, ask the prescribing physician if the dose can be reduced or taken on a different schedule to relieve these adverse effects.

Use in Children

Central nervous system stimulants are not recommended for ADHD in children younger than 6 years of age or as anorexiants in children younger than 12 years of age. When used, dosage should be carefully monitored to avoid excessive CNS stimulation, anorexia, and insomnia. Suppression of weight and height have been reported, and growth should be monitored at regular intervals during drug therapy. In children with psychosis or Tourette syndrome, CNS stimulants may exacerbate symptoms.

In ADHD, careful documentation of baseline symptoms over approximately 1 month is necessary to establish the diagnosis and evaluate outcomes of treatment. This can be done by videotapes of behavior; observations and ratings by clinicians familiar with ADHD; and by interviewing the child, parents, or caretakers. Some authorities believe that this condition is overdiagnosed and that stimulant drugs are prescribed unnecessarily. Guidelines for treatment of ADHD include the following:

1. Counseling and psychotherapy (eg, parental counseling or family therapy) are recommended along with drug therapy for effective treatment and realistic expectations of outcomes.
2. Young children may not require treatment until starting school. Then, the goal of drug therapy is to control symptoms, facilitate learning, and promote social development.
3. Drug therapy is indicated when symptoms are moderate to severe; are present for several months; and interfere in social, academic, or behavioral functioning. When possible, drug therapy should be omitted or reduced in dosage when children are not in school.
4. Methylphenidate is the most commonly used drug. It is usually given daily, including weekends, for the first 3 to 4 weeks to allow caregivers to assess beneficial and adverse effects. Desirable effects may include improvement in behavior, attention span, and quality and quantity of school work, and better relationships with other children and family members. Adverse effects include appetite suppression and weight loss, which may be worse during the first 6 months of therapy.
5. Drug holidays (stopping drug administration) are controversial. Some clinicians say they are indicated only if no significant problems occur during the drug-free period and are not recommended for most children. Other clinicians believe they are desirable when children are not in school (eg, summer) and necessary periodically to re-evaluate the child's condition. Dosage adjustments are often needed at least annually as the child grows and hepatic metabolism slows. In addition, the drug-free periods decrease weight loss and growth suppression.

Use in Older Adults

Central nervous system stimulants should be used cautiously in older adults. As with most other drugs, slowed metabolism and excretion increase the risks of accumulation and toxicity. Older adults are likely to experience anxiety, nervousness, insomnia, and mental confusion from excessive CNS stimulation. In addition, older adults often have cardiovascular disorders (eg, angina, arrhythmias, hypertension) that may be aggravated by the cardiac-stimulating effects of the drugs.

NURSING ACTIONS

Central Nervous System Stimulants

NURSING ACTIONS	RATIONALE/EXPLANATION
1. **Administer accurately**	
a. Give amphetamines and methylphenidate early in the day, at least 6 hours before bedtime.	To avoid interference with sleep. If insomnia occurs, give the last dose of the day at an earlier time or decrease the dose.
b. For children with attention deficit-hyperactivity disorder (ADHD), give amphetamines and methylphenidate before meals.	To minimize the drugs' appetite-suppressing effects and risks of interference with nutrition and growth.
2. **Observe for therapeutic effects**	Therapeutic effects depend on the reason for use.
a. Fewer "sleep attacks" with narcolepsy	
b. Improved behavior and performance of cognitive and psychomotor tasks with ADHD	
c. Increased mental alertness and decreased fatigue	

(continued)

NURSING ACTIONS	RATIONALE/EXPLANATION
3. Observe for adverse effects	Adverse effects may occur with acute or chronic ingestion of excessive amounts of coffee and with other forms of central nervous system (CNS) stimulant drugs.
a. Excessive CNS stimulation—hyperactivity, nervousness, insomnia, anxiety, tremors, convulsions, psychotic behavior	These reactions are more likely to occur with large doses.
b. Cardiovascular effects—tachycardia, other arrhythmias, hypertension	These reactions are caused by the sympathomimetic effects of the drugs.
c. Gastrointestinal effects—anorexia, weight loss, nausea, diarrhea, constipation	
4. Observe for drug interactions	
a. Drugs that *increase* effects of amphetamines:	
(1) Alkalinizing agents (eg, antacids)	Drugs that increase the alkalinity of the gastrointestinal tract increase intestinal absorption of amphetamines, and urinary alkalinizers decrease urinary excretion. Increased absorption and decreased excretion serve to potentiate drug effects.
(2) Monoamine oxidase (MAO) inhibitors	Potentiate amphetamines by slowing drug metabolism. These drugs thereby increase the risks of headache, subarachnoid hemorrhage, and other signs of a hypertensive crisis. The combination may cause death and should be avoided.
b. Drugs that *decrease* effects of amphetamines:	
(1) Acidifying agents	Urinary acidifying agents (eg, ammonium chloride) increase urinary excretion and lower blood levels of amphetamines. Decreased absorption and increased excretion serve to decrease drug effects.
(2) Antipsychotic agents	Decrease or antagonize the excessive CNS stimulation produced by amphetamines. Chlorpromazine (Thorazine) or haloperidol (Haldol) is sometimes used in treating amphetamine overdose.
c. Drugs that *increase* effects of doxapram:	
(1) MAO inhibitors; sympathomimetic or adrenergic drugs (eg, epinephrine, norepinephrine)	Synergistic vasopressor effects may occur.
d. Drugs that *decrease* effects of doxapram:	
(1) Barbiturates	These CNS depressant drugs (sedative-hypnotics) may be used to manage excessive CNS stimulation caused by doxapram overdosage.

 REVIEW AND APPLICATION EXERCISES

1. What kinds of behaviors may indicate narcolepsy?

2. What kinds of behaviors may indicate ADHD?

3. What is the rationale for treating narcolepsy and ADHD with CNS stimulants?

4. What are the major adverse effects of CNS stimulants, and how may they be minimized?

5. Do you think children taking CNS stimulants for ADHD should have drug-free periods? Justify your answer.

SELECTED REFERENCES

Block, S.L. (1998). Attention deficit disorder. *Pediatric Clinics of North America, 45,* 1053–1083.

Drug facts and comparisons. (Updated monthly). St. Louis: Facts and Comparisons.

Findling, R.L. & Dogin, J.W. (1998). Psychopharmacology of ADHD: Children and adolescents. *Journal of Clinical Psychiatry, 59*(Suppl 7), 42–49.

Hoffman, B.B. & Lefkowitz, R.J. (1996). Catecholamines, sympathomimetic drugs, and adrenergic receptor antagonists. In J.G. Hardman, L.E. Limbird, P.B. Molinoff, & R.W. Ruddon (Eds.), *Goodman & Gilman's The pharmacological basis of therapeutics*, 9th ed., pp. 199–248. New York: McGraw-Hill.

Theesen, K.A. & Dopheide, J.A. (1997). Disorders of childhood. In J.T. DiPiro, R.L. Talbert, P.E. Hayes, G.C. Yee, G.R. Matzke, B.G. Wells, & L.M. Posey (Eds.), *Pharmacotherapy: A pathophysiologic approach*, 3rd ed., pp. 1301–1310. Stamford, CT: Appleton & Lange.

Wender, P.H. (1998). Pharmacotherapy of attention-deficit/hyperactivity disorder in adults. *Journal of Clinical Psychiatry, 59*(Suppl 7), 76–79.

Drugs Affecting the Autonomic Nervous System

17

Physiology of the Autonomic Nervous System

Objectives

After studying this chapter, the student will be able to:

1. Identify physiologic effects of the sympathetic nervous system.

2. Differentiate subtypes and functions of sympathetic nervous system receptors.

3. Identify physiologic effects of the parasympathetic nervous system.

4. Differentiate subtypes and functions of parasympathetic nervous system receptors.

5. Describe signal transduction and the intracellular events that occur when receptors of the autonomic nervous system are stimulated.

6. State names and general characteristics of drugs affecting the autonomic nervous system.

AUTONOMIC NERVOUS SYSTEM

The autonomic nervous system (ANS) is a branch of the central nervous system (CNS) regulated mainly by centers in the hypothalamus, brain stem, and spinal cord. These centers serve to alter and integrate activities of the ANS, which has both central and peripheral components. The ANS automatically, without conscious thought or effort, regulates many body functions. These functions can be described broadly as mechanisms designed to maintain a constant internal environment (homeostasis), to respond to stress or emergencies, and to repair body tissues.

Nerve impulses are generated and transmitted in the ANS as they are in the CNS (see Chap. 5). Autonomic nerve impulses are transmitted to body tissues through two major subdivisions of the ANS: the *sympathetic nervous sys-*

tem (SNS) and the *parasympathetic nervous system* (PNS). More specifically, nerve impulses are carried through preganglionic fibers, ganglia, and postganglionic fibers. Preganglionic impulses travel from the CNS to ganglia (clusters of cell bodies of postganglionic fibers located outside the brain and spinal cord); postganglionic impulses travel from ganglia to effector tissues of the heart, blood vessels, glands, other visceral organs, and smooth muscle (Fig. 17-1).

The main neurotransmitters of the ANS are acetylcholine and norepinephrine (see Chap. 5). Acetylcholine is synthesized from acetylcoenzyme A and choline and released at preganglionic fibers of both the SNS and PNS and at postganglionic fibers of the PNS. The nerve fibers that secrete acetylcholine are called cholinergic fibers. Norepinephrine is synthesized from the amino acid tyrosine by a series of enzymatic conversions that also produce

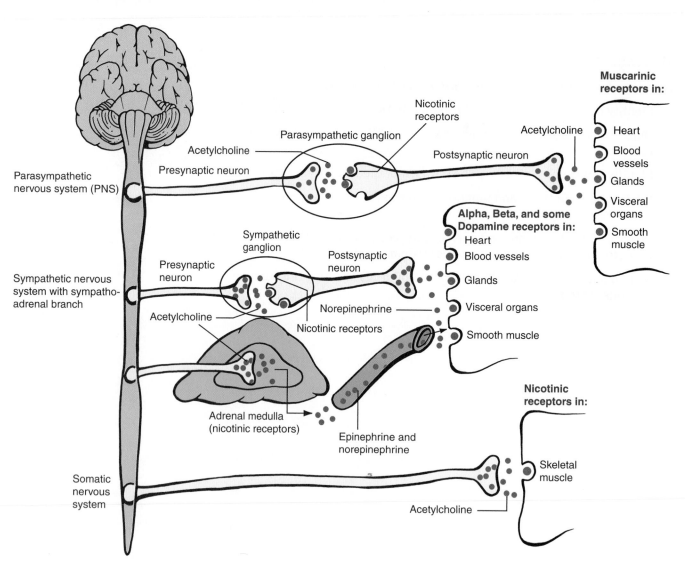

FIGURE 17–1 Organization of the autonomic and somatic nervous systems.

dopamine and epinephrine (ie, tyrosine → dopamine → norepinephrine → epinephrine). Norepinephrine is the end product, except in the adrenal medulla, where most of the norepinephrine is converted to epinephrine. Norepinephrine is released at postganglionic fibers of the SNS. Nerve fibers secreting norepinephrine are called adrenergic fibers.

Acetylcholine and norepinephrine act on receptors in body organs and tissues to cause parasympathetic or sympathetic effects, respectively. Stimulation of both systems causes excitatory effects in some organs but inhibitory effects in others. However, most organs are predominantly controlled by one system. The two divisions of the ANS are usually antagonistic in their actions on a particular organ. When the sympathetic system excites a particular organ, the parasympathetic system often inhibits it. For example, sympathetic stimulation of the heart causes an increased rate and force of myocardial contraction; parasympathetic stimulation decreases rate and force of contraction, thereby resting the heart. Exceptions to this antagonistic action include sweating and regulation of arteriolar blood vessel diameter, which is controlled by the SNS.

When receptors located on target tissues are stimulated by a ligand (a drug, hormone, or neurotransmitter that binds to a receptor), this initiates a cascade of intracellular events known as signal transduction. The ligand that binds the receptor is the so-called *first messenger*. In most cases, this ligand–receptor interaction activates a cell membrane-bound G protein and an effector enzyme that then activate a molecule inside the cell called a *second messenger*. This second messenger is the link between events that are occurring outside the cell (ie, receptor activation by the ligand) and resulting events that will occur inside the cell, such as opening ion channels, stimulating other enzymes, and increasing intracellular calcium levels. These intracellular events ultimately produce the physiologic responses to neurotransmitter and hormone release or drug administration. Figure 17-2 illustrates the intracellular events of signal transduction that occur when an adrenergic beta receptor is stimulated by epinephrine.

Sympathetic Nervous System

The SNS is stimulated by physical or emotional stress, such as strenuous exercise or work, pain, hemorrhage, intense emotions, and temperature extremes. Increased capacity for vigorous muscle activity in response to a perceived threat, whether real or imaginary, is often called the *fight-or-flight* reaction. Specific body responses include:

1. Increased arterial blood pressure and cardiac output
2. Increased blood flow to the brain, heart, and skeletal muscles; decreased blood flow to viscera, skin, and other organs not needed for fight-or-flight

3. Increased rate of cellular metabolism—increased oxygen consumption and carbon dioxide production
4. Increased breakdown of muscle glycogen for energy
5. Increased blood sugar
6. Increased mental activity and ability to think clearly
7. Increased muscle strength
8. Increased rate of blood coagulation
9. Increased rate and depth of respiration
10. Pupil dilation to aid vision
11. Increased sweating. (Note that acetylcholine is the neurotransmitter for this sympathetic response. This is a deviation from the normal postganglionic neurotransmitter, which is norepinephrine.)

These responses are protective mechanisms designed to help the person cope with the stress or get away from it. The intensity and duration of responses depend on the amounts of norepinephrine and epinephrine present. Norepinephrine is synthesized in adrenergic nerve endings and released into the synapse (the gap between nerve cells in a chain) when adrenergic nerve endings are stimulated. It exerts intense but brief effects on presynaptic and postsynaptic adrenergic receptors. Then, most of the norepinephrine is taken up again by the nerve endings and reused as a neurotransmitter; the remainder diffuses into surrounding tissue fluids and blood, or it is metabolized by monoamine oxidase (MAO) or catechol-O-methyltransferase (COMT).

Norepinephrine also functions as a hormone, along with epinephrine. In response to adrenergic nerve stimulation, norepinephrine and epinephrine are secreted into the bloodstream by the adrenal medullae and transported to all body tissues. They are continually present in arterial blood in amounts that vary according to the degree of stress present and the ability of the adrenal medullae to respond to stimuli. The larger proportion of the circulating hormones (approximately 80%) is epinephrine. These catecholamines exert the same effects as those caused by direct stimulation of the SNS. However, the effects last longer because the hormones are removed from the blood more slowly. These hormones are metabolized mainly in the liver by the enzymes MAO and COMT.

Dopamine is also an adrenergic neurotransmitter and catecholamine. In the brain, dopamine is essential for normal function (see Chap. 5); in peripheral tissues, its main effects are on the heart and blood vessels.

Adrenergic Receptors

When norepinephrine and epinephrine act on body cells that respond to sympathetic nerve or catecholamine stimulation, they interact with two distinct adrenergic receptors, alpha and beta. Norepinephrine acts mainly on alpha receptors; epinephrine acts on both alpha and beta receptors. These receptors have been further subdivided into $alpha_1$, $alpha_2$, $beta_1$, and $beta_2$ receptors. A $beta_3$ receptor

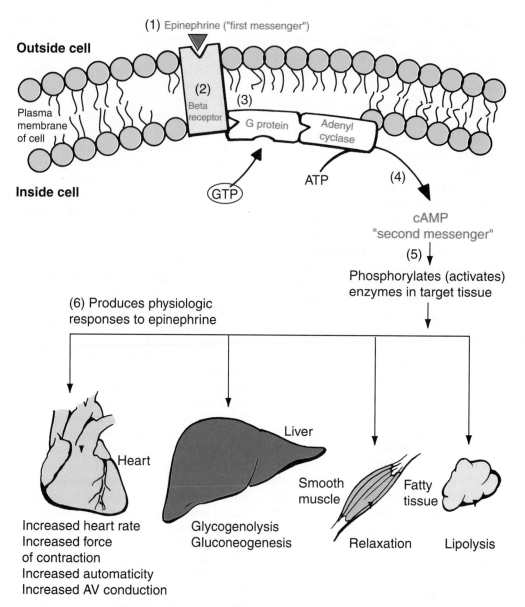

FIGURE 17–2 Signal transduction mechanism for an adrenergic beta receptor. Epinephrine, the "first messenger," interacts with a beta receptor (2). This hormone-receptor complex activates a G protein, which reacts with a guanosine triphosphate (GTP) (3). The activated G protein then activates the enzyme adenyl cyclase, which (4) catalyzes the conversion of adenosine triphosphate (ATP) to cyclic adenosine monophosphate (cAMP), the "second messenger." (5) cAMP activates enzymes, which bring about the biologic responses to epinephrine (6).

has been cloned, and animal studies suggest that drugs targeted to this receptor may augment heat production or thermogenesis and increase energy expenditure. Several compounds are being tested to treat obesity, hyperglycemia, and the problem of insulin resistance in diabetes. There are no beta$_3$ agonist compounds approved by the Food and Drug Administration for human use.

When dopamine acts on body cells that respond to adrenergic stimulation, it can activate alpha$_1$ and beta$_1$ receptors as well as dopaminergic receptors. Only dopamine can activate dopaminergic receptors. Dopamine receptors are located in the brain, in blood vessels of the kidneys and other viscera, and probably in presynaptic sympathetic nerve terminals. Activation (agonism) of these receptors may result in stimulation or inhibition of cellular function. Like alpha and beta receptors, dopamine receptors are divided into several subtypes (D$_1$ to D$_5$), and specific effects depend on which subtype of receptor is activated. Table 17-1 describes the location of adrenergic receptors in the body and the response that occurs when each receptor is stimulated.

The intracellular events (of signal transduction) after stimulation of adrenergic receptors are thought to include the following mechanisms:

Alpha$_1$ receptors: The binding of adrenergic substances to receptor proteins in the cell membrane of

TABLE 17-1	Adrenergic Receptors	
Type	Location	Effects of Stimulation
Alpha$_1$	Blood vessels	Vasoconstriction
	Heart	Increased force of contraction; arrhythmias
	Intestinal smooth muscle	Relaxation
	Liver	Glycogenolysis, gluconeogenesis
	Genitourinary smooth muscle	Contraction
	Eye	Blinking, mydriasis
Alpha$_2$	Nerve endings	Inhibit release of norepinephrine
	Vascular smooth muscle	Vasoconstriction
	Pancreatic beta cells	Inhibit insulin secretion
	Platelets	Aggregation
Beta$_1$	Heart	Increased heart rate, force of contraction, automaticity, and rate of atrioventricular conduction
	Kidney	Increased renin release
Beta$_2$	Bronchioles	Bronchodilation
	Blood vessels	Vasodilation
	Gastrointestinal tract	Decreased motility and tone
	Liver	Glycogenolysis, gluconeogenesis
	Urinary bladder	Relaxed detrusor muscle
	Pregnant uterus	Relaxation
Dopamine	Blood vessels of heart, kidney, other viscera	Vasodilation

smooth muscle cells is thought to open ion channels, allow calcium ions to move into the cell, and produce muscle contraction (eg, vasoconstriction, gastrointestinal and bladder sphincter contraction).

Alpha$_2$ receptors: In the brain, some of the norepinephrine released into the synaptic cleft between neurons returns to the nerve endings from which it was released and stimulates presynaptic alpha$_2$ receptors. This negative feedback causes less norepinephrine to be released by subsequent nerve impulses. The result is decreased sympathetic outflow and an antiadrenergic effect. The probable mechanism is that the calcium required for neurotransmitter release from storage vesicles is prevented from entering the presynaptic nerve cell.

In peripheral tissues, alpha$_2$ receptors are probably postsynaptic and have a variety of functions when stimulated by norepinephrine, epinephrine, or dopamine. However, their specific effects on the intracellular mechanisms of body cells have not been clearly elucidated.

Beta$_1$ and beta$_2$ receptors: Activation of these receptors stimulates activity of adenyl cyclase, an enzyme in cell membranes. Adenyl cyclase, in turn, stimu-

lates formation of cyclic adenosine monophosphate (cAMP). cAMP serves as a second messenger and can initiate any of several different intracellular actions, with specific actions depending on the type of cell. cAMP is rapidly degraded by an enzyme called phosphodiesterase to 5′ adenosine monophosphate (AMP). Drugs such as theophylline inhibit phosphodiesterase and increase cAMP concentrations, resulting in bronchodilation (see Chap. 47).

Dopaminergic receptors D$_1$ and D$_5$: Activation of these receptors is thought to stimulate the production of cAMP, as does activation of beta$_1$ and beta$_2$ receptors.

Dopaminergic receptor D$_2$: Activation of this receptor is thought to inhibit formation of cAMP and to alter calcium and potassium ion currents. D$_3$ and D$_4$ receptors are subgrouped with D$_2$ receptors, but the effects of their activation have not been clearly delineated.

The number and the binding activity of receptors may be altered. These phenomena are most clearly understood with beta receptors. For example, when chronically exposed to high concentrations of substances that stimulate their function, the receptors decrease in number and become less efficient in stimulating adenyl cyclase. The resulting decrease in beta-adrenergic responsiveness is called desensitization or down-regulation of receptors.

Conversely, when chronically exposed to substances that block their function, the receptors may increase in number and become more efficient in stimulating adenyl cyclase. The resulting increase in beta-adrenergic responsiveness (called hypersensitization or up-regulation) may lead to an exaggerated response when the blocking substance is withdrawn.

Parasympathetic Nervous System

Functions stimulated by the PNS are often described as resting, reparative, or vegetative functions. They include digestion, excretion, cardiac deceleration, anabolism, and near vision.

Approximately 75% of all parasympathetic nerve fibers are in the vagus nerves. These nerves supply the thoracic and abdominal organs; their branches go to the heart, lungs, esophagus, stomach, small intestine, the proximal half of the colon, the liver, gallbladder, pancreas, and the upper portions of the ureters. Other parasympathetic fibers supply pupillary sphincters and ciliary muscles; lacrimal, nasal, submaxillary, and parotid glands; descending colon and rectum; lower portions of the ureters and bladder; and genitalia.

Specific body responses to parasympathetic stimulation include:

1. Dilation of blood vessels in the skin; no particular effect on systemic blood vessels
2. Decreased heart rate, possibly bradycardia

3. Increased secretion of digestive enzymes and motility of the gastrointestinal tract
4. Constriction of smooth muscle of bronchi
5. Increased secretions from glands in the lungs, stomach, intestines, and skin (sweat glands)
6. Constricted pupils (from contraction of the sphincter muscle of the iris) and accommodation to near vision (from contraction of the ciliary muscle of the eye)
7. Contraction of smooth muscle in the urinary bladder
8. Contraction of skeletal muscle
9. No apparent effects on blood coagulation, blood sugar, mental activity, or muscle strength

These responses are regulated by acetylcholine, a neurotransmitter in the brain, ANS, and neuromuscular junctions. Acetylcholine is formed in cholinergic nerve endings from choline and acetylcoenzyme A; the reaction is catalyzed by choline acetyltransferase. After its release from the nerve ending, acetylcholine acts briefly (milliseconds), then is rapidly metabolized by acetylcholinesterase (an enzyme present in the nerve ending and on the surface of the receptor organ). Acetylcholinesterase splits the active acetylcholine into inactive acetate and choline; the choline is taken up again by the presynaptic nerve terminal and reused. Acetylcholine exerts excitatory effects at nerve synapses and nerve–muscle junctions and inhibitory effects at some peripheral sites such as the heart.

Cholinergic Receptors

When acetylcholine acts on body cells that respond to parasympathetic nerve stimulation, it interacts with two types of cholinergic receptors: nicotinic and muscarinic. Nicotinic receptors are located in motor nerves and skeletal muscle. When they are activated by acetylcholine, the cell membrane depolarizes and produces muscle contraction. Muscarinic receptors are located in most internal organs, including the cardiovascular, respiratory, gastrointestinal, and genitourinary systems. When muscarinic receptors are activated by acetylcholine, the affected cells may be excited or inhibited in their functions. These receptors have been further subdivided, with two types of nicotinic and five types of muscarinic receptors identified.

Although the subtypes of cholinergic receptors have not been as well characterized as those of the adrenergic receptors, the intracellular events (of signal transduction) after stimulation are thought to include the following mechanisms:

Muscarinic$_1$ receptors: Activation of these receptors results in a series of processes during which phospholipids in the cell membrane and inside the cell are broken down. One of the products of phospholipid metabolism is inositol phosphate. The inositol phosphate acts as a second messenger to increase the intracellular concentration of calcium. Calcium also acts as a second messenger and functions to activate several intracellular enzymes, initiate contraction of smooth muscle cells, and increase secretions of exocrine glands.

Muscarinic$_2$ receptors: Activation of these receptors results in inhibition of adenyl cyclase in the heart, smooth muscle, and brain. As a result, less cAMP is formed to act as a second messenger and stimulate intracellular activity. The overall consequence is inhibition of affected cells.

Muscarinic$_3$ receptors: Activation apparently causes the same cascade of intracellular processes as with activation of the muscarinic$_1$ receptors.

Muscarinic$_4$ and muscarinic$_5$ receptors: These two subtypes have been identified, but their locations and functions have not been delineated.

Nicotinic$_1$ receptors: These receptors are located on presynaptic nerve fibers. Their activation promotes the release of acetylcholine in the cerebral cortex and enhances the transmission of nerve impulses at all parasympathetic and sympathetic ganglia. They also promote the release of epinephrine from the adrenal medullae.

Nicotinic$_2$ receptors: These are located at neuromuscular junctions in skeletal muscle. Their activation causes muscle contraction.

CHARACTERISTICS OF AUTONOMIC DRUGS

Many drugs are used clinically because of their ability to stimulate or block activity of the SNS or PNS. Drugs that stimulate activity act like endogenous neurotransmitter substances; drugs that block activity prevent the action of both endogenous substances and stimulating drugs.

Drugs that act on the ANS usually affect the entire body rather than certain organs and tissues. Drug effects depend on which branch of the ANS is involved and whether it is stimulated or inhibited by drug therapy. Thus, knowledge of the physiology of the ANS is required if drug effects are to be understood and predicted. In addition, it is becoming increasingly important to understand receptor activity and the consequences of stimulation or inhibition. More drugs are being developed to stimulate or inhibit particular subtypes of receptors. This is part of the continuing effort to design drugs that act more selectively on particular body tissues and decrease adverse effects on other body tissues. For example, drugs such as terbutaline have been developed to stimulate beta$_2$ receptors in the respiratory tract and produce bronchodilation (a desired effect) with decreased stimulation of beta$_1$ receptors in the heart (an adverse effect).

The terminology used to describe autonomic drugs is often confusing because different terms are used to refer to the same phenomenon. Thus, *sympathomimetic, ad-*

renergic, and *alpha-* and *beta-adrenergic agonists* are used to describe a drug that has the same effects on the human body as stimulation of the SNS. *Parasympathomimetic*, *cholinomimetic*, and *cholinergic* are used to describe a drug that has the same effects on the body as stimulation of the PNS. There are also drugs that oppose or block stimulation of these systems. *Sympatholytic*, *antiadrenergic*, and *alpha-* and *beta-adrenergic blocking drugs* inhibit sympathetic stimulation. *Parasympatholytic*, *anticholinergic*, and *cholinergic blocking drugs* inhibit parasympathetic stimulation. This book uses the terms *adrenergic*, *antiadrenergic*, *cholinergic*, and *anticholinergic*.

REVIEW AND APPLICATION EXERCISES

1. What are the major differences between the sympathetic and parasympathetic branches of the ANS?
2. What are the major SNS and PNS neurotransmitters?
3. What are the locations and functions of SNS receptors?
4. What is meant when drugs are described as adrenergic, sympathomimetic, antiadrenergic, sympatholytic, cholinergic, or anticholinergic?

SELECTED REFERENCES

Carroll, E.W. & Curtis, R.L. (1998). In C.M. Porth (Ed.), *Pathophysiology: Concepts of altered health states*, 5th ed., pp. 870–878. Philadelphia: Lippincott Williams & Wilkins.

Ganong, W.F. (1997). *Review of medical physiology*, 18th ed. Stamford, CT: Appleton & Lange.

Himms-Hagen, J. & Danforth, E. (1996). The potential role of B_3 adreno-receptor agonists in the treatment of obesity and diabetes. *Current Opinion in Endocrinology and Diabetes, 3*(1), 59–65.

Lefkowitz, R.J., Hoffman, B.R., & Taylor, P. (1996). Neurotransmission: The autonomic and somatic motor nervous systems. In J.G. Hardman, L.E. Limbird, P.B. Molinoff, & R.W. Ruddon (Eds.), *Goodman & Gilman's The pharmacological basis of therapeutics*, 9th ed., pp. 105–139. New York: McGraw-Hill.

Piano, M.R. & Huether, S.E. (1998). Mechanisms of hormonal regulation. In K.L. McCance & S.E. Huether (Eds.), *Pathophysiology: The biologic basis for disease in adults and children*, 3rd ed., pp. 629–632. St. Louis: Mosby.

18

Adrenergic Drugs

Objectives

After studying this chapter, the student will be able to:

1. Differentiate effects of stimulation of alpha- and beta-adrenergic receptors.

2. List characteristics of adrenergic drugs in terms of effects on body tissues, indications for use, adverse effects, nursing process implications, principles of therapy, and observation of client responses.

3. Discuss use of epinephrine to treat anaphylactic shock, acute bronchospasm, and cardiac arrest.

4. Identify clients at risk of experiencing adverse effects with adrenergic drugs.

5. List commonly used over-the-counter preparations that contain adrenergic drugs.

6. Discuss principles of therapy and nursing process for using adrenergic drugs in special populations.

7. Describe signs and symptoms of toxicity due to noncatecholamine adrenergic drugs.

8. Discuss treatment of overdose with these drugs.

9. Teach the client about safe, effective use of adrenergic drugs.

Jill, 8 years old, is brought to the clinic for allergy desensitization. She is starting on a new concentration of allergy extract today. After her injection, as usual, you ask her to remain in the waiting room for 30 minutes. After 20 minutes, her mother comes to get you. Jill is restless, her voice is high-pitched, she feels odd, and her respiration rate has increased to 30 breaths per minute.

Reflect on:

▶ What data would you collect next?

▶ How could you differentiate anaphylaxis from anxiety?

▶ If Jill were experiencing an anaphylactic reaction, what would be the treatment of choice?

DESCRIPTION

Adrenergic (sympathomimetic) drugs produce effects similar to those produced by stimulation of the sympathetic nervous system (see Chap. 17) and therefore have widespread effects on body tissues. Some of the drugs are exogenous formulations of the naturally occurring neurotransmitters and hormones (eg, norepinephrine, epinephrine, dopamine); others are chemical relatives.

Specific effects depend mainly on the client's health status when a drug is given and the drug's activation of particular adrenergic receptors. Major therapeutic uses and adverse effects stem from drug effects on the heart, blood vessels, and lungs. The drugs discussed in this chapter are those with multiple effects and clinical uses (epinephrine, ephedrine and pseudoephedrine, isoproterenol, phenylephrine, and phenylpropanolamine). Because epinephrine, ephedrine, and phenylpropanolamine stimulate both alpha- and beta-adrenergic receptors, these drugs have widespread effects on body tissues and multiple clinical uses. Isoproterenol stimulates beta-adrenergic receptors (both $beta_1$ and $beta_2$) and may be used in the treatment of several clinical conditions. Phenylephrine stimulates alpha-adrenergic receptors and is used to induce vasoconstriction in several conditions.

Other adrenergic drugs act mainly on specific adrenergic receptors or are given topically to produce more selective therapeutic effects and fewer adverse effects. These drugs have relatively restricted clinical indications and are discussed more extensively elsewhere (Drugs Used in Hypotension and Shock, Chap. 54; Bronchodilating and Other Antiasthmatic Drugs, Chap. 47; Nasal Decongestants, Antitussives, Mucolytics, and Cold Remedies, Chap. 49; and Drugs Used in Ophthalmic Conditions, Chap. 65). Table 18-1 lists commonly used adrenergic drugs in relation to adrenergic receptor activity and clinical use.

Mechanisms of Action and Effects

Adrenergic (sympathomimetic) drugs have three mechanisms of action. For the most part, adrenergic drugs combine directly with postsynaptic alpha- or beta-adrenergic receptors on the surface membrane of body cells. The drug–receptor complex then alters the cell membrane's permeability to ions or intracellular enzymes to stimulate intracellular metabolism and production of other enzymes, structural proteins, energy, and other products required for cell function and reproduction. Epinephrine, isoproterenol, norepinephrine, and phenylephrine are examples of direct-acting adrenergic drugs. Some adrenergic drugs (eg, phenylpropanolamine) exert indirect effects on adrenergic receptors by first releasing a catecholamine from its storage site, which in turn stimulates the alpha and beta receptors. The third mechanism of adrenergic drug action

TABLE 18-1 Adrenergic Drugs

Generic/Trade Name	Major Clinical Uses
Alpha and Beta Activity	
Dopamine (Intropin)	Hypotension and shock
Epinephrine (Adrenalin)	Allergic reactions, cardiac arrest, hypotension and shock, local vasoconstriction, bronchodilation, cardiac stimulation, ophthalmic conditions
Ephedrine	Bronchodilation, cardiac stimulation, nasal decongestion
Alpha Activity	
Norepinephrine (Levophed)	Hypotension and shock
Metaraminol (Aramine)	Hypotension and shock
Naphazoline hydrochloride (Privine)	Nasal decongestion
Oxymetazoline hydrochloride (Afrin)	Nasal decongestion
Phenylephrine (Neo-Synephrine)	Hypotension and shock, nasal decongestion, ophthalmic conditions
Phenylpropanolamine hydrochloride (Propagest, Dexatrim)	Nasal decongestion, appetite suppression
Propylhexedrine (Benzedrex)	Nasal decongestion
Tetrahydrozoline hydrochloride (Tyzine, Visine)	Nasal decongestion, local vasoconstriction in the eye
Tuaminoheptane (Tuamine)	Nasal decongestion
Xylometazoline hydrochloride (Otrivin)	Nasal decongestion
Beta Activity	
Albuterol (Proventil)	Bronchodilation
Bitolterol (Tornalate)	Bronchodilation
Dobutamine (Dobutrex)	Cardiac stimulation
Isoproterenol (Isuprel)	Bronchodilation, cardiac stimulation
Isoetharine (Bronkosol)	Bronchodilation
Metaproterenol (Alupent)	Bronchodilation
Pirbuterol (Maxair)	Bronchodilation
Salmeterol (Serevent)	Bronchodilation
Terbutaline (Brethine)	Bronchodilation

is called mixed acting and is a combination of direct and indirect receptor stimulation. Ephedrine and pseudoephedrine are examples of mixed-acting adrenergic drugs. Drugs that activate $alpha_2$ receptors on presynaptic nerve fibers do not produce a sympathetic effect. These drugs inhibit the release of additional norepinephrine and exert a sympatholytic response in the body (see Chap. 19).

Because most body tissues have both alpha and beta receptors, the effects of adrenergic drugs depend on each drug's activation of particular receptors and the number of affected receptors in a particular body tissue. Some drugs act on both types of receptors; some act more selectively on certain subtypes of receptors. Activation of alpha₁ receptors in blood vessels results in vasoconstriction, which then raises blood pressure and decreases nasal congestion. Activation of beta₁ receptors in the heart results in cardiac stimulation (increased force of myocardial contraction and increased heart rate). Activation of beta₂ receptors in the lungs results in bronchodilation, and activation of beta₂ receptors in blood vessels results in vasodilation (increased blood flow to the heart, brain, and skeletal muscles, the tissues needed to aid the "fight-or-flight" response). Many newer adrenergic drugs (eg, beta₂ receptor agonists used as bronchodilators in asthma and other bronchoconstrictive disorders) were developed specifically to be more selective.

In addition to the cardiac, vascular, and pulmonary effects, other effects of adrenergic drugs include contraction of gastrointestinal (GI) and urinary sphincters, lipolysis, decreased GI tone, changes in renin secretion, uterine relaxation, hepatic glycogenolysis and gluconeogenesis, and decreased secretion of insulin.

Indications for Use

Clinical indications for the use of adrenergic drugs stem mainly from their effects on the heart, blood vessels, and bronchi. They are often used as emergency drugs in the treatment of acute cardiovascular, respiratory, and allergic disorders.

In cardiac arrest and Stokes-Adams syndrome (heart block), they may be given as cardiac stimulants. In hypotension and shock, they may be given to increase blood pressure. In hemorrhagic or hypovolemic shock, the drugs are second-line agents that may be used if adequate fluid volume replacement does not restore sufficient blood pressure and circulation to maintain organ perfusion.

In bronchial asthma and other obstructive pulmonary diseases, the drugs are given as bronchodilators to relieve bronchoconstriction and bronchospasm. In upper respiratory infections, including the common cold and sinusitis, they may be given orally or applied topically to the nasal mucosa for decongestant effects.

In allergic disorders, the drugs are given for vasoconstricting or decongestant effects to relieve edema in the respiratory tract, skin, and other tissues. Thus, they may be used to treat allergic rhinitis, acute hypersensitivity (anaphylactoid reactions to drugs, animal serums, insect stings, and other allergens), serum sickness, urticaria, and angioneurotic edema.

Other clinical uses include relaxation of uterine musculature and inhibition of uterine contractions in preterm labor. They may be added to intraspinal and local anesthetics to prolong anesthesia. Topical uses include application to skin and mucous membranes for vasoconstriction and hemostatic effects, and to the eyes for vasoconstriction and mydriasis.

Contraindications to Use

Contraindications to using adrenergic drugs include cardiac arrhythmias, angina pectoris, hypertension, hyperthyroidism, cerebrovascular disease, narrow-angle glaucoma, and hypersensitivity to the drug or any component (some preparations contain sulfites, to which some people are allergic). They are also contraindicated with local anesthesia of distal areas with a single blood supply (eg, fingers, toes, nose, ears) because of potential tissue damage and sloughing from vasoconstriction. They should not be given during the second stage of labor because they may delay progression. The drugs should be used with caution in clients with anxiety, insomnia, and psychiatric disorders because of their stimulant effects on the central nervous system (CNS) and in older adults because of their cardiac- and CNS-stimulating effects.

INDIVIDUAL ADRENERGIC DRUGS

Epinephrine (Adrenalin) is the prototype of adrenergic drugs. When given systemically, the effects may be therapeutic or adverse, depending on the reason for use and route of administration. Specific effects include:

1. Increased systolic blood pressure, due primarily to increased force of myocardial contraction and vasoconstriction in skin, mucous membranes, and kidneys
2. Vasodilation and increased blood flow to skeletal muscles, heart, and brain
3. Vasoconstriction in peripheral blood vessels. This allows shunting of blood to the heart and brain, with increased perfusion pressure in the coronary and cerebral circulations. This action is thought to be the main beneficial effect in cardiac arrest and cardiopulmonary resuscitation (CPR).
4. Increased heart rate and possibly arrhythmias due to stimulation of conducting tissues in the heart. Reflex bradycardia may occur when blood pressure is raised.
5. Relaxation of GI smooth muscle
6. Relaxation or dilation of bronchial smooth muscle
7. Increased glucose, lactate, and fatty acids in the blood due to metabolic effects
8. Inhibition of insulin secretion
9. Miscellaneous effects, including increased total leukocyte count, increased rate of blood coagulation, and decreased intraocular pressure in wide-angle glaucoma. When given locally, the main effect is vasoconstriction.

Epinephrine stimulates both alpha and beta receptors. At usual doses, beta-adrenergic effects on the heart and vascular and other smooth muscles predominate. However, at high doses, alpha-adrenergic effects (eg, vasoconstriction) predominate. As the prototype of adrenergic drugs, effects and clinical indications for epinephrine are the same as for adrenergic drugs. In addition, epinephrine is the adrenergic drug of choice for relieving the acute bronchospasm and laryngeal edema of anaphylactic shock, the most serious allergic reaction. Epinephrine is used in cardiac arrest for its cardiac stimulant and peripheral vasoconstrictive effects. It also is added to local anesthetics for vasoconstrictive effects, which prolong the action of the local anesthetic drug, prevent systemic absorption, and minimize bleeding.

Epinephrine should be used with caution in infants and children; syncope has occurred with use in asthmatic children. Epinephrine is the active ingredient in over-the-counter (OTC) inhalation products for asthma (AsthmaNefrin, Primatene Mist, Bronkaid Mist, others). These products should not be used on a regular basis, especially by people who have heart disease or are elderly. These preparations have a short duration of action, which promotes frequent and excessive use. They also lose their effectiveness with prolonged use and may cause adverse effects.

Epinephrine is not given orally because it is destroyed by enzymes in the GI tract and liver. It may be given by inhalation, injection, or topical application. Numerous epinephrine solutions are available for various uses and routes of administration. Solutions vary widely in the amount of drug they contain. They must be used correctly to avoid potentially serious hazards. When given by intravenous (IV) injection, epinephrine raises blood pressure, stimulates the heart to increase the force and rate of ventricular contraction; relaxes smooth muscle of the bronchi; and constricts arterioles in skin, mucosa, and most viscera. It also increases blood sugar and liver glycogenolysis.

Epinephrine crosses the placenta but not the blood–brain barrier. When given by injection, it acts rapidly but has a short duration of action. For acute asthma attacks, subcutaneous (SC) administration usually produces bronchodilation within 5 to 10 minutes; maximal effects may occur within 20 minutes. Most epinephrine is rapidly metabolized in the liver to inactive metabolites, which are then excreted in the urine. The small amount that is not metabolized is deactivated by reuptake at synaptic receptor sites. Epinephrine is excreted in breast milk.

Sus-Phrine is an aqueous suspension of epinephrine that is given SC only. Some of the epinephrine is in solution and acts rapidly; some is suspended in crystalline form for slower absorption and relatively prolonged activity.

Epinephrine Injection, 1:1000 (1 mg/mL) Aqueous Solution

ROUTES AND DOSAGE RANGES

Adults: Intramuscular (IM), or SC: 0.3–0.5 mg q20min to q4h if necessary
   IV: Dilute 1.0 mg with 10 mL sodium chloride injection for a final concentration 1:10,000 or 0.1 mg/mL. Give 0.5 to 1.0 mg (5 to 10 mL) of this solution IV.

Children: SC: 0.01 mg/kg q20min to q4h if necessary. Do not exceed 0.5 mg in a single dose.

Epinephrine Inhalation, 1:100 (1%) Aqueous Solution

ROUTE AND DOSAGE RANGES

Adults: Oral inhalation by aerosol, nebulizer, or intermittent positive-pressure breathing machine (not a preferred route of administration for epinephrine). Care must be taken to avoid confusing the 1:100 solution for inhalation with the 1:1000 solution for injection. Inadvertent injection of the 1:100 aqueous solution for inhalation could be fatal.

Epinephrine Nasal Solution, 1:1000 (0.1%) Solution

ROUTES AND DOSAGE RANGES

Adults: Topical application to nasal mucosa: 1 or 2 drops of an 0.1% nasal solution per nostril q4–6h. Topical application to skin and mucous membranes for hemostasis: use a 1:50,000–1:1000 solution, or 1:500,000–1:50,000 solution mixed with local anesthetic.

Sus-Phrine Injection, 1:200 (5 mg/mL) Suspension

ROUTE AND DOSAGE RANGES

Adults: SC only, 0.1 mL initially, maximum dose 0.3 mL (0.5–1.5 mg); do not repeat for at least 6 h
Children: SC 0.005 mL/kg, maximum dose 0.15 mL

Ephedrine is a mixed-acting adrenergic drug that acts by stimulating alpha and beta receptors and causing release of norepinephrine. Its actions are less potent but longer lasting than those of epinephrine. Ephedrine produces more CNS stimulation than other adrenergic drugs. It may be used in the treatment of bronchial asthma to prevent bronchospasm, but it is less effective than epinephrine for acute bronchospasm and respiratory distress.

Ephedrine can be given orally or parenterally. When given orally, therapeutic effects occur within 1 hour and last 3 to 5 hours. When given SC, it acts in approximately 20 minutes and effects last approximately 60 minutes; with intramuscular administration, it acts in approximately 10 to 20 minutes and effects last less than 60 minutes. Ephedrine is excreted unchanged in the urine. Acidic urine increases the rate of drug elimination.

Ephedrine is a common ingredient in OTC antiasthma tablets (Bronkaid, Primatene, others). The tablets contain 12.5 to 25 mg of ephedrine and 100 to 130 mg of theophylline, a xanthine bronchodilator. Other clinical uses include shock associated with spinal or epidural anesthesia, Stokes-Adams syndrome (sudden attacks of unconsciousness caused by heart block), allergic disorders, nasal congestion, and eye disorders.

Pseudoephedrine (Sudafed) is a related drug with similar actions. It is used for bronchodilating and nasal decongestant effects. Pseudoephedrine is given orally and is available OTC alone and as an ingredient in several multi-ingredient sinus, allergy, and cold remedies. Pseudoephedrine is eliminated primarily in the urine. Its elimination may be slowed by alkaline urine, which promotes drug reabsorption in the renal tubules.

Ephedrine

ROUTE AND DOSAGE RANGES

Adults: Asthma: oral (PO) 25–50 mg q4h
   Hypotension: IM, SC, or IV 25–50 mg. Do not exceed 150 mg/24 h.
   Nasal congestion: Nose drops of 0.25% solution; nasal jelly 1%; or PO 25–50 mg q4h.
Children 6–12 y: PO 6.25–12.5 mg q4–6h.
Children 2–6 y: PO 0.3–0.5 mg/kg q4–6h.

Pseudoephedrine

ROUTE AND DOSAGE RANGES

Adults: PO 60 mg three or four times a day. Do not exceed 240 mg in 24 h.
Children 6–12 y: PO 30 mg q6h. Do not exceed 120 mg in 24 h.
Children 2–5 y: PO 15 mg q6h. Do not exceed 60 mg in 24 h.

Isoproterenol (Isuprel) is a synthetic catecholamine that acts on $beta_1$- and $beta_2$-adrenergic receptors. Its main actions are to stimulate the heart, dilate blood vessels in skeletal muscle, and relax bronchial smooth muscle. Compared with epinephrine, its cardiac stimulant effects are similar, but it does not affect alpha receptors and therefore does not cause vasoconstriction. It is well absorbed when given by injection or as an aerosol. However, absorption is unreliable with sublingual and oral preparations, so their use is not recommended. It is metabolized more slowly than epinephrine by the enzyme catechol-*O*-methyltransferase (COMT). It is not well metabolized by monoamine oxidase (MAO), which may account for its slightly longer duration of action than epinephrine. Isoproterenol may be used as a cardiac stimulant in heart block and cardiogenic shock and as a bronchodilator in respiratory conditions characterized by bronchospasm. However, $beta_2$-selective agonists (eg, albuterol, others) are preferred for bronchodilating effects because they cause less cardiac stimulation. Too-frequent use may lead to tolerance and decreased bronchodilating effects.

ROUTES AND DOSAGE RANGES

Adults: Cardiac arrhythmias and resuscitation: IV 0.02–0.06 mg bolus followed by 5 µg/min infusion titrated according to clinical response; SC 0.15–0.2 mg
   Bronchospasm during anesthesia: IV 0.01–0.02 mg of diluted solution initially (1 mL of 1:5000 solu-

tion, diluted to 10 mL with sodium chloride or 5% dextrose injection for a final concentration of 1:50,000), repeated PRN
   Bronchodilation: inhalation by nebulizer, 5–15 deep inhalations of a mist of 1:200 solution, repeated in 10–30 min if necessary; by oxygen aerosol, up to 0.5 mL of 1:200 solution or 0.3 mL of 1:100 solution with oxygen flow at 4 L/min for 15–20 min; measured-dose inhalers (Mistometer, Medihaler), 1 or 2 inhalations (second inhalation is given 2–5 min after first). These treatments should usually be given no more often than q4h.
   Sublingual tablets, 10–15 mg 3 or 4 times a day, maximum 60 mg/d; not a recommended route because absorption is unpredictable
Children: Bronchodilation, inhalation, generally the same as for adults, with adult supervision; do not exceed 0.25 mL of 1:200 solution for each 10–15-min treatment; sublingual, 5–10 mg 3 or 4 times a day, maximum 30 mg/d; not a preferred route because of erratic absorption

Phenylephrine (Neo-Synephrine, others) is a synthetic drug that acts on alpha-adrenergic receptors to produce vasoconstriction. Vasoconstriction decreases cardiac output and renal perfusion and increases peripheral vascular resistance and blood pressure. There is little cardiac stimulation because phenylephrine does not activate $beta_1$ receptors in the heart or $beta_2$ receptors in blood vessels. Phenylephrine may be given to raise blood pressure in hypotension and shock. Compared with epinephrine, phenylephrine produces longer-lasting elevation of blood pressure (20 to 50 minutes with injection). When given systemically, phenylephrine produces a reflex bradycardia; this effect may be used therapeutically to relieve paroxysmal atrial tachycardia. Other uses include local application for nasal decongestant and mydriatic effects. Various preparations are available for different uses. Phenylephrine is often an ingredient in prescription and nonprescription cold and allergy remedies. It is excreted primarily in the urine.

ROUTES AND DOSAGE RANGES

Adults: Hypotension and shock, IM, SC 1–10 mg; IV 0.1–0.5 mg diluted in sodium chloride injection and given slowly, or 10 mg diluted in 500 mL 5% dextrose injection or sodium chloride and infused slowly, according to blood pressure readings
   Nasal congestion, nasal solutions of 0.125%, 0.25%, 0.5%, or 1.0% Do not use for more than 5 continuous days of treatment.
   Mydriasis, ophthalmic solutions of 2.5% or 10%. Instill one drop. May be repeated in 10–60 min as needed.
Phenylpropanolamine (Acutrim, Dexatrim) indirectly stimulates both alpha and beta receptors, causing vasoconstriction, increased blood pressure, and cardiac stimulation. Its clinical uses stem mainly from its nasal

decongestant and appetite-suppressing actions. It is a common ingredient in OTC cold and allergy remedies and is the active ingredient in most OTC appetite suppressants. For obesity, phenylpropanolamine should be used no longer than 8 to 12 weeks, and calorie restriction and safety precautions should be strictly followed. Severe hypertension and stroke may occur with overuse.

Phenylpropanolamine is readily absorbed from the GI tract; peak plasma levels and half-life depend on the drug formulation (immediate vs. sustained release). Most is excreted unchanged in urine. Most OTC preparations are long acting.

ROUTE AND DOSAGE RANGES

Adults: Decongestant: 25 mg q4h or 50 mg q8h, not to exceed 150 mg/d
  Anorexiant: PO immediate-release formulations, 25 mg 3 times daily 30 min before meals
  PO timed-release, 75 mg once daily in morning
  PO precision-release (16-h duration), 75 mg after breakfast

NURSING PROCESS

Assessment

Assess the client's status in relation to the following conditions:

- **Allergic disorders.** It is standard procedure to question a client about allergies on initial contact or admission to a health care agency. If the client reports a previous allergic reaction, try to determine what caused it and what specific symptoms occurred. It may be helpful to ask if swelling, breathing difficulty, or hives (urticaria) occurred. With anaphylactic reactions, severe respiratory distress (from bronchospasm and laryngeal edema) and profound hypotension (from vasodilation) may occur.
- **Asthma.** If the client is known to have asthma, assess the frequency of attacks, the specific signs and symptoms experienced, the precipitating factors, the actions taken to obtain relief, and the use

of bronchodilators or other medications on a long-term basis. With acute bronchospasm, respiratory distress is clearly evidenced by loud, rapid, gasping, wheezing respirations. Acute asthma attacks may be precipitated by exposure to allergens or respiratory infections. When available, check arterial blood gas reports for the adequacy of oxygen–carbon dioxide gas exchange. Hypoxemia ($\downarrow Po_2$), hypercarbia ($\uparrow Pco_2$), and acidosis ($\downarrow pH$) may occur with acute bronchospasm.

- **Chronic obstructive pulmonary disorders.** Emphysema and chronic bronchitis are characterized by bronchoconstriction and dyspnea with exercise or at rest. Check arterial blood gas reports when available. Hypoxemia, hypercarbia, and acidosis are likely with chronic bronchoconstriction. Acute bronchospasm may be superimposed on the chronic bronchoconstrictive disorder, especially with a respiratory infection.
- **Cardiovascular status.** Assess for conditions that are caused or aggravated by adrenergic drugs (eg, angina, hypertension, tachyarrhythmias).

Nursing Diagnoses

- Impaired Gas Exchange related to bronchoconstriction
- Altered Tissue Perfusion related to hypotension and shock or vasoconstriction with drug therapy
- Altered Nutrition: Less than Body Requirements related to anorexia
- Sleep Pattern Disturbance: Insomnia, nervousness
- Noncompliance: Overuse
- Risk for Injury related to cardiac stimulation (arrhythmias, hypertension)
- Knowledge Deficit: Drug effects and safe usage

Planning/Goals

The client will:

- Receive or self-administer drugs accurately
- Experience relief of symptoms for which adrenergic drugs are given
- Comply with instructions for safe drug use

Nursing Notes: Apply Your Knowledge

Jack Newton, a healthy 46-year-old, develops seasonal allergies. He self-medicates his allergy symptoms with over-the-counter ephedrine (Bronkaid) for approximately 4 weeks before going to his physician. When the nurse takes his vital signs, he is surprised that his blood pressure is 160/92 and his pulse is 102. How does ephedrine, an adrenergic agent, relieve allergy symptoms? What side effects are common?

How Can You Avoid This Medication Error?

You are working in a clinic when a patient has a sudden, severe episode of laryngeal edema and hypotension. The physician shouts an order for epinephrine 0.1 mg IV stat. Your stock supply provides epinephrine 1 mg/mL. You draw up 1 mL into a syringe and hand it to the physician for IV administration.

- Demonstrate knowledge of adverse drug effects to be reported
- Avoid preventable adverse drug effects
- Avoid combinations of adrenergic drugs

Interventions

Use measures to prevent or minimize conditions for which adrenergic drugs are required:

- Decrease exposure to allergens. Allergens include cigarette smoke, foods, drugs, air pollutants, plant pollens, insect venoms, and animal dander. Specific allergens must be determined for each person.
- For clients with chronic lung disease, use measures to prevent respiratory infections. These include interventions to aid removal of respiratory secretions, such as adequate hydration, ambulation, deep-breathing and coughing exercises, and chest physiotherapy. Immunizations with pneumococcal pneumonia vaccine (a single dose) and influenza vaccine (annually) are also strongly recommended.
- When administering substances known to produce hypersensitivity reactions (penicillin and other antibiotics, allergy extracts, vaccines, local anesthetics), observe the recipient carefully for at least 30 minutes after administration. Have adrenergic and other emergency drugs and equipment readily available in case a reaction occurs.

Evaluation

- Observe for increased blood pressure and improved tissue perfusion when a drug is given for hypotension and shock or anaphylaxis.
- Interview and observe for improved breathing and arterial blood gas reports when a drug is given for bronchoconstriction or anaphylaxis.
- Interview and observe for decreased nasal congestion.

CLIENT TEACHING GUIDELINES
Adrenergic Drugs

General Considerations

✔ Take no other medications without the physician's knowledge and approval. Many over-the-counter (OTC) cold remedies and appetite suppressants contain adrenergic drugs. Use of these along with prescribed adrenergic drugs can result in overdose and serious cardiovascular or central nervous system problems. In addition, adrenergic drugs interact with numerous other drugs to increase or decrease effects; some of these interactions may be life threatening.

✔ Tell your health care provider if you are pregnant, breast-feeding, taking any other prescription or OTC drugs, or if you are allergic to sulfite preservatives.

✔ Use these drugs only as directed. The potential for abuse is high, especially for the client with asthma or other chronic lung disease who is seeking relief from labored breathing. Some of these drugs are prescribed for long-term use, but excessive use does not increase therapeutic effects. Instead, it causes tolerance and decreased benefit from usual doses and increases the incidence and severity of adverse reactions.

✔ Frequent cardiac monitoring, checks of flow rate, blood pressure, urine output, and so on are necessary if you are receiving intravenous adrenergic drugs for cardiac stimulation or vasopressor effects. These measures increase the safety and benefits of drug therapy rather than indicate the presence of a critical condition. Ask your nurse if you have concerns about your condition.

✔ You may feel anxious or tense; have difficulty sleeping; and experience palpitations, blurred vision, headache, tremor, dizziness, and pallor. These are effects of the medication. Use of relaxation techniques to promote rest and decrease muscle tension may be helpful.

✔ Use caution when driving or performing activities requiring alertness, dexterity, and good vision.

✔ Report adverse reactions such as fast pulse, palpitations, and chest pain so that drug dosage can be reevaluated and therapy changed if needed.

Self-administration

✔ Do not use topical decongestants longer than 3 to 5 days. Long-term use may be habit forming. Burning on use and rebound congestion after the dose wears off are common. Stop using the medication gradually.

✔ Stinging may occur when using ophthalmic preparations. Do not wear soft contact lenses while using ophthalmic adrenergic drugs; discoloration of the lenses may occur. Report blurred vision, headache, palpitations, and muscle tremors to your health care provider.

✔ Follow guidelines for use of your inhaler. Do not increase the dosage or frequency; tolerance may occur. Report chest pain, dizziness, or failure to obtain relief of symptoms. Saliva and sputum may be discolored pink with isoproterenol.

✔ Learn to self-administer an injection of epinephrine if you have severe allergies. Always carry your injection kit with you. Seek immediate medical care after self-injection of epinephrine.

PRINCIPLES OF THERAPY

Drug Selection and Administration

The choice of drug, dosage, and route of administration depends largely on the reason for use. IV or SC epinephrine is the drug of choice in anaphylactic shock. Isoproterenol by oral inhalation may be used for producing bronchodilation. However, a selective beta$_2$ agonist is preferred because it causes less cardiac stimulation. Adrenergic drugs are given IV only for emergencies, such as cardiac arrest, severe arterial hypotension, circulatory shock, and anaphylactic shock. No standard doses of individual adrenergic drugs are always effective; the dosage must be individualized according to the client's response. This is especially true in emergencies, but it also applies to long-term use.

Use in Specific Situations

Because adrenergic drugs are often used in crises, they must be readily available in all health care settings (eg, hospitals, long-term care facilities, physicians' offices). All health care personnel should know where emergency drugs are stored.

Anaphylaxis

Epinephrine is the drug of choice for the treatment of anaphylaxis. It relieves bronchospasm, laryngeal edema, and hypotension. In conjunction with its alpha (vasoconstriction) and beta (cardiac stimulation, bronchodilation) effects, epinephrine acts as a physiologic antagonist of histamine and other bronchoconstricting and vasodilating substances released during anaphylactic reactions. People susceptible to severe allergic responses should carry a syringe of epinephrine at all times. Epipen and Epipen Jr. are prefilled autoinjection syringes for self-administration of Adrenalin in an emergency situation.

Victims of anaphylaxis who have been taking beta-adrenergic blocking drugs (eg, propranolol [Inderal]) do not respond as readily to epinephrine as those not taking a beta-blocker. Larger doses of epinephrine and large amounts of IV fluids may be required. Adjunct medications that may be useful in treating severe cases of anaphylaxis include corticosteroids, norepinephrine, and aminophylline. Antihistamines are not very useful because histamine plays a minor role in causing anaphylaxis, compared with leukotrienes and other inflammatory mediators.

Cardiopulmonary Resuscitation

Epinephrine is one of the first drugs administered during CPR and is the adrenergic drug of choice. Its most important action is constriction of peripheral blood vessels. This shunts blood to the central circulation and increases blood flow to the heart and brain. It is also given for asystole to stimulate electrical and mechanical activity to produce myocardial contraction. This effect is also thought to result from its vasoconstrictive action. The specific effects of epinephrine depend largely on the dose and route of administration. The optimal dose in CPR has not been established. Traditional doses are relatively conservative (eg, 0.5 to 1 mg every 3 to 5 minutes). More recently, some studies and some authorities indicate that higher doses (eg, 2 to 5 mg or up to 0.1 mg/kg every 3 to 5 minutes) may be more effective, possibly because of a more intense vasopressor response.

Hypotension and Shock

In hypotension and shock, initial efforts involve identifying and treating the cause when possible. Such treatments include blood transfusions, fluid and electrolyte replacement, treatment of infection, and use of positive inotropic drugs to treat heart failure. If these measures are ineffective in raising the blood pressure enough to maintain tissue perfusion, vasopressor drugs may be used. The usual goal of vasopressor drug therapy is to maintain tissue perfusion and a mean arterial pressure of at least 80 to 100 mm Hg.

Nasal Congestion

Adrenergic drugs are given topically and systemically to constrict blood vessels in nasal mucosa and decrease the nasal congestion associated with the common cold, allergic rhinitis, and sinusitis. Topical agents are effective, undergo little systemic absorption, are available OTC, and are widely used. However, overuse leads to decreased effectiveness (tolerance), irritation of nasal mucosa, and rebound congestion. These effects can be minimized by using small doses only when necessary and for no longer than 3 to 5 days.

Oral agents have a slower onset of action than topical ones but may last longer. They also may cause more adverse effects. Adverse effects may occur with usual therapeutic doses and are especially likely with high doses. Most worrisome are cardiac and CNS stimulation. Commonly used oral agents are pseudoephedrine, phenylpropanolamine, and ephedrine. Pseudoephedrine seems to be the safest of the three in relation to risks of hypertension and cerebral hemorrhage (stroke). Phenylpropanolamine and ephedrine may cause hypertension even in normotensive people, with higher risks in hypertensive people. Hypertensive clients should avoid these drugs if possible.

Management of Toxicity and Overdose

Unlike catecholamines, which are quickly cleared from the body, excess use of noncatecholamine adrenergic drugs (phenylpropanolamine, phenylephrine, ephedrine, and pseudoephedrine) can lead to overdose and toxicity. These drugs are an ingredient in OTC products such as nasal decongestants, cold preparations, and appetite suppressants. Ephedrine and ephedra-containing herbal preparations (eg, MaHuang and Herbal Ecstasy) are often abused as an alternative to amphetamines or to aid in rapid weight loss.

Phenylpropanolamine, phenylephrine, and ephedrine have a narrow therapeutic index with toxic doses only two to three times greater than the therapeutic dose. Pseudoephedrine toxicity occurs with doses four to five times greater than the normal therapeutic dose.

The primary clinical manifestation of noncatecholamine adrenergic drug toxicity is severe hypertension, which may lead to headache, confusion, seizures, and intracranial hemorrhage. Reflex bradycardia, atrioventricular block, and myocardial infarction have also been associated with phenylpropanolamine toxicity.

Treatment involves maintaining an airway and assisting with ventilation if needed. Activated charcoal may be administered early in treatment. Hypertension is treated with vasodilators such as phentolamine or nitroprusside. Beta blockers are not used alone to treat hypertension without first administering a vasodilator, to avoid a paradoxical increase in blood pressure.

Dialysis and hemoperfusion are not effective in clearing these drugs from the body. Urinary acidification may enhance elimination of ephedrine, pseudoephedrine and phenylpropanolamine. However, this technique is not routinely used because of the risk of renal damage from myoglobin deposition in the kidney.

Use in Children

Adrenergic agents are used to treat asthma, hypotension, shock, cardiac arrest, and anaphylaxis in children; however, guidelines for safe and effective use of adrenergic drugs in children are not well established. Children are very sensitive to drug effects, including cardiac and CNS stimulation, and recommended doses usually should not be exceeded.

The main use of epinephrine in children is for treatment of bronchospasm due to asthma or allergic reactions. Parenteral epinephrine may cause syncope when given to asthmatic children. Isoproterenol is rarely given parenterally, but if given, the first dose should be approximately half that of an adult's, and later doses should be based on the response to the first dose. There is little reason to use the inhalation route because in children, as in adults, selective beta$_2$ agonists such as albuterol are preferred for bronchodilation in asthma.

Phenylephrine is most often used to relieve congestion of the upper respiratory tract and may be given topically, as nose drops. Doses must be carefully measured. Rebound nasal congestion occurs with overuse. Phenylpropanolamine is a common ingredient in OTC cold remedies. Dosage guidelines should be followed carefully, and the drugs should be inaccessible to young children. Phenylpropanolamine also is the active ingredient in OTC appetite suppressants. These should not be used for weight reduction in children.

Use in Older Adults

Adrenergic agents are used to treat asthma, hypotension, shock, cardiac arrest, and anaphylaxis in older adults. These drugs stimulate the heart to increase rate and force of contraction and blood pressure. Because older adults often have chronic cardiovascular conditions (eg, angina, arrhythmias, congestive heart failure, coronary artery disease, hypertension, peripheral vascular disease) that are aggravated by adrenergic drugs, careful monitoring by the nurse is required.

Adrenergic drugs are often prescribed as bronchodilators and decongestants in older adults. Therapeutic doses increase the workload of the heart and may cause symptoms of impaired cardiovascular function; overdoses may cause severe cardiovascular dysfunction, including life-threatening arrhythmias.

The drugs also cause CNS stimulation. With therapeutic doses, anxiety, restlessness, nervousness, and insomnia often occur in older adults. Overdoses may cause hallucinations, convulsions, CNS depression, and death.

Adrenergics are ingredients in OTC asthma remedies, cold remedies, nasal decongestants, and appetite suppressants. Cautious use of these preparations is required for older adults. They should not be taken concurrently with prescription adrenergic drugs because of the high risk of overdose and toxicity.

Ophthalmic preparations of adrenergic drugs also should be used cautiously. For example, phenylephrine is used as a vasoconstrictor and mydriatic. Applying larger-than-recommended doses to the normal eye or usual doses to the traumatized, inflamed, or diseased eye may result in enough systemic absorption of the drug to cause increased blood pressure and other adverse effects.

Use in Renal Impairment

Adrenergic drugs exert effects on the renal system that may cause problems for clients with renal impairment. For example, adrenergic drugs with alpha$_1$ activity cause constriction of renal arteries, thereby diminishing renal blood flow and urine production. These drugs also constrict urinary sphincters, causing urinary retention and painful urination, especially in men with prostatic hyperplasia.

Many adrenergic drugs and their metabolites are eliminated by the renal system. In the presence of renal disease, these compounds may accumulate and cause increased adverse effects.

Finally, phenylpropanolamine can cause interstitial nephritis, which may lead to acute renal failure.

Use in Hepatic Impairment

The liver is rich in the enzymes MAO and COMT, which are responsible for metabolism of circulating epinephrine and other adrenergic drugs (eg, norepinephrine, dopamine, and isoproterenol). However, other tissues in the body also possess these enzymes and are capable of metabolizing natural and synthetic catecholamines. Any unchanged drug can be excreted in the urine. Many noncatecholamine adrenergic drugs are excreted largely unchanged in the urine. Therefore, liver disease is not usually considered a contraindication to administering adrenergic drugs.

Use in Critical Illness

Adrenergic drugs are an important component of the emergency drug box. They are essential for treating hypotension, shock, asystole and other dysrhythmias, acute bronchospasm, and anaphylaxis. Although they may save the life of a critically ill client, use of adrenergic drugs may result in secondary health problems that require monitoring and intervention. These include:

1. Potential for vasopressor action of adrenergic drug to result in diminished renal perfusion and decreased urine output
2. Potential for adrenergic drugs with beta$_1$ activity to induce irritable cardiac dysrhythmias
3. Potential for adrenergic drugs with beta$_1$ activity to increase myocardial oxygen requirements.
4. Potential for adrenergic drugs with vasopressor action to decrease perfusion to the liver with subsequent liver damage

5. Hyperglycemia, hypokalemia, and hypophosphatemia due to beta$_1$-adrenergic effects
6. Severe hypertension and reflex bradycardia
7. Tissue necrosis after extravasation

Occurrence of any of these adverse effects may complicate the already complex care of the critically ill client. Careful assessment and prompt nursing intervention are essential in caring for the critically ill client experiencing these health problems.

 Home Care

Adrenergic drugs are often used in the home setting. Frequently prescribed drugs include bronchodilators and nasal decongestants. OTC drugs with the same effects are also commonly used for asthma, allergic rhinitis, cold symptoms, and appetite suppression for weight control. A major function of the home care nurse is to teach clients to use the drugs correctly (especially metered-dose inhalers), to report excessive CNS or cardiac stimulation to a health care provider, and not to take OTC drugs with the same or similar ingredients as prescription drugs.

Excessive adverse effects are probably most likely to occur in children and older adults. Older adults often have other illnesses that may be aggravated by adrenergic drugs, or take other drugs, the effects of which may be altered by concomitant use of adrenergics.

NURSING ACTIONS	Adrenergic Drugs

NURSING ACTIONS	RATIONALE/EXPLANATION
1. Administer accurately **a.** Check package inserts or other references if not absolutely sure about the preparation or concentration and method of administration for an adrenergic drug.	The many different preparations and concentrations available for various routes of administration increase the risk of medication error unless extreme caution is used. Preparations for intravenous, subcutaneous, inhalation, ophthalmic, or nasal routes must be used by the designated route only.
b. To give epinephrine subcutaneously, use a tuberculin syringe, aspirate, and massage the injection site.	The tuberculin syringe is necessary for accurate measurement of the small doses usually given (often less than 0.5 mL). Aspiration is necessary to avoid inadvertent intravenous (IV) administration of the larger, undiluted amount of drug intended for subcutaneous use. Massaging the injection site accelerates drug absorption and thus relief of symptoms.
c. Give Sus-Phrine subcutaneously only, and shake well before using (both vial and syringe).	Sus-Phrine is a suspension preparation of epinephrine, and suspensions must not be given IV. Rotating or shaking the container ensures that the medication is evenly distributed throughout the suspension.

(continued)

NURSING ACTIONS	RATIONALE/EXPLANATION
d. For inhalation, be sure to use the correct drug concentration, and use the nebulizing device properly.	Inhalation medications are often administered by clients themselves or by respiratory therapists if intermittent positive-pressure breathing is used. The nurse may need to demonstrate and supervise self-administration initially.
e. Do *not* give epinephrine and isoproterenol at the same time or within 4 hours of each other.	Both of these drugs are potent cardiac stimulants, and the combination could cause serious cardiac arrhythmias. However, they have synergistic bronchodilating effects, and doses can be alternated and given safely if the drugs are given no more closely together than 4 hours.
f. For IV injection of epinephrine, dilute 1 ml of 1:1000 solution to a total volume of 10 mL with sodium chloride injection, or use a commercial preparation of 1:10,000 concentration. Use parenteral solutions of epinephrine only if clear. Epinephrine is unstable in alkaline solutions.	Dilution increases safety of administration. A solution that is brown or contains a precipitate should not be used. Discoloration indicates chemical deterioration of epinephrine. Do not administer at same time sodium bicarbonate is being administered.
g. For IV infusion of isoproterenol and phenylephrine:	
(1) Administer in an intensive care unit when possible.	These drugs are given IV in emergencies, during which the client's condition must be carefully monitored. Frequent recording of blood pressure and pulse and continuous electrocardiographic monitoring are needed.
(2) Use only clear drug solutions	A brownish color or precipitate indicates deterioration, and such solutions should not be used.
(3) Dilute isoproterenol in 500 mL of 5% dextrose injection. Phenylephrine can be diluted in 5% dextrose injection or 0.9% sodium chloride solution. Do not add the drug until ready to use.	Mixing solutions when ready for use helps to ensure drug stability. Note that drug concentration varies with the amount of drug and the amount of IV solution to which it is added.
(4) Use an infusion device to regulate flow rate accurately.	Flow rate usually requires frequent adjustment according to blood pressure measurements. An infusion device helps to regulate drug administration, so wide fluctuations in blood pressure are avoided.
(5) Use a "piggyback" IV apparatus.	Only one bottle contains an adrenergic drug, and it can be regulated or discontinued without disruption of the primary IV line.
(6) Start the adrenergic drug solution slowly and increase flow rate according to the client's response (eg, blood pressure, color, mental status). Slow or discontinue gradually as well.	To avoid abrupt changes in circulation and blood pressure
h. When giving adrenergic drugs as eye drops or nose drops, do not touch the dropper to the eye or nose.	Contaminated droppers can be a source of bacterial infection.
2. Observe for therapeutic effects	These depend on the reason for use.
a. When the drug is used as a bronchodilator, observe for absence or reduction of wheezing, less labored breathing, and decreased rate of respirations.	Indicates prevention or relief of bronchospasm. Acute bronchospasm is usually relieved within 5 minutes by injected or inhaled epinephrine or inhaled isoproterenol.

(continued)

NURSING ACTIONS	RATIONALE/EXPLANATION
b. When epinephrine is given in anaphylactic shock, observe for decreased tissue edema and improved breathing and circulation.	Epinephrine injection usually relieves laryngeal edema and bronchospasm within 5 minutes and lasts for approximately 20 minutes.
c. When isoproterenol or phenylephrine is given in hypotension and shock, observe for increased blood pressure, stronger pulse, and improved urine output, level of consciousness, and color.	These are indicators of improved circulation.
d. When a drug is given nasally for decongestant effects, observe for decreased nasal congestion and ability to breathe through the nose.	The drugs act as vasoconstrictors to reduce engorgement of nasal mucosa.
e. When given as eye drops for vasoconstrictor effects, observe for decreased redness. When giving for mydriatic effects, observe for pupil dilation.	
3. Observe for adverse effects	Adverse effects depend to some extent on the reason for use. For example, cardiovascular effects are considered adverse reactions when the drugs are given for bronchodilation. Adverse effects occur with usual therapeutic doses and are more likely to occur with higher doses.
a. Cardiovascular effects—cardiac arrhythmias, hypertension	Tachycardia and hypertension are common; if severe or prolonged, myocardial ischemia or heart failure may occur. Premature ventricular contractions and other serious arrhythmias may occur. Propranolol (Inderal) or another beta blocker may be given to decrease heart rate and hypertension resulting from overdosage of adrenergic drugs. Phentolamine (Regitine) may be used to decrease severe hypertension.
b. Excessive central nervous system (CNS) stimulation—nervousness, anxiety, tremor, insomnia	These effects are more likely to occur with ephedrine or high doses of other adrenergic drugs. Sometimes, a sedative-type drug is given concomitantly to offset these effects.
c. Rebound nasal congestion, rhinitis, possible ulceration of nasal mucosa	These effects occur with excessive use of nasal decongestant drugs.
d. Renal toxicity	Phenylpropanolamine may cause drug-induced interstitial nephritis.
4. Observe for drug interactions	
a. Drugs that *increase* effects of adrenergic drugs:	Most of these drugs increase incidence or severity of adverse reactions.
(1) Anesthetics, general (eg, halothane)	Increased risk of cardiac arrhythmias. Potentially hazardous.
(2) Anticholinergics (eg, atropine)	Increased bronchial relaxation. Also increased mydriasis and therefore contraindicated with narrow-angle glaucoma.
(3) Antidepressants, tricyclic (eg, amitriptyline [Elavil])	Increased pressor response with intravenous epinephrine
(4) Antihistamines	May increase pressor effects

(continued)

NURSING ACTIONS	RATIONALE/EXPLANATION
(5) Cocaine	Increases pressor and mydriatic effects by inhibiting uptake of norepinephrine by nerve endings. Cardiac arrhythmias, convulsions, and acute glaucoma may occur.
(6) Digoxin	Sympathomimetics, especially beta-adrenergics like epinephrine and isoproterenol, increase the likelihood of cardiac arrhythmias due to ectopic pacemaker activity.
(7) Doxapram (Dopram)	Increased pressor effect
(8) Ergot alkaloids (eg, Gynergen)	Increased vasoconstriction. Extremely high blood pressure may occur. There also may be decreased perfusion of fingers and toes.
(9) Monoamine oxidase (MAO) inhibitors (eg, isocarboxazid [Marplan])	Contraindicated. The combination may cause death. When these drugs are given concurrently with adrenergic drugs, there is danger of cardiac arrhythmias, respiratory depression, and acute hypertensive crisis with possible intracranial hemorrhage, convulsions, coma, and death. Effects of MAO inhibitors may not occur for several weeks after treatment is started and may last up to 3 weeks after the drug is stopped. Every client taking MAO inhibitors should be warned against taking any other medication without the advice of a physician or pharmacist.
(10) Methylphenidate (Ritalin)	Increased pressor and mydriatic effects. The combination may be hazardous in glaucoma.
(11) Thyroid preparations (eg, Synthroid)	Increased adrenergic effects, resulting in increased likelihood of arrhythmias
(12) Xanthines (in caffeine-containing substances, such as coffee, tea, cola drinks; theophylline)	Synergistic bronchodilating effect. Sympathomimetics with CNS-stimulating properties (eg, ephedrine, isoproterenol) may produce excessive CNS stimulation with cardiac arrhythmias, emotional disturbances, and insomnia.
(13) Beta-adrenergic blocking agents (eg, propranolol [Inderal])	May augment hypertensive response to epinephrine (see also b[4] below)
b. Drugs that *decrease* effects of adrenergics:	
(1) Anticholinesterases (eg, neostigmine [Prostigmin], pyridostigmine [Mestinon]) and other cholinergic drugs	Decrease mydriatic effects of adrenergics; thus, the two groups should not be given concurrently in ophthalmic conditions
(2) Antihypertensives (eg, methyldopa [Aldomet])	Generally antagonize pressor effects of adrenergics, which act to increase blood pressure while antihypertensives act to lower it
(3) Antipsychotic drugs (eg, haloperidol [Haldol], chlorpromazine [Thorazine])	Block the vasopressor action of epinephrine. Therefore, epinephrine should not be used to treat hypotension induced by these drugs.
(4) Beta-adrenergic blocking agents (eg, propranolol [Inderal])	Decrease bronchodilating effects of adrenergics and may exacerbate asthma. Contraindicated with asthma.
(5) Phentolamine (Regitine)	Antagonizes vasopressor effects of adrenergics

Nursing Notes: Apply Your Knowledge

Answer: As an adrenergic agent, ephedrine stimulates both alpha and beta receptors. Stimulation of alpha receptors causes vasoconstriction of vessels in the nasal passage, thus decreasing nasal congestion. Side effects are produced when beta receptors are stimulated, increasing heart rate and blood pressure. When high doses of these medications are taken, or normal doses are used by people with cardiovascular problems, the side effects can be serious.

How Can You Avoid This Medication Error?

Answer: In this situation, the wrong dose of epinephrine, which could be lethal, is being administered to the patient. IV epinephrine must be diluted to a concentration of 1:10,000 (0.1 mg/mL). In an emergency situation, it is easy to pick up the concentration of epinephrine that is intended for intramuscular or subcutaneous use. Labeling on these preparations should include "Not for IV Use" because there is not time to calculate dosage and dilute the solution in an emergency.

REVIEW AND APPLICATION EXERCISES

1. How do adrenergic drugs act to relieve symptoms of acute bronchospasm, anaphylaxis, cardiac arrest, hypotension and shock, and nasal congestion?

2. Which adrenergic receptors are stimulated by administration of epinephrine?

3. Why is it important to have epinephrine and other adrenergic drugs readily available in all health care settings?

4. Which adrenergic drug is the drug of choice to treat acute anaphylactic reactions?

5. Why is inhaled epinephrine not a drug of choice for long-term treatment of asthma and other bronchoconstrictive disorders?

6. What are the major adverse effects of adrenergic drugs?

7. Why are clients with cardiac arrhythmias, angina pectoris, hypertension, or diabetes mellitus especially likely to experience adverse reactions to adrenergic drugs?

8. For a client who reports frequent use of OTC asthma remedies and cold remedies, what teaching is needed to increase client safety?

9. Mentally rehearse nursing interventions for various emergency situations (anaphylaxis, acute respiratory distress, cardiac arrest) in terms of medications and equipment needed and how to obtain them promptly.

10. What signs and symptoms occur with overdose of noncatecholamine adrenergic drugs? What interventions are needed to treat the toxicity?

SELECTED REFERENCES

DiPiro, J.T. & Stafford, C.T. (1997). Allergic and pseudoallergic drug reactions. In J.T. DiPiro, R.L. Talbert, G.C. Yee, G.R. Matzke, B.G. Wells, & L.M. Posey (Eds.), *Pharmacotherapy: A pathophysiologic approach*, 3rd ed., pp. 1675–1688. Stamford, CT: Appleton & Lange.

Drug facts and comparisons. (Updated monthly). St. Louis: Facts and Comparisons.

Ganong, W.F. (1997). *Review of medical physiology*, 18th ed. Stamford, CT: Appleton & Lange.

Hoffman, B.B. & Lefkowitz, R.J. (1996). Catecholamines, sympathomimetic drugs, and adrenergic receptor antagonists. In J.G. Hardman, L.E. Limbird, P.B. Molinoff, & R.W. Ruddon (Eds.), *Goodman and Gilman's The pharmacological basis of therapeutics*, 9th ed., pp. 199–248. New York: McGraw-Hill.

Jones, L.A. (1997). Pharmacotherapy of cardiopulmonary resuscitation. In J.T. DiPiro, R.L. Talbert, G.C Yee, G.R. Matzke, B.G. Wells, & L.M. Posey (Eds.), *Pharmacotherapy: A pathophysiologic approach*, 3rd ed., pp. 181–193. Stamford, CT: Appleton & Lange.

Kelly, H.W. & Kamada, A.K. (1997). Asthma. In J.T. DiPiro, R.L. Talbert, G.C Yee, G.R. Matzke, B.G. Wells, & L.M. Posey (Eds.), *Pharmacotherapy: A pathophysiologic approach*, 3rd ed., pp. 553–590. Stamford, CT: Appleton & Lange.

Lefkowitz, R.J., Hoffman, B.B., & Taylor, P. (1996). Neurotransmission: The autonomic and somatic motor nervous systems. In J.G. Hardman, L.E. Limbird, P.B. Molinoff, & R.W. Ruddon (Eds.), *Goodman and Gilman's The pharmacological basis of therapeutics*, 9th ed., pp. 105–139. New York: McGraw-Hill.

Olson, K.R. (Ed.). (1999). *Poisoning and drug overdose*. 3rd ed. Stamford, CT: Appleton & Lange.

19

Antiadrenergic Drugs

Objectives

After studying this chapter, the student will be able to:

1. List characteristics of antiadrenergic drugs in terms of effects on body tissues, indications for use, nursing process implications, principles of therapy, and observation of client response.

2. Discuss alpha$_1$-adrenergic blocking agents and alpha$_2$-adrenergic agonists in terms of indications for use, adverse effects, and selected other characteristics.

3. Compare and contrast beta-adrenergic blocking agents in terms of cardioselectivity, indications for use, adverse effects, and selected other characteristics.

4. Teach clients about safe, effective use of antiadrenergic drugs.

5. Discuss principles of therapy and nursing process for using antiadrenergic drugs in special populations.

Joe Moore, 56 years of age, comes to the clinic with complaints of chest pain with exertion. His vital signs are B/P 194/88, pulse 92, respiration 18. His primary provider prescribes a selective beta blocker, atenolol (Tenormin), and schedules a follow-up visit in 2 weeks.

Reflect on:

▶ Why a beta blocker is ordered for this patient.

▶ What are the advantages of using a selective rather that a nonselective beta blocker?

▶ What side effects are likely when a patient is started on atenolol?

▶ Describe a teaching plan for this patient.

DESCRIPTION

Antiadrenergic or sympatholytic drugs decrease or block the effects of sympathetic nerve stimulation, endogenous catecholamines (eg, epinephrine), and adrenergic drugs. The drugs are chemically diverse and have a wide spectrum of pharmacologic activity, with specific effects depending mainly on the client's health status when a drug is given and the drug's binding with particular adrenergic receptors. Included here are clonidine and related centrally active antiadrenergic drugs, which are used primarily in the treatment of hypertension, and peripherally active agents (alpha- and beta-adrenergic blocking agents), which are used to treat various cardiovascular and other disorders. A few uncommonly used antiadrenergic drugs for hypertension are included in Chapter 55.

A basal level of sympathetic tone is necessary to maintain normal body functioning, including regulation of blood pressure, blood glucose, and stress response. Therefore, the goal of antiadrenergic drug therapy is to suppress pathologic stimulation, not the normal, physiologic response to activity, stress, and other stimuli.

Mechanisms of Action and Effects

Most antiadrenergic drugs have antagonist (blocking) effects in which they combine with $alpha_1$, $beta_1$, $beta_2$, or a combination of receptors in peripheral tissues and prevent adrenergic (sympathomimetic) effects. Clonidine and related drugs have agonist effects at presynaptic $alpha_2$ receptors in the brain. This means that some of the norepinephrine released by the presynaptic nerve cell into the synapse returns to the presynaptic site and activates $alpha_2$ receptors. This results in a negative feedback type of mechanism that decreases the release of additional norepinephrine. Thus, the overall effect is decreased sympathetic outflow from the brain and antiadrenergic effects on peripheral tissues (ie, decreased activation of alpha and beta receptors by norepinephrine throughout the body).

Alpha-Adrenergic Agonists and Blocking Agents

Alpha$_2$-adrenergic agonists inhibit the release of norepinephrine in the brain, thereby decreasing the effects of sympathetic nervous system stimulation throughout the body. A major clinical effect is decreased blood pressure. Although clinical effects are attributed mainly to drug action at presynaptic $alpha_2$ receptors in the brain, postsynaptic $alpha_2$ receptors in the brain and peripheral tissues (eg, vascular smooth muscle) may also be involved. Activation of $alpha_2$ receptors in the pancreatic islets suppresses insulin secretion.

Alpha$_1$-adrenergic blocking agents occupy $alpha_1$-adrenergic receptor sites in smooth muscles and glands innervated by sympathetic nerve fibers. These drugs act primarily in the skin, mucosa, intestines, and kidneys to prevent alpha-mediated vasoconstriction. Specific effects include dilation of arterioles and veins, increased local blood flow, decreased blood pressure, constriction of pupils, and increased motility of the gastrointestinal tract. Alpha-adrenergic antagonists may activate reflexes that oppose the fall in blood pressure by increasing heart rate and cardiac output and causing fluid retention.

The drugs also can prevent alpha-mediated contraction of smooth muscle in nonvascular tissues. For example, benign prostatic hyperplasia (BPH) is characterized by obstructed urine flow because the enlarged prostate gland presses on the urethra. The drugs can decrease urinary retention and improve urine flow by inhibiting contraction of muscles in the prostate and urinary bladder.

Nonselective alpha-adrenergic blocking agents occupy peripheral $alpha_1$ receptors to cause vasodilation and $alpha_2$ receptors to cause cardiac stimulation. Consequently, decreased blood pressure is accompanied by tachycardia and perhaps other arrhythmias.

Beta-Adrenergic Blocking Drugs

Beta-adrenergic blocking agents occupy beta-adrenergic receptor sites and prevent the receptors from responding to sympathetic nerve impulses, circulating catecholamines, and beta-adrenergic drugs (Fig. 19-1). Specific effects include:

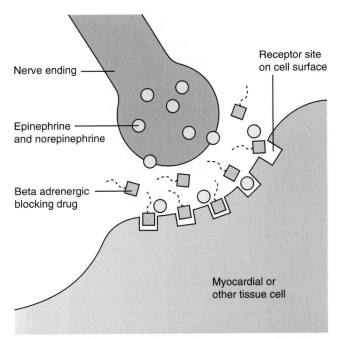

FIGURE 19-1 Beta-adrenergic blocking agents prevent epinephrine and norepinephrine from occupying receptor sites on cell membranes. This action alters cell functions normally stimulated by epinephrine and norepinephrine, according to the number of receptor sites occupied by the beta-blocking drugs. (Adapted by J. Harley from *Encyclopedia Britannica Medical and Health Annual.* [1983]. Chicago, Encyclopedia Britannica.)

1. Decreased heart rate (negative chronotropy)
2. Decreased force of myocardial contraction (negative inotropy)
3. Decreased cardiac output at rest and with exercise
4. Slowed conduction through the atrioventricular (AV) node
5. Decreased automaticity of ectopic pacemakers
6. Decreased blood pressure in supine and standing positions
7. Bronchoconstriction from blockade of beta$_2$ receptors in bronchial smooth muscle. This effect occurs primarily in people with asthma or other chronic lung diseases.
8. Less effective metabolism of glucose (decreased glycogenolysis) when needed by the body, especially in people taking beta-blocking agents along with antidiabetic drugs. These clients may experience more severe and prolonged hypoglycemia. In addition, early symptoms of hypoglycemia (eg, tachycardia) may be blocked, delaying recognition of the hypoglycemia.

Indications for Use

Alpha-Adrenergic Agonists and Blocking Agents

Alpha$_2$ agonists are used in the treatment of hypertension. Clonidine has been tested for numerous other indications, including treatment of alcohol withdrawal and opioid dependence, treatment of drug-induced akathisia, tic disorders, and attention deficit-hyperactivity disorder, but is not approved by the Food and Drug Administration (FDA) for these purposes. Alpha$_1$-adrenergic blocking agents are used in the treatment of hypertension and BPH. Nonselective alpha-blocking agents are not used as antihypertensive drugs except in hypertension caused by excessive catecholamines. Excessive catecholamines may result from overdosage of adrenergic drugs or from pheochromocytoma, a rare tumor of the adrenal medulla that secretes epinephrine and norepinephrine and causes hypertension, tachycardia, and cardiac arrhythmias. Although the treatment of choice for pheochromocytoma is surgical excision, alpha-adrenergic blocking drugs are useful adjuncts. They are given before and during surgery, usually in conjunction with beta blockers. Alpha blockers also are used in vascular diseases characterized by vasospasm, such as Raynaud's disease and frostbite, in which they improve blood flow. Phentolamine also can be used to prevent tissue necrosis from extravasation of potent vasoconstrictors (eg, norepinephrine, dopamine) into subcutaneous tissues.

Beta-Adrenergic Blocking Drugs

Clinical indications for use of beta-blocking agents are mainly cardiovascular disorders (ie, angina pectoris, cardiac tachyarrhythmias, hypertension, and myocardial infarction) and glaucoma. In angina, beta blockers decrease myocardial contractility, cardiac output, heart rate, and blood pressure. These effects decrease myocardial oxygen demand (cardiac workload), especially in response to activity, exercise, and stress. In arrhythmias, drug effects depend on the sympathetic tone of the heart (ie, the degree of adrenergic stimulation of the heart that the drug must block or overcome). The drugs slow the sinus rate and prolong conduction through the AV node, thereby slowing the ventricular response rate to supraventricular tachyarrhythmias.

In hypertension, the actions by which the drugs lower blood pressure are unclear. Possible mechanisms include reduced cardiac output, inhibition of renin, and inhibition of sympathetic nervous system stimulation in the brain. However, the drugs effective in hypertension do not consistently demonstrate these effects—in other words, a drug may lower blood pressure without reducing cardiac output or inhibiting renin, for example. After myocardial infarction, the drugs help protect the heart from reinfarction and decrease mortality rates over several years. A possible mechanism is preventing or decreasing the incidence of catecholamine-induced arrhythmias.

In glaucoma, the drugs reduce intraocular pressure by binding to beta-adrenergic receptors in the ciliary body of the eye and decreasing formation of aqueous humor.

Propranolol (Inderal) is the prototype of beta-adrenergic blocking agents. It is also the oldest and most extensively studied beta blocker. In addition to its use in the treatment of hypertension, arrhythmias, angina pectoris, and myocardial infarction, propranolol is used in hypertrophic obstructive cardiomyopathies, in which it improves exercise tolerance; pheochromocytoma, in which it decreases tachycardia and arrhythmias but must be used along with an alpha-adrenergic blocking agent; hyperthyroidism, in which it decreases heart rate, cardiac output, and tremor; and prevention of migraine headaches by an unknown mechanism (it is not helpful in acute attacks of migraine). The drug also relieves palpitation and tremor associated with anxiety, but it is not approved for clinical use as an antianxiety drug.

Contraindications to Use

Alpha$_2$ agonists are contraindicated in clients with hypersensitivity to the drugs, and methyldopa is also contraindicated in clients with active liver disease. Alpha-adrenergic blocking agents are contraindicated in angina pectoris, myocardial infarction, and stroke. Beta-adrenergic blocking agents are contraindicated in bradycardia, heart block, and asthma and other allergic or pulmonary conditions characterized by bronchoconstriction. Although new research has shown that beta blockers can be beneficial to clients with mild to moderate chronic heart failure, the drugs have not been proven safe for people older than 80 years of age or those with severe heart failure.

INDIVIDUAL ANTIADRENERGIC DRUGS

These drugs are described in the following sections; trade names, clinical indications, and dosage ranges are listed in Tables 19-1 and 19-2.

Alpha-Adrenergic Agonists and Blocking Agents

Alpha$_2$-adrenergic agonists include clonidine, guanabenz, guanfacine, and methyldopa. These drugs produce similar therapeutic and adverse effects but differ in their pharmacokinetics and frequency of administration. Oral **clonidine** reduces blood pressure within 1 hour, reaches peak plasma levels in 3 to 5 hours, and has a plasma half-life of

TABLE 19-1 Alpha-Adrenergic Agonists and Blocking Agents

Generic/Trade Name	Clinical Indications	Routes and Dosage Ranges
Alpha$_2$-Agonists		
Clonidine (Catapres)	Hypertension	PO 0.1 mg 2 times daily initially, gradually increased if necessary. Average maintenance dose, 0.2–0.8 mg/d. Transdermal 0.1-mg patch every 7 d initially; increase every 7–14 d to 0.2 mg or 0.3 mg if necessary. Maximum dose, two 0.3-mg patches every 7 d.
Guanabenz (Wytensin)	Hypertension	PO 4 mg twice daily, increased by 4–8 mg/d every 1–2 wk if necessary to a maximal dose of 32 mg twice daily.
Guanfacine (Tenex)	Hypertension	PO 1 mg daily at bedtime, increased to 2 mg after 3–4 wk, then to 3 mg if necessary.
Methyldopa (Aldomet)	Hypertension	*Adults:* PO 250 mg 2 or 3 times daily initially, increased gradually at intervals of not less than 2 d until blood pressure is controlled or a daily dose of 3 g is reached. *Children:* PO 10 mg/kg/d in 2 to 4 divided doses initially, increased or decreased according to response. Maximal dose, 65 mg/kg/d or 3 g daily, whichever is less.
Alpha$_1$-Blocking Agents		
Doxazosin (Cardura)	Hypertension BPH	PO 1 mg once daily initially, increased to 2 mg, then to 4, 8, and 16 mg if necessary.
Prazosin (Minipress)	Hypertension BPH	PO 1 mg 2 to 3 times daily initially, increased if necessary to a total daily dose of 20 mg in divided doses. Average maintenance dose, 6–15 mg/d.
Tamsulosin HCl (Flomax)	BPH	PO 0.4 mg/d after same meal each day. Dose may be increased if needed after 2–4 wk trial period.
Terazosin (Hytrin)	Hypertension BPH	PO 1 mg at bedtime initially, increased gradually to maintenance dose, usually 1–5 mg once daily
Nonselective Alpha-Blocking Agents		
Phenoxybenzamine (Dibenzyline)	Hypertension caused by pheochromocytoma Raynaud's disorder Frostbite	PO 10 mg daily initially, gradually increased by 10 mg every 4 d until therapeutic effects are obtained or adverse effects become intolerable; optimum dosage level usually reached in 2 wk; usual maintenance dose 20–60 mg/d
Phentolamine (Regitine)	Hypertension caused by pheochromocytoma Prevention of tissue necrosis from extravasation of vasoconstrictive drugs	*Before and during surgery for pheochromocytoma:* IV, IM 5–20 mg as needed to control blood pressure *Prevention of tissue necrosis:* IV 10 mg in each liter of IV solution containing a potent vasoconstrictor *Treatment of extravasation:* SC 5–10 mg in 10 mL saline, infiltrated into the area within 12 h

BPH, benign prostatic hyperplasia; IM, intramuscular; IV, intravenous; PO, oral; SC, subcutaneous.

TABLE 19-2 **Beta-Adrenergic Blocking Agents**

Generic/Trade Name	Clinical Indications	Routes and Dosage Ranges
Nonselective Blocking Agents		
Carteolol (Cartrol, Ocupress)	Hypertension Glaucoma	PO: Initially, 2.5 mg once daily, gradually increased to a maximum daily dose of 10 mg if necessary. Usual maintenance dose, 2.5–5 mg once daily. Extend dosage interval to 48 h for a creatinine clearance of 20–60 mL/min and to 72 h for a creatinine clearance below 20 mL/min.
Levobunolol (Betagan)	Glaucoma	Topically to affected eye, 1 drop twice daily
Metipranolol (OptiPranolol)	Glaucoma	Topically to each eye, 1 drop once or twice daily
Penbutolol (Levatol)	Hypertension	PO 20 mg once daily
Propranolol (Inderal)	Hypertension	PO 40 mg twice daily initially, may be increased to 120–240 mg daily in divided doses Sustained release capsules, PO 80 mg once daily, may be increased to 120–160 mg once daily Maximal daily dose, 640 mg
	Angina pectoris	PO 80–320 mg in two to four divided doses Sustained release, PO 80–160 mg once daily Maximal daily dose, 320 mg
	Dysrhythmias	PO 10–30 mg, q6–8h Life-threatening dysrhythmias, IV 1–3 mg at a rate not to exceed 1 mg/min with electrocardiographic and blood-pressure monitoring
	Myocardial infarction	PO 180–240 mg daily in three or four divided doses Maximal daily dose, 240 mg
	Hypertrophic subaortic stenosis	PO 20–40 mg daily in three or four divided doses Sustained release, PO 80–160 mg once daily
	Migraine prophylaxis	PO 80–240 mg daily in divided doses Sustained release, PO 80 mg once daily
Nadolol (Corgard)	Hypertension Angina pectoris	Hypertension, PO 40 mg once daily initially, gradually increased. Usual daily maintenance dose, 80–320 mg Angina, PO 40 mg once daily initially, increased by 40–80 mg at 3- to 7-d intervals. Usual daily maintenance dose, 80–240 mg
Pindolol (Visken)	Hypertension	PO 5 mg twice daily initially, increased by 10 mg every 3–4 wk, to a maximal daily dose of 60 mg
Sotalol (Betapace)	Cardiac arrhythmias	PO 80–160 mg twice daily
Timolol (Blocadren, Timoptic)	Hypertension Myocardial infarction Glaucoma	Hypertension, PO 10 mg twice daily initially, increased at 7-d intervals to a maximum of 60 mg/d in 2 divided doses; usual maintenance dose, 20–40 mg daily Myocardial infarction, PO 10 mg twice daily Glaucoma, topically to eye, 1 drop of 0.25% or 0.5% solution (Timoptic) in each eye twice daily
Cardioselective Blocking Agents		
Acebutolol (Sectral)	Hypertension Ventricular arrhythmias	Hypertension, PO 400 mg daily in 1 or 2 doses; usual maintenance dose, 400–800 mg daily Arrhythmias, PO 400 mg daily in 2 divided doses; usual maintenance dose, 600–1200 mg daily
Atenolol (Tenormin)	Hypertension Angina pectoris Myocardial infarction	Hypertension, PO 50–100 mg daily Angina, PO 50–100 mg daily, increased to 200 mg daily if necessary Myocardial infarction, IV 5 mg over 5 min, then 5 mg 10 min later, then 50 mg PO 10 min later, then 50 mg 12 h later. Thereafter, PO 100 mg daily, in 1 or 2 doses, for 6–9 d or until discharge from hospital
Betaxolol (Betoptic, Kerlone)	Glaucoma Hypertension	Topically to each eye, 1 drop twice daily Hypertension, PO 10–20 mg daily
Bisoprolol (Zebeta)	Hypertension	PO 5–20 mg once daily
Esmolol (Brevibloc)	Supraventricular tachyarrhythmias	IV 50–200 μg/kg per minute; average dose, 100 μg/kg per minute, titrated to effect with close monitoring of client's condition
Metoprolol (Lopressor)	Hypertension Myocardial infarction	Hypertension, PO 100 mg daily in single or divided doses, increased at 7-d or longer intervals; usual maintenance dose, 100–450 mg/d Myocardial infarction, early treatment, IV 5 mg every 2 min for total of 3 doses (15 mg), then 50 mg PO q6h for 48 h, then 100 mg PO twice daily. Myocardial infarction, late treatment, PO 100 mg twice daily, at least 3 months, up to 1–3 y

TABLE 19-2	**Beta-Adrenergic Blocking Agents (*continued*)**	
Generic/Trade Name	Clinical Indications	Routes and Dosage Ranges
Alpha–Beta-blocking Agents **Carvedilol** (Coreg)	Hypertension	PO 6.25 mg twice daily for 7–14 d, then increase to 12.5 mg twice daily if necessary for 7–14 d, then increase to 25 mg twice daily if necessary (maximum dose).
Labetalol (Trandate, Normodyne)	Hypertension, including hypertensive emergencies	PO 100 mg twice daily IV 20 mg over 2 min then 40–80 mg every 10 min until desired blood pressure achieved or 300 mg given IV infusion 2 mg/min (eg, add 200 mg of drug to 250 mL 5% dextrose solution for a 2 mg/3 mL concentration)

IV, intravenous; PO, oral.

approximately 12 to 16 hours (longer with renal impairment). Approximately half the oral dose is metabolized in the liver; the remainder is excreted unchanged in urine. With transdermal clonidine, therapeutic plasma levels are reached in 2 to 3 days and last 1 week. **Guanabenz** action occurs within 1 hour, peaks within 2 to 4 hours, and lasts 6 to 8 hours. It is metabolized extensively; very little unchanged drug is excreted in urine. **Guanfacine** is well absorbed and widely distributed, with approximately 70% bound to plasma proteins. Peak plasma levels occur in 1 to 4 hours and the half-life is 10 to 30 hours. Approximately half is metabolized and the metabolites and unchanged drug are excreted in urine. Because of its longer half-life, guanfacine can be given once daily. **Methyldopa** is an older drug with low to moderate absorption, peak plasma levels in 2 to 4 hours, and peak antihypertensive effects in approximately 2 days. When discontinued, blood pressure rises in approximately 2 days. Intravenous administration reduces blood pressure in 4 to 6 hours and lasts 10 to 16 hours. Methyldopa is metabolized to some extent in the liver but is largely excreted in urine. In clients with renal impairment, blood pressure–lowering effects may be pronounced and prolonged because of slower excretion. In addition to the adverse effects that occur with all these drugs, methyldopa also may cause hemolytic anemia and hepatotoxicity (eg, jaundice, hepatitis).

Alpha₁-adrenergic antagonists include doxazosin, prazosin, terazosin, and tamsulosin. **Prazosin**, the prototype, is well absorbed after oral administration and reaches peak plasma concentrations in 1 to 3 hours; action lasts approximately 4 to 6 hours. The drug is highly bound to plasma proteins and the plasma half-life is approximately 2 to 3 hours. It is extensively metabolized in the liver and its metabolites are excreted by the kidneys. **Doxazosin** and **terazosin** are similar to prazosin but have longer half-lives (doxazosin, 10 to 20 hours; terazosin, approximately 12 hours) and durations of action (doxazosin, up to 36 hours; terazosin, 18 hours or longer). Prazosin must be taken in multiple doses; doxazosin and terazosin may usually be taken once daily to control hypertension.

Tamsulosin is the first alpha₁ antagonist designed specifically to treat BPH. It blocks alpha₁ receptors in the male genitourinary system, producing smooth muscle relaxation in the prostate gland and bladder neck. Urinary flow rate is improved and symptoms of BPH are reduced. Because of the specificity of tamsulosin for receptors in the genitourinary system, this drug causes less orthostatic hypotension than other alpha₁ antagonists. After oral administration, greater than 90% of tamsulosin is absorbed. Administration with food decreases bioavailability by 30%. Tamsulosin is highly protein bound and is metabolized by the liver; approximately 10% of the drug is excreted unchanged in the urine. An advantage of tamsulosin is the ability to start the drug at the recommended dosage. Most of the alpha₁ antagonists must be gradually increased to the recommended dosage. Common side effects include abnormal ejaculation and dizziness.

Nonselective alpha-adrenergic blocking agents include phenoxybenzamine and phentolamine. **Phenoxybenzamine** is long acting; effects of a single dose persist for 3 to 4 days. **Phentolamine** is similar to phenoxybenzamine but more useful clinically. Phentolamine is short acting; effects last only a few hours and can be reversed by an alpha-adrenergic stimulant drug, such as norepinephrine (Levophed).

Beta-Adrenergic Blocking Drugs

Numerous beta-blocking agents are marketed in the United States. Although they produce similar effects, they differ in several characteristics, including clinical indications for use, receptor selectivity, intrinsic sympathomimetic activity, membrane-stabilizing ability, lipid solubility, routes of excretion, routes of administration, and duration of action.

Clinical Indications

Most beta blockers are approved for the treatment of hypertension. A beta blocker may be used alone or with another antihypertensive drug, such as a diuretic. Labetalol is also approved for treatment of hypertensive emergencies. Atenolol, metoprolol, nadolol, and propranolol are approved as antianginal agents; acebutolol, esmolol, propranolol, and sotalol are approved as antiarrhythmic agents. Atenolol, metoprolol, propranolol, and timolol are used to prevent myocardial infarction or reinfarction. Betaxolol, carteolol, and timolol (Timoptic) are used for hypertension and glaucoma; levobunolol and metipranolol are used only for glaucoma.

Beta blockers have traditionally been considered contraindicated in clients with heart failure because of their ability to decrease cardiac function. A growing number of studies, however, are showing that beta blockers are useful not only in the treatment of mild to moderate cases of chronic heart failure, but in reducing the risk of sudden death in these clients. The only beta blocker approved by the FDA to treat heart failure is carvedilol. Treatment should begin with a low dose of the beta blocker, administered concurrently with an angiotensin-converting enzyme (ACE) inhibitor. The purpose of the ACE inhibitor is to counteract any initial worsening of the heart failure symptoms due to beta blocker therapy. It is unclear exactly how beta blockers benefit clients with heart failure. Possible mechanisms of action include blockade of the damaging effects of sympathetic stimulation on the heart, beta receptor up-regulation, decreased sympathetic stimulation due to decreased plasma norepinephrine and antiarrhythmic effects, and improved diastolic function by lengthening diastolic filling time.

Receptor Selectivity

Carteolol, levobunolol, metipranolol, penbutolol, nadolol, pindolol, propranolol, sotalol, and timolol are nonselective beta blockers. The term *nonselective* indicates that the drugs block both beta$_1$ (cardiac) and beta$_2$ (mainly smooth muscle in the bronchi and blood vessels) receptors. Blockade of beta$_2$ receptors is associated with adverse effects such as bronchoconstriction, peripheral vasoconstriction, and interference with glycogenolysis.

Acebutolol, atenolol, betaxolol, bisoprolol, esmolol, and metoprolol are cardioselective agents, which means they have more effect on beta$_1$ receptors than on beta$_2$ receptors. As a result, they may cause less bronchospasm, less impairment of glucose metabolism, and less peripheral vascular insufficiency. These drugs are preferred when beta blockers are needed by clients with asthma or other bronchospastic pulmonary disorders, diabetes mellitus, or peripheral vascular disorders. However, cardioselectivity is lost at higher doses because most organs have both beta$_1$ and beta$_2$ receptors rather than one or the other exclusively.

Labetalol and carvedilol block alpha$_1$ receptors to cause vasodilation and beta$_1$ and beta$_2$ receptors to cause all the effects of the nonselective agents. Both alpha- and beta-adrenergic blocking actions contribute to antihypertensive effects, but it is unclear whether these drugs have any definite advantage over other beta blockers. They may cause less bradycardia but more postural hypotension than other beta-blocking agents, and they may cause less reflex tachycardia than other vasodilators.

Intrinsic Sympathomimetic Activity

Drugs with this characteristic (ie, acebutolol, carteolol, penbutolol, and pindolol) have a chemical structure similar to that of catecholamines. As a result, they can block some beta receptors and stimulate others. Consequently, these drugs are less likely to cause bradycardia and may be useful for clients experiencing bradycardia with other beta-blockers.

Membrane-Stabilizing Activity

Several beta blockers have a membrane-stabilizing effect sometimes described as quinidine-like (ie, producing myocardial depression). Because the doses required to produce this effect are much higher than those used for therapeutic effects, this characteristic is considered clinically insignificant.

Lipid Solubility

The more lipid-soluble beta blockers were thought to penetrate the central nervous system (CNS) more extensively and cause adverse effects, such as confusion, depression, hallucinations, and insomnia. Some clinicians state that this characteristic is important only in terms of drug usage and excretion in certain disease states. Thus, a water-soluble, renally excreted beta blocker may be preferred in clients with liver disease, and a lipid-soluble, hepatically metabolized drug may be preferred in clients with renal disease.

Routes of Elimination

Most beta-blocking agents are metabolized in the liver. Atenolol, carteolol, nadolol, and an active metabolite of acebutolol are excreted by the kidneys, and dosage must be reduced in the presence of renal failure.

Routes of Administration

Most beta blockers can be given orally. Atenolol, esmolol, labetalol, metoprolol, and propranolol also can be given intravenously, and ophthalmic solutions are applied topically to the eye. Betaxolol, carteolol, and timolol are available in oral and ophthalmic forms.

Duration of Action

Acebutolol, atenolol, bisoprolol, carteolol, penbutolol, and nadolol have long serum half-lives and can usually be given once daily. Carvedilol, labetalol, metoprolol, pindolol, sotalol, and timolol are usually given twice daily. Propranolol required administration several times daily until development of a sustained-release capsule allowed once-daily dosing.

Nursing Notes: Apply Your Knowledge

Ms. Viola Green, 36 years of age, was prescribed propranolol (Inderal) to treat a newly diagnosed mitral valve prolapse. She has been healthy except for multiple allergies and asthma. Ms. Green calls the consulting nurse to report that her asthma has deteriorated since she started on the Inderal and she wonders if she might be allergic to this new medication. How would you advise her?

NURSING PROCESS

Assessment

* Assess the client's condition in relation to disorders in which antiadrenergic drugs are used. Because most of the drugs are used to treat hypertension, assess blood pressure patterns over time, when possible, including antihypertensive drugs used and the response obtained. With other cardiovascular disorders, check blood pressure for elevation and pulse for tachycardia or arrhythmia, and determine the presence or absence of chest pain, migraine headache, or hyperthyroidism. If the client reports or medical records indicate one or more of these disorders, assess for specific signs and symptoms. With BPH, assess for signs and symptoms of urinary retention and difficulty voiding.

* Assess for conditions that contraindicate the use of antiadrenergic drugs.
* Assess vital signs to establish a baseline for later comparisons.
* Assess for use of prescription and nonprescription drugs that are likely to increase or decrease effects of antiadrenergic drugs.
* Assess for lifestyle habits that are likely to increase or decrease effects of antiadrenergic drugs (eg, ingestion of caffeine or nicotine).

Nursing Diagnoses

* Decreased Cardiac Output related to drug-induced postural hypotension (alpha$_2$ agonists, alpha$_1$ and nonselective alpha-blocking agents, and beta blockers) and heart failure (beta blockers)
* Impaired Gas Exchange related to drug-induced bronchoconstriction with beta blockers
* Sexual Dysfunction in men related to impotence and decreased libido
* Fatigue related to decreased cardiac output
* Noncompliance related to adverse drug effects or inadequate understanding of drug regimen
* Risk for Injury related to hypotension, dizziness, sedation
* Knowledge Deficit: Drug effects and safe usage

Planning/Goals

The client will:
* Receive or self-administer drugs accurately

CLIENT TEACHING GUIDELINES
Alpha$_2$ Agonists and Alpha-Blocking Agents

General Considerations

✔ Have your blood pressure checked regularly. Report high or low values to your health care provider.

✔ The adverse reactions of palpitations, weakness, and dizziness usually disappear with continued use. However, they may recur with conditions promoting vasodilation (dosage increase, exercise, high environmental temperatures, ingesting alcohol or a large meal).

✔ To prevent falls and injuries, if the above reactions occur, sit down or lie down immediately and flex arms and legs. Change positions slowly, especially from supine to standing.

✔ Do not drive a car or operate machinery if drowsy or dizzy from medication.

✔ Do not stop the drugs abruptly. Hypertension, possibly severe, may develop.

✔ With methyldopa, report any signs of abdominal pain, nausea, vomiting, diarrhea, or jaundice to your health care provider. Regular blood tests are needed to make sure the medication is working as it should.

✔ Do not take over-the-counter or other medications without the physician's knowledge. Many drugs interact to increase or decrease the effects of antiadrenergic drugs.

Self-administration

✔ Sedation and first-dose syncope may be minimized by taking all or most of the prescribed dose at bedtime.

✔ When using the clonidine transdermal patch, select a hairless area on the upper arm or torso for the application. The patch is changed once a week.

✔ Avoid alcohol use with these medications because excessive drowsiness may occur.

CLIENT TEACHING GUIDELINES
Beta-Blocking Agents

General Considerations

✔ Count your pulse daily and report to a health care provider if under 50 for several days in succession. This information helps to determine if the drug therapy needs to be altered to avoid more serious adverse effects.

✔ Report weight gain (more than 2 pounds within a week), ankle edema, shortness of breath, or excessive fatigue. These are signs of heart failure. If they occur, the drug will be stopped.

✔ Report fainting spells, excessive weakness, or difficulty in breathing. Beta-blocking drugs decrease the usual adaptive responses to exercise or stress. Syncope may result from hypotension, bradycardia, or heart block; its occurrence probably indicates stopping or decreasing the dose of the drug.

✔ Do not stop taking the drugs abruptly. Stopping the drugs suddenly may cause or aggravate chest pain (angina).

✔ Do not take over-the-counter or other medications without the physician's knowledge. Many drugs interact to increase or decrease the effects of beta-blocking agents.

Self-administration

✔ Consistently take the drug at the same time each day with or without food. This maintains consistent therapeutic blood levels.

✔ Do not crush or chew long-acting forms of these medications.

- Experience relief of symptoms for which antiadrenergic drugs are given
- Comply with instructions for safe drug usage
- Avoid stopping antiadrenergic drugs abruptly
- Demonstrate knowledge of adverse drug effects to be reported
- Avoid preventable adverse drug effects
- Keep appointments for blood pressure monitoring and other follow-up activities

Interventions

Use measures to prevent or decrease the need for antiadrenergic drugs. Because the sympathetic nervous system is stimulated by physical and emotional stress, efforts to decrease stress may indirectly decrease the need for drugs to antagonize sympathetic effects. Such efforts may include the following:

- Helping the client stop or decrease cigarette smoking. Nicotine stimulates the CNS and the sympathetic nervous system to cause tremors, tachycardia, and elevated blood pressure.
- Teaching measures to relieve pain, anxiety, and other stresses

- Counseling regarding relaxation techniques
- Helping the client avoid temperature extremes
- Helping the client avoid excessive caffeine in coffee or other beverages
- Helping the client develop a reasonable balance among rest, exercise, work, and recreation
- Recording vital signs at regular intervals in hospitalized clients to monitor for adverse effects
- Helping with activity or ambulation as needed to prevent injury from dizziness

Evaluation

- Observe for decreased blood pressure when antiadrenergic drugs are given for hypertension.
- Interview regarding decreased chest pain when beta blockers are given for angina.
- Interview and observe for signs and symptoms of adverse drug effects (eg, edema, tachycardia with alpha agonists and blocking agents; bradycardia, congestive heart failure, bronchoconstriction with beta blockers).
- Interview regarding knowledge and use of drugs.

How Can You Avoid This Medication Error?

Inderal, 40 mg bid, has been effectively controlling John Morgan's hypertension for 3 years. He is admitted to a medical unit for tests. In the morning he is NPO. The stock supply of intravenous (IV) Inderal provides 1 mg per 0.5 mL. You administer 20 cc of Inderal IV over 5 minutes for his morning dose.

PRINCIPLES OF THERAPY

Alpha-Adrenergic Agonists and Blocking Agents

1. When an alpha$_1$-blocking agent (doxazosin, prazosin, or terazosin) is given for hypertension, "first-dose syncope" may occur from hypotension. This

reaction can be prevented or minimized by starting with a low dose, increasing the dose gradually, and giving the first dose at bedtime. In addition, the decreased blood pressure stimulates reflex mechanisms to raise blood pressure (increase heart rate and cardiac output, fluid retention) so that a diuretic may be needed.

2. A client diagnosed with BPH should be evaluated for prostatic cancer before starting drug therapy, because the signs and symptoms of the two conditions are similar. The two conditions may also coexist.

3. When an alpha$_2$ agonist is given for hypertension, it is very important not to stop the drug abruptly because of the risk of rebound hypertension. To discontinue clonidine, for example, the dose should be gradually reduced over 2 to 4 days.

4. When phenoxybenzamine is given on a long-term basis, dosage must be carefully individualized. Because the drug is long acting and accumulates in the body, dosage is small initially and gradually increased at intervals of approximately 4 days. Several weeks may be required for full therapeutic benefit, and drug effects persist for several days after the drug is discontinued. If circulatory shock develops from overdosage or hypersensitivity, norepinephrine (Levophed) can be given to overcome the blockade of alpha-adrenergic receptors in arterioles and to raise blood pressure. Epinephrine is contraindicated because it stimulates both alpha- and beta-adrenergic receptors, resulting in increased vasodilation and hypotension.

Beta-Adrenergic Blocking Drugs

1. For most people, a nonselective beta blocker that can be taken once or twice daily is acceptable. For others, the choice of a beta-blocking agent depends largely on the client's condition and response to the drugs. For example, cardioselective drugs are preferred for clients with pulmonary disorders and diabetes mellitus; a drug with intrinsic sympathomimetic activity may be preferred for those who experience significant bradycardia with beta blockers lacking this property.

2. Dosage of beta-blocking agents must be individualized because of wide variations in plasma levels from comparable doses. Variations are attributed to initial metabolism in the liver, the extent of binding to plasma proteins, and the degree of beta-adrenergic stimulation that the drugs must overcome. In general, low doses should be used initially and increased gradually until therapeutic or adverse effects occur. Adequacy of dosage or extent of beta blockade can be assessed by determining whether the heart rate increases in response to exercise.

3. When a beta blocker is used to prevent myocardial infarction, it should be started as soon as the client is hemodynamically stable after a definite or suspected acute myocardial infarction. The drug should be continued for at least 2 years.

4. Beta-blocking drugs should not be discontinued abruptly. Long-term blockade of beta-adrenergic receptors increases the receptors' sensitivity to epinephrine and norepinephrine when the drugs are discontinued. There is a risk of severe hypertension, angina, arrhythmias, and myocardial infarction from the increased or excessive sympathetic nervous system stimulation. Thus, dosage should be tapered and gradually discontinued to allow beta-adrenergic receptors to return to predrug density and sensitivity. An optimal tapering period has not been defined. Some authorities recommend 1 to 2 weeks; others recommend reducing dosage over approximately 10 days to 30 mg/day of propranolol (or an equivalent amount of other drugs) and continuing this amount at least 2 weeks before the drug is stopped completely.

5. Opinions differ regarding use of beta blockers before anesthesia and major surgery. On the one hand, the drugs block arrhythmogenic properties of some general inhalation anesthetics; on the other hand, there is a risk of excessive myocardial depression. If feasible, the drug may be tapered gradually and discontinued (at least 48 hours) before surgery. If the drug is continued, the lowest effective dosage should be given. If emergency surgery is necessary, the effects of beta blockers can be reversed by administration of beta receptor stimulants, such as dobutamine or isoproterenol.

6. Various drugs may be used to treat adverse effects of beta blockers. Atropine can be given for bradycardia, digoxin and diuretics for heart failure, vasopressors for hypotension, and bronchodilator drugs for bronchoconstriction.

Genetic or Ethnic Considerations

Most studies involve adults with hypertension and compare drug therapy responses between African Americans and whites. Findings indicate that monotherapy with alpha$_1$ blockers and combined alpha and beta blockers is equally effective in the two groups. However, monotherapy with beta blockers is less effective in African Americans than in whites. When beta blockers are used in African Americans, they should usually be part of a multidrug treatment regimen, and higher doses may be required. In addition, labetalol, an alpha and beta blocker, has been shown to be more effective in the African-American population than propranolol, timolol, or metoprolol.

Several studies indicate that Asians achieve higher blood levels of beta blockers with given doses and in general need much smaller doses than whites. This increased sensitivity to the drugs may result from slower metabolism and excretion.

Use in Children

Alpha-adrenergic agonists and blocking agents have not been established as safe and effective in children.

Beta-adrenergic blocking agents are used in children for disorders similar to those occurring in adults. However, safety and effectiveness have not been established, and manufacturers of most of the drugs do not recommend pediatric use or doses. The drugs are probably contraindicated in young children with resting heart rates below 60 beats per minute.

When a beta blocker is given, general guidelines include the following:

1. Dosage should be adjusted for body weight.
2. Monitor responses closely. Children are more sensitive to adverse drug effects than adults.
3. If given to infants (up to 1 year of age) with immature liver function, blood levels may be higher and accumulation is more likely even when doses are based on weight.
4. When monitoring responses, remember that heart rate and blood pressure vary among children according to age and level of growth and development. They also differ from those of adults.
5. Children are more likely to have asthma than adults. Thus, they may be at greater risk of drug-induced bronchoconstriction.

Propranolol is probably the most frequently used beta blocker in children. Intravenous administration is not recommended. The drug is given orally for hypertension, and dosage should be individualized. The usual dosage range is 2 to 4 mg/kg/day in two equal doses. Dosage calculated from body surface area is not recommended because of excessive blood levels of drug and greater risk of toxicity. As with adults, dosage should be tapered gradually over 1 to 3 weeks. The drug should not be stopped abruptly.

Use in Older Adults

Alpha$_2$-adrenergic agonists (clonidine and related drugs) may be used to treat hypertension in older adults; alpha$_1$-adrenergic antagonists (prazosin and related drugs) may be used to treat hypertension and BPH. Dosage of these drugs should be reduced because older adults are more likely to experience adverse drug effects, especially with impaired renal or hepatic function. As with other populations, these drugs should not be stopped suddenly. Instead, they should be tapered in dosage and discontinued gradually, over 1 to 2 weeks.

Beta-adrenergic blocking agents are commonly used in older adults for angina, arrhythmias, hypertension, and glaucoma. With hypertension, beta blockers are not recommended for monotherapy because older adults may be less responsive than younger adults. Thus, the drugs are probably most useful as second drugs (with diuretics) in clients who require multidrug therapy and clients who also have angina pectoris or another disorder for which a beta blocker is indicated.

Whatever the circumstances for using beta blockers in older adults, use them cautiously and monitor responses closely. Older adults are likely to have disorders that place them at high risk of adverse drug effects, such as heart failure and other cardiovascular conditions, renal or hepatic impairment, and chronic pulmonary disease. Thus, they may experience bradycardia, bronchoconstriction, and hypotension to a greater degree than younger adults. Dosage usually should be reduced because of decreased hepatic blood flow and subsequent slowing of drug metabolism. As with administration in other populations, beta blockers should be tapered in dosage and discontinued over 1 to 3 weeks to avoid myocardial ischemia and other potentially serious adverse cardiovascular effects.

Use in Renal Impairment

Centrally acting alpha$_2$ agonists such as clonidine, guanabenz, and methyldopa are eliminated by a combination of liver metabolism and renal excretion. Renal impairment may result in slower excretion of these medications with subsequent accumulation and increased adverse effects.

Alpha$_1$-adrenergic antagonists such as prazosin, terazosin, doxazosin, and tamsulosin are eliminated primarily by liver metabolism and biliary excretion. Therefore, renal impairment is not a contraindication to use of these medications.

Many beta blockers are eliminated primarily in the urine and pose potentially serious problems for the client with renal failure. In renal failure, the dosage of acebutolol, atenolol, carteolol, and nadolol must be reduced because they are eliminated mainly through the kidneys. The dosage of acebutolol and nadolol should be reduced if creatinine clearance is under 50 mL/minute; the dosage of atenolol should be decreased if the creatinine clearance is under 35 mL/minute. With carteolol, the same amount is given per dose, but the interval between doses is extended to 48 hours for a creatinine clearance of 20 to 60 mL/minute and to 72 hours for a creatinine clearance below 20 mL/minute.

Use in Liver Impairment

Caution must be used when administering centrally acting alpha$_2$-adrenergic agonists such as clonidine, guanabenz, and methyldopa to clients with liver impairment.

These medications rely on hepatic metabolism as well as renal elimination to clear the body. Furthermore, methyldopa has been associated with liver disorders such as hepatitis and hepatic necrosis.

Alpha$_1$-adrenergic medications such as prazosin, terazosin, doxazosin, and tamsulosin rely heavily on liver metabolism and biliary excretion to clear the body. Liver impairment may result in increased drug levels and adverse effects. In the presence of hepatic disease (eg, cirrhosis) or impaired blood flow to the liver (eg, reduced cardiac output from any cause), dosage of some beta blockers such as propranolol, metoprolol, and timolol should be substantially reduced because these drugs are extensively metabolized in the liver. The use of atenolol or nadolol is preferred in liver disease because both are eliminated primarily by the kidneys.

Use in Critical Illness

Antiadrenergic drugs are one of several families of medications that may be used to treat urgent or malignant hypertension. An alpha$_2$ agonist such as clonidine might be prescribed under such conditions. A loading dose of clonidine 0.2 mg followed by 0.1 mg hourly until the diastolic pressure falls below 110 mm Hg may be administered. Do not exceed 0.7 mg when using clonidine to treat malignant hypertension.

Beta blockers may be used in the treatment of acute myocardial infarction. Early administration of a beta blocker after an acute myocardial infarction results in a lower incidence of reinfarction, ventricular arrhythmias, and mortality. These results have been demonstrated with several different agents; however, those with intrinsic sympathomimetic activity are not prescribed for this purpose.

Clients must be carefully monitored for hypotension and heart failure when receiving beta blockers after a myocardial infarction.

 Home Care

Antiadrenergic drugs are commonly used in the home setting, mainly to treat chronic disorders in adults. With alpha$_1$-adrenergic blocking agents, the home care nurse may need to teach clients ways to avoid orthostatic hypotension. Most clients probably take these medications for hypertension. However, some older men with BPH take one of these drugs to aid urinary elimination. For an older man taking one of these drugs, the home care nurse must assess the reason for use to teach the client and monitor for drug effects.

With beta-adrenergic blocking agents, the home care nurse may need to assist clients and caregivers in assessing for therapeutic and adverse drug effects. It is helpful to have the client or someone else in the household count and record the radial pulse daily, preferably approximately the same time interval before or after taking a beta blocker. Several days of a slow pulse should probably be reported to the health care provider who prescribed the beta blocker, especially if the client also has excessive fatigue or signs of heart failure.

If wheezing respirations (indicating bronchoconstriction) develop in a client taking a nonselective beta blocker, the client or the home care nurse must consult the prescribing physician about changing to a cardioselective beta blocker. If a client has diabetes mellitus, the home care nurse must interview and observe the client for alterations in blood sugar control, especially increased episodes of hypoglycemia. If a client has hypertension, the home care nurse must teach the client to avoid over-the-counter (OTC) asthma and cold remedies, decongestants, and appetite suppressants because these drugs act to increase blood pressure and may reduce the benefits of antiadrenergic medications. In addition, OTC analgesics such as ibuprofen, ketoprofen, and naproxen may raise blood pressure by causing retention of sodium and water.

NURSING ACTIONS	Antiadrenergic Drugs

NURSING ACTIONS	RATIONALE/EXPLANATION
1. Administer accurately	
a. With alpha$_2$ agonists:	
(1) Give all or most of a dose at bedtime, when possible.	To minimize daytime drowsiness and sedation
(2) Apply the clonidine skin patch to a hairless, intact area on the upper arm or torso; then apply adhesive overlay securely. Do not cut or alter the patch. Remove a used patch and fold its adhesive edges together before discarding. Apply a new patch in a new site.	To promote effectiveness and safe usage

(continued)

NURSING ACTIONS	RATIONALE/EXPLANATION
b. With alpha₁-blocking agents:	
(1) Give the first dose of doxazosin, prazosin, or terazosin at bedtime.	To prevent fainting from severe orthostatic hypotension
c. With beta-adrenergic blocking agents:	
(1) Check blood pressure and pulse frequently, especially when dosage is being increased.	To monitor therapeutic effects and the occurrence of adverse reactions. Some clients with heart rates between 50 and 60 beats per minute may be continued on a beta blocker if hypotension or escape arrhythmias do not develop.
(2) See Table 19-2 and manufacturers' literature regarding intravenous (IV) administration.	Specific instructions vary with individual drugs.
2. Observe for therapeutic effects	
a. With alpha₂ agonists and alpha-blocking agents:	
(1) With hypertension, observe for decreased blood pressure.	With most of the drugs, blood pressure decreases within a few hours. However, antihypertensive effects with clonidine skin patches occur 2–3 days after initial application (overlap with oral clonidine or other antihypertensive drugs may be needed) and persist 2–3 days when discontinued.
(2) With benign prostatic hyperplasia, observe for improved urination.	The client may report a larger stream, less nocturnal voiding, and more complete emptying of the bladder.
(3) In pheochromocytoma, observe for decreased pulse rate, blood pressure, sweating, palpitations, and blood sugar.	Because symptoms of pheochromocytoma are caused by excessive sympathetic nervous system stimulation, blocking stimulation with these drugs produces a decrease or absence of symptoms.
(4) In Raynaud's disease or frostbite, observe affected areas for improvement in skin color and temperature and in the quality of peripheral pulses.	These conditions are characterized by vasospasm, which diminishes blood flow to the affected part. The drugs improve blood flow by vasodilation.
3. Observe for adverse effects	Adverse effects are usually extensions of therapeutic effects.
a. With alpha₂ agonists and alpha-blocking agents:	
(1) Hypotension	Hypotension may range from transient postural hypotension to a more severe hypotensive state resembling shock. "First-dose syncope" may occur with prazosin and related drugs.
(2) Sedation, drowsiness	Sedation can be minimized by increasing dosage slowly and giving all or most of the daily dose at bedtime.
(3) Tachycardia	Tachycardia occurs as a reflex mechanism to increase blood supply to body tissues in hypotensive states.

(continued)

NURSING ACTIONS	RATIONALE/EXPLANATION
(4) Edema	These drugs promote retention of sodium and water. Concomitant diuretic therapy may be needed to maintain antihypertensive effects with long-term use.
b. With beta-blocking agents:	
(1) Bradycardia and heart block	These are extensions of the therapeutic effects, which slow conduction of electrical impulses through the atrioventricular node, particularly in clients with compromised cardiac function.
(2) Congestive heart failure—edema, dyspnea, fatigue	Caused by reduced force of myocardial contraction
(3) Bronchospasm—dyspnea, wheezing	Caused by drug-induced constriction of bronchi and bronchioles. It is more likely to occur in people with bronchial asthma or other obstructive lung disease.
(4) Fatigue and dizziness, especially with activity or exercise	These symptoms occur because the usual sympathetic nervous system stimulation in response to activity or stress is blocked by drug action.
(5) Central nervous system (CNS) effects—depression, insomnia, vivid dreams, and hallucinations	The mechanism by which these effects are produced is unknown.
4. Observe for drug interactions	
a. Drugs that *increase* effects of alpha-antiadrenergic agents:	
(1) Other antihypertensive drugs	Additive antihypertensive effects
(2) CNS depressants	Additive sedation and drowsiness
(3) Nonsteroidal anti-inflammatory drugs	Additive sodium and water retention, possible edema
(4) Epinephrine	Epinephrine increases the hypotensive effects of phenoxybenzamine and phentolamine and should not be given to treat shock caused by these drugs. Because epinephrine stimulates both alpha- and beta-adrenergic receptors, the net effect is vasodilation and a further drop in blood pressure.
b. Drugs that *decrease* effects of alpha-antiadrenergic agents:	
(1) Alpha adrenergics (eg, norepinephrine [Levophed])	Norepinephrine is a strong vasoconstricting agent and is the drug of choice for treating shock caused by overdosage of, or hypersensitivity to, phenoxybenzamine or phentolamine.
(2) Estrogens, oral contraceptives, nonsteroidal anti-inflammatory drugs	These drugs may cause sodium and fluid retention and thereby decrease antihypertensive effects of alpha-antiadrenergic drugs.
c. Drugs that *increase* effects of beta-adrenergic blocking agents (eg, propranolol):	
(1) Other antihypertensives	Synergistic antihypertensive effects. Clients who do not respond to beta blockers or vasodilators

(continued)

NURSING ACTIONS	RATIONALE/EXPLANATION
	alone may respond well to the combination. Also, beta blockers prevent reflex tachycardia, which usually occurs with vasodilator antihypertensive drugs.
(2) Phenoxybenzamine or phentolamine	Synergistic effects to prevent excessive hypertension before and during surgical excision of pheochromocytoma
(3) Chlorpromazine, cimetidine, furosemide	Increase plasma levels by slowing hepatic metabolism
(4) Digoxin	Additive bradycardia, heart block
(5) Phenytoin	Potentiates cardiac depressant effects of propranolol
(6) Quinidine	The combination may be synergistic in treating cardiac arrhythmias. However, additive cardiac depressant effects also may occur (bradycardia, decreased force of myocardial contraction [negative inotropy], decreased cardiac output).
(7) Verapamil, IV	IV verapamil and IV propranolol should never be used in combination because of additive bradycardia and hypotension.
d. Drugs that *decrease* effects of beta-adrenergic blocking agents:	
(1) Antacids	Decrease absorption of several oral beta blockers from the gastrointestinal tract
(2) Atropine	Increases heart rate and may be used to counteract excessive bradycardia caused by beta blockers
(3) Isoproterenol	Stimulates beta-adrenergic receptors and therefore antagonizes effects of beta-blocking agents. Isoproterenol also can be used to counteract excessive bradycardia.

Nursing Notes: Apply Your Knowledge

Answer: Although she is probably not allergic to the Inderal, this new medication is responsible for her breathing difficulties. Inderal is a nonselective beta blocker, which means that it blocks beta₁ and beta₂ receptors. Blocking the beta₂ receptor causes bronchial constriction. Clients with asthma are likely to become symptomatic when this occurs. Selective beta blockers, which primarily block beta₁ receptors, should be used for any clients with a history of asthma or chronic obstructive pulmonary disease. In high doses, even selective beta blockers can cause bronchoconstriction in high-risk patients.

How Can You Avoid This Medication Error?

Answer: This would be a lethal mistake. Inderal is greatly affected by the first-pass effect, so the normal IV dose is significantly less than the normal oral dose. When a patient is NPO, an order needs to be obtained to change the route of administration. The nurse should question administering 20 cc of a medication IV push. Normal IV push doses are usually 1 to 2 cc.

REVIEW AND APPLICATION EXERCISES

1. How do alpha$_2$ agonists and alpha$_1$-blocking agents decrease blood pressure?

2. What are safety factors in administering and monitoring the effects of alpha$_2$ agonists and alpha$_1$-blocking agents?

3. Why should a client be cautioned against stopping alpha$_2$ agonists and alpha$_1$-blocking agents abruptly?

4. What are the main mechanisms by which beta blockers relieve angina pectoris?

5. How are beta blockers thought to be "cardioprotective" in preventing repeat myocardial infarctions?

6. What are some noncardiovascular indications for the use of propranolol?

7. What are the main differences between cardioselective and nonselective beta blockers?

8. Why are cardioselective beta blockers preferred for clients with asthma or diabetes mellitus?

9. List at least five adverse effects of beta blockers.

10. Explain the drug effects that contribute to each adverse reaction.

11. What signs, symptoms, or behaviors would lead you to suspect adverse drug effects?

12. Do the same adverse effects occur with beta blocker eye drops that occur with systemic drugs? If so, how may they be prevented or minimized?

13. What information needs to be included in teaching clients about beta blocker therapy?

14. What is the risk of abruptly stopping a beta blocker drug rather than tapering the dose and gradually discontinuing, as recommended?

15. How can beta blockers be both therapeutic and nontherapeutic for heart failure?

SELECTED REFERENCES

Carroll, E.W. & Curtis, R.L. (1998) Organization and control of neural function. In C.M. Porth (Ed.), *Pathophysiology: Concepts of altered health states*, 5th ed., pp. 833–878. Philadelphia: Lippincott Williams & Wilkins.

Dargie, H.S. & Lechat, P.C. (1999). The cardiac insufficiency bisoprolol study II (CIBIS-II): A randomised trial. *Lancet, 353*(2), 9–13.

Drug facts and comparisons. (Updated monthly). St. Louis: Facts and Comparisons.

Hawkins, D.W., Bussey, H.I., & Prisant, L.M. (1997). Hypertension. In J.T. DiPiro, R.L. Talbert, G.C. Yee, G.R. Matzke, B.G. Wells, & L.M. Posey (Eds.), *Pharmacotherapy: A pathophysiologic approach*, 3rd ed., pp. 195–218. Stamford, CT: Appleton & Lange.

Hoffman, B.B. & Lefkowitz, R.J. (1996). Catecholamines, sympathomimetic drugs, and adrenergic receptor antagonists. In J.G. Hardman, L.E. Limbird, R.B. Molinoff, & R.W. Ruddon (Eds.), *Goodman and Gilman's The pharmacological basis of therapeutics*, 9th ed., pp. 199–248. New York: McGraw-Hill.

Johnson, J.A., & Lalonde, R.L. (1997). Congestive heart failure. In J.T. DiPiro, R.L. Talbert, G.C. Yee, G.R. Matzke, B.G. Wells, & L.M. Posey (Eds), *Pharmacotherapy: A pathophysiologic approach*, 3rd ed., pp. 219–256. Stamford, CT: Appleton & Lange.

Krumholz, H.M. (1999). Commentary: B-blockers for mild to moderate heart failure. *Lancet, 353*(2), 2–3.

Kudzma, E.C. (1999). Culturally competent drug administration. *American Journal of Nursing, 99*(8), 46–51.

Sorenson, S.J. & Abel, S.R. (1996). Comparison of the ocular beta-blockers. *Annals of Pharmacotherapy, 30*, 43–54.

Stewart, S.M. (1998). Alterations in structure and function of the male genitourinary system. In C.M. Porth (Ed.), *Pathophysiology: Concepts of altered health states*, 5th ed., pp. 1159–1174. Philadelphia: Lippincott Williams & Wilkins.

Stringer, K.A. & Lopez, L.M. (1997). Acute myocardial infarction. In J.T. DiPiro, R.L. Talbert, G.C. Yee, G.R. Matzke, B.G. Wells, & L.M. Posey (Eds.), *Pharmacotherapy: A pathophysiologic approach*, 3rd ed., pp. 295–322. Stamford, CT: Appleton & Lange.

VirSci Corporation (1997). Tamsulosin for benign prostatic hyperplasia. *Medical Sciences Bulletin, 9*(240) (http://pharminfonet.com).

20

Cholinergic Drugs

Objectives

After studying this chapter, the student will be able to:

1. Describe effects and indications for use of selected cholinergic drugs.

2. Discuss drug therapy of myasthenia gravis.

3. Discuss drug therapy of Alzheimer's disease.

4. Discuss atropine and pralidoxime as antidotes for cholinergic drugs.

5. Describe major nursing care needs of clients receiving cholinergic drugs.

6. Discuss principles of therapy for using cholinergic drugs in special populations.

7. Describe signs, symptoms, and treatment of overdose with cholinergic drugs.

8. Teach clients about safe, effective use of cholinergic drugs.

Jamie, a 14-year-old, was diagnosed with myasthenia gravis 3 years ago and has been well managed on neostigmine (Prostigmin), an anticholinesterase agent. His mother calls the clinic and, clearly upset, reports the following symptoms that Jamie is experiencing: severe headache, drooling, and one fainting episode. Jamie states he "just doesn't feel right."

Reflect on:

▶ Review the underlying pathophysiology of myasthenia gravis. Explain how Prostigmin alters neurotransmitters to manage this condition. (Hint: think first how the parasympathetic nervous system is altered and how balance could be restored.)

▶ Contrast the symptoms of cholinergic crisis (too much Prostigmin) with myasthenic crisis (undertreatment). Which seems to fit with Jamie's symptoms?

▶ What additional data would you collect to help arrive at a diagnosis before treatment?

▶ Discuss appropriate medical and pharmacologic management of Jamie.

DESCRIPTION

Cholinergic drugs, also called parasympathomimetics and cholinomimetics, stimulate the parasympathetic nervous system in the same manner as acetylcholine (see Chap. 17). Some drugs act directly to stimulate cholinergic receptors; others act indirectly by slowing acetylcholine metabolism at autonomic nerve synapses and terminals. Selected drugs are discussed here in relation to their use in myasthenia gravis; primary degenerative dementia, Alzheimer's type; and urinary retention.

In normal neuromuscular function, acetylcholine is released from nerve endings and binds to nicotinic receptors on cell membranes of muscle cells to cause muscle contraction. Myasthenia gravis is an autoimmune disorder in which autoantibodies are thought to destroy nicotinic receptors for acetylcholine on skeletal muscle. As a result, acetylcholine is less able to stimulate muscle contraction, and muscle weakness occurs.

In normal brain function, acetylcholine is an essential neurotransmitter and plays an important role in cognitive functions, including memory storage and retrieval. Alzheimer's disease, the most common type of dementia in adults, is characterized by abnormalities in the cholinergic, serotonergic, noradrenergic, and glutamatergic neurotransmission systems (see Chap. 5). In the cholinergic system, there is a substantial loss of neurons that secrete acetylcholine in the brain and decreased activity of choline acetyltransferase, the enzyme required for synthesis of acetylcholine.

Acetylcholine stimulates cholinergic receptors in the urinary system to promote normal urination. Cholinergic stimulation results in contraction of the detrusor muscle and relaxation of the urinary sphincter to facilitate emptying the urinary bladder.

Mechanisms of Action and Effects

Direct-acting cholinergic drugs are synthetic derivatives of choline. They are lipid insoluble and do not readily enter the central nervous system; thus, their effects occur primarily in the periphery. These drugs can exert their therapeutic effects because they are highly resistant to metabolism by acetylcholinesterase, the enzyme that normally metabolizes acetylcholine. Their action is longer than that of acetylcholine. They have widespread systemic effects when they combine with muscarinic receptors in cardiac muscle, smooth muscle, exocrine glands, and the eye. Specific effects include:

1. Decreased heart rate, vasodilation, and unpredictable changes in blood pressure
2. Increased tone and contractility in gastrointestinal (GI) smooth muscle, relaxation of sphincters, increased salivary gland and GI secretions
3. Increased tone and contractility of smooth muscle (detrusor) in the urinary bladder and relaxation of the sphincter

4. Increased tone and contractility of bronchial smooth muscle
5. Increased respiratory secretions
6. Constriction of pupils (miosis) and contraction of ciliary muscle, resulting in accommodation for near vision.

Indirect-acting cholinergic or *anticholinesterase drugs* decrease the inactivation of acetylcholine in the synapse by the enzyme acetylcholinesterase. Acetylcholine can then accumulate in the synapse and enhance the activation of postsynaptic muscarinic and nicotinic receptors. This improves cholinergic neurotransmission in the brain and the force of muscle contraction in peripheral tissues.

Anticholinesterase drugs are classified as either reversible or irreversible inhibitors of acetylcholinesterase. The reversible inhibitors exhibit a moderate duration of action and have several therapeutic uses, as described later. The irreversible inhibitors produce prolonged effects and are highly toxic. These agents are used primarily as poisons (ie, insecticides and nerve gases). Their only therapeutic use is in the treatment of glaucoma (see Chap. 65).

Indications for Use

Cholinergic drugs have limited but varied uses. A direct-acting drug, bethanechol, is used to treat urinary retention and postoperative abdominal distention due to hypoperistalsis. The anticholinesterase agents are used in the diagnosis and treatment of myasthenia gravis and to reverse the action of nondepolarizing neuromuscular blocking agents (eg, tubocurarine and related drugs) used in surgery (see Chap. 14). The drugs do not reverse the neuromuscular blockade produced by depolarizing agents, such as succinylcholine. In addition, tacrine and donepezil are anticholinesterase agents approved for treatment of Alzheimer's disease. Cholinergic drugs may also be used to treat glaucoma (see Chap. 65).

Contraindications to Use

These drugs are contraindicated in urinary or GI tract obstruction, asthma, peptic ulcer disease, coronary artery disease, hyperthyroidism, pregnancy, and inflammatory abdominal conditions. Tacrine is also contraindicated in previous users in whom jaundice or a serum bilirubin level above 3 mg/dL developed.

INDIVIDUAL CHOLINERGIC DRUGS

Direct-Acting Cholinergics

Bethanechol (Urecholine) is a synthetic derivative of choline. Because the drug produces smooth muscle contractions, it should not be used in obstructive conditions.

Because oral bethanechol is not well absorbed from the GI tract, oral doses are much larger than subcutaneous (SC) doses. Because severe adverse effects may occur with intramuscular (IM) or intravenous (IV) administration, the drug is not given by these routes.

ROUTE AND DOSAGE RANGES

Adults: Oral (PO) 10–50 mg two to four times per day; maximum single dose 50 mg, SC 2.5–5 mg three or four times per day

Children: PO 0.2 mg/kg three times per day, SC 0.05 mg/kg three times per day

Reversible Indirect-Acting Cholinergics (Anticholinesterases)

Neostigmine (Prostigmin) is the prototype anticholinesterase agent. It is used for long-term treatment of myasthenia gravis and as an antidote for tubocurarine and other nondepolarizing skeletal muscle relaxants used in surgery. Neostigmine is poorly absorbed from the GI tract; consequently, oral doses are much larger than parenteral doses. When it is used for long-term treatment of myasthenia gravis, resistance to its action may occur, and larger doses may be required.

ROUTE AND DOSAGE RANGES

Adults: Myasthenia gravis, PO 15–30 mg q4h while awake

Exacerbation of myasthenia gravis, IM, SC 0.25–2 mg q2–3h

Prevention and treatment of urinary retention, IM, SC 0.25–0.5 mg q4–6h (up to 2 or 3 d)

Children: Myasthenia gravis, PO 0.3–0.6 mg/kg q3–4h while awake

Exacerbation of myasthenia gravis, IM, SC 0.01–0.04 mg/kg q2–3h

Donepezil (Aricept) is used to treat mild to moderate Alzheimer's disease. Like tacrine (see later), donepezil increases acetylcholine in the brain by inhibiting its metabolism. The drug is well absorbed after oral administration and absorption is unaffected by food. It is highly bound (96%) to plasma proteins. It is metabolized in the liver to several metabolites, some of which are pharmacologically active; metabolites and some unchanged drug are excreted mainly in urine. Adverse effects include nausea, vomiting, diarrhea, bradycardia, and possible aggravation of asthma, peptic ulcer disease, and chronic obstructive pulmonary disease. Unlike tacrine, donepezil does not cause liver toxicity.

ROUTE AND DOSAGE RANGES

Adults: PO 5 mg daily at bedtime for 4–6 wk, then increase to 10 mg once daily, if necessary

Edrophonium (Tensilon) is a short-acting cholinergic drug used to diagnose myasthenia gravis, to differentiate between myasthenic crisis and cholinergic crisis, and to reverse the neuromuscular blockade produced by nondepolarizing skeletal muscle relaxants. It is given IM or IV by a physician who remains in attendance. Atropine, an antidote, and life support equipment, such as ventilators and endotracheal tubes, must be available when the drug is given.

ROUTE AND DOSAGE RANGES

Adults: Diagnosis of myasthenia gravis, IV 2–4 mg initially; may be repeated and increased up to a total dose of 10 mg if no response is elicited by smaller amounts after 45 sec; or IM 10 mg as a single dose

Differential diagnosis of myasthenic crisis or cholinergic crisis, IV 1–2 mg

Children: Diagnosis of myasthenia gravis, IV 0.2 mg/kg

Diagnosis in infants, IM 0.1 mg/kg

Ambenonium (Mytelase) is a long-acting drug used for the treatment of myasthenia gravis. It is used less often than neostigmine and pyridostigmine. It may be useful in clients who are allergic to bromides, however, because the other drugs are both bromide salts. Ambenonium may be useful for myasthenic clients on ventilators because it is less likely to increase respiratory secretions than other anticholinesterase drugs.

ROUTE AND DOSAGE RANGES

Adults: PO 5 mg initially, increased to 10–30 mg tid or qid. Dosage varies considerably, depending on client; dosage range, 5–75 mg/d

Children: PO 0.1 mg/kg initially, increased if necessary to 0.4 mg/kg q4h while awake

Physostigmine salicylate (Antilirium) is the only anticholinesterase capable of crossing the blood–brain barrier. It is sometimes used as an antidote for overdosage of anticholinergic drugs ("atropine poisoning"), including tricyclic antidepressants. However, its potential for causing serious adverse effects limits its usefulness. Some preparations of physostigmine are used in the treatment of glaucoma.

ROUTE AND DOSAGE RANGES

Adults: IV, IM 0.5–2 mg; give slowly IV, no faster than 1 mg/min. Rapid administration may cause bradycardia, respiratory distress, and seizures.

Pyridostigmine (Mestinon) is similar to neostigmine in actions, uses, and adverse effects. It may have a longer duration of action than neostigmine and is the maintenance drug of choice for clients with myasthenia gravis. An added advantage is the availability of a slow-release form, which is effective for 8 to 12 hours. When this form is taken at bedtime, the client does not have to take other medications during the night and does not awaken too weak to swallow.

ROUTE AND DOSAGE RANGES

Adults: PO 60–120 mg q3–4h when awake; maximal single dose, 180 mg; or one Timespan tablet (180 mg) at bedtime. Up to 1500 mg daily may be necessary.

IM (exacerbations of myasthenia gravis or when oral administration is contraindicated) 2 mg

Children: PO 1–2 mg/kg q3–4h when awake
　　Newborns whose mothers have myasthenia gravis,
　　IM 0.05–0.15 mg/kg

Tacrine (Cognex) is a centrally acting anticholinesterase agent approved for treatment of clients with mild to moderate Alzheimer's disease. The drug does not cure the disease, but it may delay progression in some clients. Tacrine is well absorbed after oral administration and reaches peak plasma levels in 1 to 2 hours. It is approximately 50% protein bound, is extensively metabolized in the liver, is excreted in the urine, and has an elimination half-life of 2 to 4 hours. The initial enthusiasm for tacrine has declined because of inconsistent clinical trial results and the occurrence of hepatotoxicity.

ROUTE AND DOSAGE RANGES

Adults: PO 40 mg/d (10 mg qid) for 6 wk, during which aminotransferase levels are monitored weekly; after 6 wk, increase dose to 80 mg/d (20 mg qid). If the client tolerates the drug and alanine aminotransferase (ALT) levels are within normal limits, increase the daily dose by 10 mg every 6 wk to a total of 120–160 mg/d.

NURSING PROCESS

Assessment

Assess the client's condition in relation to disorders for which cholinergic drugs are used:

- In clients known to have myasthenia gravis, assess for muscle weakness. This may be manifested by ptosis (drooping) of the upper eyelid and diplopia (double vision) caused by weakness of the eye muscles. More severe disease may be indicated by difficulty in chewing, swallowing, and speaking; accumulation of oral secretions, which the client may be unable to expectorate or swallow; decreased skeletal muscle activity, including impaired chest expansion; and eventual respiratory failure.
- In clients with possible urinary retention, check for bladder distention and time and amount of previous urination, and assess fluid intake.
- In clients with Alzheimer's disease, assess for abilities and limitations in relation to memory, cognitive functioning, self-care activities, and pre-existing conditions that may be aggravated by a cholinergic drug.

Nursing Diagnoses

- Altered Urinary Elimination: Incontinence
- Ineffective Breathing Pattern related to bronchoconstriction
- Ineffective Airway Clearance related to increased respiratory secretions

Nursing Notes: Apply Your Knowledge

Jill and her boyfriend ate mushrooms they picked while hiking. They were admitted to the hospital later that afternoon with acute cholinergic poisoning. Describe the signs and symptoms they likely exhibited. What antidote do you think was given, and why?

- Self Care Deficit related to muscle weakness or cognitive impairment
- Knowledge Deficit: Drug administration and effects
- Risk for Injury related to adverse drug effects
- Sensory-Perceptual Alteration: Diplopia

Planning/Goals

The client will:

- Verbalize or demonstrate correct drug administration
- Improve in self-care abilities
- Regain usual patterns of urinary elimination
- Maintain effective oxygenation of tissues
- Report adverse drug effects
- For clients with myasthenia gravis, at least one family member will verbalize or demonstrate correct drug administration, symptoms of too much or too little drug, and emergency care procedures.
- For clients with dementia, a caregiver will verbalize or demonstrate correct drug administration and knowledge of adverse effects to be reported to a health care provider.

Interventions

- Use measures to prevent or decrease the need for cholinergic drugs. Ambulation, adequate fluid intake, and judicious use of opioid analgesics or other sedative-type drugs help prevent postoperative urinary retention. In myasthenia gravis, muscle weakness is aggravated by exercise and improved by rest. Therefore, scheduling activities to avoid excessive fatigue and to allow adequate rest periods may be beneficial.
- With tacrine, assist and teach caregivers to:
  ○ Maintain a quiet, stable environment and daily routines to decrease confusion (eg, verbal or written reminders and simple directions, adequate lighting, calendars, personal objects within view and reach).
  ○ Avoid altering dosage or stopping the drug without consulting the prescribing physician.
  ○ Be sure that clients keep appointments for supervision and blood tests.

○ Report signs and symptoms (ie, skin rash, jaundice, light-colored stools) that may indicate hepatotoxicity.

○ Notify surgeons about tacrine therapy. Exaggerated muscle relaxation may occur if succinylcholine-type drugs are given.

- Before giving cholinergic drugs for bladder atony and urinary retention, be sure there is no obstruction in the urinary tract.
- For long-term use, assist clients and families to establish a schedule of drug administration that best meets the client's needs.
- With myasthenia gravis, recommend that one or more family members be trained in cardiopulmonary resuscitation.

Evaluation

- Observe and interview about the adequacy of urinary elimination.
- Observe abilities and limitations in self-care.

- Question the client and at least one family member of clients with myasthenia gravis about correct drug usage, symptoms of underdosage and overdosage, and emergency care procedures.
- Question caregivers of clients with dementia about the client's level of functioning and response to medication.

PRINCIPLES OF THERAPY

Use in Myasthenia Gravis

Guidelines for the use of anticholinesterase drugs in myasthenia gravis include the following:

1. Drug dosage should be increased gradually until maximal benefit is obtained. Larger doses are often required with increased physical activity, emotional stress, and infections, and sometimes premenstrually.

CLIENT TEACHING GUIDELINES
Cholinergic Drugs

General Considerations

✔ Cholinergic drugs used for urinary retention usually act within 60 minutes after administration. Be sure bathroom facilities are available.

✔ Wear a medical alert identification device if taking long-term cholinergic drug therapy for myasthenia gravis, hypotonic bladder, or Alzheimer's disease.

✔ Atropine 0.6 mg IV may be administered for overdose of cholinergic drugs.

✔ Record symptoms of myasthenia gravis and effects of drug therapy, especially when drug therapy is initiated and medication doses are being titrated. The amount of medication required to control symptoms of myasthenia gravis varies greatly and the physician needs this information to adjust the dosage correctly.

✔ Do not overexert yourself if you have myasthenia gravis. Rest between activities. Although the dose of medication may be increased during periods of increased activity, it is desirable to space activities to obtain optimal benefit from the drug, at the lowest possible dose, with the fewest adverse effects.

✔ Report increased muscle weakness, difficulty breathing, or recurrence of myasthenic symptoms to the physician. These are signs of drug underdosage (myasthenic crisis) and indicate a need to increase or change drug therapy.

✔ Report adverse reactions, including abdominal cramps, diarrhea, excessive oral secretions, difficulty in breathing, and muscle weakness. These are signs of drug overdosage (cholinergic crisis) and require immediate discontinuation of drugs and treatment by the physician. Respiratory failure can result if this condition is not recognized and treated properly.

✔ Clients taking tacrine need weekly monitoring of liver aminotransferase levels for 18 weeks when initiating therapy and weekly for 6 weeks after any increase in dose. Caregivers should report any signs or symptoms of adverse drug reactions such as nausea, vomiting, diarrhea, rash, jaundice, or change in the color of stools. The drug should not be suddenly discontinued.

✔ If dizziness or syncope occurs when taking tacrine or donepezil, ambulation should be supervised to avoid injury.

Self- or Caregiver Administration

✔ Take drugs as directed on a regular schedule to maintain consistent blood levels and control of symptoms.

✔ *Do not* chew or crush sustained-release medications.

✔ Take oral cholinergics on an empty stomach to lessen nausea and vomiting. Also, food decreases absorption of tacrine by up to 40%.

✔ Ensure adequate fluid intake if vomiting or diarrhea occurs as a side effect of cholinergic medications.

2. Some clients with myasthenia gravis cannot tolerate optimal doses of anticholinesterase drugs unless atropine is given to decrease the severity of adverse reactions due to muscarinic activation. However, atropine should be given only if necessary because it may mask the sudden increase of side effects. This increase is the first sign of overdose.

3. Drug dosage in excess of the amount needed to maintain muscle strength and function can produce a cholinergic crisis. A cholinergic crisis is characterized by excessive stimulation of the parasympathetic nervous system. If early symptoms are not treated, hypotension and respiratory failure may occur. At high doses, anticholinesterase drugs weaken rather than strengthen skeletal muscle contraction because excessive amounts of acetylcholine accumulate at motor end plates and reduce nerve impulse transmission to muscle tissue.

  a. *Treatment for cholinergic crisis* includes withdrawal of anticholinesterase drugs, administration of atropine, and measures to maintain respiration. Endotracheal intubation and mechanical ventilation may be necessary due to profound skeletal muscle weakness (including muscles of respiration), which is not counteracted by atropine.

  b. *Differentiating myasthenic crisis from cholinergic crisis* may be difficult because both are characterized by respiratory difficulty or failure. It is necessary to differentiate between them, however, because they require *opposite* treatment measures. Myasthenic crisis requires more anticholinesterase drug, whereas cholinergic crisis requires discontinuing any anticholinesterase drug the client has been receiving. The physician may be able to make an accurate diagnosis from signs and symptoms and their timing in relation to medication; that is, signs and symptoms having their onset within approximately 1 hour after a dose of anticholinesterase drug are more likely to be caused by cholinergic crisis (too much drug). Signs and symptoms beginning 3 hours or more after a drug dose are more likely to be caused by myasthenic crisis (too little drug).

  c. If the differential diagnosis cannot be made on the basis of signs and symptoms, the client can be intubated, mechanically ventilated, and observed closely until a diagnosis is possible. Still another way to differentiate between the two conditions is for the physician to inject a small dose of IV edrophonium. If the edrophonium causes a dramatic improvement in breathing, the diagnosis is myasthenic crisis; if it makes the client even weaker, the diagnosis is cholinergic crisis. Note, however, that edrophonium or any other pharmacologic agent should be administered only after endotracheal intubation and controlled ventilation have been instituted.

4. Some people acquire partial or total resistance to anticholinesterase drugs after taking them for months or years. Therefore, do not assume that drug therapy that is effective initially will continue to be effective over the long-term course of the disease.

Use in Children

Bethanechol is occasionally used, but safety and effectiveness for children younger than 8 years of age have not been established. Neostigmine is used to treat myasthenia gravis and to reverse neuromuscular blockade after general anesthesia but is not recommended for urinary retention. Other indirect-acting cholinergic drugs are used only in the treatment of myasthenia gravis. Precautions and adverse effects are the same for children as for adults.

Use in Older Adults

Indirect-acting cholinergic drugs may be used in myasthenia gravis, Alzheimer's disease, or overdoses of atropine and other centrally acting anticholinergic drugs (eg, those used for parkinsonism). Older adults are more likely to experience adverse drug effects because of age-related physiologic changes and superimposed pathologic conditions.

Use in Renal Impairment

Because bethanechol and other cholinergic drugs increase pressure in the urinary tract by stimulating detrusor muscle contraction and relaxation of urinary sphincters, they are contraindicated for clients with urinary tract obstructions or weaknesses in the bladder wall. Administering a cholinergic drug to these people might result in rupture of the bladder.

Some aspects of the pharmacokinetics of cholinergic drugs are unknown. Many of the drugs are degraded enzymatically by cholinesterases. However, a few (eg, neostigmine and pyridostigmine) undergo hepatic metabolism and tubular excretion in the kidneys. Renal impairment may result in accumulation and increased adverse effects, especially with chronic use.

Use in Hepatic Impairment

The hepatic metabolism of neostigmine and pyridostigmine may be impaired by liver disease, resulting in an increase in adverse effects.

Tacrine is contraindicated by liver disease. Approximately 20% to 50% of clients experience an increase in liver aminotransferase levels after beginning therapy with tacrine. Most enzyme elevation occurs in the first 18 weeks of therapy and is more common in female clients. When tacrine is started, serum ALT should be monitored weekly for 18 weeks. Then, if values are within normal limits and signs of liver damage do not occur, the test can be done every 3 months. Immediate withdrawal of the medication usually restores liver enzymes to normal levels with no permanent liver injury.

Use in Critical Illness

Cholinergic drugs have several specific uses in critical illness. These include:

1. Use of neostigmine, pyridostigmine, and edrophonium to reverse neuromuscular blockade (skeletal muscle paralysis) caused by nondepolarizing muscle relaxants.
2. Anticholinesterase drugs are used to treat myasthenic crisis and improve muscle strength.
3. Physostigmine may be used in severe cases as an antidote to anticholinergic poisoning with drugs such as atropine or tricyclic antidepressants.

Management of Cholinergic Drug Overdose

Atropine, an anticholinergic drug, is a specific antidote to cholinergic agents. The drug and equipment for injection should be readily available whenever cholinergic drugs are given. It is important to note that atropine reverses only the muscarinic effects of cholinergic drugs. It does not reverse the nicotinic effects (skeletal muscle weakness or paralysis) of the indirect cholinergic drugs.

Management of Overdose of Irreversible Anticholinesterase Agents

Exposure to toxic doses of anticholinesterase agents such as organophosphate insecticides (malathion, parathion) or nerve gases (sarin, tabun, soman) produces a cholinergic crisis characterized by excessive cholinergic (muscarinic) stimulation and neuromuscular blockade. This cholinergic crisis occurs because the irreversible anticholinesterase poison binds to the enzyme acetylcholinesterase and inactivates it. Consequently, acetylcholine remains in cholinergic synapses and causes excessive stimulation of muscarinic and nicotinic receptors.

Emergency treatment includes decontamination procedures such as removing contaminated clothing, flushing poison from skin and eyes, and use of activated charcoal and lavage to remove ingested poison from the GI tract. Pharmacologic treatment includes administering atropine to counteract the muscarinic effects of the poison (eg, salivation, urination, defecation, bronchial secretions, laryngospasm, bronchospasm).

To relieve the neuromuscular blockade, a second drug, pralidoxime, is needed. Pralidoxime (Protopam), a cholinesterase reactivator, is a specific antidote for overdose with irreversible anticholinesterase agents. Pralidoxime treats toxicity by causing the anticholinesterase poison to release the enzyme acetylcholinesterase. The reactivated acetylcholinesterase can then degrade excess acetylcholine at the cholinergic synapses, including the neuromuscular junction. Pralidoxime cannot cross the blood–brain barrier, and therefore is effective only in the peripheral areas of the body. Pralidoxime must be given as soon after the poisoning as possible. If too much time passes, the bond between the irreversible anticholinesterase agent and acetylcholinesterase becomes stronger and pralidoxime is unable to release the enzyme from the poison. This phenomenon is called *aging*. Treatment of anticholinesterase overdose may also require use of diazepam to control seizures. Mechanical ventilation may be necessary to treat respiratory paralysis.

 Home Care

Medications to treat long-term conditions such as myasthenia gravis or Alzheimer's disease are often administered in the home setting. Often the person using the drugs may have difficulty with self-administration. The client with myasthenia gravis may have problems with diplopia or diminished muscle strength that make it difficult to self-administer medications. The client with Alzheimer's disease may have problems with remembering to take medications and may easily underdose or overdose himself. It is important to work with responsible family members in such cases to ensure accurate drug administration.

NURSING ACTIONS	Cholinergic Drugs

NURSING ACTIONS	RATIONALE/EXPLANATION
1. **Administer accurately** **a.** Give oral bethanechol before meals.	If given after meals, nausea and vomiting may occur because the drug stimulates contraction of muscles in the gastrointestinal (GI) tract. *(continued)*

NURSING ACTIONS	RATIONALE/EXPLANATION
b. Give parenteral bethanechol by the subcutaneous route *only*.	Intramuscular (IM) and intravenous (IV) injections may cause acute, severe hypotension and circulatory failure. Cardiac arrest may occur.
c. With pyridostigmine and other drugs for myasthenia gravis, give at regularly scheduled intervals.	For consistent blood levels and control of symptoms
d. Give tacrine on an empty stomach, 1 hour before or 2 hours after a meal, if possible, at regular intervals around the clock (eg, q6h). Give with meals if GI upset occurs.	Food decreases absorption and decreases serum drug levels by 30% or more. Regular intervals increase therapeutic effects and decrease adverse effects.
2. Observe for therapeutic effects	
a. When the drug is given for postoperative hypoperistalsis, observe for bowel sounds, passage of flatus through the rectum, or a bowel movement.	These are indicators of increased GI muscle tone and motility.
b. When bethanechol or neostigmine is given for urinary retention, micturition usually occurs within approximately 60 minutes. If it does not, urinary catheterization may be necessary.	
c. When the drug is given in myasthenia gravis, observe for increased muscle strength as shown by: (1) Decreased or absent ptosis of eyelids (2) Decreased difficulty with chewing, swallowing, and speech (3) Increased skeletal muscle strength, increased tolerance of activity, less fatigue	With neostigmine, onset of action is 2–4 hours after oral administration and 10–30 minutes after injection. Duration is approximately 3–4 hours. With pyridostigmine, onset of action is approximately 30–45 minutes after oral use, 15 minutes after IM injection, and 2–5 minutes after IV injection. Duration is approximately 4–6 hours. The long-acting form of pyridostigmine lasts 8–12 hours.
d. With tacrine and donepezil, observe for improvement in memory and cognitive functioning in activities of daily living.	Improved functioning is most likely to occur in patients with mild to moderate dementia.
3. Observe for adverse effects	Adverse effects occur with usual therapeutic doses but are more likely with large doses. They are caused by stimulation of the parasympathetic nervous system.
a. Central nervous system effects—convulsions, dizziness, drowsiness, headache, loss of consciousness	
b. Respiratory effects—increased secretions, bronchospasm, laryngospasm, respiratory failure	
c. Cardiovascular effects—arrhythmias (bradycardia, tachycardia, atrioventricular block), cardiac arrest, hypotension, syncope	These may be detected early by regular assessment of blood pressure and heart rate. Bradycardia is probably the most likely arrhythmia to occur.
d. GI effects—nausea and vomiting, diarrhea, increased peristalsis, abdominal cramping, increased secretions (ie, saliva, gastric and intestinal secretions)	GI effects commonly occur.
e. Other effects—increased frequency and urgency of urination, increased sweating, miosis, skin rash	Skin rashes are most likely to occur from formulations of neostigmine or pyridostigmine that contain bromide.

(continued)

NURSING ACTIONS	RATIONALE/EXPLANATION

4. Observe for drug interactions
   a. Drug that *increases* effects of tacrine:
      (1) Cimetidine
	Slows metabolism of tacrine in the liver, thereby increasing risks of accumulation and adverse effects

b. Drugs that *decrease* effects of cholinergic agents: (1) Anticholinergic drugs (eg, atropine)	Antagonize effects of cholinergic drugs (miosis, increased tone and motility in smooth muscle of the GI tract, bronchi, and urinary bladder, bradycardia). Atropine is the specific antidote for overdosage with cholinergic drugs.
(2) Antihistamines	Most antihistamines have anticholinergic properties that antagonize effects of cholinergic drugs.

Nursing Notes: Apply Your Knowledge

Answer: Excessive stimulation of the parasympathetic nervous system causes decreased heart rate and cardiac contractility, hypotension, bronchial constriction, excessive saliva and mucus production, nausea, vomiting, diarrhea, and abdominal cramping. Because these symptoms are a result of excessive stimulation of cholinergic receptors, treatment includes administration of an anticholinergic drug such as atropine.

REVIEW AND APPLICATION EXERCISES

1. What are the actions of cholinergic drugs?
2. Which neurotransmitter is involved in cholinergic (parasympathetic) stimulation?
3. When a cholinergic drug is given to treat myasthenia gravis, what is the expected effect?
4. What is the difference between cholinergic crisis and myasthenic crisis? How are they treated?
5. When tacrine is given to treat Alzheimer's disease, what is the desired effect?

6. Is a cholinergic drug the usual treatment of choice for urinary bladder atony or hypotonicity? Why or why not?
7. What are the adverse effects of cholinergic drugs?
8. How are overdoses of cholinergic drugs treated?

SELECTED REFERENCES

Carroll, E.W. & Curtis, R.L. (1998). Organization and control of neural function. In C.M. Porth (Ed.), *Pathophysiology: Concepts of altered health states*, 5th ed., pp. 833–878. Philadelphia: Lippincott Williams & Wilkins.

Drug facts and comparisons. (Updated monthly). St. Louis: Facts and Comparisons.

Eggert. A., Crismon, M.L., & Ereshefsky, L. (1997). Alzheimer's disease. In J.T. DiPiro, R.L. Talbert, G.C. Yee, G.R. Matzke, B.G. Wells, & L.M. Posey (Eds.), *Pharmacotherapy: A pathophysiologic approach*, 3rd ed., pp. 1325–1344. Stamford, CT: Appleton & Lange.

Eisenhauer, L.A., Nichols, L.W., Spencer, R.T., & Bergan, F.W. (1998). *Clinical pharmacology and nursing management*, 5th ed., pp. 248–283. Philadelphia: Lippincott Williams & Wilkins.

Girolami, U.D., Anthony, D.C., & Frosch, M.P. (1999). Peripheral nerve and skeletal muscle. In R.S. Cotran, V. Kumar, & T. Collins (Eds.), *Pathologic basis of disease*, 6th ed., p. 1289. Philadelphia: W.B. Saunders.

Girolami, U.D., Anthony, D.C., & Frosch, M.P. (1999). The central nervous system. In R.S. Cotran, V. Kumar, & T. Collins (Eds.), *Pathologic basis of disease*, 6th ed., pp. 1329–1333. Philadelphia: W.B. Saunders.

Olson, K.R. (Ed.). (1999). *Poisoning and drug overdose*, 3rd ed. Stamford, CT: Appleton & Lange.

21

Anticholinergic Drugs

Objectives

After studying this chapter, the student will be able to:

1. List characteristics of anticholinergic drugs in terms of effects on body tissues, indications for use, nursing process implications, observation of client response, and teaching clients.

2. Discuss atropine as the prototype of anticholinergic drugs.

3. Discuss clinical disorders/symptoms for which anticholinergic drugs are used.

4. Describe the mechanism by which atropine relieves bradycardia.

5. Review anticholinergic effects of antipsychotics, tricyclic antidepressants, and antihistamines.

6. Discuss principles of therapy and nursing process for using anticholinergic drugs in special populations.

7. Describe the signs and symptoms of atropine or anticholinergic drug overdose and its treatment.

8. Teach clients about the safe, effective use of anticholinergic drugs.

George Wilson, 76 years of age, has been treated for depression with amitriptyline (Elavil) for 5 years. He is admitted to the hospital for elective surgery, after which he becomes acutely confused. The physician prescribes haloperidol (Haldol) PRN to control severe agitation. You note in the drug reference text that both these medications have anticholinergic side effects.

Reflect on:

▶ Important assessments to detect anticholinergic effects.

▶ How anticholinergic side effects can be especially significant for the elderly.

▶ Developing a plan to minimize or manage anticholinergic effects for this client.

DESCRIPTION

Anticholinergic drugs, also called cholinergic blocking and parasympatholytic agents, block the action of acetylcholine on the parasympathetic nervous system (PNS). Usual doses block muscarinic cholinergic receptors in the brain, secretory glands, heart, and smooth muscle; large doses may block nicotinic receptors in skeletal muscle (see Chap. 17). The prototype drug is **atropine**, and this drug class includes belladonna alkaloids, their derivatives, and many synthetic substitutes.

Atropine and scopolamine are tertiary amines and therefore are able to cross cell membranes readily. They are well absorbed from the gastrointestinal (GI) tract and conjunctiva, and they cross the blood–brain barrier. Tertiary amines are excreted in the urine. Some belladonna derivatives and synthetic anticholinergics are quaternary amines. These drugs carry a positive charge and are lipid insoluble. Consequently, they do not readily cross cell membranes. They are poorly absorbed from the GI tract and do not cross the blood–brain barrier. Quaternary amines are excreted largely in the feces. Table 21-1 lists common tertiary amine and quaternary amine anticholinergic drugs.

Mechanism of Action and Effects

These drugs act by occupying receptor sites at parasympathetic nerve endings, thereby leaving fewer receptor sites free to respond to acetylcholine. Parasympathetic response is absent or decreased, depending on the number of receptors blocked by anticholinergic drugs and the underlying degree of parasympathetic activity. Overall, anticholinergic drugs have widespread effects on the body, including smooth muscle relaxation, decreased glandular secretions, and mydriasis. Specific effects on body tissues and organs include:

1. **Central nervous system (CNS) stimulation followed by depression,** which may result in coma and death. This is most likely to occur with large doses of anticholinergic drugs that cross the blood–brain barrier (atropine, scopolamine, and antiparkinson agents).

2. **Decreased cardiovascular response to parasympathetic (vagal) stimulation that slows heart rate.** Atropine is the anticholinergic drug most used for its cardiovascular effects. Usual clinical doses may produce a slight and temporary decrease in heart rate; moderate to large doses (0.5 to 1 mg) increase heart rate. This effect may be therapeutic in bradycardia or adverse in other types of heart disease. Atropine usually has little or no effect on blood pressure. Large doses cause facial flushing because of dilation of blood vessels in the neck.

3. **Bronchodilation and decreased respiratory tract secretions.** Bronchodilating effects result from blocking the bronchoconstrictive effects of acetylcholine.

4. **Antispasmodic effects in the GI tract due to decreased muscle tone and motility.** The drugs have little inhibitory effect on gastric acid secretion with usual doses, and insignificant effects on pancreatic and intestinal secretions.

5. **Mydriasis and cycloplegia in the eye.** Normally, anticholinergics do not change intraocular pressure, but with glaucoma, they may increase intraocular pressure. When the pupil is fully dilated, photophobia may be bothersome, and reflexes to light and accommodation may disappear.

6. **Miscellaneous effects** include decreased secretions from salivary and sweat glands; relaxation of ureters, urinary bladder, and the detrusor muscle; and relaxation of smooth muscle in the gallbladder and bile ducts.

The clinical usefulness of anticholinergic drugs is limited by their widespread effects. Consequently, several synthetic drugs have been developed in an effort to increase selectivity of action on particular body tissues, especially to retain the antispasmodic and antisecretory effects of atropine while eliminating its adverse effects. This effort has been less than successful—all the synthetic drugs produce atropine-like adverse effects when given in sufficient dosage.

One group of synthetic drugs is used for antispasmodic effects in GI disorders (Table 21-2). These drugs are quaternary amine compounds, which do not readily cross the blood–brain barrier. They are less likely to cause CNS effects than the natural alkaloids, which readily enter the CNS.

Another group of synthetic drugs includes centrally active anticholinergics used in the treatment of Parkinson's disease (see Chap. 12). They balance the relative cholinergic dominance that causes the movement disorders associated with parkinsonism.

TABLE 21-1	**Common Tertiary Amine and Quaternary Amine Anticholinergic Drugs**
Tertiary Amines	**Quaternary Amines**
Atropine	Glycopyrrolate (Robinul)
Benztropine (Cogentin)	Ipratropium (Atrovent)
Biperiden (Akineton)	Methscopolamine (Pamine)
Dicyclomine hydrochloride (Bentyl)	Propantheline bromide (Pro-Banthine)
Flavoxate (Urispas)	
L-Hyoscyamine (Anaspaz)	
Oxybutynin (Ditropan)	
Procyclidine (Kemadrin)	
Scopolamine	
Tolterodine (Detrol)	
Trihexyphenidyl (Artane)	

TABLE 21-2	Synthetic Anticholinergic-Antispasmodics Used in Gastrointestinal Disorders		
		Routes and Dosage Ranges	
Generic/Trade Name	**Adults**		**Children**
Dicyclomine hydrochloride (Bentyl)	PO, IM 10–20 mg 3–4 times daily		PO, IM 10 mg 3–4 times daily Infants: 5 mg 3–4 times daily
Glycopyrrolate (Robinul)	PO 1–2 mg 3 times daily initially, 1 mg 2 times daily for maintenance IM, IV, SC 0.1–0.2 mg 3–4 times daily at 4-h intervals		Dosage not established
Propantheline bromide (Pro-Banthine)	PO 15 mg 3 times daily before meals and 30 mg at bedtime		PO 1.5 mg/kg per day in 4 divided doses

IM, intramuscular; IV, intravenous; PO, oral; SC, subcutaneous.

Indications for Use

Anticholinergic drugs are used for disorders in many body systems. Clinical indications for use of anticholinergic drugs include GI, genitourinary, ophthalmic and respiratory disorders, bradycardia, and Parkinson's disease. They also are used before surgery and bronchoscopy.

- **GI disorders** in which anticholinergics have been used include peptic ulcer disease, gastritis, pylorospasm, diverticulitis, ileitis, and ulcerative colitis. These conditions are often characterized by excessive gastric acid and abdominal pain because of increased motility and spasm of GI smooth muscle. In peptic ulcer disease, more effective drugs have been developed, and anticholinergics are rarely used. The drugs are weak inhibitors of gastric acid secretion even in maximal doses (which usually produce intolerable adverse effects). Although they do not heal peptic ulcers, they may relieve abdominal pain by relaxing GI smooth muscle.

  Anticholinergics may be helpful in treating irritable colon or colitis, but they may be contraindicated in chronic inflammatory disorders (eg, diverticulitis, ulcerative colitis) or acute intestinal infections (eg, bacterial, viral, amebic). Other drugs are used to decrease diarrhea and intestinal motility in these conditions.

- In **genitourinary disorders,** anticholinergic drugs may be given for their antispasmodic effects on smooth muscle to relieve the symptoms of urinary incontinence and frequency that accompany an overactive bladder. In infections such as cystitis, urethritis, and prostatitis, the drugs decrease the frequency and pain of urination. The drugs are also given to increase bladder capacity in enuresis, paraplegia, or neurogenic bladder.

- In **ophthalmology,** anticholinergic drugs are applied topically for mydriatic and cycloplegic effects to aid examination or surgery. They are also used to treat some inflammatory disorders. Anticholinergic preparations used in ophthalmology are discussed further in Chapter 65.

- In **respiratory disorders** characterized by bronchoconstriction (ie, asthma, chronic bronchitis), ipratropium (Atrovent) may be given by inhalation for bronchodilating effects (see Chap. 47).

- In **cardiology,** atropine may be given to increase heart rate in bradycardia and heart block characterized by hypotension and shock.

- In **Parkinson's disease,** anticholinergic drugs are given for their central effects in decreasing salivation, spasticity, and tremors. They are used mainly in clients who have minimal symptoms, who do not respond to levodopa, or who cannot tolerate levodopa because of adverse reactions or contraindications. An additional use of anticholinergic drugs is to relieve Parkinson-like symptoms that occur with older antipsychotic drugs.

- **Before surgery,** anticholinergics are given to prevent vagal stimulation and potential bradycardia, hypotension, and cardiac arrest. They are also given to reduce respiratory tract secretions, especially in head and neck surgery and **bronchoscopy.**

Contraindications to Use

Contraindications to the use of anticholinergic drugs include any condition characterized by symptoms that would be aggravated by the drugs. Some of these are prostatic hypertrophy, myasthenia gravis, hyperthyroidism,

Nursing Notes: Apply Your Knowledge

Scott Andrews is scheduled for a bronchoscopy. Before this procedure, you have been ordered to give him Valium and atropine. Explain the rationale of giving an anticholinergic agent as a preoperative medication.

glaucoma, tachyarrhythmias, myocardial infarction, and heart failure unless bradycardia is present. They should not be given in hiatal hernia or other conditions contributing to reflux esophagitis because the drugs delay gastric emptying, relax the cardioesophageal sphincter, and increase esophageal reflux.

INDIVIDUAL ANTICHOLINERGIC DRUGS

Belladonna Alkaloids and Derivatives

Atropine, the prototype of anticholinergic drugs, produces the same effects and has the same clinical indications for use and the same contraindications as those described earlier. In addition, it is used as an antidote for an overdose of cholinergic drugs and exposure to insecticides that have cholinergic effects.

Atropine is a naturally occurring belladonna alkaloid that can be extracted from the belladonna plant or prepared synthetically. It is usually prepared as atropine sulfate, a salt that is very soluble in water. It is well absorbed from the GI tract and distributed throughout the body. It crosses the blood–brain barrier to enter the CNS, where large doses produce stimulant effects and toxic doses produce depressant effects. Atropine is also absorbed systemically when applied locally to mucous membranes. The drug is rapidly excreted in the urine. Pharmacologic effects are of short duration except for ocular effects, which may last for several days.

ROUTES AND DOSAGE RANGES

Adults: GI disorders, oral (PO), subcutaneous (SC) 0.3–1.2 mg q4–6h

Before surgery, intramuscular (IM) 0.4–0.6 mg in a single dose 45–60 min before anesthesia

Bradyarrhythmias, intravenous (IV) 0.4–1 mg q1–2h PRN

Bronchoconstriction, 0.025 mg/kg diluted with 3–5 mL saline and given by nebulizer three or four times per day

Topically to eye, one drop of 1% or 2% ophthalmic solution

Children: GI disorders, SC 0.01 mg/kg of body weight q4–6h

Before surgery, IM 0.4 mg for children 3–14 y, less for younger children and infants

Bradyarrhythmias, IV 0.01–0.03 mg/kg of body weight

Bronchoconstriction, 0.05 mg/kg diluted with 3–5 mL saline and given by nebulizer three or four times per day

Topically to eye, one drop of 0.5% or 1% ophthalmic solution

Belladonna tincture is a mixture of alkaloids in an aqueous-alcohol solution. It is most often used in GI disorders for antispasmodic effect. It is an ingredient in several drug mixtures.

ROUTE AND DOSAGE RANGE

Adults: PO 0.6–1 mL three or four times per day
Children: PO 0.03 mL/kg per day in three or four divided doses

Homatropine hydrobromide (Homapin) is a semisynthetic derivative of atropine used as eye drops to produce mydriasis and cycloplegia. Homatropine may be preferable to atropine because ocular effects do not last as long.

ROUTE AND DOSAGE RANGES

Adults: Topically to eye, 1 drop of 5% ophthalmic solution every 5 min for two or three doses for refraction; 1 drop of 2% to 5% solution two or three times per day for uveitis

Hyoscyamine (Anaspaz) is a belladonna alkaloid used in GI and genitourinary disorders characterized by spasm, increased secretion, and increased motility. It has the same effects as other atropine-like drugs.

ROUTE AND DOSAGE RANGES

Adults: PO 0.125–0.25 mg q6–8h until symptoms are controlled; IM, SC, IV 0.25–0.5 mg q6–12h until symptoms are controlled
Children: PO 0.062–0.125 mg q6–8h for children 2–10 y; half this dosage for children <2 y

Scopolamine is similar to atropine in uses, adverse effects, and peripheral effects but different in central effects. When given parenterally, scopolamine depresses the CNS and causes amnesia, drowsiness, euphoria, relaxation, and sleep. Effects of scopolamine appear more quickly and disappear more readily than those of atropine. Scopolamine also is used in motion sickness. It is available as oral tablets and as a transdermal adhesive disc that is placed behind the ear. The disc (Transderm-V) protects against motion sickness for 72 hours.

ROUTES AND DOSAGE RANGES

Adults: Before surgery, IM 0.4 mg
Motion sickness, PO 0.25–0.8 mg 1 h before travel; transdermally 1 disc q72h
Mydriasis, topically to the eye, 1 drop of 0.2% to 0.25% ophthalmic solution, repeated PRN
Children: Before surgery, 6 mo–3 y, IM 0.1–0.15 mg; 3–6 y, IM 0.15–0.2 mg; 6–12 y, 0.2–0.3 mg
Mydriasis, same as for adults

Centrally Acting Anticholinergics Used in Parkinson's Disease

Older anticholinergic drugs such as atropine are rarely used to treat Parkinson's disease because of their undesirable peripheral effects (eg, dry mouth, blurred vision, photophobia, constipation, urinary retention, and tachycardia). Newer, centrally acting synthetic anticholinergic drugs are more selective for muscarinic receptors in the CNS and are designed to produce fewer undesirable side effects.

Trihexyphenidyl (Artane) is used in the treatment of parkinsonism and extrapyramidal reactions caused by some antipsychotic drugs. Trihexyphenidyl relieves smooth muscle spasm by a direct action on the muscle and by inhibiting the PNS. The drug supposedly has fewer side effects than atropine, but approximately half the recipients report mouth dryness, blurring of vision, and other side effects common to anticholinergic drugs. Trihexyphenidyl requires the same precautions as other anticholinergic drugs and is contraindicated in glaucoma. **Biperiden** (Akineton) and **procyclidine** (Kemadrin) are chemical derivatives of trihexyphenidyl and have similar actions, uses, and adverse effects.

Trihexyphenidyl

ROUTE AND DOSAGE RANGES

Adults: Parkinsonism, PO 2 mg two or three times per day initially, gradually increased until therapeutic effects or severe adverse effects occur

Drug-induced extrapyramidal reactions, PO 1 mg initially, gradually increased to 5–15 mg/d in divided doses

Biperiden

ROUTES AND DOSAGE RANGES

Adults: Parkinsonism, PO 2 mg three or four times per day

Drug-induced extrapyramidal reactions, IM 2 mg, repeated q30 min, if necessary; maximum of four consecutive doses in 24 h

Children: Drug-induced extrapyramidal reactions, IM 0.04 mg/kg, repeated as above, if necessary

Procyclidine

ROUTE AND DOSAGE RANGES

Adults: Parkinsonism, PO 5 mg twice daily initially, gradually increased to 5 mg three or four times per day, if necessary

Drug-induced extrapyramidal reactions, PO 2–2.5 mg three times per day, gradually increased to 10–20 mg/d, if necessary

Benztropine (Cogentin) is a synthetic drug with both anticholinergic and antihistaminic effects. Its anticholinergic activity approximates that of atropine. A major clinical use is to treat acute dystonic reactions caused by antipsychotic drugs and to prevent their recurrence in clients receiving long-term antipsychotic drug therapy. It also may be given in small doses to supplement other antiparkinson drugs. In full dosage, adverse reactions are common.

ROUTES AND DOSAGE RANGES

Adults: PO 0.5–1 mg at bedtime, initially, gradually increased to 4–6 mg/d if required and tolerated

Drug-induced extrapyramidal reactions PO, IM, IV 1–4 mg once or twice per day

Urinary Antispasmodics

Flavoxate (Urispas) was developed specifically to counteract spasm in smooth muscle tissue of the urinary tract. It has anticholinergic, local anesthetic, and analgesic effects. Thus, the drug relieves dysuria, urgency, frequency, and pain with genitourinary infections, such as cystitis and prostatitis.

ROUTE AND DOSAGE RANGE

Adults and children 12 y or older: PO 100–200 mg three or four times per day. Reduce dose when symptoms improve.

Children <12 y: Dosage not established

Oxybutynin (Ditropan) has direct antispasmodic effects on smooth muscle and anticholinergic effects. It increases bladder capacity and decreases frequency of voiding in clients with neurogenic bladder.

ROUTE AND DOSAGE RANGE

Adults: PO 5 mg two or three times per day; maximum dose 5 mg four times per day

Children >5 y: PO 5 mg twice a day; maximum dose 5 mg three times per day

Tolterodine (Detrol) is a competitive antimuscarinic, anticholinergic agent able to inhibit bladder contraction, decrease detrusor muscle pressure, and delay the urge to void. It is used to treat urinary frequency, urgency, and urge incontinence. Tolterodine is more selective for muscarinic receptors in the urinary bladder than other areas of the body, such as the salivary glands, and therefore anticholinergic side effects are less marked.

ROUTE AND DOSAGE RANGE

Adults: PO initially 2 mg twice a day with or without food. Reduced doses of 1 mg PO twice a day are recommended for those with reduced hepatic function.

NURSING PROCESS

Assessment

- Assess the client's condition in relation to disorders for which anticholinergic drugs are used (ie, check for bradycardia or heart block, diarrhea, dysuria, abdominal pain, and other disorders). If the client reports or medical records indicate a specific disorder, assess for signs and symptoms of that disorder (eg, Parkinson's disease).
- Assess for disorders in which anticholinergic drugs are contraindicated (eg, glaucoma, prostatic hypertrophy, reflux esophagitis, myasthenia gravis, hyperthyroidism).
- Assess use of other drugs with anticholinergic effects, such as antihistamines (histamine-1 receptor antagonists [see Chap. 48]), antipsychotic agents, and tricyclic antidepressants.

Nursing Diagnoses

- Altered Urinary Elimination: Decreased bladder tone and urine retention
- Constipation related to slowed GI function
- Altered Thought Processes: Confusion, disorientation, especially in older adults
- Knowledge Deficit: Drug effects and accurate usage
- Risk for Injury related to drug-induced blurred vision and photophobia
- Risk for Noncompliance related to adverse drug effects
- Risk for Altered Body Temperature: Hyperthermia

Planning/Goals

The client will:

- Receive or self-administer the drugs correctly
- Experience relief of symptoms for which anticholinergic drugs are given
- Be assisted to avoid or cope with adverse drug effects on vision, thought processes, bowel and bladder elimination, and heat dissipation.

Interventions

Use measures to decrease the need for anticholinergic drugs. For example, with peptic ulcer disease, teach the client to avoid factors known to increase gastric secretion and GI motility (alcohol; cigarette smoking; caffeine-containing beverages, such as coffee, tea, and cola drinks; ulcerogenic drugs, such as aspirin). Late evening snacks also should be avoided because increased gastric acid secretion occurs approximately 90 minutes after eating and may cause pain and awakening from sleep. Although milk was once considered an "ulcer food," it contains protein and calcium, which promote acid secretion, and is a poor buffer of gastric acid. Thus, drinking large amounts of milk should be avoided.

Evaluation

- Interview and observe in relation to safe, accurate drug administration.
- Interview and observe for relief of symptoms for which the drugs are given.
- Interview and observe for adverse drug effects.

CLIENT TEACHING GUIDELINES
Anticholinergic Drugs

General Considerations

✔ Do not take other drugs without the physician's knowledge. In addition to some prescribed antidepressants, antihistamines, and antipsychotic drugs with anticholinergic properties, over-the-counter sleeping pills and antihistamines have anticholinergic effects. Taking any of these concurrently could cause overdosage or excessive anticholinergic effects.

✔ Use measures to minimize risks of heat exhaustion and heat stroke:
  ✔ Wear light, cool clothing in warm climates or environments.
  ✔ Maintain fluid and salt intake if not contraindicated.
  ✔ Limit exposure to direct sunlight.
  ✔ Limit physical activity.
  ✔ Take frequent cool baths.
  ✔ Ensure adequate ventilation, with fans or air conditioners if necessary.
  ✔ Avoid alcoholic beverages.

✔ Use sugarless chewing gum and hard candy, if not contraindicated, to relieve mouth dryness.

✔ Carry out good dental hygiene practices (eg, regular brushing of teeth) to prevent dental caries and loss of teeth that may result from drug-induced xerostomia (dry mouth from decreased saliva production). This is more likely to occur with long-term use of these drugs.

✔ To prevent injury due to blurring of vision or drowsiness, avoid potentially hazardous activities (eg, driving or operating machinery).

✔ To reduce sensitivity to light (photophobia), dark glasses can be worn outdoors in strong light.

✔ Contact lens wearers who experience dry eyes may need to use an ophthalmic lubricating solution.

✔ When using anticholinergic ophthalmic preparations, if eye pain occurs, stop using the medication and contact your physician or health care provider. This may be a warning sign of undiagnosed glaucoma.

✔ Notify your physician or health care provider if urinary retention or constipation occurs.

✔ Tell your physician or health care provider if you are pregnant or breastfeeding or allergic to sulfite preservatives or any other atropine compound.

Self-administration

✔ Take anticholinergic drugs for gastrointestinal disorders 30 minutes before meals and at bedtime.

✔ Safeguard anticholinergic medications from children because they are especially sensitive to atropine poisoning.

✔ To prevent constipation, use a diet high in fiber. Include whole grains, fruits, and vegetables in your daily menu. Also, drink 2 to 3 quarts of fluid a day and exercise regularly.

PRINCIPLES OF THERAPY

Use in Specific Conditions

Renal or Biliary Colic

Atropine is sometimes given with morphine or meperidine to relieve the severe pain of renal or biliary colic. It acts mainly to decrease the spasm-producing effects of the opioid analgesics. It has little antispasmodic effect on the involved muscles and is not used alone for this purpose.

Preoperative Use in Clients With Glaucoma

Glaucoma is usually listed as a contraindication to anticholinergic drugs because the drugs impair outflow of aqueous humor and may cause an acute attack of glaucoma (increased intraocular pressure). However, anticholinergic drugs can be given safely before surgery to clients with open-angle glaucoma (80% of clients with primary glaucoma) if they are receiving miotic drugs, such as pilocarpine. If anticholinergic preoperative medication is needed in clients predisposed to angle closure, the hazard of causing acute glaucoma can be minimized by also giving pilocarpine eye drops and acetazolamide (Diamox).

Gastrointestinal Disorders

When anticholinergic drugs are given for GI disorders, larger doses may be given at bedtime to prevent pain and awakening during sleep.

Parkinsonism

When these drugs are used in parkinsonism, small doses are given initially and gradually increased. This regimen decreases adverse reactions.

Extrapyramidal Reactions

When used in drug-induced extrapyramidal reactions (parkinson-like symptoms), these drugs should be prescribed only if symptoms occur. They should not be used routinely to prevent extrapyramidal reactions because fewer than half the clients taking antipsychotic drugs experience such reactions. Most drug-induced reactions last approximately 3 months and do not recur if anticholinergic drugs are discontinued at that time. (An exception is tardive dyskinesia, which does not respond to anticholinergic drugs and may be aggravated by them.)

Muscarinic Agonist Poisoning

Atropine is the antidote for poisoning by muscarinic agonists such as certain species of mushrooms, cholinergic agonist drugs, cholinesterase inhibitor drugs, and insecticides containing organophosphates. Symptoms of muscarinic poisoning include salivation, lacrimation, visual disturbances, bronchospasm, diarrhea, bradycardia, and hypotension. Atropine blocks the poison from interacting with the muscarinic receptor, thus reversing the toxic effects.

Asthma

Oral anticholinergics are not used to treat asthma and other chronic obstructive pulmonary diseases because of their tendency to thicken secretions and form mucus plugs in airways. Ipratropium (Atrovent) may be given by inhalation to produce bronchodilation without thickening of respiratory secretions.

Treatment of Atropine or Anticholinergic Overdosage

Overdosage of atropine or other anticholinergic drugs produces the usual pharmacologic effects in a severe and exaggerated form. The anticholinergic overdose syndrome is characterized by hyperthermia; hot, dry, flushed skin; dry mouth; mydriasis; delirium; tachycardia; ileus; and urinary retention. Myoclonic movements and choreoathetosis may be seen. Seizures, coma, and respiratory arrest may also occur. Treatment involves use of activated charcoal to absorb ingested poison. Hemodialysis, hemoperfusion, peritoneal dialysis, and repeated doses of charcoal are not effective in removing anticholinergic agents.

Physostigmine salicylate (Antilirium), an acetylcholinesterase inhibitor, is a specific antidote. It is usually given IV at a slow rate of injection. Adult dosage is 2 mg (no more than 1 mg/minute); child dosage is 0.5 to 1 mg (no more than 0.5 mg/minute). Rapid administration may cause bradycardia, hypersalivation (with subsequent respiratory distress), and seizures. Repeated doses may be given if life-threatening arrhythmias, convulsions, or coma occur. Diazepam (Valium) or a similar drug may be given for excessive CNS stimulation (delirium, excitement). Ice bags, cooling blankets, and tepid sponge baths may help reduce fever. Artificial ventilation and cardiopulmonary resuscitative measures are used if excessive depression of the CNS causes coma and respiratory failure. Infants, children, and the elderly are especially susceptible to the toxic effects of anticholinergic agents.

Use in Children

Systemic anticholinergics, including atropine, glycopyr-rolate (Robinul), and scopolamine, are given to children of all ages for essentially the same effects as for adults. The antispasmodic agents are also used. Flavoxate is not recommended for children younger than 12 years, and oxybutynin is not recommended for children younger than 5 years of age.

The drugs cause the same adverse effects in children as in adults. However, they may be more severe because children are especially sensitive to the drugs. Facial flushing is common in children, and a skin rash may occur.

Ophthalmic anticholinergic drugs are used for cyclo-plegia and mydriasis before eye examinations and surgical procedures. They should be used only with close medical supervision. Cyclopentolate (Cyclogyl) and tropicamide (Mydriacyl) have been associated with behavioral disturbances and psychotic reactions in children. Tropicamide also has been associated with cardiopulmonary collapse.

Use in Older Adults

Anticholinergic drugs are given for the same purposes as in younger adults. In addition to the primary anticholinergic drugs, many others that are commonly prescribed for older adults have high anticholinergic activity. These include many antihistamines (histamine-1 receptor antagonists), tricyclic antidepressants, and antipsychotic drugs.

Older adults are especially likely to have significant adverse reactions because of slowed drug metabolism and the frequent presence of several disease processes. Some common adverse effects and suggestions for reducing their impact are:

- **Blurred vision.** The client may need help with ambulation, especially with stairs or other potentially hazardous environments. Remove obstacles and hazards when possible.
- **Confusion.** Provide whatever assistance is needed to prevent falls and other injuries.
- **Heat stroke.** Help to avoid precipitating factors, such as strenuous activity and high environmental temperatures.
- **Constipation.** Encourage or assist with an adequate intake of high-fiber foods and fluids and adequate exercise when feasible.
- **Urinary retention.** Encourage adequate fluid intake and avoid high doses of the drugs. Men should be examined for prostatic hypertrophy.
- **Hallucinations and other psychotic symptoms.** These are most likely to occur with the centrally active anticholinergics given for Parkinson's disease or drug-induced extrapyramidal effects, such as trihexyphenidyl or benztropine. Dosage of these drugs should be carefully regulated and supervised.

Use in Renal Impairment

Anticholinergic agents that have a tertiary amine structure, such as atropine, are eliminated by a combination of hepatic metabolism and renal excretion. In the presence of renal impairment, they may accumulate and cause increased adverse effects. Quaternary amines are eliminated largely in the feces and are less affected by renal impairment.

Use in Hepatic Impairment

Because some anticholinergic drugs are metabolized by the liver, they may accumulate and cause adverse effects in the presence of hepatic impairment.

Use in Critical Illness

Atropine is an important drug in the emergency drug box. According to Advanced Cardiac Life Support guidelines, atropine is the first drug to be administered in the emergency treatment of bradyarrhythmias. Atropine 0.5 to 1 mg should be administered IV every 5 minutes and may be repeated up to 2 to 3 mg (0.03 to 0.04 mg/kg total dose). For clients with asystole, 1 mg of atropine is administered IV and repeated every 3 to 5 minutes if asystole persists, up to 0.4 mg/kg. Administration of atropine in doses less than 0.5 mg should be avoided because this may result in a paradoxical bradycardia. Atropine may be administered by endotracheal tube in clients without an intravenous access. The recommended dose is 1 to 2 mg diluted with sterile water or normal saline, not to exceed 10 mL total volume.

Abuse of Anticholinergic Agents

Anticholinergic drugs have potential intoxicating effects. Abuse of these drugs may produce euphoria, disorientation, hallucinations, and paranoia in addition to the classic anticholinergic adverse reactions.

 Home Care

Anticholinergic medications are commonly used in home care with children and adults. Children and elderly adults are probably most likely to experience adverse effects of these drugs and should be monitored carefully. With elderly clients, the home care nurse needs to assess medication regimens for combinations of drugs with anticholinergic effects, especially if mental confusion develops or worsens. The home care nurse may also need to teach elderly clients or caregivers that the drugs prevent sweating and heat loss and increase risks of heat stroke if precautions to avoid overheating are not taken.

NURSING ACTIONS — Anticholinergic Drugs

NURSING ACTIONS	RATIONALE/EXPLANATION
1. Administer accurately	
a. For gastrointestinal disorders, give most oral anticholinergic drugs approximately 30 min before meals and at bedtime.	To allow the drugs to reach peak antisecretory effects by the time ingested food is stimulating gastric acid secretion. Bedtime administration helps prevent awakening with abdominal pain.
b. When given before surgery, parenteral preparations of atropine can be mixed in the same syringe with several other common preoperative medications, such as meperidine (Demerol), morphine, oxymorphone (Numorphan), and promethazine (Phenergan).	The primary reason for mixing medications in the same syringe is to decrease the number of injections and thus decrease client discomfort. Note, however, that extra caution is required when mixing drugs to be sure that the dosage of each drug is accurate. Also, if any question exists regarding compatibility with another drug, it is safer not to mix the drugs, even if two or three injections are required.
c. When applying topical atropine solutions or ointment to the eye, be sure to use the correct concentration and blot any excess from the inner canthus.	Atropine ophthalmic preparations are available in several concentrations (usually 1%, 2%, and 3%). Excess medication should be removed so the drug will not enter the nasolacrimal (tear) ducts and be absorbed systemically through the mucous membrane of the nasopharynx or be carried to the throat and swallowed.
d. If propantheline is to be given intravenously, dissolve the 30-mg dose of powder in no less than 10 mL of sterile water for injection.	Parenteral administration is reserved for clients who cannot take the drug orally.
e. Instruct clients to swallow oral propantheline tablets, not to chew them.	The tablets have a hard sugar coating to mask the bitter taste of the drug.
f. Parenteral glycopyrrolate can be given through the tubing of a running intravenous infusion of physiologic saline or lactated Ringer's solution.	
2. Observe for therapeutic effects	Therapeutic effects depend primarily on the reason for use. Thus, a therapeutic effect in one condition may be a side effect or an adverse reaction in another condition.
a. When a drug is given for *peptic ulcer disease* or other gastrointestinal disorders, observe for decreased abdominal pain.	Relief of abdominal pain is due to the smooth muscle relaxant or antispasmodic effect of the drug.
b. When the drug is given for *diagnosing or treating eye disorders,* observe for pupil dilation (mydriasis) and blurring of vision (cycloplegia).	Note that these ocular effects are side effects when the drugs are given for problems not related to the eyes.
c. When the drug is given for *symptomatic bradycardia,* observe for increased pulse rate.	These drugs increase heart rate by blocking action of the vagus nerve.
d. When the drug is given for *urinary tract disorders,* such as cystitis or enuresis, observe for decreased frequency of urination. When the drug is given for *renal colic due to stones,* observe for decreased pain.	Anticholinergic drugs decrease muscle tone and spasm in the smooth muscle of the ureters and urinary bladder.

(*continued*)

NURSING ACTIONS	RATIONALE/EXPLANATION
e. When the centrally acting anticholinergics are given for *Parkinson's disease*, observe for decrease in tremor, salivation, and drooling.	Decreased salivation is a therapeutic effect with parkinsonism but an adverse reaction in most other conditions.
3. Observe for adverse effects	These depend on reasons for use and are dose related.
a. Tachycardia	Tachycardia may occur with usual therapeutic doses because anticholinergic drugs block vagal action, which normally slows heart rate. Tachycardia is not likely to be serious except in clients with underlying heart disease. For example, in clients with angina pectoris, prolonged or severe tachycardia may increase myocardial ischemia to the point of causing an acute attack of angina (chest pain) or even myocardial infarction. In clients with congestive heart failure, severe or prolonged tachycardia can increase the workload of the heart to the point of causing acute heart failure or pulmonary edema.
b. Excessive central nervous system (CNS) stimulation (tremor, restlessness, confusion, hallucinations, delirium) followed by excessive CNS depression (coma, respiratory depression)	These effects are more likely to occur with large doses of atropine because atropine crosses the blood-brain barrier. Large doses of trihexyphenidyl (Artane) also may cause CNS stimulation.
c. Sedation and amnesia with scopolamine or benztropine (Cogentin)	This may be a therapeutic effect but becomes an adverse reaction if severe or if the drug is given for another purpose. Benztropine has anticholinergic and antihistaminic properties. Apparently, drowsiness and sedation are caused by the antihistaminic component.
d. Constipation or paralytic ileus	These effects are the result of decreased gastrointestinal motility and muscle tone. Constipation is more likely with large doses or parenteral administration. Paralytic ileus is not likely unless the drugs are given to clients who already have decreased gastrointestinal motility.
e. Decreased oral and respiratory tract secretions, which cause mouth dryness and thick respiratory secretions	Mouth dryness is more annoying than serious in most cases and is caused by decreased salivation. However, clients with chronic lung disease, who usually have excessive secretions, tend to retain them with the consequence of frequent respiratory tract infections.
f. Urinary retention	This reaction is caused by loss of bladder tone and is most likely to occur in elderly men with enlarged prostate glands. Thus, the drugs are usually contraindicated with prostatic hypertrophy.
g. Hot, dry skin; fever; heat stroke	These effects are due to decreased sweating and impairment of the normal heat loss mechanism. Fever may occur with any age group. Heat stroke is more likely to occur with cardiovascular disease, strenuous physical activity, and high environmental temperatures, especially in elderly people.

(continued)

NURSING ACTIONS	RATIONALE/EXPLANATION
h. Ocular effects-mydriasis, blurred vision, photophobia	These are adverse effects when anticholinergic drugs are given for conditions not related to the eyes.
4. Observe for drug interactions **a.** Drugs that *increase* effects of anticholinergic drugs: Antihistamines, disopyramide, phenothiazines, thioxanthene agents, and tricyclic antidepressants	These drugs have anticholinergic properties and produce additive anticholinergic effects.
b. Drugs that *decrease* effects of anticholinergic drugs: Cholinergic drugs	These drugs counteract the inhibition of gastrointestinal motility and tone induced by atropine. They are sometimes used in atropine overdose.

Nursing Notes: Apply Your Knowledge

Answer: Although anticholinergic medications are no longer used routinely as preoperative medication, they are still used in some preoperative situations when decreased secretions in the respiratory tract are important. Also, anticholinergic agents block excessive vagal stimulation by the parasympathetic nervous system, which can occur after administration of some anesthetics or muscle relaxants (eg, succinylcholine) or after manipulation of the pharynx or trachea. Vagal stimulation causes bradycardia and hypotension, and in severe cases can result in cardiac arrest.

How Can You Avoid This Medication Error?

Answer: To prevent possible complications, more information must be obtained from Mr. Miller before the scopolamine patch can be safely administered. If Mr. Miller has closed-angle glaucoma, administering an anticholinergic agent could result in a significant rise in intraocular pressure and visual impairment. If it cannot be determined whether Mr. Miller has open-angle or closed-angle glaucoma, the drug should be held. Anticholinergic medications should be used cautiously with clients who have BPH because these drugs can cause urinary retention. Anticholinergic medications increase heart rate, which may not be advisable for many clients with heart disease.

REVIEW AND APPLICATION EXERCISES

1. How do anticholinergic drugs exert their therapeutic effects?
2. What are indications for use and contraindications for anticholinergic drugs?
3. What is the effect of anticholinergic drugs on heart rate, and what is the mechanism for this effect?
4. Under what circumstances is it desirable to administer atropine before surgery, and why?
5. What are adverse effects of anticholinergic drugs?
6. What treatment measures are indicated for a client with an overdose of a drug with anticholinergic effects?
7. Name two other commonly used drug groups that have anticholinergic effects.
8. What nursing observations and interventions are needed to increase client safety and comfort during anticholinergic drug therapy?

SELECTED REFERENCES

American Heart Association. (1997–99). *Advanced cardiac life support.* R.O. Cummins (Ed.).

Brown, J.H. & Taylor, P. (1996). Muscarinic receptor agonists and antagonists. In J.G. Hardman, L.E. Limbird, P.B. Molinoff, & R.W. Ruddon (Eds.), *Goodman & Gilman's The pharmacological basis of therapeutics,* 9th ed., pp. 141–160. New York: McGraw-Hill.

Carroll, E.W. & Curtis, R.L. (1998). Organization and control of neural function. In C.M. Porth (Ed.), *Pathophysiology: Concepts of altered health status,* 5th ed., pp. 870–877. Philadelphia: Lippincott Williams & Wilkins.

Crabtree, B.L. & Polles, A. (1997). Substance-related disorders. In J.T. Dipiro, R.L. Talbert, G.C. Yee, G.R. Matzke, B.G. Wells, and L.M. Posey (Eds.), *Pharmacotherapy: A pathophysiologic approach,* 3rd ed., pp. 1345–1365. Stamford, CT: Appleton & Lange.

Drug facts and comparisons. (Updated monthly). St. Louis: Facts and Comparisons.

Ganong, W.F. (1997). *Review of medical physiology,* 18th ed. Stamford, CT: Appleton & Lange.

Jones, L.A. (1997). Pharmacotherapy of cardiopulmonary resuscitation. In J.T. Dipiro, R.L. Talbert, G.C. Yee, G.R. Matzke, B.G. Wells, & L.M. Posey (Eds.), *Pharmacotherapy: A pathophysiologic approach,* 3rd ed., pp. 181–193. Stamford, CT: Appleton & Lange.

Kelly, H.W. & Kamada, A.K., (1997). Asthma. In J.T. Dipiro, R.L. Talbert, G.C. Yee, G.R. Matzke, B.G. Wells, and L.M. Posey (Eds.), *Pharmacotherapy: A pathophysiologic approach,* 3rd ed., pp. 553–590. Stamford, CT: Appleton & Lange.

Olson, K.R. (Ed.). (1999). *Poisoning and drug overdose,* 3rd ed. Stamford, CT: Appleton & Lange.

Drugs Affecting the Endocrine System

22

Physiology of the Endocrine System

Objectives

After studying this chapter, the student will be able to:

1. Discuss the relationship between the endocrine system and the central nervous system.

2. Describe general characteristics and functions of hormones.

3. Differentiate steroid and protein hormones in relation to site of action and pharmacokinetics.

4. Discuss hormonal action at the cellular level.

5. Describe the second messenger roles of cyclic adenosine monophosphate and calcium within body cells.

6. Differentiate between physiologic and pharmacologic doses of hormonal drugs.

THE ENDOCRINE SYSTEM

The endocrine system participates in the regulation of essentially all body activities, including metabolism of nutrients and water, reproduction, growth and development, and adapting to changes in internal and external environments. The major organs of the endocrine system are the hypothalamus, pituitary, thyroid, parathyroids, pancreas, adrenals, ovaries, and testes. These tissues function through *hormones*, substances that are synthesized and secreted into body fluids by one group of cells and have physiologic effects on other body cells. Hormones act as chemical messengers to transmit information between body cells and organs. Most hormones from the traditional endocrine glands are secreted into the bloodstream and act on distant organs.

In addition to the major endocrine organs, other tissues also produce hormones. These endocrine-like cells intermingle with nonendocrine cells in various organs. Their hormones are secreted into tissue fluids and act locally on nearby cells, as in the following examples:

Gastrointestinal mucosa produces hormones that are important in the digestive process (eg, gastrin, enterogastrone, secretin, and cholecystokinin).

The kidneys produce erythropoietin, a hormone that stimulates the bone marrow to produce red blood cells.

White blood cells produce cytokines that function as messengers among leukocytes in inflammatory and immune processes.

Many body tissues produce prostaglandins and leukotrienes, which have a variety of physiologic effects.

Neoplasms also may produce hormones. In endocrine tissues, neoplasms may be an added source of the hormone normally produced by the organ. In nonendocrine tissues, various hormones may be produced. For example, lung tumors may produce corticotropin (adrenocorticotropic hormone [ACTH]), antidiuretic hormone, or parathyroid hormone; kidney tumors may produce parathyroid hormone. The usual effects are those of excess hormone secretion.

This chapter focuses on the traditional endocrine organs and their hormones. Specific organs are discussed in the following chapters; general characteristics of the endocrine system and hormones are described in the following sections and in Box 22-1.

ENDOCRINE SYSTEM–NERVOUS SYSTEM INTERACTIONS

The endocrine and nervous systems are closely connected, anatomically and physiologically, and work in harmony to integrate and regulate body functions. In general, the ner-

---

BOX 22–1 MAJOR HORMONES AND THEIR GENERAL FUNCTIONS

Anterior pituitary hormones are growth hormone (also called somatotropin), corticotropin, thyroid-stimulating hormone, follicle-stimulating hormone, luteinizing hormone, and prolactin. Most of these hormones function by stimulating secretion of other hormones.

Posterior pituitary hormones are antidiuretic hormone (ADH or vasopressin) and oxytocin. ADH helps maintain fluid balance; oxytocin stimulates uterine contractions during childbirth.

Adrenal cortex hormones, commonly called corticosteroids, include the glucocorticoids, such as cortisol, and the mineralocorticoids, such as aldosterone. Glucocorticoids influence carbohydrate storage, exert anti-inflammatory effects, suppress corticotropin secretion, and increase protein catabolism. Mineralocorticoids help regulate electrolyte balance, mainly by promoting sodium retention and potassium loss. The adrenal cortex also produces sex hormones. The adrenal medulla hormones are epinephrine and norepinephrine (see Chap. 17).

Thyroid hormones include triiodothyronine (T$_3$ or liothyronine) and tetraiodothyronine (T$_4$ or thyroxine). These hormones regulate the metabolic rate of the body and greatly influence growth and development.

Parathyroid hormone, also called parathormone or PTH, regulates calcium and phosphate metabolism.

Pancreatic hormones are insulin and glucagon, which regulate the metabolism of glucose, lipids, and proteins.

Ovarian hormones (female sex hormones) are estrogens and progesterone. Estrogens promote growth of specific body cells and development of most female secondary sexual characteristics. Progesterone helps prepare the uterus for pregnancy and the mammary glands for lactation.

Testicular hormone (male sex hormone) is testosterone, which regulates development of masculine characteristics.

Placental hormones are chorionic gonadotropin, estrogen, progesterone, and human placental lactogen, all of which are concerned with reproductive functions.

vous system regulates rapid muscular and sensory activities by secreting substances that act as neurotransmitters, circulating hormones, and local hormones (eg, norepinephrine, epinephrine). The endocrine system regulates slow metabolic activities by secreting hormones that control cellular metabolism, transport of substances across cell membranes, and other functions (eg, reproduction, growth and development, secretion).

The main connecting link between the nervous system and the endocrine system is the hypothalamus, which responds to nervous system stimulation by producing hormones. Thus, secretion of almost all hormones from the pituitary gland is controlled by the hypothalamus. Special nerve fibers originating in the hypothalamus and ending in the posterior pituitary gland control secretions of the posterior pituitary. The hypothalamus secretes hormones called *releasing* and *inhibitory factors*, which regulate functions of the anterior pituitary. The anterior pituitary, in turn, secretes hormones that act on target tissues, usually to stimulate production of other hormones. For example, hypothalamic corticotropin-releasing hormone stimulates the anterior pituitary to produce corticotropin, and corticotropin, in turn, stimulates the adrenal cortex to produce cortisol. This complex interrelationship is often referred to as the *hypothalamic–pituitary–adrenocortical* axis. It functions by a *negative feedback* system, in which hormone secretion is stimulated when hormones are needed and inhibited when they are not needed. The hypothalamic–pituitary–thyroid axis also functions by a negative feedback mechanism.

GENERAL CHARACTERISTICS OF HORMONES

Hormones are extremely important in regulating body activities. Their normal secretion and function help to maintain the internal environment and determine response and adaptation to the external environment. Hormones participate in complex interactions with other hormones and nonhormone chemical substances in the body to influence every aspect of life. Although hormones are usually studied individually, virtually all endocrine functions are complex processes that are influenced by more than one hormone.

Although hormones circulating in the bloodstream reach essentially all body cells, some (eg, growth hormone, thyroid hormone) affect almost all cells, whereas others affect specific "target" tissues (eg, corticotropin stimulates the adrenal cortex). In addition, *one hormone can affect different tissues* (eg, ovarian estrogen can act on ovarian follicles to promote their maturation, on the endometrial lining of the uterus to stimulate its growth and cyclic changes, on breast tissue to stimulate growth of milk ducts, and on

the hypothalamic–pituitary system to regulate its own secretion), or *several hormones can affect a single tissue or function* (eg, catecholamines, glucagon, secretin, and prolactin regulate lipolysis [release of fatty acids from adipose tissue]).

Several hormones are secreted in cyclic patterns. For example, ACTH, cortisol, and growth hormone are secreted in 24-hour (circadian) cycles, whereas estrogen and progestin secretion is related to the 28-day menstrual cycle.

Hormone Pharmacokinetics

Protein-derived hormones (amines, amino acids, peptides, and polypeptides) are synthesized, stored, and released into the bloodstream in response to a stimulus. The steroid hormones, which are synthesized in the adrenal cortex and gonads from cholesterol, are released as they are synthesized. Most hormones are constantly present in the blood; plasma concentrations vary according to body needs, the rate of synthesis and release, and the rate of metabolism and excretion.

Protein-derived hormones usually circulate in an unbound, active form. Steroid and thyroid hormones are transported by specific carrier proteins synthesized in the liver. (Some drugs may compete with a hormone for binding sites on the carrier protein. If this occurs, hormone effects are enhanced because more unbound, active molecules are available to act on body cells.)

Hormones must be continuously inactivated to prevent their accumulation and excessive effects. Several mechanisms operate to eliminate hormones from the body. The water-soluble, protein-derived hormones have a short duration of action and are inactivated by enzymes mainly in the liver and kidneys. The lipid-soluble steroid and thyroid hormones have a longer duration of action because they are bound to plasma proteins. Once released by the plasma proteins, these hormones are conjugated in the liver to inactive forms and then excreted in bile or urine. A third, less common mechanism is inactivation by enzymes at receptor sites on target cells.

Hormone Action at the Cellular Level

Hormones modify rather than initiate cellular reactions and functions. Once hormone molecules reach a responsive cell, they bind with receptors in the cell membrane (eg, catecholamines and protein hormones) or inside the cell (eg, steroid and thyroid hormones). The number of hormone receptors and the affinity of the receptors for the hormone are the major determinants of target cell response to hormone action.

The main target organs for a given hormone contain large numbers of receptors. However, the number of receptors may be altered by various conditions. For example, receptors may be increased (called *up-regulation*) when there are low levels of hormone. This allows the cell to obtain more of the needed hormone than it can obtain with fewer receptors. Receptors may be decreased (called *down-regulation*) when there are excessive amounts of hormone. This mechanism protects the cell by making it less responsive to excessive hormone levels. Receptor up-regulation and down-regulation occur with chronic exposure to abnormal levels of hormones. In addition, receptor proteins may be decreased by inadequate formation or antibodies that destroy them. Thus, receptors are constantly being synthesized and degraded, so the number of receptors may change within hours. Receptor affinity for binding with hormone molecules probably changes as well.

After binding occurs, the resulting hormone–receptor complex initiates intracellular biochemical reactions, depending on the particular hormone and the type of cell. Many hormones act as a "first messenger" to the cell, and the hormone–receptor complex activates a "second messenger." The second messenger then activates intracellular structures to produce characteristic cellular functions and products. Steroid hormones from the adrenal cortex, ovaries, and testes stimulate target cells to synthesize various proteins (eg, enzymes, transport and structural proteins) needed for normal cellular function.

Second Messenger Systems

Three major second messenger systems, cyclic adenosine monophosphate (cAMP), calcium–calmodulin, and phospholipid products, are described in this section.

Cyclic AMP is the second messenger for many hormones, including corticotropin, catecholamines, glucagon, thyroid-stimulating hormone, follicle-stimulating hormone, luteinizing hormone, parathyroid hormone, secretin, and antidiuretic hormone. It is formed by the action of the enzyme adenyl cyclase on adenosine triphosphate, a component of all cells and the main source of energy for cellular metabolism. Once formed, cAMP activates a series of enzyme reactions that alter cell function. The amount of intracellular cAMP is increased by hormones that activate adenyl cyclase (eg, the pituitary hormones, calcitonin, glucagon, parathyroid hormone) and decreased by hormones that inactivate adenyl cyclase (eg, angiotensin, somatostatin). Cyclic AMP is inactivated by phosphodiesterase enzymes.

Calcium is the second messenger for angiotensin II, a strong vasoconstrictor that participates in control of arterial blood pressure, and for gonadotropin-releasing hormone. The postulated sequence of events is that hormone binding to receptors increases intracellular calcium. The calcium binds with an intracellular regulatory protein called calmodulin. The calcium–calmodulin complex activates protein kinases, which then regulate contractile structures of the cell, cell membrane permeability, and intracellular enzyme activity. Specific effects include contraction of smooth muscle, changes in the secretions produced by secreting cells, and changes in ciliary action in the lungs.

Phospholipid products are mainly involved with local hormones. Phospholipids are major components of the cell membrane portion of all body cells. Some local hormones activate cell membrane receptors and transform them into phospholipase C, an enzyme that causes some of the phospholipids in cell membranes to split into smaller molecules (eg, inositol triphosphate and diacylglycerol). These products then act as second messengers to intracellular structures. Inositol triphosphate mobilizes intracellular calcium ions and the calcium ions then fulfill their functions as second messengers, as described previously. Diacylglycerol activates an enzyme, protein kinase C, which is important in cell reproduction. Also, the lipid component of diacylglycerol is arachidonic acid, the precursor for prostaglandins, leukotrienes, and other local hormones with extensive effects.

Steroid Stimulation of Protein Synthesis

Steroid hormones are lipid soluble and therefore cross cell membranes easily. Once inside the cell cytoplasm, the hormone molecules bind with specific receptor proteins. The hormone–receptor complex then enters the nucleus of the cell where it activates nucleic acids (DNA and RNA) and the genetic code to synthesize new proteins.

Hormonal Disorders

Abnormal secretion and function of hormones, even minor alterations, can impair physical and mental health. Malfunction of an endocrine organ is usually associated with hyposecretion, hypersecretion, or inappropriate secretion of its hormones. Any malfunction can produce serious disease or death.

Hypofunction

Hypofunction may be associated with a variety of circumstances, including the following:

1. A congenital defect may result in the absence of an endocrine gland, the presence of an abnormally developed gland, or the absence of an enzyme required for glandular synthesis of its specific hormone.
2. The endocrine gland may be damaged or destroyed by impaired blood flow, infection or inflammation, autoimmune disorders, or neoplasms.
3. The endocrine gland may atrophy and become less able to produce its hormone because of aging, drug therapy, disease, or unknown reasons.
4. The endocrine gland may produce adequate hormone, but the hormone may not be able to function normally because of receptor defects (not enough receptors or the receptors present are unable to bind with the hormone).

5. Even if there is adequate hormone and adequate binding to receptors, intracellular metabolic processes (eg, enzyme function, protein synthesis, energy production) may not respond appropriately.

Hyperfunction

Hyperfunction is usually characterized by excessive hormone production. Excessive amounts of hormone may occur from excessive stimulation and enlargement of the endocrine gland, from a hormone-producing tumor of the gland, or from a hormone-producing tumor of non-endocrine tissues (eg, some primary lung tumors produce antidiuretic hormone and adrenocorticotropic hormone).

GENERAL CHARACTERISTICS OF HORMONAL DRUGS

1. Hormones given for therapeutic purposes include natural hormones from human or animal sources and synthetic hormones. Many of the most important hormones have been synthesized, and these preparations may have more potent and prolonged effects than the naturally occurring hormones.

2. Hormones are given for physiologic or pharmacologic effects. *Physiologic* use involves giving small doses as a replacement or substitute for the amount secreted by a normally functioning endocrine gland. Such use is indicated only when a gland cannot secrete an adequate amount of hormone. Examples of physiologic use include insulin administration in diabetes mellitus and adrenal corticosteroid administration in Addison's disease. *Pharmacologic* use involves relatively large doses for effects greater than

physiologic effects. For example, adrenal corticosteroids are widely used for anti-inflammatory effects in endocrine and nonendocrine disorders.

3. Hormones are powerful drugs that produce widespread therapeutic and adverse effects.

4. Administration of one hormone may alter effects of other hormones. These alterations result from the complex interactions among hormones.

5. Hormonal drugs are more often given for disorders resulting from endocrine gland hypofunction than for those related to hyperfunction.

 REVIEW AND APPLICATION EXERCISES

1. How do hormones function in maintaining homeostasis?

2. What is the connection between the nervous system and the endocrine system?

3. What is meant by a negative feedback system?

4. Because classic hormones are secreted into blood and circulated to essentially all body cells, why do they not affect all body cells?

5. What are the functions and characteristics of the pituitary gland?

SELECTED REFERENCES

Guyton, A.C. & Hall, J.E. (1996). *Textbook of medical physiology*, 9th ed. Philadelphia: W.B. Saunders.

Porth, C.M. (Ed.). (1998). Mechanisms of endocrine control. In *Pathophysiology: Concepts of altered health states*, 5th ed., pp. 775–783. Philadelphia: Lippincott Williams & Wilkins.

23

Hypothalamic and Pituitary Hormones

Objectives

After studying this chapter, the student will be able to:

1. Describe clinical uses of major pituitary hormones.

2. Differentiate characteristics and functions of anterior and posterior pituitary hormones.

3. Discuss limitations of hypothalamic and pituitary hormones as therapeutic agents.

4. State major nursing considerations in the care of clients receiving specific hypothalamic and pituitary hormones.

John, 11 years of age, is brought to the pediatric nurse practitioner for his annual sports physical. His mother voices concerns about John's short stature and questions you about the use of growth hormone. You note that John is in the 25th percentile for height and the 50th percentile for weight.

Reflect on:

▶ Additional assessment questions to ask John and his mother.

▶ Factors that might influence their desire for increased height and the use of growth hormone to accomplish this.

▶ If John uses growth hormone, outline some of the disadvantages and side effects.

DESCRIPTION

The hypothalamus and pituitary gland (hypophysis) interact to control most metabolic functions of the body and to maintain homeostasis. They are anatomically connected by the hypophyseal stalk. The hypothalamus controls secretions of the pituitary gland. The pituitary gland, in turn, regulates secretions or functions of other body tissues, called *target* tissues. The pituitary gland is actually two glands, each with different structures and functions. The anterior pituitary (adenohypophysis) is composed of different types of glandular cells that synthesize and secrete different hormones. The posterior pituitary (neurohypophysis) is anatomically an extension of the hypothalamus and is composed largely of nerve fibers. It does not manufacture any hormones itself but stores and releases hormones synthesized in the hypothalamus.

Hypothalamic Hormones

The hypothalamus produces a releasing hormone (also called factor) or an inhibiting hormone that corresponds to each of the major hormones of the anterior pituitary gland. Specifically, they are:

1. **Corticotropin-releasing hormone,** which causes release of corticotropin, also called adrenocorticotropic hormone (ACTH), in response to stress and threatening stimuli.
2. **Growth hormone-releasing factor,** which causes release of growth hormone in response to low blood levels of the hormone.
3. **Growth hormone release-inhibiting hormone** (somatostatin), which inhibits release of growth hormone. Somatostatin is found in many tissues other than the hypothalamus and inhibits many functions other than release of growth hormone. Additional inhibitions include secretion of thyroid-stimulating hormone (TSH or thyrotropin), prolactin, corticotropin, pancreatic secretions (insulin, glucagon, others), gastrointestinal (GI) secretions (gastrin, cholecystokinin, secretin, vasoactive intestinal peptide), GI motility, bile flow, and mesenteric blood flow.
4. **Thyrotropin-releasing hormone** (TRH), which causes release of TSH in response to stress, such as exposure to cold.
5. **Gonadotropin-releasing hormone** (GnRH), which causes release of follicle-stimulating hormone (FSH) and luteinizing hormone (LH).
6. **Prolactin-releasing factor,** which is active during lactation after childbirth.
7. **Prolactin-inhibitory factor** (PIF), which is active at times other than during lactation.

Pituitary Hormones

The anterior pituitary gland produces seven hormones. Two of these, growth hormone and prolactin, act directly on their target tissues; the other five act indirectly by stimulating target tissues to produce other hormones.

1. **Corticotropin,** also called ACTH, stimulates the adrenal cortex to produce adrenocorticosteroids. Secretion is controlled by the hypothalamus and by plasma levels of cortisol, the major adrenocorticosteroid. When plasma levels are adequate for body needs, the anterior pituitary does not release corticotropin (negative feedback mechanism).
2. **Growth hormone,** also called somatotropin, stimulates growth of all body tissues that are capable of responding. It promotes an increase in cell size and number, largely by affecting metabolism of carbohydrate, protein, fat, and bone tissue. Deficient growth hormone in children produces dwarfism, a condition marked by severely decreased linear growth and, frequently, severely delayed mental, emotional, dental, and sexual growth as well. Excessive growth hormone in preadolescent children produces gigantism, resulting in heights of 8 or 9 feet if untreated. Excessive growth hormone in adults produces acromegaly.
3. **Thyrotropin,** also called TSH, regulates secretion of thyroid hormones. Thyrotropin secretion is controlled by a negative feedback mechanism in proportion to metabolic needs. Thus, increased thyroid hormones in body fluids inhibit secretion of thyrotropin by the anterior pituitary and of TRH by the hypothalamus.
4. **FSH,** one of the gonadotropins, stimulates functions of sex glands. It is produced by the anterior pituitary gland of both sexes beginning at puberty. FSH acts on the ovaries in a cyclical fashion during the reproductive years, stimulating growth of ovarian follicles. These follicles then produce estrogen, which prepares the endometrium for implantation of a fertilized ovum. FSH acts on the testes to stimulate the production and growth of sperm (spermatogenesis), but it does not stimulate secretion of male sex hormones.
5. **LH** (also called *interstitial cell-stimulating hormone*) is another gonadotropin that stimulates hormone production by the gonads of both sexes. LH is important in the maturation and rupture of the ovarian follicle (ovulation). After ovulation, LH acts on the cells of the collapsed sac to produce the corpus luteum, which then produces progesterone during the last half of the menstrual cycle. When blood progesterone levels rise, a negative feedback effect is exerted on hypothalamic and anterior pituitary secretion of gonadotropins. Decreased pituitary secretion of LH causes the corpus luteum to die and

stop producing progesterone. Lack of progesterone causes slough and discharge of the endometrial lining as menstrual flow. (Of course, if the ovum has been fertilized and attached to the endometrium, menstruation does not occur.)

In men, LH stimulates the Leydig's cells in the spaces between the seminiferous tubules. These cells then secrete androgens, mainly testosterone.

6. **Prolactin** plays a part in milk production by nursing mothers. It is not usually secreted in nonpregnant women because of the hypothalamic hormone PIF. During late pregnancy and lactation, various stimuli, including suckling, inhibit the production of PIF, and thus prolactin is synthesized and released.

7. **Melanocyte-stimulating hormone** plays a role in skin pigmentation, but its function in humans is not clearly delineated.

The posterior pituitary gland stores and releases two hormones that are synthesized by nerve cells in the hypothalamus:

1. **Antidiuretic hormone** (ADH), also called vasopressin, functions to regulate water balance. When ADH is secreted, it makes renal tubules more permeable to water. This allows water in renal tubules to be reabsorbed into the plasma and so conserves body water. In the absence of ADH, little water is reabsorbed, and large amounts are lost in the urine.

Antidiuretic hormone is secreted when body fluids become concentrated (high amounts of electrolytes in proportion to the amount of water) and when blood volume is low. In the first instance, ADH causes reabsorption of water, dilution of extracellular fluids, and restoration of normal osmotic pressure. In the second instance, ADH raises blood volume and arterial blood pressure toward homeostatic levels.

2. **Oxytocin** functions in childbirth and lactation. It initiates uterine contractions at the end of gestation to induce childbirth, and it causes milk to move from breast glands to nipples so the infant can obtain the milk by suckling.

THERAPEUTIC LIMITATIONS

There are few approved clinical uses for hypothalamic hormones and pituitary hormones. Drug formulations of some hypothalamic hormones are relatively new and clinical experience with their use is limited; there are several reasons why pituitary hormones are not used extensively. First, other effective agents are available for some potential uses. When there is a deficiency of target gland hormones (eg, adrenocorticosteroids, thyroid hormones, male or female sex hormones), it is usually more convenient and effective to administer those hormones instead of the anterior pituitary hormones that stimulate their

secretion. Second, some pituitary hormones must be obtained from natural sources, which tends to be inconvenient and expensive. For example, corticotropin, thyrotropin, and ADH are obtained from the pituitary glands of domestic animals slaughtered for food; gonadotropins are obtained from the urine of pregnant or menopausal women. A third reason for the infrequent use of pituitary hormones is that most conditions in which pituitary hormones are indicated are uncommon.

Despite their limitations, hypothalamic and pituitary hormones perform important functions when indicated for clinical use.

INDIVIDUAL HORMONAL AGENTS

Hypothalamic Hormones

Gonadorelin acetate (Lutrepulse), gonadorelin hydrochloride (Factrel), and nafarelin (Synarel) are synthetic equivalents of GnRH. The acetate salt is used to induce ovulation in women with hypothalamic amenorrhea. The hydrochloride salt is used in diagnostic tests of gonadotropic functions of the anterior pituitary. Nafarelin is used in the treatment of endometriosis. For specific instructions regarding administration, consult current literature from the drug manufacturer.

Gonadorelin Acetate
ROUTE AND DOSAGE RANGE

Adults: Intravenous (IV) using special pump, 5 μg every 90 min for approximately 21 d

Gonadorelin Hydrochloride
ROUTE AND DOSAGE RANGE

Adults: Subcutaneous (SC), IV 100 μg

Nafarelin
ROUTE AND DOSAGE RANGE

Adults: One spray (200 μg) in one nostril in the morning and one spray in the other nostril in the evening (total daily dose, 400 μg), starting between the second and fourth days of the menstrual cycle

Octreotide (Sandostatin) has pharmacologic actions similar to those of somatostatin. Indications for use include acromegaly, in which it reduces blood levels of growth hormone and insulin-like growth factor-1; carcinoid tumors, in which it inhibits diarrhea and flushing; and in vasoactive intestinal peptide tumors, in which it relieves diarrhea (by decreasing GI secretions and motility). It is also used to treat diarrhea in acquired immunodeficiency syndrome and other conditions. The drug can be given IV, but is most often given SC and may be self-administered. Dosage needs to be reduced in elderly persons.

ROUTES AND DOSAGE RANGES

Adults: Acromegaly, SC 50–100 µg three times daily

Carcinoid tumors, SC 100–600 µg daily in 2 to 4 divided doses; average dose 300 µg daily

Intestinal tumors, SC 200–300 µg daily in 2 to 4 divided doses

Diarrhea, IV, SC 50 µg two to three times daily initially, then adjusted according to response

Protirelin (Thypinone) is a synthetic equivalent of natural TRH. It is used for diagnostic tests of thyroid, pituitary, and hypothalamic function. For specific test methodology and interpretation, consult the drug manufacturers' instructions.

ROUTES AND DOSAGE RANGES

Adults: IV 200–500 µg, injected over 15–30 sec, with client supine and remaining supine for at least 15 min

Children, 6–16 y: 7 µg/kg, up to a maximum dose of 500 µg

Infants and children up to 6 y: Dosage not established

Anterior Pituitary Hormones

Corticotropin (ACTH, Acthar) is obtained from porcine pituitary glands. Corticotropin is composed of 39 amino acids, 24 of which exert the characteristic physiologic effects. Because it is a protein substance, corticotropin is destroyed by proteolytic enzymes in the digestive tract and must therefore be given parenterally. Corticotropin has a short duration of action and must be administered frequently. There are, however, repository preparations (Cortrophin-Gel, Cortrophin-Zinc) that are slowly absorbed, have a longer duration of action, and can be given once daily.

Corticotropin is given to stimulate synthesis of hormones by the adrenal cortex (glucocorticoids, mineralocorticoids, sex hormones). It is not effective unless the adrenal cortex can respond. Adrenocortical response is variable, and dosage of corticotropin must be individualized. When corticotropin therapy is being discontinued, dosage is gradually reduced to avoid the steroid withdrawal syndrome, characterized by muscle weakness, fatigue, and hypotension. Corticotropin is also used in laboratory tests of adrenal function.

Cosyntropin (Cortrosyn) is a synthetic drug with biologic activity similar to that of corticotropin. It is used as a diagnostic test in suspected adrenal insufficiency.

Corticotropin

ROUTES AND DOSAGE RANGES

Adults: Therapeutic use, intramuscular (IM), SC 20 units four times per day

Diagnostic use, IM 40–80 units daily for 1–3 d; IV 10–25 units in 500 mL of 5% dextrose or 0.9% sodium chloride solution, infused over 8 h once a day. A continuous infusion with 40 units q12h for 48 h may also be used.

Cortrophin-Gel

ROUTE AND DOSAGE RANGE

Adults: Therapeutic use, IM 40–80 units q24–72h

Diagnostic use, IM 40–80 units/d for 1–3 d

Cosyntropin

ROUTES AND DOSAGE RANGE

Adults: Diagnostic use, IM, IV 0.25 mg (equivalent to 25 units ACTH)

Growth hormone is synthesized from bacteria by recombinant DNA technology. Two forms are available. Somatropin (Humatrope) contains the same number and sequence of amino acids as pituitary-derived human growth hormone. Somatrem (Protropin) is the same except it contains one additional amino acid, methionine. The drugs are therapeutically equivalent to endogenous growth hormone produced by the pituitary gland. The only clinical use of the drugs is for children whose growth is impaired by a deficiency of endogenous growth hormone. The drugs are ineffective when impaired growth results from other causes or after puberty, when epiphyses of the long bones have closed. Dosage should be individualized according to response. Excessive administration can cause excessive growth (gigantism).

Somatrem

ROUTE AND DOSAGE RANGE

Children: IM, up to 0.1 mg/kg three times per week

Somatropin

ROUTE AND DOSAGE RANGE

Children: IM, up to 0.06 mg/kg three times per week

Human chorionic gonadotropin (HCG [Follutein]) is a placental hormone obtained from the urine of pregnant women. In men, HCG produces physiologic effects similar to those of the naturally occurring LH. HCG is used clinically to evaluate the ability of the Leydig's cells to produce testosterone and to treat cryptorchidism (undescended testicle) in preadolescent boys. Excessive doses or prolonged administration can lead to sexual precocity, edema, and breast enlargement caused by oversecretion of testosterone and possibly estrogen. In women, HCG is used in combination with menotropins to induce ovulation in the treatment of infertility.

ROUTE AND DOSAGE RANGES

Adults and preadolescent boys: Cryptorchidism and male hypogonadism, IM 500–4000 units two or three times per week for several weeks

To induce ovulation, IM 5000–10,000 units in one dose, 1 d after treatment with menotropins

Menotropins (Pergonal), a gonadotropin preparation obtained from the urine of postmenopausal women, contains both FSH and LH. It is usually combined with HCG to induce ovulation in the treatment of infertility caused by lack of pituitary gonadotropins.

ROUTE AND DOSAGE RANGE

Adults: IM 1 ampule (75 units FSH and 75 units LH) daily for 9–12 d, followed by HCG to induce ovulation

Thyrotropin (Thytropar) is obtained from bovine pituitary glands. It is used as a diagnostic agent to distinguish between primary hypothyroidism (caused by a thyroid disorder) and secondary hypothyroidism (caused by pituitary malfunction). If thyroid hormones in serum are elevated after the administration of thyrotropin, then the hypothyroidism is secondary to inadequate pituitary function. Thyrotropin must be used cautiously in clients with coronary artery disease, congestive heart failure, or adrenocortical insufficiency.

ROUTES AND DOSAGE RANGES

Adults: IM, SC 10 units daily for 1–3 d, followed by ^{131}I in 18–24 h. Thyroid uptake of iodine is measured 24 h after iodine administration. Accumulation is greater in hypopituitarism than in primary hypothyroidism.

Posterior Pituitary Hormones

Desmopressin acetate (DDAVP, Stimate) is a synthetic analogue of ADH. A major clinical use is the treatment of neurogenic diabetes insipidus, a disorder characterized by a deficiency of ADH and the excretion of large amounts of dilute urine. Diabetes insipidus may be idiopathic, hereditary, or acquired as a result of trauma, surgery, tumor, infection, or other conditions that impair the function of the hypothalamus or posterior pituitary. Parenteral desmopressin is also used as a hemostatic in clients with hemophilia A or mild to moderate von Willebrand's disease (type 1). The drug is effective in controlling spontaneous or trauma-induced bleeding and intraoperative and postoperative bleeding when given 30 minutes before the procedure.

ROUTES AND DOSAGE RANGES

Adults: Diabetes insipidus, intranasally 0.1–0.4 mL/d, usually in two divided doses
Hemophilia A, von Willebrand's disease, IV 0.3 µg/kg in 50 mL sterile saline, infused over 15–30 min
Children 3 mo–2 y: Diabetes insipidus, intranasally 0.05–0.3 mL/d in one or two doses
Children weighing >10 kg: Hemophilia A, von Willebrand's disease, same as adult dosage
Children weighing ≤10 kg: Hemophilia A, von Willebrand's disease, IV 0.3 µg/kg in 10 mL of sterile saline

Lypressin is a synthetic vasopressin that is given intranasally rather than by injection. It is used only for controlling the excessive water loss of diabetes insipidus caused by inadequate function of the posterior pituitary gland.

ROUTE AND DOSAGE RANGE

Adults: Intranasal spray, one or two sprays to one or both nostrils, three or four times per day

Vasopressin (Pitressin) is available as a synthetic preparation. Until lypressin was developed, vasopressin was the most widely used drug for diabetes insipidus caused by hypofunction of the posterior pituitary gland. Vasopressin has a short duration of action (a few hours), which is a disadvantage when long-term treatment of diabetes insipidus is necessary. Vasopressin tannate is a long-acting oil suspension that also must be injected; its effects last 1 to 3 days. Vasopressin has a vasoconstrictor effect and is used in the treatment of bleeding esophageal varices.

ROUTES AND DOSAGE RANGES

Adults: IM, SC, intranasally on cotton pledgets, 0.25–0.5 mL (5–10 units) two or three times per day
Children: IM, SC, intranasally on cotton pledgets, 0.125–0.5 mL (2.5–10 units) three or four times per day

Oxytocin (Pitocin) is a synthetic drug that exerts the same physiologic effects as the posterior pituitary hormone. Thus, it promotes uterine contractility and is used clinically to induce labor and in the postpartum period to control bleeding. Oxytocin must be used only when clearly indicated and when the recipient can be supervised by well-trained personnel, as in a hospital.

ROUTES AND DOSAGE RANGES

Adults: Induction of labor, IV 1-mL ampule (10 units) in 1000 mL of 5% dextrose injection (10 units/1000 mL = 10 milliunits/mL), infused at 0.2–2 milliunits/min initially, then regulated according to frequency and strength of uterine contractions
Prevention or treatment of postpartum bleeding, IV 10–40 units in 1000 mL of 5% dextrose injection, infused at 125 mL/h (40 milliunits/min) or 0.6–1.8 units (0.06–0.18 mL) diluted in 3–5 mL sodium chloride injection and injected slowly; IM 0.3–1 mL (3–10 units)

NURSING PROCESS

Assessment

Assess for disorders for which hypothalamic and pituitary hormones are given:

- For children with impaired growth, assess height and weight (actual and compared with growth charts) and diagnostic x-ray reports of bone age.
- For clients with diabetes insipidus, assess baseline blood pressure, weight, ratio of fluid intake to urine output, urine specific gravity, and laboratory reports of serum electrolytes.

- For clients with diarrhea, assess number and consistency of stools per day as well as hydration status.

Nursing Diagnoses

- Knowledge Deficit: Drug administration and effects
- Altered Growth and Development
- Anxiety related to multiple injections
- Risk for Injury: Adverse drug effects

Planning/Goals

The client will:

- Experience relief of symptoms without serious adverse effects
- Take or receive the drug accurately
- Comply with procedures for monitoring and follow-up

Interventions

- For children receiving growth hormone, assist the family to set reasonable goals for increased height and weight and to comply with accurate drug administration and follow-up procedures (periodic x-rays to determine bone growth and progress toward epiphyseal closure, recording height and weight at least weekly).
- For clients with diabetes insipidus, assist them to develop a daily routine to monitor their response to drug therapy (eg, weigh themselves, monitor fluid intake and urine output for approximately equal amounts, or check urine specific gravity (should be at least 1.015) and replace fluids accordingly.

Evaluation

- Interview and observe for compliance with instructions for taking the drug(s).
- Observe for relief of symptoms for which pituitary hormones were prescribed.

Nursing Notes: Apply Your Knowledge

After surgery for a brain tumor, you note that Mr. Willis has excessive, dilute urine output (8000 mL/24 h). The physician diagnoses deficient antidiuretic hormone production and prescribes lypressin (Diapid), a synthetic vasopressin. What assessment data will indicate that this medication is effective?

PRINCIPLES OF THERAPY

1. Hypothalamic hormones are rarely used in most clinical practice settings. The drugs should be prescribed by physicians who are knowledgeable about endocrinology and administered according to current manufacturers' literature.
2. Most drug therapy with pituitary hormones is given to replace or supplement naturally occurring hormones in situations involving inadequate function of the pituitary gland (hypopituitarism). Conditions resulting from excessive amounts of pituitary hormones (hyperpituitarism) are more often treated with surgery or irradiation.
3. Diagnosis of suspected pituitary disorders should be thorough to promote more effective treatment, including drug therapy.
4. Even though manufacturers recommend corticotropin for treatment of diseases that respond to glucocorticoids, corticotropin is less predictable and less convenient than glucocorticoids and has no apparent advantages over them.
5. Dosage of any pituitary hormone must be individualized because responsiveness of affected tissues varies.

NURSING ACTIONS   Hypothalamic and Pituitary Hormones

NURSING ACTIONS	RATIONALE/EXPLANATION
1. **Administer accurately** **a.** Read the manufacturer's instructions and drug labels carefully before drug preparation and administration.	These hormone preparations are given infrequently and often require special techniques of administration.
2. **Observe for therapeutic effects**	Therapeutic effects vary widely, depending on the particular pituitary hormone given and the reason for use.

(continued)

NURSING ACTIONS	RATIONALE/EXPLANATION
a. With gonadorelin, observe for ovulation or decreased symptoms of endometriosis and absence of menstruation.	Therapeutic effects depend on the reason for use. Note that different formulations are used to stimulate ovulation and treat endometriosis.
b. With corticotropin, therapeutic effects stem largely from increased secretion of adrenal cortex hormones, especially the glucocorticoids, and include anti-inflammatory effects (see Chap. 24).	Corticotropin is usually not recommended for the numerous nonendocrine inflammatory disorders that respond to glucocorticoids. Administration of glucocorticoids is more convenient and effective than administration of corticotropin.
c. With chorionic gonadotropin and menotropins given in cases of female infertility, ovulation and conception are therapeutic effects.	
d. With chorionic gonadotropin given in cryptorchidism, the therapeutic effect is descent of the testicles from the abdomen to the scrotum.	
e. With growth hormone, observe for increased skeletal growth and development.	Indicated by appropriate increases in height and weight.
f. With antidiuretics (desmopressin, lypressin, and vasopressin), observe for decreased urine output, increased urine specific gravity, decreased signs of dehydration, decreased thirst.	These effects indicate control of diabetes insipidus.
g. With oxytocin given to induce labor, observe for the beginning or the intensifying of uterine contractions.	
h. With oxytocin given to control postpartum bleeding, observe for a firm uterine fundus and decreased vaginal bleeding.	
i. With octreotide given for diarrhea, observe for decreased number and fluidity of stools.	Octreotide is often used to control diarrhea associated with a number of conditions.
3. Observe for adverse effects	
a. With gonadorelin, observe for headache, nausea, lightheadedness, and local edema, pain and pruritus after subcutaneous injections.	Systemic reactions occur infrequently.
b. With protirelin, observe for hypotension, nausea, headache, lightheadedness, anxiety, drowsiness.	Although adverse effects occur in about 50% of patients, they are usually minor and of short duration.
c. With corticotropin, observe for sodium and fluid retention, edema, hypokalemia, hyperglycemia, osteoporosis, increased susceptibility to infection, myopathy, behavioral changes.	These adverse reactions are in general the same as those produced by adrenal cortex hormones. Severity of adverse reactions tends to increase with dosage and duration of corticotropin administration.
d. With human chorionic gonadotropin given to preadolescent boys, observe for sexual precocity, breast enlargement, and edema.	Sexual precocity results from stimulation of excessive testosterone secretion at an early age.
e. With growth hormone, observe for mild edema, headache, localized muscle pain, weakness, hyperglycemia.	Adverse effects are not common. Another adverse effect may be development of antibodies to the drug, but this does not prevent its growth-stimulating effects.
f. With menotropins, observe for symptoms of ovarian hyperstimulation, such as abdominal	Adverse effects can be minimized by frequent pelvic examinations to check for ovarian enlargement and

(*continued*)

NURSING ACTIONS	RATIONALE/EXPLANATION
discomfort, weight gain, ascites, pleural effusion, oliguria, and hypotension.	by laboratory measurement of estrogen levels. Multiple gestation (mostly twins) is a possibility and is related to ovarian overstimulation.
g. With desmopressin, observe for headache, nasal congestion, nausea, and occasionally a slight increase in blood pressure. A more serious adverse reaction is water retention and hyponatremia.	Adverse reactions usually occur only with high dosages and tend to be relatively mild. Water intoxication (headache, nausea, vomiting, confusion, lethargy, coma, convulsions) may occur with any antidiuretic therapy if excessive fluids are ingested.
h. With lypressin, observe for headache and congestion of nasal passages, dyspnea and coughing (if the drug is inhaled), and water intoxication if excessive amounts of lypressin or fluid are taken.	Adverse effects are usually mild and occur infrequently with usual doses.
i. With vasopressin, observe for water intoxication; chest pain, myocardial infarction, increased blood pressure; abdominal cramps, nausea, and diarrhea.	With high doses, vasopressin constricts blood vessels, especially coronary arteries, and stimulates smooth muscle of the gastrointestinal tract. Special caution is necessary in clients with heart disease, asthma, or epilepsy.
j. With oxytocin, observe for excessive stimulation or contractility of the uterus, uterine rupture, and cervical and perineal lacerations.	Severe adverse reactions are most likely to occur when oxytocin is given to induce labor and delivery.
k. With octreotide, observe for arrhythmias, bradycardia, diarrhea, headache, hyperglycemia, injection site pain, and symptoms of gallstones.	These are more common effects, especially in those receiving octreotide for acromegaly.
4. **Observe for drug interactions**	
a. Drugs that *decrease* effects of protirelin (ie, thyrotropin response): Aspirin (2 g or more per day), glucocorticoids (pharmacologic doses), levodopa, thyroid hormones	
b. Drugs that *increase* effects of vasopressin: General anesthetics, chlorpropamide (Diabinese)	Potentiate vasopressin
c. Drug that *decreases* effects of vasopressin: Lithium	Inhibits the renal tubular reabsorption of water normally stimulated by vasopressin
d. Drugs that *increase* effects of oxytocin: (1) Estrogens	With adequate estrogen levels, oxytocin increases uterine contractility. When estrogen levels are low, the effect of oxytocin is reduced.
(2) Vasoconstrictors or vasopressors (eg, ephedrine, epinephrine, norepinephrine)	Severe, persistent hypertension with rupture of cerebral blood vessels may occur because of additive vasoconstrictor effects. This is a potentially lethal interaction and should be avoided.

Nursing Notes: Apply Your Knowledge

Answer: Lypressin replaces the antidiuretic hormone that acts to decrease urine output. If this medication is effective, you would expect to see a decrease in urine output. The urine will appear less dilute (may be pale yellow rather than clear) and have a higher specific gravity. Keep accurate intake and output records on Mr. Willis, record daily weights, and monitor specific gravity.

REVIEW AND APPLICATION EXERCISES

1. What hormones are secreted by the hypothalamus and pituitary, and what are their functions?

2. What are the functions and clinical uses of ADH, growth hormone, and oxytocin?

3. What are adverse effects of the hypothalamic and pituitary hormones used in clinical practice?

SELECTED REFERENCES

Ascoli, M. & Segaloff, D.L. (1996). Adenohypophyseal hormones and their hypothalamic releasing factors. In J.G. Hardman, L.E. Limbird, P.B. Molinoff, & R.W. Ruddon (Eds.), *Goodman & Gilman's The pharmacological basis of therapeutics*, 9th ed., pp. 1363–1382. New York: McGraw-Hill.

Drug facts and comparisons. (Updated monthly). St. Louis: Facts and Comparisons.

Guyton, A.C. & Hall. J.E. (1996). *Textbook of medical physiology*, 9th ed. Philadelphia: W.B. Saunders.

Porth, C.M. (Ed.). (1998). *Pathophysiology: Concepts of altered health states*, 5th ed. Philadelphia: Lippincott Williams & Wilkins.

24

Corticosteroids

Objectives

After studying this chapter, the student will be able to:

1. Review physiologic effects of endogenous corticosteroids.

2. List at least five clinical indications for use of exogenous corticosteroids.

3. Differentiate between physiologic and pharmacologic doses of corticosteroids.

4. Differentiate between short-term and long-term corticosteroid therapy.

5. List at least 10 adverse effects of long-term corticosteroid therapy.

6. Explain the pathophysiologic basis of adverse effects.

7. State the rationale for giving corticosteroids topically when possible rather than systemically.

8. Use other drugs and interventions to decrease the need for corticosteroids.

9. Discuss the use of corticosteroids in selected populations and conditions.

10. Apply the nursing process with a client receiving long-term systemic corticosteroid therapy, including teaching needs.

Sally, 15 years of age, was hospitalized with ulcerative colitis 2 days ago. When you enter her room, she is crying and does not look up. You sit down quietly beside her. Finally, she begins to tell you her fears. "The doctor says I have to go on steroids for my ulcerative colitis. I remember this girl in middle school who had a kidney transplant and had to take steroids. She gained lots of weight and her face became round and fat. I don't want that to happen to me."

Reflect on:

▶ The developmental level of a 15-year-old.

▶ The impact a chronic illness or long-term use of corticosteroids would have for an adolescent.

▶ What you could say in this situation that might be helpful. Provide rationale.

▶ What you should not say in this situation. Provide rationale.

Corticosteroids, also called *glucocorticoids* or *steroids*, are hormones produced by the adrenal cortex. These hormones affect almost all body organs and are extremely important in maintaining homeostasis when secreted in normal amounts. Disease results from inadequate or excessive secretion. Exogenous corticosteroids are used as drugs in a variety of disorders. Their use must be closely monitored because the drugs produce profound therapeutic and adverse effects. To understand the effects of corticosteroids used as drugs, it is necessary to understand physiologic effects and other characteristics of the endogenous hormones.

ENDOGENOUS CORTICOSTEROIDS

The adrenal cortex produces approximately 30 steroid hormones, which are divided into glucocorticoids, mineralocorticoids, and adrenal sex hormones. Glucocorticoids are important in metabolic, inflammatory, and immune processes. Mineralocorticoids are important in maintaining fluid and electrolyte balance. The adrenal sex hormones have little effect on normal body function.

Chemically, all corticosteroids are derived from cholesterol and have similar chemical formulas. Despite their similarities, however, slight differences in structure cause them to have different functions.

Secretion of Corticosteroids

Corticosteroid secretion is controlled by the hypothalamus, anterior pituitary, and adrenal cortex (the hypothalamic–pituitary–adrenal, or HPA, axis). Various stimuli (eg, low plasma levels of corticosteroids, pain, anxiety, trauma, illness, anesthesia) activate the system. These stimuli cause the hypothalamus to secrete corticotropin-releasing hormone (CRH). CRH stimulates the anterior pituitary to secrete corticotropin, and corticotropin stimulates the adrenal cortex to secrete corticosteroids.

The rate of corticosteroid secretion is usually maintained within relatively narrow limits but changes according to need. When plasma corticosteroid levels rise to an adequate level, secretion of corticosteroids slows or stops. The mechanism by which the hypothalamus and anterior pituitary are informed that no more corticosteroids are needed is called a *negative feedback mechanism*.

This negative feedback mechanism is normally very important, but it does not work during stress responses. The stress response activates the sympathetic nervous system (SNS) to produce more epinephrine and norepinephrine and the adrenal cortex to produce as much as 10 times the normal amount of cortisol. The synergistic interaction of these hormones increases the person's ability to respond to stress. However, the increased SNS activity continues to stimulate cortisol production and over-

rules the negative feedback mechanism. Excessive and prolonged corticosteroid secretion damages body tissues.

Corticosteroids are secreted directly into the bloodstream, where they are approximately 90% bound to plasma proteins (approximately 80% to an alpha globulin called transcortin or corticosteroid-binding globulin and approximately 10% to albumin). The remaining 10%, which has a plasma half-life of approximately 1.5 hours, is unbound and biologically active.

Corticosteroids are metabolized in the liver. Most metabolites (approximately 75%) are excreted in the urine, the remainder in bile and feces. Metabolism is slowed by hepatic disease, and excretion is slowed by renal disease. In these conditions, corticosteroids may accumulate and cause signs and symptoms of hypercortism.

Glucocorticoids

The term *corticosteroids* actually means all secretions of the adrenal cortex, but it is most often used to designate the glucocorticoids. Glucocorticoids include cortisol, corticosterone, and cortisone. *Cortisol* accounts for at least 95% of glucocorticoid activity, and approximately 10 to 25 mg are secreted daily. *Corticosterone* has a small amount of activity, and approximately 1.5 to 4 mg are secreted daily. *Cortisone* has little activity and is secreted in minute quantities. *Glucocorticoids* are secreted cyclically, with the largest amount being produced in the early morning and the smallest amount during the evening hours (in people with a normal day–night schedule). At the cellular level, glucocorticoids account for most of the characteristics and physiologic effects of the corticosteroids (Box 24-1).

Mineralocorticoids

Mineralocorticoids play a vital role in maintaining fluid and electrolyte balance. *Aldosterone* is the main mineralocorticoid and is responsible for approximately 90% of mineralocorticoid activity. Characteristics and physiologic effects of aldosterone are summarized in Box 24-2.

Adrenal Sex Hormones

The adrenal cortex secretes male (androgens) and female (estrogens and progesterone) sex hormones. The adrenal sex hormones are insignificant compared with those produced by the testes and ovaries. Adrenal androgens, secreted continuously in small quantities by both sexes, are responsible for most of the physiologic effects exerted by the adrenal sex hormones. They increase protein synthesis (anabolism), which increases the mass and strength of muscle and bone tissue; they affect development of male secondary sex characteristics; and they increase hair growth and libido in women. Excessive secretion of

BOX 24-1 EFFECTS OF GLUCOCORTICOIDS ON BODY PROCESSES AND SYSTEMS

Carbohydrate Metabolism

- ↑Formation of glucose (gluconeogenesis) by breaking down protein into amino acids. The amino acids are then transported to the liver, where they are acted on by enzymes that convert them to glucose. The glucose is then returned to the circulation for use by body tissues or storage in the liver as glycogen.
- ↓Cell use of glucose, especially in muscle cells. This is attributed to a ↓effect of insulin on the proteins that normally transport glucose into cells and by ↓numbers and functional capacity of insulin receptors.
- Both the ↑production and ↓use of glucose promote higher levels of glucose in the blood (hyperglycemia) and may lead to diabetes mellitus. These actions also increase the amount of glucose stored as glycogen in the liver, skeletal muscles, and other tissues.

Protein Metabolism

- ↑Breakdown of protein into amino acids (catabolic effect); ↑rate of amino acid transport to the liver and conversion to glucose.
- ↓Rate of new protein formation from dietary and other amino acids (antianabolic effect)
- The combination of ↑breakdown of cell protein and ↓protein synthesis leads to protein depletion in virtually all body cells except those of the liver. Thus, glycogen stores in the body are ↑ and protein stores are ↓.

Lipid Metabolism

- ↑Breakdown of adipose tissue into fatty acids; the fatty acids are transported in the plasma and used as a source of energy by body cells.
- ↑Oxidation of fatty acids within body cells

Inflammatory and Immune Responses

- ↓Inflammatory response. Inflammation is the normal bodily response to tissue damage and involves three stages. First, a large amount of plasma-like fluid leaks out of capillaries into the damaged area and becomes clotted. Second, leukocytes migrate into the area. Third, tissue healing occurs, largely by growth of fibrous scar tissue. Normal or physiologic amounts of glucocorticoids probably do not significantly affect inflammation and healing, but large amounts of glucocorticoids inhibit all three stages of the inflammatory process.

  More specifically, corticosteroids stabilize lysosomal membranes (and thereby prevent the release of inflammatory proteolytic enzymes), ↓capillary permeability (and thereby ↓leakage of fluid and proteins into the damaged tissue), ↓the accumulation of neutrophils and macrophages at sites of inflammation (and thereby impair phagocytosis of pathogenic microorganisms and waste products of cellular metabolism), and ↓production of inflammatory chemicals, such as interleukin-1, prostaglandins, and leukotrienes, by injured cells.

- ↓Immune response. The immune system normally protects the body from foreign invaders, and several immune responses overlap inflammatory responses, including phagocytosis. In addition, the immune response stimulates the production of antibodies and activated lymphocytes to destroy the foreign substance. Glucocorticoids impair protein synthesis, including the production of antibodies; ↓the numbers of circulating lymphocytes, eosinophils, and macrophages; and ↓amounts of lymphoid tissue. These effects help to account for the immunosuppressive and antiallergic actions of the glucocorticoids.

Cardiovascular System

- Help to regulate arterial blood pressure by modifying vascular smooth muscle tone, by modifying myocardial contractility, and by stimulating renal mineralocorticoid and glucocorticoid receptors.
- ↑The response of vascular smooth muscle to the pressor effects of catecholamines and other vasoconstrictive agents.

Nervous System

- Physiologic amounts help to *maintain normal nerve excitability;* pharmacologic amounts ↓nerve excitability, slow activity in the cerebral cortex, and alter brain wave patterns.
- ↓Secretion of corticotropin-releasing hormone by the hypothalamus and of corticotropin by the anterior pituitary gland. This results in suppression of further glucocorticoid secretion by the adrenal cortex (negative feedback system).

Musculoskeletal System

- Maintain muscle strength when present in physiologic amounts but cause muscle atrophy (from protein breakdown) when present in excessive amounts.
- ↓Bone formation and growth and ↑bone breakdown. Glucocorticoids also ↓intestinal absorption and ↑renal excretion of calcium. These effects contribute to bone demineralization (osteoporosis) in adults and to ↓linear growth in children.

Respiratory System

- Maintain open airways. Glucocorticoids do not have direct bronchodilating effects, but help to maintain and restore responsiveness to the bronchodilating

(continued)

BOX 24–1 EFFECTS OF GLUCOCORTICOIDS ON BODY PROCESSES AND SYSTEMS (*continued*)

effects of endogenous catecholamines, such as epinephrine.
- Stabilize mast cells and other cells to inhibit the release of bronchoconstrictive and inflammatory substances, such as histamine.

Gastrointestinal System
- ↓Viscosity of gastric mucus. This effect may ↓protective properties of the mucus and contribute to the development of peptic ulcer disease.

↑-increase/increased; ↓-decrease/decreased.

---

adrenal androgens in women causes masculinizing effects (eg, hirsutism, acne, breast atrophy, deepening of the voice, and amenorrhea). Female sex hormones are secreted in small amounts and normally exert few physiologic effects. Excessive secretion may produce feminizing effects in men (eg, breast enlargement, decreased hair growth, voice changes).

Disorders of the Adrenal Cortex

Disorders of the adrenal cortex involve increased or decreased production of corticosteroids, especially cortisol as the primary glucocorticoid and aldosterone as the primary mineralocorticoid. These disorders include the following:

- **Primary adrenocortical insufficiency (Addison's disease)** is associated with destruction of the adrenal cortex by disorders such as tuberculosis, cancer, or hemorrhage; with atrophy of the adrenal cortex caused by autoimmune disease or prolonged administration of exogenous corticosteroids; and with surgical excision of the adrenal glands. In this condition, there is inadequate production of both cortisol and aldosterone.
- **Secondary adrenocortical insufficiency**, produced by inadequate secretion of corticotropin, is most often caused by prolonged administration of corticosteroids. This condition is largely a glucocorticoid deficiency; mineralocorticoid secretion is not significantly impaired.
- **Congenital adrenogenital syndromes and adrenal hyperplasia** result from deficiencies in one or more enzymes required for cortisol production. Low plasma levels of cortisol lead to excessive corticotropin secretion, which then leads to excessive adrenal secretion of androgens and hyperplasia.
- **Androgen-producing tumors** of the adrenal cortex, which are usually benign, produce masculinizing effects.
- **Adrenocortical hyperfunction** (Cushing's disease) may result from excessive corticotropin or a primary adrenal tumor. Adrenal tumors may be benign or malignant. Benign tumors often produce one corticosteroid normally secreted by the adrenal cortex, but malignant tumors often secrete several corticosteroids.
- **Hyperaldosteronism** is a rare disorder caused by adenoma or hyperplasia of the adrenal cortex cells that produce aldosterone. It is characterized by hypokalemia, hypernatremia, hypertension, thirst, and polyuria.

BOX 24–2 EFFECTS OF MINERALOCORTICOIDS ON BODY PROCESSES AND SYSTEMS

- The overall physiologic effects are to conserve sodium and water and eliminate potassium. Aldosterone increases sodium reabsorption from kidney tubules, and water is reabsorbed along with the sodium. When sodium is conserved, another cation must be excreted to maintain electrical neutrality of body fluids; thus, potassium is excreted. This is the only potent mechanism for controlling the concentration of potassium ions in extracellular fluids.
- Secretion of aldosterone is controlled by several factors, most of which are related to kidney function. In general, secretion is increased when the potassium level of extracellular fluid is high, the sodium level of extracellular fluid is low, the renin–angiotensin system of the kidneys is activated, or the anterior pituitary gland secretes corticotropin.
- Inadequate secretion of aldosterone causes hyperkalemia, hyponatremia, and extracellular fluid volume deficit (dehydration). Hypotension and shock may result from decreased cardiac output. Absence of mineralocorticoids causes death.
- Excessive secretion of aldosterone produces hypokalemia, hypernatremia, and extracellular fluid volume excess (water intoxication). Edema and hypertension may result.

EXOGENOUS CORTICOSTEROIDS (GLUCOCORTICOID DRUGS)

When corticosteroids are administered from sources outside the body, they are given mainly for replacement or therapeutic purposes. Replacement involves small doses to correct a deficiency state and restore normal function. Therapeutic purposes involve relatively large doses to exert pharmacologic effects. Drug effects involve extension of the physiologic effects of endogenous corticosteroids and new effects that do not occur with small, physiologic doses. The most frequently desired effects are anti-inflammatory, immunosuppressive, antiallergic, and antistress. These are glucocorticoid effects. Mineralocorticoid and androgenic effects are usually considered adverse reactions. Additional characteristics of therapeutic corticosteroids include the following:

- All adrenal corticosteroids are available as drug preparations, as are many synthetic derivatives developed by altering the basic steroid molecule in efforts to increase therapeutic effects while minimizing adverse effects. These efforts have been most successful in decreasing mineralocorticoid activity.

- The drugs are palliative; they control many symptoms but do not cure underlying disease processes. In chronic disorders, they may enable a client to continue the usual activities of daily living and delay disability. However, the disease may continue to progress and long-term use of corticosteroids inevitably produces adverse effects.

- Drug effects vary, so a specific effect may be considered therapeutic in one client but adverse in another. For example, an increased blood sugar level is therapeutic for the client with adrenocortical insufficiency or an islet cell adenoma of the pancreas, but an adverse reaction for most clients, especially for those with diabetes mellitus. In addition, some clients respond more favorably or experience adverse reactions more readily than others taking equivalent doses. This is partly caused by individual differences in the rate at which corticosteroids are metabolized.

- Administration of exogenous corticosteroids suppresses the HPA axis. This decreases secretion of corticotropin, which, in turn, causes atrophy of the adrenal cortex and decreased production of endogenous adrenal corticosteroids. Daily administration of physiologic doses (approximately 10 to 20 mg of hydrocortisone or its equivalent) or administration of pharmacologic doses (more than 10 to 20 mg of hydrocortisone or its equivalent) for approximately 2 weeks suppresses the HPA axis. HPA recovery usually occurs within a few weeks or months after corticosteroids are discontinued, but may take a year or longer. During that time, supplemental corticosteroids are usually needed during stressful situations (eg, fever, illness, surgical procedures) to improve the client's ability to respond to stress and prevent acute adrenocortical insufficiency.

- **Hydrocortisone**, the exogenous equivalent of endogenous cortisol, is the prototype of corticosteroid drugs. When a new corticosteroid is developed, it is compared with hydrocortisone to determine its potency in producing anti-inflammatory and antiallergic responses, increasing deposition of liver glycogen, and suppressing secretion of corticotropin.

- Anti-inflammatory activity of glucocorticoids is approximately equal when the drugs are given in equivalent doses. Mineralocorticoid activity is intermediate to high in the older drugs, cortisone and hydrocortisone, and low in newer agents.

- Many glucocorticoids are available for use in different clinical problems, and routes of administration vary. Several of these drugs can be given by more than one route; others can be given only orally or topically. For intramuscular (IM) or intravenous (IV) injections, sodium phosphate or sodium succinate salts are used because they are most soluble in water. For intra-articular or intralesional injections, acetate salts are used because they have low solubility in water and provide prolonged local action.

Mechanisms of Action

Like endogenous glucocorticoids, exogenous drug molecules act at the cellular level by binding to glucocorticoid receptors in target tissues. The receptors are small proteins located in intracellular cytoplasm. The drug–receptor complex then moves to the cell nucleus where it influences genetically controlled aspects of cellular synthesis. Because the genes vary in different types of body cells, glucocorticoid effects also vary, depending on the specific cells being targeted. For example, supraphysiologic concentrations of glucocorticoids induce the synthesis of lipolytic and proteolytic enzymes and other specific proteins in various tissues. Overall, corticosteroids have multiple mechanisms of action and effects, including the following:

- **Inhibiting arachidonic acid metabolism**. Normally, when a body cell is injured or activated by various stimuli, the enzyme phospholipase A_2 causes the phospholipids in cell membranes to release arachidonic acid. Free arachidonic acid is then metabolized to produce proinflammatory prostaglandins and leukotrienes (see Chap. 1). At sites of inflammation, corticosteroids induce the synthesis of proteins called lipocortins. Lipocortins suppress the activation of phospholipase A_2, thereby decreasing the release of arachidonic acid and the formation of prostaglandins and leukotrienes.

- **Inhibiting the production of interleukin-1 and other cytokines**. This action also contributes to the anti-inflammatory and immunosuppressant effects of glucocorticoids.

- **Strengthening or stabilizing biologic membranes**. This inhibits capillary permeability and thus prevents leakage of fluid into the injured area and development of edema. It further inhibits release of bradykinin, histamine, lysosomal enzymes, and perhaps other substances that normally cause vasodilation and tissue irritation.
- **Impairing phagocytosis**. The drugs inhibit the ability of phagocytic cells to leave the bloodstream and move into the injured or inflamed tissue.
- **Impairing lymphocytes.** The drugs inhibit the ability of these immune cells to increase in number and perform their functions, including antibody production
- **Inhibiting tissue repair**. The drugs inhibit the growth of new capillaries, fibroblasts, and collagen needed for tissue repair.

Indications for Use

Corticosteroids are extensively used to treat many different disorders. Except for replacement therapy in deficiency states, the use of corticosteroids is largely empiric. Because the drugs affect virtually every aspect of inflammatory and immune responses, they are used in the treatment of a broad spectrum of diseases with an inflammatory or immunologic component.

Corticosteroid preparations applied topically in ophthalmic and dermatologic disorders are discussed in Chapters 65 and 66, respectively. The corticosteroids discussed in this chapter (Table 24-1) are primarily those given systemically, topically to nasal and oral mucosa, or by local injection in potentially serious or disabling disorders. These disorders include the following:

- **Allergic** disorders, such as allergic reactions to drugs, serum and blood transfusions, and dermatoses with an allergic component
- **Collagen** disorders, such as systemic lupus erythematosus, scleroderma, and periarteritis nodosa. Collagen is the basic structural protein of connective tissue, tendons, cartilage, and bone, and it is therefore present in almost all body tissues and organ systems. The collagen disorders are characterized by inflammation of various body tissues. Signs and symptoms depend on which body tissues or organs are affected and the severity of the inflammatory process.
- **Dermatologic** disorders that may be treated with systemic corticosteroids include acute contact dermatitis, erythema multiforme, herpes zoster (prophylaxis of postherpetic neuralgia), lichen planus, pemphigus, skin rashes caused by drugs, and toxic epidermal necrolysis.
- **Endocrine** disorders, such as adrenocortical insufficiency and congenital adrenal hyperplasia. Cortico-

steroids are given to replace or substitute for the natural hormones (both glucocorticoids and mineralocorticoids) in cases of insufficiency and to suppress corticotropin when excess secretion causes adrenal hyperplasia. These conditions are rare and account for only a small percentage of corticosteroid usage.

- **Gastrointestinal** disorders, such as ulcerative colitis and regional enteritis (Crohn's disease)
- **Hematologic** disorders, such as idiopathic thrombocytopenic purpura or acquired hemolytic anemia
- **Hepatic** disorders characterized by edema, such as cirrhosis and ascites
- **Neoplastic** disease, such as acute and chronic leukemias, Hodgkin's disease, other lymphomas, and multiple myeloma. The effectiveness of corticosteroids in these conditions probably stems from their ability to suppress lymphocytes and other lymphoid tissue.
- **Neurologic** conditions, such as cerebral edema, brain tumor, and myasthenia gravis
- **Ophthalmic** disorders, such as optic neuritis, sympathetic ophthalmia, and chorioretinitis
- **Organ or tissue transplants and grafts** (eg, kidney, heart, bone marrow). Corticosteroids suppress cellular and humoral immune responses (see Chap. 42) and help prevent rejection of transplanted tissue. Drug therapy is continued as long as the transplanted tissue is in place (usually lifelong).
- **Renal** disorders characterized by edema, such as the nephrotic syndrome
- **Respiratory** disorders, such as asthma, status asthmaticus, chronic obstructive pulmonary disease (COPD), and inflammatory disorders of nasal mucosa (rhinitis). In asthma, corticosteroids increase the number of beta-adrenergic receptors and increase or restore responsiveness of beta receptors to beta-adrenergic bronchodilating drugs. In asthma, COPD, and rhinitis, the drugs decrease mucus secretion and inflammation.
- **Rheumatic** disorders, such as ankylosing spondylitis, acute and chronic bursitis, acute gouty arthritis, rheumatoid arthritis, and osteoarthritis
- **Shock**. Corticosteroids are clearly indicated only for shock resulting from adrenocortical insufficiency (addisonian crisis), which may mimic hypovolemic or septic shock. Several studies demonstrate that the drugs are not beneficial in treating septic shock. In anaphylactic shock resulting from an allergic reaction, corticosteroids may increase or restore cardiovascular responsiveness to adrenergic drugs.

Contraindications to Use

Corticosteroids are contraindicated in systemic fungal infections and in people who are hypersensitive to drug

(*text continues on page 332*)

TABLE 24-1   **Corticosteroids***

Generic/Trade Name	Routes and Dosage Ranges	Anti-inflammatory Dose Equivalent to 20 mg of Hydrocortisone (mg)	Mineralocorticoid Activity	Duration of Action (h)
Glucocorticoids				
Beclomethasone Oral inhalation (Beclovent, Vanceril)	*Adults:* 2 oral inhalations (84 μg) 3–4 times daily (maximal daily dose is 20 inhalations or 840 μg) *Children 6–12 y:* 1–3 oral inhalations (42–84 μg) 3–4 times daily (maximal daily dose is 10 inhalations or 420 μg)			
Nasal inhalation (Beconase, Vancenase)	*Adults and children ≥ 12 y:* 1 nasal inhalation (42 μg) in each nostril 2–4 times daily (total dose 168–336 μg/d) *Children 6–12 y:* 1 nasal inhalation in each nostril 3 times daily (252 μg/d) *Children <6 y:* Not recommended			
Betamethasone (Celestone)	*Adults:* PO 6–7.2 mg daily initially, depending on the disease being treated, gradually reduced to lowest effective maintenance dose	0.6	Low	48
Betamethasone acetate and sodium phosphate (Celestone Soluspan)	*Adults:* IM 1–2 mL (3-6 mg each of betamethasone acetate and betamethasone phosphate) Intra-articular injection 0.25-2 mL Soft-tissue injection 0.25-1.0 mL			
Budesonide (Rhinocort) Nasal inhalation	*Adults and children ≥ 6 y:* Initially 256 μg daily (2 sprays each nostril morning and evening or 4 sprays each nostril every morning). When symptoms are controlled, reduce dosage to lowest effective maintenance dose.			
Cortisone (Cortone)	Chronic adrenocortical insufficiency, PO 15–30 mg daily Congenital adrenal hyperplasia, PO 15–50 mg daily Anti-inflammatory effects, PO 25–50 mg daily for mild, chronic disorders; 125–300 mg daily in 4 or more doses for acute, life-threatening disease Anti-inflammatory effects, IM 75–300 mg daily for serious disease	25	High	12
Dexamethasone (Decadron)	PO 0.75–9 mg daily in 2–4 doses. Dosages in higher ranges are used for serious disease (leukemia, pemphigus)	0.75	Low	48
Dexamethasone acetate	IM 8–16 mg (1–2 mL) in single dose, repeated every 1–3 wk if necessary Intralesional 0.8–1.6 mg (0.1–0.2 mL) Intra-articular or soft tissue injection, 4–16 mg (0.5–2 mL), repeated every 1–3 wk if necessary			
Dexamethasone sodium phosphate	IM, IV 0.5–9 mg, depending on severity of the disease Intra-articular, soft-tissue injection 0.2–6 mg, depending on size of affected area or joint			
(Decadron Turbinaire)	Intranasal, 2 sprays in each nostril 2–3 times daily			
(Decadron Respihaler)	2–3 inhalations 3–4 times daily			
Dexamethasone/ lidocaine (Decadron with Xylocaine)	Soft tissue injection, 0.5–0.75 mL			

(continued)

TABLE 24-1)   **Corticosteroids*** (*continued*)

Generic/Trade Name	Routes and Dosage Ranges	Anti-inflammatory Dose Equivalent to 20 mg of Hydrocortisone (mg)	Mineralocorticoid Activity	Duration of Action (h)
Flunisolide 　Oral inhalation 　(Aerobid) 　Nasal inhalation 　(Nasalide)	*Adults:* 2 oral inhalations (500 µg) twice daily *Children 6–15 y:* Same as adults *Adults:* 2 sprays (50 µg) in each nostril 2 times daily (total dose 200 µg/d); maximal daily dose is 8 sprays in each nostril (400 µg/d) *Children 6–14 y:* 1 spray (25 µg) in each nostril 3 times daily or 2 sprays (50 µg) in each nostril 2 times daily (total dose 150–200 µg/d); maximal daily dose 4 sprays in each nostril (200 µg/d)			
Fluticasone (Flonase) 　Nasal inhalation	*Adults:* Initially 200 µg daily (2 sprays each nostril once daily or 1 spray each nostril twice daily). After a few days, reduce dosage to 100 µg daily (1 spray each nostril once daily) for maintenance therapy. *Adolescents ≥12 y:* 100 µg daily (1 spray per nostril once daily)			
Hydrocortisone 　(Hydrocortone, 　Cortef)	Chronic adrenocortical insufficiency, PO 10–20 mg daily in 3–4 doses Chronic nonfatal diseases, PO 20–40 mg daily in 3–4 doses Congenital adrenal hyperplasia, PO 10–30 mg daily in 3–4 doses Chronic, potentially fatal diseases, PO 60–120 mg daily in 3–4 doses Acute, nonfatal diseases, PO 60–120 mg daily in 3–4 doses Acute life-threatening diseases, PO 100–240 mg daily in at least 4 divided doses Disorders other than shock, IV 100–500 mg initially, repeated if necessary Intra-articular injections, 5–50 mg depending on size of joint Soft tissue injection, 25–75 mg Rectally, one enema (100 mg) nightly for 21 d or until optimal response is obtained	20	Intermediate	18
Methylprednisolone 　(Medrol) Methylprednisolone 　sodium succinate 　(Solu-Medrol)	PO 4–48 mg daily initially, gradually reduced to lowest effective level IM 40–120 mg as needed IV 100–250 mg q4–6h for shock; 10–40 mg as needed for other conditions Intra-articular and soft tissue injection, 4–80 mg as needed, depending on size of the affected area Intralesional injection, 20–60 mg Rectally, 40 mg as retention enema 3–7 times weekly for 2 or more wk	4	Low	18–36
Prednisolone (Sterane, Delta-Cortef) Prednisolone acetate 　(Fernisolone, others) Prednisolone 　sodium phosphate 　(Hydeltrasol)	PO 5–60 mg daily initially, adjusted for maintenance IM 4–60 mg daily initially, adjusted for maintenance Intra-articular or soft tissue injection, 4–60 mg daily, depending on the disease IM 4–60 mg daily initially, adjusted for maintenance	5	Intermediate	18–36

(*continued*)

TABLE 24-1) **Corticosteroids*** (*continued*)

Generic/Trade Name	Routes and Dosage Ranges	Anti-inflammatory Dose Equivalent to 20 mg of Hydrocortisone (mg)	Mineralocorticoid Activity	Duration of Action (h)
	Emergencies, IV 20–100 mg, repeated if necessary, to a maximal daily dose of 400 mg. When the client's condition improves, 10–20 mg in single doses may be given.			
	Intra-articular or soft tissue injection, 2–30 mg from once every 3–5 d to once every 2–3 wk			
Prednisolone sodium succinate (Meticortelone soluble)	IM 4–60 mg daily initially, adjusted for maintenance			
	Emergencies, IV 20–100 mg, repeated if necessary to a maximal daily dose of 480 mg. When the client's condition improves, 10–20 mg in single doses may be given.			
Prednisolone tebutate (Hydeltra-TBA)	Intra-articular or soft tissue injection, 4–60 mg daily, depending on the disease			
Prednisone (Deltasone)	PO 5–60 mg daily initially, reduced for maintenance	5	Intermediate	18–30
Triamcinolone (Aristocort, Kenacort)	PO 4–48 mg daily initially; dosage reduced for maintenance	4	Low	18–36
Triamcinolone acetonide (Kenalog-40)	IM (deep) 2.5–60 mg daily, depending on the disease. When the client's condition improves, dosage should be reduced and oral therapy instituted when feasible			
	Intra-articular or intrabursal injection, 2.5–15 mg every 1–8 wk depending on the size of the joint and the disease being treated			
	Soft tissue injection, 5–48 mg			
Oral inhalation (Azmacort)	*Adults:* 2 oral inhalations (200 μg) 3 times daily			
	Children: 1–2 oral inhalations (100–200 μg) 3 times daily			
Nasal inhalation (Nasacort)	*Adults and children >12 y:* 2 sprays (110 μg) in each nostril once daily (total dose 220 μg/d). May increase to maximal daily dose of 440 μg.			
Triamcinolone diacetate (Aristocort diacetate, Kenacort diacetate)	PO 4–48 mg daily initially; dosage reduced for maintenance			
	IM (deep) 20–80 mg initially			
	Intra-articular injection, 2.5–80 mg every 1–8 wk, depending on size of joint or affected area			
	Soft tissue injection, 5–48 mg			
Triamcinolone hexacetonide (Aristospan)	Intra-articular injection, 2.5–80 mg every 1–8 wk, depending on size of joint or affected area			
Mineralocorticoid				
Fludrocortisone (Florinef)	Chronic adrenocortical insufficiency, PO 0.05–0.1 mg daily			
	Salt-losing adrenogenital syndromes, PO 0.1–0.2 mg daily			

IM, intramuscular; IV, intravenous; PO, oral.
* Ophthalmic and dermatologic preparations are discussed in Chapters 65 and 66, respectively.

formulations. They should be used with caution in clients at risk for infections (they may decrease resistance), clients with infections (they may mask signs and symptoms so that infections become more severe before they are recognized and treated), diabetes mellitus (they cause or increase hyperglycemia), peptic ulcer disease, inflammatory bowel disorders, hypertension, congestive heart failure, and renal insufficiency.

(text continues on page 336)

Nursing Notes: Apply Your Knowledge

Kim Wilson, 62 years of age, was admitted for elective abdominal surgery. Her medication history reveals daily use of prednisone. Individualize a postoperative plan of care for Kim considering her chronic steroid use.

NURSING PROCESS

Assessment Related to Initiation of Corticosteroid Therapy

- For a client expected to receive short-term corticosteroid therapy, the major focus of assessment is the extent and severity of symptoms. Such data can then be used to evaluate the effectiveness of drug therapy.
- For a client expected to receive long-term, systemic corticosteroid therapy, a thorough assessment is needed. This may include diagnostic tests for diabetes mellitus, tuberculosis, and peptic ulcer disease because these conditions may develop from or be exacerbated by administration of corticosteroid drugs. If one of these conditions is present, corticosteroid therapy must be altered and other drugs given concomitantly.
- If acute infection is found on initial assessment, it should be treated with appropriate antibiotics either before corticosteroid drugs are started or concomitantly with corticosteroid therapy. This is necessary because corticosteroids may mask symptoms of infection and impair healing. Thus, even minor infections can become serious if left untreated during corticosteroid therapy. If infection occurs during long-term corticosteroid therapy, appropriate antibiotic therapy (as determined by culture of the causative microorganism and antibiotic sensitivity studies) is again indicated. Also, increased doses of corticosteroids are usually indicated to cope with the added stress of the infection.

Assessment Related to Previous or Current Corticosteroid Therapy

Initial assessment of every client should include information about previous or current treatment with systemic corticosteroids. This can usually be determined by questioning the client or reviewing medical records.

- If the nurse determines that the client has taken corticosteroids in the past, additional information is needed about the specific drug and dosage taken, the purpose and length of therapy, and when therapy was stopped. Such information is necessary for planning nursing care. If the client had an acute illness and received an oral or injected corticosteroid for approximately 1 week or received corticosteroids by local injection or application to skin lesions, no special nursing care is likely to be required. If, however, the client took systemic corticosteroids 2 weeks or longer during the past year, nursing observations must be especially vigilant. Such a client may be at higher risk for development of acute adrenocortical insufficiency during stressful situations. If the client is having surgery, corticosteroid therapy is restarted either before or on the day of surgery and continued, in decreasing dosage, for a few days after surgery. In addition to anesthesia and surgery, potentially significant sources of stress include hospitalization, various diagnostic tests, concurrent infection or other illnesses, and family problems.

  If the client is currently taking a systemic corticosteroid drug, again the nurse must identify the drug, the dosage and schedule of administration, the purpose for which the drug is being taken, and the length of time involved. Once this basic information is obtained, the nurse can further assess client status and plan nursing care. Some specific factors include the following:

  - If the client will undergo anesthesia and surgery, expect that higher doses of corticosteroids will be given for several days. This may be done by changing the drug, the route of administration, and the dosage. Specific regimens vary according to type of anesthesia, surgical procedure, client condition, physician preference, and other variables. A client having major abdominal surgery may be given 300 to 400 mg of hydrocortisone (or the equivalent dosage of other agents) on the day of surgery and then be tapered back to maintenance dosage within a few days.
  - Note that additional corticosteroids may be given in other situations as well. One extra

dose may be adequate for a short-term stress situation, such as an angiogram or other invasive diagnostic test.

- Using all available data, assess the likelihood of the client's having acute adrenal insufficiency (sometimes called adrenal crisis).
- Assess for signs and symptoms of adrenocortical excess and adverse drug effects.
- Assess for signs and symptoms of the disease for which long-term corticosteroid therapy is being given.

Nursing Diagnoses

- Body Image Disturbance related to cushingoid changes in appearance
- Altered Nutrition: Less Than Body Requirements related to protein and potassium losses
- Altered Nutrition: More Than Body Requirements related to sodium and water retention and hyperglycemia
- Altered Tissue Perfusion related to atherosclerosis and hypertension
- Fluid Volume Excess related to sodium and water retention
- Risk for Injury related to adverse drug effects of impaired wound healing; increased susceptibility to infection; weakening of skin and muscles; osteoporosis, gastrointestinal ulceration, diabetes mellitus, hypertension, and acute adrenocortical insufficiency
- Ineffective Individual Coping related to chronic illness and long-term drug therapy
- Ineffective Individual Coping related to drug-induced mood changes, irritability, insomnia
- Knowledge Deficit related to disease process and corticosteroid drug therapy

Planning/Goals

The client will:

- Receive or take the drug correctly
- Receive and practice measures to decrease the need for corticosteroids and minimize adverse effects
- Be monitored regularly for adverse drug effects
- Keep appointments for follow-up care
- Be assisted to cope with body image changes
- Verbalize or demonstrate essential drug information

Interventions

For clients on long-term, systemic corticosteroid therapy, use supplementary drugs as ordered and nondrug measures to decrease dosage and adverse effects of corticosteroid drugs. Some specific measures include the following:

- Help clients to set reasonable goals of drug therapy. For example, partial relief of symptoms may be better than complete relief if the latter requires larger doses or longer periods of treatment with systemic drugs.
- In clients with bronchial asthma and COPD, other treatment measures should be continued during corticosteroid therapy. With asthma, the corticosteroid needs to be given on a regular schedule; inhaled bronchodilators can usually be taken as needed.
- In clients with rheumatoid arthritis, rest, physical therapy, and salicylates or other nonsteroid anti-inflammatory drugs are continued. Systemic corticosteroid therapy is reserved for severe, acute exacerbations when possible.
- Help clients to identify stressors and to find ways to modify or avoid stressful situations when possible. For example, most clients probably do not think of extreme heat or cold or minor infections as significant stressors. They can be, however, for people taking corticosteroid drugs. This assessment of potential stressors must be individualized because a situation viewed as stressful by one client may not be stressful to another.
- Encourage activity, if not contraindicated, to slow demineralization of bone (osteoporosis). This is especially important in postmenopausal women who are not taking replacement estrogens, because they are very susceptible to osteoporosis. Walking is preferred if the client is able. Range-of-motion exercises are indicated in immobilized or bedfast people. Also, bedfast clients taking corticosteroid drugs should have their positions changed frequently because these drugs thin the skin and increase the risk of pressure ulcers. This risk is further increased if edema also is present.
- Dietary changes may be beneficial in some clients. Salt restriction may help prevent hypernatremia, fluid retention, and edema. Foods high in potassium may help prevent hypokalemia. A diet high in protein, calcium, and vitamin D may help to prevent osteoporosis. Increased intake of vitamin C may help to decrease bleeding in the skin and soft tissues.
- Avoid exposing the client to potential sources of infection by washing hands frequently, using aseptic technique when changing dressings, keeping health care personnel and visitors with colds

or other infections away from the client, and following other appropriate measures. Reverse or protective isolation of the client is sometimes indicated, commonly for those who have had organ transplants and are receiving corticosteroids to help prevent rejection of the transplanted organ.

- Handle tissues very gently during any procedures (eg, bathing, assisting out of bed, venipunctures). Because long-term corticosteroid therapy weakens the skin and bones, there are risks of skin damage and fractures with even minor trauma.

Evaluation

- Interview and observe for relief of symptoms for which corticosteroids were prescribed.
- Interview and observe for accurate drug administration.
- Interview and observe for use of nondrug measures indicated for the condition being treated.
- Interview and observe for adverse drug effects on a regular basis.
- Interview regarding drug knowledge and effects to be reported to health care providers.

CLIENT TEACHING GUIDELINES
Long-term Corticosteroids

General Considerations

✔ In most instances, corticosteroids are used to relieve symptoms; they do not cure the underlying disease process. However, they can improve comfort and quality of life.

✔ When taking an oral corticosteroid (eg, prednisone) for longer than 2 weeks, it is extremely important to take the drug as directed. Missing a dose or two, stopping the drug, changing the amount or time of administration, or taking extra drug (except as specifically directed during stress situations) or any other alterations may result in complications. Some complications are relatively minor; several are serious, even life threatening. When these drugs are being discontinued, the dosage is gradually reduced over several weeks. **They must not be stopped abruptly.**

✔ Wear a special medical alert bracelet or tag or carry an identification card stating the drug being taken; the dosage; the physician's name, address, and telephone number; and instructions for emergency treatment. If an accident or emergency situation occurs, health care providers must know about corticosteroid drug therapy to give additional amounts during the stress of the emergency.

✔ Report to all health care providers consulted that corticosteroid drugs are being taken or have been taken within the past year. Current or previous corticosteroid therapy can influence treatment measures, and such knowledge increases the ability to provide appropriate treatment.

✔ Maintain regular medical supervision. This is extremely important so that the physician can detect adverse reactions, evaluate disease status, and evaluate drug response and indications for dosage change, as well as other responsibilities that can be carried out only with personal contact between the physician and the client.

Periodic blood tests, x-ray studies, and other tests may be performed during long-term corticosteroid therapy.

✔ Take no other drugs, prescription or nonprescription, without notifying the physician who is supervising corticosteroid therapy. Corticosteroid drugs influence reactions to many other drugs, and many other drugs interact with corticosteroids either to increase or decrease their effects. Thus, taking other drugs can decrease the expected therapeutic benefits or increase the incidence or severity of adverse reactions.

✔ Avoid exposure to infection when possible. Avoid crowds and people known to have an infection. Also, wash hands frequently and thoroughly. These drugs increase the likelihood of infection, so preventive measures are necessary. Also, if infection does occur, healing is likely to be slow.

✔ Practice safety measures to avoid accidents (eg, falls and possible fractures due to osteoporosis, cuts or other injuries because of delayed wound healing, soft tissue trauma because of increased tendency to bruise easily).

✔ Weigh frequently when starting corticosteroid therapy and at least weekly during long-term maintenance. An initial weight gain is likely to occur and is usually attributed to increased appetite. Later weight gains may be caused by fluid retention.

✔ Ask the physician about the amount and kind of activity or exercise needed. As a general rule, being as active as possible helps to prevent or delay osteoporosis, a common adverse reaction. However, increased activity may not be desirable for everyone. A client with rheumatoid arthritis, for example, may become too active when drug therapy relieves joint pain and increases mobility.

(continued)

CLIENT TEACHING GUIDELINES
Long-term Corticosteroids (*continued*)

✔ Follow instructions for other measures used in treatment of the particular condition (eg, other drugs and physical therapy for rheumatoid arthritis). Such measures may allow smaller doses of corticosteroids and decrease adverse reactions.

✔ Because the corticosteroid impairs the ability to respond to stress, dosage may need to be temporarily increased with illness, surgery, or other stressful situations. Clarify with the physician predictable sources of stress and the amount of drug to be taken if the stress cannot be avoided.

✔ In addition to stressful situations, report sore throat, fever, or other signs of infection; weight gain of 5 lbs. or more in a week; or swelling in the ankles or elsewhere. These symptoms may indicate adverse drug effects and changes in corticosteroid therapy may be indicated.

✔ Muscle weakness and fatigue or disease symptoms may occur when drug dosage is reduced, withdrawn, or omitted (eg, the nondrug day of alternate-day therapy). Although these symptoms may cause some discomfort, they should be tolerated if possible rather than increasing the corticosteroid dose. If severe, of course, dosage or time of administration may have to be changed.

✔ Dietary changes may be helpful in reducing some adverse effects of corticosteroid therapy. Decreasing salt intake (eg, by not adding table salt to foods and avoiding obviously salty foods, such as many snack foods and prepared sandwich meats) may help decrease swelling. Eating high-potassium foods, such as citrus fruits and juices or bananas, may help prevent potassium loss. An adequate intake of calcium, protein, and vitamin D (meat and dairy products are good sources) may help to prevent or delay osteoporosis. Vitamin C (eg, from citrus fruits) may help to prevent excessive bruising.

✔ Do not object when your physician reduces your dose of oral corticosteroid, with the goal of stopping the drug entirely or continuing with a smaller dose. Long-term therapy should be used only when necessary because of the potential for serious adverse effects, and the lowest effective dose should be given.

✔ With local applications of corticosteroids, there is usually little systemic absorption and few adverse effects, compared with oral or injected drugs. When effective in relieving symptoms, it is better to use a local than a systemic corticosteroid. In some instances, combined systemic and local application allows administration of a lesser dose of the systemic drug.

Commonly used local applications are applied topically to skin disorders, by oral inhalation for asthma, and by nasal inhalation for allergic rhinitis. Although long-term use is usually well tolerated, systemic toxicity can occur if excess corticosteroid is inhaled or if occlusive dressings are used over skin lesions. Thus, a corticosteroid for local application must be applied correctly and not overused.

✔ Corticosteroids are *not* the same as the steroids often abused by athletes and body builders.

Self- or Caregiver Administration

✔ Take an oral corticosteroid with a meal or snack to decrease gastrointestinal upset.

✔ If taking the medication once a day or every other day, take before 9 AM; if taking multiple doses, take at evenly spaced intervals throughout the day.

✔ Report to the physician if unable to take a dose orally because of vomiting or some other problem. In some circumstances, the dose may need to be given by injection.

✔ If taking an oral corticosteroid in tapering doses, be sure to follow instructions exactly to avoid adverse effects.

✔ When applying a corticosteroid to skin lesions, do not apply more often than ordered and do not cover with an occlusive dressing unless specifically instructed to do so.

✔ With an intranasal corticosteroid, use on a regular basis (usually once or twice daily) for the best anti-inflammatory effects.

✔ With an oral inhalation corticosteroid, use on a regular schedule for anti-inflammatory effects (the drug is *not* effective in relieving acute asthma attacks or shortness of breath and should not be used "as needed" for that purpose) and use metered-dose inhalers as follows:
1. Shake canister thoroughly.
2. Place canister between lips (both open and pursed lips have been recommended) or outside lips.
3. Exhale completely.
4. Activate canister while taking a slow, deep breath.
5. Hold breath for 10 seconds or as long as possible.
6. Wait at least 1 minute before taking additional inhalations.
7. Rinse mouth after inhalations to decrease the incidence of oral thrush.
8. Rinse mouthpiece at least once per day.

PRINCIPLES OF THERAPY

Risk–Benefit Factors

1. Because corticosteroid drugs can cause serious adverse reactions, indications for their clinical use should be as clear-cut as possible. They are relatively safe for short-term treatment of self-limiting conditions, such as allergic reactions or acute exacerbations of chronic conditions. Long-term use of pharmacologic doses (more than 10 to 20 mg of hydrocortisone daily or its equivalent) produces adverse reactions. For this reason, long-term corticosteroid therapy should be reserved for life-threatening conditions or severe, disabling symptoms that do not respond to treatment with more benign drugs or other measures. Both physician and client should be convinced that the anticipated benefits of long-term therapy are worth the risks.

2. The goal of corticosteroid therapy is usually to reduce symptoms to a tolerable level. Total suppression of symptoms may require excessively large doses and produce excessive adverse effects.

Drug Selection

Choice of corticosteroid drug is influenced by many factors, including the purpose for use, characteristics of specific drugs, desired route of administration, characteristics of individual clients, and expected side effects. Some guidelines for rational drug choice include the following:

1. **Adrenocortical insufficiency**, whether caused by Addison's disease, adrenalectomy, or inadequate corticotropin, requires replacement of both glucocorticoids and mineralocorticoids. Hydrocortisone and cortisone are usually the drugs of choice because they have greater mineralocorticoid activity compared with other corticosteroids. If additional mineralocorticoid activity is required, fludrocortisone is most convenient because it can be given orally.

2. **Nonendocrine disorders**, in which anti-inflammatory, antiallergic, antistress, and immunosuppressive effects are desired, can be treated by a corticosteroid drug with primarily glucocorticoid activity. Prednisone is often the glucocorticoid of choice. It has less mineralocorticoid activity than hydrocortisone and is less expensive than newer synthetic glucocorticoids.

3. **Respiratory disorders**. Beclomethasone (Vanceril), flunisolide (Aerobid), fluticasone (Flonase), and triamcinolone (Azmacort) are corticosteroids formulated to be given by oral or nasal inhalation. Their use replaces, prevents, delays, or decreases use of systemic drugs and thereby decreases risks

of serious adverse effects. High doses or frequent use may suppress adrenocortical function.

4. **Cerebral edema** associated with brain tumors, craniotomy, or head injury. Dexamethasone (parenterally or orally) is considered the corticosteroid of choice because it is thought to penetrate the blood–brain barrier more readily and achieve higher concentrations in cerebrospinal fluids and tissues. It also has minimal sodium- and water-retaining properties. With brain tumors, the drug is more effective in metastatic lesions and glioblastomas than astrocytomas and meningiomas.

5. **Acute, life-threatening situations** require a drug that can be given parenterally, usually IV. This limits the choice of drugs because not all are available in injectable preparations. Hydrocortisone, dexamethasone, and methylprednisolone are among those that may be given parenterally.

Dosage Factors

Dosage of corticosteroid drugs must be individualized because it is influenced by many factors, such as the specific drug to be given, the desired route of administration, the reason for use, expected adverse effects, and client characteristics. In general, the smallest effective dose should be given for the shortest effective time. Dosage guidelines include the following:

1. Dosage must be individualized according to the severity of the disorder being treated, whether the disease is acute or chronic, and the client's response to drug therapy. If life-threatening disease is present, high doses are usually given until acute symptoms are brought under control. Then, dosage is gradually reduced until a maintenance dose is determined or the drug is discontinued. If the disease is not life threatening, the physician may still choose to prescribe relatively high doses initially and reduce to maintenance doses.

2. Physiologic doses (approximately 10 to 20 mg of hydrocortisone or its equivalent daily) are given to replace or substitute for endogenous adrenocortical hormone. Pharmacologic doses (supraphysiologic amounts) are usually required for anti-inflammatory, antiallergic, antistress, and immunosuppressive effects.

3. Compared with hydrocortisone, newer drugs are more potent on a weight basis but are equipotent in anti-inflammatory effects when given in equivalent doses (see Table 24-1). Statements of equivalency with hydrocortisone are helpful in evaluating new drugs, comparing different drugs, and changing drugs or dosages. However, dosage equivalents usually apply only to drugs given orally or IV. When the drugs are given by other routes, equivalency relationships are likely to be changed.

4. Dosage for children is calculated according to severity of disease rather than weight.

5. For people receiving chronic corticosteroid therapy, dosage must be increased during periods of stress. Although an event that is stressful for one client may not be stressful for another, some common sources of stress for most people include surgery and anesthesia, infections, anxiety, and extremes of temperature. Some guidelines for corticosteroid dosage during stress include the following:

   a. During *minor or relatively mild illness* (viral upper respiratory infection, any febrile illness, strenuous exercise, gastroenteritis with vomiting and diarrhea, minor surgery), doubling the daily maintenance dose is usually adequate. Once the stress period is over, dosage may be reduced abruptly to the usual maintenance dose.

   b. During *major stress or severe illness*, even larger doses are necessary. For example, a client undergoing abdominal surgery may require 300 to 400 mg of hydrocortisone on the day of surgery. This dose can gradually be reduced to usual maintenance doses within approximately 5 days if postoperative recovery is uncomplicated. As a general rule, it is better to administer excessive doses temporarily than to risk inadequate doses and adrenal insufficiency. The client also may require sodium chloride and fluid replacement, antibiotic therapy if infection is present, and supportive measures if shock occurs.

      An acute stress situation of short duration, such as traumatic injury or invasive diagnostic tests (eg, angiography), can usually be treated with a single dose of approximately 100 mg of hydrocortisone immediately after the injury or before the diagnostic test.

   c. Many chronic diseases that require long-term corticosteroid therapy are characterized by exacerbations and remissions. Dosage of corticosteroids usually must be increased during acute flare-ups of disease symptoms but can then be decreased gradually to maintenance levels.

6. With long-term corticosteroid therapy, periodic attempts to reduce dosage are desirable to decrease adverse effects. One way is gradually to reduce the dose until symptoms worsen, indicating the minimally effective dose.

Route of Administration

Corticosteroid drugs can be given by several different routes to achieve local or systemic effects. When feasible, they should be given locally rather than systemically to prevent or decrease systemic toxicity. When corticosteroids must be given systemically, the oral route is preferred. Parenteral administration is indicated only for clients who are seriously ill or unable to take oral medications.

Scheduling Guidelines

Scheduling of drug administration is more important with corticosteroids than with most other drug classes. Most adverse effects occur with long-term administration of high doses. A major adverse reaction is suppression of the HPA axis and subsequent loss of adrenocortical function. Although opinions differ, the following schedules are often recommended to prevent or minimize HPA suppression:

1. **Short-term use (approximately 1 week) in acute situations:** Corticosteroids can be given in relatively large, divided doses for approximately 48 to 72 hours until the acute situation is brought under control. At times, also, continuous IV infusions may be given. After acute symptoms subside or 48 to 72 hours have passed, the dosage is tapered so that a slightly smaller dose is given each day until the drug can be discontinued completely. Such a regimen may be useful in allergic reactions, contact dermatitis, exacerbations of chronic conditions (eg, bronchial asthma), and stressful situations such as surgery.

2. **Replacement therapy in cases of chronic adrenocortical insufficiency:** Daily administration is required. The entire daily dose can be taken each morning, between 6 and 9 AM. This schedule simulates normal endogenous corticosteroid secretion.

3. **Other chronic conditions**: Alternate-day therapy (ADT), in which a double dose is taken every other morning, is usually preferred. This schedule allows rest periods so that adverse effects are decreased while anti-inflammatory effects continue.

   a. ADT seems to be as effective as more frequent administration in most clients with bronchial asthma, ulcerative colitis, and other conditions for which long-term corticosteroid therapy is prescribed.

   b. ADT is used only for maintenance therapy (ie, clinical signs and symptoms are controlled initially with more frequent drug administration). ADT can be started once symptoms have subsided and stabilized.

   c. ADT does not retard growth in children, as do other schedules.

   d. ADT probably decreases susceptibility to infection.

   e. Intermediate-acting glucocorticoids, such as prednisone, prednisolone, and methylprednisolone, are the drugs of choice for ADT.

   f. ADT is not usually indicated in clients who have received long-term corticosteroid therapy. First, these clients already have maximal HPA suppression, so a major advantage of ADT is lost. Second, if they are transferred to ADT, recurrence of symptoms and considerable discomfort may occur on days when drugs are omitted. Clients with severe disease and very painful or disabling symptoms also may experience severe discomfort with ADT.

Use in Specific Conditions

Allergic Rhinitis

Allergic rhinitis (also called seasonal rhinitis or hay fever and perennial rhinitis) is a common problem for which corticosteroids are given by nasal spray, once or twice daily. Therapeutic effects usually occur within a few days with regular use. Systemic adverse effects are minimal with recommended doses but may occur with higher doses, including adrenocortical insufficiency from HPA suppression.

Arthritis

Corticosteroids are the most effective drugs for rapid relief of the pain, edema, and restricted mobility associated with acute episodes of joint inflammation. They are usually given on a short-term basis. When inflammation is limited to three or fewer joints, the preferred route of drug administration is by injection directly into the joint. Intra-articular injections relieve symptoms in approximately 2 to 8 weeks, and several formulations are available for this route. However, these drugs do not prevent disease progression and joint destruction. As a general rule, a joint should not be injected more often than three times yearly because of risks of infection and damage to intra-articular structures from the injections and from overuse when pain is relieved.

Asthma

Corticosteroids are commonly used in the treatment of asthma for anti-inflammatory and other effects. In acute asthma attacks or status asthmaticus unrelieved by an inhaled beta-adrenergic bronchodilator, high doses of systemic corticosteroids are given orally or IV along with the bronchodilator for approximately 5 to 10 days. Although these high doses suppress the HPA axis, the suppression only lasts for 1 to 3 days and other serious adverse effects are avoided. Thus, systemic corticosteroids are used in short courses as needed and not for long-term treatment. People who regularly use inhaled corticosteroids also need high doses of systemic drugs during acute attacks because aerosols are not effective. As soon as acute symptoms subside, dosage should be tapered to the lowest effective maintenance dose or the drug should be discontinued.

In chronic asthma, inhaled corticosteroids are drugs of first choice. This recommendation evolved from increased knowledge about the importance of inflammation in the pathophysiology of asthma and the development of aerosol corticosteroids that are effective with minimal adverse effects because there is little systemic absorption with recommended doses. Inhaled drugs may be given alone or with systemic drugs. In general, inhaled corticosteroids can replace oral drugs when daily dosage of the oral agent has been tapered to 10 to 15 mg of prednisone or the equivalent dosage of other agents. When a client is being switched from an oral to an inhaled corticosteroid, the inhaled drug should be started during tapering of the oral drug, approximately 1 or 2 weeks before discontinuing or reaching the lowest anticipated dose of the oral drug. When a client requires a systemic corticosteroid, coadministration of an aerosol allows smaller doses of the systemic corticosteroid. Although the inhaled drugs can cause suppression of the HPA axis and adrenocortical function, especially at higher doses, they are much less likely to do so than systemic drugs.

In addition to their anti-inflammatory effects, corticosteroids also increase the effects of adrenergic bronchodilators that are given in asthma and other disorders to prevent or treat bronchoconstriction and bronchospasm. They perform this important function by increasing the number and responsiveness of beta-adrenergic receptors and preventing the tolerance usually associated with chronic administration of adrenergic bronchodilators. Research studies indicate increased responsiveness to beta-adrenergic bronchodilators within 2 hours and increased numbers of beta receptors within 4 hours of corticosteroid administration.

Cancer

Corticosteroids are commonly used in the treatment of lymphomas, lymphocytic leukemias, and multiple myeloma. In these disorders, corticosteroids inhibit cell reproduction and are cytotoxic to lymphocytes. In addition to their anticancer effects in hematologic malignancies, corticosteroids are beneficial in treatment of several signs and symptoms that often accompany cancer. Although the mechanisms of action are unknown and drug/dosage regimens vary widely, corticosteroids are used to treat anorexia, nausea and vomiting, cerebral edema and inflammation associated with brain metastases or radiation of the head, spinal cord compression, pain and edema related to pressure on nerves or bone metastases, graft-versus-host disease after bone marrow transplantation, and other disorders. Clients tend to feel better when taking corticosteroids, although the basic disease process may be unchanged. The following are some guidelines for corticosteroid therapy of cancer and associated symptoms:

Primary central nervous system (CNS) lymphomas. Formerly considered rare tumors of older adults, these tumors are being diagnosed more often in younger clients. They are usually associated with chronic immunosuppression from immunosuppressant drugs or from acquired immunodeficiency syndrome (AIDS). Many of these lymphomas are very sensitive to corticosteroids and therapy is indicated once the diagnosis is established.

Other CNS tumors. Corticosteroid therapy may be useful in both supportive and definitive treatment of brain and spinal cord tumors; neurologic signs and symptoms often improve dramatically within 24 to 48 hours. Corticosteroids help to relieve symptoms by controlling edema around the tumor, at operative sites, and at sites receiving radiation therapy. Some clients can be tapered off corticosteroids after surgical or radiation therapy; others require continued therapy to manage neurologic symptoms. Adverse effects of long-term corticosteroid therapy may include mental changes ranging from mild agitation to psychosis and steroid myopathy, which may be confused with tumor progression. Mental symptoms usually improve if drug dosage is reduced and resolve if the drug is discontinued; steroid myopathy may persist for weeks or months.

Chemotherapy-induced emesis. Corticosteroids have strong antiemetic effects; the mechanism is unknown. One effective regimen combines an oral or IV dose of dexamethasone (10 to 20 mg) with a serotonin antagonist or metoclopramide and is given immediately before the chemotherapeutic drug. This regimen is the treatment of choice for chemotherapy with cisplatin, which is a strongly emetic drug.

Chronic Obstructive Pulmonary Disease

Corticosteroids are more helpful in acute exacerbations than in stable disease. However, oral corticosteroids may improve pulmonary function and symptoms in some clients. For a client with inadequate relief from a bronchodilator, a trial of a corticosteroid (eg, prednisone 20 to 40 mg each morning for 5 to 7 days) may be justified. Treatment should be continued only if there is significant improvement. As in other conditions, the lowest effective dose is needed to minimize adverse drug effects.

Inhaled corticosteroids can also be tried. They produce minimal adverse effects, but their effectiveness in COPD has not been clearly demonstrated.

Inflammatory Bowel Disease

Crohn's disease and ulcerative colitis often require periodic corticosteroid therapy. With moderate Crohn's disease, clients are usually given oral prednisone, 40 mg daily, until symptoms subside. With severe disease, clients often require hospitalization, IV fluids for hydration, and parenteral corticosteroids until symptoms subside.

With ulcerative colitis, corticosteroids are usually used when aminosalicylates are not effective or when symptoms are more severe. Initially, hydrocortisone enemas may be effective. If not effective, oral prednisone 20 to 60 mg daily may be given until symptoms subside. In clients with severe disease, oral prednisone may be required initially. Once remission of symptoms is achieved, the dose can be tapered by 2.5 to 5 mg/day each week to a dose of 20 mg. Then, tapering may be slowed to 2.5 to 5 mg/day every other week. As with Crohn's disease, clients with severe ulcerative colitis often require hospitalization and parenteral corticosteroids. One regimen uses IV hydrocortisone 300 mg/day or the equivalent dose of another drug. When the client's condition improves, oral prednisone can replace the IV corticosteroid.

Prevention of Acute Adrenocortical Insufficiency

Suppression of the HPA axis may occur with corticosteroid therapy and may lead to life-threatening inability to increase cortisol secretion when needed to cope with stress. It is most likely to occur with abrupt withdrawal of systemic corticosteroid drugs. The risk of HPA suppression is high with systemic drugs given for more than a few days, although clients vary in degree and duration of suppression with comparable doses, and the minimum dose and duration of therapy that cause suppression are unknown.

When the drugs are given for replacement therapy, adrenal insufficiency is lifelong and drug administration must be continued. When the drugs are given for purposes other than replacement and then discontinued, the HPA axis usually recovers within several weeks to months, but may take a year or longer. Several strategies have been developed to minimize HPA suppression and risks of acute adrenal insufficiency, including:

- Administer a systemic corticosteroid during high-stress situations (eg, moderate or severe illness, trauma, or surgery) to clients who have received pharmacologic doses for 2 weeks within the previous year or who receive long-term systemic therapy (ie, are steroid dependent).
- Give short courses of systemic therapy for acute disorders, such as asthma attacks, then decrease the dose or stop the drug within a few days.
- Gradually taper the dose of any systemic corticosteroid. Although specific guidelines for tapering dosage have not been developed, higher doses and longer durations of administration in general require slower tapering, possibly over several weeks. The goal of tapering may be to stop the drug or to decrease the dosage to the lowest effective amount.
- Use local rather than systemic therapy when possible, alone or in combination with low doses of systemic drugs. Numerous preparations are available for local application, including aerosols for oral or nasal inhalation, formulations for topical application to the skin, eyes, and ears, and drugs for intra-articular injections.
- Use ADT, which involves titrating the daily dose to the lowest effective maintenance level, then giving a double dose every other day.

How Can You Avoid This Medication Error?

Jane Wright has been receiving high-dose corticosteroid therapy (hydrocortisone 80 mg bid) for the last month. You receive an order to taper the steroid dose as follows: decrease hydrocortisone dose 20 mg each day for 3 days, then decrease by 10 mg per day and give only qd. You are caring for Jane on the third day after this order was written. You administer 40 mg for her morning dose.

Use in Children

Corticosteroids are used for the same conditions in children as in adults; a common use is for treatment of asthma. With severe asthma, continual drug therapy with relatively high doses may be required. A major concern with children is growth retardation, which can occur with small doses and administration by inhalation. Many children have a growth spurt when the drug is discontinued, but drug effects on adult stature are unknown.

Parents and health care providers can monitor drug effects, recording height and weight weekly. ADT is less likely to impair normal growth and development than daily administration. In addition, for both systemic and inhaled corticosteroids, each child's dose should be titrated to the lowest effective amount.

Use in Older Adults

Corticosteroids are used for the same conditions in older adults as in younger ones. Older adults are especially likely to have conditions that are aggravated by the drugs (eg, congestive heart failure, hypertension, diabetes mellitus, arthritis, osteoporosis, increased susceptibility to infection, and concomitant drug therapy that increases risks of gastrointestinal ulceration and bleeding). Consequently, risk–benefit ratios of corticosteroid therapy should be carefully considered, especially for long-term therapy.

When used, lower doses are usually indicated because of decreased muscle mass, plasma volume, hepatic metabolism, and renal excretion in older adults. In addition, therapeutic and adverse responses should be monitored regularly by a health care provider (eg, blood pressure, serum electrolytes, and blood glucose levels at least every 6 months).

Use in Renal Impairment

Corticosteroids should be used with caution because of slowed excretion, with possible accumulation and signs and symptoms of hypercorticism. In renal transplantation, corticosteroids are extensively used, along with other immunosuppressive drugs, to prevent or treat rejection reactions. In these clients, as in others, adverse effects of systemic corticosteroids may include infections, hypertension, glucose intolerance, obesity, cosmetic changes, bone loss, growth retardation in children, cataracts, pancreatitis, peptic ulcerations, and psychiatric disturbances. Dosages should be minimized and the drugs can be withdrawn in some clients.

Use in Hepatic Impairment

Metabolism of corticosteroids is slowed by severe hepatic disease, so that corticosteroids may accumulate and cause signs and symptoms of hypercorticism. In addition, clients with liver disease should be given prednisolone rather than prednisone. Liver metabolism of prednisone is required to convert it to its active form, prednisolone.

Use in Critical Illness

Corticosteroids have been extensively used in the treatment of serious illness, with much usage empiric. Some guidelines regarding their use in various critical illnesses include the following:

Adrenal insufficiency is the most clear-cut indication for use of a corticosteroid, and even a slight impairment of the adrenal response during severe illness can be lethal if corticosteroid therapy is not provided. For example, hypotension is a common symptom in critically ill clients and hypotension caused by adrenal insufficiency may mimic either hypovolemic or septic shock. If adrenal insufficiency is the cause of the hypotension, administration of corticosteroids can eliminate the need for vasopressor drugs to maintain adequate tissue perfusion.

However, adrenal insufficiency may not be recognized because hypotension and other symptoms also occur with many illnesses. The normal response to critical illness (eg, pain, hypovolemia) is increased and prolonged secretion of cortisol. If this does not occur, or if too little cortisol is produced, a state of adrenal insufficiency exists. One way to evaluate a client for adrenal insufficiency is a test in which a baseline serum cortisol level is measured, after which corticotropin is given IV to stimulate cortisol production, and the serum cortisol level is measured again in approximately 30 to 60 minutes. Test results are hard to interpret in seriously ill clients, however, because serum cortisol concentrations that would be normal in normal subjects may be low in this population. In addition, a lower-than-expected rise in serum cortisol levels may indicate a normal HPA axis that is already maximally stimulated, or interference with the ability of the adrenal cortex to synthesize cortisol. Thus, a critically ill client may have a limited ability to increase cortisol production in response to stress.

In any client suspected of having adrenal insufficiency, a single IV dose of corticosteroid seems justified. If the client does have adrenal insufficiency, the dose may prevent immediate death and allow time for other diagnostic and therapeutic measures. If the client does not have adrenal insufficiency, the single dose is not harmful.

Acute respiratory failure in clients with COPD. Some studies support the use of IV methylprednisolone. Thus, if other medications do not produce adequate bronchodilation, it seems reasonable to try an IV corticosteroid during the first 72 hours of the illness. However, corticosteroid therapy increases the risks of pulmonary infection.

Adult respiratory distress syndrome (ARDS). Although corticosteroids have been widely used, several well-controlled studies demonstrate that the drugs are not beneficial in early treatment or in prevention of ARDS. Thus, corticosteroids should be used in these clients only if there are other specific indications.

Sepsis. Large, well-controlled, multicenter studies have shown no beneficial effect from the use of corticosteroids in gram-negative bacteremia, sepsis, or septic shock. In addition, they do not prevent development of ARDS or multiple organ dysfunction syndrome or decrease mortality in clients with sepsis. In addition, clients receiving corticosteroid therapy for other conditions are at risk for development of sepsis

because the drugs impair the ability of white blood cells to leave the bloodstream and reach a site of infection.

AIDS. Adrenal insufficiency is being increasingly recognized in this population and clients should be assessed and treated for it, if indicated. In addition, corticosteroid therapy improves survival and decreases risks of respiratory failure with pneumocystosis, a common cause of death in clients with AIDS. The recommended regimen is prednisone 40 mg twice daily for 5 days, then 40 mg once daily for 5 days, then 20 mg daily until completion of treatment for pneumocystosis. The effect of corticosteroids on risks for development of other opportunistic infections or neoplasms is unknown.

 Home Care

Corticosteroids are extensively used in the home setting, by all age groups, for a wide variety of disorders, and by most routes of administration. Because of potentially serious adverse effects, especially with oral drugs, it is extremely important that these drugs be used as prescribed. A major responsibility of the home care nurse is to teach, demonstrate, supervise, monitor, or do whatever is needed to facilitate correct use. In addition, the home care nurse needs to teach clients and caregivers interventions to minimize adverse effects of these drugs.

(*text continues on page 344*)

NURSING ACTIONS	Corticosteroid Drugs
NURSING ACTIONS	**RATIONALE/EXPLANATION**
1. Administer accurately **a.** Read the drug label carefully to be certain of having the correct preparation for the intended route of administration.	Many corticosteroid drugs are available in several different preparations. For example, hydrocortisone is available in formulations for intravenous (IV) or intramuscular (IM) administration, for intra-articular injection, and for topical application in creams and ointments of several different strengths. These preparations cannot be used interchangeably without causing potentially serious adverse reactions and decreasing therapeutic effects. Some drugs are available for only one use. For example, several preparations are for topical use only; beclomethasone is prepared only for oral and nasal inhalation.
b. With oral corticosteroid drugs, give with or after meals.	Opinion seems divided regarding the effectiveness of this scheduling in relation to meals. The rationale is to decrease gastric irritation and prevent (*continued*)

NURSING ACTIONS	RATIONALE/EXPLANATION
	development or aggravation of peptic ulcer disease. Corticosteroid drugs have long been considered ulcerogenic, but there is no valid evidence to substantiate this claim. Many physicians prescribe antacids to be given at the same time as the corticosteroid drug.
c. For IV or IM administration:	
(1) Follow the manufacturer's directions on the drug vial for the type and amount of diluent to add.	Instructions vary with specific preparations.
(2) Give direct IV injection over at least 1 min.	To increase safety of administration
(3) Follow the manufacturer's directions for diluting and administering by continuous IV infusions.	Instructions vary with specific preparations.
d. For oral inhalation of a corticosteroid, check the instruction leaflet that accompanies the inhaler. If the client also is receiving a bronchodilator, administer it first.	Giving a bronchodilating drug by inhalation before giving the corticosteroid increases penetration of the corticosteroid into the tracheobronchial tree and increases its therapeutic effectiveness.
2. Observe for therapeutic effects	The primary objective of corticosteroid therapy is to relieve signs and symptoms, because the drugs are not curative. Therefore, therapeutic effects depend largely on the reason for use.
a. With adrenocortical insufficiency, observe for absence or decrease of weakness, weight loss, anorexia, nausea, vomiting, hyperpigmentation, hypotension, hypoglycemia, hyponatremia, and hyperkalemia.	These signs and symptoms of impaired metabolism do not occur with adequate replacement of corticosteroids.
b. With rheumatoid arthritis, observe for decreased pain and edema in joints, greater capacity for movement, and increased ability to perform usual activities of daily living.	
c. With asthma and chronic obstructive pulmonary disease, observe for decrease in respiratory distress and increased tolerance of activity.	
d. With skin lesions, observe for decreasing inflammation.	
e. When the drug is given to suppress the immune response to organ transplants, therapeutic effect is the absence of signs and symptoms indicating rejection of the transplanted tissue.	
3. Observe for adverse effects	These are uncommon with replacement therapy but common with long-term administration of the pharmacologic doses used for many disease processes. Adverse reactions may affect every body tissue and organ.
a. Adrenocortical insufficiency—fainting, weakness, anorexia, nausea, vomiting, hypotension, shock, and if untreated, death	This reaction is likely to occur in clients receiving daily corticosteroid drugs who encounter stressful situations. It is caused by drug-induced suppression of the hypothalamic–pituitary–adrenal axis,

(continued)

NURSING ACTIONS	RATIONALE/EXPLANATION
	which makes the client unable to respond to stress by increasing adrenocortical hormone secretion.
b. Adrenocortical excess (hypercorticism or Cushing's disease)	Most adverse effects result from excessive corticosteroids.
(1) "Moon face," "buffalo hump" contour of shoulders, obese trunk, thin extremities	This appearance is caused by abnormal fat deposits in cheeks, shoulders, breasts, abdomen, and buttocks. These changes are more cosmetic than physiologically significant. However, the alterations in self-image can lead to psychological problems. These changes cannot be prevented, but they may be partially reversed if corticosteroid therapy is discontinued or reduced in dosage.
(2) Diabetes mellitus—glycosuria, hyperglycemia, polyuria, polydipsia, polyphagia, impaired healing, and other signs and symptoms	Corticosteroid drugs can cause hyperglycemia and diabetes mellitus or aggravate preexisting diabetes mellitus by their effects on carbohydrate metabolism.
(3) Central nervous system effects—euphoria, psychological dependence, nervousness, insomnia, depression, personality and behavioral changes, aggravation of pre-existing psychiatric disorders	Some clients enjoy the drug-induced euphoria so much that they resist attempts to withdraw the drug or decrease its dosage
(4) Musculoskeletal effects—osteoporosis, pathologic fractures, muscle weakness and atrophy, decreased linear growth in children	Demineralization of bone produces thin, weak bones that fracture easily. Fractures of vertebrae, long bones, and ribs are relatively common, especially in postmenopausal women and immobilized clients. Myopathy results from abnormal protein metabolism. Decreased growth in children results from impaired bone formation and protein metabolism.
(5) Cardiovascular, fluid, and electrolyte effects—fluid retention, edema, hypertension, congestive heart failure, hypernatremia, hypokalemia, metabolic alkalosis	These effects result largely from mineralocorticoid activity, which causes retention of sodium and water. They are more likely to occur with older corticosteroids, such as hydrocortisone and prednisone.
(6) Gastrointestinal effects—nausea, vomiting, possible peptic ulcer disease, increased appetite, obesity	
(7) Increased susceptibility to infection and delayed wound healing	Caused by suppression of normal inflammatory and immune processes and impaired protein metabolism
(8) Menstrual irregularities, acne, excessive facial hair	Caused by excessive sex hormones, primarily androgens
(9) Ocular effects—increased intraocular pressure, glaucoma, cataracts	
(10) Integumentary effects—skin becomes reddened, thinner, has stretch marks, and is easily injured	
4. Observe for drug interactions	
a. Drugs that *increase* effects of corticosteroids:	

(continued)

NURSING ACTIONS	RATIONALE/EXPLANATION
(1) Adrenergics (eg, epinephrine), anticholinergics (eg, atropine), tricyclic antidepressants (eg, amitriptyline [Elavil]), antihistamines, and meperidine	Potentiation of increased intraocular pressure. The combinations are hazardous in glaucoma and should be avoided if possible.
(2) Diuretics	Excessive potassium depletion may occur because both diuretics and corticosteroids can cause hypokalemia.
(3) Estrogens	Potentiate glycosuria and anti-inflammatory effects of hydrocortisone but not those of dexamethasone, methylprednisolone, prednisolone, or prednisone
(4) Salicylates	May potentiate all effects of corticosteroids by displacing the drug from plasma protein binding sites
b. Drugs that *decrease* effects of corticosteroids:	
(1) Antihistamines, barbiturates, chloral hydrate, phenytoin, rifampin	These drugs induce microsomal enzymes in the liver and increase the rate at which corticosteroids are metabolized or deactivated.

Nursing Notes: Apply Your Knowledge

Answer: Kim's prednisone should not be stopped before surgery. In fact, the dose may be increased because of the physiologic stress of the surgery. Check with the surgeon to clarify preoperative and postoperative steroid orders. Side effects of steroid use are significant for the postoperative patient. Wound healing is delayed because the inflammatory response is impaired. Carefully inspect the incision for dehiscence and know that staples or sutures may remain in place for a longer period of time. Signs of infection (fever, elevated white blood cell count, purulent drainage) may be absent or diminished even when an infection is present. Assess for fluid and electrolyte imbalances (sodium and fluid retention) during the postoperative period, as well as gastrointestinal irritation.

How Can You Avoid This Medication Error?

Answer: By the third day, the dose should be 20 mg (first day 60 mg; second day 40 mg), so this medication error occurred because the wrong dose was administered. This taper order is not written clearly. Clarify with the physician the dosage for each day and have him or her write the order indicating the dosage for day 1, day 2, day 3, and so forth. When administering a dose that is adjusted daily, it helps to look at how much was administered the previous days to double-check the dosage to be administered.

REVIEW AND APPLICATION EXERCISES

1. What are the main characteristics and functions of cortisol?

2. What is the difference between glucocorticoid and mineralocorticoid components of corticosteroids?

3. How do glucocorticoids affect body metabolism?

4. What is meant by the HPA axis?

5. What are the mechanisms by which exogenous corticosteroids may cause adrenocortical insufficiency and excess?

6. What are adverse effects associated with chronic use of systemic corticosteroids?

7. For a client on long-term systemic corticosteroid therapy, why is it important to taper the dose and gradually discontinue the drug rather than stop it abruptly?

8. Why is alternate-day administration of a systemic corticosteroid preferred when possible?

9. What are the main differences between administering corticosteroids in adrenal insufficiency and in other disorders?

10. When a corticosteroid is given by inhalation to clients with asthma or other bronchoconstrictive disorder, what is the expected effect?

SELECTED REFERENCES

Brenner, Z.R. & Cannito, M. (1998). Administering steroids. *Nursing, 28*(3), 34–38.

Brestel, E.P. & Van Dyke, K. (1997). Antiinflammatory and antirheumatic drugs. In C.R. Craig & R.E. Stitzel (Eds.), *Modern pharmacology with clinical applications*, 5th ed., pp. 455–469. Boston: Little, Brown & Company.

Drug facts and comparisons. (Updated monthly). St. Louis: Facts and Comparisons.

Gums, J.G. & Wilt, V.M. (1997). Disorders of the adrenal gland. In J.T. DiPiro, R.L. Talbert, P.E. Hayes, G.C. Yee, G.R. Matzke, B.G. Wells, & L.M. Posey (Eds.), *Pharmacotherapy: A pathophysiologic approach*, 3rd ed., pp. 1547–1564. Stamford, CT: Appleton & Lange.

Guyton, A.C. & Hall, J.E. (1996). *Textbook of medical physiology*, 9th ed. Philadelphia: W.B. Saunders.

Kelley, W.N. (Ed.) (1997). *Textbook of internal medicine*, 3rd ed. Philadelphia: Lippincott-Raven.

Kelly, H.W. & Kamada, A.K. (1997). Asthma. In J.T. DiPiro, R.L. Talbert, P.E. Hayes, G.C. Yee, G.R. Matzke, B.G. Wells, & L.M. Posey (Eds.), *Pharmacotherapy: A pathophysiologic approach*, 3rd ed., pp. 553–588. Stamford, CT: Appleton & Lange.

Lamberts, S.W.J., Bruining, H.A., & DeJong, F.H. (1997). Corticosteroid therapy in severe illness. *New England Journal of Medicine, 337*(18), 1285–1292.

Porth, C.M. (1998). Alterations in endocrine control of growth and metabolism. In C.M. Porth (Ed.), *Pathophysiology: Concepts of altered health states*, 5th ed., pp. 785–803. Philadelphia: Lippincott Williams & Wilkins.

Rubin, R.P. (1997). Adrenocortical hormones and drugs affecting the adrenal cortex. In C.R. Craig & R.E. Stitzel (Eds.), *Modern pharmacology with clinical applications*, 5th ed., pp. 721–735. Boston: Little, Brown & Company.

Schimmer, B.P. & Parker, K.L. (1996). Adrenocorticotropic hormone; adrenocortical steroids and their synthetic analogs; inhibitors of the synthesis and actions of adrenocortical hormones. In J.G. Hardman, L.E. Limbird, P.B. Molinoff, & R.W. Ruddon (Eds.), *Goodman & Gilman's The pharmacological basis of therapeutics*, 9th ed., pp. 1459–1485. New York: McGraw-Hill.

25

Thyroid and Antithyroid Drugs

Objectives

After studying this chapter, the student will be able to:

1. Describe physiologic effects of thyroid hormone.

2. Identify effects of hyposecretion and hypersecretion of thyroid hormone.

3. Describe characteristics, uses, and effects of thyroid drugs.

4. Describe characteristics, uses, and effects of antithyroid drugs.

5. Discuss the influence of thyroid and antithyroid drugs on the metabolism of other drugs.

6. Teach clients self-care activities related to the use of thyroid and antithyroid drugs.

Mary Sanchez, 55 years of age, is diagnosed with chronic (Hashimoto's) thyroiditis and is to begin treatment with levothyroxine (Synthroid) 0.1 mg daily. You are the nurse in the clinic and responsible for teaching Ms. Sanchez about her hypothyroidism and thyroid replacement therapy.

Reflect on:

▶ Signs and symptoms of hypothyroidism and its impact on functional abilities.

▶ Priority information that should be given to Ms. Sanchez during the brief (10-minute) time allotted.

▶ How you will need to individualize teaching if Ms. Sanchez's ability to speak and read English is limited.

▶ Necessary follow-up for Ms. Sanchez's hypothyroidism and drug management.

DESCRIPTION AND USES

The thyroid gland produces three hormones: thyroxine, triiodothyronine, and calcitonin. Thyroxine contains four atoms of iodine and is also called T_4. Triiodothyronine contains three atoms of iodine and is called T_3. Compared with thyroxine, triiodothyronine is more potent and has a more rapid onset but shorter duration of action. Despite these minor differences, the two hormones produce the same physiologic effects and have the same actions and uses. Calcitonin functions in calcium metabolism and is discussed in Chapter 26.

Production of thyroxine and triiodothyronine depends on the presence of iodine and tyrosine in the thyroid gland. Plasma iodide is derived from dietary sources and from the metabolic breakdown of thyroid hormone, which allows some iodine to be reused. The thyroid gland extracts iodide from the circulating blood, concentrates it, and secretes enzymes that change the chemically inactive iodide to free iodine atoms. Tyrosine is an amino acid derived from dietary protein. It forms the basic structure of thyroglobulin. In a series of chemical reactions, iodine atoms become attached to tyrosine to form the thyroid hormones T_3 and T_4. Once formed, the hormones are stored within the chemically inactive thyroglobulin molecule.

Thyroid hormones are released into the circulation when the thyroid gland is stimulated by thyroid-stimulating hormone (thyrotropin or TSH) from the anterior pituitary gland. Because the thyroglobulin molecule is too large to cross cell membranes, proteolytic enzymes break down the molecule so the active hormones can be released. After their release from thyroglobulin, the hormones become largely bound to plasma proteins. Only the small amounts left unbound are biologically active. The bound thyroid hormones are released to tissue cells very slowly. Once in the cells, the hormones combine with intracellular proteins so they are again stored. They are released slowly within the cell and used over a period of days or weeks. Once used by the cells, the thyroid hormones release the iodine atoms. Most of the iodine is reabsorbed and used to produce new thyroid hormones; the remainder is excreted in the urine.

Thyroid hormones control the rate of cellular metabolism and thereby influence the functioning of virtually every cell in the body. The heart, skeletal muscle, liver, and kidneys are especially responsive to the stimulating effects of thyroid hormones. The brain, spleen, and gonads are less responsive. Thyroid hormones are required for normal growth and development and are considered especially critical for brain and skeletal development and maturation. These hormones are thought to act mainly by controlling intracellular protein synthesis. Some specific physiologic effects include:

- Increased rate of cellular metabolism and oxygen consumption with a resultant increase in heat production
- Increased heart rate, force of contraction, and cardiac output (increased cardiac workload)
- Increased carbohydrate metabolism
- Increased fat metabolism, including increased lipolytic effects of other hormones and metabolism of cholesterol to bile acids
- Inhibition of pituitary secretion of TSH

THYROID DISORDERS

Thyroid disorders requiring drug therapy are goiter, hypothyroidism, and hyperthyroidism. Hypothyroidism and hyperthyroidism produce opposing effects on body tissues, depending on the levels of circulating thyroid hormone. Specific effects and clinical manifestations are listed in Table 25-1.

Simple Goiter

Simple goiter is an enlargement of the thyroid gland resulting from iodine deficiency. Inadequate iodine decreases thyroid hormone production. To compensate, the anterior pituitary gland secretes more TSH, which causes the thyroid to enlarge and produce more hormone. If the enlarged gland secretes enough hormone, thyroid function is normal and the main consequences of the goiter are disfigurement, psychological distress, dyspnea, and dysphagia. If the gland cannot secrete enough hormone despite enlargement, hypothyroidism results. Simple or endemic goiter is a common condition in some geographic areas. It is uncommon in the United States, largely because of the widespread use of iodized table salt.

Treatment of simple goiter involves giving iodine preparations and thyroid hormones to prevent further enlargement and promote regression in gland size. Large goiters may require surgical excision.

Hypothyroidism

Primary hypothyroidism occurs when disease or destruction of thyroid gland tissue causes inadequate production of thyroid hormones. Causes of primary hypothyroidism include chronic (Hashimoto's) thyroiditis, an autoimmune disorder, and treatment of hyperthyroidism with antithyroid drugs, radiation therapy, or surgery. Secondary hypothyroidism occurs when there is decreased TSH from the anterior pituitary gland.

Congenital hypothyroidism (cretinism) occurs when a child is born without a thyroid gland or with a poorly functioning gland. Cretinism is uncommon in the United States but may occur with a lack of iodine in the mother's diet. Symptoms are rarely present at birth, but develop gradually during infancy and early childhood and include poor growth and development, lethargy and inactivity, feeding problems, slow pulse, subnormal temperature, and

TABLE 25-1	Thyroid Disorders and Their Effects on Body Systems

Hypothyroidism	Hyperthyroidism
Cardiovascular Effects	
Increased capillary fragility	Tachycardia
Decreased cardiac output	Increased cardiac output
Decreased blood pressure	Increased blood volume
Decreased heart rate	Increased systolic blood pressure
Cardiac enlargement	Cardiac arrhythmias
Congestive heart failure	Congestive heart failure
Anemia	
More rapid development of atherosclerosis and its complications (eg, coronary artery and peripheral vascular disease)	
Central Nervous System Effects	
Apathy and lethargy	Nervousness
Emotional dullness	Emotional instability
Slow speech, perhaps slurring and hoarseness as well	Restlessness
Hypoactive reflexes	Anxiety
Forgetfulness and mental sluggishness	Insomnia
Excessive drowsiness and sleeping	Hyperactive reflexes
Metabolic Effects	
Intolerance of cold	Intolerance of heat
Subnormal temperature	Low-grade fever
Increased serum cholesterol	Weight loss despite increased appetite
Weight gain	
Gastrointestinal Effects	
Decreased appetite	Increased appetite
Constipation	Abdominal cramps
	Diarrhea
	Nausea and vomiting
Muscular Effects	
Weakness	Weakness
Fatigue	Fatigue
Vague aches and pains	Muscle atrophy
	Tremors
Integumentary Effects	
Dry, coarse, and thickened skin	Moist, warm, flushed skin due to vasodilation and increased sweating
Puffy appearance of face and eyelids	Hair and nails soft
Dry and thinned hair	
Thick and hard nails	
Reproductive Effects	
Prolonged menstrual periods	Amenorrhea or oligomenorrhea
Infertility or sterility	
Decreased libido	
Miscellaneous Effects	
Increased susceptibility to infection	Dyspnea
Increased sensitivity to narcotics, barbiturates, and anesthetics due to slowed metabolism of these drugs	Polyuria
	Hoarse, rapid speech
	Increased susceptibility to infection
	Excessive perspiration
	Localized edema around the eyeballs, which produces characteristic eye changes, including exophthalmos

constipation. If the disorder is untreated until the child is several months old, permanent mental retardation is likely to result.

Adult hypothyroidism produces variable signs and symptoms, depending on the amount of circulating thyroid hormone. Initially, manifestations are mild and vague. They usually increase in incidence and severity over time as the thyroid gland gradually atrophies and functioning glandular tissue is replaced by nonfunctioning fibrous connective tissue (see Table 25-1).

Regardless of the cause of hypothyroidism and the age at which it occurs, the specific treatment is replacement of thyroid hormone from an exogenous source. Synthetic levothyroxine is the drug of choice.

The main clinical indication for use of thyroid drugs is hypothyroidism manifested by signs and symptoms and diagnostic tests of thyroid function. They also may be used to suppress secretion of TSH by the anterior pituitary gland.

Hyperthyroidism

Hyperthyroidism is characterized by excessive secretion of thyroid hormone. It may be associated with Graves' disease, nodular goiter, thyroiditis, overtreatment with thyroid drugs, functioning thyroid carcinoma, and pituitary adenoma that secretes excessive TSH. Hyperthyroidism usually involves an enlarged thyroid gland that has an increased number of cells and an increased rate of secretion. The hyperplastic thyroid gland may secrete 5 to 15 times the normal amount of thyroid hormone. As a result, body metabolism is greatly increased. Specific physiologic effects and clinical manifestations of hyperthyroidism are listed in Table 25-1. These effects vary, depending on the amount of circulating thyroid hormone, and they usually increase in incidence and severity with time if hyperthyroidism is not treated.

Thyroid storm or thyrotoxic crisis is a rare but severe complication characterized by extreme symptoms of hyperthyroidism, such as severe tachycardia, fever, dehydration, heart failure, and coma. It is most likely to occur in clients with hyperthyroidism that has been inadequately treated, especially when stressful situations occur (eg, trauma, infection, surgery, emotional upsets).

Treatment

Hyperthyroidism is treated with antithyroid drugs, radioactive iodine, surgery, or a combination of these methods. The drugs act by decreasing production or release of thyroid hormones. Radioactive iodine emits rays that destroy thyroid gland tissue. Subtotal thyroidectomy involves surgical excision of thyroid tissue. All these methods reduce the amount of thyroid hormones circulating in the bloodstream.

The antithyroid drugs include the thioamide derivatives (propylthiouracil and methimazole) and iodine preparations. The thioamide drugs inhibit synthesis of thyroid hormone, are inexpensive and relatively safe, and they do not damage the thyroid gland. These drugs may be used as the primary treatment (for which they may be given 6 months to 2 years) or to decrease blood levels of thyroid hormone before radioactive iodine therapy or surgery.

Radioactive iodine is a frequently used treatment. It is safe, effective, inexpensive, and convenient. One disadvantage is hypothyroidism, which usually develops within a few months and requires lifelong thyroid hormone replacement therapy. Another disadvantage is the delay in therapeutic benefits. Results may not be apparent for 3 months or longer, during which time severe hyperthyroidism must be brought under control with one of the thioamide antithyroid drugs. Other iodine preparations are not used in long-term treatment of hyperthyroidism. They are indicated when a rapid clinical response is needed, as in thyroid storm and acute hyperthyroidism, or to prepare a hyperthyroid person for thyroidectomy. A thioamide drug is given to produce a euthyroid state, and an iodine preparation is given to reduce the size and vascularity of the thyroid gland to reduce the risk of excessive bleeding.

Iodine preparations inhibit the release of thyroid hormones and cause them to be stored within the gland. They reduce blood levels of thyroid hormones more quickly than thioamide drugs or radioactive iodine. Maximal effects are reached in approximately 10 to 15 days of continuous therapy, and this is probably the primary advantage. Disadvantages, however, include the following:

- They may produce goiter, hyperthyroidism, or both.
- They cannot be used alone. Therapeutic benefits are temporary, and symptoms of hyperthyroidism may reappear and even be intensified if other treatment methods are not also used.
- Radioactive iodine cannot be used effectively for a prolonged period in a client who has received iodine preparations. Even if the iodine preparation is discontinued, the thyroid gland is saturated with iodine and does not attract enough radioactive iodine for treatment to be effective. Also, if radioactive iodine is given later, acute hyperthyroidism is likely to result because the radioactive iodine causes the stored hormones to be released into the circulation.
- Although giving a thioamide drug followed by an iodine preparation is standard preparation for thyroidectomy, the opposite sequence of administration is unsafe. If the iodine preparation is given first and followed by propylthiouracil or methimazole, the client is likely to experience acute hyperthyroidism because the thioamide causes release of the stored thyroid hormones.

Subtotal thyroidectomy is effective in relieving hyperthyroidism but also has several disadvantages. First, preparation for surgery requires several weeks of drug therapy. Second, there are risks involved in anesthesia and surgery and potential postoperative complications. Third, there is a high risk of eventual hypothyroidism. For these reasons, surgery is usually used for clients with large goiters or contraindications to other treatments.

Propranolol is used as an adjunctive drug in the treatment of hyperthyroidism. It relieves tachycardia, cardiac palpitations, excessive sweating, and other symptoms. Propranolol is especially helpful during the several weeks required for therapeutic results from antithyroid drugs or from radioactive iodine administration.

INDIVIDUAL DRUGS

Thyroid Agents (Drugs Used in Hypothyroidism)

Levothyroxine (Synthroid, Levothroid) is a synthetic preparation of T_4. It is a potent form that contains a uniform amount of hormone and can be given parenterally.

Compared with liothyronine, levothyroxine has a slower onset and longer duration of action. Levothyroxine is considered the drug of choice for long-term treatment of hypothyroidism.

ROUTES AND DOSAGE RANGES

Adults: Oral (PO) 0.05–0.1 mg/d initially, increased every 1–3 wk until the desired response is obtained; usual maintenance dose is 0.1–0.2 mg/d
Myxedema coma, intravenous (IV) 0.2–0.5 mg (0.1 mg/mL) in a single dose; 0.1–0.3 mg may be repeated on the second day if necessary

Older adults, clients with cardiac disorders, and clients with hypothyroidism of long duration: PO 0.0125–0.025 mg/d for 6 wk, then dose is doubled every 6–8 wk until the desired response is obtained
Myxedema coma, same as adult dosage

Children: PO no more than 0.05 mg/d initially, then increased by 0.05–0.1 mg every 2 wk until the desired response is obtained; usual dosage range is 0.3–0.4 mg/d
Myxedema coma, same as adult dosage

Liothyronine (Cytomel, Triostat) is a synthetic preparation of T_3. Compared with levothyroxine, liothyronine has a more rapid onset and a shorter duration of action. Consequently, it may be more likely to produce high concentrations in blood and tissues and cause adverse reactions. Also, it requires more frequent administration if used for long-term treatment of hypothyroidism. Only the IV formulation (Triostat) is used in treating myxedema coma.

ROUTES AND DOSAGE RANGES

Adults: PO 25 µg/d initially, increased by 12.5–25 µg every 1–2 wk until desired response is obtained
Myxedema coma, IV 25–50 µg initially, then adjust dosage according to clinical response. Usual dosage, 65–100 µg/d, with doses at least 4 h apart and no more than 12 h apart

Older adults: PO 2.5–5 µg/d for 3–6 wk, then doubled every 6 wk until the desired response is obtained
Myxedema coma, IV 10–20 µg initially, then adjusted according to clinical response

Children: PO 5 µg/d initially, increased by 5 µg/d every 3–4 d until the desired response is obtained. Doses as high as 20–80 µg may be required in cretinism
Myxedema coma, dosage, safety, and effectiveness have not been established

Liotrix (Euthroid, Thyrolar) contains levothyroxine and liothyronine in a 4 : 1 ratio, resembling the composition of natural thyroid hormone. Euthroid and Thyrolar are available in strengths ranging from 15 to 180 mg in thyroid equivalency.

ROUTE AND DOSAGE RANGES

Adults: PO 15–30 mg/d initially, increased gradually every 1–2 wk until response is obtained

Older adults, clients with cardiac disorders, and clients with hypothyroidism of long duration: PO one fourth to one half the usual adult dose initially, doubled every 8 wk if necessary

Children: PO same as adult dosage, increased every 2 wk if necessary

Antithyroid Agents (Drugs Used in Hyperthyroidism)

Propylthiouracil is the prototype of the thioamide antithyroid drugs. It can be used alone to treat hyperthyroidism, as part of the preoperative preparation for thyroidectomy, before or after radioactive iodine therapy, and in the treatment of thyroid storm or thyrotoxic crisis. Propylthiouracil acts by inhibiting production of thyroid hormones and peripheral conversion of T_4 to the more active T_3. It does not interfere with release of thyroid hormones previously produced and stored. Thus, therapeutic effects do not occur for several days or weeks until the stored hormones have been used. **Methimazole** (Tapazole) is similar to propylthiouracil in actions, uses, and adverse reactions.

Propylthiouracil

ROUTE AND DOSAGE RANGES

Adults: PO 300–400 mg/d in divided doses q8h, until the client is euthyroid; then 100–150 mg/d in three divided doses, given for maintenance

Children >10 y: PO 150–300 mg/d in divided doses q8h; usual maintenance dose, 100–300 mg/d in two divided doses, q12h

Children 6–10 y: 50–150 mg/d in divided doses q8h
Neonatal thyrotoxicosis, 10 mg/kg/d in divided doses

Methimazole

ROUTE AND DOSAGE RANGES

Adults: PO 15–60 mg/d initially, in divided doses q8h until the client is euthyroid; maintenance, 5–15 mg/d in two or three doses

Children: PO 0.4 mg/kg/d initially, in divided doses q8h; maintenance dose, one half initial dose

Strong iodine solution (Lugol's solution) and **saturated solution of potassium iodide** (SSKI) are iodine preparations sometimes used in short-term treatment of hyperthyroidism. The drugs inhibit release of thyroid hormones, causing them to accumulate in the thyroid gland. Lugol's solution is usually used to treat thyrotoxic crisis and to decrease the size and vascularity of the thyroid gland before thyroidectomy. SSKI is more often used as an expectorant but may be given as preparation for thyroidectomy. Iodine preparations should not be followed by propylthiouracil, methimazole, or radioactive iodine because the latter drugs cause release of stored thyroid hormone and may precipitate acute hyperthyroidism.

Strong Iodine Solution

ROUTE AND DOSAGE RANGES

Adults and children: PO 2–6 drops three times per day for 10 d before thyroidectomy

Potassium Iodide Solution

ROUTE AND DOSAGE RANGES

Adults and children: PO 5 drops three times per day for 10 d before thyroidectomy

Sodium iodide ^{131}**I** (Iodotope) is a radioactive isotope of iodine. The thyroid gland cannot differentiate between regular iodide and radioactive iodide, so it picks up the radioactive iodide from the circulating blood. As a result, small amounts of radioactive iodide can be used as a diagnostic test of thyroid function, and larger doses are used therapeutically to treat hyperthyroidism. Therapeutic doses act by emitting beta and gamma rays, which destroy thyroid tissue and thereby decrease production of thyroid hormones. It is also used to treat thyroid cancer.

Radioactive iodide is usually given in a single dose on an outpatient basis. For most clients, no special radiation precautions are necessary. If a very large dose is given, the client may be isolated for 8 days, which is the half-life of radioactive iodide. Therapeutic effects are delayed for several weeks or up to 6 months. During this time, symptoms may be controlled with thioamide drugs or propranolol. Radioactive iodide is usually given to middle-aged and elderly people; it is contraindicated during pregnancy and lactation.

ROUTES AND DOSAGE RANGES

Adults and children: PO, IV, dosage as calculated by a radiologist trained in nuclear medicine

Propranolol (Inderal) is an antiadrenergic, not an antithyroid, drug. It does not affect thyroid function, hormone secretion, or hormone metabolism. It is most often used to treat cardiovascular conditions, such as arrhythmias, angina pectoris, and hypertension. When given to clients with hyperthyroidism, propranolol blocks beta-adrenergic receptors in various organs and thereby controls symptoms of hyperthyroidism resulting from excessive stimulation of the sympathetic nervous system. These symptoms include tachycardia, palpitations, excessive sweating, tremors, and nervousness. Propranolol is useful for controlling symptoms during the delayed response to thioamide drugs and radioactive iodine, before thyroidectomy, and in treating thyrotoxic crisis. When the client becomes euthyroid and hyperthyroid symptoms are controlled by definitive treatment measures, propranolol should be discontinued.

ROUTE AND DOSAGE RANGE

Adults: PO 40–160 mg/d in divided doses

Nursing Notes: Apply Your Knowledge

Ms. Sanchez has been taking Synthroid for approximately 2 years. She switched to a generic brand of levothyroxine 2 months ago. When she returns to the clinic, she is complaining of fatigue, weight gain, dry skin, and cold intolerance. What do you suggest?

NURSING PROCESS

Assessment

- Assess for signs and symptoms of thyroid disorders (see Table 25-1). During the course of treatment with thyroid or antithyroid drugs, the client's blood level of thyroid hormone may range from low to normal to high. At either end of the continuum, signs and symptoms may be dramatic and obvious. As blood levels change toward normal as a result of treatment, signs and symptoms become less obvious. If presenting signs and symptoms are treated too aggressively, they may change toward the opposite end of the continuum and indicate adverse drug effects. Thus, each client receiving a drug that alters thyroid function must be assessed for indicators of hypothyroidism, euthyroidism, and hyperthyroidism.
- Check laboratory reports for serum TSH (normal = 0.5 to 5 µU/mL) when available. An elevated serum TSH is the first indication of primary hypothyroidism and commonly occurs in middle-aged women, even in the absence of other signs and symptoms. Serum TSH is used to monitor response to drugs that alter thyroid function.

Nursing Diagnoses

- Decreased Cardiac Output related to disease- or drug-induced hypothyroidism
- Altered Nutrition: Less Than Body Requirements with hyperthyroidism
- Altered Nutrition: More Than Body Requirements with hypothyroidism
- Body Image Disturbance related to weight gain with hypothyroidism or weight loss and exophthalmos with hyperthyroidism
- Ineffective Individual Coping related to disease process and long-term drug therapy
- Constipation with hypothyroidism, diarrhea with hyperthyroidism
- Ineffective Thermoregulation related to changes in metabolism rate and body heat production
- Knowledge Deficit: Disease process and drug therapy

Planning/Goals

The client will:

- Achieve normal blood levels of thyroid hormone
- Receive or take drugs accurately
- Experience relief of symptoms of hypothyroidism or hyperthyroidism
- Be assisted to cope with symptoms until therapy becomes effective
- Avoid preventable adverse drug effects
- Be monitored regularly for therapeutic and adverse responses to drug therapy

Interventions

Use nondrug measures to control symptoms, increase effectiveness of drug therapy, and decrease adverse reactions. Some areas for intervention include the following:

- **Environmental temperature.** Regulate for the client's comfort, when possible. Clients with *hypothyroidism* are very intolerant of cold owing to their slow metabolism rate. Chilling and shivering should be prevented because of added strain on the heart. Provide blankets and warm clothing as needed. Clients with *hyperthyroidism* are very intolerant of heat and perspire excessively owing to their rapid metabolism rate. Provide cooling baths and lightweight clothing as needed.
- **Diet.** Despite a poor appetite, *hypothyroid* clients are often overweight. Thus, a low-calorie, weight-reduction diet may be indicated. In addition, an increased intake of high-fiber foods is usually needed to prevent constipation as a result of decreased gastrointestinal secretion and motility. Despite a good appetite, *hyperthyroid* clients are often underweight because of rapid metabolism rates. They often need extra calories and nutri-

ents to prevent tissue breakdown. These can be provided by extra meals and snacks. The client may wish to avoid highly seasoned and high-fiber foods because they may increase diarrhea.

- **Fluids.** With *hypothyroidism*, clients need an adequate intake of low-calorie fluids to prevent constipation. With *hyperthyroidism*, clients need large amounts of fluids (3000–4000 mL/day) unless contraindicated by cardiac or renal disease. The fluids are needed to eliminate heat and waste products produced by the hypermetabolic state. Much of the client's fluid loss is visible as excessive perspiration and urine output.
- **Activity.** With *hypothyroidism*, encourage activity to maintain cardiovascular, respiratory, gastrointestinal, and musculoskeletal function. With *hyperthyroidism*, encourage rest and quiet, nonstrenuous activity. Because clients differ in what they find restful, this must be determined with each one. A quiet room, reading, and soft music may be helpful. Mild sedatives are often given. The client is caught in the dilemma of needing rest because of the high metabolic rate but being unable to rest because of nervousness and excitement.
- **Skin care.** *Hypothyroid* clients are likely to have edema and dry skin. When edema is present, inspect pressure points, turn often, and avoid trauma when possible. Edema increases risks of skin breakdown and decubitus ulcer formation. Also, increased capillary fragility increases the likelihood of bruising from seemingly minor trauma. When skin is dry, use soap sparingly and lotions and other lubricants freely.
- **Eye care.** *Hyperthyroid* clients may have exophthalmos. In mild cases, use measures to protect the eye. For example, dark glasses, local lubri-

CLIENT TEACHING GUIDELINES
Levothyroxine

General Considerations

✔ Thyroid hormone is required for normal body functioning and for life. When a person's thyroid gland is unable to produce enough thyroid hormone, levothyroxine is used as a synthetic substitute. Thus, levothyroxine therapy for hypothyroidism is lifelong; stopping it may lead to life-threatening illness.

✔ Periodic tests of thyroid function are needed.

✔ Dosage adjustments are made according to clinical response and results of thyroid function tests.

✔ Do not switch from one brand name to another; effects may be different.

Self-administration

✔ Take every morning, preferably before breakfast, for best absorption.

✔ Take approximately the same time each day for more consistent blood levels and more normal body metabolism.

✔ Report chest pain, heart palpitations, nervousness, or insomnia. These adverse effects may indicate that drug dosage needs to be reduced.

✔ Consult a health care provider before taking over-the-counter drugs that stimulate the heart or cause nervousness (eg, asthma remedies, cold remedies, decongestants).

cants, and patching of the eyes at night may be needed. Diuretic drugs and elevating the head of the bed may help reduce periorbital edema and eyeball protrusion. If the eyelids cannot close, they are sometimes taped shut to avoid corneal abrasion. In severe exophthalmos, the preceding measures are taken and large doses of corticosteroids are usually given.

Evaluation

- Interview and observe for compliance with instructions for taking medications.
- Observe for relief of symptoms.
- Check laboratory reports for normal blood levels of thyroid hormones.
- Interview and observe for adverse drug effects.
- Check appointment records for compliance with follow-up procedures.

How Can You Avoid This Medication Error?

Gina Sinatro takes Synthroid 0.1 mg once daily. Your stock supply contains Synthroid 100 µg per tablet. To administer the morning dose, the nurse gives Ms. Sinatro 10 tablets.

PRINCIPLES OF THERAPY

Thyroid Drugs

Drug Selection

Levothyroxine is considered the drug of choice for thyroid hormone replacement because of uniform potency, once-daily dosing, and low cost.

Dosage Factors

Dosage is influenced by the choice of drug, the client's age, the client's general condition, severity and duration of hypothyroidism, and clinical response to drug therapy. Specific factors include the following:

1. Dosage must be individualized to approximate the amount of thyroid hormone needed to make up the deficit in endogenous hormone production.
2. As a general rule, initial dosage is relatively small. Dosage is gradually increased at approximately 2-week intervals in most clients until an optimum response is obtained, and symptoms are relieved. Maintenance dosage for long-term therapy is based on the client's clinical status and periodic measurement of serum TSH.
3. Infants requiring thyroid hormone replacement need relatively large doses. After thyroid drugs are started, the maintenance dosage is determined by periodic radioimmunoassay of serum T_4 and by periodic x-ray studies to follow bone development.
4. Clients who are elderly or have cardiovascular disease are given small initial doses. Also, increments are smaller and made at longer intervals, usually approximately 8 weeks. The primary reason for cautious thyroid replacement in such clients is the high risk of adverse effects on the cardiovascular system.

Hypothyroidism and the Metabolism of Other Drugs

Changes in the rate of body metabolism affect the metabolism of various drugs. Most drugs given to a client with hypothyroidism have a prolonged effect because drug metabolism in the liver is delayed and the glomerular filtration rate of the kidneys is decreased. Also, drug absorption from the gastrointestinal system or a parenteral injection site may be slowed. As a result, dosage of many other drugs should be reduced, including digoxin and

---

CLIENT TEACHING GUIDELINES
Propylthiouracil or Methimazole

General Considerations

✔ These drugs are sometimes called antithyroid drugs because they are given to decrease the production of thyroid hormone by an overactive thyroid gland.

✔ These drugs must be taken for 1 year or longer to decrease thyroid hormone levels to normal.

✔ Periodic tests of thyroid function and drug dosage adjustments are needed.

✔ Ask the physician if it is necessary to avoid or restrict amounts of seafood or iodized salt. These sources of iodide may need to be reduced or omitted during antithyroid drug therapy.

Self-administration

✔ When taking multiple doses each day, take at regular intervals around the clock.

✔ Report fever, sore throat, unusual bleeding or bruising, headache, skin rash, yellowing of the skin, or vomiting. If these adverse effects occur, drug dosage may need to be reduced or the drug may need to be discontinued.

✔ Consult a health care provider before taking over-the-counter drugs. Some drugs contain iodide, which can increase the likelihood of goiter and the risk of adverse reactions from excessive doses of iodide. For example, some cough syrups, asthma medications, and multivitamins may contain iodide.

insulin. In addition, people with hypothyroidism are especially likely to experience respiratory depression and myxedema coma with opioid analgesics and other sedating drugs. These drugs should be avoided, but, if considered necessary, they are given very cautiously and in dosages of approximately one third to one half the usual dose. Even then, clients must be observed very closely for respiratory depression.

Once thyroid replacement therapy is started and stabilized, the client becomes euthyroid, has a normal rate of metabolism, and can tolerate usual doses of most drugs if other influencing factors are not present. On the other hand, excessive doses of thyroid drugs may produce hyperthyroidism and a greatly increased rate of metabolism. In this instance, larger doses of most other drugs are necessary to produce the same effects. Rather than increasing dosage of other drugs, however, dosage of thyroid drugs should be reduced so the client is euthyroid again.

Duration of Replacement Therapy

Thyroid replacement therapy in the client with hypothyroidism is lifelong. Medical supervision is needed frequently during early treatment and at least annually after the client's condition has stabilized and maintenance dosage has been determined.

Adrenal Insufficiency

If adrenal insufficiency is present in a client who needs thyroid drugs, that insufficiency must be corrected by giving corticosteroid drugs before starting thyroid replacement because thyroid hormones increase tissue metabolism and tissue demands for adrenocortical hormones. If adrenal insufficiency is not treated first, administration of thyroid hormone may cause acute adrenocortical insufficiency.

Antithyroid Drugs

Dosage Factors

Dosage of the thioamide antithyroid drugs is relatively large until a euthyroid state is reached, in approximately 6 to 8 weeks. A maintenance dose, in the smallest amount that prevents recurrent symptoms of hyperthyroidism, is then given for 1 year or longer. Dosage should be decreased if the thyroid gland enlarges or signs and symptoms of hypothyroidism occur.

Duration of Antithyroid Therapy

No clear-cut guidelines exist regarding duration of antithyroid drug therapy because exacerbations and remissions occur. It is usually continued until the client is euthyroid for 6 to 12 months. Diagnostic tests to evaluate thyroid function or a trial withdrawal then may be implemented to determine whether the client is likely to remain euthyroid without further drug therapy. If the drug is to be discontinued, this is usually done gradually over weeks or months.

Use in Pregnancy

Iodine preparations and thioamide antithyroid drugs are contraindicated during pregnancy because they can lead to goiter and hypothyroidism in the fetus or newborn.

Hyperthyroidism and the Metabolism of Other Drugs

Treatment of hyperthyroidism changes the rate of body metabolism, including the rate of metabolism of many drugs. During the hyperthyroid state, drug metabolism may be very rapid, and higher doses of most drugs may be necessary to achieve therapeutic results. When the client becomes euthyroid, the rate of drug metabolism is decreased. Consequently, doses of all medications should be evaluated and probably reduced to avoid severe adverse reactions.

Iodine Ingestion and Hyperthyroidism

Iodine is present in foods (especially seafood) and in contrast dyes used for gallbladder and other radiologic procedures. Ingestion of large amounts of iodine from these sources may result in goiter and hyperthyroidism.

Use in Children

For *hypothyroidism* in children, replacement therapy is required because thyroid hormone is essential for normal growth and development. As in adults, levothyroxine is the drug of choice in children and dosage needs may change with growth. For congenital hypothyroidism (cretinism), drug therapy should be started within 6 weeks of birth and continued for life. Initially, the recommended dose is 10 to 15 μg/kg/day. Then, maintenance doses for long-term therapy vary with the child's age and weight, usually decreasing over time to a typical adult dose at 11 to 20 years of age. To monitor drug effects on growth, height and weight should be recorded and compared with growth charts at regular intervals. Adverse drug effects are similar to those seen in adults, and children should be monitored closely.

For *hyperthyroidism* in children, a thioamide antithyroid drug (propylthiouracil or methimazole) is used. Potential risks of adverse effects are similar to those in adults. Because radioactive iodine may cause cancer and chromosome damage in children, it should be used only for hyperthyroidism that cannot be controlled by other antithyroid drugs or surgery.

Use in Older Adults

Signs and symptoms of thyroid disorders may mimic those of other disorders that often occur in older adults (eg, congestive heart failure). Therefore, a thorough physical examination and diagnostic tests of thyroid function are necessary before starting any type of treatment.

For *hypothyroidism*, levothyroxine is given. Thyroid replacement hormone increases the workload of the heart and may cause serious adverse effects in older adults, especially those with cardiovascular disease. Cardiac effects also may be increased in clients receiving bronchodilators or other cardiac stimulants. To decrease adverse effects, the drugs should be given in small initial dosages (eg, 25 μg/day) and increased by 25 μg/day at monthly intervals until euthyroidism is attained. Then, a client may be maintained on that dose of levothyroxine for a lifetime or the dose may need to be reduced as the client gets older. Periodic measurements of serum TSH levels are indicated to monitor drug therapy, and doses can be adjusted when indicated.

Blood pressure and pulse should be monitored regularly. As a general rule, the drug should not be given if the resting heart rate is more than 100 beats per minute.

For *hyperthyroidism*, propylthiouracil or methimazole may be used, but radioactive iodine is often preferred because it is associated with fewer adverse effects than other antithyroid drugs or surgery. Clients should be monitored closely for hypothyroidism, which usually develops within a year after receiving treatment for hyperthyroidism.

(*text continues on page 358*)

NURSING ACTIONS	Thyroid and Antithyroid Drugs

NURSING ACTIONS	RATIONALE/EXPLANATION
1. Administer accurately **a.** With thyroid drugs: (1) Administer in a single daily dose, usually before breakfast.	This allows peak drug activity during daytime hours and is less likely to interfere with sleep.
(2) Check the pulse rate before giving the drug. If the rate is over 100 per minute or if any changes in cardiac rhythm are noted, consult the physician before giving the dose.	Tachycardia or other cardiac arrhythmias may indicate adverse cardiac effects. Dosage may need to be reduced or the drug stopped temporarily.
(3) Do not switch among various brands or generic forms of the drug.	Differences in bioavailability have been identified among available products. Changes in preparations may alter dosage and therefore symptom control.
b. With antithyroid and iodine drugs: (1) Administer q8h.	All these drugs have rather short half-lives and must be given frequently and regularly to maintain therapeutic blood levels. In addition, if iodine preparations are not given every 8 h, symptoms of hyperthyroidism may recur.
(2) Dilute iodine solutions in a full glass of fruit juice or milk, if possible and have the client drink the medication through a straw.	Dilution of the drug reduces gastric irritation and masks the unpleasant taste. Using a straw prevents staining the teeth.
2. Observe for therapeutic effects **a.** With thyroid drugs, observe for: (1) Increased energy and activity level, less lethargy and fatigue (2) Increased alertness and interest in surroundings (3) Increased appetite (4) Increased pulse rate and temperature (5) Decreased constipation (6) Reversal of coarseness and other changes in skin and hair	Therapeutic effects result from a return to normal metabolic activities and relief of the symptoms of hypothyroidism. Therapeutic effects may be evident as early as 2 or 3 d after drug therapy is started or delayed up to approximately 2 wk. All signs and symptoms of myxedema should disappear in approximately 3 to 12 wk.

(continued)

NURSING ACTIONS	RATIONALE/EXPLANATION
(7) With cretinism, increased growth rate (record height periodically)	
(8) With myxedema, diuresis, weight loss, and decreased edema	
(9) Decreased serum cholesterol and possibly decreased creatine phosphokinase, lactate dehydrogenase, and aspartate aminotransferase	These tests are often elevated with myxedema and may return to normal when thyroid replacement therapy is begun.
b. With antithyroid and iodine drugs, observe for:	
(1) Slower pulse rate	With propylthiouracil and methimazole, some therapeutic effects are apparent in 1 or 2 wk, but euthyroidism may not occur for 6 or 8 wk.
(2) Slower speech	With iodine solutions, therapeutic effects may be apparent within 24 h. Maximal effects occur in approximately 10 to 15 d. However, therapeutic effects may not be sustained. Symptoms may reappear if the drug is given longer than a few weeks, and they may be more severe than initially.
(3) More normal activity level (slowing of hyperactivity)	
(4) Decreased nervousness	
(5) Decreased tremors	
(6) Improved ability to sleep and rest	
(7) Weight gain	
3. Observe for adverse effects	
a. With thyroid drugs, observe for tachycardia and other cardiac arrhythmias, angina pectoris, myocardial infarction, congestive heart failure, nervousness, hyperactivity, insomnia, diarrhea, abdominal cramps, nausea and vomiting, weight loss, fever, intolerance to heat.	Most adverse reactions stem from excessive doses, and signs and symptoms produced are the same as those occurring with hyperthyroidism. Excessive thyroid hormones make the heart work very hard and fast in attempting to meet tissue demands for oxygenated blood and nutrients. Symptoms of myocardial ischemia occur when the myocardium does not get an adequate supply of oxygenated blood. Symptoms of congestive heart failure occur when the increased cardiac workload is prolonged. Cardiovascular problems are more likely to occur in clients who are elderly or who already have heart disease.
b. With propylthiouracil and methimazole, observe for:	
(1) Hypothyroidism—bradycardia, congestive heart failure, anemia, coronary artery and peripheral vascular disease, slow speech and movements, emotional and mental dullness, excessive sleeping, weight gain, constipation, skin changes, and others	
(2) Blood disorders—leukopenia, agranulocytosis, hypoprothrombinemia	Leukopenia may be difficult to evaluate because it may occur with hyperthyroidism and with antithyroid drugs. Agranulocytosis occurs rarely but is the most severe adverse reaction; the earliest symptoms are likely to be sore throat and fever. If these occur, report them to the physician immediately.
(3) Integumentary system—skin rash, pruritus, alopecia	

(continued)

NURSING ACTIONS	RATIONALE/EXPLANATION

(4) Central nervous system—headache, dizziness, loss of sense of taste, drowsiness, paresthesias

(5) Gastrointestinal system—nausea, vomiting, abdominal discomfort, gastric irritation, cholestatic hepatitis

(6) Other—lymphadenopathy, edema, joint pain, drug fever

c. With iodine preparations, observe for:

   Adverse effects are uncommon with short-term use.

(1) Iodism—metallic taste, burning in mouth, soreness of gums, excessive salivation, gastric or respiratory irritation, rhinitis, headache, redness of conjunctiva, edema of eyelids

(2) Hypersensitivity—acneiform skin rash, pruritus, fever, jaundice, angioedema, serum sickness

   Allergic reactions rarely occur.

(3) Goiter with hypothyroidism

   Uncommon but may occur in adults and newborns whose mothers have taken iodides for long periods

4. Observe for drug interactions

a. Drugs that *increase* effects of thyroid hormones:

(1) Antidepressants (tricyclic), epinephrine

   These drugs primarily increase catecholamines. When combined with thyroid hormones, excessive cardiovascular stimulation may occur and cause myocardial ischemia, cardiac arrhythmias, hypertension, and other adverse cardiovascular effects.

(2) Phenobarbital, phenytoin

   Potentiate thyroid drugs by displacement from plasma protein-binding sites or by slowing liver metabolism.

b. Drugs that *decrease* effects of thyroid hormones:

(1) Antihypertensives

   These agents decrease the cardiovascular effects of catecholamines (epinephrine and norepinephrine) and thyroid hormone, so angina pectoris is less likely to occur.

(2) Cholestyramine resin (Questran)

   This drug decreases gastrointestinal absorption of thyroid hormones. Cholestyramine binds T_4 and T_3 almost irreversibly. If it is necessary to give these drugs concurrently, give the resin at least 4 or 5 h before or after giving the thyroid drug.

(3) Estrogens, including oral contraceptives containing estrogens

   Estrogens inhibit thyroid hormones by increasing thyroxine-binding globulin. This increases the amount of bound, inactive thyroid hormones in clients with hypothyroidism. This decreased effect does not occur in clients with adequate thyroid hormone secretion because the increased binding is offset by increased T_4 production. Women taking oral contraceptives may need larger doses of thyroid

(continued)

NURSING ACTIONS	RATIONALE/EXPLANATION
	hormone replacement than would otherwise be needed.
(4) Propranolol (Inderal)	This drug decreases cardiac effects of thyroid hormones. It is used in hyperthyroidism to reduce tachycardia and other symptoms of excessive cardiovascular stimulation.
c. Drugs that *increase* effects of antithyroid drugs:	
(1) Chlorpromazine, sulfonamides, oral anti-diabetic drugs, xanthines	Increased risk of goiter
(2) Lithium	Acts synergistically to produce hypothyroidism

Nursing Notes: Apply Your Knowledge

Answer: For most drugs, substituting generic brands is safe and economical. For some drugs, the bioavailability (amount of drug absorbed into the bloodstream) differs significantly for generic brands. This is true for thyroid preparations. Ms. Sanchez is experiencing signs of hypothyroidism because her blood levels have fallen below the therapeutic range since she started taking generic thyroid. In this situation, the cost benefit of taking generic drugs may be offset by the higher dose required to achieve therapeutic levels.

How Can You Avoid This Medication Error?

Answer: To convert from milligrams to micrograms, use the conversion factor of 1 mg = 1000 µg. When doing the computation, 0.1 mg converts to 100 µg, and thus one tablet should have been administered. Always question the dosage when more than 2 tablets are given.

 REVIEW AND APPLICATION EXERCISES

1. Where is TSH produced, and what is its function?
2. What is the role of thyroid hormones in maintaining body functions?

3. What signs and symptoms are associated with hypothyroidism?
4. In primary hypothyroidism, are blood levels of TSH increased or decreased?
5. What is the drug of first choice for treating hypothyroidism?
6. What are adverse effects of drug therapy for hypothyroidism?
7. What signs and symptoms are associated with hyperthyroidism?
8. Which drugs reduce blood levels of thyroid hormone in hyperthyroidism, and how do they act?
9. What are adverse effects of drug therapy for hyperthyroidism?
10. When propranolol is used in the treatment of hyperthyroidism, what are its expected effects?
11. What is the effect of thyroid disorders on metabolism of other drugs?

SELECTED REFERENCES

Drug facts and comparisons. (Updated monthly). St. Louis: Facts and Comparisons.

Guyton, A.C. & Hall, J.E. (1996). *Textbook of medical physiology*, 9th ed. Philadelphia: W.B. Saunders.

Porth, C.M. (Ed.). (1998). Mechanisms of endocrine control. *Pathophysiology: Concepts of altered health states*, 5th ed., pp. 785–803. Philadelphia: Lippincott Williams & Wilkins.

Reasner, C.A. II & Talbert R.L. (1997). Thyroid disorders. In J.T. DiPiro, R.L. Talbert, P.E. Hayes, G.C. Yee, G.R. Matzke, B.G. Wells & L.M. Posey (Eds.), *Pharmacotherapy: A pathophysiologic approach*, 3rd ed., pp. 1521–1546. Stamford, CT: Appleton & Lange.

Utiger, R.D. (1997). Disorders of the thyroid gland. In W.N. Kelley (Ed.), *Textbook of internal medicine*, 3rd ed., pp. 2204–2218. Philadelphia: Lippincott-Raven.

26

Hormones That Regulate Calcium and Bone Metabolism

Objectives

After studying this chapter, the student will be able to:

1. Describe the roles of parathyroid hormone, calcitonin, and vitamin D in regulating calcium metabolism.

2. Identify populations at risk for development of hypocalcemia.

3. Discuss prevention and treatment of hypocalcemia.

4. Identify clients at risk for development of hypercalcemia.

5. Discuss recognition and management of hypercalcemia as a medical emergency.

6. Discuss the use of calcium and vitamin D supplements, calcitonin, and bisphosphonate drugs in the treatment of osteoporosis.

You are working at a community center, providing health promotion and disease prevention programs for older adults who live independently in the community. You are planning an osteoporosis prevention workshop.

Reflect on:

▶ Risk factors for osteoporosis.

▶ Nonpharmacologic management strategies to reduce osteoporosis risk.

▶ Methods to increase calcium intake via diet or medications.

▶ Benefits of estrogen replacement therapy for postmenopausal women.

▶ How medication classes, such as bisphosphonates and selective estrogen receptor modulators, work to prevent osteoporosis in high-risk people.

OVERVIEW

Calcium and bone metabolism are regulated by three hormones: parathyroid hormone (PTH), calcitonin, and vitamin D, which act to maintain normal serum levels of calcium. When serum calcium levels are decreased, hormonal mechanisms are activated to raise them; when they are elevated, mechanisms act to lower them (Fig. 26-1). Overall, the hormones alter absorption of dietary calcium from the gastrointestinal tract, movement of calcium from bone to serum, and excretion of calcium through the kidneys.

Disorders of calcium and bone metabolism include hypocalcemia, hypercalcemia, osteoporosis, Paget's disease, and bone breakdown associated with breast cancer and multiple myeloma. Drugs used to treat these disorders are mainly those to alter serum calcium levels or to strengthen bone. To aid understanding of these drugs, characteristics of the hormones, calcium, phosphorus, bone metabolism, and selected disorders are described.

Parathyroid Hormone

Parathyroid hormone secretion is stimulated by low serum calcium levels and inhibited by normal or high levels (a negative feedback system). Because phosphate is closely related to calcium in body functions, PTH also regulates phosphate metabolism. In general, when serum calcium levels go up, serum phosphate levels go down, and vice versa. Thus, an inverse relationship exists between calcium and phosphate.

When the serum calcium level falls below the normal range, PTH raises the level by acting on bone, intestines, and kidneys. In bone, breakdown is increased, so that calcium moves from bone into the serum. In the intestines, there is increased absorption of calcium ingested in food (PTH activates vitamin D, which increases intestinal absorption). In the kidneys, there is increased reabsorption of calcium in the renal tubules and less urinary excretion. The opposite effects occur with phosphate (ie, PTH decreases serum phosphate and increases urinary phosphate excretion).

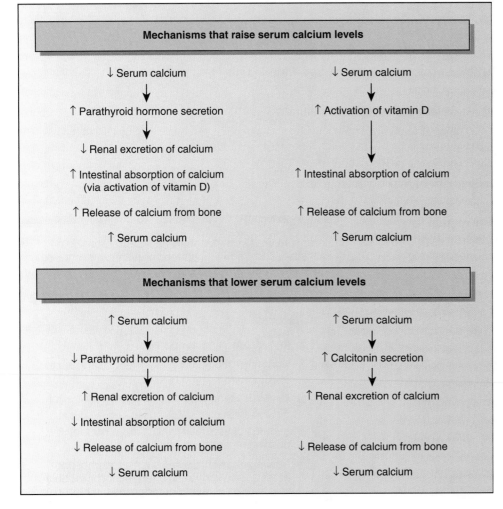

FIGURE 26–1 Hormonal regulation of serum calcium levels. When serum calcium levels are low (hypocalcemia), there is increased secretion of parathyroid hormone and increased activation of vitamin D. These mechanisms lead to decreased loss of calcium in the urine, increased absorption of calcium from the intestine, and increased resorption of calcium from bone. These mechanisms work together to raise serum calcium levels to normal.

When serum calcium levels are high (hypercalcemia), there is decreased secretion of parathyroid hormone and increased secretion of calcitonin. These mechanisms lead to increased loss of calcium in the urine, decreased absorption of calcium from the intestine, and decreased resorption of calcium from bone. These mechanisms lower serum calcium levels to normal.

Disorders of parathyroid function are related to deficient production of PTH (hypoparathyroidism) or excessive production (hyperparathyroidism). Hypoparathyroidism is most often caused by removal of or damage to the parathyroid glands during neck surgery. Hyperparathyroidism is most often caused by a tumor or hyperplasia of a parathyroid gland. It also may result from ectopic secretion of PTH by malignant tumors (eg, carcinomas of the lung, pancreas, kidney, ovary, prostate gland, or bladder). Clinical manifestations and treatment of hypoparathyroidism are the same as those of hypocalcemia; clinical manifestations of hyperparathyroidism are those of hypercalcemia.

Calcitonin

Calcitonin is a hormone from the thyroid gland whose secretion is controlled by the concentration of ionized calcium in the blood flowing through the thyroid gland. When the serum level of ionized calcium is increased, secretion of calcitonin is increased. The function of calcitonin is to lower serum calcium in the presence of hypercalcemia, which it does by decreasing movement of calcium from bone to serum and increasing urinary excretion of calcium. Calcitonin's action is rapid but of short duration. Thus, it has little effect on long-term calcium metabolism.

Vitamin D (Calciferol)

Vitamin D is a fat-soluble vitamin that includes both ergocalciferol (obtained from foods) and cholecalciferol (formed by exposure of skin to sunlight). It functions as a hormone and plays an important role in calcium and bone metabolism. The main action of vitamin D is to raise serum calcium levels by increasing intestinal absorption of calcium and mobilizing calcium from bone. It also promotes bone formation by providing adequate serum concentrations of minerals. Vitamin D is not physiologically active in the body. It must be converted to an intermediate metabolite in the liver, then to an active metabolite (1,25-dihydroxyvitamin D or calcitriol) in the kidneys. PTH and adequate hepatic and renal function are required to produce the active metabolite.

Deficiency of vitamin D causes inadequate absorption of calcium and phosphorus. This, in turn, leads to low levels of serum calcium and stimulation of PTH secretion. In children, this sequence of events produces inadequate mineralization of bone (rickets), a rare condition in the United States. In adults, vitamin D deficiency causes osteomalacia, a condition characterized by decreased bone density and strength.

Calcium and Phosphorus

Calcium and phosphorus are discussed together because they are closely related physiologically. These mineral nutrients are found in many of the same foods, from which they are absorbed together. They are regulated by PTH and excreted through the kidneys. They are both required in cellular structure and function and, as calcium phosphate, in formation and maintenance of bones and teeth. Their characteristics and functions are summarized in Box 26-1.

BOX 26-1 CHARACTERISTICS AND FUNCTIONS OF CALCIUM AND PHOSPHORUS

Calcium

Calcium is the most abundant cation in the body. Approximately 99% is located in the bones and teeth; the rest is in the extracellular fluid and soft tissues. Approximately half of serum calcium is bound, mostly to serum proteins, and is physiologically inactive. The other half is ionized and physiologically active. Ionized calcium can leave the vascular compartment and enter cells, where it participates in intracellular functions. An adequate amount of free (ionized) calcium is required for normal function of all body cells.

Calcium is obtained from the diet, but only 30% to 50% is absorbed from the small intestine; the rest is lost in feces. Absorption is increased in the presence of vitamin D, lactose, moderate amounts of fat, and high pro-

tein intake; increased acidity of gastric secretions; and a physiologic need. Absorption is inhibited by vitamin D deficiency; a high-fat diet; the presence of oxalic acid (from beet greens, chard), which combines with calcium to form insoluble calcium oxalate in the intestine; alkalinity of intestinal secretions, which leads to formation of insoluble calcium phosphate; diarrhea or other conditions of rapid intestinal motility, which do not allow sufficient time for absorption; and immobilization.

Calcium is lost from the body in feces, urine, and sweat. Even when there is deficient intake, approximately 150 mg are lost daily through the intestines (in mucosal and biliary secretions and sloughed intestinal cells). In lactating women, relatively large amounts are lost in breast milk.

(continued)

BOX 26–1   CHARACTERISTICS AND FUNCTIONS OF CALCIUM AND PHOSPHORUS (*continued*)

Functions

- Calcium participates in many metabolic processes, including the regulation of:
  - Cell membrane permeability and function
  - Nerve cell excitability and transmission of impulses (eg, it is required for release of neurotransmitters at synapses)
  - Contraction of cardiac, skeletal, and smooth muscle
  - Conduction of electrical impulses in the heart
  - Blood coagulation and platelet adhesion processes
  - Hormone secretion
  - Enzyme activity
  - Catecholamine release from the adrenal medulla,
  - Release of chemical mediators (eg, histamine from mast cells)
- Calcium is required for building and maintaining bones and teeth. Bone calcium is composed mainly of calcium phosphate and calcium carbonate. In addition to these bound forms, a small amount of calcium is available for exchange with serum. This acts as a reserve supply of calcium. Calcium is constantly shifting between bone and serum as bone is formed and broken down. When serum calcium levels become low, calcium moves into serum.

Requirements and Sources

The calcium requirement of normal adults is approximately 1000 mg daily. Increased daily amounts are needed by growing children (1200 mg), pregnant or lactating women (1200 mg), and postmenopausal women who do not take replacement estrogens (1500 mg to prevent osteoporosis).

The best sources of calcium are milk and milk products. Three 8-oz glasses of milk daily contain approximately the amount needed by healthy adults. Calcium in milk is readily used by the body because milk also contains lactose and vitamin D, both of which are involved in calcium absorption. Other sources of calcium include vegetables (eg, broccoli, spinach, kale, mustard greens) and seafood (eg, clams, oysters).

Phosphorus

Phosphorus is one of the most important elements in normal body function. Most phosphorus is combined with calcium in bones and teeth as calcium phosphate (approximately 80%). The remainder is distributed in every body cell and in extracellular fluid. It is combined with carbohydrates, lipids, proteins, and various other compounds.

Phosphorus is obtained from the diet, and approximately 70% of dietary phosphorus is absorbed from the gastrointestinal (GI) tract. The most efficient absorption occurs when calcium and phosphorus are ingested in approximately equal amounts. Because this equal ratio is present in milk, milk is probably the best source of phosphorus. In general, factors that increase or decrease calcium absorption act the same way on phosphorus absorption. Vitamin D enhances, but is not essential for, phosphorus absorption. Large amounts of calcium or aluminum in the GI tract may combine with phosphate to form insoluble compounds and thereby decrease absorption of phosphorus.

Phosphorus is lost from the body primarily in urine. In people with acute or chronic renal failure, phosphorus intake is restricted because excretion is impaired.

Functions

Phosphorus, most of which is located intracellularly as the phosphate ion, performs many metabolic functions:

- It is an essential component of deoxyribonucleic acid, ribonucleic acid, and other nucleic acids in body cells. Thus, it is required for cell reproduction and body growth.
- It combines with fatty acids to form phospholipids, which are components of all cell membranes in the body. This reaction also prevents buildup of excessive amounts of free fatty acids.
- It forms a phosphate buffer system, which helps to maintain acid–base balance. When excess hydrogen ions are present in kidney tubules, phosphate combines with them and allows their excretion in urine. At the same time, bicarbonate is retained by the kidneys and contributes to alkalinity of body fluids. Although there are other buffering systems in the body, failure of the phosphate system leads to metabolic acidosis (retained hydrogen ions or acid and lost bicarbonate ions or base).
- It is necessary for cell use of glucose and production of energy.
- It is necessary for proper function of several B vitamins (ie, the vitamins function as coenzymes in various chemical reactions only when combined with phosphate).

Requirements and Sources

Daily requirements for phosphorus are approximately 800 mg for normal adults and 1200 mg for growing children and pregnant or lactating women. Phosphorus is widely available in foods. Good sources are milk and other dairy products, meat, poultry, fish, eggs, and nuts. There is little risk of phosphorus deficiency with an adequate intake of calcium and protein.

Bone Metabolism

Bone is mineralized connective tissue that functions as structural support and a reservoir for calcium, phosphorus, magnesium, sodium, and carbonate. The role of bone in maintaining serum calcium levels takes precedence over its structural function (that is, bone may be weakened or destroyed as calcium leaves bone and enters serum).

Bone tissue is constantly being formed and broken down in a process called remodeling. During childhood, adolescence, and early adulthood, formation usually exceeds breakdown (resorption) as the person attains adult height and peak bone mass. After approximately 35 years of age, resorption is greater than formation. Hormonal deficiencies, some diseases, and some medications (eg, glucocorticoids) can also increase resorption, resulting in loss of bone mass and osteoporosis.

Calcium and Bone Disorders

The calcium disorders are hypocalcemia and hypercalcemia, either of which can be life threatening. The bone disorders discussed in this chapter are those characterized by increased resorption of calcium and loss of bone mass. These disorders weaken bone and lead to fractures, pain, and disability. Calcium and selected bone disorders are described in Box 26-2.

DRUGS USED FOR CALCIUM AND BONE DISORDERS

Drugs from several groups are used to treat calcium and bone disorders. Calcium and vitamin D supplements are

---

BOX 26–2 CALCIUM AND BONE DISORDERS

Hypocalcemia

Hypocalcemia is an abnormally low blood calcium level (ie, <8.5 mg/dL). It may be caused by inadequate intake of calcium and vitamin D, numerous disorders (eg, diarrhea or malabsorption syndromes that cause inadequate absorption of calcium and vitamin D, hypoparathyroidism, renal failure, severe hypomagnesemia, hypermagnesemia, acute pancreatitis, rhabdomyolysis, tumor lysis syndrome, vitamin D deficiency), and several drugs (eg, cisplatin, cytosine arabinoside, foscarnet, ketoconazole, pentamidine, and agents used to treat hypercalcemia). Hypocalcemia associated with renal failure is caused by two mechanisms. First, inability to excrete phosphate in urine leads to accumulation of phosphate in the blood (hyperphosphatemia). Because phosphate levels are inversely related to calcium levels, hyperphosphatemia induces hypocalcemia. Second, when kidney function is impaired, vitamin D conversion to its active metabolite is impaired. This results in decreased intestinal absorption of calcium.

Clinical manifestations are characterized by increased neuromuscular irritability, which may progress to tetany. Tetany is characterized by numbness and tingling of the lips, fingers, and toes; twitching of facial muscles; spasms of skeletal muscle; carpopedal spasm; laryngospasm; and convulsions. In young children, hypocalcemia may be manifested by convulsions rather than tetany and erroneously diagnosed as epilepsy. This may be a serious error because anticonvulsant drugs used for epilepsy may further decrease serum calcium levels. Severe hypocalcemia may cause lethargy or confusion.

Hypercalcemia

Hypercalcemia is an abnormally high blood calcium level (ie, >10.5 mg/dL). It may be caused by hyperparathyroidism, hyperthyroidism, malignant neoplasms, vitamin D or vitamin A intoxication, aluminum intoxication, prolonged immobilization, adrenocortical insufficiency, and ingestion of thiazide diuretics, estrogens, and lithium. In hospitalized clients, cancer is a common cause, especially carcinomas (of the breast, lung, head and neck, or kidney) and multiple myeloma. Cancer stimulates bone resorption or breakdown, which increases serum calcium levels. Increased urine output leads to fluid volume deficit. This leads, in turn, to increased reabsorption of calcium in renal tubules and decreased renal excretion of calcium. Decreased renal excretion potentiates hypercalcemia.

Clinical manifestations are caused by the decreased ability of nerves to respond to stimuli and the decreased ability of muscles to contract and relax. Hypercalcemia has a depressant effect on nerve and muscle function. Gastrointestinal problems with hypercalcemia include anorexia, nausea, vomiting, constipation, and abdominal pain. Central nervous system problems include apathy, depression, poor memory, headache, and drowsiness. Severe hypercalcemia may produce lethargy, syncope, disorientation, hallucinations, coma, and death. Other signs and symptoms include weakness and decreased tone in skeletal and smooth muscle, dysphagia, polyuria, polyphagia, and cardiac arrhythmias. In addition, calcium may be deposited in various tissues, such as the conjunctiva, cornea, and kidneys. Calcium deposits in the kidneys (renal calculi) may lead to irreversible damage and impairment of function.

(continued)

BOX 26-2   CALCIUM AND BONE DISORDERS (continued)

Osteoporosis

Osteoporosis is characterized by decreased bone density (osteopenia) and weak, fragile bones that often lead to fractures, pain, and disability. Although any bones may be affected, common fracture sites are the vertebrae of the lower dorsal and lumbar spines, wrists, and hips.

Risk factors include female sex, advanced age, small stature, lean body mass, white or Asian race, positive family history, low calcium intake, menopause, sedentary lifestyle, nulliparity, smoking, excessive ingestion of alcohol or caffeine, high protein intake, high phosphate intake, hyperthyroidism, and chronic use of certain medications (eg, corticosteroids, phenytoin). Postmenopausal women who do not take estrogen replacement therapy are at high risk because of estrogen deficiency, age-related bone loss, and a low peak bone mass. Osteoporosis occurs in men but less often than in women. Both men and women who take high doses of corticosteroids are at high risk because the drugs demineralize bone. In addition, renal transplant recipients can acquire osteoporosis from corticosteroid therapy, decreased renal function, increased parathyroid hormone secretion, and cyclosporine immunosuppressant therapy.

Osteopenia or early osteoporosis may be present and undetected unless radiography or a bone density measurement is done. If detected, treatment is needed to slow bone loss. If undetected or untreated, clinical manifestations of osteoporosis include shortened stature (a measurable loss of height), back pain, spinal deformity, or a fracture. Fractures often occur with common bending or lifting movements or falling.

Paget's Disease

Paget's disease is an inflammatory skeletal disease that affects older people. Its etiology is unknown. It is characterized by a high rate of bone turnover and results in bone deformity and pain. It is treated with non-narcotic analgesics and drugs that decrease bone resorption (eg, bisphosphonates, calcitonin).

---

used to treat hypocalcemia and to prevent and treat osteoporosis. These agents are described in the following sections; names and dosages of individual drug preparations are listed in Table 26-1. Drugs used for hypercalcemia include bisphosphonates, calcitonin, corticosteroids, 0.9% sodium chloride intravenous (IV) infusion, and others. Those used for osteoporosis inhibit bone breakdown and demineralization and include bisphosphonates, calcitonin, estrogens, and antiestrogens. These drugs are described in the following sections; indications for use and dosages are listed in Table 26-2.

Bisphosphonates

Alendronate (Fosamax), **etidronate** (Didronel), **pamidronate** (Aredia), **risedronate** (Actonel), and **tiludronate** (Skelid) are drugs that bind to bone and inhibit calcium resorption from bone. Although indications for use vary among the drugs, they are used mainly in the treatment of hypercalcemia and osteoporosis. Etidronate also inhibits bone mineralization and may cause osteomalacia. Newer bisphosphonates do not have this effect.

These drugs are poorly absorbed from the intestinal tract and must be taken on an empty stomach, with water, at least 30 minutes before any other fluid, food, or medication. The drugs are not metabolized; most of the drug that is not bound to bone is excreted in the urine.

Calcitonin

Calcitonin-salmon (Calcimar, Miacalcin) is used in the treatment of hypercalcemia, Paget's disease, and osteoporosis. In hypercalcemia, calcitonin lowers serum calcium levels by inhibiting bone resorption. It is most likely to be effective in hypercalcemia caused by hyperparathyroidism, prolonged immobilization, or certain malignant neoplasms. In acute hypercalcemia, calcitonin may be used along with other measures to lower serum calcium levels rapidly. A single injection of calcitonin decreases serum calcium levels in approximately 2 hours; effects last approximately 6 to 8 hours.

In Paget's disease, calcitonin slows the rate of bone turnover, improves bone lesions on radiologic examination, and relieves bone pain. In osteoporosis, calcitonin prevents further bone loss in the presence of adequate calcium and vitamin D. In addition, calcitonin helps to control pain in clients with osteoporosis or metastatic bone disease. Both subcutaneous injections and intranasal administration relieve pain within 1 to 12 weeks. The drug is given daily initially, then decreased to 50 to 100 IU two to three times a week. The mechanism by which pain is reduced is unknown.

Calcitonin-human (Cibacalcin) is a synthetic preparation used in Paget's disease. Compared with calcitonin-salmon, calcitonin-human is more likely to cause nausea and facial flushing and less likely to cause antibody formation and allergic reactions.

TABLE 26-1 **Drugs Used in Hypocalcemia and Osteoporosis**

Generic/Trade Name	Routes and Dosage Ranges	
	Adults	Children
Calcium Preparations		
Calcium carbonate precipitated (40% calcium) (Os-Cal 500)	PO 1–1.5 g three times daily with meals (maximal daily dose, 8 g)	
Calcium chloride (10 mL of 10% solution contains 273 mg [13.6 mEq] of calcium)	IV 500 mg–1 g (5–10 mL of 10% solution) every 1–3 d, depending on clinical response or serum calcium measurements.	IV 0.2 mL/kg, up to 1–10 mL/d
Calcium citrate (21% calcium) (Citracal)	1–2 tablets (200 mg calcium per tablet) two to four times daily	
Calcium glubionate (6% calcium) (Neo-Calglucon)	PO 15 ml three times daily Pregnancy or lactation, PO 15 mL four times daily	PO 10 mL three times daily
Calcium gluceptate (8% calcium)	IV 5–20 mL IM 2–5 mL	IM 2–5 mL
Calcium gluconate (9% calcium)	PO 1–2 g three or four times daily IV 5–20 mL of 10% solution	PO, IV 500 mg/kg/d in divided doses
Calcium lactate (13% calcium)	PO 1–3 g three times daily with meals	PO 500 mg/kg/d in divided doses
Calcium phosphate dibasic (30% calcium) (Dical-D)	PO 0.5–1.5 g two or three times daily with meals	Dosage not established
Calcium phosphate tribasic (39% calcium) (Posture)	1–2 tablets (600 mg calcium per tablet) two to four times daily	
Vitamin D Preparations		
Calcifediol (Calderol)	PO 50–100 µg daily	Dosage not established
Calcitriol (Rocaltrol)	PO 0.25 µg daily initially, then adjusted according to serum calcium levels (usual daily maintenance dose 0.5–1 µg)	
Cholecalciferol (Delta-D)	PO 400–1000 IU daily	Dosage not established
Dihydrotachysterol (Hytakerol)	PO 0.8–2.4 mg daily, then decreased for maintenance according to serum calcium levels (usual daily maintenance dose, 0.2–1.0 mg)	
Ergocalciferol (vitamin D) (Drisdol)	PO 50,000–200,000 units daily initially (average daily maintenance dose, 25,000–100,000 units)	
Paracalcitol (Zemplar)	IV, during dialysis, 0.04–0.1 µg/kg no more often than every other day initially; increased by 2–4 µg at 2- to 4-week intervals, if necessary. Reduce dosage or interrupt therapy if hypercalcemia occurs.	Dosage not established

IM, intramuscular; IV, intravenous; PO, oral.

Calcium Preparations

For acute, symptomatic hypocalcemia, a calcium salt (usually calcium gluconate) is given IV. For asymptomatic, less severe, or chronic hypocalcemia, an oral preparation (eg, calcium carbonate) is given. These preparations differ mainly in the amounts of calcium they contain and the routes by which they may be given.

Even when serum calcium levels are normal, calcium supplements may be needed by people who do not get enough calcium in their diets. Most diets are thought to be deficient in calcium for all age groups, but especially for young women and older adults. Calcium supplements are also used in the prevention and treatment of osteoporosis.

Corticosteroids

Glucocorticoids (see Chap. 24) are used in the treatment of hypercalcemia due to malignancies or vitamin D intoxication. These drugs lower serum calcium by inhibiting cytokine release, by direct cytolytic effects on some tumor cells, by inhibiting calcium absorption from the intestine,

TABLE 26-2 **Drugs Used in Hypercalcemia and Selected Bone Disorders**

Generic/Trade Name	Indications for Use	Routes and Dosage Ranges
Bisphosphonates		
Alendronate (Fosamax)	Prevention and treatment of osteoporosis in postmenopausal women Paget's disease	Prevention, PO 5 mg once daily Treatment, PO 10 mg once daily Paget's disease, PO 40 mg daily for 6 mo. The course of therapy may be repeated if necessary.
Etidronate (Didronel)	Paget's disease Heterotopic ossification Hypercalcemia of malignancy	Paget's disease, PO 5 mg/kg/d for up to 6 mo; may be repeated if symptoms recur. Heterotopic ossification caused by spinal cord injury, PO 20 mg/kg/d for 2 wk, then 10 mg/kg/d for 10 wk Heterotopic ossification associated with total hip replacement, PO 20 mg/kg/d for 1 mo before and 3 mo after surgery Hypercalcemia of malignancy, IV 7.5 mg/kg/d, in at least 250 mL of 0.9% sodium chloride solution and infused over at least 2 h, daily for 3 d
Pamidronate (Aredia)	Hypercalcemia of malignancy Osteolytic lesions of breast cancer metastases or multiple myeloma Paget's disease	Hypercalcemia, IV 60 mg over 4 h; 90 mg over 24 h Osteolytic bone metastases, IV 90 mg over 2 h every 3–4 wk Paget's disease, IV 30 mg over 4 h, daily for 3 doses Osteolytic bone lesions of multiple myeloma, IV 90 mg over 4 h, once monthly
Risedronate (Actonel)	Paget's disease	PO 30 mg once daily for 2 mo
Tiludronate (Skelid)	Paget's disease	PO 400 mg once daily for 3 mo
Calcitonin		
Calcitonin-human (Cibacalcin)	Paget's disease	SC 0.5 mg/d
Calcitonin-salmon (Calcimar, Miacalcin)	Hypercalcemia Paget's disease Postmenopausal osteoporosis	Hypercalcemia, SC, IM 4 IU/kg q12h; can be increased after 1 or 2 d to 8 IU/kg q12h; maximum dose, 8 IU/kg q6h Paget's disease, SC, IM 50–100 IU/d Postmenopausal osteoporosis, SC, IM 100 IU/d; nasal spray (Miacalcin) 200 IU/d
Miscellaneous Agents		
Furosemide (Lasix)	Hypercalcemia	*Adults*: IV 80–100 mg q2h until a diuretic response is obtained or other treatment measures are initiated *Children*: IV 20–40 mg q4h until a diuretic response is obtained or other treatment measures are initiated
Gallium (Ganite)	Malignancy-related, symptomatic hypercalcemia unresponsive to adequate hydration	IV 200 mg/m^2, diluted in 1000 mL of 0.9% sodium chloride or 5% dextrose, over 24h, daily for 5 d
Plicamycin (Mithracin)	Malignancy-related, symptomatic hypercalcemia unresponsive to other treatment measures	IV 25 µg/kg/d for 3 or 4 d, repeated at intervals of 1 wk or more if necessary
Phosphate salts (Neutra-Phos)	Hypercalcemia	PO 1–2 tablets three or four times daily, or contents of 1 capsule mixed with 75 mL of water four times daily
Prednisone or Hydrocortisone	Hypercalcemia	Prednisone PO 20–50 mg bid (or equivalent dose of another glucocorticoid) for 5–10 d, then tapered to the minimum dose required to prevent hypercalcemia Hydrocortisone IM, IV 100–500 mg/d
0.9% Sodium chloride injection	Acute hypercalcemia	4–6 L/d

IM, intramuscular; IV, intravenous; PO, oral; SC, subcutaneous.

and by increasing calcium excretion in the urine. Hydrocortisone or prednisone is often used; serum calcium levels decrease in approximately 5 to 10 days. After the serum calcium level stabilizes, dosage should be gradually reduced to the minimum needed to control symptoms of hypercalcemia. High dosage or prolonged administration leads to serious adverse reactions.

Estrogens and Antiestrogens

Estrogens are discussed here in relation to osteoporosis; see Chapter 28 for other uses and dosages. Estrogen replacement therapy (ERT) is the treatment of choice for preventing postmenopausal osteoporosis. It is most beneficial immediately after menopause, when a period of accelerated bone loss occurs. Mechanisms by which ERT protects against bone loss and fractures are thought to include decreased bone breakdown, increased calcium absorption from the intestine, and increased calcitriol (the active form of vitamin D) concentration.

Progestins are used with estrogens in women with an intact uterus because of the increased risk of endometrial cancer with estrogen therapy alone. The combination is called hormone replacement therapy (HRT). Although progestins alone delay bone loss, HRT seems no more beneficial than estrogens alone. Raloxifene (Evista) and tamoxifen act like estrogen in some body tissues and prevent the action of estrogen in other body tissues. Raloxifene is classified as a selective estrogen receptor modulator and is approved for prevention of postmenopausal osteoporosis. It has estrogenic effects in bone tissue, thereby decreasing bone breakdown and increasing bone mass density. It has antiestrogen effects in uterine and breast tissue. Tamoxifen, which is classified as an antiestrogen, is used to prevent and treat breast cancer. It also has estrogenic effects and can be used to prevent osteoporosis and cardiovascular disease, although it is not approved for these uses. Tamoxifen may help prevent osteoporosis in clients with breast cancer. In postmenopausal osteoporosis, these drugs are recommended for those women who are unable or unwilling to take ERT or HRT.

Vitamin D Preparations

Vitamin D is used in chronic hypocalcemia if calcium supplements alone cannot maintain serum calcium levels within normal range. It is also used to prevent deficiency states and treat hypoparathyroidism and osteoporosis. Although authorities agree that dietary intake is better than supplements, some suggest a vitamin D supplement for people who ingest less than the recommended amount (400 IU daily for those aged 6 months to 24 years; 200 IU for those 25 years of age and older). In addition, the recommended amount for older adults may be too low, especially for those who receive little exposure to sunlight, and

dosage needs for all age groups may be greater during winter, when there is less sunlight. If used, vitamin D supplements should be taken cautiously and not overused; excessive amounts can cause serious problems, including hypercalcemia.

Miscellaneous Drugs for Hypercalcemia

Furosemide (Lasix) is a loop diuretic (see Chap. 56) that increases calcium excretion in urine by preventing its reabsorption in renal tubules. Although it can be given IV for rapid effects in acute hypercalcemia, opinions seem divided regarding its use. Some recommend its use once extracellular fluid volume has been restored and saline diuresis occurs with IV infusion of several liters of 0.9% sodium chloride. Others recommend its use only if evidence of fluid overload or heart failure develops. Thiazide diuretics are contraindicated in clients with hypercalcemia because they *decrease* urinary excretion of calcium.

Gallium (Ganite), like calcitonin, alendronate, etidronate, and pamidronate, inhibits calcium resorption from bone. It is used to treat hypercalcemia of malignancy that does not respond to hydration. It is excreted mainly by the kidneys.

Phosphate salts (Neutra-Phos) inhibit intestinal absorption of calcium and increase deposition of calcium in bone. Oral salts are effective in the treatment of hypercalcemia of any etiology. A potential adverse reaction to phosphates is calcification of soft tissues due to deposition of calcium phosphate. This can lead to severe impairment of function in the kidneys and other organs. Phosphates should be given only when hypercalcemia is accompanied by hypophosphatemia (serum phosphorus <3 mg/dL) and renal function is normal, to minimize the risk of soft tissue calcification. Serum calcium, phosphorus, and creatinine should be monitored frequently and the dose should be reduced if serum phosphorus exceeds 4.5 mg/dL or the product of serum calcium and phosphorus (measured in milligrams per deciliter) exceeds 60. Neutra-Phos is an oral combination of sodium phosphate and potassium phosphate.

Plicamycin (Mithracin) lowers serum calcium levels by blocking calcium resorption from bone. It is used to treat malignancy-associated hypercalcemia that does not respond to hydration and diuretics. Calcium levels start to decline within 12 hours after a dose and reach their lowest levels in 2 to 4 days.

Sodium chloride (0.9%) injection (normal saline) is an IV solution containing water, sodium, and chloride. It is included here because it is the treatment of choice for hypercalcemia and is usually effective. The sodium contained in the solution inhibits the reabsorption of calcium in renal tubules and thereby increases urinary excretion of calcium. The solution also relieves the dehydration caused by vomiting and polyuria, and it dilutes the calcium concentration of serum and urine. Several liters are given daily. The client should be monitored closely for signs of fluid overload and serum calcium, magnesium, and potassium levels should be measured every 6 to 12 hours. Large amounts of magnesium and potassium are lost in the urine and adequate replacement is essential.

Nursing Notes: Apply Your Knowledge

Ms. Sadie Evans had a subtotal thyroidectomy 2 days ago. When you perform your morning assessment, she complains of tingling in her fingers. What additional data should be collected at this time?

NURSING PROCESS

Assessment

- Assess for risk factors and manifestations of hypocalcemia and calcium deficiency:
  - Assess dietary intake of dairy products, other calcium-containing foods, and vitamin D.
  - Check serum calcium reports for abnormal values. The normal total serum calcium level is approximately 8.5 to 10.5 mg/dL (SI units 2.2 to 2.6 mmol/L). Approximately half of the total serum calcium (eg, 4 to 5 mg/dL) should be free ionized calcium, the physiologically active form. To interpret serum calcium levels accurately, serum albumin levels and acid–base status must be considered. Low serum albumin decreases the total serum level of calcium by decreasing the amount of calcium that is bound to protein. However, the ionized concentration is normal. Metabolic and respiratory alkalosis increase binding of calcium to serum proteins, thereby maintaining normal total serum calcium but decreasing the ionized values. Conversely, metabolic and respiratory acidosis decrease binding and therefore increase the concentration of ionized calcium.
  - Check for *Chvostek's sign*: Tap the facial nerve just below the temple, in front of the ear. If facial muscles twitch, hyperirritability of the nerve and potential tetany are indicated.
  - Check for *Trousseau's sign*: Constrict blood circulation in an arm (usually with a blood pressure cuff) for 3 to 5 minutes. This produces ischemia and increased irritability of peripheral nerves, which causes spasms of the lower arm and hand muscles (carpopedal spasm) if tetany is present.

- Assess for conditions in which hypercalcemia is likely to occur (eg, cancer, prolonged immobilization, vitamin D overdose).
- Observe for signs and symptoms of hypercalcemia in clients at risk. Electrocardiogram changes indicative of hypercalcemia include a shortened Q-T interval and an inverted T wave.
- Assess for risk factors and manifestations of osteoporosis, especially in postmenopausal women and men and women on chronic corticosteroid therapy:
  - If risk factors are identified, ask if preventive measures are being used (eg, increasing calcium intake, exercise, medications)
  - If the client is known to have osteoporosis, ask about duration and severity of symptoms, age of onset, location, whether fractures have occurred, what treatments have been done, and response to treatments.
- If Paget's disease is suspected, assess for an elevated serum alkaline phosphatase and abnormal bone scan reports.

Nursing Diagnoses

- Altered Nutrition: Less Than Body Requirements with hypocalcemia
- Knowledge Deficit: Recommended daily amounts and dietary sources of calcium and vitamin D
- Knowledge Deficit: Rational use of vitamin and mineral supplements
- Knowledge Deficit: Disease process and drug therapy for hypocalcemia
- Knowledge Deficit: Disease process and drug therapy for hypercalcemia
- Knowledge Deficit: Disease process and drug therapy for osteoporosis
- Risk for Injury: Tetany, sedation, seizures from hypocalcemia
- Risk for Injury: Hypercalcemia related to overuse of supplements
- Risk for Injury: Hypocalcemia from aggressive treatment of hypercalcemia
- Constipation with oral calcium supplements
- Altered Thought Processes: Confusion with hypercalcemia
- Fluid Volume Excess related to large amounts of 0.9% sodium chloride solution used to treat acute hypercalcemia
- Anxiety related to disease process and treatment

Planning/Goals

The client will:

- Achieve and maintain normal serum levels of calcium

- Increase dietary intake of calcium-containing foods to prevent or treat osteoporosis
- Use calcium or vitamin D supplements in recommended amounts
- Comply with instructions for safe drug use
- Be monitored closely for therapeutic and adverse effects of drugs used to treat hypercalcemia
- Comply with procedures for follow-up treatment of hypocalcemia, hypercalcemia, or osteoporosis
- Avoid preventable adverse effects of treatment for acute hypocalcemia or hypercalcemia

Interventions

Assist all clients in meeting the recommended daily requirements of calcium and vitamin D. With an adequate protein and calcium intake, enough phosphorus also is obtained.

- The best dietary source is milk and other dairy products, including yogurt.
- Unless contraindicated by the client's condition, recommend that adults drink at least two 8-oz glasses of milk daily. This furnishes approximately half the daily calcium requirement; the remainder will probably be obtained from other foods.
- Children need approximately four glasses of milk or an equivalent amount of calcium in milk and other foods to support normal growth and development.
- Pregnant and lactating women also need approximately four glasses of milk or their equivalents to meet increased needs. Vitamin and mineral supplements are often prescribed during these periods. However, some supplements contain only 250 mg of a calcium salt (equivalent to 8 oz of

CLIENT TEACHING GUIDELINES
Drugs for Osteoporosis

General Considerations

✔ Osteoporosis involves weak bones that fracture easily and may cause pain and disability.

✔ Important factors in prevention and treatment include an adequate intake of calcium and vitamin D (from the diet, from supplements, or a combination of both sources), regular weight-bearing exercise, estrogen replacement therapy for postmenopausal women, and drugs that can slow bone loss.

✔ It is better to obtain calcium and vitamin D from foods such as milk and other dairy products. Approximately 1000 to 1500 mg of calcium and 400 IU of vitamin D are recommended daily.

✔ If unable to get sufficient dietary calcium and vitamin D, consider supplements of these nutrients. Consult a health care provider about the types and amounts. For example, a daily multivitamin and mineral supplement may contain adequate amounts when added to dietary intake. If taking other supplements, avoid those containing bone meal because they may contain lead and other contaminants that are toxic to the human body. Do not take more than the recommended amounts of supplements; overuse can cause serious, life-threatening problems.

✔ For women who refuse or hesitate to take estrogens, health care providers must emphasize that the benefits in bone and cardiovascular protection outweigh potential adverse effects.

✔ Besides estrogen replacement therapy, the main drug approved for prevention and treatment of osteoporosis is alendronate (Fosamax). This drug helps to prevent

the loss of calcium from bone, thereby strengthening bone and reducing the risks of fractures.

✔ For people at high risk for development of osteoporosis (eg, postmenopausal women who do not take estrogen, men and women who take an oral or inhaled corticosteroid such as prednisone or fluticasone [Flonase], or those being treated for osteoporosis, a baseline measurement of bone mineral density and periodic follow-up measurements are needed. This is a noninvasive test that does not involve any injections or device insertions.

Self-administration

✔ If taking a calcium supplement, calcium carbonate 500 mg twice daily is often recommended. This can be obtained from an inexpensive over-the-counter antacid called Tums, which contains 200 mg of calcium per tablet.

✔ Do not take a calcium supplement with an iron preparation, tetracycline, ciprofloxacin, or phenytoin. Instead, take the drugs at least 2 hours apart to avoid calcium interference with absorption of the other drugs.

✔ If taking both a calcium supplement and alendronate, take the calcium at least 2 hours after the alendronate. Calcium, antacids, and other drugs interfere with absorption of alendronate.

✔ Take alendronate with 6 to 8 oz of water at least 30 minutes before any food, other fluid, or other medication. Beverages other than water and foods decrease absorption and effectiveness.

✔ Take alendronate in an upright position and do not lie down for at least 30 minutes. This helps prevent esophageal irritation and stomach upset.

milk). This amount does not go very far in meeting a requirement of approximately 1200 mg.

- Postmenopausal women who take estrogens need at least the usual adult amount (1000 mg). Those who do not take estrogens need at least 1500 mg to prevent or minimize osteoporosis.
- For clients who avoid or minimize their intake of dairy products because of the calories, identify low-calorie sources, such as skim milk and low-fat yogurt.
- Milk that has been fortified with vitamin D is the best food source. Exposure of skin to sunlight is also needed to supply adequate amounts of vitamin D.
- For people who are unable or unwilling to ingest sufficient calcium, a supplement may be needed to prevent osteoporosis.

Assist clients with hypercalcemia to decrease formation of renal calculi by forcing fluids to approximately 3000 to 4000 mL/day and preventing urinary tract infections.

Evaluation

- Check laboratory reports of serum calcium levels for normal values.
- Interview and observe for relief of symptoms of hypocalcemia, hypercalcemia, or osteoporosis.
- Interview and observe intake of calcium-containing foods.
- Question about normal calcium requirements and how to meet them.
- Interview and observe for accurate drug usage and compliance with follow-up procedures.
- Interview and observe for therapeutic and adverse drug effects.

PRINCIPLES OF THERAPY

Management of Hypocalcemia

Treatment of hypocalcemia includes giving a calcium preparation and perhaps vitamin D.

1. Acute, severe hypocalcemia is a medical emergency and requires IV administration of calcium. One regimen suggests calcium gluconate 10% solution (10 mL = 1 g), 20 mL over 10 minutes, followed by an infusion of 6 g in 500 mL of D_5W over 4 to 6 hours. Infusion rate is titrated to avoid symptoms of hypocalcemia and maintain normal serum calcium levels (as measured every 4 to 6 hours). Once stabilized, treatment is aimed toward the underlying cause or preventing recurrence, and the IV infusion can be tapered. Serum magnesium levels should also be measured, and, if hypomagnesemia is pres-

ent, it must be treated before treatment of hypocalcemia can be effective.

2. For less acute situations or for long-term treatment of chronic hypocalcemia, oral calcium supplements are preferred. Vitamin D is given also if a calcium preparation alone cannot maintain serum calcium levels within a normal range.

3. Calcium deficits caused by inadequate dietary intake affect bone tissue rather than serum calcium levels. Calcium supplements can decrease bone loss and fractures, especially in women, including those who take replacement estrogens. Calcium carbonate contains the most elemental calcium by weight (40%) and is inexpensive. It is available in the nonprescription antacid called Tums.

4. If hypocalcemia is caused by diarrhea or malabsorption, treatment of the underlying condition decreases loss of calcium from the body and increases absorption.

5. When vitamin D is given to treat hypocalcemia, dosage is determined by frequent measurement of serum calcium levels. Usually, higher doses are given initially, then decreased for maintenance therapy.

6. Calcium salts and vitamin D are combined in a number of commercial preparations promoted as dietary supplements for children and for women during pregnancy and lactation. There is no evidence that these fixed amounts of calcium and vitamin D meet the dietary needs of most people. Therefore, calcium and vitamin D should be prescribed individually. Also, these mixtures are not indicated for maintenance therapy in chronic hypocalcemia.

7. Calcium preparations and digoxin have similar effects on the myocardium. Therefore, if calcium is given to a digitalized client, the risks of digitalis toxicity and cardiac arrhythmias are increased. This combination must be used very cautiously.

8. Oral calcium preparations decrease effects of oral tetracycline drugs by combining with the antibiotic and preventing its absorption. They should not be given at the same time or within 2 to 3 hours of each other.

Management of Hypercalcemia

Clients at risk for hypercalcemia should be monitored for early signs and symptoms so treatment can be started before severe hypercalcemia develops. Treatment depends largely on the cause and severity.

1. When hypercalcemia is caused by a tumor of parathyroid tissue, the usual treatment is surgical excision. When it is caused by malignant tumor, treatment of the tumor with surgery, irradiation, or chemotherapy may reduce production of PTH. When it is caused by excessive intake of vitamin D,

the vitamin D preparation should be stopped immediately.

2. Acute hypercalcemia is a medical emergency. It is treated with interventions that increase calcium excretion in the urine and decrease resorption of calcium from bone into the serum. For severe symptoms or a serum calcium level above 12 mg/dL, the priority is rehydration. This need can be met by IV saline infusion (0.9% or 0.45% NaCl) 4000 mL/day or more if kidney function is adequate. After rehydration, furosemide may be given IV to increase renal excretion of calcium and prevent fluid overload. Because sodium, potassium, and water are also lost in the urine, these must be replaced in the IV fluids.

   With mild hypercalcemia, most clients respond to the aforementioned treatment, and further drug therapy is not needed. With moderate to severe hypercalcemia, pamidronate may be the drug of choice. When pamidronate is given in a single IV infusion containing 60 or 90 mg, serum calcium levels decrease within 2 days, reach their lowest levels in approximately 7 days, and remain lower for 2 weeks or longer. Treatment can be repeated if hypercalcemia recurs. Phosphates should not be used unless hypophosphatemia is present. They are also contraindicated in clients with persistent urinary tract infections and an alkaline urine because calcium phosphate kidney stones are likely to form in such cases.

3. Chronic hypercalcemia requires treatment of the underlying disease process and measures to control serum calcium levels (eg, a high fluid intake and mobilization to help retain calcium in bone). Oral phosphate administration may help if other measures are ineffective.

4. Serum calcium levels should be measured periodically to monitor effects of therapy.

5. For clients with severely impaired renal function in whom hypercalcemia develops, hemodialysis or peritoneal dialysis with a calcium-free solution is effective and safe.

6. For clients receiving a calcium channel blocker (see Chap. 53), the drug may be less effective in the presence of hypercalcemia.

Prevention of Osteoporosis

Preventive measures should be implemented for all age groups because bone loss can be slowed, but new, strong bone cannot be created with current knowledge and resources.

1. In all age groups, preventive efforts include a consistently adequate dietary intake of calcium to promote normal bone development and maintenance. In children, adolescents, and young adults, an adequate calcium intake promotes bone growth and peak bone mass. A well-stocked "reservoir" means that, in later years when bone loss exceeds formation, more bone can be lost before osteoporosis develops. In postmenopausal women and men older than 40 years of age, an adequate calcium intake may slow the development of osteoporosis and fractures. Although dietary intake is much preferred, a supplement may be needed to ensure a daily intake of 1000 to 1500 mg, especially in adolescent girls, frail elderly, and those receiving corticosteroids.

2. Regular exercise is also important in all age groups. Vigorous, weight-bearing exercise helps to promote and maintain strong bone; inactivity promotes bone weakening and loss.

3. Women who smoke should be encouraged to stop. Smoking decreases the amount of active estrogen in the body and thus accelerates bone loss.

4. Estrogen replacement therapy (plus progesterone in those with an intact uterus) is probably the best preventive measure for postmenopausal women. Which estrogen preparation should be given and for how long has not been established. Conjugated estrogens (eg, Premarin) have been used in most studies; 0.625 mg daily is considered adequate for "bone protection." If ERT is stopped, the rate of bone loss accelerates. Thus, lifetime therapy may be needed. ERT is contraindicated in women with active estrogen-dependent cancers.

5. Alendronate (Fosamax), in a dose of 5 mg daily, is approved by the Food and Drug Administration (FDA) for prevention of osteoporosis.

6. Raloxifene (Evista) is approved for prevention of postmenopausal osteoporosis in women who are unable or unwilling to take ERT.

7. An adequate intake of vitamin D helps to prevent osteoporosis, but supplementation is probably not indicated unless a deficiency can be demonstrated. Serum calcitriol can be measured in clients at risk for vitamin D deficiency, including elderly adults and those on chronic corticosteroid therapy.

8. Preventive measures are needed for clients on chronic corticosteroid therapy (eg, prednisone 7.5 mg daily, equivalent amounts of other systemic drugs, or high doses of inhaled drugs). For both men and women, most of the preceding guidelines apply (eg, calcium supplements, regular exercise). In addition, low doses and nonsystemic routes help prevent osteoporosis and other adverse effects. For men, corticosteroids decrease testosterone levels by approximately one half, and replacement therapy may be needed.

Management of Osteoporosis

Once bone loss is evident (from diagnostic tests of bone density or occurrence of fractures), several interventions may help slow further skeletal bone loss or prevent fractures. Drugs used to treat osteoporosis decrease the rate of bone breakdown and thus slow the rate of bone loss.

1. As with prevention, those diagnosed with osteoporosis need adequate calcium and vitamin D (at least the recommended dietary allowance), whether obtained from the diet or from supplements. Pharmacologic doses of vitamin D are sometimes used to treat clients with serious osteoporosis. If such doses are used, caution should be exercised because excessive amounts of vitamin D can cause hypercalcemia and hypercalciuria.

2. Regular exercise is needed. Numerous studies indicate that regular physical activity helps to reduce bone loss and fractures.

3. Women who smoke should be encouraged to stop because smoking has effects similar to those of menopause (estrogen deficiency and accelerated bone loss).

4. In menopausal women, ERT is the most beneficial treatment and should usually be used along with any other measures (see Prevention of Osteoporosis, earlier). For women with an intact uterus, combined estrogen and progesterone therapy (HRT) is needed.

5. Alendronate (Fosamax), in a dose of 10 mg daily, is FDA approved for treatment of osteoporosis in postmenopausal women. The drug can increase bone mineral density, reduce risks of vertebral fractures, and slow progression of vertebral deformities and loss of height.

6. Treatment of men is similar to that of women except that testosterone replacement may be needed rather than estrogen.

7. With corticosteroid-induced osteoporosis, multiple treatment measures may be needed, including increased dietary and supplemental calcium and possibly vitamin D, hormone replacement, corticosteroid dosage reduction, exercise, and calcitonin or other drugs to slow skeletal bone loss.

Use in Children

Hypocalcemia is uncommon in children. However, inadequate calcium in the diet is thought to be common, especially in girls. Inadequate calcium and exercise in children are risk factors for eventual osteoporosis. If hypocalcemia or dietary calcium deficiency develops, principles of using calcium or vitamin D supplements are the same as those in adults. Children should be monitored closely for signs and symptoms of adverse effects, including hypercalcemia. Hypercalcemia is probably most likely to occur in children with a malignant tumor. Guidelines for treating hypercalcemia in children are essentially the same as those for adults, with drug dosages adjusted. Safety, effectiveness, and dosages of etidronate, gallium, and pamidronate have not been established.

Use in Older Adults

Hypocalcemia is uncommon because calcium moves from bone to blood to maintain normal serum levels. However, calcium deficiency commonly occurs because of long-term dietary deficiencies of calcium and vitamin D, impaired absorption of calcium from the intestine, lack of exposure to sunlight, and impaired liver or kidney metabolism of vitamin D to its active form. These and other factors lead to demineralization and weakening of bone (osteoporosis) and an increased risk of fractures. Postmenopausal women are at high risk for development of osteoporosis. Although osteoporosis also develops in older men, it occurs less often, at a later age, and to a lesser extent than in older women. Thus, older adults need to continue their dietary intake of dairy products and other calcium-containing foods. Estrogen replacement drugs and calcium supplements are recommended for postmenopausal women to prevent or treat osteoporosis.

With hypercalcemia, treatment usually requires large amounts of IV 0.9% sodium chloride (eg, 150 to 200 mL/hour). Older adults often have chronic cardiovascular disorders that may be aggravated by this treatment. They should be monitored closely for signs of fluid overload, congestive heart failure, pulmonary edema, and hypertension.

Use in Renal Impairment

If vitamin D therapy is needed to treat osteomalacia in clients with renal impairment, calcitriol (Rocaltrol) or dihydrotachysterol is preferred. Calcitriol is the active form of vitamin D and thus requires no metabolism; dihydrotachysterol is a synthetic compound that is metabolized in the liver but not in the kidneys.

None of the bisphosphonate drugs is recommended for use in severe renal impairment (eg, serum creatinine >5 mg/dL or creatinine clearance <30 mL/minute). With alendronate, dosage does not need to be reduced in mild to moderate impairment (eg, creatinine clearance 35 to 60 mL/minute). Etidronate should be used cautiously with mild renal impairment and is contraindicated with severe renal impairment. Pamidronate was nephrotoxic in animal studies. If it is used to treat hypercalcemia in clients with renal impairment, renal function should be closely monitored. Gallium nitrate is contraindicated in clients with severe renal impairment.

Use in Hepatic Impairment

If vitamin D therapy is needed for a client with impaired liver function, calcifediol (Calderol) is preferred because it does not require liver metabolism.

NURSING ACTIONS	Drugs Used in Calcium and Bone Disorders

NURSING ACTIONS	RATIONALE/EXPLANATION
1. Administer accurately	
a. With calcium preparations:	
(1) Give oral preparations 30 min before meals or at bedtime.	To increase absorption
(2) Give intravenous (IV) preparations slowly, over at least 2 min, check pulse and blood pressure closely, and monitor the electrocardiogram (ECG) if possible.	Arrhythmias and hypotension may occur. Hypercalcemia is indicated on the ECG by a prolonged Q-T interval associated with an inverted T wave.
(3) Do not mix IV preparations with any other drug in the same syringe.	Calcium reacts with some other drugs and forms a precipitate.
b. With bisphosphonates:	
(1) Give alendronate with 6–8 oz of plain water, at least 30 min before the first food, beverage, or medication of the day.	To promote absorption and decrease esophageal irritation
(2) Give oral etidronate on an empty stomach, as a single dose or in divided doses. Avoid giving within 2 h of ingesting dairy products, antacids, or vitamin or mineral preparations.	If gastrointestinal (GI) symptoms occur with the single dose, divided doses may relieve them. Substances containing calcium or other metals decrease absorption of etidronate.
(3) Give IV etidronate, gallium, and pamidronate according to the manufacturers' instructions.	The drugs require reconstitution, diluting with IV fluids, and specific time intervals of administration.
c. Give calcitonin at bedtime.	To decrease nausea and discomfort from flushing
d. With phosphate salts, mix powder forms with water for oral administration. See package inserts for specific instructions.	
2. Observe for therapeutic effects	
a. With calcium preparations, observe for:	
(1) Relief of symptoms of neuromuscular irritability and tetany, such as decreased muscle spasms and decreased paresthesias	
(2) Serum calcium levels within the normal range (8.5–10.5 mg/dL)	
(3) Absence of Chvostek's and Trousseau's signs	
b. With calcitonin, corticosteroids, or pamidronate for hypercalcemia, observe for:	
(1) Decreased serum calcium level	Calcitonin lowers serum calcium levels in approximately 2 h after injection and effects last 6–8 h. Corticosteroids require 10–14 d to lower serum calcium. Pamidronate lowers serum calcium within 2 d.
(2) Decreased signs and symptoms of hypercalcemia	

(continued)

NURSING ACTIONS	RATIONALE/EXPLANATION
c. With alendronate for osteoporosis, observe for improved bone mass density and absence of fractures.	Early osteopenia and osteoporosis are asymptomatic. Measurement of bone mass density is the only way to quantify bone loss.
3. Observe for adverse effects	
a. With calcium preparations, observe for hypercalcemia:	
(1) GI effects—anorexia, nausea, vomiting, abdominal pain, constipation	
(2) Central nervous system effects—apathy, poor memory, depression, drowsiness, disorientation	
(3) Other effects—weakness and decreased tone in skeletal and smooth muscles, dysphagia, polyuria, polydipsia, cardiac dysrhythmias	
(4) Serum calcium >10.5 mg/dL	
b. With vitamin D preparations, observe for hypervitaminosis D and hypercalcemia (see above).	This is most likely to occur with chronic ingestion of 50,000 or more units of vitamin D daily. In children, accidental ingestion may lead to acute toxicity.
c. With drug therapy of hypercalcemia, observe for hypocalcemia.	Hypocalcemia may occur with vigorous treatment of hypercalcemia, especially with etidronate, gallium, and pamidronate. This can be minimized by monitoring serum calcium levels frequently and adjusting drug dosages and other treatments.
d. With calcitonin, observe for nausea, vomiting, tissue irritation at administration sites, and allergic reactions.	Adverse reactions are usually mild and transient. Nasal administration produces greater client compliance than injections, with few adverse effects.
e. With pamidronate, observe for:	Adverse effects were reported more often with osteolytic bone lesions of multiple myeloma and may have been related to the multiple myeloma or its treatment.
(1) GI effects—anorexia, nausea, vomiting, constipation	
(2) Cardiovascular effects—fluid overload, hypertension	
(3) Electrolyte imbalances—hypokalemia, hypomagnesemia, hypophosphatemia	
(4) Musculoskeletal effects—muscle and joint pain	
(5) Miscellaneous effects—fever, tissue irritation at IV insertion site, pain, anemia	
f. With etidronate, observe for anorexia, nausea, diarrhea, bone pain, fever, fluid overload, and increased serum creatinine.	Adverse effects are more frequent and more severe at higher doses. The drug is nephrotoxic and should not be used in clients with renal failure.
g. With gallium, observe for renal impairment, as indicated by increasing blood urea nitrogen and serum creatinine levels.	Nephrotoxicity reportedly develops in approximately 12% of recipients.
h. With plicamycin, observe for bone marrow depression, nausea, vomiting, and impaired liver function.	These reactions are much less likely to occur with the small doses used for hypercalcemia than with the large doses used for malignant neoplasms.

(continued)

NURSING ACTIONS	RATIONALE/EXPLANATION
i. With phosphates, observe for nausea, vomiting, and diarrhea.	
j. With alendronate, observe for: (1) GI effects—abdominal distention, acid regurgitation, dysphagia, esophagitis, flatulence (2) Other effects—headache, musculoskeletal pain, decreased serum calcium and phosphate	Adverse effects are usually minor with the doses taken for prevention or treatment of osteoporosis, if the drug is taken as directed. More severe effects may occur with the higher doses taken for Paget's disease.
4. Observe for drug interactions	
a. Drug that *increases* effects of calcium: (1) Vitamin D	Increases intestinal absorption of calcium from both dietary and supplemental drug sources
b. Drug that *decrease* effects of calcium: (1) Adrenocorticosteroids (prednisone, others), calcitonin, plicamycin, and phosphates	These drugs lower serum calcium levels by various mechanisms. They are used in the treatment of hypercalcemia.
(2) Antacids	Oral calcium preparations are more soluble and better absorbed in an acid medium. Antacids decrease acidity of gastric secretions and therefore may decrease absorption of calcium.
(3) Laxatives	These drugs decrease absorption of calcium from the intestinal tract by increasing motility. This allows less time for calcium absorption.
c. Drugs that *increase* effects of vitamin D: Thiazide diuretics	Thiazide diuretics administered to hypoparathyroid clients may cause hypercalcemia (potentiate vitamin D effects).
d. Drugs that *decrease* effects of vitamin D: (1) Anticonvulsants (eg, phenytoin [Dilantin], primidone [Mysoline], phenobarbital)	These drugs accelerate and change the metabolism of vitamin D in the liver. As a result, vitamin D deficiency, hypocalcemia, and rickets or osteomalacia are likely to develop in clients receiving anticonvulsant drugs for seizure disorders. These problems can be prevented by increasing intake of vitamin D.
(2) Cholestyramine resin (Questran)	May decrease intestinal absorption of calcitriol (Rocaltrol)
(3) Mineral oil	Mineral oil is a fat and therefore combines with fat-soluble vitamins, such as vitamin D, and prevents their absorption from the gastrointestinal tract.
e. Drugs that alter effects of calcitonin: (1) Testosterone and other androgens *increase* effects (2) Parathyroid hormone *decreases* effects	Androgens and calcitonin have additive effects on calcium retention and inhibition of bone resorption (movement of calcium from bone to serum). Parathyroid hormone antagonizes or opposes calcitonin. Parathyroid hormone *increases* serum calcium concentration, whereas calcitonin *decreases* it.
f. Drugs that *increase* nephrotoxic effects of gallium:	These drugs are nephrotoxic alone and cause additive nephrotoxicity when combined.

(*continued*)

NURSING ACTIONS	RATIONALE/EXPLANATION
(1) Aminoglycoside antibiotics (eg, gentamicin) (2) Amphotericin B (3) Other nephrotoxic drugs	
g. Drugs that *increase* effects of plicamycin: Antineoplastic drugs that cause bone marrow depression (see Chap. 64)	Additive bone marrow depression may occur.
h. Drugs that *decrease* effects of phosphate salts: Antacids containing aluminum and magnesium	Aluminum and magnesium may combine with phosphate and thereby prevent its absorption and therapeutic effect.
i. Drugs that *decrease* effects of alendronate and other oral bisphosphonates: Antacids and calcium supplements	These drugs interfere with absorption of the bisphosphonates and should be taken at least 2 h after the bisphosphonate.

Nursing Notes: Apply Your Knowledge

Answer: Tingling may be a symptom of hypocalcemia. Hypocalcemia can occur in Ms. Evans because, during her thyroid surgery, the parathyroid glands that maintain calcium balance could have been damaged or inadvertently removed. Assess Chvostek's sign by tapping on Ms. Evans' face just above the temple, observing for twitching, which indicates hypocalcemia. Trousseau's sign can be assessed by constricting circulation in the arm by inflating a blood pressure cuff and observing for spasms of the lower arm and hand. Serum calcium levels should be obtained and compared with previous readings. Normal values are 8.5 to 10.5 mg/d and must be adjusted when albumin levels are low. Report hypocalcemia or signs of tetany to the physician so that calcium replacement can be promptly administered.

► REVIEW AND APPLICATION EXERCISES

1. What are the major physiologic functions of calcium?
2. What is the normal serum level of calcium?
3. What are some nursing interventions to prevent hypocalcemia?
4. What signs and symptoms may indicate hypocalcemia?
5. How is hypocalcemia treated?
6. What signs and symptoms may indicate hypercalcemia?
7. How is hypercalcemia treated?
8. Why is it important to have an adequate intake of calcium and vitamin D throughout life?
9. What are the main elements of prevention and treatment of osteoporosis?

SELECTED REFERENCES

Dagogo-Jack, S. (1998). Mineral and metabolic bone disease. In C.F. Carey, H.H. Lee, & K.F. Woeltje (Eds.), *The Washington manual of medical therapeutics*, 29th ed., pp. 441–455. Philadelphia: Lippincott Williams & Wilkins.

Dowd, R. & Cavalieri, R.J. (1999). Help your patient live with osteoporosis. *American Journal of Nursing 99*(4), 55–60.

Drug facts and comparisons. (Updated monthly). St. Louis: Facts and Comparisons.

Khovidhunkit, W. & Shoback, D.M. (1999). Clinical effects of raloxifene hydrochloride in women. *Annals of Internal Medicine 130*, 431–439.

Lyles, K.W. (1997). Osteoporosis: Pathophysiology, clinical presentation and management. In W.N. Kelley (Ed.), *Textbook of internal medicine*, 3rd ed., pp. 2536–2541. Philadelphia: Lippincott-Raven.

Marcus, R. (1996). Agents affecting calcification and bone turnover. In J.G. Hardman, L.E. Limbird, P.B. Molinoff, and R.W. Ruddon (Eds.), *Goodman & Gilman's The pharmacological basis of therapeutics*, 9th ed., pp. 1519–1546. New York: McGraw-Hill.

O'Connell, M.B. & Bauwens, S.F. (1997). Osteoporosis and osteomalacia. In J.T. DiPiro, R.L. Talbert, P.E. Hayes, G.C. Yee, G.R. Matzke, B.G. Wells, & L.M. Posey (Eds.), *Pharmacotherapy: A pathophysiologic approach*, 3rd ed., pp. 1689–1716. Stamford, CT: Appleton & Lange.

Porth, C.M. (Ed.). (1998). *Pathophysiology: Concepts of altered health states*, 5th ed. Philadelphia: Lippincott Williams & Wilkins.

Schultz, N.J. & Chitwood-Dagner, K.K. (1997). Body electrolyte homeostasis. In J.T. DiPiro, R.L. Talbert, P.E. Hayes, G.C. Yee, G.R. Matzke, B.G. Wells, & L.M. Posey (Eds.), *Pharmacotherapy: A pathophysiologic approach*, 3rd ed., pp. 1105–1137. Stamford, CT: Appleton & Lange.

27

Antidiabetic Drugs

Objectives

After studying this chapter, the student will be able to:

1. Describe major effects of endogenous insulin on body tissues.

2. Discuss regular, NPH and Lente insulins in terms of mechanism of action, indications for use, route of administration, and duration of action.

3. Differentiate characteristics of regular insulin and insulin lispro.

4. Discuss the relationships among diet, exercise, and drug therapy in controlling diabetes.

5. Differentiate types of oral antidiabetic agents in terms of mechanisms of action, indications for use, adverse effects, and nursing process implications.

6. Explain the benefits of maintaining glycemic control in preventing complications of diabetes.

7. State reasons for combinations of insulin and oral agents or two types of oral agents.

8. Assist clients or caregivers in learning how to manage diabetes care, including administration of antidiabetic medications.

9. Collaborate with nurse diabetes educators, dietitians, and others in teaching self-care activities to clients with diabetes.

You are assigned to care for Ellen Rodriguez, a 13-year-old, who was admitted to the intensive care unit 12 hours ago in acute ketoacidosis. Her blood glucose level has stabilized after emergency treatment. She lives with her mother (a single parent) and five younger siblings in public housing within the Latino community. The diagnosis of diabetes mellitus is completely unexpected. Her mother asks why Ellen has to take shots, because her aunt did just fine on pills.

Ellen will be discharged in 2 to 3 days on insulin, glucose monitoring before meals and at bedtime, and a diabetic diet. Use the following questions to think about and plan Ellen's care.

▶ Visualize yourself as Ellen and try to verbalize how you might feel. Now visualize yourself as Ellen's mother and again try to explain how you are feeling. Compare and contrast these two pictures.

▶ Reflect on developmental and socioeconomic factors that need to be considered when planning Ellen's care.

▶ Role play how you might answer Ellen's mother's question concerning why her daughter needs to inject insulin rather than take pills to manage her diabetes.

▶ Before discharge, you have three teaching sessions of approximately 30 minutes each. Prioritize essential teaching and describe your teaching plan for Ellen.

▶ Discuss appropriate postdischarge follow-up to continue diabetic teaching and monitor compliance with prescribed management strategies.

There are two types of antidiabetic drugs: insulin and oral agents. Because these drugs are used to lower blood glucose, they are also called hypoglycemic or antihyperglycemic agents. Diabetes mellitus is a common, complex disorder. To understand clinical use of antidiabetic drugs, it is necessary to understand the characteristics of endogenous insulin, diabetes mellitus, and the drugs.

ENDOGENOUS INSULIN

Insulin is a protein hormone secreted by beta cells in the pancreas. The average adult pancreas secretes a basal amount of 1 to 2 units/hour and additional amounts (approximately 4 to 6 units/hour) after meals or when the blood sugar level exceeds 100 mg/dL, with an average daily secretion of about 40 to 60 units. In a fasting state, serum insulin levels are low and stored glucose and amino acids are used for energy needs of tissues that require glucose. After a meal, serum insulin levels increase in a few minutes, peak in approximately 30 minutes, and decrease to baseline levels in approximately 3 hours.

Insulin is secreted into the portal circulation and transported to the liver, where approximately half is used or degraded. The other half reaches the systemic circulation, where it circulates mainly in an unbound form and is transported to most body cells.

At the cellular level (Fig. 27-1), insulin binds with and activates receptors on the cell membranes of approximately 80% of body cells. Liver, muscle, and adipose cells have many insulin receptors and are primary tissues for insulin action. After insulin–receptor binding occurs, cell membranes become highly permeable to glucose and allow rapid entry of glucose into the cells. The cell membranes also become more permeable to amino acids, fatty acids, and electrolytes such as potassium, magnesium, and phosphate ions. Cellular metabolism is altered by the movement of these substances into the cells, activation of some enzymes and inactivation of others, movement of proteins between cellular compartments, changes in the amounts of proteins produced, and perhaps other mechanisms. Overall, the changes in cellular metabolism stimulate anabolic effects (eg, utilization and storage of glucose, amino acids, and fatty acids) and inhibit catabolic processes (eg, breakdown of glycogen, fat, and protein). After binding to insulin and entering the cell, receptors may be degraded or recycled back to the cell surface.

Insulin is cleared from circulating blood in approximately 10 to 15 minutes because of rapid binding to peripheral tissues or metabolic breakdown. The insulin that does not combine with receptors is metabolized in the liver, kidneys, plasma, and muscles. In the kidneys, insulin is filtered by the glomeruli and reabsorbed by the tubules, which also degrade it. Severe renal impairment slows the clearance of insulin from the blood.

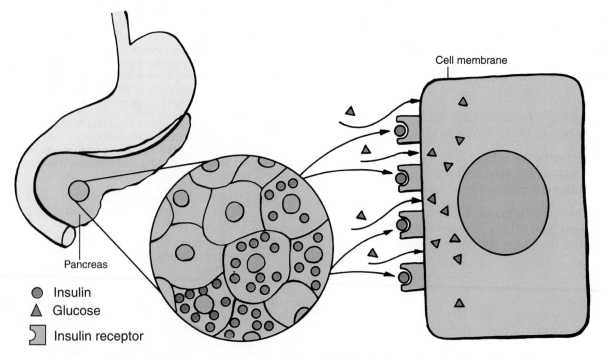

FIGURE 27–1   Normal glucose metabolism. Once insulin binds with receptors on the cell membrane, glucose can move into the cell, promoting cellular metabolism and energy production.

Physiologically, insulin plays a major role in metabolism of carbohydrate, fat, and protein (Box 27-1). These foodstuffs are broken down into molecules of glucose, lipids, and amino acids, respectively. The molecules enter the cells and are converted to energy for cellular activities. The energy can be used immediately or converted to storage forms for later use. When carrying out its metabolic functions, the overall effect of insulin is to lower blood glucose levels, primarily by the following mechanisms:

1. In the liver, insulin acts to *decrease* breakdown of glycogen (glycogenolysis), formation of new glucose from fatty acids and amino acids (gluconeogenesis), and formation of ketone bodies (ketogenesis). At the same time, it acts to *increase* synthesis and storage of glycogen and fatty acids.
2. In adipose tissue, insulin acts to *decrease* breakdown of fat (lipolysis) and to *increase* production of glycerol and fatty acids.
3. In muscle tissue, insulin acts to *decrease* protein breakdown and amino acid output and to *increase* amino acid uptake, protein synthesis, and glycogen synthesis.

Regulation of Insulin Secretion

Insulin, the only hormone that decreases blood sugar, plays a major role in regulating the amount of glucose available for cellular metabolism and energy needs, during both fasting and feeding. The complex process of insulin secretion involves coordination of numerous factors, including various nutrients, gastrointestinal (GI) and pancreatic hormones, and the autonomic nervous system.

Factors that stimulate insulin secretion include glucose (the major stimulus), amino acids, fatty acids, ketone bodies, and stimulation of beta$_2$-adrenergic receptors or vagal nerves. Oral glucose is more effective than intravenous (IV) glucose in stimulating insulin secretion because glucose or food in the digestive tract induces the release of GI hormones (eg, gastrin, secretin, cholecystokinin, gastric inhibitory peptide) and stimulates vagal activity. Other hormones that raise blood glucose levels and stimulate insulin secretion include glucagon, cortisol, growth hormone, estrogen, and progesterone. Excessive, prolonged endogenous secretion or administration of pharmacologic preparations of these hormones can exhaust the abil-

---

BOX 27–1   EFFECTS OF INSULIN ON METABOLISM

Carbohydrate Metabolism
- Insulin increases glucose transport into the liver, skeletal muscle, adipose tissue, the heart, and some smooth muscle organs, such as the uterus; it must be present for muscle and fat tissues to use glucose for energy. It does not increase glucose transport into brain cells, red blood cells, intestinal mucosal cells, or tubular epithelial cells of the kidney.
- Insulin regulates glucose metabolism and homeostasis. The main goal of glucose metabolism is to produce energy for cellular functions. If excess glucose is present after this need is met, it is converted to glycogen and stored for future energy needs or converted to fat and stored. The excess glucose transported to liver cells is converted to fat only after glycogen stores are saturated. When insulin is absent or blood glucose levels are low, these stored forms of glucose can be reconverted. The liver is especially important in restoring blood sugar levels by breaking down glycogen or by forming new glucose.

Fat Metabolism
- Insulin promotes transport of glucose into fat cells. Once inside the cell, glucose is broken down. One of the breakdown products is alpha-glycerophosphate, which combines with fatty acids to form triglycerides. This is the mechanism by which insulin promotes fat storage.

- When insulin is lacking, fat is not stored in the fat cells. Instead, it is released into the bloodstream in the form of free fatty acids. Blood concentrations of other lipids (triglycerides, cholesterol, phospholipids) are also increased. The high blood lipid concentration probably accounts for the atherosclerosis that tends to develop early and progress more rapidly in people with diabetes mellitus. Also, when more fatty acids are released than the body can use as fuel, some fatty acids are converted into ketones. Excessive amounts of ketones produce acidosis and coma.

Protein Metabolism
- Insulin increases the total amount of body protein by increasing transport of amino acids into cells and synthesis of protein within the cells. The basic mechanism of these effects is unknown.
- Insulin potentiates the effects of growth hormone.
- Lack of insulin causes protein depletion and breakdown into amino acids. These amino acids are released into the bloodstream and transported to the liver for energy or gluconeogenesis. These proteins are not replaced by synthesis of new proteins. The overall consequences of protein wasting include abnormal functioning of many body organs, severe weakness, and weight loss.

ity of pancreatic beta cells to produce insulin and thereby cause or aggravate diabetes mellitus.

Factors that inhibit insulin secretion include stimulation of pancreatic alpha$_2$-adrenergic receptors and stress conditions such as hypoxia, hypothermia, surgery, or severe burns.

DIABETES MELLITUS

Diabetes mellitus is a chronic systemic disease characterized by metabolic and vascular abnormalities. Metabolic problems occur early in the disease process and are related to changes in the metabolism of carbohydrate, fat, and protein. A major clinical manifestation of disordered metabolism is hyperglycemia.

Vascular problems include development and progression of atherosclerosis throughout the body and changes in small blood vessels, which especially affect the retina and kidney. Clinical manifestations of vascular disorders may include hypertension, myocardial infarction, stroke, retinopathy, blindness, nephropathy, and peripheral vascular disease.

Classifications

The two major classifications are type 1 and type 2. Although both types are characterized by hyperglycemia, they differ significantly in onset, course, treatment, and pathologic changes. Secondary diabetes may be induced by certain disease processes, certain drugs, and pregnancy.

Type 1
Type 1 diabetes results from an autoimmune disorder that destroys pancreatic beta cells. Hyperglycemia and other symptoms usually develop when approximately 10% to 20% of functioning beta cells remain, but may occur at any time during the progressive loss of beta cells if acute illness or stress increases the body's demand for insulin beyond the capacity of the remaining beta cells to secrete insulin. Eventually, all the beta cells are destroyed, and no insulin is produced.

Type 1 diabetes may occur at any age but usually starts before 20 years of age. It usually has a sudden onset; produces severe symptoms; is difficult to control; produces a high incidence of complications, such as diabetic ketoacidosis (DKA) and renal failure; and requires administration of exogenous insulin. Approximately 10% of people with diabetes have type 1.

Type 2
Type 2 diabetes is characterized by hyperglycemia and insulin resistance. The hyperglycemia results from increased production of glucose by the liver and decreased uptake of glucose in muscle and fat. Insulin resistance means that insulin is present but unable to work effectively (ie, inhibit hepatic production of glucose and cause glucose to move from the bloodstream into liver, muscle, and fat cells). Most insulin resistance is attributed to impaired insulin action at the cellular level. Postreceptor, intracellular mechanisms may be responsible.

Type 2 diabetes may occur at any age but usually starts after 40 years of age. Compared with type 1, it usually has a gradual onset, produces less severe symptoms initially, is easier to control, causes less DKA and renal failure but more myocardial infarctions and strokes, and does not necessarily require exogenous insulin because endogenous insulin is still produced by pancreatic beta cells. Approximately 90% of people with diabetes have type 2; 20% to 30% of them require exogenous insulin.

Type 2 is a heterogenous disease, and etiology probably involves multiple factors such as a genetic predisposition and environmental factors. Obesity is a major cause. With obesity and chronic ingestion of excess calories, along with a sedentary lifestyle, more insulin is required. The increased need leads to prolonged stimulation and eventual "fatigue" of pancreatic beta cells. As a result, the cells become less responsive to elevated blood sugar levels and less able to produce enough insulin to meet metabolic needs. Thus, insulin is secreted but is inadequate or ineffective, especially when insulin demand is increased by obesity, pregnancy, aging, or other factors.

In the United States, African Americans, Hispanics, and Native Americans are at high risk for development of type 2 diabetes.

Signs and Symptoms

Most signs and symptoms of diabetes mellitus stem from a lack of effective insulin and the subsequent metabolic abnormalities. The incidence and severity of clinical manifestations are correlated with the amount of effective insulin, and they may be precipitated by infection, rapid growth, pregnancy, or other factors that increase demand for insulin. Most early manifestations result from disordered carbohydrate metabolism, which causes excess glucose to accumulate in the blood (hyperglycemia). Hyperglycemia produces glucosuria, which, in turn, produces polydipsia, polyuria, dehydration, and polyphagia.

Glucosuria usually appears when the blood glucose level is approximately twice the normal value and the kidneys receive more glucose than can be reabsorbed. However, renal threshold varies, and the amount of glucose lost in the urine does not accurately reflect blood glucose. In very young people, glucose tends to appear in urine at much lower or even normal blood glucose levels. In older people, the ability of the kidneys to excrete excess glucose from the blood is decreased. Therefore, some older people can have rather high blood glucose levels with little or no glucose appearing in the urine.

When large amounts of glucose are present, water is pulled into the renal tubule. This results in a greatly increased urine output (polyuria). The excessive loss of fluid in urine (osmotic diuresis) leads to increased thirst (polydipsia) and, if fluid intake is inadequate, to fluid volume deficit (dehydration). Dehydration also occurs because high blood glucose levels increase osmotic pressure in the bloodstream, and fluid is pulled out of the cells in the body's attempt to regain homeostasis.

Polyphagia (increased appetite) occurs because the body cannot use ingested foods. Many people with diabetes lose weight because of abnormal metabolism.

Complications

Complications of diabetes mellitus are common and potentially disabling or life threatening. Diabetes is a leading cause of myocardial infarction, stroke, blindness, leg amputation, and kidney failure. These complications result from hyperglycemia and other metabolic abnormalities that accompany a lack of effective insulin. The metabolic abnormalities associated with hyperglycemia can cause early, acute complications, such as DKA or hyperosmolar hyperglycemic nonketotic coma (HHNC) (Box 27-2). Eventually, metabolic abnormalities lead to damage in blood vessels and other body tissues.

Macrovascular changes, mainly atherosclerosis, are associated with such complications as myocardial infarction and stroke. Atherosclerosis develops in people with diabetes at an earlier age and it progresses more rapidly and becomes more severe than in people who do not have diabetes. Microvascular changes are associated with nephropathy, retinopathy, and peripheral neuropathy. Diabetic retinopathy is related to the duration of diabetes. Approximately 50% of diabetic people have some degree of retinopathy after 10 years, approximately 80% to 90% after 20 years. Other complications include musculoskeletal disorders, increased numbers and severity of infections, and complications of pregnancy in women with diabetes. All of these complications can be decreased by controlling hyperglycemia and normalizing metabolic processes.

BOX 27–2   ACUTE COMPLICATIONS OF DIABETES MELLITUS

Diabetic Ketoacidosis (DKA)

This life-threatening complication occurs with severe insulin deficiency. In the absence of insulin, glucose cannot be used by body cells for energy and fat is mobilized from adipose tissue to furnish a fuel source. The mobilized fat circulates in the bloodstream, from which it is extracted by the liver and broken down into glycerol and fatty acids. The fatty acids are further changed in the liver to ketones (acetoacetic acid, acetone, beta-hydroxybutyric acid), which then enter the bloodstream and are circulated to body cells for metabolic conversion to energy, carbon dioxide, and water.

These metabolic abnormalities produce clinical signs and symptoms rather rapidly because ketones are produced more rapidly than body cells can use them. Ketone accumulation produces acidemia (a drop in blood pH and an increase in blood hydrogen ions). The body attempts to buffer the acidic hydrogen ions by exchanging them for intracellular potassium ions. Hydrogen ions enter body cells, and potassium ions leave the cells to be excreted in the urine. Another attempt to remove excess acid involves the lungs. Deep, labored respirations, called Kussmaul respirations, eliminate more carbon dioxide and prevent formation of carbonic acid. A third attempt to regain homeostasis involves the kidneys, which excrete some of the ketones, thereby producing acetone in the urine.

Diabetic ketoacidosis worsens as the compensatory mechanisms fail. Clinical signs and symptoms vary and become progressively more severe. Early ones include blurred vision, anorexia, nausea and vomiting, thirst, and polyuria. Later ones include drowsiness, which progresses to stupor and coma, Kussmaul breathing, dehydration and other signs of fluid and electrolyte imbalances, and decreased blood pressure, increased pulse, and other signs of shock.

Two major causes of DKA are omission of insulin (eg, on sick days) and illnesses such as infection, trauma, myocardial infarction, or stroke.

Hyperosmolar Hyperglycemic Nonketotic Coma (HHNC)

This is another type of diabetic coma that is potentially life threatening. It is relatively rare and carries a high mortality rate. The term *hyperosmolar* refers to an excessive amount of glucose, electrolytes, and other solutes in the blood in relation to the amount of water.

Like DKA, HHNC is characterized by hyperglycemia, which leads to osmotic diuresis and resultant thirst, polyuria, dehydration, and electrolyte losses, as well as neurologic signs ranging from drowsiness to stupor to coma. Additional clinical problems may include hypovolemic shock, thrombosis, renal problems, or stroke. In contrast to DKA, hyperosmolar coma occurs in people with previously unknown or mild diabetes, usually after an illness; occurs in hyperglycemic conditions other than diabetes (eg, severe burns, corticosteroid drug therapy); and does not cause ketosis.

HYPOGLYCEMIC DRUGS

Insulin

Insulin is described in this section, and individual insulins are listed in Table 27-1.

- Exogenous insulin used to replace endogenous insulin has the same effects as the pancreatic hormone.

- The primary clinical indication for insulin is treatment of diabetes mellitus. Insulin is the only effective treatment for type 1 diabetes because pancreatic beta cells are unable to secrete endogenous insulin and metabolism is severely impaired. Insulin is required for type 2 diabetic clients who cannot control their disease with diet, weight control, and oral agents. It may be needed by anyone with diabetes during times of stress, such as illness, infection, or surgery.

TABLE 27-1 **Insulins**

Generic/Trade Name	Characteristics	Routes and Dosage Ranges	Action (h)		
			Onset	Peak	Duration
Short-acting Insulin					
Insulin injection (Regular Iletin II, Humulin R, Novolin R)	1. A clear liquid solution with the appearance of water 2. The hypoglycemic drug of choice for diabetics experiencing acute or emergency situations, diabetic ketoacidosis, hyperosmolar nonketotic coma, severe infections or other illnesses, major surgery, and pregnancy 3. The only insulin preparation that can be given IV	SC, dosage individualized according to blood glucose levels. For sliding scale, 5–20 units before meals and bedtime, depending on blood glucose levels IV, dosage individualized. For ketoacidosis, regular insulin may be given by direct injection, intermittent infusion, or continuous infusion. One regimen involves an initial bolus injection of 10–20 units followed by a continuous low-dose infusion of 2–10 units/h, based on hourly blood and urine glucose levels	½–1	2–3	5–7
Intermediate-acting Insulins					
Isophane insulin suspension (NPH, NPH Iletin II, Humulin N, Novolin N)	1. Commonly used for long-term administration 2. Modified by addition of protamine (a protein) and zinc 3. A suspension with a cloudy appearance when correctly mixed in the drug vial 4. Given *only* SC 5. Not recommended for use in acute situations 6. Hypoglycemic reactions are more likely to occur during mid-to-late afternoon	SC, dosage individualized. Initially, 7–26 units may be given once or twice daily.	1–1½	8–12	18–24
Insulin zinc suspension (Lente Iletin II, Lente L, Humulin L, Novolin L)	1. Modified by addition of zinc 2. May be used interchangeably with NPH insulin 3. A suspension with a cloudy appearance when correctly mixed in the drug vial 4. Given *only* SC	SC, dosage individualized. Initially, 7–26 units may be given once or twice daily.	1–2	8–12	18–24
Long-acting Insulin					
Extended insulin zinc suspension (Humulin U Ultralente)	1. Modified by addition of zinc and formation of large crystals, which are slowly absorbed 2. Hypoglycemic reactions are frequent and likely to occur during sleep.	SC, dosage individualized. Initially, 7–26 units may be given once daily	4–8	10–30	36 plus

(continued)

TABLE 27-1 **Insulins (*continued*)**

Generic/Trade Name	Characteristics	Routes and Dosage Ranges	Action (h)		
			Onset	Peak	Duration
Insulin Mixtures **NPH 70%** **Regular 30%** (Humulin 70/30, Novolin 70/30)	1. Stable mixture 2. Onset, peak, and duration of action same as individual components	SC, dosage individualized			
NPH 50% **Regular 50%** (Humulin 50/50)	See Humulin 70/30, above	SC, dosage individualized			
Insulin Analog **Insulin lispro** (Humalog)	1. A synthetic insulin of recombinant DNA origin, created by reversing two amino acids 2. Has a faster onset and a shorter duration of action than human regular insulin 3. Intended for use with a longer-acting insulin	SC, dosage individualized, 15 min before meals	¼	½–1½	6–8

IV, intravenous; SC, subcutaneous.

Insulin also is used to control diabetes induced by chronic pancreatitis, surgical excision of pancreatic tissue, hormones and other drugs, and pregnancy (gestational diabetes). In nondiabetic clients, insulin is used to prevent or treat hyperglycemia induced by IV hyperalimentation solutions and to treat hyperkalemia. In hyperkalemia, an IV infusion of insulin and dextrose solution causes potassium to move from the blood into the cells; it does not eliminate potassium from the body.

- The only clear-cut contraindication to the use of insulin is hypoglycemia, because of the risk of brain damage (Box 27-3). Pork insulin is contraindicated in clients allergic to the animal protein.

Available insulins are pork insulin and human insulin. Pork insulin differs from human insulin by one amino acid. Human insulin is synthesized in the laboratory with recombinant deoxyribonucleic acid techniques using strains of *Escherichia coli* or yeast or by modifying pork insulin to replace the single different amino acid. The name *human insulin* means that the synthetic product is identical to endogenous insulin (ie, has the same number and sequence of amino acids). It is not derived from the human pancreas.

An insulin analog called *insulin lispro* (Humalog) is also available. It is identical to human insulin except for the reversal of two amino acids (lysine and proline). Insulin lispro is absorbed more rapidly and has a shorter half-life after subcutaneous (SC) injection than regular human insulin. As a result, it is similar to physiologic insulin secretion after a meal, more effective at decreasing postprandial hyperglycemia, and less likely to cause hypoglycemia before the next meal. Injection just before a meal produces hypoglycemic effects similar to those of an injection of conventional regular insulin given 30 minutes before a meal. Other insulin analogs are being developed.

- Insulin cannot be given orally because it is a protein that is destroyed by proteolytic enzymes in the GI tract. It is given only parenterally, most often SC.
- Insulins differ in onset and duration of action. They are usually categorized as short, intermediate, or long acting. Short-acting insulins have a rapid onset and a short duration of action. Intermediate- and long-acting insulins are modified by adding protamine (a large, insoluble protein), zinc, or both to slow absorption and prolong drug action. Mixtures of 70% isophane insulin (NPH) and 30% regular insulin (eg, Humulin 70/30) or 50% each (Humulin 50/50) are available. The mixtures are more convenient and may be more accurately measured when both an intermediate- and a short-acting insulin are needed.
- U-100 is the main insulin concentration in the United States. This means that it contains 100 units of insulin per milliliter of solution. U-100 insulin can be accurately measured only in a syringe designed for use with U-100 insulin.
- Insulin absorption is delayed or decreased when it is injected into SC tissue with lipodystrophy or other lesions, when circulatory problems (eg, edema or hypotension) are present, by insulin-binding antibodies (which develop after 2 or 3 months of insulin administration), and by injecting cold (ie, refrigerated) insulin.

BOX 27-3　HYPOGLYCEMIA: CHARACTERISTICS AND MANAGEMENT

Hypoglycemia may occur with insulin or oral sulfonylureas. When hypoglycemia is suspected, the blood glucose level should be measured if at all possible, although signs and symptoms and the plasma glucose level at which they occur vary from person to person. Hypoglycemia is usually defined as a blood glucose below 60 to 70 mg/dL and is especially dangerous at approximately 40 mg/dL or below. Central nervous system effects of hypoglycemia may lead to accidental injury or permanent brain damage; cardiovascular effects may lead to cardiac arrhythmias or myocardial infarction. Causes of hypoglycemia include:

- Intensive insulin therapy (ie, continuous subcutaneous [SC] infusion or three or more injections daily).
- Omitting or delaying meals
- An excessive or incorrect dose of insulin or an oral agent that causes hypoglycemia
- Altered sensitivity to insulin
- Decreased clearance of insulin or an oral agent (eg, with renal insufficiency)
- Decreased glucose intake
- Decreased production of glucose in the liver
- Giving an insulin injection intramuscularly (IM) rather than SC
- Drug interactions that decrease blood glucose levels
- Increased physical exertion
- Ethanol ingestion

Hormones That Raise Blood Sugar

Normally, when hypoglycemia occurs, several hormones (glucagon, epinephrine, growth hormone, and cortisol) work to restore and maintain blood glucose levels. Glucagon and epinephrine, the dominant counter-regulatory hormones, act rapidly because they are activated as soon as blood glucose levels start declining. Growth hormone and cortisol act more slowly, approximately 2 hours after hypoglycemia occurs.

People with diabetes who develop hypoglycemia may have impaired secretion of these hormones, especially those with type 1 diabetes. Decreased secretion of glucagon is often evident in clients who have had diabetes for 5 years or longer. Decreased secretion of epinephrine also occurs in people who have been treated with insulin for several years. Decreased epinephrine decreases tachycardia, a common sign of hypoglycemia, and may delay recognition and treatment.

The Conscious Client

When hypoglycemic reactions occur, treatment consists of immediate administration of a rapidly absorbed carbohydrate. For the conscious client who is able to swallow, the carbohydrate is given orally. Foods and fluids that provide approximately 15 g of carbohydrate include:

- Two sugar cubes or 1 to 2 teaspoons of sugar, syrup, honey, or jelly
- Two or three small pieces of candy or approximately eight Lifesaver candies
- 4 oz of fruit juice, such as orange, apple, or grape
- 4 oz of ginger ale
- Coffee or tea with 2 teaspoons of sugar added
- Commercial glucose products (eg, Glutose, B-D Glucose). These products must be swallowed to be effective.

Symptoms usually subside within 15 to 20 minutes. If they do not subside, the patient should take another 10 to 15 g of oral carbohydrate. *If acarbose or miglitol has been taken with insulin or a sulfonylurea and a hypoglycemic reaction occurs, glucose (oral or intravenous [IV]) or glucagon must be given for treatment.* Sucrose (table sugar) and other oral carbohydrates do not relieve hypoglycemia because the presence of acarbose or miglitol prevents their digestion and absorption from the gastrointestinal tract.

The Unconscious Client

For the unconscious client, carbohydrate cannot be given orally because of the risks of aspiration. Therefore, the treatment choices involve parenteral glucose or glucagon.

If the client is in a health care facility where medical help is readily available, IV glucose in a 25% or 50% solution is the treatment of choice. It acts rapidly to raise blood glucose levels and arouse the client. If the client is at home or elsewhere, glucagon may be given if available and there is someone to inject it. A family member or roommate may be taught to give glucagon SC or IM. It can also be given IV. The usual adult dose is 0.5 to 1 mg. Glucagon is a pancreatic hormone that increases blood sugar by converting liver glycogen to glucose. It is effective only when liver glycogen is present. Some clients cannot respond to glucagon because glycogen stores are depleted by such conditions as starvation, adrenal insufficiency, or chronic hypoglycemia. The hyperglycemic effect of glucagon occurs more slowly than that of IV glucose and is of relatively brief duration. If the client does not respond to one or two doses of glucagon within 20 minutes, IV glucose is indicated.

Caution is needed in the treatment of hypoglycemia. Although the main goal of treatment is to relieve hypoglycemia and restore the brain's supply of glucose, a secondary goal is to avoid overtreatment and excessive hyperglycemia. The client having a hypoglycemic re-

(continued)

- Temperature extremes can cause loss of potency. Insulin retains potency up to 36 months under refrigeration and approximately 18 to 24 months at room temperature. At high temperatures (approximately 100°F or 37.8°C), insulin loses potency in approximately 2 months. If frozen, insulin remains potent but tends to clump or precipitate. This prevents withdrawal of an accurate dose, and the vial should be discarded.

Oral Hypoglycemic Drugs

There are five types of oral antidiabetic agents, all of which may be used to treat type 2 diabetes that is not controlled by diet and exercise. The drugs lower blood sugar by different mechanisms (Fig. 27-2) and may be used in various combinations for additive effects. Some are also combined with insulin. These drugs are further described in the following sections; dosages of individual drugs are listed in Table 27-2.

Sulfonylureas

- The sulfonylureas are the oldest and largest group of oral agents. They lower blood glucose mainly by increasing secretion of insulin. They may also increase peripheral use of glucose, decrease production of glucose in the liver, increase the number of insulin receptors, or alter postreceptor actions to

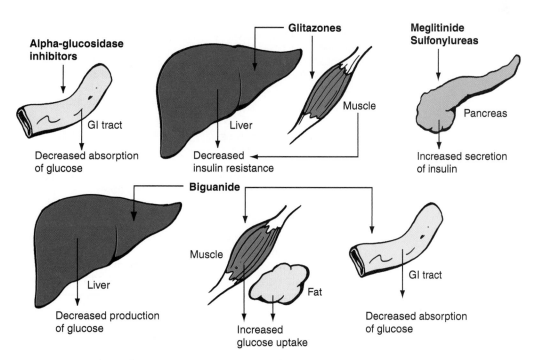

FIGURE 27–2 Actions of oral antidiabetic drugs. The drugs lower blood sugar by decreasing absorption or production of glucose, by increasing secretion of insulin, or by increasing the effectiveness of available insulin (decreasing insulin resistance).

TABLE 27-2   **Oral Drugs For Diabetes Mellitus**

Generic/Trade Name	Characteristics	Routes and Dosage Ranges
Sulfonylureas, Second Generation		
Glimepiride (Amaryl)	Onset of action about 1 h; peak, 2–3 h	PO, initially 1–2 mg once daily, with breakfast or first main meal. Maximum starting dose 2 mg or less. Maintenance dose 1–4 mg once daily. After a dose of 2 mg is reached, increase dose in increments of 2 mg or less at 1- to 2-week intervals, based on blood glucose levels. Maximum recommended dose, 8 mg once daily. In combination with insulin, PO 8 mg once daily with the first main meal.
Glipizide (Glucotrol)	Onset of action, approximately 1–1.5 h; duration 10–16 h	PO, initially 5 mg daily in a single dose, 30 min before breakfast. Maximum dose, 40 mg daily. In elderly, may start with 2.5 mg daily
Glyburide (DiaBeta, Micronase, Glynase Pres Tab)	Onset of action approximately 2–4 h; duration 24 h. Glynase is better absorbed, acts faster (onset about 1 h; duration 24 h), and is given in smaller doses than other forms of glyburide.	PO, initially 2.5–5 mg daily in a single dose, with breakfast. Maximum dose, 20 mg daily. Glynase PO initially 1.5–3 mg daily with breakfast. Maximum dose, 12 mg daily.
Alpha-Glucosidase Inhibitors		
Acarbose (Precose)	Delays digestion of carbohydrate foods when acarbose and food are present in GI tract at the same time	PO, initially 25 mg, three times daily with first bite of main meals; increase at 4- to 8-week intervals to a maximum dose of 50 mg three times daily (for patients weighing under 60 kg) if necessary, depending on 1-h postprandial blood glucose levels and tolerance. Clients weighing more than 60 kg may need doses up to 100 mg three times daily (the maximum dose).
Miglitol (Glyset)	Delays digestion of carbohydrates in the GI tract	PO, initially 25 mg three times daily with the first bite of each main meal, gradually increased if necessary. Maximum dose, 100 mg three times daily
Biguanide		
Metformin (Glucophage)	Older adults are at higher risk for development of lactic acidosis, a rare but potentially fatal reaction. Thus, smaller doses and monitoring of renal function are recommended.	PO, initially 500 mg twice daily, with morning and evening meals; increase dose in increments of 500 mg/d every 2–3 weeks if necessary, up to a maximum of 3000 mg daily, based on patient tolerance and blood glucose levels. In elderly patients, do not increase to maximum dose.
Glitazones		
Pioglitazone (Actos)	Increases effects of insulin; may be used alone or with insulin, metformin, or a sulfonylurea	PO 15–30 mg once daily
Rosiglitazone (Avandia)	Increases effects of insulin; may be used alone or with metformin	PO 4–8 mg once daily , in one dose or two divided doses
Meglitinide		
Repaglinide (Prandin)	Onset of action, within 30 min; peak, 1 h; duration approximately 3–4 h	PO 1–2 mg 15–30 min. before each meal; increased to 4 mg before meals if necessary. Maximum dose, 16 mg daily. Omit a dose if skip a meal; add a dose if add a meal.

GI, gastrointestinal; PO, oral.

increase tissue responsiveness to insulin. Because the drugs stimulate pancreatic beta cells to produce more insulin, they are effective only when functioning pancreatic beta cells are present.

- First-generation sulfonylureas, which include acetohexamide, chlorpropamide, tolazamide, and tolbutamide, have largely been replaced by the second-generation sulfonylureas, and are not discussed further. The second-generation drugs, glipizide, glyburide, and glimepiride, are similar in therapeutic and adverse effects. The main adverse effect is hypoglycemia (see Box 27-3).
- The sulfonylureas are chemically related to sulfonamide antibacterial drugs; well absorbed with oral administration; more than 90% bound to plasma proteins; and metabolized in the liver to inactive metabolites, which are excreted primarily by the kidneys (except for glyburide, which is excreted approximately 50% in urine and 50% in bile).
- Glimepiride is the only sulfonylurea that is approved by the Food and Drug Administration (FDA) for combination therapy with insulin, although others would presumably produce the same effects. In addition, when hyperglycemia is not controlled by diet and a single drug, a sulfonylurea may be given along with acarbose, miglitol, or metformin.
- Sulfonylureas are contraindicated in clients with hypersensitivity to them, with severe renal or hepatic impairment, and during pregnancy. They are unlikely to be effective during periods of stress, such as major surgery, severe illness, or infection. Insulin is usually required in these circumstances.

Alpha-Glucosidase Inhibitors

- Acarbose and miglitol inhibit alpha-glucosidase enzymes (eg, sucrase, maltase, amylase) in the GI tract and thereby delay digestion of complex carbohydrates into glucose and other simple sugars. As a result, glucose absorption is delayed and there is a smaller increase in blood glucose levels after a meal.
- The drugs are metabolized in the GI tract by digestive enzymes and intestinal bacteria. Some of the metabolites are absorbed systemically and excreted in urine; plasma concentrations are increased in the presence of renal impairment.
- One of the drugs may be given alone or combined with a sulfonylurea. They are also combined with insulin and other oral agents.
- These drugs are contraindicated in clients with hypersensitivity, DKA, hepatic cirrhosis, inflammatory or malabsorptive intestinal disorders, and severe renal impairment.

Biguanide

- Metformin increases the use of glucose by muscle and fat cells, decreases hepatic glucose production,

and decreases intestinal absorption of glucose. It is preferably called an antihyperglycemic rather than a hypoglycemic agent because it does not cause hypoglycemia, even in large doses, when used alone.
- It is absorbed from the small intestine, circulates without binding to plasma proteins, and has a serum half-life of 1.3 to 4.5 hours. It is not metabolized in the liver and is excreted unchanged in the urine.
- Metformin may be used alone or in combination with a sulfonylurea or repaglinide.
- It is contraindicated in clients with diabetes complicated by fever, severe infections, severe trauma, major surgery, acidosis, or pregnancy (insulin is indicated in these conditions). It is also contraindicated in clients with serious hepatic or renal impairment, cardiac or respiratory insufficiency, hypoxia, or a history of lactic acidosis because these conditions may increase production of lactate and the risk of potentially fatal lactic acidosis.

Glitazones

- These drugs—pioglitazone and rosiglitazone—are also called thiazolidinediones and insulin sensitizers.
- They decrease insulin resistance, a major factor in the pathophysiology of type 2 diabetes. The drugs stimulate receptors on muscle, fat, and liver cells. This stimulation increases or restores the effectiveness of circulating insulin and results in increased uptake of glucose by peripheral tissues and decreased production of glucose by the liver.
- The drugs may be used as monotherapy with diet and exercise or in combination with insulin or a sulfonylurea.
- The drugs are contraindicated in clients with active liver disease or a serum alanine aminotransferase (ALT) >2.5 times the upper limit of normal. They are also contraindicated in clients who are hypersensitive to them.

Meglitinide

- Repaglinide is a nonsulfonylurea that lowers blood sugar by stimulating pancreatic secretion of insulin.
- It can be used as monotherapy with diet and exercise or in combination with metformin. It may be especially useful for clients with renal impairment because it is minimally excreted by the kidneys.
- It is well absorbed from the GI tract; peak plasma level occurs within 1 hour. It has a plasma half-life of approximately 1 hour and is highly bound (>98%) to plasma proteins. It is metabolized to inactive metabolites that are excreted mainly in feces.
- Repaglinide is metabolized and removed from the bloodstream within 3 to 4 hours after a dose. This decreases the workload of pancreatic beta cells

(ie, decreases duration of beta cell stimulation), allows serum insulin levels to return to normal before the next meal, and decreases risks of hypoglycemic episodes.

- It is taken 15 to 30 minutes before a meal. If a meal is skipped, the drug dose should be skipped; if a meal is added, a drug dose should be added.

NURSING PROCESS

Assessment

Assess the client's knowledge, attitude, and condition in relation to diabetes, the prescribed treatment plan, and complications. Assessment data should include past manifestations of the disease process and the client's response to them, present status, and potential problem areas.

- *Historic data* include age at onset of diabetes, prescribed control measures and their effectiveness, the ease or difficulty of complying with the prescribed treatment, occurrence of complications such as ketoacidosis, and whether other disease processes have interfered with diabetes control.

- *Assess the client's current status*, including subjective and objective information related to the following areas:
  - **Diet.** Ask about the prescribed nutritional plan, if the client consults a nutritionist, who prepares the food, what factors help in following the diet, what factors interfere with following the diet, the current weight and whether there has been a recent change. If a dietitian is available, ask one to assess the client's dietary practices and needs.
  - **Activity.** Ask the client to describe usual activities of daily living, including those related to work, home, and recreation and whether he or she participates in a regular exercise program. If so, ask for more information about what, how often, how long, and so forth. If not, teaching is needed because exercise is extremely important in diabetes management.
  - **Medication.** If the client takes insulin, ask what kind, how much, who administers it, usual time of administration, sites used for injections, if a hypoglycemic reaction to insulin has ever been experienced, and if so, how it was handled. This information helps to assess knowledge, usual practices, and teaching needs. If the client takes an oral antidiabetic drug, ask the name, dosage, and time taken.

  - **Monitoring methods.** Testing the blood for glucose and the urine for ketones (eg, when blood sugar is elevated or when ill and unable to eat) are the two main methods of monitoring glycemic control. Ask about the method used, the frequency of testing, and the pattern of results. If possible, observe the client performing and interpreting an actual test to assess accuracy.
  - **Skin and mucous membranes.** Inspect for signs of infection and any other lesions. Infections often occur in the axillary and groin areas because these areas have large numbers of microorganisms. Periodontal disease (pyorrhea) may be manifested by inflammation and bleeding of the gums. Women with diabetes are susceptible to monilial vaginitis and infections under the breasts. Check the sites of insulin injection for atrophy (dimpling or indentation), hypertrophy (nodules or lumps), and fibrosis (hardened areas). Check the lower leg for brown spots; these are caused by small hemorrhages into the skin and may indicate widespread changes in the blood vessels.

    Problems are especially likely to develop in the feet from infection, trauma, pressure, vascular insufficiency, and neuropathy. Therefore, inspect the feet for calluses, ulcers, and signs of infection. When such problems develop, sensory impairment from neuropathy may delay detection and impaired circulation may delay healing. Check pedal pulses, color, and temperature in both feet to evaluate arterial blood flow. Ankle edema may indicate venous insufficiency or impaired cardiac function.
  - **Eyes.** Ask if the client has experienced any difficulties with vision and if eyes are examined regularly. Diabetic clients are prone to development of retinopathy, cataracts, and possibly glaucoma.
  - **Cardiovascular system.** Clients with diabetes have a high incidence of atherosclerosis, which makes them susceptible to hypertension, angina pectoris, myocardial infarction, peripheral vascular disease, and stroke. Therefore, check blood pressure and ask about chest pain and pain in the legs with exercise (intermittent claudication).
  - **Genitourinary system.** People with diabetes often have kidney and bladder problems. Assess for signs of urinary tract infection; albumin, white blood cells, or blood in urine; edema; increased urination at night; difficulty voiding; generalized itching; easy bleeding and bruising; fatigue; and muscular weakness. Im-

potence may develop in men and is attributed to neuropathy.

- Assess blood sugar reports for abnormal levels. Two or more fasting blood glucose levels greater than 126 mg/dL or two random levels greater than 200 mg/dL are diagnostic of diabetes. Decreased blood sugar levels are especially dangerous at 40 mg/dL or below.
- Assess the glycosylated hemoglobin (also called glycated hemoglobin and HbA_{1c}) level when available. This test indicates glucose bound to hemoglobin in red blood cells (RBCs) when RBCs are exposed to hyperglycemia. The binding is irreversible and lasts for the lifespan of RBCs (approximately 120 days). The test reflects the average blood sugar during the previous 2 to 3 months. The goal is usually less than 7% (the range for people without diabetes is approximately 4% to 6%). The test should be done every 3 to 6 months.

  Test results are not affected by several factors that alter blood sugar levels, such as time of day, food intake, exercise, recently administered antidiabetic drugs, emotional stress, or client cooperation. The test is especially useful with children, those whose diabetes is poorly controlled, those who do not test blood glucose regularly, and those who change their usual habits before a scheduled appointment with a health care provider so that their blood sugar control appears better than it actually is.

Nursing Diagnoses

- Altered Tissue Perfusion related to atherosclerosis and vascular impairment
- Sensory/Perceptual Alterations related to impaired vision
- Sensory/Perceptual Alterations related to neuropathy, especially in the legs
- Ineffective Individual Coping related to chronic illness and required treatment
- Anxiety: Managing a chronic illness, finger sticks, insulin injections
- Risk for Injury: Trauma, infection, hypoglycemia, hyperglycemia
- Noncompliance related to inability or unwillingness to manage the disease process and required treatment
- Knowledge Deficit: Disease process and management
- Knowledge Deficit: Administration and effects of antidiabetic drugs
- Knowledge Deficit: Interrelationships among diet, exercise, and antidiabetic drugs
- Knowledge Deficit: Management of hypoglycemia, "sick days," and other complications

Planning/Goals

The client will:

- Learn self-care activities at an individualized pace
- Manage drug therapy to prevent or minimize hypoglycemia and other adverse effects
- Develop a consistent pattern of diet and exercise
- Use available resources to learn about the disease process and how to manage it
- Take antidiabetic drugs accurately
- Self-monitor blood glucose and urine ketones appropriately
- Keep appointments for follow-up and monitoring procedures by a health care provider

Interventions

Use nondrug measures to improve control of diabetes and to help prevent complications.

- Assist the client in maintaining the prescribed diet. Specific measures vary but may include teaching the client and family about the importance of diet, referring the client to a dietitian, and helping the client identify and modify factors that decrease compliance with the diet. If the client is obese, assist in developing a program to lose weight and then maintain weight at a more nearly normal level.
- Assist the client to develop and maintain a regular exercise program.
- Perform and interpret blood tests for glucose accurately, and assist clients and family members to do so. Self-monitoring of blood glucose levels allows the client to see the effects of diet, exercise, and hypoglycemic medications on blood glucose levels and may promote compliance.

  Several products are available for home glucose monitoring. All involve obtaining a drop of capillary blood from a finger with a sterile lancet. The blood is placed on a semipermeable membrane that contains a reagent. The amount of blood glucose can be read visually or with various machines (eg, Accu-Chek Glucometer). The latter method is more accurate but less convenient and more expensive than visual reading.
- Test urine for ketones when the client is sick, when blood glucose levels are above 200 mg/dL, and when episodes of nocturnal hypoglycemia are suspected. Also teach clients and family members to test urine when indicated.
- Promote early recognition and treatment of problems by observing for signs and symptoms of urinary tract infection, peripheral vascular disease, vision changes, ketoacidosis, hypoglycemia, and others. Teach clients and families to observe for these conditions and report their occurrence.

- Discuss the importance of regular visits to health care facilities for blood sugar measurements, weights, blood pressure measurements, and eye examinations.
- Perform and teach correct foot care. Have the client observe the following safeguards: avoid going barefoot, to prevent trauma to the feet; wear correctly fitted shoes; wash the feet daily with warm water, dry well, inspect for any lesions or pressure areas, and apply lanolin if the skin is dry; wear cotton or wool socks because they are more absorbent than synthetic materials, such as nylon; cut toenails straight across and only after the feet have been soaked in warm water and washed thoroughly. Teach the client to avoid use of hot water bottles or electric heating pads, cutting toenails if vision is impaired, use of strong antiseptics on the feet, and cutting corns or calluses. Also teach the client to report any lesions on the feet to the physician.

- Help clients keep up with newer developments in diabetes care by providing information, sources of information, consultations with specialists, and other resources. However, do not overwhelm a newly diagnosed diabetic client with sudden and excessive information or assume that a long-term diabetic client does not need information.

Evaluation

- Check blood sugar reports regularly for normal or abnormal values.
- Check glycosylated hemoglobin reports when available.
- Interview and observe for therapeutic and adverse responses to antidiabetic drugs.
- Interview and observe for compliance with prescribed treatment.
- Interview clients and family members about the frequency and length of hospitalizations for diabetes mellitus.

CLIENT TEACHING GUIDELINES
Antidiabetic Drugs

General Considerations

✔ Learn as much as you can about diabetes and its management. Few other diseases require as much adaptation in activities of daily living, and you must be well informed to control the disease, minimize complications, and achieve an optimal quality of life. Although much information is available from health care providers (physicians, nurses, diabetes nurse educators, nutritionists), an additional major resource is the

American Diabetes Association
1660 Duke St.
Alexandria, VA 22314
1-800-ADA-DISC
http://www.diabetes.org

✔ Diet, weight control, and exercise are extremely important in managing diabetes. Maintaining normal weight and avoiding excessive caloric intake decrease the need for medication and decrease the workload of the pancreas. Exercise helps body tissues use insulin better, which means that glucose moves out of the bloodstream and into muscles and other body tissues. This promotes more normal blood glucose levels and decreases long-term complications of diabetes.

✔ Take any antidiabetic medication as prescribed. If unable to take a medication, notify a health care provider. To control blood sugar most effectively, medications are balanced with diet and exercise. If you take insulin, you need to know what type(s) you are taking, how to obtain

more, how to store it, and how to get syringes. Insulin lispro (Humalog) is the only commonly used insulin that requires a prescription. Other insulins and supplies for injection are available at drugstores. Keep several days' supply of insulin and syringes on hand to allow for weather or other conditions that might prevent replacement of insulin or other supplies when needed.

✔ You need to know the signs and symptoms of high blood sugar (hyperglycemia): increased blood glucose and excessive thirst, hunger, and urine output. Persistent hyperglycemia may indicate a need to change some aspect of the treatment program, such as diet or medication.

✔ You need to know the symptoms of low blood sugar (hypoglycemia): sweating, nervousness, hunger, weakness, tremors, and mental confusion. Hypoglycemia may indicate too much medication or exercise or too little food. Treatment is a rapidly absorbed source of sugar, which usually reverses symptoms within 10 to 20 minutes. If you are alert and able to swallow, take approximately 4 oz of fruit juice, 4 to 6 oz of a sugar-containing soft drink, a piece of fruit or approximately ⅓ cup of raisins, two to three glucose tablets (5 grams each), a tube of glucose gel, 1 cup of skim milk, tea or coffee with 2 teaspoons of sugar, or eight Lifesaver candies. Avoid taking so much sugar that hyperglycemia occurs.

If you take acarbose (Precose) or miglitol (Glyset) along with insulin or a sulfonylurea (eg, glimepiride, glipizide, or

(continued)

CLIENT TEACHING GUIDELINES
Antidiabetic Drugs (continued)

glyburide) and a hypoglycemic reaction occurs, you must take some form of glucose (or glucagon) for treatment. Sucrose (table sugar) and other oral carbohydrates do not relieve hypoglycemia because the presence of acarbose or miglitol prevents their digestion and absorption from the gastrointestinal (GI) tract.

✔ You need to have a family member or roommate instructed in recognizing and managing hypoglycemia in case you are unable to obtain or swallow a source of glucose. If you take insulin, glucagon should be available in the home and a caregiver should know how to give it.

✔ The best way to prevent, delay, or decrease the severity of diabetes complications is to maintain blood sugar at a normal or near-normal level. Other measures include regular visits to health care providers, preferably a team of specialists in diabetes care; regular vision and glaucoma testing; and special foot care. In addition, if you have hypertension, treatment can help prevent heart attacks and strokes.

✔ Take only drugs prescribed by a physician who knows you have diabetes. Avoid other prescriptions and over-the-counter drugs unless these are discussed with the physician treating the diabetes because adverse reactions and interactions may occur. For example, nasal decongestants (alone or in cold remedies) and asthma medications may cause tachycardia and nervousness, which may be interpreted as hypoglycemia. In addition, liquid cold remedies and cough syrups may contain sugar and raise blood glucose levels. Aspirin may increase the likelihood of hypoglycemia.

✔ Test blood regularly for glucose. A schedule individualized to your needs is best. Testing should be done more often when medication dosages are changed or when you are ill.

✔ Reduce insulin dosage or eat extra food if you expect to exercise more than usual. Specific recommendations should be individualized and worked out with health care providers in relation to the type of exercise.

✔ Ask for written instructions about managing "sick days" and call your physician if unsure about what you need to do. Although each person needs individualized instructions, some general guidelines include the following:

  ✔ If you take insulin, glimepiride, glipizide, glyburide, or repaglinide, continue to take the usual dose. Additional insulin also may be needed, especially if ketosis develops. Ketones in the urine indicate insulin deficiency or insulin resistance.

  ✔ Check blood glucose levels at least four times daily; test urine for ketones when the blood glucose level exceeds 250 mg/dL or with each urination. If unable to test urine, have someone else do it.

  ✔ Rest, keep warm, do not exercise, and keep someone with you if possible.

  ✔ If unable to eat solid food, take easily digested liquids or semiliquid foods. Approximately 15 g of carbohydrate every 1 to 2 hours is usually enough and can be provided by ½ cup of apple juice, applesauce, cola, cranberry juice, eggnog, Cream of Wheat cereal, custard, vanilla ice cream, regular gelatin, or frozen yogurt.

  ✔ Drink 2 to 3 quarts of fluids daily, especially if you have a fever. Water, tea, broths, clear soups, diet soda, or carbohydrate-containing fluids are acceptable.

  ✔ Record the amount of fluid intake as well as the number of times you urinate, vomit, or have loose stools.

  ✔ Seek medical attention if a premeal blood glucose level is more than 250 mg/dL, if urine ketones are present, if you have fever above 100°F, if you have several episodes of vomiting or diarrhea, or if you experience other severe symptoms such as difficulty in breathing, chest pain, severe abdominal pain, or severe dehydration.

Self-administration

✔ Use correct techniques for injecting insulin:

  ✔ Wash hands; wash injection site, if needed.

  ✔ Draw up insulin in a good light, being very careful to draw up the correct dose. If you have trouble seeing the syringe markers, get a magnifier or ask someone else to draw up the insulin.

  ✔ Instructions may vary about cleaning the top of the insulin vial and the injection site with an alcohol swab and about pulling back on the plunger after injection to see if any blood enters the syringe. These techniques have been commonly used, but many diabetes experts do not believe they are necessary.

  ✔ Inject straight into the fat layer under the skin, at a 90-degree angle. If very thin, pinch up a skin-fold and inject at a 45-degree angle.

  ✔ Rotate injection sites. Your health care provider may suggest a rotation plan. Many people rotate between the abdomen and the thighs. Insulin is absorbed fastest from the abdomen. Do not inject insulin within 2 inches of the "belly button" or into any skin lesions.

  ✔ If it is necessary to mix two insulin preparations, ask for specific instructions about the technique and then follow it consistently. There is a risk of inaccurate dosage of both insulins unless measured very carefully.

  ✔ Change insulin dosage only if instructed to do so and the circumstances are specified.

  ✔ Carry sugar, candy, or a commercial glucose preparation for immediate use if a hypoglycemic reaction occurs.

✔ Take oral drugs as directed. Recommendations usually include the following:

(continued)

CLIENT TEACHING GUIDELINES
Antidiabetic Drugs (continued)

✔ Take glipizide or glyburide approximately 30 minutes before meals; take glimepiride with breakfast or the first main meal.
✔ Take acarbose or miglitol with the first bite of each main meal. The drugs need to be in the GI tract with food because they act by decreasing absorption of sugar in the food. Starting with a small dose and increasing it gradually helps to prevent bloating, "gas pains," and diarrhea.
✔ Take metformin with meals to decrease stomach upset.
✔ Take repaglinide 15 to 30 minutes before meals (2, 3, or 4 times daily). Doses may vary from 0.5 to 4.0 mg, depending on fasting blood glucose levels. Dosage changes should be at least 1 week apart. If you skip a

meal, you should skip that dose of repaglinide; if you eat an extra meal, you should take an extra dose.
✔ Take pioglitazone and rosiglitazone without regard to meals.
✔ If you take glimepiride, glipizide, glyburide, or repaglinide, alone or in combination with other antidiabetic drugs, be prepared to handle hypoglycemic reactions (as with insulin, above). Acarbose, miglitol, metformin, pioglitazone, and rosiglitazone do not cause hypoglycemia when taken alone. Do not skip meals and snacks. This increases the risk of hypoglycemic reactions.
✔ If you exercise vigorously, you may need to decrease your dose of antidiabetic drug or eat more. Ask for specific instructions related to the type and frequency of the exercise.

PRINCIPLES OF THERAPY

Goals of Therapy

For most clients, the goals of treatment are to maintain blood glucose at normal or near-normal levels; promote near-normal metabolism of carbohydrate, fat, and protein; prevent acute and long-term complications; and prevent hypoglycemic episodes.

There is strong evidence that strict control of blood sugar decreases complications. A few years ago, the Diabetes Control and Complications Trial demonstrated that adequate glycemic control could delay the onset and slow progression of complications associated with microvascular disease (eg, nephropathy, retinopathy, and possibly neuropathy) in people with type 1 diabetes. A more recent study, the United Kingdom Prospective Diabetes Study (UKPDS) demonstrated similar results in people with type 2 diabetes. In fact, the UKPDS showed a 25% decrease in microvascular complications in clients receiving intensive therapy compared with those receiving conventional therapy. It also showed that aggressive treatment of blood pressure decreased strokes, heart failure, and diabetes-related deaths.

In addition to glycemic control, other measures can be used to help prevent end-stage renal disease. Administration of angiotensin-converting enzyme (ACE) inhibitors (eg, captopril) has protective effects on the kidneys in both type 1 and type 2 diabetes and in both normotensive and hypertensive people. Although ACE inhibitors are also used in the treatment of hypertension, their ability to delay nephropathy seems to be independent of antihypertensive effects. Additional measures to preserve renal function include effective treatment of hypertension, limited intake of dietary protein, prompt treatment of urinary tract infections, and avoidance of nephrotoxic drugs when possible.

Treatment Regimens

When possible, it is desirable to have an interdisciplinary diabetes care team (eg, physician, nurse diabetes educator, dietitian, and perhaps others) work with the client to design, monitor, and revise an individualized treatment plan. This is especially important for clients with newly diagnosed diabetes to assist them in learning to manage their disease and make appropriate lifestyle changes.

The best regimen for a particular client depends on the type of diabetes, the client's age and general condition, and the client's ability and willingness to comply with the prescribed therapy. In type 1 diabetes, the only effective treatment measures are insulin, diet, and exercise. In type 2, the initial treatment of choice is diet, exercise, and weight control. If this regimen is ineffective, oral agents or insulin may be added.

Guidelines for Insulin Therapy

Choice of Preparation

When insulin therapy is indicated, the physician may choose from several preparations that vary in composition, onset, duration of action, and other characteristics. Some factors to be considered include the following:

• Human insulin is preferred for newly diagnosed type 1 diabetes, gestational diabetes, poorly controlled diabetes, and clients having surgery or an illness that requires short-term insulin therapy. Human insulin is less likely to cause allergic reactions and insulin antibody formation.
• Isophane insulin (NPH) or insulin zinc suspension (Lente) is often used for long-term insulin therapy. NPH is more commonly used.
• Regular insulin (insulin injection) has a rapid onset of action and can be given IV. Therefore, it is the insulin

of choice during acute situations, such as DKA, severe infection or other illness, and surgical procedures.

- For many clients, a combination of regular insulin and an intermediate-acting insulin, most often NPH, provides more consistent control of blood glucose levels. Although several regimens are used, a common one is a mixture of regular and NPH insulins administered before the morning and evening meals. A commercial mixture is more convenient and probably more accurate than a mixture prepared by a client or caregiver, if the proportions of insulins are appropriate for the client.
- For clients with local or systemic manifestations of insulin allergy, the insulin of choice is human insulin.
- Insulin lispro may be used instead of SC regular insulin in most situations, but safe usage requires both health care providers and clients to be aware of its differences.

Dosage Factors

Dosage of insulin must be individualized according to blood glucose levels. The goal is to alleviate symptoms of hyperglycemia and reestablish metabolic balance without causing hypoglycemia. An initial dose of approximately 0.5 to 1 unit/kg/day may be started and then adjusted to maintain blood glucose levels (tested before meals and at bedtime) of 80 to 140 mg/dL. However, many factors influence blood glucose response to exogenous insulin and therefore influence insulin requirements.

- Factors that increase insulin requirements include weight gain; increased caloric intake; pregnancy; decreased activity; acute infections; hyperadrenocorticism (Cushing's disease); primary hyperparathyroidism; acromegaly; hypokalemia; and drugs such as corticosteroids, epinephrine, levothyroxine, and thiazide diuretics. Clients who are obese may require approximately 2 units/kg/day because of resistance to insulin in peripheral tissues.
- Factors that decrease insulin requirements include weight reduction; decreased caloric intake; increased physical activity; development of renal insufficiency; stopping administration of corticosteroids, epinephrine, levothyroxine, and diuretics; hypothyroidism; hypopituitarism; recovery from hyperthyroidism; recovery from acute infections; and the "honeymoon period," which sometimes occurs with type 1 diabetes.

Nursing Notes: Apply Your Knowledge

Your patient is managing his diabetes with the following split-dose insulin regimen:

Before breakfast (8 AM) 32 units of NPH
Before dinner (6 PM) 10 units of NPH

Using Table 27-1, calculate when this patient is most likely to experience hypoglycemia.

People who need less than 0.5 unit/kg/day may produce some endogenous insulin or their tissues may be more responsive to insulin because of exercise and good physical conditioning. Renal insufficiency decreases dosage requirements because less insulin is metabolized in the kidneys than with normal renal function. The honeymoon period, characterized by recovery of beta cell function and temporary production of insulin, may occur after diabetes is first diagnosed. Insulin requirements may decrease rapidly, and if the dosage is not decreased, severe hypoglycemic reactions may occur.

- In acute situations, dosage of regular insulin needs frequent adjustments based on measurements of blood glucose. When insulin is given IV in a continuous infusion, approximately 20% to 30% binds to the IV fluid container and the plastic infusion set.
- Dosage of insulin for long-term therapy is determined by blood glucose levels at various times of the day and adjusted when indicated (eg, because of illness or changes in physical activity). Titrating insulin dosage may be difficult and time consuming; it requires cooperation and collaboration between clients and health care providers.
- Insulin pumps have advantages and disadvantages and are used by relatively few people. These devices allow continuous SC administration of regular insulin. A basal amount of insulin is injected (eg, 1 unit/hour or a calculated fraction of the dose used previously) continuously, with bolus injections before meals. This method of insulin administration maintains more normal blood glucose levels and avoids wide fluctuations. Candidates for insulin pumps include clients with diabetes that is poorly controlled with other methods and those who are able and willing to care for the devices properly.

Timing of Insulin Administration

Many clients who take insulin seem to need at least two injections daily to control hyperglycemia. A common regimen is one half to two thirds of the total daily dose in the morning, before breakfast, and the remaining one half or one third before the evening meal or at bedtime. With regular insulin before meals, it is very important that the medication be injected 30 to 45 minutes before meals so that the insulin will be available when blood sugar increases after meals. With insulin lispro before meals, it is very important to inject the medication approximately 15 minutes before eating. If the client does not eat within 15 minutes, hypoglycemia may occur.

Selection of Subcutaneous Sites for Insulin Injections

Several factors affect insulin absorption from injection sites, including the site location, environmental temperature, and exercise or massage. Research studies indicate that insulin is absorbed fastest from the abdomen, followed by the deltoid, thigh, and hip. Because of these differences, many clinicians recommend rotating injection sites *within* areas (eg, using several sites in the abdomen before moving to another area) on a daily basis. This technique decreases rotations *between* areas and promotes more consistent blood glucose levels. With regard to temperature, insulin is absorbed more rapidly in warmer sites and environments. In relation to exercise, people who exercise should avoid injecting insulin into SC tissue near the muscles to be used. The increased blood flow that accompanies exercise promotes rapid absorption and may lead to hypoglycemia.

Timing of Food Intake

Clients receiving insulin need food at the peak action time of the insulin and at bedtime. The food is usually taken as a between-meal and a bedtime snack. These snacks help prevent hypoglycemic reactions between meals and at night. When hypoglycemia occurs during sleep, recognition and treatment may be delayed. This delay may allow the reaction to become more severe.

Management of Diabetic Ketoacidosis

Insulin therapy is a major component of any treatment program for DKA. Clients with DKA have a deficiency in the total amount of insulin in the body and a resistance to the action of the insulin that is available, probably owing to acidosis, hyperosmolality, infection, and other factors. To be effective, insulin therapy must be individualized according to frequent measurements of blood glucose. Low doses, given by continuous IV infusion, are preferred in most circumstances.

Additional measures include identification and treatment of conditions that precipitate DKA, administration of IV fluids to correct hyperosmolality and dehydration, administration of potassium supplements to restore and maintain normal serum potassium levels, and administration of sodium bicarbonate to correct metabolic acidosis. Infection is one of the most common and important causes of DKA. If no obvious source of infection is identified, cultures of blood, urine, and throat swabs are recommended. When infection is identified, antibacterial drug therapy may be indicated.

Intravenous fluids, possibly the most important first step in treating DKA, usually consist of 0.9% sodium chloride, an isotonic solution. Hypotonic solutions are usually avoided because they allow intracellular fluid shifts and may cause cerebral, pulmonary, and peripheral edema.

Although serum potassium levels may be normal at first, they fall rapidly after insulin and IV fluid therapy are begun. Decreased serum potassium levels are caused by expansion of extracellular fluid volume, movement of potassium into cells, and continued loss of potassium in the urine as long as hyperglycemia persists. For these reasons, potassium supplements are usually added to IV fluids. Because both hypokalemia and hyperkalemia can cause serious cardiovascular disturbances, dosage of potassium supplements must be based on frequent measurements of serum potassium levels. Also, continuous or frequent electrocardiogram monitoring is recommended.

Severe acidosis can cause serious cardiovascular disturbances, which usually stem from peripheral vasodilation and decreased cardiac output with hypotension and shock. Acidosis usually can be corrected by giving fluids and insulin; sodium bicarbonate may be given if the pH is less than 7.2. If used, sodium bicarbonate should be given slowly and cautiously. Rapid alkalinization can cause potassium to move into body cells faster than it can be replaced IV. The result may be severe hypokalemia and cardiac arrhythmias. Also, giving excessive amounts of sodium bicarbonate can produce alkalosis.

Treatment of the Unconscious Client

When a person with diabetes becomes unconscious and it cannot be determined whether the unconsciousness is caused by DKA or by hypoglycemia due to the effects of insulin (ie, by measuring blood glucose levels), the client should be treated for hypoglycemia. If hypoglycemia is the cause of unconsciousness, giving some form of glucose may avert brain damage, which results from severe, prolonged hypoglycemia. If DKA is the cause of unconsciousness, giving glucose does not harm the client. Sudden unconsciousness in a client who takes insulin is most likely to result from an insulin reaction; DKA usually develops gradually over several days or even weeks.

Hyperosmolar Hyperglycemic Nonketotic Coma

Treatment of HHNC is similar to that of DKA in that insulin, IV fluids, and potassium supplements are major components. Regular insulin is given by continuous IV infusion, and dosage is individualized according to frequent measurements of blood glucose levels. IV fluids are given to correct the profound dehydration and hyperosmolality, and potassium is given IV to replace the large amounts lost in urine during a hyperglycemic state.

Perioperative Insulin Therapy

Clients with diabetes who undergo major surgery have increased risks of both surgical and diabetic complications. Risks associated with surgery and anesthesia are greater if diabetes is not well controlled and complications of diabetes (eg, hypertension, nephropathy, vascular damage) are already evident. Hyperglycemia and poor metabolic control are associated with increased susceptibility to infection, poor wound healing, and fluid and electrolyte imbalances. Risks of diabetic complications are increased because the stress of surgery increases insulin requirements and may precipitate DKA. Metabolic responses to stress include increased secretion of catecholamines, cortisol, glucagon, and growth hormone, all of which increase blood sugar levels. In addition to hyperglycemia, protein breakdown, lipolysis, ketogenesis, and insulin resistance occur. The risk of hypoglycemia is also increased.

The goals of treatment are to avoid hypoglycemia, severe hyperglycemia, ketoacidosis, and fluid and electrolyte imbalances. In general, mild hyperglycemia (eg, blood glucose levels between 150 and 250 mg/dL) is considered safer for the client than hypoglycemia, which may go unrecognized during anesthesia and surgery. Because surgery is a stressful event that increases blood glucose levels and the body's need for insulin, insulin therapy is usually required.

The goal of insulin therapy is to avoid ketosis from inadequate insulin and hypoglycemia from excessive insulin. Specific actions to reach this goal depend largely on the severity of diabetes and the type of surgical procedure. Diabetes should be well controlled before any type of surgery. Minor procedures usually require little change in the usual treatment program; major operations usually require a different medication regimen.

As a general rule, regular, short-acting insulin is used with major surgery or surgery requiring general anesthesia. For clients who use an intermediate-acting insulin, a different regimen using regular insulin in doses approximating the usual daily requirement is needed. For clients who usually manage their diabetes with diet alone or with diet and oral medications, insulin therapy may be started. Human insulin is preferred for temporary use to minimize formation of insulin antibodies. Small doses are usually required.

For elective major surgery, clients should be scheduled early in the day to avoid prolonged fasting. In addition, most authorities recommend omitting usual doses of insulin on the day of surgery and oral antidiabetic medications for 1 or 2 days before surgery. While the client is receiving nothing by mouth, before and during surgery, IV insulin is usually given. Along with the insulin, clients need adequate sources of carbohydrate. This is usually supplied by IV solutions of 5% or 10% dextrose.

After surgery, IV insulin and dextrose may be continued until the client is able to eat and drink. Regular insulin also can be given SC every 4 to 6 hours, with frequent blood glucose measurements. Oral fluids and foods that contain carbohydrate should be resumed as soon as possible. When meals are fully tolerated, the preoperative insulin or oral medication regimen can be resumed. Additional regular insulin can be given for elevated blood glucose and ketones, if indicated.

Guidelines for Using Oral Antidiabetic Drugs

Sulfonylureas

- Sulfonylureas are not effective in all clients with type 2 diabetes mellitus. Even when carefully selected, many clients experience primary or secondary treatment failure. Primary failure involves a lack of initial response to the drugs. Secondary failure means that a therapeutic response occurs when the drugs are first given, but the drugs eventually become ineffective.

How Can You Avoid This Medication Error?

Mrs. Julliet, who has been insulin dependent for 15 years, is admitted to your unit for elective surgery. She usually takes 20 units of NPH every morning. Her physician writes the following orders after surgery regarding her insulin and diet.

[handwritten orders]
Cl liq → diet as Tol
80 NPH insulin AC dinner
Sliding Scale Coverage
201–250   5 u Reg
251–300   100 Reg
300–351   120 Reg
> 351   Call MD

By dinner, Mrs. Julliet's postoperative condition has stabilized. She is taking clear liquids and has not experienced any nausea. Her 5 PM blood glucose level was 116 mg/dL. The nurse orders her a full liquid tray for dinner and gives her 80 units of NPH insulin at 5:30 PM.

Identify the error that has occurred.

What could the nurse have done to prevent it?

What could the physician have done to prevent it?

After the error has occurred, what needs to be done to keep the patient safe?

The reasons for secondary failure are unclear but may include decreased compliance with diet and exercise instructions, failure to take the drugs as prescribed, or decreased ability of the pancreatic beta cells to produce more insulin in response to the drugs.

- These drugs must be used cautiously in clients with impaired renal or hepatic function.

- Dosage of sulfonylureas is usually started at low amounts and increased gradually until the fasting blood glucose level is 110 mg/dL or less. The lowest dose that achieves normal levels of both fasting and postprandial blood sugars is recommended.

- Sulfonylureas are not recommended for use during pregnancy because the drugs may cause fetal hypoglycemia and even death. Also, an increased risk of congenital anomalies is possible. A third reason is the risk that overt diabetes will develop in women with gestational diabetes because the drugs stimulate an already overstimulated pancreas.

Alpha-Glucosidase Inhibitors

- Compared with other oral agents, the important differences are that these drugs do not alter insulin secretion and do not cause hypoglycemia.

- Acarbose and miglitol should be taken at the beginning of a meal so they will be present in the GI tract with food and able to block digestion of carbohydrates.

- Starting with low doses and increasing them gradually may help decrease GI upset (eg, bloating, flatulence, diarrhea) and promote client compliance.

- Clients taking acarbose and miglitol should continue their diet, exercise, and blood glucose testing routines. During initiation and dosage titration, the client's response can be monitored by measuring 1-hour postprandial blood glucose levels. During long-term therapy, measurement of glycosylated hemoglobin is recommended approximately every 3 months to evaluate glycemic control. The goal of treatment is to lower the postprandial blood glucose and glycosylated hemoglobin levels to normal or near normal.

Biguanide

- Renal function should be assessed before starting metformin and at least annually during long-term therapy. The drug should not be given initially if renal impairment is present; it should be stopped if renal impairment occurs during treatment.
- As with other antidiabetic drugs, clients taking metformin should continue their diet, exercise, and blood glucose testing regimens. During initiation and dosage titration, the client's response can be monitored by measuring blood glucose levels. During long-term therapy, measurement of glycosylated hemoglobin is recommended approximately every 3 months to evaluate glycemic control. The goal of treatment is to lower the fasting blood glucose and the glycosylated hemoglobin levels to normal or near normal.
- Parenteral radiographic contrast media containing iodine (eg, Cholografin, Hypaque, Omnipaque) may cause renal failure, and they have been associated with lactic acidosis in clients receiving metformin. Metformin should be discontinued at least 48 hours before diagnostic tests are performed with these materials and should not be resumed for at least 48 hours after the tests are done and tests indicate renal function is normal.

Glitazones

Liver function tests (eg, serum aminotransferase enzymes) should be checked before starting therapy and periodically thereafter.

Combination Drug Therapy for Type 2 Diabetes

Combination drug therapy is an increasing trend in type 2 diabetes that is not controlled by diet and exercise or by diet, exercise, and single-drug therapy. Useful combinations include drugs with different mechanisms of action, and the potential for rational combinations has greatly increased with the development of newer types of antidiabetic drugs. However, clinical experience with some combinations is limited, and guidelines for optimal therapy are still being defined. Most studies have involved combinations of two drugs; some three-drug combinations are also being used. All combination therapy should

be monitored with periodic measurements of fasting plasma glucose and glycosylated hemoglobin levels. If adequate glycemic control is not achieved, oral drugs may need to be discontinued and insulin therapy started. Two-drug combinations include the following:

- **Insulin plus a sulfonylurea**. Advantages include lower fasting blood glucose levels, decreased glycosylated hemoglobin levels, increased secretion of endogenous insulin, smaller daily doses of insulin, and no significant change in body weight. The role of insulin lispro (Humalog) in combination therapy is not clear. One regimen, called BIDS, uses bedtime insulin, usually NPH, with a daytime sulfonylurea, usually glyburide.
- **Insulin plus pioglitazone**. Pioglitazone increases the effectiveness of insulin, whether endogenous or exogenous.
- **Sulfonylurea plus acarbose or miglitol**. This combination is FDA approved for clients who do not achieve adequate glycemic control with one of the drugs alone.
- **Sulfonylurea plus metformin**. Glimepiride is FDA approved for this combination.
- **Sulfonylurea plus a glitazone**. The sulfonylurea increases insulin and the glitazone increases insulin effectiveness.
- **Metformin plus repaglinide**. If one of the drugs alone does not produce adequate glycemic control, the other one may be added. Dosage of each drug should be titrated to the minimal dose required to achieve the desired effects.

Effects of Illness on Diabetes Care

Various illnesses develop in people with diabetes that may affect diabetes control in several ways. First, illness causes a stress response. Part of the stress response is increased secretion of glucagon, epinephrine, growth hormone, and cortisol, hormones that raise blood glucose levels (by stimulating gluconeogenesis and inhibiting insulin action) and cause ketosis (by stimulating lipolysis and ketogenesis). Second, if the illness makes a person unable or unwilling to eat, hypoglycemia can occur. Third, if the illness affects GI function (eg, causes vomiting or diarrhea), the person may be unable to drink enough fluids to prevent dehydration and electrolyte imbalance. In addition, hyperglycemia induces an osmotic diuresis that increases dehydration and electrolyte imbalances.

As a result of these potentially serious effects, an illness that would be minor in people without diabetes may become a major illness or medical emergency in people with diabetes. Everyone involved should be vigilant about recognizing and seeking prompt treatment for any illness. In addition, clients with diabetes (or their caregivers) should be taught how to adjust their usual regimens to maintain metabolic balance and prevent severe complications. The main goal during illness is to prevent complications such as severe hyperglycemia, dehydration, and DKA.

Use in Children

Type 1 Diabetes

Insulin is the only drug indicated for use in type 1 diabetes. It is required as replacement therapy because children cannot produce insulin. Factors that influence management and insulin therapy include the following:

- Effective management requires a consistent schedule of meals, snacks, blood glucose monitoring, insulin injections and dose adjustments, and exercise. Such a schedule is difficult to maintain in children, but extremely important in promoting normal growth and development. A major factor in optimal treatment is a supportive family in which at least one member is thoroughly educated about the disease and its management. Less-than-optimal treatment can lead to stunted growth; delayed puberty; and early development of complications such as retinopathy, nephropathy, or neuropathy.

- Infections and other illnesses may cause wide fluctuations in blood glucose levels and interfere with metabolic control. For example, some infections cause hypoglycemia; others, especially chronic infections, may cause hyperglycemia and insulin resistance and may precipitate ketoacidosis. As a result, insulin requirements may vary widely during illness episodes and should be based on blood glucose and urine ketone levels. Hypoglycemia often develops in young children, partly because of anorexia and smaller glycogen reserves.

- During illness, children with type 1 diabetes are highly susceptible to dehydration, and an adequate fluid intake is very important. Many clinicians recommend sugar-containing liquids (eg, regular sodas, clear juices, regular gelatin desserts) if blood glucose values are lower than 250 mg/dL. When blood glucose values are above 250 mg/dL, diet soda, unsweetened tea, and other fluids without sugar should be given.

- For infants and toddlers who weigh less than 10 kg or require less than 5 units of insulin per day, a diluted insulin can be used because such small doses are hard to measure in a U-100 syringe. The most common dilution is U-10, and a diluent is available from insulin manufacturers. Vials of diluted insulin should be clearly labeled and discarded after 1 month.

- Rotation of injection sites is important in infants and young children because of the relatively small areas for injection at each anatomic site and to prevent lipodystrophy.

- Young children usually adjust to injections and blood glucose monitoring better when the parents express less anxiety about these vital procedures.

- Avoiding hypoglycemia is a major goal in infants and young children because of potentially damaging effects on growth and development. For example, the brain and spinal cord do not develop normally without an available source of glucose. Animal studies indicate that prolonged hypoglycemia results in decreased brain weight, numbers of neurons, and protein content. Myelinization of nerve cells is also decreased. Because complex motor and intellectual functions require an intact central nervous system, frequent, severe, or prolonged hypoglycemia can be a serious problem in infants, toddlers, and preschoolers. In addition, recognition of hypoglycemia may be delayed because signs and symptoms are vague and the children may be unable to communicate them to parents or caregivers. Because of these difficulties, most pediatric diabetologists recommend maintaining blood glucose levels between 100 and 200 mg/dL to prevent hypoglycemia. In addition, *the bedtime snack and blood glucose measurement should never be skipped.*

- Signs and symptoms of hypoglycemia in older children are similar to those in adults (eg, hunger, sweating, tachycardia). In young children, hypoglycemia may be manifested by changes in behavior, including severe hunger, irritability, and lethargy. In addition, mental functioning may be impaired in all age groups, even with mild hypoglycemia. Anytime hypoglycemia is suspected, blood glucose should be tested.

- Adolescents with type 1 diabetes may resist adhering to their prescribed treatment regimens, and effective management may be especially difficult during this developmental period. Adolescents and young adults with type 1 diabetes may delay, omit, or decrease dosage of insulin to fit in socially (eg, by eating more, sleeping in, or drinking alcohol) or to control their weight. Omitting or decreasing insulin dosage may lead to repeated episodes of ketoacidosis.

Type 2 Diabetes

Type 2 diabetes is being increasingly identified in children. This trend is attributed mainly to obesity and inadequate exercise because most children with type 2 diabetes are seriously overweight and have poor eating habits. In addition, most are members of high-risk ethnic groups (eg, African American, Native American, or Hispanic) and have relatives with diabetes. These children are at high risk for development of serious complications during early adulthood, such as myocardial infarction during their fourth decade. Management involves exercise, weight loss, and a more healthful diet.

Use in Older Adults

General precautions for safe and effective use of antidiabetic drugs apply to older adults, including close monitoring of blood glucose levels. In addition, older adults may have impaired vision or other problems that decrease their ability to perform needed tasks (eg, self-administration of insulin, monitoring blood glucose levels, managing diet and exercise). They also may have other disorders and may take other drugs that complicate management of diabetes. For example, renal insufficiency may increase risks of adverse effects with antidiabetic drugs and treatment with thiazide diuretics, corticosteroids, estrogens, and other drugs may cause hyperglycemia, thereby increasing dosage requirements for antidiabetic drugs.

With oral sulfonylureas, drugs with a short duration of action and inactive metabolites are considered safer, especially with impaired liver or kidney function. Therapy usually should start with a low dose, which is then increased or decreased according to blood glucose levels and clinical response.

There has been little clinical experience with newer antidiabetic drugs in older adults. The insulin analog (Humalog) appears to have some advantages over conventional insulin. Acarbose, miglitol, and metformin may not be as useful in older adults as in younger ones because of the high prevalence of impaired renal function. These drugs are relatively contraindicated in clients with renal insufficiency because they have a longer half-life and may accumulate. With metformin, dosage should be based on periodic tests of renal function and the drug should be stopped if renal impairment occurs (ie, serum creatinine increases) or if serum lactate increases. In addition, dosage should not be titrated to the maximum amount recommended for younger adults. During clinical trials with repaglinide, no differences in therapeutic or adverse effects were found between clients older than 65 and those younger than 65 years of age.

Use in Renal Impairment

Insulin. Frequent monitoring of blood glucose levels and dosage adjustments may be needed. It is difficult to predict dosage needs because, on the one hand, less insulin is degraded by the kidneys (normally, approximately 25%) and this may lead to higher blood levels of insulin if dosage is not reduced. On the other hand, muscles and possibly other tissues are less sensitive to insulin and this insulin resistance may result in an increased blood glucose level if dosage is not increased. Overall, vigilance is required to prevent dangerous hypoglycemia, especially in clients whose renal function is unstable or worsening.

Sulfonylureas. These drugs and most of their metabolites are excreted by the kidneys. Renal impairment may lead to accumulation and hypoglycemia. These drugs should be used cautiously, with close monitoring of renal function, in clients with mild to moderate renal impairment, and are contraindicated in severe renal impairment.

Alpha-glucosidase inhibitors. These drugs are excreted by the kidneys and accumulate in clients with renal impairment. However, dosage reduction is not helpful because the drugs act locally, within the GI tract.

Metformin. Renal function should be assessed before starting metformin and at least annually during long-term therapy. The drug should not be given initially if renal impairment is present; it should be stopped if renal impairment occurs during treatment.

Repaglinide. Initial dosage adjustment are not needed, but increments should be made cautiously in clients with renal impairment or renal failure requiring hemodialysis.

Use in Hepatic Impairment

Insulin. There may be higher blood levels of insulin in clients with hepatic impairment because less insulin may be degraded. Careful monitoring of blood glucose levels and insulin dosage reductions may be needed to prevent hypoglycemia.

Sulfonylureas. These drugs should be used cautiously in clients with hepatic impairment, and liver function should be monitored. They are metabolized in the liver and hepatic impairment may result in higher serum drug levels and inadequate release of hepatic glucose in response to hypoglycemia. With glipizide, initial dosage should be reduced in clients with liver failure. Glyburide may cause hypoglycemia in clients with liver disease.

Alpha-glucosidase inhibitors. Acarbose is metabolized in the GI tract and miglitol is not metabolized. Thus, no precautions are recommended with hepatic impairment.

Metformin. This drug is not recommended for use in clients with clinical or laboratory evidence of hepatic impairment because risks of lactic acidosis may be increased.

Repaglinide. Serum drug levels are higher, for a longer period of time, in clients with moderate to severe hepatic impairment. The drug should be used cautiously and dosage increments should be made more slowly, at longer intervals.

Glitazones. Troglitazone (Rezulin), the first drug of this group, was taken off the market because of serious hepatotoxicity. Although pioglitazone and rosiglitazone are not expected to cause serious hepatotoxicity, caution is advised. Liver enzymes should be measured before starting a glitazone and the drug should *not* be given to clients with active liver disease or a serum alanine aminotransferase (ALT) >2.5 times the upper limit of normal. Once glitazone therapy is initiated, liver enzymes should be measured every two months for 1 year, then periodically.

Use in Critical Illness

Insulin is more likely to be used in critical illness than any of the oral agents. Reasons include greater ability to titrate dosage needs in clients who are often debilitated and unstable, with varying degrees of cardiovascular, liver, and kidney impairment. One important consideration with IV insulin therapy is that 30% or more of a dose may adsorb into the container of IV fluid or the plastic infusion sets. In addition, many critically ill clients are unable to take oral drugs.

Overall, critically ill clients are at risk for development of serious hypoglycemia, especially if they are debilitated, sedated, or unable to recognize and communicate symptoms. Vigilant monitoring is essential for any client who has diabetes and a critical illness.

 ## Home Care

Most diabetes care is delivered in ambulatory care settings or in the home, and any client with diabetes may need home care. Hospitalization usually occurs only for complications, and clients are quickly discharged if pos-sible. The home care nurse may need to assist clients of multiple age groups to learn self-care and assist caregivers to support client efforts or actively participate in diabetes management. Some aspects of the nursing role include mobilizing and coordinating health care providers and community resources, teaching and supporting clients and caregivers, monitoring the client's health status and progress in disease management, and preventing or solving problems.

The person with diabetes has a tremendous amount of information to learn about living with this disease on a day-to-day basis. For most clients, the goal of diabetes education is self-care in terms of diet, exercise, medication administration, blood glucose monitoring, and prevention, recognition, and treatment of complications. For some clients, a parent or caregiver may assume most of the responsibility for diabetes management. Because of the amount and complexity of information, a multidisciplinary health care team that includes a nurse diabetes educator is preferred in home care as in other settings. The role of the home care nurse may include initial teaching or reinforcement and follow-up of teaching done by others.

(*text continues on page 406*)

NURSING ACTIONS **Antidiabetic Drugs**

NURSING ACTIONS	RATIONALE/EXPLANATION
1. Administer accurately	
a. With insulin:	
(1) Store the insulin vial in current use and administer insulin at room temperature. Refrigerate extra vials.	Cold insulin is more likely to cause lipodystrophy, local sensitivity reactions, discomfort, and delayed absorption. Insulin preparations are stable for months at room temperature if temperature extremes are avoided.
(2) Avoid freezing temperatures (32°F) or high temperatures (95°F or above).	Extremes of temperature decrease insulin potency and cause clumping of the suspended particles of modified insulins (all except regular insulin). This clumping phenomenon causes inaccurate dosage even if the volume is accurately measured.
(3) Use only an insulin syringe calibrated to measure U-100 insulin.	For accurate measurement of the prescribed dose.
(4) With NPH and Lente insulins, be sure they are mixed to a uniform cloudy appearance before drawing up a dose.	These insulin preparations are suspensions, and the components separate on standing. Unless the particles are resuspended in the solution and distributed evenly, dosage will be inaccurate.
(5) When regular and NPH insulins must be mixed, prepare as follows:	It is important that the insulins be drawn up in the same sequence every time. Most authorities recom-

(continued)

NURSING ACTIONS	RATIONALE/EXPLANATION
(a) Draw into the insulin syringe the amount of air equal to the total amount of both insulins. (b) Draw up the regular insulin first. Inject the equivalent portion of air, and aspirate the ordered dose. (c) With the NPH vial, insert the remaining air (avoid injecting regular insulin into the NPH vial), and aspirate the ordered dose. (d) Expel air bubbles, if present, and verify that the correct dosage is in the syringe.	mend that regular insulin *always* be drawn up first. This avoids contamination of the regular insulin with the NPH. Because regular insulin combines with excess protamine in NPH, the concentration of regular insulin is changed when they are mixed. Following the same sequence also leaves the same type of insulin in the needle and syringe (dead space) every time. Although dead space is not usually considered a significant factor with available insulin syringes, it may be with small doses.
(e) Administer the combined insulins *consistently* within 15 min of mixing or after a longer period; that is, do not give one dose within 15 min of mixing and another 2 h or days after mixing.	As stated previously, regular insulin combines with excess protamine when combined with NPH insulin. This reaction, which occurs within 15 min of mixing, alters the amount of regular insulin present. After approximately 15 min, the mixture is stable for approximately 1 month at room temperature and 3 months when refrigerated. Thus, to administer the same dose consistently, the mixture must be given at approximately the same time interval after mixing. NPH and regular insulins are most often combined.
(6) Rotate injection sites systematically, and use all available sites. These include the thighs, abdomen, upper back, upper arms, and buttocks unless some of these locations are contraindicated.	Frequent injection in the same site can cause tissue fibrosis, erratic absorption, and deposits of unabsorbed insulin. Also, if insulin is usually injected into fibrotic tissue where absorption is slow, injection into healthy tissue may result in hypoglycemia because of more rapid absorption. Further, deposits of unabsorbed insulin may initially lead to hyperglycemia. If dosage is increased to control the apparent hyperglycemia, hypoglycemia may occur. In addition, a sudden increase in physical activity is likely to increase subcutaneous blood circulation, causing rapid absorption of insulin.
(7) Rotate sites within the same anatomic area (eg, abdomen) until all sites are used. Avoid random rotation between the abdomen and thigh or arm, for example.	Rates of absorption differ among anatomic sites, and random rotation increases risks of hypoglycemic reactions. Some authorities recommend giving all insulin injections in the abdomen.
(8) Inject insulin at a 90-degree angle into a subcutaneous pocket created by raising subcutaneous tissue away from muscle tissue. Avoid intramuscular injection.	Injection into a subcutaneous pocket is thought to produce less tissue irritation and better absorption than injection into subcutaneous tissue. Intramuscular injection should not be used because of rapid absorption.
b. With oral sulfonylureas: Give a single daily dose approximately 30 min before breakfast; give a second daily dose approximately 30 min before the evening meal.	To promote absorption and effective plasma levels. Most of these drugs are given once or twice daily.
c. With acarbose and miglitol: Give at the beginning of each main meal, three times daily.	These drugs must be in the gastrointestinal (GI) tract when carbohydrate foods are ingested.

(continued)

NURSING ACTIONS	RATIONALE/EXPLANATION
d. With metformin: Give two daily doses with morning and evening meals; give three daily doses with meals.	Giving with food decreases GI upset
e. With pioglitazone and rosiglitazone: Give once daily, without regard to meals	
f. With repaglinide: Give 15–30 min before meals. If the client does not eat a meal, omit that dose; if the client eats an extra meal, give an extra dose.	Dosage is individualized according to the levels of fasting blood glucose and glycosylated hemoglobin.
2. Observe for therapeutic effects	
a. Improved blood glucose levels (fasting, preprandial and postprandial) and glycosylated hemoglobin levels	The general goal of antidiabetic drug therapy is normal or near-normal blood glucose levels. However, specific targeted levels for individuals vary depending on intensity of treatment, risks of hypoglycemia, and other factors. Improved metabolic control can prevent or delay complications.
b. Absent or decreased ketones in urine (N = none)	In diabetes, ketonuria indicates insulin deficiency and impending diabetic ketoacidosis if preventive measures are not taken. Thus, always report the presence of ketones. In addition, when adequate insulin is given, ketonuria decreases. Ketonuria does not often occur with type 2 diabetes.
c. Absent or decreased pruritus, polyuria, polydipsia, polyphagia, and fatigue	These signs and symptoms occur in the presence of hyperglycemia. When blood sugar levels are lowered with antidiabetic drugs, they tend to subside.
d. Decreased complications of diabetes	
3. Observe for adverse effects	
a. With insulin and oral sulfonylureas:	
(1) Hypoglycemia	Hypoglycemia is more likely to occur with insulin than with oral agents and at peak action times of the insulin being used (eg, 2–3 h after injection of regular insulin; 8–12 h after injection of NPH or Lente insulins).
(a) Sympathetic nervous system activation—tachycardia, palpitations, nervousness, weakness, hunger, perspiration	The sympathetic nervous system is activated as part of the stress response to low blood glucose levels. Epinephrine and other hormones act to raise blood glucose levels.
(b) Central nervous system impairment—mental confusion, incoherent speech, blurred vision, double vision, headache, convulsions, coma	There is an inadequate supply of glucose for normal brain function.
b. With insulin:	
(1) Local insulin allergy—erythema, induration, itching at injection sites	Allergic reactions are less common with increased use of human insulin and decreased use of animal insulins.
(2) Systemic allergic reactions—skin rash, dyspnea, tachycardia, hypotension, angioedema, anaphylaxis	Infrequent; anaphylaxis is rare. If a severe systemic reaction occurs, skin testing and desensitization are usually required even if patients are switched from animal to human insulin.
(3) Lipodystrophy—atrophy and "dimpling" at injection site; hypertrophy at injection site	These changes in subcutaneous fat occur from too-frequent injections into the same site. They are less likely to occur with human insulin.

(continued)

NURSING ACTIONS	RATIONALE/EXPLANATION
c. With oral sulfonylureas:	
(1) Hypoglycemia—see above	Hypoglycemia occurs less commonly with oral agents than with insulin. It is more likely to occur in patients who are elderly, debilitated, or who have impaired renal and hepatic function.
(2) Allergic skin reactions—skin rash, urticaria, erythema, pruritus	These reactions may subside with continued use of the drug. If they do not subside, the drug should be discontinued.
(3) GI upset—nausea, heartburn	These are the most commonly reported adverse effects. If severe, reducing drug dosage usually relieves.
(4) Miscellaneous—fluid retention and hyponatremia; facial flushing if alcohol is ingested; hematologic disorders (hemolytic or aplastic anemia, leukopenia, thrombocytopenia, others)	These are less common adverse effects.
d. With acarbose and miglitol:	
GI symptoms—flatulence, diarrhea, abdominal pain	These are commonly reported. They are caused by the presence of undigested carbohydrate in the lower GI tract and usually subside with continued therapy.
e. With metformin:	
(1) GI effects—anorexia, nausea, vomiting, diarrhea, abdominal discomfort, decreased intestinal absorption of folate and vitamin B_{12}	GI symptoms are the most frequently reported adverse effects. They may be minimized by increasing drug dosage slowly and taking the drug with meals.
(2) Hypoglycemia	Hypoglycemia is uncommon when metformin is taken as the sole antidiabetic drug but may occur if taken with a sulfonylurea. It also occurs if taken with alcohol.
(3) Allergic skin reactions—eczema, pruritus, erythema, urticaria	
(4) Lactic acidosis—drowsiness, malaise, respiratory distress, bradycardia and hypotension (if severe), blood lactate levels above 5 mmol/L, blood pH below 7.35	A rare but serious adverse effect (approximately 50% fatal). Most likely with renal or hepatic impairment, advanced age, or hypoxia. This is a medical emergency that requires hospitalization for treatment. Hemodialysis is effective in correcting acidosis and removing metformin.
	Lactic acidosis may be prevented by monitoring plasma lactate levels and stopping the drug if they exceed 3 mmol/L. Other reasons to stop the drug include patients experiencing decreased renal or hepatic function, a prolonged fast, or a very low calorie diet. The drug should be stopped immediately if a patient has a myocardial infarction or septicemia.
f. With pioglitazone and rosiglitazone:	
(1) Upper respiratory infections—pharyngitis, sinusitis	The drugs were generally well tolerated in clinical trials. However, there is a potential for hepatotoxicity. They are structurally similarly to trogli-

(*continued*)

NURSING ACTIONS	RATIONALE/EXPLANATION
(2) Headache	tazone, a drug that was taken off the market because of hepatotoxicity.
(3) Edema	
(4) Anemia	
g. With repaglinide:	
(1) Hypoglycemia	If occurs, usually of mild to moderate intensity.
(2) Rhinitis, respiratory infection, influenza symptoms	These were the most commonly reported during clinical drug trials.
4. Observe for drug interactions	
a. Drugs that *increase* effects of insulin:	
(1) Oral sulfonylurea hypoglycemic agents	These agents are increasingly being used with insulin in the treatment of some patients with type 2 diabetes. The risks of hypoglycemia are probably greater with the combination but depend on the dosage of each drug and other factors that affect blood glucose levels.
(2) Alcohol	Increased hypoglycemia. Ethanol inhibits gluconeogenesis (in people with or without diabetes).
(3) Beta-adrenergic blocking agents (eg, propranolol, others)	These drugs increase hypoglycemia by inhibiting the effects of catecholamines on gluconeogenesis and glycogenolysis (effects that normally raise blood glucose levels in response to hypoglycemia). They also may mask signs and symptoms of hypoglycemia (eg, tachycardia, tremors) that normally occur with a hypoglycemia-induced activation of the sympathetic nervous system.
(4) Monoamine oxidase (MAO) inhibitors	These drugs may significantly potentiate and prolong insulin-induced hypoglycemia. Such a combination is hazardous and should be used very cautiously, if at all.
(5) Salicylates	Salicylates increase risks of hypoglycemia by increasing insulin secretion.
b. Drugs that *decrease* effects of insulin:	These drugs are often called *diabetogenic* because of their tendencies to raise blood sugar levels.
(1) Corticosteroids (eg, hydrocortisone)	Antagonize hypoglycemic effects, produce hyperglycemia.
(2) Diuretics (especially thiazide diuretics, such as hydrochlorothiazide)	These drugs antagonize hypoglycemic effects of insulin and may cause hyperglycemia.
(3) Epinephrine	This adrenergic drug tends to raise blood glucose levels and thereby antagonize hypoglycemic effects of insulin.
(4) Glucagon	In small doses, glucagon is used to counteract hypoglycemia induced by insulin. Glucagon raises blood glucose levels by converting liver glycogen to glucose.
(5) Oral contraceptives	Tend to raise blood glucose levels and thereby antagonize insulin effects. Insulin dosage may need to be increased.

(*continued*)

NURSING ACTIONS	RATIONALE/EXPLANATION
(6) Phenytoin (Dilantin)	Inhibits insulin secretion and may cause severe hyperglycemia.
(7) Propranolol (Inderal)	May inhibit insulin release
(8) Thyroid preparations (eg, levothyroxine [Synthroid])	May cause hyperglycemia
c. Drugs that *increase* effects of oral sulfonylureas:	
(1) Acarbose, miglitol, metformin, and pioglitazone	Either of these drugs may be used concomitantly with a sulfonylurea to improve glycemic control in patients with type 2 diabetes. There is an increased risk of hypoglycemia with the combination.
(2) Acidifying agents (eg, ascorbic acid) and probenecid (Benemid)	Increase effects by slowing the rate of urinary excretion.
(3) Alcohol	Additive hypoglycemia. If alcohol use is chronic and heavy, oral hypoglycemic agents may be metabolized more rapidly and *hyperglycemia* may occur.
(4) Allopurinol (Zyloprim), cyclophosphamide (Cytoxan), MAO inhibitors, sulfinpyrazone (Anturane); tetracyclines	Increase hypoglycemia, mechanisms unclear
(5) Anticoagulants, oral	Increase hypoglycemia by slowing metabolism of oral antidiabetic agents and possibly by decreasing their urinary excretion.
(6) Insulin	Additive hypoglycemia
(7) Salicylates (eg, aspirin) and sulfonamides	Increase hypoglycemia by displacing oral sulfonylureas from protein-binding sites
d. Drugs that *decrease* effects of oral sulfonylureas:	
(1) Alcohol	Heavy, chronic intake of alcohol induces metabolizing enzymes in the liver. This increases the rate of metabolism of oral sulfonylureas, shortens their half-lives, and may produce hyperglycemia.
(2) Beta-blocking agents	Decrease hypoglycemic effects, possibly by decreasing release of insulin in the pancreas
(3) Corticosteroids, diuretics, epinephrine, estrogens, and oral contraceptives	These drugs have hyperglycemic effects.
(4) Glucagon	Raises blood glucose levels. It is used to treat severe hypoglycemia induced by insulin or oral antidiabetic agents.
(5) Nicotinic acid	Large doses have a hyperglycemic effect.
(6) Phenytoin (Dilantin)	Inhibits insulin secretion and has hyperglycemic effects
(7) Rifampin	Increases the rate of metabolism of oral antidiabetic agents by inducing liver-metabolizing enzymes
(8) Thyroid preparations	Antagonize the hypoglycemic effects of oral antidiabetic drugs

(*continued*)

NURSING ACTIONS	RATIONALE/EXPLANATION
e. Drugs that *decrease* effects of acarbose and miglitol:	
(1) Digestive enzymes	Decrease effects and should not be used concomitantly
(2) Intestinal adsorbents (eg, charcoal)	Decrease effects and should not be used concomitantly
f. Drugs that *increase* effects of metformin:	
(1) Alcohol	Increases risk of hypoglycemia and lactic acidosis. Patients should avoid acute and chronic ingestion of excessive alcohol.
(2) Cimetidine	Increases risk of hypoglycemia. Cimetidine interferes with metabolism and increases blood levels of metformin.
(3) Furosemide	Increases blood levels of metformin
(4) Nifedipine	Apparently increases absorption of metformin
(5) Sulfonylurea hypoglycemic agents	The combination of these drugs is used therapeutically to improve control of hyperglycemia in type 2 diabetes but it also increases risk of hypoglycemia.
g. Drug that *increases* effects of pioglitazone:	Decreases metabolism of pioglitazone and may increase adverse effects
(1) Ketoconazole	
h. Drugs that *increase* effects of repaglinide:	
(1) Nonsteroidal anti-inflammatory drugs and other agents that are highly bound to plasma proteins	May displace repaglinide from binding sites, therefore increasing its blood level
(2) Beta blockers	
(3) Cimetidine, erythromycin, ketoconazole, miconazole	May inhibit hepatic metabolism of repaglinide and increase its blood levels
(4) Sulfonamides	
i. Drugs that *decrease* effects of repaglinide:	
(1) Adrenergics, corticosteroids, estrogens, niacin, oral contraceptives, thiazide diuretics	May cause hyperglycemia
(2) Carbamazepine, rifampin	Induce drug-metabolizing enzymes in liver, which leads to faster inactivation of repaglinide

Nursing Notes: Apply Your Knowledge

Answer: NPH is an intermediate-acting insulin that usually peaks 8 to 12 hours after administration. Hypoglycemia is most likely to occur before meals. The morning NPH is most likely to cause hypoglycemia before dinner and the evening NPH is likely to cause hypoglycemia after midnight, so diabetics need to eat an evening snack.

How Can You Avoid This Medication Error?

Answer:

Identify the error that occurred. The wrong dose of NPH insulin was administered.

What could the nurse have done to prevent the error? With a sound understanding of diabetes, the nurse should recognize that 80 units is a very high dose to administer to a postoperative client who is on clear liquids and has a blood sugar of 116 mg/dL. This could result in severe hypoglycemia. The nurse should question this dosage for this client. Insulin doses should always be double-checked by another nurse. If this had been done, perhaps the second nurse might have questioned the high dose.

What could the physician have done to prevent it? The physician needs to write medication orders clearly. His writing can be easily misinterpreted to be 80 rather than 8 units since units is not written out and the U looks like 0.

After the error has occurred, what needs to be done to keep the patient safe? Monitor blood glucose levels frequently (eg, q2h), especially when the NPH insulin is peaking. Have the patient inform you immediately if she experiences any signs and symptoms of hypoglycemia. Keep her IV patent and IV dextrose available should her blood sugar fall quickly.

REVIEW AND APPLICATION EXERCISES

1. What is the function of insulin in normal cellular metabolism?

2. What is the effect of insulin on blood glucose levels?

3. What are the effects of cortisol, epinephrine, glucagon, and growth hormone on blood glucose levels?

4. What are the major differences between type 1 and type 2 diabetes?

5. What are advantages and disadvantages of human insulin preparations?

6. What is the rationale for maintaining near-normal blood glucose levels?

7. What is the major risk of maintaining near-normal blood glucose levels?

8. At what blood glucose range is brain damage most likely to occur?

9. Compare regular, lispro, NPH, and Lente insulins in terms of onset, peak, and duration of action.

10. In a diabetic client with typical signs and symptoms, distinguish between manifestations of hyperglycemia and hypoglycemia.

11. Contrast the five types of oral hypoglycemic agents in terms of mechanisms of action, indications for use, contraindications to use, and adverse effects.

12. For an adult client newly diagnosed with type 2 diabetes, outline interventions to assist the client in learning self-care.

13. Prepare a teaching plan for a client starting insulin therapy and for a client starting an oral hypoglycemic drug.

SELECTED REFERENCES

American Diabetes Association. (1999). Insulin administration. *Diabetes Care, 22*(Suppl. 1), S83–S86.

Barrett, A., Licking, E., & Rae-Dupree, J. (1999). New weapons to cut diabetes' toll. *Business Week, March 29,* 58–60.

Buse, J.B. (1999). Overview of current therapeutic options in type 2 diabetes. *Diabetes Care, 22*(Suppl. 3), C65–C69.

Colman, E.G., Goldberg, A.P., & Katzel, L.I. (1997). Approach to the elderly patient with hyperglycemia and diabetes mellitus. In W.N. Kelley (Ed.), *Textbook of internal medicine,* 3rd ed., pp. 2488–2494. Philadelphia: Lippincott-Raven.

Cziraky, M.J., Mehra, I.V., Wilson, M.D., & Bakris, G.L. (1996). Current issues in treating the hypertensive patient with diabetes: Focus on diabetic nephropathy. *Annals of Pharmacotherapy, 30,* 791–798.

Davis, S.N. & Granner, D.K. (1996). Insulin, oral hypoglycemic agents, and the pharmacology of the endocrine pancreas. In J.G. Hardman, L.E. Limbird, P.B. Molinoff, & R.W. Ruddon (Eds.), *Goodman & Gilman's The pharmacological basis of therapeutics,* 9th ed., pp. 1487–1517. New York: McGraw-Hill.

Drug facts and comparisons. (Updated monthly). St Louis: Facts and Comparisons.

Fleming, D.R. (1999). Challenging traditional insulin injection practices. *American Journal of Nursing, 99*(2), 72–74.

Freeland, B.S. (1998). Diabetic ketoacidosis. *American Journal of Nursing, 98*(8), 52.

Guyton, A.C. & Hall, J.E. (1996). *Textbook of medical physiology,* 9th ed. Philadelphia: W.B. Saunders.

Guven, S. & Kuenzi, J. (1998). Diabetes mellitus. In C.M. Porth (Ed.), *Pathophysiology: Concepts of altered health states,* 5th ed., pp. 805–830. Philadelphia: Lippincott Williams & Wilkins.

Hernandez, D. (1998). Microvascular complications of diabetes: Nursing assessment and intervention. *American Journal of Nursing, 98*(6), 26–31.

Kappel, C. & Dills, D.G. (1998). Type 2 diabetes: Update on therapy. *Comprehensive Therapy, 24,* 319–326.

Maffeo, R. (1997). Helping families cope with type 1 diabetes. *American Journal of Nursing, 97*(6), 36–39.

Noble, S.L., Johnston, E., & Walton, B. (1998). Insulin lispro: A fast-acting insulin analog. *American Family Physician, 57,* 279–286.

Orland, M.J. (1998). Diabetes mellitus and related disorders. In C.F.Carey, H.H. Lee, & K.F. Woeltje (Eds.), *The Washington manual of medical therapeutics,* 29th ed., pp. 396–417. Philadelphia: Lippincott Williams & Wilkins.

Portyansky, E. (1998). New treatment strategies take aim at type 2 diabetes. *Drug Topics* (Suppl., Oct.), S12–S14.

Reusch, J.E. (1998). Focus on insulin resistance in type 2 diabetes: Therapeutic implications. *The Diabetes Educator, 24*(2), 188–193.

Savinetti-Rose, B. & Bommer, L. (1997). Understanding continuous subcutaneous insulin infusion therapy. *American Journal of Nursing, 97*(3), 42–48.

Setter, S.M. & Campbell, R.K. (1998). Type 1 diabetes: New treatment options and strategies for care. *Drug Topics* (Suppl., Oct.), S4–S10.

Skyler, J.S. (1997). Approach to hyperglycemia in the patient with diabetes mellitus. In W.N. Kelley (Ed.), *Textbook of internal medicine,* 3rd ed., pp. 2155–2165. Philadelphia: Lippincott-Raven.

28

Estrogens, Progestins, and Oral Contraceptives

Objectives

After studying this chapter, the student should be able to:

1. Discuss effects of endogenous estrogens and progestins.

2. Describe benefits of postmenopausal hormone replacement therapy.

3. Differentiate between estrogen replacement therapy and hormone replacement therapy.

4. Describe adverse effects associated with estrogens, progestins, and oral contraceptives.

5. Apply nursing process with clients taking estrogens, progestins, and oral contraceptives.

Sally Chow, a perimenopausal woman, has concerns about hormone replacement therapy (HRT). She seeks information from you to help her make an informed choice whether to use HRT.

Reflect on:

▶ Benefits of HRT for the postmenopausal woman.

▶ Possible adverse effects of HRT for the post-menopausal woman.

▶ Teaching strategies helpful in teaching Ms. Chow about HRT.

▶ As a nurse, your role in assisting Ms. Chow in her decision-making process.

Estrogens and progestins are female sex hormones produced primarily by the ovaries and secondarily by the adrenal cortices in nonpregnant women. Small amounts of estrogens are also synthesized in the liver, kidney, brain, skeletal muscle, testes, and adipose tissue. In normal premenopausal women, estrogen synthesis in adipose tissue may be a significant source of the hormone. Some evidence indicates that a minimum body weight (approximately 105 lbs.) and fat content (16% to 24%) are required for initiation and maintenance of the menstrual cycle. This view is supported by the observation that women with anorexia nervosa, chronic disease, or malnutrition and those who are long-distance runners usually have amenorrhea. With anorexia nervosa, regaining weight and body mass usually reestablishes normal menstrual patterns.

Small amounts of progesterone are secreted by the testes and adrenal glands. In men and postmenopausal women, the peripheral sites produce all endogenous estrogen. Almost no progesterone is synthesized in postmenopausal women.

Like other steroid hormones, estrogens and progestins are synthesized from cholesterol. The ovaries and adrenal glands can manufacture cholesterol or extract it from the blood. Through a series of chemical reactions, cholesterol is converted to progesterone, then to the androgens, testosterone and androstenedione. These male sex hormones are used by the ovaries to produce estrogens. After formation, the hormones are secreted into the bloodstream in response to stimulation by the anterior pituitary gonadotropic hormones, follicle-stimulating hormone (FSH) and luteinizing hormone (LH). In the bloodstream, the hormones combine with serum proteins and are transported to target tissues where they enter body cells. They cross cell membranes easily because of their steroid structure and lipid solubility. Once inside the cells, they bind to estrogen or progestin receptors and regulate intracellular protein synthesis. Estrogen can enhance target tissue responses to progesterone by increasing progesterone receptors. Progesterone seems to inhibit tissue responses to estrogen by decreasing estrogen receptors.

ESTROGENS

Three ovarian estrogens (estradiol, estrone, and estriol) are secreted in significant amounts. Estradiol is the major estrogen because it exerts more estrogenic activity than the other two combined. The main function of the estrogens is to promote growth in tissues related to reproduction and sexual characteristics in the woman. More specific effects of estrogens on body tissues are described in Box 28-1.

In nonpregnant women, between puberty and menopause, estrogens are secreted in a monthly cycle called the menstrual cycle. During the first half of the cycle, before ovulation, estrogens are secreted in progressively larger amounts. During the second half of the cycle, estrogens and progesterone are secreted in increasing amounts until approximately 2 days before the onset of menstruation. At that time, secretion of both hormones decreases abruptly. When the endometrial lining of the uterus loses its hormonal stimulation, it is discharged vaginally as menstrual flow.

During pregnancy, the placenta produces large amounts of estrogen, mainly estriol. The increased estrogen causes enlargement of the uterus and breasts, growth of glandular tissue in the breasts, and relaxation of ligaments and joints in the pelvis. All these changes are necessary for growth and birth of the fetus.

Finally, estrogens are inactivated in the liver. They are conjugated with glucuronic acid or sulfuric acid, which makes them water soluble and readily excreted through the kidneys. Metabolites are also formed in the gastrointestinal tract, brain, skin, and other steroid target tissues. Approximately 80% of the conjugates are excreted in urine, with the remainder excreted in bile, where they may be reabsorbed and recirculated (enterohepatic recirculation) before they are eliminated from the body.

PROGESTERONE

Progesterone is a progestin concerned almost entirely with reproduction. In the nonpregnant woman, progesterone is secreted by the corpus luteum during the last half of the menstrual cycle, after ovulation. This hormone continues the changes in the endometrial lining of the uterus begun by estrogens during the first half of the menstrual cycle. These changes provide for implantation and nourishment of a fertilized ovum. When fertilization does not take place, the levels of estrogen and progesterone decrease, and menstruation occurs.

If the ovum is fertilized, progesterone acts to maintain the pregnancy. The corpus luteum produces progesterone during the first few weeks of gestation. Then, the placenta produces the progesterone needed to maintain the endometrial lining of the uterus. In addition to its effects on the uterus, progesterone prepares the breasts for lactation by promoting development of milk-producing cells. Milk is not secreted, however, until the cells are further stimulated by prolactin from the anterior pituitary gland. Progesterone also may help maintain pregnancy by decreasing uterine contractility. This, in turn, decreases the risk of spontaneous abortion.

Progesterone, in general, has opposite effects on lipid metabolism compared with estrogen. That is, progestins decrease high-density lipoprotein (HDL) cholesterol and increase low-density lipoprotein (LDL) cholesterol, both of which increase risks of cardiovascular disease. Physiologic progesterone increases insulin levels but does not usually impair glucose tolerance. However, long-term administration of potent synthetic progestins such as norgestrel may decrease glucose tolerance and make diabetes mellitus more difficult to control. Like estrogen, progesterone is metabolized in the liver.

BOX 28–1 EFFECTS OF ENDOGENOUS ESTROGENS

Breasts

- Stimulate growth at puberty by causing deposition of fat, formation of connective tissue, and construction of ducts. These ducts become part of the milk-producing apparatus after additional stimulation by progesterone.

Sexual Organs

- Enlarge the fallopian tubes, uterus, vagina, and external genitalia at puberty, when estrogen secretion increases greatly.
- Cause the endometrial lining of the uterus to proliferate and develop glands that later nourish the implanted ovum when pregnancy occurs.
- Increase resistance of the epithelial lining of the vagina to trauma and infection.

Skeleton

- Stimulate skeletal growth so that, beginning at puberty, height increases rapidly for several years. Estrogen then causes the epiphyses to unite with the shafts of the long bones, and linear growth is halted. This effect of estrogen is stronger than the similar effect of testosterone in the male. Consequently, women stop growing in height several years earlier than men and on the average are shorter than men.
- Conserve calcium and phosphorus for healthy bones and teeth. This action promotes bone formation and decreases bone loss.
- Broaden the pelvis in preparation for childbirth.

Skin and Subcutaneous Tissue

- Increase vascularity in the skin. This leads to greater skin warmth and likelihood of bleeding in women.

- Cause deposition of fat in subcutaneous tissue, especially in the breasts, thighs, and buttocks, which produces the characteristic female figure.

Anterior Pituitary Gland

- Decrease pituitary secretion of follicle-stimulating hormone and increase secretion of luteinizing hormone when blood levels are sufficiently high (negative feedback mechanism).

Metabolism

- Affect metabolism of both reproductive and nonreproductive tissues. Estrogen receptors are found in female reproductive organs, breast tissue, bone, the brain, liver, heart, and blood vessels. They are also found in various tissues in men.
- Increase protein anabolism, bone growth, and epiphyseal closure in young girls.
- Decrease bone resorption.
- Increase sodium and water retention, serum triglycerides, and high-density lipoproteins (HDL or "good" cholesterol because of cardioprotective effects).
- Decrease low-density lipoproteins (LDL or "bad" cholesterol because of cardiotoxic effects).
- Increase the amount of cholesterol in bile and thereby increase gallstone formation.

Blood Coagulation

- Enhance coagulation by increasing blood levels of several clotting factors, including prothrombin and factors VII, IX, and X, and probably increase platelet aggregation.

ESTROGENS AND PROGESTINS USED AS DRUGS

- When estrogens and progestins are given from exogenous sources as drugs for therapeutic purposes, they produce the same effects as endogenous (naturally occurring) hormones.
- Several preparations of estrogens and progestins are available for various purposes and routes of administration:
  - *Naturally occurring, nonconjugated estrogens* (estradiol, estrone) *and natural progesterone* are given intramuscularly because they are rapidly metabolized if given orally. Some crystalline suspensions of estrogens and oil solutions of both estrogens and progesterone prolong drug action by slowing absorption.
  - *Conjugated estrogens* (eg, Premarin) and some synthetic derivatives of natural estrogens (eg, ethinyl estradiol) and natural progesterone (eg, norethindrone) are chemically modified to be effective with oral administration. The most widely used synthetic steroidal estrogen is ethinyl estradiol, which is used in oral contraceptives (OCs). Ethinyl estradiol is better absorbed with oral administration and has a longer half-life than natural estrogen. It is excreted primarily in feces.
  - *Nonsteroidal, synthetic preparations* are usually given orally or topically. They are chemically altered to slow their metabolism in the liver. They are also less bound to serum proteins than the naturally occurring hormones.
- Most OCs consist of a synthetic estrogen (eg, ethinyl estradiol) and a synthetic progestin (eg, norethindrone). Monophasic contraceptives contain fixed

amounts of both components. Biphasics and triphasics contain either fixed amounts of estrogen and varied amounts of progestins or varied amounts of both estrogens and progestins. Biphasic and triphasic preparations mimic normal variations of hormone secretion, decrease the total dosage of hormones, and may decrease adverse effects.

These contraceptives are dispensed in containers with color-coded tablets that must be taken in the correct sequence. Dispensers with 28 tablets contain seven inactive or placebo tablets of a third color. A few contraceptive products contain a progestin only. These are not widely used because they are less effective in preventing pregnancy and are more likely to cause vaginal bleeding irregularities, which makes them less acceptable to many women.

Mechanisms of Action

The precise mechanisms by which estrogens and progestins produce their effects is unknown. Estrogens circulate briefly in the bloodstream before reaching target cells, where they enter the cells and combine with receptor proteins in cell cytoplasm. The estrogen–receptor complex then interacts with deoxyribonucleic acid (DNA) to produce ribonucleic acid and new DNA. These substances stimulate cell reproduction and production of various proteins. Progestins also diffuse freely into cells, where they bind to progesterone receptors.

Oral contraceptives act by several mechanisms. First, they inhibit hypothalamic secretion of gonadotropin-releasing hormone, which inhibits pituitary secretion of FSH and LH. When these gonadotropic hormones are absent, ovulation and therefore conception cannot occur. Second, the drugs produce cervical mucus that resists penetration of spermatozoa into the upper reproductive tract. Third, the drugs interfere with endometrial maturation and reception of ova that are released and fertilized. These overlapping mechanisms make the drugs highly effective in preventing pregnancy.

Indications for Use

Estrogens

- **As replacement therapy in deficiency states**. Deficiency states usually result from hypofunction of the pituitary gland or the ovaries and may occur anytime during the life cycle. For example, in the adolescent girl with delayed sexual development, estrogen can be given to produce the changes that normally occur at puberty. In the woman of reproductive age (approximately 12 to 45 years of age), estrogens are sometimes used in menstrual disorders, including amenorrhea and abnormal uterine bleeding due to estrogen deficiency.
- **As a component in birth control pills**. An estrogen, combined with a progestin, is used widely in the 12-

to 45-year age group to control fertility. If pregnancy does occur, estrogens are contraindicated because their use during pregnancy has been associated with the occurrence of vaginal cancer in female offspring and possible harmful effects on male offspring.
- **During menopause**. Estrogens are given to relieve atrophic vaginitis and vasomotor instability, which produces "hot flashes."
- **In postmenopausal women**. Estrogens are given to prevent or treat osteoporosis and to prevent cardiovascular disease (eg, myocardial infarction, stroke). When estrogen is given to women with a uterus, a progestin is also given to prevent endometrial cancer.

Progestins

Progestins are most often used in combination with an estrogen, in oral contraceptive pills and hormone replacement therapy (HRT) in postmenopausal women. In HRT, the purpose of a progestin is to prevent endometrial cancer. Progestins also are used to suppress ovarian function in dysmenorrhea, endometriosis, and uterine bleeding. These uses of oral progestins are extensions of the physiologic actions of progesterone on the neuroendocrine control of ovarian function and on the endometrium.

Hormonal Contraceptives

The primary clinical indication for the use of hormonal contraceptives is to control fertility and prevent pregnancy. Some products are used as postcoital contraceptives after unprotected sexual intercourse. These preparations also are used to treat various menstrual disorders, such as amenorrhea and dysmenorrhea.

Contraindications to Use

Because of their widespread effects on body tissues and reported adverse reactions, estrogens, progestins, and OCs are contraindicated in:

- Known or suspected pregnancy, because damage to the fetus may result
- Thromboembolic disorders, such as thrombophlebitis, deep vein thrombosis, or pulmonary embolism
- Known or suspected cancers of breast or genital tissues, because the drugs may stimulate tumor growth. An exception is the use of estrogens for treatment of metastatic breast cancer in women at least 5 years postmenopause.
- Undiagnosed vaginal or uterine bleeding
- Fibroid tumors of the uterus
- Active liver disease or impaired liver function
- History of cerebrovascular disease, coronary artery disease, thrombophlebitis, hypertension, or conditions predisposing to these disease processes
- Women older than 35 years of age who smoke cigarettes. These women have a greater risk of thrombo-

embolic disorders if they take OCs, possibly because of increased platelet aggregation with estrogen ingestion and cigarette smoking. In addition, estrogen increases hepatic production of blood clotting factors.

- Family history of breast or reproductive system cancer

INDIVIDUAL ESTROGENS, PROGESTINS, AND ORAL CONTRACEPTIVES

Table 28-1 lists the clinical indications, routes of administration, and dosages of estrogens. Table 28-2 provides the clinical indications, routes of administration, and

TABLE 28-1　Estrogens

Generic/Trade Name	Routes and Dosage Ranges for Various Indications			
	Menopausal Symptoms	Female Hypogonadism	Prevention of Osteoporosis	Other
Conjugated estrogens (synthetic) (Cenestin)	PO 0.625–1.25 mg daily			
Conjugated estrogens (Premarin)	PO 0.3–1.25 mg daily for 21 d followed by 7 d without the drug	PO 2.5–7.5 mg daily in divided doses, cyclically, 20 d on, 10 d off the drug	PO 0.625 mg daily for 21 d, then 7 d without the drug	Dysfunctional uterine bleeding: IM or intravenous for emergency use, 25 mg, repeated in 6–12 h if necessary Atrophic vaginitis: topically, 2.4 g of vaginal cream inserted daily
Dienestrol (DV)				Atrophic or senile vaginitis: topically, vaginal cream applied two or three times daily for approximately 2 wk, then reduced to three times weekly
Esterified estrogens (Estratab)	PO 0.3–1.25 mg daily for 21 d, then 7 d without the drug	PO 2.5–7.5 mg daily in divided doses, for 21 d, then 7 d without the drug		
Estradiol (Estrace)	PO 1–2 mg daily for 3 wk, then 1 wk off or daily Monday through Friday, none on Saturday or Sunday		PO 0.5 mg daily for 23 d and no drug for 5 d each month	
Estradiol cypionate (Depo-Estradiol)	IM 1–5 mg every 3–4 wk	IM 1.5–2 mg at monthly intervals		
Estradiol transdermal system (Estraderm)	Topically to skin, 1 patch one or two times weekly for 3 wk followed by 1 wk off (cyclically)	Same as for menopause	0.05 mg daily	
Estradiol valerate (Delestrogen)	IM 10–20 mg every 4 wk	IM 10–20 mg every 4 wk		
Estrone	IM 0.1–0.5 mg weekly in single or divided doses	IM 0.1–2 mg weekly		Dysfunctional uterine bleeding: IM 2–4 mg daily for several days until bleeding is controlled, followed by progestin for 1 wk
Estropipate (Ogen)	PO 0.625–5 mg daily, cyclically	PO 1.25–7.5 mg daily for 3 wk, followed by an 8- to 10-d rest period. Repeat as needed.	PO 0.625 mg daily 25 d, no drug 6 d each month	Ovarian failure: same dosage as for female hypogonadism Atrophic vaginitis: topically, 1–2 g vaginal cream daily
Ethinyl estradiol (Estinyl)	PO 0.02–0.05 mg daily, cyclically	PO 0.05 mg one to three times daily for 2 wk with addition of progestin for last 2 wk of month		

IM, intramuscular; PO, oral.

TABLE 28-2   **Progestins**

| Generic/Trade Name | Routes and Dosage Ranges for Various Indications | | | |
	Menstrual Disorders	Endometriosis	Endometrial Cancer	Other
Hydroxyproges-terone caproate (Hylutin)	Amenorrhea, dysfunctional uterine bleeding: IM 375 mg. If no bleeding after 21 d, begin cyclic therapy with estradiol and repeat every 4 wk for 4 cycles			Uterine adenocarcinoma: IM 1 g or more initially; repeat one or more times each week (maximum, 7 g/wk). Stop when relapse occurs or after 12 wk with no response. Test for endogenous estrogen production: IM 250 mg, repeated in 4 wk. Bleeding 7–14 d after injection indicates endogenous estrogen.
Medroxyproges-terone acetate (Depo-Provera, Provera)	Dysfunctional uterine bleeding: PO 5–10 mg daily for 5–10 d beginning on 16th or 21st d of cycle		IM 400–1000 mg weekly until improvement, then 400 mg monthly	
Megestrol acetate (Megace)	Amenorrhea: PO 5–10 mg daily for 5–10 d		PO 40–320 mg daily in four divided doses for at least 2 mo	Breast cancer: PO 160 mg daily in four divided doses for at least 2 months Contraception: See Table 28–3
Norethindrone acetate (Aygestin)	Amenorrhea, dysfunctional uterine bleeding: PO 2.5–10 mg daily, starting on 5th d of menstrual cycle and ending on 25th d	PO 5 mg daily for 2 wk, increased by 2.5 mg daily every 2 wk to dose of 15 mg. Then give 10–15 mg daily for maintenance.		
Progesterone	Amenorrhea, dysfunctional uterine bleeding: IM 5–10 mg for 6–8 consecutive d			

IM, intramuscular; PO, oral.

dosages of progestins. Oral contraceptive agents are listed in Table 28-3.

NURSING PROCESS

Assessment

Before drug therapy is started, clients need a thorough history and physical examination, including measurements of blood pressure, serum cholesterol, and triglycerides. These parameters must be monitored periodically as long as the drugs are taken.

- Assess for conditions in which estrogens and progestins are used (eg, menstrual disorders, menopausal symptoms).
- Assess for conditions that increase risks of adverse effects or are contraindications for hormonal therapy (eg, thromboembolic disorders, pregnancy).

- Record blood pressure with each outpatient contact or regularly with hospitalized clients. Increases are likely in premenopausal women, especially with OCs, but are unlikely in postmenopausal women who are receiving physiologic replacement doses.
- Check laboratory reports of cholesterol and triglyceride levels when available.
- Assess diet and presence of cigarette smoking. A high-fat diet increases the risks of gallbladder disease and perhaps other problems; cigarette smoking clearly increases risks of cardiovascular disease in women older than 35 years of age who take OCs.
- Assess the client's willingness to comply with instructions about drug therapy and follow-up procedures.
- Assess for signs and symptoms of thromboembolic disorders regularly. These are most likely to occur in women older than 35 years of

TABLE 28-3   Oral and Other Contraceptives

Trade Name	Phase	Estrogen (μg)	Progestin (mg)
Monophasics			
Brevicon		Ethinyl estradiol 35	Norethindrone 0.5
Demulen 1/35		Ethinyl estradiol 35	Ethynodiol diacetate 1
Demulen 1/50		Ethinyl estradiol 50	Ethynodiol diacetate 1
Desogen		Ethinyl estradiol 30	Desogestrel 0.15
Genora 1/35		Ethinyl estradiol 35	Norethindrone 1
Genora 1/50		Mestranol 50	Levonorgestrel 0.15
Levlen		Ethinyl estradiol 30	Levonorgestrel 0.15
Loestrin 21 1.5/30		Ethinyl estradiol 30	Norethindrone 1.5
Loestrin Fe 1/20		Ethinyl estradiol 20	Norethindrone 1
Loestrin Fe 1.5/30		Ethinyl estradiol 30	Norethindrone 1.5
Lo/Ovral		Ethinyl estradiol 30	Norethindrone 0.3
Modicon		Ethinyl estradiol 35	Norethindrone 0.5
N.E.E. 1/35		Ethinyl estradiol 35	Norethindrone 0.5
Nelova 0.5/35E		Ethinyl estradiol 35	Norethindrone 0.5
Nelova 1/35E		Ethinyl estradiol 35	Norethindrone 1
Nelova 1/50M		Mestranol 50	Norethindrone 1
Nordette		Ethinyl estradiol 30	Norethindrone 1
Norethin 1/35E		Ethinyl estradiol 35	Norethindrone 1
Norethin 1/50		Mestranol 50	Norethindrone 1
Norinyl 1 + 35		Ethinyl estradiol 35	Norethindrone 1
Norinyl 1 + 50		Mestranol 50	Norethindrone 1
Ortho-Cept		Ethinyl estradiol 30	Desogestrel 0.15
Ortho-Cyclen		Ethinyl estradiol 35	Norgestimate 0.25
Ortho-Novum 1/35		Ethinyl estradiol 35	Norethindrone 1
Ovcon-35		Ethinyl estradiol 35	Norethindrone 0.4
Ovral		Ethinyl estradiol 50	Norethindrone 0.5
Biphasics			
Jenest-28	I: 10 d	Ethinyl estradiol 35	Norethindrone 0.5
	II: 11 d	Ethinyl estradiol 35	Norethindrone 1
Nelova 10/11	I: 10 d	Ethinyl estradiol 35	Norethindrone 0.5
	II: 11 d	Ethinyl estradiol 35	Norethindrone 1
Ortho-Novum 10/11	I: 10 d	Ethinyl estradiol 35	Norethindrone 0.5
	II: 11 d	Ethinyl estradiol 35	Norethindrone 1
Triphasics			
Ortho-Novum 7/7/7	I: 7 d	Ethinyl estradiol 35	Norethindrone 0.5
	II: 7 d	Ethinyl estradiol 35	Norethindrone 0.75
	III: 7 d	Ethinyl estradiol 35	Norethindrone 1
Ortho Tri-Cyclen	I: 7 d	Ethinyl estradiol 35	Norgestimate 0.18
	II: 9 d	Ethinyl estradiol 35	Norgestimate 0.215
	III: 5 d	Ethinyl estradiol 35	Norgestimate 0.25
Tri-Levlen	I: 6 d	Ethinyl estradiol 30	Levonorgestrel 0.05
	II: 5 d	Ethinyl estradiol 40	Levonorgestrel 0.75
	III: 10 d	Ethinyl estradiol 30	Levonorgestrel 0.125
Tri-Norinyl	I: 7 d	Ethinyl estradiol 35	Norethindrone 0.5
	II: 9 d	Ethinyl estradiol 35	Norethindrone 1
	III: 5 d	Ethinyl estradiol 35	Norethindrone 0.5
Triphasil	I: 6 d	Ethinyl estradiol 30	Levonorgestrel 0.05
	II: 5 d	Ethinyl estradiol 40	Levonorgestrel 0.075
	III: 10 d	Ethinyl estradiol 30	Levonorgestrel 0.125
Progestin-Only Products			
Depo-Provera			Medroxyprogesterone 1.50
Micronor			Norethindrone 0.35
Norplant Subdermal System			Levonorgestrel 216
Nor-QD			Norethindrone 0.35
Ovrette			Norgestrel 0.075
Progestasert intrauterine			Progesterone 38

age who take OCs and women or men who take large doses for cancer; they have not been associated with postmenopausal estrogen replacement therapy (ERT).

Nursing Diagnoses

- Body Image Disturbance in women, related to effects of hormone deficiency states
- Body Image Disturbance in men, related to feminizing effects and impotence from female hormones
- Altered Tissue Perfusion related to thromboembolic effects of oral contraceptives
- Fluid Volume Excess related to sodium and water retention
- Knowledge Deficit: Effects of hormonal therapy
- Risk for Injury related to increased risks of hypertension and gallbladder disease

Planning/Goals

The client will:

- Be assisted to cope with self-concept and body image changes
- Take the drugs accurately, for the length of time prescribed
- Experience relief of symptoms for which the drugs are given
- Avoid preventable adverse drug effects
- Keep appointments for monitoring of drug effects
- Avoid postmenopausal cardiovascular disease and fractures from osteoporosis

Interventions

- Assist clients of childbearing age to choose an appropriate contraceptive method. If the choice is an estrogen–progestin combination, help the client take it accurately.
- Help postmenopausal women plan for adequate calcium and vitamin D in the diet and adequate weight-bearing exercise to maintain bone strength.
- Assist clients in obtaining follow-up health care when indicated.

Evaluation

- Interview and observe for compliance with instructions for taking the drugs.
- Interview and observe for therapeutic and adverse drug effects.

PRINCIPLES OF THERAPY

Need for Continuous Supervision

Because estrogens, progestins, and OCs are often taken for years and may cause adverse reactions, clients taking these drugs need continued medical supervision. Before the drugs are given, a complete medical history; a physical examination, including breast and pelvic examinations and a Pap smear; urinalysis; and weight and blood pressure measurements are recommended. These examinations should be repeated periodically, at least annually, as long as the client is taking the drugs.

Drug Selection Factors

Choice of preparation depends on the reason for use, desired route of administration, and duration of action. Conjugated estrogen (eg, Premarin) is a commonly used oral estrogen and medroxyprogesterone (eg, Provera) is a commonly used oral progestin.

The choice of combination OCs may be determined by the progestin component. Some progestins are more likely to cause weight gain, acne, and changes in blood lipids that increase risks of myocardial infarction or stroke. These adverse effects are attributed mainly to the androgenic activity of the progestin, and some progestins have more androgenic effects than others. Progestins with the least androgenic activity are desogestrel and norgestimate; those with intermediate activity include norethindrone and ethynodiol diacetate; and norgestrel has the highest androgenic effects. In addition, there are long-acting progestin contraceptive preparations such as IM depot medroxyprogesterone (Depo-Provera) that lasts approximately 3 months per injection, intrauterine progesterone that lasts 1 year, and levonorgestrel subcutaneous implants (Norplant) that last 5 years.

Dosage Factors

Although dosage needs vary with clients and the conditions for which the drugs are prescribed, a general rule is to use the smallest effective dose for the shortest effective time. Estrogens are usually given cyclically. In one regimen, the drug is taken for 3 weeks, then omitted for 1 week; in another, it is omitted the first 5 days of each month. These regimens more closely resemble normal secretion of estrogen and avoid prolonged stimulation of body tissues. A progestin may be added for 10 days each month.

CLIENT TEACHING GUIDELINES
Oral Contraceptives

General Considerations

✔ Seek information about the use of oral contraceptives.

✔ Oral contraceptives are very effective at preventing pregnancy, but they do *not* prevent transmission of sexually transmitted diseases (eg, acquired immunodeficiency syndrome, chlamydia, gonorrhea).

✔ See a health care provider every 6 to 12 months for blood pressure measurement, breast and pelvic examinations, and other care as indicated. This is very important to monitor for adverse drug effects such as high blood pressure, gallbladder disease, and blood clotting disorders.

✔ Do not smoke cigarettes. Cigarette smoking increases risks of blood clots in the legs, lungs, heart, or brain. The blood clots may cause heart attack, stroke, or other serious diseases.

✔ Several medications may reduce the effectiveness of oral contraceptives (ie, increase the likelihood of pregnancy). These include several antibiotics (eg, ampicillin, isoniazid, nitrofurantoin, rifampin, penicillin V, sulfonamides, tetracyclines) and antiseizure medications (eg, carbamazepine, phenobarbital, phenytoin). Inform all health care providers who prescribe medications for you that you are taking a birth control pill.

✔ Be prepared to use an alternative method of birth control if a dose is missed, if you are unable to take the oral contraceptive because of illness, or if you have an infection for which an antibiotic is prescribed. For example, use a different method of birth control while taking an antibiotic and for the remainder of that cycle.

✔ Avoid pregnancy for approximately 3 to 6 months after the drugs are stopped.

Self-administration

✔ Read, keep, and follow instructions in the package inserts that are dispensed with the drugs. These inserts provide information about safe and effective use of the drugs.

✔ Take oral contraceptives with meals or food or at bedtime to decrease nausea.

✔ Take about the same time every day to maintain effective blood levels and establish a routine so that missed doses are less likely. Missing one dose may allow pregnancy to occur. If you forget to take one pill, take it as soon as you remember. If you do not remember until the next scheduled pill, you can take two pills at once. If you miss two pills in a row, you may take two pills for the next 2 days. If you miss more than two pills, notify your health care provider.

✔ Use sunscreen and protective clothing when outdoors. The drugs may cause photosensitivity, with increased likelihood of sunburn after short periods of exposure.

✔ Weigh weekly and report sudden weight gain. The drugs may cause fluid retention; decreasing salt intake may be helpful.

✔ Report any unusual vaginal bleeding; calf tenderness, redness, or swelling; chest pain; weakness or numbness in an arm or leg; or sudden difficulty with seeing or talking.

CLIENT TEACHING GUIDELINES
Estrogen Replacement Therapy

General Considerations

✔ Estrogen replacement therapy has numerous benefits for postmenopausal women. In addition to relieving symptoms of menopause, it helps to prevent heart attack, stroke, and osteoporosis.

✔ Maintain medical supervision at least annually to check blood pressure, breasts, pelvis, and other areas for possible adverse reactions when these drugs are taken for long periods.

✔ Women who have not had a hysterectomy should take both estrogen and progestin; the progestin component (eg, Provera) prevents endometrial cancer, an adverse effect of estrogen-only therapy.

✔ Women with diabetes should report increased blood glucose levels.

Self-administration

✔ Take estrogens and progestins with food or at bedtime to decrease nausea, a common adverse reaction.

✔ Apply skin patch estrogen (eg, Estraderm) to clean, dry skin, preferably the abdomen. Press the patch tightly approximately 10 seconds to get a good seal and rotate sites so that at least a week passes between applications to a site.

✔ Weigh weekly and report sudden weight gain. Fluid retention and edema may occur and produce weight gain.

✔ Report any unusual vaginal bleeding.

Use in Specific Situations

Contraception

Estrogen and progestin contraceptive preparations are nearly 100% effective in preventing pregnancy. Some guidelines for their use include the following:

- Numerous oral contraceptive preparations are available, with different components and different doses of components, so that a preparation can be chosen to meet individual needs. Most OCs contain an estrogen and a progestin. The estrogen dose is usually 30 to 35 μg. Smaller amounts (eg, 20 μg) may be adequate for small or underweight women; larger amounts (eg, 50 μg) may be needed for large or overweight women. When estrogen is contraindicated, a progestin-only OC may be used.

- Current products contain small amounts of estrogen and cause fewer adverse effects than earlier products. Despite the decreased estrogen dosage, OCs may still be safest when given to nonsmoking women younger than 35 years of age who do not have a history of thromboembolic problems, diabetes mellitus, hypertension, or migraine.

- Assess each client's need and desire for OCs, as well as her willingness to comply with the prescribed regimen. Assessment information includes the client's knowledge about OCs and other methods of birth control. Compliance involves the willingness to take the drugs as prescribed, to have examinations of breasts and pelvis and blood pressure measurements every 6 to 12 months, and to stop the oral contraceptive periodically (other contraceptive methods can be used during these periods). Assessment also includes identifying clients in whom OCs are contraindicated or who are at increased risk for adverse reactions.

- The most effective and widely used OCs are estrogen–progestin combinations (see Table 28-3). Effects of estrogen components are similar when prescribed in equipotent doses, but progestins differ in progestogenic, estrogenic, antiestrogenic, and androgenic activity. Consequently, adverse effects may differ to some extent, and a client may be able to tolerate one OC better than another.

- Oral contraceptives decrease effects of oral anticoagulants, insulin and oral sulfonylureas, antihypertensive drugs, and drugs used to lower serum cholesterol. If OCs are used concurrently with these drug groups, dosage of these groups may need to be increased. If OCs are discontinued, dosage of the other drugs may need to be decreased.

Postcoital Contraception

Postcoital contraception may be used to avoid pregnancy after unprotected sexual intercourse, especially for victims of rape or incest or women whose physical or mental health is threatened by pregnancy. It is very effective if started within 24 hours and no later than 72 hours after exposure. The mechanism of action is unclear, but the drugs are thought to interfere with tubal transport or endometrial implantation of the ovum.

Although no drug has been approved by the Food and Drug Administration for postcoital contraception, Ovral (containing 50 μg of ethinyl estradiol and 0.5 mg of norgestrel) is prescribed by some health care providers. The usual regimen is 2 tablets initially and 2 more tablets 12 hours later. Levonorgestrel 75 mg is also effective; one dose is taken as soon as possible and a second dose 12 hours later. These are high doses and common adverse effects are nausea and vomiting. Antiemetic medication or repeating vomited doses may be needed.

Menopause

Menopause usually occurs when women are 48 to 55 years of age. A women who has not menstruated for a full year is considered menopausal, although symptoms of estrogen deficiency and irregular periods start approximately 4 years before final cessation. Physiologic menopause results from the gradual cessation of ovarian function and the resultant decrease in estrogen levels. Surgical menopause results from excision of both ovaries and the sudden loss of ovarian estrogen. Although estrogens from the adrenal cortex and other sites are still produced, the amount is insufficient to prevent estrogen deficiency.

ERT or HRT prevents vasomotor instability ("hot flashes") and other menopausal symptoms. A commonly prescribed regimen is a conjugated estrogen (eg, Premarin) 0.625 mg to 1.25 mg daily for 25 days of each month, with a progestin, such as Provera, 10 mg daily for 10 days of each month, on days 15 to 25 of the cycle. The main function of the progestin is to decrease the risk of endometrial cancer; thus, it is not needed by women who have had a hysterectomy. Another regimen uses estradiol as a transdermal patch (Estraderm), which releases the drug slowly, provides more consistent blood levels than oral formulations, and is applied weekly. A newer synthetic conjugated estrogen (Cenestin) is also approved for short-term treatment of hot flashes and sweating; it is not approved for long-term use in preventing cardiovascular disease or osteoporosis in postmenopausal women.

Nursing Notes: Apply Your Knowledge

Jane Smily, an adolescent, calls the clinic because she forgot to take her birth control pill yesterday. What effect will this have on the therapeutic effects of the birth control pills? How should you advise her? What teaching can you provide that will help her remember to take her birth control pills regularly?

Prevention of Cardiovascular Disease in Postmenopausal Women

Postmenopausal women are at high risk of cardiovascular disease (eg, myocardial infarction, stroke) and death. Possible reasons include abnormalities in blood coagulation factors, blood lipids, and the endothelial lining of blood vessel walls. These abnormalities increase formation of blood clots and atherosclerotic plaque. In addition, hypertension is more prevalent.

Numerous studies indicate that ERT reduces cardiovascular disease and related mortality by 50% or more, and most authorities believe the benefits of ERT greatly outweigh the risks. Until studies clearly demonstrated cardiovascular benefits of ERT, there was concern because of thromboembolic disorders in women taking OCs (pharmacologic doses of estrogens and progestins). However, evidence indicates that the small doses used for physiologic replacement do not increase risks of hypertension, myocardial infarction, stroke, or venous thrombosis in women without other risk factors, such as those older than 35 years of age who smoke.

Protective effects are attributed to improvements in blood lipid levels (ie, increases in HDL cholesterol and decreases in LDL cholesterol), antiatherosclerotic effects on the endothelial lining and the arterial wall (ie, increased prostacyclin production, with resultant vasodilation and decreased platelet adhesiveness), improved glucose metabolism (ie, fasting blood glucose levels are unchanged or lower), and direct effects on cardiac function (ie, increased left ventricular diastolic filling and stroke volume output). Blood pressure is usually unchanged or lower, because ERT does not raise blood pressure in normotensive women.

Adverse effects of ERT include increased plasma triglyceride levels, retention of sodium and water, increased risk of cholelithiasis, vaginal spotting and bleeding, breast tenderness and enlargement, pedal edema, and weight gain.

Estrogen replacement therapy is recommended for women who have had a hysterectomy. The optimal estrogen preparation and duration of therapy for cardiovascular protection have not been established. In long-term studies, most clients used conjugated estrogens (mainly Premarin 0.625 mg daily for 3 weeks of each month) in doses similar to those used for prevention of osteoporosis.

For women with an intact uterus, a progestin should also be given to prevent endometrial cancer from the estrogen. When a progestin is added, cardiovascular protective effects may be decreased or lost because progestins have opposite effects on blood lipids. Thus, the lowest effective doses should be given. Medroxyprogesterone is commonly used (10 mg for 10 to 14 days each month or 2.5 to 5 mg daily). Progestins are also associated with most adverse effects of combination therapy such as withdrawal bleeding and mood changes. Combination therapy is often called HRT.

Prevention and Treatment of Osteoporosis

Estrogen replacement therapy is the most effective method of preventing or treating osteoporosis and preventing fractures in postmenopausal women (see Chap. 26). Estrogenic effects in preventing bone loss include decreased bone resorption (breakdown), increased intestinal absorption of calcium, and increased calcitriol concentration. Calcitriol is the active form of vitamin D, which is required for absorption of calcium.

The best estrogen compounds for osteoporosis are unknown. Most long-term studies used conjugated estrogens (eg, Premarin), 0.625 mg daily or cyclically (3 weeks of each month). Other regimens thought to be equally effective include ethinyl estradiol 0.02 mg, estropipate 0.625 mg, esterified estrogens 0.625 mg, estradiol 0.5 mg, and transdermal estradiol 0.05 mg/day.

Estrogens are more effective in preventing bone loss than restoring bone after loss has occurred. Thus, maximum benefit is gained by starting ERT soon after menopause. Therapy should be continued for years, probably for life, because bone loss resumes when ERT is discontinued.

For women with an intact uterus, a progestin should also be given to prevent endometrial cancer. Estrogen alone for longer than 6 months increases the risk of endometrial cancer up to 10-fold; concomitant progestin therapy for at least 10 to 14 days per month usually eliminates this risk. Medroxyprogesterone 10 mg for 10 to 14 days of the month or 2.5 to 5 mg daily are commonly used regimens. Although progestins retard bone loss when given alone, giving them with estrogen seems no more protective of bone than estrogen alone.

Common adverse effects include vaginal spotting and bleeding, breast tenderness and enlargement, pedal edema, and weight gain. There is also an increased risk of gallbladder disease. With the small, physiologic doses used for ERT/HRT, the thromboembolic events that occurred with the early estrogen/progestin OCs have not been reported.

Despite the clear benefits of ERT/HRT, some women refuse or are reluctant to take ERT/HRT. Some stop therapy, often because of vaginal bleeding. Dosage may need to be adjusted to control vaginal bleeding.

ERT/HRT is more effective if the client consumes adequate calcium in the diet and participates in weight-bearing exercises. Fractures may still occur if bone demineralization was severe before therapy was begun.

Use in Children

There is little information about effects of estrogens in children, and the drugs are not indicated for use. Because the drugs cause epiphyseal closure, they should be used with caution before completion of bone growth and attainment of adult height. When hormonal contraceptives are given to adolescent girls, the smallest effective doses should be used, as in other populations.

Use in Older Adults

Estrogens alone or estrogens and progestins are commonly used in postmenopausal women, whether menopause is physiologic or surgically induced by excision of both ovaries. Progestins reduce the risk of endometrial cancer in women who have not had hysterectomies.

Use in Hepatic Impairment

Estrogens are contraindicated in impaired liver function, liver disease, or liver cancer. Impaired liver function may lead to impaired estrogen metabolism with resultant accumulation and adverse effects. In addition, women who have had jaundice during pregnancy have an increased risk of recurrence if they take an estrogen-containing oral contraceptive. Any client in whom jaundice develops while taking estrogen should stop the drug. Because jaundice may indicate liver damage, the cause should be investigated.

Progestins are contraindicated in clients with impaired liver function or liver disease.

 Home Care

Estrogens, progestins, and OCs are usually self-administered at home. The home care nurse may encounter clients or family members taking one of the drugs when visiting the home for another purpose. Teaching or assisting clients to take the drugs as prescribed may be needed. In addition, clients may need encouragement to keep appointments for follow-up supervision and monitoring of blood pressure. When visiting families that include adolescent girls or young women, the nurse may need to teach about birth control or preventing osteoporosis by improving diet and exercise patterns.

NURSING ACTIONS | **Estrogens, Progestins, and Oral Contraceptives**

NURSING ACTIONS	RATIONALE/EXPLANATION
1. **Administer accurately**	
a. Give oral estrogens, progestins, and contraceptive preparations after meals or at bedtime.	To decrease nausea, a common adverse reaction
b. With aqueous suspensions to be given intramuscularly, roll the vial between the hands several times.	To be sure that drug particles are evenly distributed through the liquid vehicle
c. Give oil preparations deeply into a large muscle mass, preferably gluteal muscles.	
2. **Observe for therapeutic effects**	Therapeutic effects vary, depending on the reason for use.
a. With estrogens:	
(1) When given for menopausal symptoms, observe for decrease in hot flashes and vaginal problems.	
(2) When given for amenorrhea, observe for menstruation.	
(3) When given for female hypogonadism, observe for menstruation, breast enlargement, axillary and pubic hair, and other secondary sexual characteristics.	
b. With progestins:	
(1) When given for menstrual disorders, such as abnormal uterine bleeding, amenorrhea, dysmenorrhea, premenstrual discomfort, and endometriosis, observe for relief of symptoms.	

(continued)

NURSING ACTIONS	RATIONALE/EXPLANATION
3. Observe for adverse effects	
a. With estrogens:	
(1) Menstrual disorders—breakthrough bleeding, dysmenorrhea, amenorrhea, exacerbation of endometriosis	Estrogen drugs may alter hormonal balance.
(2) Gastrointestinal system—nausea, vomiting, abdominal cramps, bloating, cholestatic jaundice, colitis, acute pancreatitis	Nausea commonly occurs but usually subsides within 1 to 2 wk of continued therapy. When high doses of estrogens are used as postcoital contraceptives, nausea and vomiting may be severe enough to require administration of antiemetic drugs.
(3) Cardiovascular system—thromboembolic conditions such as thrombophlebitis, pulmonary embolism, cerebral thrombosis, and coronary thrombosis; edema and weight gain	Thromboembolic disorders were associated with earlier oral contraceptive pills, which contained larger amounts of estrogen than those currently used. The only population groups now considered at high risk for thromboembolic disorders are women older than 35 y who take oral contraceptives, even low-estrogen preparations, and men or women who receive large does of estrogens for treatment of cancer.
	Edema and weight gain are caused by fluid retention.
(4) Central nervous system—headache, migraine, dizziness, mental depression, convulsions	Estrogens may cause or aggravate migraine in some women; the mechanism is unknown.
(5) Cancer—endometrial and possibly breast cancer	When estrogens are used alone in postmenopausal women, they cause endometrial hyperplasia and may cause endometrial cancer. This effect can be prevented by also giving a progestin, which opposes the effects of estrogen on the endometrium.
	Opinions differ regarding estrogens as a cause of breast cancer. Most studies indicate little risk; a few indicate some risk, especially with high doses for prolonged periods (ie, 10 y or longer).
b. With progestins:	
(1) Menstrual disorders—breakthrough bleeding	Irregular vaginal bleeding is a common adverse effect that decreases during the first year of use. This is a major reason that some women do not want to take progestin-only contraceptives.
(2) Cardiovascular system—decreased high-density lipoprotein and increased low-density lipoprotein cholesterol	These adverse effects on plasma lipids potentially increase the risks of cardiovascular disease. Long-term effects of progestins on thrombosis and other cardiovascular disorders are unclear because these drugs have not been investigated as much as combined estrogen–progestin oral contraceptives.
(3) Gastrointestinal system—nausea, increased or decreased weight	Nausea may be decreased by taking with food.
(4) Endocrine system—impaired glucose tolerance	Impaired glucose tolerance may occur, especially in people with diabetes mellitus.
(5) Central nervous system—drowsiness, insomnia, mental depression	
(6) Miscellaneous effects—edema, weight gain	

(continued)

NURSING ACTIONS	RATIONALE/EXPLANATION
c. Combined estrogen and progestin oral contraceptives:	
(1) Gastrointestinal effects—nausea, others	Nausea can be minimized by taking the drugs with food or at bedtime.
(2) Cardiovascular effects—thromboembolism, myocardial infarction, stroke, hypertension	These effects occurred with earlier oral contraceptives, which contained larger amounts of estrogen than those currently used, and are much less common in most people who take low-dose preparations. However, for women older than 35 y who smoke, there is an increased risk of myocardial infarction and other cardiovascular disorders even with low-dose pills.
(3) Gallbladder disease—cholelithiasis and cholecystitis	Women who use oral contraceptives are two to three times as likely to develop gallstones as non-users. This is attributed to increased concentration of cholesterol in bile acids, which leads to decreased solubility and increased precipitation of stones.
(4) Miscellaneous—edema, weight gain, headache	
4. Observe for drug interactions	
a. Drugs that *decrease* effects of estrogens, progestins, and oral contraceptives:	
(1) Anticonvulsants, barbiturates, rifampin	Decrease effects by inducing enzymes that accelerate metabolism of estrogens and progestins
(2) Antimicrobials—ampicillin, chloramphenicol, neomycin, nitrofurantoin, penicillin V, sulfonamides, tetracyclines	By disrupting the normal bacterial flora of the gastrointestinal tract, antimicrobial drugs may decrease or eliminate enterohepatic circulation of estrogens and their conjugates. This action may decrease effectiveness of the contraceptive or cause breakthrough bleeding.

Nursing Notes: Apply Your Knowledge

Answer: Factors such as the number of doses omitted and the time of the month such omission occurred may affect whether skipped doses could alter therapeutic drug levels. If Jane remembers a skipped dose within hours, instruct her just to take the pill late. If a longer period of time elapses (eg, over 48 hours), instruct Jane not to take all the missed doses at once and to check with her health care provider. Alternative forms of birth control may be required for the rest of the cycle.

Teach Jane to take her birth control pills at the same time each day, in association with a daily task or ritual (eg, after breakfast, after brushing teeth before bed). Advise her to notify any health care provider she is taking birth control pills when other medications are prescribed. Drug interactions can occur with some other drugs. Antibiotics, which childbearing women may often require, can decrease the effectiveness of oral contraceptives.

 REVIEW AND APPLICATION EXERCISES

1. What are the reproductive and nonreproductive functions of estrogens?
2. What are the functions of progestins?
3. What is considered the major mechanism of action of oral contraceptives?
4. What are adverse effects of oral contraceptives, and how can they be prevented or minimized?
5. Why should postmenopausal women seriously consider estrogen replacement therapy?

SELECTED REFERENCES

Bucci, K.K. & Carson, D.S. (1997). Contraception. In J.T. DiPiro, R.L. Talbert, P.E. Hayes, G.C. Yee, G.R. Matzke, B.G. Wells, & L.M. Posey (Eds.), *Pharmacotherapy: A pathophysiologic approach*, 3rd ed., pp. 1601–1620. Stamford, CT: Appleton & Lange.

Drug facts and comparisons. (Updated monthly). St. Louis: Facts and Comparisons.

Guyton, A.C. & Hall, J.E. (1996). *Textbook of medical physiology*, 9th ed. Philadelphia: W.B. Saunders.

Lip, G.Y.H, Blann, A.D., Jones, A.F., & Beevers, D.G. (1997). Effects of hormone-replacement therapy on hemostatic factors, lipid factors, and endothelial function in women undergoing surgical menopause: Implications for prevention of atherosclerosis. *American Heart Journal, 134*, 764–771.

Mehring, P.M. (1998). Structure and function of the female reproductive system. In C.M. Porth (Ed.), *Pathophysiology: Concepts of altered health states*, 5th ed., pp. 1175–1186. Philadelphia: Lippincott Williams & Wilkins.

Mullins, P.M., Pugh, M.C., & Moore, A.O. (1997). Hormonal replacement therapy. In J.T. DiPiro, R.L. Talbert, P.E. Hayes, G.C. Yee, G.R. Matzke, B.G. Wells, & L.M. Posey (Eds.), *Pharmacotherapy: A pathophysiologic approach*, 3rd ed., pp. 1635–1646. Stamford, CT: Appleton & Lange.

Strobl, J.S. (1997). Estrogens, progestins, and antiestrogens. In C.R. Craig & R.E. Stitzel (Eds.), *Modern pharmacology with clinical applications*, 5th ed., pp. 737–747. Boston: Little, Brown.

Williams, C.L. & Stancel, G.M. (1996). Estrogens and progestins. In J.G. Hardman, L.E. Limbird, P.B. Molinoff, and R.W. Ruddon (Eds.), *Goodman & Gilman's The pharmacological basis of therapeutics*, 9th ed., pp. 1411–1440. New York: McGraw-Hill.

29

Androgens and Anabolic Steroids

Objectives

After studying this chapter, the student will be able to:

1. Discuss effects of endogenous androgens.

2. Discuss uses and effects of exogenous androgens and anabolic steroids.

3. Describe potential consequences of abusing anabolic steroids.

You are a nurse working in a rural high school. The wrestling coach asks you to talk with his wrestling team about anabolic steroids.

Reflect on:

▶ Why adolescents might want to use anabolic steroids.

▶ Potential dangers of anabolic steroid use.

▶ Confusion regarding the difference between anabolic steroids and corticosteroids.

▶ Strategies that might be effective in limiting the use of anabolic steroids among young athletes.

ANDROGENS

Androgens are male sex hormones secreted by the testes in men, the ovaries in women, and the adrenal cortices of both sexes. Like the female sex hormones, the naturally occurring male sex hormones are steroids synthesized from cholesterol. The sex organs and adrenal glands can produce cholesterol or remove it from the blood. Cholesterol then undergoes a series of conversions to progesterone, androgenic prehormones, and finally testosterone. The androgens produced by the ovaries have little androgenic activity and are used mainly as precursor substances for the production of naturally occurring estrogens. The adrenal glands produce approximately five androgens, including androstenedione and dehydroepiandrosterone, but these ordinarily have little masculinizing effect.

ANABOLIC STEROIDS

Anabolic steroids are synthetic drugs with increased anabolic activity and decreased androgenic activity compared with testosterone. They were developed during attempts to modify testosterone so that its tissue-building and growth-stimulating effects could be retained while its masculinizing effects could be eliminated or reduced.

TESTOSTERONE

Testosterone is normally the only important male sex hormone. It is secreted by the Leydig's cells in the testes in response to stimulation by luteinizing hormone from the anterior pituitary gland. The main functions of testosterone are related to the development of male sexual characteristics, reproduction, and metabolism (Box 29-1).

After testosterone is secreted by the testes, most of it binds reversibly to plasma proteins. It then circulates in the bloodstream for a half hour or less before it becomes attached to tissues or is broken down into inactive products. The portion that is attached to tissues enters the cells and is changed to dihydrotestosterone. The dihydrotestosterone binds with receptors in the cell and stimulates increased production of protein by the cell. The portion that does not become attached to tissues is converted into androsterone and dehydroepiandrosterone by the liver. These are conjugated with glucuronic or sulfuric acid and excreted in the bile or urine.

ABUSE OF ANDROGENIC AND ANABOLIC STEROID DRUGS

These drugs, especially the anabolic steroids, are widely abused in attempts to enhance muscle development, muscle strength, and athletic performance. Because of

their abuse potential, the drugs are Schedule III controlled substances. Although nonprescription sales of the drugs are illegal, they are apparently easily obtained.

Athletes are considered a high-risk group because some start taking the drugs in their early teenage years and continue for years. Abusers usually take massive doses and often take several drugs or combine injectable and oral drugs for maximum effects. The large doses produce potentially serious adverse effects in several body tissues:

- **Liver disorders** include benign and malignant neoplasms, cholestatic hepatitis and jaundice, and peliosis hepatis, a disorder in which blood-filled cysts develop in the liver and may lead to hemorrhage or liver failure.
- **Central nervous system disorders** include aggression, hostility, combativeness, and dependence characterized by preoccupation with drug use, inability to stop taking the drugs, and withdrawal symptoms similar to those that occur with alcohol, cocaine, and narcotics.
- **Reproductive system disorders** include testicular atrophy, low sperm counts, and impotence in men. They include menstrual irregularities, baldness, hirsutism, and deepening of the voice in women.
- **Metabolic disorders** include increased serum cholesterol, with increased risk of cardiovascular disease and retention of fluids, with edema and other imbalances. Fluid and electrolyte retention contribute to the increased weight associated with drug use.
- **Dermatologic disorders** include moderate to severe acne in both sexes, depending on drug dosage.

Many of these adverse effects persist several months after the drugs are stopped and may be irreversible. Names of anabolic steroids include nandrolone (Durabolin, Deca-Durabolin), oxandrolone (Oxandrin), oxymetholone (Anadrol-50), and stanazolol (Winstrol).

CHARACTERISTICS OF ANDROGENIC AND ANABOLIC STEROID DRUGS

Routes and dosage ranges of individual androgens are listed in Table 29-1.

- When male sex hormones or androgens are given from exogenous sources for therapeutic purposes, they produce the same effects as the naturally occurring hormones.
- Male sex hormones given to women antagonize or reduce the effect of female sex hormones. Thus, administration of testosterone to women can suppress menstruation and cause atrophy of the endometrial lining of the uterus.
- Most exogenous androgens are given intramuscularly or orally. Naturally occurring androgens are given by injection because they are rapidly metabolized by the liver if given orally. Some esters of testosterone have been modified to slow the rate of metabolism and

---

BOX 29–1   EFFECTS OF TESTOSTERONE ON BODY TISSUES

Fetal Development

Large amounts of chorionic gonadotropin are produced by the placenta during pregnancy. Chorionic gonadotropin is similar to luteinizing hormone (LE) from the anterior pituitary gland. It promotes development of the interstitial or Leydig's cells in fetal testes, which then secrete testosterone. Testosterone production begins approximately the second month of fetal life. When present, testosterone promotes development of male sexual characteristics, such as the penis, scrotum, prostate gland, seminal vesicles, and seminiferous tubules, and suppresses development of female sexual characteristics. In the absence of testosterone, the fetus develops female sexual characteristics.

Testosterone also provides the stimulus for the descent of the testes into the scrotum. This normally occurs after the seventh month of pregnancy, when the fetal testes are secreting relatively large amounts of testosterone. If the testes do not descend before birth, administration of testosterone or gonadotropic hormone, which stimulates testosterone secretion, produces descent in most cases.

Adult Development

Little testosterone is secreted in boys until 11 to 13 years of age. At the onset of puberty, testosterone secretion increases rapidly and remains at a relatively high level until about 50 years of age, after which it gradually declines.

- The testosterone secreted at puberty acts as a growth hormone to produce enlargement of the penis, testes, and scrotum until approximately 20 years of age. The prostate gland, seminal vesicles, seminiferous tubules, and vas deferens also increase in size and functional ability. Under the combined influence of testosterone and follicle-stimulating hormone (FSH) from the anterior pituitary gland, sperm production is initiated and maintained throughout the man's reproductive life.

- **Skin.** Testosterone increases skin thickness and activity of the sebaceous glands. Acne in the male adolescent is attributed to the increased production of testosterone.
- **Voice.** The larynx enlarges and deepens the voice of the adult man.
- **Hair.** Testosterone produces the distribution of hair growth on the face, limbs, and trunk typical of the adult man. In men with a genetic trait toward baldness, large amounts of testosterone cause alopecia (baldness) of the scalp.
- **Skeletal muscles.** Testosterone is largely responsible for the larger, more powerful muscles of men. This characteristic is caused by the effects of testosterone on protein metabolism. Testosterone helps the body retain nitrogen, form new amino acids, and build new muscle protein. At the same time, it slows the loss of nitrogen and amino acids formed by the constant breakdown of body tissues. Overall, testosterone increases protein anabolism (buildup) and decreases protein catabolism (breakdown).
- **Bone.** Testosterone makes bones thicker and longer. After puberty, more protein and calcium are deposited and retained in bone matrix. This causes a rapid rate of bone growth. The height of a male adolescent increases rapidly for a time, then stops as epiphyseal closure occurs. This happens when the cartilage at the end of the long bones in the arms and legs becomes bone. Further lengthening of the bones is then prevented.

Anterior Pituitary Function

High blood levels of testosterone decrease secretion of FSH and LH from the anterior pituitary gland. This, in turn, decreases testosterone production.

---

thus prolong action. Testosterone transdermal systems are also available.

- All synthetic anabolic steroids are weak androgens. Consequently, giving these drugs for anabolic effects also produces masculinizing effects. This characteristic limits the clinical usefulness of these drugs in women and children. Profound changes in growth and sexual development may occur if these drugs are given to young children.

Mechanism of Action

Androgenic and anabolic drugs penetrate the cell membrane and bind to receptor proteins in the cell cytoplasm. The steroid–receptor complex is then transported to the nucleus, where it activates ribonucleic and deoxyribonucleic acid production and stimulates cellular synthesis of protein.

Indications for Use

With male sex hormones, the most clear-cut indication for use is to treat androgen deficiency states (eg, hypogonadism, cryptorchidism, impotence, oligospermia) in boys and men. Hypogonadism may result from hypothalamic-pituitary or testicular dysfunction. In prepubertal boys, administration of the drugs stimulates the development of masculine characteristics. In postpubertal men who become androgen deficient, the hormones reestablish and maintain masculine characteristics and functions.

TABLE 29-1 Androgens

Generic/Trade Name	Routes and Dosage Ranges	
	Hypogonadism	Other
Testosterone aqueous (Histerone, others)	IM 25–50 mg two to three times weekly PO 10–40 mg daily Buccal tablets 5–20 mg daily	Cryptorchidism: PO 30 mg daily; buccal tablets, 15 mg daily
Testosterone cypionate (Depo-Testosterone)	IM 50–200 mg every 2–4 wk	
Testosterone enanthate (Delatestryl)	IM 50–200 mg every 2–4 wk	
Testosterone transdermal systems (Androderm, Testoderm)	Apply two Androderm systems (dose of 5 mg) nightly to back, abdomen, upper arm or thigh; apply Testoderm (one 6-mg system) to scrotal sac daily	
Testolactone (Teslac)		Breast cancer: PO 250 mg four times daily
Fluoxymesterone (Halotestin)	PO 5–20 mg daily	
Methyltestosterone (Oreton methyl)		Cryptorchidism: PO 30 mg daily; buccal tablets, 15 mg daily
Danazol (Danocrine)		Endometriosis: PO 800 mg daily in two divided doses for 3–9 mo Fibrocystic breast disease: PO 100–400 mg daily in two divided doses for 3–6 mo

IM, intramuscular; PO, oral.

In women, danazol (Danocrine) may be used to prevent or treat endometriosis, fibrocystic breast disease, or hereditary angioedema. Anabolic steroids are more often abused for body-building purposes than used for therapeutic effects.

Contraindications to Use

Androgens and anabolic steroids are contraindicated during pregnancy (because of possible masculinizing effects on a female fetus), in clients with preexisting liver disease, and in men with prostate gland disorders. Men with enlarged prostates may have additional enlargement, and men with prostatic cancer may experience tumor growth. Although not contraindicated in children, these drugs must be used very cautiously and with x-rays approximately every 6 months to evaluate bone growth.

NURSING PROCESS

Assessment

Before drug therapy is started, clients need a thorough history and physical examination. Periodic monitoring of the client's condition is needed throughout drug therapy.

- Assess for conditions in which androgens are used (eg, deficiency states).

- Assess for conditions that increase risks of adverse effects or are contraindications (eg, pregnancy, liver disease, prostatic hypertrophy).
- Check laboratory reports of liver function tests (the drugs may cause cholestatic jaundice and liver damage), serum electrolytes (the drugs may cause sodium and water retention), and serum lipids (the drugs may increase levels and aggravate atherosclerosis).
- Assess weight and blood pressure regularly. These may be elevated by retention of sodium and water with resultant edema, especially in clients with congestive heart failure.
- For children, check x-ray reports of bone growth status initially and approximately every 6 months while the drugs are being taken.
- Assess the client's attitude toward taking male sex hormones.
- Assess the client's willingness to comply with instructions for taking the drugs and follow-up procedures.

Nursing Diagnoses
- Body Image Disturbance in women related to masculinizing effects and menstrual irregularities
- Sexual Dysfunction in men related to impotence and changes in libido
- Ineffective Individual Coping related to use of androgens and anabolic steroids for nonmedical purposes

- Knowledge Deficit: Physiologic and psychological consequences of overuse and abuse of the drugs to enhance athletic performance
- Noncompliance: Overuse
- Fluid Volume Excess related to sodium and water retention
- Risk for Injury: Liver disease and other serious adverse drug effects
- Risk for Violence: Directed at Others related to feelings of aggression and hostility in those who take large doses

Planning/Goals

The client will:

- Use the drugs for medical purposes only
- Receive or take the drugs as prescribed
- Avoid overuse and abuse of drugs for body building
- Be counseled regarding effects of overuse and abuse if identified as being at risk (eg, athletes, especially weight lifters and football players)
- Avoid preventable adverse drug effects
- Comply with monitoring and follow-up procedures

Interventions

- Assist clients to use the drug correctly.
- Assist clients to reduce sodium intake if edema develops.
- Record weight and blood pressure at regular intervals.

- Participate in school or community programs to inform children, parents, coaches, athletic trainers, and others of the risks of inappropriate use of androgens and anabolic steroids.

Evaluation

- Interview and observe for compliance with instructions for taking prescribed drugs.
- Interview and observe for therapeutic and adverse drug effects.
- Question athletes about illegal use of the drugs.
- Observe athletes for increased weight and behavioral changes that may indicate drug abuse.

PRINCIPLES OF THERAPY

- When these drugs are given to women and prepubertal boys, good skin care is indicated to decrease the incidence and severity of acne.
- Drug therapy with androgens and anabolic steroids may be short or long term, depending on the condition in question, the client's response to treatment, and the incidence of adverse reactions. If feasible, intermittent rather than continuous therapy is recommended.
- Androgens usually potentiate oral anticoagulants, oral antidiabetic agents, and insulin. Dosage of these drugs may need to be decreased during concurrent therapy with androgens or anabolic drugs.

CLIENT TEACHING GUIDELINES
Androgens

General Considerations

✔ Take the drugs only if prescribed and as prescribed. Use by athletes for body building is inappropriate and, if not prescribed by a licensed physician, illegal.

✔ Continue medical supervision as long as the drugs are being taken.

✔ Weigh once or twice weekly and record the amount. An increase may indicate fluid retention and edema.

✔ Practice frequent and thorough skin cleansing to decrease acne, which is most likely to occur in women and children.

Self-administration

✔ Take oral preparations before or with meals, in divided doses.

✔ For buccal preparations:
  ✔ Take in divided doses.
  ✔ Place the tablet between the cheek and gum and allow to dissolve (do not swallow).
  ✔ Avoid eating, drinking, or smoking while the tablet is in place.

✔ With transdermal systems:
  ✔ Apply 2 Androderm systems nightly to clean, dry skin on back, abdomen, upper arm, or thigh. Do *not* apply to scrotum. Rotate sites, with 7 days between applications to a site. Press firmly into place for adherence.
  ✔ Apply 1 Testoderm system to clean, dry scrotal skin (shaved, for best adherence) once daily.

Use in Children

The main indication for use of androgens is for boys with established deficiency states. Because the drugs cause epiphyseal closure, hands and wrists should be x-rayed every 6 months to detect bone maturation and prevent loss of adult height. Stimulation of skeletal growth continues for approximately 6 months after drug therapy is stopped. If premature puberty occurs (precocious sexual development, enlarged penis), the drug should be stopped. The drugs may cause or aggravate acne. Scrupulous hygiene and other antiacne treatment may be needed, especially in adolescent boys.

Use in Older Adults

The main indication for use of androgens is a deficiency state in men. Older adults often have hypertension and other cardiovascular disorders that may be aggravated by the sodium and water retention associated with androgens and anabolic steroids. In men, the drugs may increase prostate size and interfere with urination, increase risk of prostatic cancer, and cause excessive sexual stimulation and priapism.

Use in Hepatic Impairment

Androgens and anabolic steroids are contraindicated in clients with preexisting liver disease. Prolonged use of high doses may cause potentially life-threatening conditions such as peliosis hepatis, hepatic neoplasms, and hepatocellular carcinoma. In addition, androgen therapy should be discontinued if cholestatic hepatitis with jaundice occurs, or if liver function tests become abnormal. Drug-induced jaundice is reversible when the medication is stopped.

NURSING ACTIONS: Androgens and Anabolic Steroids

NURSING ACTIONS	RATIONALE/EXPLANATION
1. Administer accurately	
a. Give intramuscular preparations of testosterone, other androgens and anabolic steroids deeply, preferably in the gluteal muscle.	
b. Give oral preparations before or with meals, in divided doses.	To decrease gastrointestinal disturbances
c. For buccal preparations:	
(1) Give in divided doses.	
(2) Place the tablet between the cheek and gum.	Buccal preparations must be absorbed through the mucous membranes.
(3) Instruct the client not to swallow the tablet and not to drink, chew, or smoke until the tablet is completely absorbed.	
d. With transdermal systems:	Correct site selection and application are necessary for therapeutic effects. Scrotal skin is more permeable to testosterone than other skin areas.
(1) Apply 2 Androderm systems nightly to clean, dry skin on back, abdomen, upper arm, or high. Do *not* apply to scrotum. Rotate sites, with 7 days between applications to a site. Press firmly into place for adherence.	
(2) Apply 1 Testoderm system to clean, dry scrotal skin (shaved, for best adherence) once daily.	
2. Observe for therapeutic effects	
a. When the drug is given for hypogonadism, observe for masculinizing effects, such as growth	

(continued)

NURSING ACTIONS	RATIONALE/EXPLANATION
of sexual organs, deepening of voice, growth of body hair, and acne.	
b. When the drug is given for anabolic effects, observe for increased appetite, euphoria, or statements of feeling better.	
3. Observe for adverse reactions	
a. Virilism or masculinizing effects:	
(1) In adult men with adequate secretion of testosterone—priapism, increased sexual desire, reduced sperm count, and prostate enlargement	
(2) In prepubertal boys—premature development of sex organs and secondary sexual characteristics, such as enlargement of the penis, priapism, pubic hair	
(3) In women—masculinizing effects include hirsutism, deepening of the voice, menstrual irregularities	
b. Jaundice—dark urine, yellow skin and sclera, itching	
c. Edema	More likely in clients who are elderly or who have heart or kidney disease
d. Hypercalcemia	More likely in women with advanced breast cancer
e. Difficulty voiding due to prostate enlargement	More likely in middle-aged or elderly men
f. Inadequate growth in height of children	
4. Observe for drug interactions	
a. Drugs that *decrease* effects of androgens	
(1) Barbiturates	Increase enzyme induction and rate of metabolism
(2) Calcitonin	Decreases calcium retention and thus antagonizes calcium-retaining effects of androgens

REVIEW AND APPLICATION EXERCISES

1. How does testosterone promote development of male sexual characteristics?

2. What is the major clinical indication for therapeutic use of testosterone and related androgens?

3. What is the difference between androgenic activity and anabolic activity?

4. What are the adverse effects of using large doses of anabolic steroids in body-building efforts?

5. If your 14-year-old brother said some friends were telling him to take drugs to increase muscle development and athletic ability, how would you reply? Justify your answer.

SELECTED REFERENCES

Drug facts and comparisons. (Updated monthly). St. Louis: Facts and Comparisons.

Guyton, A.C. & Hall, J.E. (1996). *Textbook of medical physiology*, 9th ed. Philadelphia: W.B. Saunders.

Wilson, J.D. (1996). Androgens. In J.G. Hardman, L.E. Limbird, P.B. Molinoff, & R.W. Ruddon (Eds.), *Goodman & Gilman's The pharmacological basis of therapeutics*, 9th ed., pp. 1441–1455. New York: McGraw-Hill.

SECTION V

Nutrients, Fluids, and Electrolytes

30

Nutritional Support Products and Drugs for Obesity

Objectives

After studying this chapter, the student should be able to:

1. Assess clients for risk factors and manifestations of fluid imbalances, undernutrition, and obesity.

2. Evaluate the types and amounts of nutrients provided in commercial products for oral and tube feedings.

3. Collaborate with nutritionists and physicians in designing and implementing nutritional support measures for undernourished or malnourished clients.

4. Minimize complications of enteral and parenteral nutrition.

5. Monitor laboratory reports that indicate nutritional status.

6. Review health consequences of obesity.

7. Assist clients who are overweight or obese to develop and maintain a realistic weight loss program.

Jamie, 2 months of age, had a gastrostomy tube placed after surgical repair of his esophagus. He is being sent home with his parents to receive tube feedings for a period of 6 to 8 weeks.

Reflect on:

▶ Questions and anxieties the parents may have.

▶ Potential impact on infant–parent bonding.

▶ Compare and contrast how tube feedings are the same and different for an infant and adult.

▶ Review priority teaching needs for Jamie's parents before discharge.

OVERVIEW

Water, carbohydrates, proteins, fats, vitamins, and minerals are required for human nutrition, to promote or maintain health, to prevent illness, and to promote recovery from illness or injury. The first four nutrients are discussed in this chapter; vitamins and minerals are discussed in the following chapters.

Water, carbohydrates, proteins, and fats are necessary for life. Water is required for cellular metabolism and excretion of metabolic waste products; approximately 2000 to 3000 mL is needed daily. Proteins are basic anatomic and physiologic components of all body cells and tissues; the recommended amount for adults is 50 to 60 g daily. Carbohydrates and fats serve primarily as sources of energy for cellular metabolism. Energy is measured in kilocalories (kcal) per gram of food oxidized in the body. Carbohydrates and proteins supply 4 kcal/g; fats supply 9 kcal/g.

Although recommended amounts of these nutrients can be used as rough estimates of clients' nutritional needs, actual requirements vary widely, depending on age, sex, size, illness, and other factors. Thus, nutritional care should be individualized. Although physicians usually order diets and nutritionists advise about dietary matters, it is often the nurse who must implement or assist others to implement nutritional care. Consequently, this chapter discusses the use of products to improve nutritional status in clients with deficiency states and special needs. It also discusses obesity and drugs to aid weight loss.

NUTRITIONAL DEFICIENCY STATES

Nutritional deficiencies result from inadequate amounts of water, carbohydrates, proteins, or fats. Treatment of deficiency states may lead to excess states. Causes and symptoms of water imbalances are listed in Table 30-1; those of protein-calorie imbalances are listed in Table 30-2.

Nurses encounter many clients who are unable to ingest adequate fluid and food because of illness. Debilitating illnesses such as cancer, acquired immunodeficiency syndrome, and chronic lung, kidney, or cardiovascular disorders often interfere with appetite and gastrointestinal (GI) function. Therapeutic drugs often cause anorexia, nausea, vomiting, diarrhea, or constipation. Nutritional deficiencies may impair the function of essentially every body organ, impair wound healing, and increase risks of infection.

NUTRITIONAL PRODUCTS

Numerous products are available to supplement or substitute for dietary intake in clients who cannot ingest, digest, absorb, or use nutrients. For example, liquid for-

TABLE 30-1 Water Imbalances

Water Deficit

Causes	Signs and Symptoms
1. Inadequate fluid intake, most likely to occur in people who are comatose, unable to swallow, or otherwise incapacitated 2. Excessive fluid loss due to vomiting, diarrhea, fever, diuretic drug therapy, high environmental temperatures, strenuous physical activity, or excessive sweating 3. A combination of 1 and 2	1. Thirst 2. Oliguria and concentrated urine 3. Weakness 4. Dry tongue and oral mucous membranes 5. Flushed skin 6. Weight loss 7. Fever 8. Increased hematocrit 9. Mental disturbances ranging from mild confusion to delirium, convulsions, and coma 10. Hypovolemic shock if the deficiency is severe or develops rapidly

Water Excess

Causes	Signs and Symptoms
1. Excessive intake, most likely to occur with excessive amounts or rapid infusion of intravenous fluids 2. Impaired excretion of fluids due to endocrine, renal, cardiovascular, or central nervous system disorders	1. Drowsiness 2. Weakness and lethargy 3. Weight gain 4. Edema 5. Low serum sodium and hematocrit 6. Disorientation 7. Circulatory overload and pulmonary edema if water excess is severe or develops rapidly

TABLE 30-2 Carbohydrate, Protein, and Fat Imbalances

Protein-Calorie Deficit

Causes	Signs and Symptoms
1. Inadequate intake of protein, carbohydrate, and fat 2. Impaired ability to digest, absorb, or use nutrients 3. Excessive losses	1. Weight loss with eventual loss of subcutaneous fat and muscle mass 2. Increased susceptibility to infection 3. Weakness and fatigability 4. Dry, scaly skin 5. Impaired healing 6. Impaired growth and development in children 7. Edema 8. Decreased hemoglobin 9. Acidosis 10. Disordered brain function 11. Coma 12. Starvation

Protein-Calorie Excess

Causes	Signs and Symptoms
1. Excessive intake, especially of carbohydrates and fats	1. Weight gain 2. Obesity

mulas are available for oral or tube feedings. Many are nutritionally complete, except for water, when given in sufficient amounts. Additional water is given to meet fluid needs. Other formulas are nutritionally incomplete but useful in certain circumstances.

Intravenous (IV) fluids are also available. Most are nutritionally incomplete and are designed for short-term use when oral or tube feedings are contraindicated. They are most useful in meeting fluid and electrolyte needs. When nutrients must be provided parenterally for more than a few days, a special formula can be given. Parenteral nutritional formulas can be designed to meet all nutritional needs or to supplement other feeding methods. Fat emulsions are usually included to supply additional calories and essential fatty acids.

Intravenous fluids and representative enteral products for infants and children and adults are listed in Tables 30-3, 30-4, and 30-5, respectively. For nutritional deficiencies due to malabsorption of carbohydrates, protein, and fat, pancreatic enzymes may be given.

PANCREATIC ENZYMES

Pancreatin is an oral preparation of pancreatic enzymes used to aid digestion and absorption of dietary carbohydrate, protein, and fat in conditions characterized by pancreatic enzyme deficiency. These conditions include (*text continues on page 436*)

TABLE 30-3	Intravenous Fluids		
Type	**Characteristics**	**Uses**	**Comments**
Dextrose injection	Available in preparations containing 2.5%, 5%, 10%, 20%, 25%, 30%, 40%, 50%, 60%, and 70% dextrose. The most frequently used concentration is 5% dextrose in water (D₅W) or sodium chloride injection. 5% dextrose in water is isotonic with blood. It provides water and 170 kcal/L. 10% dextrose solution provides twice the calories in the same volume of fluid but is hypertonic and therefore may cause phlebitis. Except for 25% or 50% solutions sometimes used to treat hypoglycemia, the higher concentrations are used in parenteral nutrition. They are hypertonic and must be given through a central or subclavian catheter.	To provide water and calories Treat hypoglycemia (eg, insulin overdose) As a component of parenteral nutritional mixtures	The dextrose in D₅W is rapidly used, leaving "free" water for excreting waste products, maintaining renal function, and maintaining urine output. Coinfusion of 10% dextrose solutions with lipid emulsions in peripheral parenteral nutrition may prevent or decrease phlebitis.
Dextrose and sodium chloride injection	Available in several concentrations Frequently used are 5% dextrose in 0.225% (also called D₅1/4 normal saline) and 5% dextrose in 0.45% sodium chloride (D₅1/2 normal saline) These provide approximately 170 kcal/L, water, sodium, and chloride.	Maintenance fluids, usually with added potassium chloride, in clients who cannot eat or drink Replacement fluids when large amounts are lost To keep IV lines open Administration of IV medications	
Crystalline amino acid solutions (Aminosyn, Freamine)	Contain essential and nonessential amino acids	As a component of peripheral or central IV parenteral nutrition, with concentrated dextrose solutions	Special formulations are available for use in patients with renal or hepatic failure.
Fat emulsions (Intralipid, Liposyn)	Provide concentrated calories and essential fatty acids Available in 10% and 20% emulsions 500 mL of 10% emulsion provides 550 calories.	As a component of peripheral or central total parenteral nutrition	More calories can be supplied with a fat emulsion than with dextrose-protein solutions alone.

IV, intravenous.

TABLE 30-4	Representative Enteral Formulas for Infants and Children

Name	Characteristics	Uses	Comments
Casec	Nutritionally incomplete Provides protein	Protein supplement for infants and children	
Enfamil, Similac, and SMA	Complete nutritional formulas for full-term infants	Alone for bottle-fed infants As a supplement for breastfed infants	These formulas are similar to human breast milk. They are deficient in iron, which may be given separately or in a formula preparation containing iron.
Enfamil Premature, Special Care Similac, and Preemie SMA	Complete nutritional formulas for preterm infants	Alone for bottle-fed or tube-fed premature infants	Nutritional needs of preterm infants differ from those of full-term infants.
Isomil Nursoy, ProSobee, and Soyalac	Hypoallergenic, milk-free formulas Contain soy protein Provide 20 calories/oz when mixed as directed Provide all other essential nutrients for normal growth and development	As milk substitutes for infants who are allergic to milk	
Lofenalac	Contains less phenylalanine than other products	For infants and children with phenylketonuria (a metabolic disorder in which phenylalanine cannot be metabolized normally)	Inadequate for complete nutrition and growth. It is recommended that approximately 85% of a child's protein needs be supplied with Lofenalac and the remaining 10% to 15% be supplied with foods containing phenylalanine, which is an essential amino acid.
Nutramigen	Nutritionally complete, hypoallergenic formula containing pre-digested protein	Infants and children who are allergic to ordinary food proteins Infants and children who have diarrhea or other GI problems	
Precision diets	Nutritionally complete, low-residue formulas for oral or tube feedings The **high-nitrogen diet** provides 125 g of protein or 20 g of nitrogen, 3000 kcal, and recommended amounts of essential vitamins and minerals in 10 3-oz servings. The **low-residue** formula contains 45 g of protein or 7.2 g of nitrogen (a maintenance amount of protein), 1900 kcal, and essential vitamins and minerals in six 3-oz servings The **isotonic** diet contains the same amounts of protein, vitamins, and minerals as the low-residue formula but is isotonic rather than hypertonic and provides 1500 kcal in six 2-oz servings.	These formulas can be given to children if the amount is calculated to provide recommended amounts of nutrients for the particular age group.	These preparations are ingested or given by tube slowly over 4 hours. Contraindicated in children with diabetes mellitus because the carbohydrate may produce hyperglycemia
PediaSure	Nutritionally complete formula for enteral use	Children 1 to 6 years of age	Amounts should be individualized.
Pregestimil	Contains easily digested protein, fat, and carbohydrate	Infants with diarrhea, food intolerances, or malabsorption syndromes	
Vivonex	Nutritionally complete diet that contains amino acids as its protein source Can be used for oral or tube feedings Requires virtually no digestion Leaves virtually no fecal residue	Children with GI disorders	The amount, concentration, and rate of administration can be adjusted to meet nutritional needs and tolerance.

GI, gastrointestinal.

TABLE 30-5	Representative Enteral Formulas for Adults		
Name	**Characteristics**	**Uses**	**Comments**
Amin-Aid	Provides amino acids, carbohydrates, and a few electrolytes	As a source of protein for clients with acute and chronic renal insufficiency in whom dietary protein must be restricted	
Casec	Nutritionally incomplete Provides protein	Protein supplement	
Citrotein, Gevral, Ensure, Isocal, and Osmolite	Provide protein, vitamins, and minerals Given orally Gevral powder can be mixed with water, milk, or other cold liquids; added to cereals; or mixed into desserts. Nutritionally complete May be given orally or by tube feeding	Dietary supplements, useful when appetite and food intake are decreased or during rapid growth periods when intake does not meet nutritional needs Supplement other sources of nutrients Serve as sole source of nutrients	2000 mL daily meets basic nutritional needs for adults.
MCT Oil	A preparation of medium-chain triglycerides More easily digested than fats contained in most foods, which are mainly long-chain triglycerides. Can be mixed with fruit juices, used with salads or vegetables, or used in cooking and baking	Clients with fat malabsorption syndromes	Limit use in clients with severe hepatic cirrhosis because it may precipitate encephalopathy and coma. Although useful as a caloric substitute for dietary fat (1 tbsp provides 115 kcal), it does not promote absorption of fat-soluble vitamins or provide essential fatty acids as the long-chain triglycerides do.
Polycose	An oral supplement used to increase caloric intake Derived from carbohydrate Available in liquid and powder May be mixed with water or other beverages and with foods	Clients on protein-, electrolyte-, or fat-restricted diets	Individualize amounts by calories needed and tolerance.
Portagen	Nutritionally complete formula that contains medium-chain triglycerides, an easily digested form of fat	Clients with fat malabsorption problems It may be used as the complete diet, as a beverage with meals, or as an addition to various recipes.	May induce coma in clients with severe hepatic cirrhosis The fat provides calories and essential fatty acids.
Precision diets	Nutritionally complete, low-residue formulas for oral or tube feedings. The **high-nitrogen diet** provides 125 g of protein or 20 g of nitrogen, 3000 kcal, and recommended amounts of essential vitamins and minerals in 10 3-oz servings. The **low-residue** formula contains 45 g of protein or 7.2 g of nitrogen (a maintenance amount of protein), 1900 kcal, and essential vitamins and minerals in six 3-oz servings. The **isotonic** diet contains the same amounts of protein, vitamins, and minerals as the low-residue formula but is isotonic rather than hypertonic and provides 1500 kcal in six 2-oz servings.		These preparations are ingested or given by tube slowly over 4 hours. The carbohydrate content may produce hyperglycemia; therefore, they should not be used in clients with diabetes mellitus.
Pulmocare and Nutrivent	These products are high in fat and low in carbohydrates because fat metabolism produces less carbon dioxide than carbohydrate metabolism.	Clients with chronic obstructive pulmonary disease or respiratory insufficiency	Clients with impaired breathing have difficulty eliminating sufficient quantities of carbon dioxide, a waste product of carbohydrate metabolism.

(continued)

TABLE 30-5 **Representative Enteral Formulas for Adults** (*continued*)

Name	Characteristics	Uses	Comments
			When carbon dioxide accumulates in the body, it may produce respiratory acidosis and respiratory failure.
Sustacal	Nutritionally complete May be given orally or by tube feeding	Supplement other sources of nutrients Serve as sole source of nutrients	
TraumaCal	High-protein formula with easily assimilated amino acids and other nutrients	Clients with severe trauma or burn injuries, to help meet nutritional needs and promote healing	
Vivonex	Nutritionally complete diet that contains amino acids as its protein source Can be used for oral or tube feedings Requires virtually no digestion Leaves virtually no fecal residue	Clients with gastrointestinal disorders	The amount, concentration, and rate of administration can be adjusted to meet nutritional needs and tolerance.

cystic fibrosis, chronic pancreatitis, pancreatectomy, and pancreatic obstruction. **Pancrelipase** (Viokase) is essentially the same as pancreatin except that it may be more effective in steatorrhea (excess fat in the feces).

Pancreatin

ROUTE AND DOSAGE RANGES

Adults: Oral (PO) 1 or 2 capsules or tablets with meals or snacks

Children: PO 1 or 2 capsules or tablets with each meal initially, increased in amount or frequency if necessary and if adverse effects do not occur

Pancrelipase

ROUTE AND DOSAGE RANGES

Adults: PO 1 to 3 capsules or tablets before or with meals or snacks; or 1 or 2 packets of powder with meals or snacks

OBESITY

Overweight and obesity are widespread in the United States and are considered major public health concerns because of their association with high rates of morbidity and mor-

tality. Overweight is defined as a body mass index (BMI) of 25 to 29.9 kg/m^2; obesity is defined as a BMI of 30 kg/m^2 or more. The BMI reflects weight in relation to height.*

Obesity, also defined as excessive body fat, may occur in any group but is more likely to occur in women, minority groups, and in the poor. It results from consistent ingestion of more calories than are used and it substantially increases risks for development of cardiovascular disease (eg, hypertension, angina pectoris, myocardial infarction, stroke), diabetes mellitus, dyslipidemia, some types of cancer, gallbladder disease, sleep apnea, and osteoarthritis of the knees. These disorders are attributed to the multiple metabolic abnormalities associated with obesity. Abdominal fat out of proportion to total body fat (also called central obesity), which often occurs in men, is considered a greater risk factor for disease and death than lower body obesity. Many people consider obesity a chronic disease.

Childhood Obesity

Overweight and obesity are common and increasing among children, especially those with overweight parents. Overweight is defined as a BMI above the 85th percentile for the age group. Studies indicate that obesity in childhood and adolescence is predictive of obesity and increased health risks in adulthood. In addition, more children are developing type 2 diabetes, which was formerly thought to occur only in adults. The increase in

How Can You Avoid This Medication Error?

Pancrelipase, a pancreatic enzyme, 2 capsules ac is ordered for John Smily. His meal times are breakfast 8:00 AM, lunch 12:00, and dinner 6:00 PM. You administer his morning dose of Pancrelipase at 9:15 AM.

*
$$BMI = \frac{Weight\ (pounds)}{Height\ (inches)^2} \times 703$$

Example: A person who weighs 150 lbs. and is 5'5" (65 inches) tall:

$$BMI = \frac{150\ lbs}{65\ in \times 65\ in} \times 703 = \frac{105,450}{4225} = 24.95$$

obesity and type 2 diabetes is mainly attributed to too much food and too little exercise.

Drugs for Obesity

Drug therapy for obesity (Table 30-6) has a problematic history because available drugs had potentially serious adverse effects, were recommended only for short-term use, and weight was rapidly regained when the drugs were stopped. Two widely used drugs, fenfluramine and dexfenfluramine, were taken off the market in 1997 because of their association with diseased heart valves and pulmonary hypertension.

Older drugs include amphetamines and similar drugs (eg, diethylpropion, mazindol, phendimetrazine, phentermine, phenylpropanolamine). Amphetamines (see Chap. 16) are not recommended because they are controlled substances with a high potential for abuse and dependence. Except for phenylpropanolamine, the amphetamine-like drugs are promoted for short-term use (8 to 12 weeks) as appetite suppressants or anorexiants. Anorexiant effects are attributed to increased levels of serotonin and catecholamines in the brain. These drugs are also controlled substances and their use is not generally recommended.

Phenylpropanolamine is an adrenergic drug (see Chap. 18) commonly used as a nasal decongestant in over-the-counter (OTC) cold remedies. It is also the active ingredient in OTC appetite suppressants (eg, Dexatrim, Acutrim). Effectiveness of the drug in weight reduction is limited, and its use has been associated with psychosis, hypertension, stroke, renal failure, cardiac arrhythmias, and death. These adverse effects have occurred with recommended doses but are especially likely with overdoses or concomitant use of other stimulants, such as caffeine.

The amphetamine-like drugs and phenylpropanolamine are central nervous system and cardiovascular stimulants and are contraindicated in cardiovascular disease, hyperthyroidism, glaucoma, and agitated states.

Two newer drugs are **sibutramine** and **orlistat**. Sibutramine mainly inhibits the reuptake of serotonin and norepinephrine in the brain. Clinical effects include increased satiety, decreased food intake, and a faster metabolism rate. Sibutramine is rapidly absorbed from the intestine and undergoes first-pass metabolism, during which active metabolites are formed. Peak plasma levels of the active metabolites occur within 3 to 4 hours. The drug is highly bound to plasma proteins and rapidly distributed to most body tissues, with the highest concentrations in the liver and kidneys. It is metabolized in the liver mainly by the cytochrome P450 enzymes. The active metabolites produced by first-pass metabolism are further metabolized to inactive metabolites, which are then excreted mainly in the urine.

Sibutramine is approved by the Food and Drug Administration for long-term use, but effects are mostly unknown beyond 1 year. The drug is not associated with cardiac valve disorders, but it does increase blood pressure and heart rate. It should be used cautiously in clients with hypertension or who take other medications that increase blood pressure and pulse rate. It should also be used cautiously in clients with narrow-angle glaucoma (may cause mydriasis) or a history of substance abuse or dependency.

Orlistat differs from other antiobesity drugs because it decreases absorption of dietary fat from the intestine (by inhibiting gastric and pancreatic lipase enzymes that normally break down fat). The drug blocks absorption of approximately 30% of the fat ingested in a meal and improves body weight and other risk factors (eg, decreases total and low-density lipoprotein [LDL] cholesterol levels). Because the drug acts within the intestine, a common adverse effect is passage of fatty stools. In addition, the drug prevents absorption of the fat-soluble vitamins, A, D, E, and K, so that supplements of these vitamins are needed.

Orlistat is intended for people who are clinically obese, not those wanting to lose a few pounds. In addition, high-fat foods still need to be decreased because total caloric

TABLE 30-6 **Drugs for Obesity**

Generic/Trade Name	Route and Dosage Range (Adults)	Status Under Controlled Substances Act
Appetite Suppressants		
Diethylpropion (Tenuate)	PO 25 mg three times daily	Schedule IV
Mazindol (Sanorex)	PO 1 mg three times daily	Schedule III
Phendimetrazine (Plegine)	PO 35 mg two or three times daily or 105 mg once daily	Schedule III
Phentermine hydrochloride (Fastin)	PO 8.0 mg three times daily or 15–37 mg daily in the morning	Schedule IV
Phentermine resin (Ionamin)	PO 15–30 mg once daily	Schedule IV
Sibutramine (Meridia)	PO 10–15 mg once daily, in the morning, with or without food	Schedule IV
Fat Blocker		
Orlistat (Xenical)	PO 1 capsule with each main meal, up to 3 capsules daily	

PO, oral.

intake is a major determinant of weight and adverse effects worsen with high fat consumption. Long-term effects of orlistat are unknown, although one study reported safe and effective use for 2 years.

NURSING PROCESS

Assessment

Assess each client for current or potential nutritional disorders. Some specific assessment factors include the following:

* What are usual drinking and eating patterns? Does fluid intake seem adequate? Does food intake seem adequate in terms of normal nutrition? Is the client financially able to purchase sufficient food? What are fluid and food likes and dislikes?
* Does the client know the basic foods for normal nutrition? Does the client view nutrition as important in maintaining health?
* Does the client appear overweight or underweight? How does current weight compare with the ideal weight for age and height? Has there been a recent change in weight (eg, unintended weight loss)?
* Does the client have symptoms, disease processes, treatment measures, medications, or diagnostic tests that are likely to interfere with nutrition? For example, many illnesses and oral medications cause anorexia, nausea, vomiting, and diarrhea.
* Are any conditions present that increase or decrease nutritional requirements?
* Check available reports of laboratory tests, such as serum albumin, complete blood count, and blood glucose. Nutritional disorders, as well as many other disorders, may cause abnormal values.

Nursing Diagnoses

* Altered Nutrition: Less Than Body Requirements related to inadequate intake
* Altered Nutrition: Less Than Body Requirements related to impaired ability to digest and absorb nutrients
* Altered Nutrition: More Than Body Requirements related to excessive intake
* Fluid Volume Deficit related to inadequate intake
* Fluid Volume Excess related to excessive intake
* Diarrhea related to enteral nutrition
* Altered Growth and Development related to nutrient deficiency
* Altered Protection related to nutrient deficiency
* Self Care Deficit: Feeding

* Body Image Disturbance related to excessive weight loss or weight gain
* Knowledge Deficit: Normal nutrition
* Knowledge Deficit: Nutritional needs during illness
* Risk for Infection related to microbial contamination of enteral formulas
* Risk for Infection related to impaired tissue integrity with parenteral therapy

Planning/Goals

The client will:

* Improve nutritional status in relation to body needs
* Maintain fluid and electrolyte balance
* Avoid complications of enteral nutrition, including aspiration, diarrhea, fluid volume deficit or excess, and infection
* Avoid complications of parenteral nutrition, including fluid volume deficit or excess and infection
* Identify the types and amounts of foods to meet nutritional needs
* Avoid overuse and abuse of anorexiant drugs

Interventions

Implement measures to prevent nutritional disorders by promoting a well-balanced diet for all clients. Depending on the client's condition, diet orders, food preferences, knowledge and attitudes about nutrition, and other factors, specific activities may include the following:

* Provide food and fluid the client is willing and able to take, at preferred times when possible.
* Assist the client to a sitting position, cut meat, open containers, feed the client, and perform other actions if indicated.
* Treat symptoms or disorders that are likely to interfere with nutrition, such as pain, nausea, vomiting, or diarrhea.
* Consult with the physician or dietitian when needed, especially when special diets are ordered. Compliance is improved when the ordered diet differs as little as possible from the usual diet. Also, preferred foods often may be substituted for disliked ones.
* Promote exercise and activity. For undernourished clients, this may increase appetite, improve digestion, and aid bowel elimination. For overweight and obese clients, exercise may decrease appetite and distract from eating behaviors as well as increase calorie expenditure.
* Minimize the use of sedative-type drugs when appropriate. Although no one should be denied pain relief, strong analgesics and other sedatives may cause drowsiness and decreased desire or

CLIENT/CAREGIVER TEACHING GUIDELINES
Nutritional Supplements and Tube Feedings

General Considerations

✔ Nutrition is extremely important in promoting health and recovery from illness. For people who are unable to take in enough nutrients because of poor appetite or illness, nutritional supplements can be very beneficial in improving their nutritional status. For example, supplemental feedings can slow or stop weight loss, increase energy and feelings of well-being, and increase resistance to infection.

✔ With oral supplements, choose one or more that the client is able and willing to take. Many are available, some in different flavors, and trying several different ones may be helpful. If a health care provider recommends one that the client does not like, ask for the names of others with comparable nutritional value.

✔ With feedings by a tube inserted into the gastrointestinal tract, taste is not a consideration. However, there may be other factors that make a formula more or less acceptable, such as the occurrence of nausea or diarrhea.

Self- or Caregiver Administration

✔ For oral supplemental feedings:
  ✔ Take or give at the preferred time and temperature, when possible. Chilling may improve taste.
  ✔ Mix powders or concentrated liquid preparations in preferred beverages, when possible. Some can be mixed with fruit juice, milk, tea, or coffee, which may improve taste and acceptability.
  ✔ Provide a variety of flavors, when possible, to improve acceptability.

✔ For tube feedings:
  ✔ Use or give with the client in a sitting position, if possible, to decrease risks of strangling and pulling formula into the lungs.
  ✔ Be sure the tube is placed correctly before each feeding. Ask a health care provider the best way of checking placement for your type of tube.

✔ Be sure the solution is room temperature. Cold formulas may cause abdominal cramping.

✔ Do not take or give more than 1 pint (500 mL) per feeding, including 2 to 3 oz of water for rinsing the tube. This helps to avoid overfilling the stomach and possible vomiting.

✔ Take or give slowly, over approximately 30 to 60 minutes. Rapid administration may cause nausea and vomiting.

✔ With continuous feedings, change containers and tubing daily. With intermittent feedings, rinse all equipment after each use, and change at least every 24 hours. Most tube feeding formulas are milk based and infection may occur if formulas become contaminated or equipment is not kept clean.

✔ Ask a health care provider about the amount of water to take or give. Most people receiving 1.5 to 2 quarts (1500 to 2000 mL) of tube feeding daily need approximately 1 quart (1000 mL) or more of water daily. However, clients' needs vary. Water can be mixed with the tube feeding formula, given after the tube feeding, or given between feedings. Be sure to include the amount of water used for rinsing the tube in the total daily amount.

✔ For giving medications by tube:
  ✔ Give liquid preparations when available. When not available, some tablets may be crushed and some capsules may be emptied and mixed with 1 to 2 tablespoons of water. Ask a health care provider which medications can safely be crushed or altered, because some (eg, long-acting or enteric-coated) can be harmful if crushed.
  ✔ Do not mix medications with the tube feeding formula because some medications may not be absorbed.
  ✔ Do not mix medications; give each one separately.
  ✔ Rinse the tube with water before and after each medication to get the medication through the tube and to keep the tube open.

---

ability to eat and drink as well as constipation and a feeling of fullness.
• Weigh clients at regular intervals.
• Use available resources to individualize nutritional care according to the client's clinical status and needs. For example, in hospitalized clients who are able to eat, consult a nutritionist about providing foods the client is able and willing to take. In hospitalized or outpatient clients who need a nutritional supplement, consult a nutritionist about choices, amounts, and costs.

• For clients receiving parenteral nutrition, monitor weight, fluid intake, urine output, vital signs, blood glucose, serum electrolytes, and complete blood count daily or weekly, according to the client's status and whether hospitalized or at home.

Evaluation
• Observe undernourished clients for quantity and quality of nutrient intake, weight gain, and

CLIENT TEACHING GUIDELINES
Drugs That Aid Weight Loss

General Considerations

✔ In addition to feeling better, health benefits of weight loss may include reduced blood pressure, reduced blood fats, less likelihood of having a heart attack or stroke, and less risk for development of diabetes mellitus.

✔ Any weight loss program should include a nutritionally adequate diet with decreased calories and increased exercise. The recommended rate of weight loss is approximately 2 to 3 lb weekly.

✔ Regular physical examinations and follow-up care are needed during weight loss programs.

✔ Diet and exercise are recommended for people who want to lose a few pounds. Medications to aid weight loss are usually recommended only for people whose health is endangered (ie, those who are overweight and have other risk factors for heart disease and those who are obese).

✔ Read package inserts and other available information about the drug being taken, who should not take the drug, instructions and precautions for safe usage, and so forth. Keep the material for later reference if questions arise. If unclear about any aspect of the information, consult a health care provider before taking the drug.

✔ Appetite-suppressant drugs (including nonprescription drugs containing phenylpropanolamine, such as Acutrim and Dexatrim) must be used correctly to avoid potentially serious adverse effects. Because these drugs stimulate the heart and the brain, adverse effects may include increased blood pressure, fast heart beat, irregular heart beat, heart attack, stroke, dizziness, nervousness, insomnia (if taken late in the day), and mental confusion. In addition, prolonged use of prescription drugs may lead to psychological dependence.

✔ Avoid over-the-counter decongestants and allergy, asthma, and cold remedies when taking an appetite suppressant. The combination can cause serious adverse effects from excessive heart and brain stimulation.

✔ Inform health care providers when taking an appetite suppressant, mainly to avoid other drugs with similar effects.

Self-administration

✔ Usually take appetite suppressants in the morning to decrease appetite during the day and avoid interference with sleep at night.

✔ Do not crush or chew sustained-release products.

✔ With sibutramine:
  ✔ Take once daily, with or without food.
  ✔ Have blood pressure and heart rate checked at regular intervals (the drug increases them).
  ✔ Notify a health care provider if a skin rash, hives, or other allergic reaction occurs.

✔ With phenylpropanolamine, follow instructions for the particular preparation:
  ✔ With immediate-release 25-mg tablets, take three times daily, a half hour before meals.
  ✔ With timed-release 75-mg tablets or capsules, take once daily in the morning.
  ✔ With precision release (16 hours), take 75 mg after breakfast.

✔ With orlistat:
  ✔ Take one capsule with each main meal, up to three capsules daily.
  ✔ Take supplements of vitamins A, D, E, and K 2 hours before or after taking orlistat. Ask a health care provider about recommended amounts.

---

improvement in laboratory tests of nutritional status (eg, serum proteins, blood sugar, electrolytes).

• Observe obese clients for food intake, weight loss, and appropriate use of exercise and anorexiant drugs.

• Observe children for quantity and quality of food intake and appropriate increases in height and weight.

• Interview and observe for signs and symptoms of complications of enteral and parenteral nutrition.

PRINCIPLES OF THERAPY

Managing Fluid Disorders

Fluid Deficiency

Treatment of fluid deficiency is aimed toward increasing intake or decreasing loss, depending on causative factors. The safest and most effective way of replacing body fluids is to give oral fluids when possible. Water is probably best, at least initially. Fluids containing large amounts of carbohydrate, fat, or protein are hypertonic and may increase fluid volume deficit if taken without sufficient water. If the client cannot take oral food or fluids for a few days or can take only limited amounts, IV fluids can be used to provide complete or supplemental amounts of fluids. Frequently used solutions include 5% dextrose in water or sodium chloride.

To meet fluid needs over a longer period, a nasogastric or other GI tube may be used to administer fluids. Fluid needs must be assessed carefully for the client receiving food and fluid only by tube. Additional water is needed after or between tube feedings. Another way of meeting long-term fluid needs when the GI tract cannot be used is parenteral nutrition. These IV solutions provide other nutrients as well as fluids.

Optimal amounts of fluid may vary greatly. For most clients, 2000 to 3000 mL daily is adequate. A person with severe heart failure or oliguric kidney disease needs smaller amounts, but someone with fever or extra losses (eg, vomiting, diarrhea) needs more.

Fluid Excess

Treatment of fluid excess is aimed toward decreasing intake and increasing loss. In acute circulatory overload or pulmonary edema, the usual treatment is to stop fluid intake (if the client is receiving IV fluids, slow the rate but keep the vein open for medication) and administer an IV diuretic. Because fluid excess may be a life-threatening emergency, prevention is better than treatment.

Managing Nutritional Deficiencies

Undernutrition impairs the function of essentially every body organ, impairs wound healing, and increases risks of infection. The goal of treatment is to provide an adequate quantity and quality of nutrients to meet tissue needs. Requirements for nutrients vary with age, level of activity, level of health or illness, and other factors that must be considered when designing appropriate therapy.

Oral Feedings

The safest and most effective way of increasing nutritional intake is by oral feedings when feasible. High-protein, high-calorie foods can be included in many diets and given as between-meal or bedtime snacks. If the client cannot ingest enough food and fluid, many of the commercial nutritional preparations can be given as between-meal supplements to increase intake of protein and calories. These preparations vary in taste and acceptability. Measures to improve taste may include chilling, serving over ice, or mixing with fruit juice or another beverage. Specific methods depend on the client's taste preferences and the available formulas. Refer to instructions, usually on the labels, for appropriate diluting and mixing of beverages.

Enteral (Tube) Feedings

When oral feeding is contraindicated but the GI tract is functioning, tube feeding has several advantages over IV fluids, especially for long-term use. First, tube feeding is usually safer, more convenient, and more economical. Second, it helps to prevent GI atrophy, maintain GI function, and maintain immune system function. Third, several tubes and placement sites are available. For example, a nasogastric tube may be used for approximately 4 weeks. For long-term feedings, a gastrostomy tube may be placed percutaneously (called percutaneous endoscopic gastrostomy) or surgically. Nasointestinal tubes are recommended for clients at risk of aspiration from gastric feedings or with gastric disorders. Except for gastrostomy tubes, the tubes should be soft and small bore to decrease trauma.

When tube feedings are the client's only source of nutrients, they should be nutritionally complete and given in amounts calculated to provide adequate water, protein, calories, vitamins, and minerals. Although tube feeding formulas vary in the volume needed for adequate intake of nutrients, any of the complete formulas can be used effectively. Other guidelines include the following:

- Once the kind and amount of formula are chosen, the method of feeding is selected. For feedings that enter the stomach, an intermittent schedule of administration every 4 to 6 hours, over 30 to 60 minutes, is usually recommended. For feedings that enter the duodenum or jejunum, a continuous drip method is required because the small bowel cannot tolerate the larger volumes of intermittent feedings. Continuous feedings require an infusion pump for accurate control of the flow rate. When used at home, enteral feedings are often given overnight to allow daytime oral feedings and more activity, if feasible, for the client.
- A common practice has been to initiate feedings with small amounts of diluted solution (ie, half strength), then increase to larger amounts and full strength. The rationale is to decrease the diarrhea and dehydration that may ensue when hypertonic solutions are given and water is drawn into the GI tract. Some authorities question the value of this regimen and prefer starting with small amounts of full-strength formulas. Isocal and Osmolite are isotonic and should be given full strength. Most formulas provide 1 kcal/mL so that caloric intake can be quickly calculated. Water can be given with, after, or between regular feedings and with medications, according to the client's fluid needs.
- Other than problems resulting from hypertonic solutions and inadequate fluid intake (diarrhea, fluid volume deficit, hypernatremia), a major complication of tube feeding is aspiration of the formula into the lungs. This is more likely to occur with unconscious clients. It can be prevented by correctly positioning clients,

verifying tube placement (before every intermittent feeding and approximately every 4 hours with continuous feedings), and giving feedings slowly.

Parenteral Feedings

Parenteral feedings are indicated when the GI tract is nonfunctioning, when enteral feedings would aggravate conditions such as inflammatory bowel diseases or pancreatitis, and when nutritional needs cannot be met by enteral feedings. For short-term use (approximately 3 to 5 days) of IV fluids, the goal is to provide adequate amounts of fluids and electrolytes and enough carbohydrate to minimize oxidation of body protein and fat for energy. The choice of specific solution depends on individual needs, but it should contain at least 5% dextrose. A frequently used solution is 5% dextrose in 0.22% sodium chloride, 2000 to 3000 mL/24 hours. Potassium chloride is often added, and vitamins may be added. These solutions are nutritionally inadequate.

Parenteral Nutrition

For long-term IV feedings (weeks to months), the goal is to provide all nutrients required for normal body functioning, including tissue growth. This goal can be met with parenteral nutrition. Basic nutritional solutions provide water, carbohydrate, protein, vitamins, and minerals. Originally, calories were supplied primarily by 25% to 50% glucose. This resulted in a hypertonic solution that had to be given in a central vein so it could be diluted rapidly. Although effective, central parenteral nutrition requires special techniques to increase safety and decrease complications. For example, a physician must insert the central IV catheter, and placement must be verified by a chest x-ray. Complications include air embolism and pneumothorax. Peripheral parenteral nutrition (PPN) was then developed. PPN, which contains 5% or 10% dextrose, can be given alone or in combination with oral or enteral feedings to increase nutrient intake.

Intravenous fat emulsions provide calories and essential fatty acids. These solutions are isotonic and may be given centrally or peripherally. When given peripherally, they are coinfused with the PPN solution. The fat emulsion is thought to protect the vein and decrease phlebitis.

Guidelines for administration of central parenteral nutrition and PPN include the following:

- Administer with an infusion pump to control the flow rate accurately. The solution must be given at a consistent rate so nutrients can be used and complications prevented. The initial flow rate is usually 50 mL/hour; flow rate is then increased as tolerated to meet nutritional requirements (approximately 1500 to 3000 mL/day). With home administration, the entire daily amount may be infused overnight.
- To prevent infection, several measures are indicated. First, the IV catheter must be inserted with aseptic technique. Second, all solutions must be prepared aseptically in a pharmacy under a laminar-flow hood. Third, use a 0.45- to 0.22-µm in-line filter. Fourth, change solution containers and tubing every 24 hours. Fifth, change the dressing at the venipuncture site every 48 hours. Most hospitals and home health agencies have established protocols regarding dressing changes. These usually include cleansing around the catheter with povidone-iodine solution (Betadine), applying povidone-iodine ointment, and reapplying an occlusive dressing. Sterile technique is used throughout.
- "Piggyback" fat emulsions into the IV line beyond the filter.

Managing Overweight or Obesity

The general goals of weight management are to assist clients to prevent further weight gain, lose weight, and maintain a lower body weight more conducive to health. People who want to lose a few pounds should be encouraged to decrease caloric intake and increase exercise. For overweight people (BMI of 25 to 29.9 kg/m^2), treatment is recommended for those with two or more risk factors (eg, hypertension, dyslipidemia, diabetes) or a high waist circumference (central obesity). For obese people (BMI of 30 kg/m^2 or above), treatment is recommended. Considerations include the following:

- Any weight reduction program needs to include a reduced-calorie diet and physical activity. Diets should consist of nutritionally sound foods in balanced meals. "Fad" diets are potentially hazardous to health and should be avoided. Exercise increases use of calories and helps preserve lean body mass during weight loss. It may also help to prevent the decreased metabolic rate that usually occurs with low-calorie diets.
- Emphasize health benefits of weight reduction. There is strong evidence that weight loss reduces risk factors for cardiovascular disease, including blood pressure, serum triglycerides, and total and LDL cholesterol. It also increases high-density lipoprotein cholesterol. In addition, in overweight and obese people without diabetes, weight loss reduces blood glucose levels and the risk for development of type 2 diabetes. For

people who already have type 2 diabetes, weight loss reduces blood levels of glucose and glycosylated hemoglobin. These effects make the diabetes easier to manage, reduce complications of diabetes, and may allow smaller doses of antidiabetic medications. In general, modest weight losses of only 5 to 10 lbs lower blood pressure and blood lipids and improve insulin resistance and glucose tolerance.

- Provide psychological support and positive reinforcement for efforts toward weight management.
- There seems to be increasing consensus that obesity is a chronic disease and that obese people should take weight loss medications on a long-term basis. Usually, however, the medications are recommended only in clients whose health is significantly endangered by obesity.
- When drug therapy is indicated, a single drug in the lowest effective dose is recommended. As with most other drugs, low doses decrease risks of adverse drug effects.
- Clients undergoing a weight loss regimen should be monitored regularly in terms of body weight, BMI, blood pressure, blood lipids, and other factors as indicated.
- A client taking an appetite suppressant who has not lost 4 lbs during the first month of treatment is unlikely to benefit from longer use of the drug.
- Maximum weight loss usually occurs during the first 6 months of drug therapy. With most available drugs, use for this long is an unlabeled use of the drug.
- After a weight loss regimen of a few months, some experts recommend letting the body adjust to the lower weight before attempting additional losses. Thus, a weight maintenance program, possibly with continued drug therapy, is indicated.
- The use of OTC appetite suppressants (eg, Dexatrim, Acutrim) is discouraged because of potentially serious adverse effects. In addition, these drugs should *never* be taken with prescription appetite suppressants.
- The National Institutes of Health do not recommend combining weight loss medications except in the context of clinical trials. This recommendation may change with orlistat, which works in the intestines and is not systemically absorbed.

Nutritional Support and Obesity in Children

Children in general need increased amounts of water, protein, carbohydrate, and fat in proportion to their size to support growth and increased physical activity. However, reports of childhood obesity and inadequate exercise abound. Therefore, the goal of nutritional support is to meet needs without promoting obesity.

With tube feedings, to prevent nausea and regurgitation, the recommended rate of administration is no more than 5 mL every 5 to 10 minutes for premature and small infants and 10 mL/minute for older infants and children. Preparation of formulas, positioning of children, and administration are the same as for adults to prevent aspiration, diarrhea, and infection.

Parenteral nutrition may be indicated in infants and children who cannot eat or be fed enterally. With newborns, especially preterm and low–birth-weight infants, parenteral nutrition is needed within approximately 3 days of birth because they have little nutritional reserve. However, lipid emulsions should be given very cautiously in preterm infants because deaths have been attributed to increased serum levels of lipids and free fatty acids. With other infants and children, parenteral nutrition may be used during medical illnesses or perioperative conditions to improve or maintain nutritional status. Overall, benefits include weight gain, increased height, increased liver synthesis of plasma proteins, and improved healing and recovery.

Treatment of childhood obesity should focus on normalizing food intake, especially fat intake, and increasing physical activity. One study indicates more success when caregivers work with the parents rather than the children themselves. None of the available weight loss drugs is indicated for use in children.

Emphasis is being placed on prevention of obesity, especially in children, adolescents, and young adults. The main elements are a more active lifestyle, a low-fat diet, regular meals, avoidance of snacking, drinking water instead of calorie-containing beverages, and decreasing the time spent watching television.

Nutritional Support and Obesity in Older Adults

Older adults are at risk for development of deficits and excesses in fluid volume. Inadequate intake is common and may result from numerous causes (eg, impaired thirst mechanism, impaired ability to obtain and drink fluids, inadequate water with tube feedings). Increased losses also occur with diuretic drugs, which are commonly prescribed for older adults. Fluid volume excess is most likely to occur with large amounts or rapid administration of IV fluids, especially in older adults with impaired cardiovascular function.

Older adults also are at risk of undernutrition in terms of protein, carbohydrate, and fat intake. Inadequate intake may result from the inability to obtain and prepare food, as well as disease processes that interfere with the ability to digest and use nutrients. When alternative feeding methods (tube feedings, IV fluids) are used, careful assessment of nutritional status is required to avoid deficits or excesses. Overweight and obesity are also common among older adults. Although caloric needs are usually decreased in older adults, primarily because of slowed metabolism and decreased physical activity, most people continue usual eating patterns. With the high incidence of atherosclerosis and cardiovascular disease in older adults, it is especially important that fat intake be reduced. Anorexiant drugs should be used very cautiously, if at all, because older adults often have cardiovascular, renal, or hepatic impairments that increase risks of adverse drug effects. The newer drug, orlistat, has not been studied in older adults.

Use in Renal Impairment

Because the kidneys excrete water and waste products of food metabolism, clients with renal impairment often have accumulation of water and urea nitrogen. As a result, these clients have special needs in relation to nutritional support. The needs differ with acute renal failure (ARF) and chronic renal failure (CRF).

With ARF, clients usually have major physiologic stress (eg, serious illness, sepsis, major surgery) that leads to metabolic disorders. These disorders include glucose intolerance (hyperglycemia and peripheral insulin resistance); accumulation of urea nitrogen, the end product of protein metabolism; and increased serum triglyceride levels from disordered fat metabolism. With CRF, clients are not usually as stressed as those with ARF. However, they often have multiple metabolic and fluid and electrolyte disorders. Those on dialysis have impaired host defense mechanisms and increased risk of infection. Undernourished clients have increased morbidity and mortality. Some considerations in nutritional support of clients with ARF and CRF are listed in the following sections.

Acute Renal Failure

- In early ARF, dietary protein is usually restricted to 20 to 30 g/day to minimize urea nitrogen production.
- In oliguric ARF, small volumes of concentrated nutrients with minimal sodium are needed.
- In nonoliguric ARF, large amounts of sodium may be lost in urine and sodium replacement may be needed.
- Enteral nutrition is preferred if possible. However, most clients are unable to tolerate enteral feedings because they are critically ill and have an ileus.
- Parenteral nutrition formulas should be carefully calculated according to nutritional status and metabolic disorders. Several amino acid solutions are formulated for clients with renal failure (eg, Aminosyn-RF, Aminess, NephrAmine, RenAmin). In addition, clients with ARF often have hyperkalemia, hyperphosphatemia, and hypermagnesemia, so that potassium, phosphorus, and magnesium should be omitted until serum levels return to normal.
- Intravenous fat emulsions should not be given to clients with ARF if serum triglyceride levels exceed 300 mg/dL.

Chronic Renal Failure

- Enteral nutritional support is usually indicated because the GI tract is functional. Normal amounts of protein (eg, 1 g/kg/day) may be given. The former recommendation that protein restriction delayed progression of renal failure and the need for dialysis is not supported by newer data.
- High-calorie, low-electrolyte enteral formulations are usually indicated. Nepro is a formulation for clients receiving dialysis; Suplena, which is lower in protein and some electrolytes than Nepro, may be used in clients who are not receiving dialysis.
- If parenteral nutrition is needed, solutions should be carefully formulated according to nutritional status, the extent of metabolic disorders, and whether the client is receiving dialysis. Several amino acid solutions are formulated for clients with renal failure (eg, Aminosyn-RF, Aminess, NephrAmine, RenAmin).
- Serum triglyceride levels should be measured before IV fat emulsions are given. Many clients with CRF have hypertriglyceridemia, which would be worsened by fat emulsions, possibly leading to pancreatitis.

In relation to drugs for weight loss and obesity, little information is available about their use in clients with renal impairment. With sibutramine, dosage reductions are not recommended with mild to moderate impairment because the drug and its active metabolites are eliminated by the liver. However, some inactive metabolites are also formed and these are excreted renally. The drug is contraindicated in clients with severe renal impairment.

Use in Hepatic Impairment

The liver is extremely important in digestion and metabolism of carbohydrates, proteins, and fat as well as storage of nutrients. Thus, clients with impaired hepatic function are often undernourished, with impaired metabolism of foodstuffs, vitamin deficiencies, and fluid and electrolyte imbalances. Depending on the disease process and the extent of liver impairment, these clients have special needs in relation to nutritional support.

- Clients with alcoholic hepatitis or cirrhosis have a high rate of metabolism and therefore need foods to supply extra energy. However, metabolic disorders interfere with the liver's ability to process and use foodstuffs.
- Disorders of glucose metabolism are common. Clients with cirrhosis often have hyperglycemia. Clients with severe hepatitis often have hypoglycemia because of impaired hepatic production of glucose and possibly impaired hepatic metabolism of insulin.
- Protein restriction is usually needed in clients with cirrhosis to prevent or treat hepatic encephalopathy, which is caused by excessive protein or excessive production of ammonia (from protein breakdown in

the GI tract). For clients able to tolerate enteral feedings (usually by GI tube), Nutrihep and Hepatic Aid II are products formulated for clients with liver failure. When peripheral or central parenteral nutrition is necessary for clients with hepatic failure and hepatic encephalopathy, HepatAmine, a special formulation of amino acids, may be used. Other amino acid preparations are contraindicated in clients with hepatic encephalopathy and coma.

- Enteral and parenteral fat preparations must be used very cautiously. Medium-chain triglycerides (eg, MCT oil), which are used to provide calories in other malnourished clients, may lead to coma in clients with advanced cirrhosis. Clients who require parenteral nutrition may develop high serum triglyceride levels and pancreatitis if given usual amounts of IV fat emulsions. If serum triglyceride levels exceed 300 mg/dL, fat emulsions should be used only to prevent a deficiency of essential fatty acids.
- Sodium and fluid restrictions are often needed to decrease edema.

In relation to drugs for weight loss and obesity, little information is available about their use in clients with hepatic impairment. Because sibutramine is metabolized in the liver, it is contraindicated in clients with severe hepatic impairment.

Use in Critical Illness

Critically ill clients often have organ failures that alter their ability to use and eliminate essential nutrients. Thus, their nutritional needs vary with the type and extent of organ impairment. In addition to renal and hepatic impairments, which were discussed previously, clients with pulmonary failure, cardiac failure, and multiple organ dysfunction syndrome (MODS) have specific needs in relation to nutritional support.

Pulmonary Impairment

- In clients with chronic obstructive pulmonary disease (COPD), major concerns are weight loss and decreasing the work of breathing. Weight loss is attributed mainly to hyperactive metabolism. However, increasing caloric intake in these clients must be done cautiously because overfeeding leads to increased carbon dioxide (CO_2) production, increased work of breathing, and perhaps respiratory acidosis. Thus, excessive carbohydrate in enteral or parenteral feedings may cause respiratory failure.
- Enteral nutrition is preferred if the GI tract is functional and accessible. Nutrivent and Pulmocare are enteral products for clients with COPD or respiratory failure and mechanical ventilation. They contain less carbohydrate and more fat than other products.

- Clients need adequate amounts of protein, but too much can increase the work of breathing and lead to muscle fatigue and respiratory failure. Moderate amounts (1 to 1.5 g/kg/day) are recommended for clients with stable COPD. Higher amounts are usually needed by clients with sepsis and respiratory failure who require mechanical ventilation.
- Enteral formulas with more concentrated calories (eg, 2 kcal/mL) may be useful for clients with adult respiratory distress syndrome (ARDS), pulmonary edema, or other conditions requiring fluid restriction.
- Parenteral nutrition is often needed because clients with pulmonary failure from severe pneumonia or septicemia may have a prolonged ileus and be unable to tolerate enteral feedings. As with enteral feedings, excessive carbohydrate must be avoided.
- Intravenous fat emulsions should be infused slowly, over 24 hours. Rapid infusion may lead to pulmonary vasoconstriction.
- Excessive amounts of sodium and fluids should be avoided with both enteral and parenteral nutrition because they may worsen impaired pulmonary function.

Cardiac Impairment

- Undernutrition may lead to decreased cardiac output and stroke volume, with resultant hypotension and bradycardia.
- Excessive amounts of nutrients or fluids may worsen heart failure by increasing cardiac workload.
- Restricting sodium and fluid intake and increasing serum albumin may decrease edema and prevent or treat congestive heart failure, which commonly occurs in clients with impaired cardiac function. Also, loop diuretics are often given to increase excretion of sodium and water.
- With enteral nutrition, concentrated products (eg, 1.5 to 2 kcal/mL) provide more calories and help with fluid restrictions.
- Parenteral nutrition is usually needed only when a superimposed illness prevents use of the GI tract. Excessive amounts of sodium and fluid or rapid administration may precipitate or worsen heart failure and should be avoided. If IV fat emulsions are used, they should be given over 24 hours because faster infusion may depress myocardial function.

Multiple Organ Dysfunction Syndrome

- Clients with MODS, who are usually in critical care units, require nutritional support because they have high rates of metabolism and tissue breakdown (catabolism). However, nutritional support is complex because a client may have a combination of renal, hepatic, pulmonary, and cardiac impairments.

Thus, it must be individualized according to the type and extent of organ impairment.

- Clients often have an ileus and GI dysfunction so that they require parenteral nutrition.
- Usual amounts of glucose are usually recommended. Clients with oliguric ARF or ARDS as part of their MODS need concentrated nutrients because fluid intake must be limited.
- During the severe physiologic stress of MODS, clients need higher-than-usual amounts of protein (eg, 1.5 to 2.5 g/kg/day) for growth, tissue maintenance and repair, and enzyme and hormone production. However, many clients may not be able to tolerate this amount because of organ impairments. For example, clients with ARF and dialysis or severe hepatic failure usually have protein intake restricted.
- Intravenous fat emulsions, a readily used source of energy, should provide 20% to 30% of calories. They also provide essential fatty acids. Some clients with MODS already have high serum triglyceride levels and are at risk for development of acute pancreatitis and further organ impairment. In these clients, IV fat emulsions are usually avoided until serum triglyceride levels are less than 300 mg/dL. In clients with MODS who receive IV fat emulsions, serum triglyceride levels should be monitored at least weekly.

 Home Care

The home care nurse is involved with nutritional matters in almost any home care setting. Because nutrition is so important to health, the home care nurse should take advantage of any opportunity for health promotion in this area. Health promotion may involve assessing the nutritional status of all members of the household, especially children, elderly adults, and those with obvious deficiencies or excesses, and providing counseling or other assistance to improve nutritional status.

For clients receiving tube feedings at home, the home care nurse may teach about the goals of treatment, administration, preparation or storage of solutions, equipment (eg, obtaining, cleaning), and monitoring responses (eg, weight, urine output).

For clients receiving parenteral nutrition at home, solutions, infusion pumps, and other equipment are often obtained from a pharmacy, home health agency, or independent company. The home care nurse may not be involved in the initial setup but is likely to participate in ongoing client care, monitoring of client responses, and supporting caregivers. In addition, the home care nurse may need to coordinate activities among physicians, IV therapy personnel, and other health care providers.

(*text continues on page 449*)

NURSING ACTIONS | **Nutritional Products and Drugs for Obesity**

NURSING ACTIONS	RATIONALE/EXPLANATION
1. Administer accurately	
a. For oral supplemental feedings:	
(1) Give at the preferred time and temperature, when possible.	To increase the likelihood the feeding will be taken. Chilling the formula may increase palatability.
(2) Mix powders or concentrated liquid preparations in preferred beverages if not contraindicated.	Some can be mixed with fruit juice, milk, tea, or coffee, which may improve taste and acceptability.
b. For intravenous (IV) feedings:	
(1) Administer fluids at the prescribed flow rate. Use an infusion control device for hyperalimentation solutions.	To administer sufficient fluids without a rapid flow rate. Rapid flow rates or large amounts of IV fluids can cause circulatory overload and pulmonary edema. In addition, hyperglycemia and osmotic diuresis may occur with hyperalimentation solutions.
(2) With IV fat emulsions, connect to the primary IV line beyond the filter; start slowly (0.5–1 mL/min) for approximately 30 minutes. If no adverse effects occur, increase rate to a maximum of 125 mL/h for the 10% solution or 60 mL/h for a 20% solution.	Lipid emulsions should not be filtered.

(continued)

NURSING ACTIONS	RATIONALE/EXPLANATION
(3) Use sterile technique when changing containers, tubings, or dressings.	To prevent infection
(4) When adding drugs, use sterile technique, and add only those drugs known to be compatible with the IV solution.	To avoid physical or chemical incompatibility
(5) Do not administer antibiotics or other drugs through central venous catheters.	To avoid incompatibilities and possible precipitation or inactivation of the drug or fluid components
c. For tube feedings:	
(1) Have the client sitting, if possible.	To decrease risks of aspirating formula into lungs
(2) Check tube placement before each feeding by aspirating stomach contents or instilling air into the tube while listening over the stomach with a stethoscope.	To prevent aspiration or accidental instillation of feedings into lungs
(3) Give the solution at room temperature.	Cold formulas may cause abdominal cramping.
(4) If giving by intermittent instillation, do not give more than 500 mL per feeding, including water for rinsing the tube.	To avoid gastric distention, possible vomiting, and aspiration into lungs
(5) Give by gravity flow (over 30–60 minutes) or infusion pump.	Rapid administration may cause nausea, vomiting, and other symptoms.
(6) With continuous feedings, change containers and tubing daily. With intermittent bolus feedings, rinse all equipment after each use, and change at least every 24 hours.	Most tube feeding formulas are milk based and provide a good culture medium for bacterial growth. Clean technique, not sterile technique, is required.
(7) Give an adequate amount of water, based on assessment of fluid needs. This may be done by mixing water with the tube feeding formula, giving it after the tube feeding, or giving it between feedings.	To avoid dehydration and promote fluid balance. Most clients receiving 1500 to 2000 mL of tube feeding formula daily will need 1000 mL or more of water daily.
(8) Rinse nasogastric tubes with at least 50 to 100 mL water after each bolus feeding or administration of medications through the tube.	To keep the tube patent and functioning. This water is included in calculation of fluid intake.
(9) When medications are ordered by tube, liquid preparations are preferred over crushed tablets or powders emptied from capsules.	Tablets or powders may stick in the tube lumen. This may mean the full dose of the medication does not reach the stomach. Also, the tube is likely to become obstructed.
d. With pancreatic enzymes, give with meals or food.	To obtain therapeutic effects, these agents must be in the small intestine when food is present.
e. With anorexiant drugs:	
(1) Give single-dose drugs in the early morning.	For maximum appetite-suppressant effects during the day
(2) Give multiple-dose preparations 30 to 60 minutes before meals and the last dose of the day about 6 hours before bedtime.	For maximum appetite-suppressant effects at mealtime and to avoid interference with sleep from the drug's stimulating effects on the central nervous system (CNS)
f. With orlistat, give one capsule with each main meal, up to three capsules daily.	The drug needs to be in the gastrointestinal tract when fat-containing foods are eaten to prevent fat absorption.

(continued)

NURSING ACTIONS	RATIONALE/EXPLANATION
2. Observe for therapeutic effects	
a. With water and other fluids, observe for fluid balance (amber-colored urine, approximately 1500 mL daily; moist mucous membranes in the oral cavity; adequate skin turgor).	
b. With nutritional formulas given orally or by tube feeding, observe for weight gain and increased serum albumin. For infants and children receiving milk substitutes, observe for decreased diarrhea and weight gain.	Therapeutic effects depend on the reason for use (ie, prevention or treatment of undernutrition).
c. With parenteral hyperalimentation, observe for weight maintenance or gain and normal serum levels of glucose, electrolytes, and protein.	These are indications of improved metabolism, nitrogen balance, and nutritional status. When parenteral hyperalimentation is used for gastrointestinal malabsorption syndromes, diarrhea and other symptoms are usually relieved when oral feedings are stopped.
d. With pancreatic enzymes, observe for decreased diarrhea and steatorrhea.	The pancreatic enzymes function the same way as endogenous enzymes to aid digestion of carbohydrate, protein, and fat.
e. With anorexiant drugs and orlistat, observe for decreased caloric intake and weight loss.	The recommended rate of weight loss is approximately 2 to 3 lb weekly.
3. Observe for adverse effects	
a. With fluids, observe for peripheral edema, circulatory overload, and pulmonary edema (severe dyspnea, crackles).	Fluid excess is most likely to occur with rapid administration or large amounts of IV fluids, especially in people who are elderly or have congestive heart failure.
b. With commercial nutritional formulas (except Osmolite and Isocal), observe for hypotension, tachycardia, increased urine output, dehydration, nausea, vomiting, or diarrhea.	These adverse reactions are usually attributed to the hyperosmolality or hypertonicity of the preparations. They can be prevented or minimized by starting with small amounts of formula, given slowly.
c. With parenteral hyperalimentation, observe for elevated blood and urine glucose levels, signs of infection (fever, inflammation at the venipuncture site), concentrated urine or high specific gravity ($\geq$1.035), hypertension, dyspnea.	These signs and symptoms indicate complications of therapy. Except for infection, they are likely to occur when the solution is given in a concentration or at a rate that delivers more glucose than can be used. This produces hyperglycemia, which in turn causes excessive amounts of fluid to be excreted in the urine (osmotic diuresis). Hyperglycemic, hyperosmolar, nonketotic coma also may occur.
d. With IV fat emulsions, observe for signs of fat embolism (dyspnea, fever, chills, pain in the chest and back), phlebitis from vein irritation, and sepsis from contamination. Hyperlipidemia and hepatomegaly also may occur.	Thrombophlebitis and sepsis are the most frequent adverse effects.
e. With anorexiant drugs, observe for:	
(1) Nervousness, insomnia, hyperactivity	These adverse effects are caused by excessive stimulation of the CNS. They are more likely to occur with large doses or too frequent administration.
(2) Hypertension	Anorexiant drugs stimulate the sympathetic nervous system and may cause or aggravate hypertension.

(continued)

NURSING ACTIONS	RATIONALE/EXPLANATION
(3) Development of tolerance to appetite-suppressant effects	This usually occurs within 4 to 6 weeks and is an indication for discontinuing drug administration. Continued administration does not maintain appetite-suppressant effects but increases incidence of adverse effects. In addition, taking large doses of the drug does not restore appetite-suppressant effects.
(4) Signs of psychological drug dependence	More likely with large doses or long-term use
f. With orlistat, observe for abdominal cramping, gas pains, diarrhea, and fatty stools.	These effects commonly occur and worsen with a high intake of dietary fat. The drug should not be used as an excuse for eating large amounts of fatty foods.
4. Observe for drug interactions with anorexiants	
a. Drugs that *increase* effects:	
(1) Antidepressants, tricyclic	May increase hypertensive effects of anorexiants
(2) Monoamine oxidase (MAO) inhibitors	Increase hypertensive effects. Anorexiants should not be given within 2 weeks of MAO inhibitors because of possible hypertensive crisis.
(3) Other CNS stimulants	Additive stimulant effects
(4) Other sympathomimetic drugs (eg, epinephrine, isoproterenol)	Additive hypertensive and other cardiovascular effects
b. Drugs that *decrease* effects:	
(1) Antihypertensive drugs	Anorexiants have blood pressure–raising effects that antagonize blood pressure–lowering effects of drugs used for hypertension.
(2) CNS depressants (eg, alcohol, chlorpromazine)	Antagonize or decrease effects

How Can You Avoid This Medication Error?

Answer: Pancreatic enzymes are usually given before meals, so that the medication will be in the small intestine to aid digestion. Giving this drug at the wrong time (more than 1 hour after eating breakfast) decreases drug effectiveness. Review your abbreviations to ensure that you can interpret drug orders correctly. Organize your day so that ac medications can be administered before eating.

Nursing Notes: Apply Your Knowledge

Answer: To obtain a ½ strength solution, the formula has to be diluted with an equal amount of water, so you will add 240 cc of tap water to 1 can of Ensure. The infusion rate is for 2000 mL per 24 hours, which calculates to an hourly rate of 83 mL/hour. Set the infusion pump to deliver 83 mL/hour.

 REVIEW AND APPLICATION EXERCISES

1. Differentiate clients who are at high risk for development of fluid imbalances.
2. When assessing a client's fluid balance, what signs and symptoms indicate fluid volume deficit or excess?
3. What are pharmacologic and nonpharmacologic interventions to restore fluid balance when an imbalance occurs?
4. For clients who are unable to ingest food, which nutrients can be provided with IV nutritional formulas?
5. What is the role of lipid emulsions in parenteral nutrition?
6. In an infant receiving parenteral nutrition, what is the best way to assess the adequacy of nutritional status?
7. In an outpatient or home care client with a protein-calorie deficit and various commercial nutritional formulas:
   Analyze the types and amounts of nutrients provided.

Choose a supplement to recommend to the client or caregiver.

Designate the amount to be taken daily for optimum nutritional status.

Suggest ways to increase palatability and client ingestion of the nutrients.

8. With an overweight or obese client who wants to lose weight, what are some nursing interventions to assist and support the client?

9. With critically ill clients, what special needs must be considered in relation to nutritional support?

SELECTED REFERENCES

Brown, R.O. & Sacks, G.S. (1997). Nutritional considerations in major organ failure. In J.T. DiPiro, R.L. Talbert, G.C. Yee, G.R. Matzke, B.G. Wells, & L.M. Posey (Eds.), *Pharmacotherapy: A pathophysiologic approach*, 3rd ed., pp. 2805–2830. Stamford, CT: Appleton & Lange.

Chessman, K.H. & Anderson, J.D. (1997). Pediatric and geriatric nutrition support. In J.T. DiPiro, R.L. Talbert, G.C. Yee, G.R. Matzke, B.G. Wells, & L.M. Posey (Eds.), *Pharmacotherapy: A pathophysiologic approach*, 3rd ed., pp. 2787–2804. Stamford, CT: Appleton & Lange.

Darby, M.K. & Loughead, J.L. (1996). Neonatal nutritional requirements and formula composition: A review. *Journal of Obstetrics, Gynecology, and Neonatal Nursing, 25*, 209–217.

Davidson, M.H., Hauptman, J., DiGirolamo, M., Foreyt, J.P., Halsted, C.H., Heber, D., et al. (1999). Weight control and risk factor reduction in obese subjects treated for 2 years with orlistat: A randomized controlled trial. *Journal of the American Medical Association, 281*, 235–242.

Drug facts and comparisons. (Updated monthly). St. Louis: Facts and Comparisons.

Dwyer, J.T., Stone, E.T., Yang, M., Feldman, H., Webber, L.S., Must, A., et al. (1998). Predictors of overweight and overfatness in a multi-ethnic pediatric population. *American Journal of Clinical Nutrition, 67*, 602–610.

Expert Panel. (1998). Clinical guidelines on the identification, evaluation, and treatment of overweight and obesity in adults: Executive summary. *American Journal of Clinical Nutrition, 68*, 899–917.

Golan, M., Weizman, A., Apter, A., & Fainara, M. (1998). Parents as the exclusive agents of change in the treatment of childhood obesity. *American Journal of Clinical Nutrition, 67*, 1130–1135.

Gunnell, D.J., Frankel, S.J., Nanchahal, K., Peters, T.J., & Smith, G.D. (1998). Childhood obesity and adult cardiovascular mortality. *American Journal of Clinical Nutrition, 67*, 1111–1118.

Janson, D.D. (1997). Enteral nutrition. In J.T. DiPiro, R.L. Talbert, G.C. Yee, G.R. Matzke, B.G. Wells, & L.M. Posey (Eds.), *Pharmacotherapy: A pathophysiologic approach*, 3rd ed., pp. 2759–2785. Stamford, CT: Appleton & Lange.

Mattox, T.W. (1997). Parenteral nutrition. In J.T. DiPiro, R.L. Talbert, G.C. Yee, G.R. Matzke, B.G. Wells, & L.M. Posey (Eds.), *Pharmacotherapy: A pathophysiologic approach*, 3rd ed., pp. 2735–2758. Stamford, CT: Appleton & Lange.

Morrissey, N.A. (1996). Gastrointestinal intubation and special nutritional management. In S.C. Smeltzer & B.G. Bare (Eds.), *Brunner and Suddarth's textbook of medical-surgical nursing*, 8th ed., pp. 859–883. Philadelphia: Lippincott-Raven.

Pinkowish, M.D. (1998). Obesity: A chronic disease. *Patient Care, 32*(16), 29–50.

Pleuss, J. (1998). Alterations in nutritional status. In C.M. Porth (Ed.), *Pathophysiology: Concepts of altered health states*, 5th ed., pp. 1243–1263. Philadelphia: Lippincott Williams & Wilkins.

Stenson, W.F. & Eisenberg, P. (1997). Parenteral and enteral nutrition. In W.N. Kelley (Ed.), *Textbook of internal medicine*, 3rd ed., pp. 890–902. Philadelphia: Lippincott-Raven.

Stunkard, A.J. & Wadden, T.A. (1997). Obesity. In W.N. Kelley (Ed.), *Textbook of internal medicine*, 3rd ed., pp. 192–198. Philadelphia: Lippincott-Raven.

Wallace, J.I. & Schwartz, R.S. (1997). Geriatric clinical nutrition including malnutrition and cachexia. In W.N. Kelley (Ed.), *Textbook of internal medicine*, 3rd ed., pp. 2554–2560. Philadelphia: Lippincott-Raven.

Williamson, D.F. (1999). Pharmacotherapy for obesity [Editorial]. *Journal of the American Medical Association, 281*, 278–280.

31

Vitamins

Objectives

After studying this chapter, the student will be able to:

1. Review functions and food sources of essential vitamins.

2. Differentiate between maintenance and therapeutic doses of vitamins.

3. Identify clients at risk for development of vitamin deficiency or excess.

4. Delineate circumstances in which therapeutic vitamins are likely to be needed.

5. Describe adverse effects associated with overdose of fat-soluble and selected water-soluble vitamins.

6. Discuss the rationale for administering vitamin K to newborns.

You have been asked to speak with a group of senior citizens, living independently in a retirement community, about vitamins and health. You have a group of about 25 who signed up for this talk as part of a general education series on "Staying Fit and Healthy After 65."

Reflect on:

▶ Teaching strategies that might enhance learning, considering the size of the group and the age of the participants.

▶ Review important vitamins, their benefits, and Recommended Dietary Allowances (RDAs).

▶ Review dietary sources to meet daily requirements.

▶ Problem-solve which nonprescription vitamins are indicated and cost-effective.

▶ Review potential problems in megadosing.

OVERVIEW

Vitamins are required for normal body metabolism. They act mainly as coenzymes to help convert carbohydrate and fat into energy and form bones and tissues. They are effective in small amounts and are mainly obtained from foods or supplements. Most nutritionists agree that a varied and well-balanced diet provides an adequate intake of vitamins for most people and that dietary sources of vitamins are in general preferred to supplement sources. However, studies indicate that most adults and children do not consume enough fruits, vegetables, cereal grains, dairy products, and other foods to consistently meet their vitamin requirements. In addition, some conditions increase requirements above the usual recommended amounts (eg, pregnancy, lactation, wound healing, various illnesses).

Many people take vitamin supplements to promote health and prevent or treat illness. These supplements can be harmful if overused. On the other hand, there is increasing information about the potential benefits of certain vitamins in preventing heart disease, cancer, and other illnesses. For example, research studies demonstrated that folic acid can prevent birth defects such as spina bifida. As a result, the Food and Drug Administration (FDA) mandated that folic acid be added to cereal grain foods. Some scientists also recommend the addition of vitamin B_{12} because folic acid can mask pernicious anemia from a B_{12} deficiency and result in permanent damage to the nervous system.

There is also a proposal to increase the recommended dietary allowance (RDA) of vitamin C. RDAs were established by the Food and Nutrition Board of the National Academy of Sciences for daily intake by healthy adults and children and are periodically revised according to newer information.

There has also been extensive discussion about the benefits of vitamins C and E and beta carotene, a precursor of vitamin A. The benefits, including prevention of cancer and cardiovascular disease, are attributed to antioxidant effects. Antioxidants inactivate oxygen free radicals, potentially toxic substances formed during normal cell metabolism, and prevent or inhibit them from damaging body cells. Fruits and vegetables are natural sources of antioxidants and at least five servings daily are recommended. Supplements of antioxidant vitamins are not recommended because more research is needed.

It seems clear that vitamins are extremely important in promoting and maintaining health and in preventing illness. The primary focus of this chapter is to review selected vitamin-related aspects of normal nutrition and provide some guidelines for personal use of or client counseling about vitamin supplements.

DESCRIPTION AND USES

Vitamins are usually classified as fat soluble (A, D, E, K) and water soluble (B complex, C). Fat-soluble vitamins are absorbed from the intestine with dietary fat, and absorption requires the presence of bile salts and pancreatic lipase. These vitamins are relatively stable in cooking. Water-soluble vitamins are readily absorbed but are also readily lost by improper cooking and storage. Vitamin D is discussed in Chapter 26 because of its major role in bone metabolism.

Table 31-1 summarizes the characteristics, functions, food sources, and recommended amounts of vitamins. Deficiency states occur with inadequate intake or disease processes that interfere with absorption or use of vitamins. Excess states occur with excessive intake of fat-soluble vitamins because these vitamins accumulate in the body. Excess states do not occur with dietary intake of

(*text continues on page 455*)

TABLE 31-1 **Vitamins as Nutrients**

	Characteristics	Functions	Recommended Dietary Allowances (RDAs)	Dietary Sources
Fat-Soluble Vitamins				
Vitamin A (Retinol)	Obtained from animal foods and plant foods that contain carotenoids (precursors of vitamin A) About one third of carotenoids are absorbed, and they become active in body functioning only after conversion to retinol in the wall of the small intestine.	Required for normal vision, growth, bone development, skin, and mucous membrane	Women: 800 RE (4000 IU) Men: 1000 RE (5000 IU) Pregnant women: 1000 RE (5000 IU) Lactating women: 1200 RE (6000 IU) Children 1–10 y: 400–700 RE (2000–3500 IU); 11 y and older: same as adults	Preformed vitamin A—meat, butter and fortified margarine, egg yolk, whole milk, cheese made from whole milk Carotenoids—turnip and collard greens, carrots, sweet potatoes, squash, apricots, peaches, cantaloupe

(continued)

TABLE 31-1 **Vitamins as Nutrients** (*continued*)

	Characteristics	Functions	Recommended Dietary Allowances (RDAs)	Dietary Sources
	Retinol, another name for preformed vitamin A, is the physiologically active form. Vitamin A activity is expressed in retinol equivalents (RE), which include both preformed vitamin A and carotenoids. 1 RE = 1 μg retinol or 6 μg beta carotene.			
Vitamin E	A group of substances called tocopherols, of which alpha-tocopherol is most biologically active Vitamin E activity is expressed in milligrams of alpha-tocopherol equivalents (alpha TE).	Thought to act as an antioxidant in preventing destruction of certain fats, including the lipid portion of cell membranes. It also may increase absorption, hepatic storage, and use of vitamin A.	Women: 8 mg alpha TE Men: 10 mg alpha TE Children up to 10 y: 3–7 mg alpha TE; 11 y and older, same as adults	Cereals, green vegetables, egg yolk, milk fat, butter, meat, vegetable oils
Vitamin K	Occurs naturally in two forms: phytonadione (K_1) found in plant foods, and menaquinone (K_2) synthesized in the intestine by bacteria Absorbed mainly from the upper intestine in the presence of bile and dietary fats	Essential for normal blood clotting. Activates precursor proteins, found in the liver, into clotting factors II, VII, IX and X.	1 μg/kg	Green leafy vegetables (spinach, kale, cabbage, lettuce), cauliflower, tomatoes, wheat bran, cheese, egg yolk, liver
Vitamin D	See Chapter 26.			

Water-Soluble Vitamins

B-COMPLEX VITAMINS

	Characteristics	Functions	Recommended Dietary Allowances (RDAs)	Dietary Sources
Biotin	Must be obtained from dietary intake. There is also some synthesis by intestinal bacteria, and a portion is absorbed.	Essential in fat and carbohydrate metabolism	Not established; provisionally set at 30–100 μg	Meat, especially liver, egg yolk, nuts, cereals; most vegetables
Cyanocobalamin (vitamin B_{12})	In addition to food sources, some is also obtained from tissue storage in the liver and from recovery of cyanocobalamin secreted in bile and reabsorbed in the small intestine.	Essential for normal metabolism of all body cells; normal red blood cells; growth; and metabolism of carbohydrate, protein, and fat	Adults: 2 μg Children: 0.7–1.4 μg Infants: 0.3–0.5 μg	Meat, especially liver, eggs, fish, cheese
Folic acid (folate)	Obtained from foods and the enterohepatic cycle. The latter provides an endogenous source, because folate is excreted in bile, reabsorbed in the small bowel, and reused. May be lost from vegetables stored at room temperature or cooked at high temperatures.	Essential for normal metabolism of all body cells, for normal red blood cells, and for growth	Women: 180 μg Men: 200 μg Pregnant women or sexually active women of childbearing age: 400 μg Lactating women: 260–280 μg Children, 1–10 y: 50–100 μg; 11–14 y, 150 μg Infants: 25–35 μg	Liver, kidney beans, fresh green vegetables (spinach, broccoli, asparagus)

(*continued*)

TABLE 31-1   **Vitamins as Nutrients (*continued*)**

	Characteristics	Functions	Recommended Dietary Allowances (RDAs)	Dietary Sources
Niacin (vitamin B_3)	Obtained from food and endogenous synthesis from tryptophan. Niacin activity is expressed in niacin equivalents (NE): 1 mg of niacin or 60 mg tryptophan = 1 NE.	Essential for glycolysis, fat synthesis, and tissue respiration. It functions as a coenzyme in many metabolic processes (after conversion to nicotinamide, the physiologically active form).	Women: 15 NE Men: 20 NE Pregnant women: 17 NE Lactating women: 20 NE Children, 1–10 y: 9-13 NE Boys, 11–14 y: 17 NE; girls, 11–14 y, 15 NE Infants: 5–6 NE	Meat, poultry, fish, peanuts
Pantothenic acid (vitamin B_5)		A component of coenzyme A and essential for cellular metabolism (intermediary metabolism of carbohydrate, fat, and protein; release of energy from carbohydrate; fatty acid metabolism; synthesis of cholesterol, steroid hormones, phospholipids, and porphyrin)	Not established. Estimated at 4–7 mg.	Eggs, liver, salmon, yeast, cauliflower, broccoli, lean beef, potatoes, tomatoes
Pyridoxine (vitamin B_6)	Occurs in three forms (pyridoxal, pyridoxine, and pyridoxamine), all of which are converted in the body to pyridoxal phosphate, the physiologically active form.	Serves as a coenzyme in many metabolic processes Functions in metabolism of carbohydrate, protein, and fat Required for formation of tryptophan and conversion of tryptophan to niacin As part of the enzyme phosphorylase, helps release glycogen from the liver and muscle tissue Functions in metabolism of the central nervous system Helps maintain cellular immunity	Women: 1.6 mg Men: 2 mg Pregnant women: 2.2 mg Lactating women: 2.1 mg Children, 1–10 y: 1–1.4 mg Boys, 11–14 y, 1.7 mg; girls, 11–14 y, 1.4 mg Infants: 0.3–0.6 mg	Yeast, wheat germ, liver and other glandular meats, whole grain cereals, potatoes, legumes
Riboflavin (vitamin B_2)		Serves as a coenzyme in metabolism Necessary for growth May function in production of corticosteroids and red blood cells and gluconeogenesis	Women: 1.3 mg Men: 1.7 mg Pregnant women: 1.6 mg Lactating women: 1.7 mg Children, 1–10 y: 0.8–1.2 mg Boys, 11–14 y: 1.5 mg; girls, 11–14 y, 1.3 mg Infants: 0.4–0.5 mg	Milk, cheddar and cottage cheese, meat, eggs, green leafy vegetables
Thiamine (vitamin B_1)		A coenzyme in carbohydrate metabolism and essential for energy production	Women: 1.1 mg Men: 1.5 mg Pregnant women: 1.5 mg Lactating women: 1.6 mg Children, 1–10 y: 0.7–1 mg Boys, 11–14 y, 1.3 mg; girls, 11–14 y, 1.1 mg Infants: 0.3–0.4 mg	Meat, poultry, fish, egg yolk, dried beans, whole-grain cereal products, peanuts

(*continued*)

	Characteristics	Functions	Recommended Dietary Allowances (RDAs)	Dietary Sources
VITAMIN C				
Vitamin C (ascorbic acid)	Dietary vitamin C is well absorbed from the intestinal tract and distributed widely in body tissues. Not stored in body to a significant extent. Once tissues are saturated with about 1500 mg, any excess is excreted in the urine.	Essential for collagen formation (collagen is a fibrous protein in connective tissue throughout the body, including skin, ligaments, cartilage, bone, and teeth) Required for wound healing and tissue repair, metabolism of iron and folic acid, synthesis of fats and proteins, preservation of blood vessel integrity, and resistance to infection	Adults: 60 mg Pregnant women: 70 mg Lactating women: 90–95 mg Children, Infancy–14 y: 30–50 mg; 15 y and older, 60 mg	Fruits and vegetables, especially citrus fruits and juices

TABLE 31-1 Vitamins as Nutrients (*continued*)

water-soluble vitamins because these vitamins are rapidly excreted in the urine. Causes and clinical manifestations of vitamin disorders are listed in Table 31-2.

VITAMIN SUPPLEMENTS

Vitamin supplements may be prescribed by health care providers, but most are probably self-prescribed. Preparations may contain one or several vitamins. The only clearcut indications for these products are prevention and treatment of vitamin deficiencies. Because vitamins are essential nutrients, some people believe that large amounts (megadoses) promote health and provide other beneficial effects. Excessive intake of vitamins causes harmful effects. Thus, "megavitamins" should never be self-prescribed. Additional characteristics include the following:

- Vitamins from supplements exert the same physiologic effects as those obtained from foods.
- Vitamin supplements do not require a physician's prescription.
- Vitamin products vary widely in number, type, and amount of specific ingredients. They cannot be used interchangeably or indiscriminately with safety.
- Preparations promoted for use as dietary supplements may contain 50% to 100% of the amounts recommended for daily intake. In healthy people who eat a well-balanced diet, nutrient needs may be exceeded.
- Preparations for therapeutic use may contain 300% to 500% of the amounts recommended for daily intake in normal circumstances. These should not contain more than recommended amounts of vitamin D, folic acid, and vitamin A.

- Synthetic vitamins have the same structure and function as natural vitamins derived from plant and animal sources. Contrary to some claims, natural vitamins are no better than synthetic vitamins and are more expensive.
- Multivitamin preparations often contain minerals as well, usually in smaller amounts than those recommended for daily intake. Large doses of minerals are toxic (see Chap. 32).

Selected vitamin preparations are listed in Table 31-3.

NURSING PROCESS

Assessment

Assess each client for current or potential vitamin disorders during an overall assessment of nutritional status. Specific assessment factors related to vitamins include the following:

- Deficiency states are more common than excess states.
- People with other nutritional deficiencies are likely to have vitamin deficiencies as well.
- Deficiencies of water-soluble vitamins (B complex and C) are more common than those of fat-soluble vitamins.
- Vitamin deficiencies are usually multiple and signs and symptoms often overlap, especially with B-complex deficiencies.
- Vitamin requirements are increased during infancy, pregnancy, lactation, fever, hyperthyroidism, and many illnesses. Thus, a vitamin intake that is

(*text continues on page 459*)

TABLE 31-2   Vitamin Imbalances

	Deficiency States		Excess States	
	Causes	Signs and Symptoms	Causes	Signs and Symptoms
Fat-Soluble Vitamins				
Vitamin A	Rarely caused by inadequate dietary intake in the United States. May occur during periods of rapid growth, with GI disorders affecting its absorption or conversion, and with liver disorders limiting conversion of beta carotene to the active form or storage of vitamin A	Night blindness Xerophthalmia, which may progress to corneal ulceration and blindness Changes in skin and mucous membranes that lead to skin lesions and infections, respiratory tract infections, and urinary calculi	Excessive intake of vitamin A, which is unlikely with dietary intake but can occur with overuse of vitamin A supplements	Anorexia Vomiting Irritability Headache Skin changes (dryness, itching, desquamation, dermatitis) Later manifestations may include fatigue, pain in muscles, bones, and joints, gingivitis, enlargement of spleen and liver, altered liver function, increased intracranial pressure, and other neurologic signs. Congenital abnormalities may occur in newborns whose mothers took excessive vitamin A during pregnancy. Acute toxicity, with increased intracranial pressure, bulging fontanels, and vomiting, may occur in infants who are given vitamin A. Plasma retinol levels above 100 µg/dL
Vitamin E	Deficiency is rare.		Excessive intake of vitamin E, which is rare with dietary intake but can occur with overuse of vitamin E supplements	Fatigue, nausea, headache, blurred vision, diarrhea
Vitamin K	Inadequate intake, absorption, or use. Rarely caused by inadequate intake after infancy. Occurs commonly in newborns owing to lack of dietary intake of vitamin K and lack of intestinal synthesis of the vitamin during the first week of life. After infancy, deficiency usually results from diseases that interfere with absorption (biliary tract and GI disorders) or use (hepatic cirrhosis and hepatitis). In alcoholics, deficiency commonly occurs and probably	Abnormal bleeding (melena, hematemesis, hematuria, epistaxis, petechiae, ecchymoses, hypovolemic shock)	Unlikely to occur from dietary intake; may occur when vitamin K is given as an antidote for oral anticoagulants	Clinical manifestations rarely occur. However, when vitamin K is given to someone who is receiving warfarin (Coumadin), the client can be made "warfarin-resistant" for 2–3 wk.

(continued)

	Causes of deficiency	Signs and symptoms of deficiency	Signs and symptoms of excess
Vitamin D	results from decreased intake and impaired use. Drug-induced deficiency occurs with oral coumarin anticoagulants and some other drugs that act as vitamin K antagonists. Also, antibiotics reduce bacterial synthesis of vitamin K in the intestine, but this is a rare cause of deficiency. See Chapter 26.		Signs and symptoms of excess states not established for most water-soluble vitamins
WATER-SOLUBLE VITAMINS			
Biotin	Inadequate intake or impaired absorption. Biotin deficiency is rare.	Anorexia Nausea Depression Muscle pain Dermatitis	Megadoses of pharmaceutical vitamin supplements
Cyanocobalamin (vitamin B_{12})	Usually impaired absorption from a lack of hydrochloric acid or intrinsic factor in the stomach	Megaloblastic or pernicious anemia: Decreased numbers of RBCs Abnormally large, immature RBCs Fatigue Dyspnea With severe deficiency, leukopenia, thrombocytopenia, cardiac arrhythmias, heart failure, or infections may occur. Neurologic signs and symptoms: Paresthesias in hands and feet Unsteady gait Depressed deep-tendon reflexes With severe deficiency, loss of memory, confusion, delusions, hallucinations, and psychosis may occur. Nerve damage may be irreversible.	
Folic acid	Inadequate diet Impaired absorption (intestinal disorders) Greatly increased requirements (pregnancy, lactation, hemolytic anemias) Ingestion of folate antagonist drugs (eg, methotrexate) Alcoholism is a common cause. It interferes with intake and absorption.	Megaloblastic anemia that cannot be distinguished from the anemia produced by B_{12} deficiency Impaired growth in children Glossitis GI problems (folic acid deficiency does not produce neurologic signs and symptoms as B_{12} deficiency does)	

TABLE 31-2 Vitamin Imbalances (*continued*)

	Deficiency States		Excess States	
	Causes	Signs and Symptoms	Causes	Signs and Symptoms
Niacin (vitamin B₃)	Inadequate diet or impaired absorption	Pellagra: Erythematous skin lesions GI problems (stomatitis, glossitis, enteritis, diarrhea) Central nervous system problems (headache, dizziness, insomnia, depression, memory loss) With severe deficiency, delusions, hallucinations, and impairment of peripheral motor and sensory nerves may occur.	Large doses (2–6 g daily) used to treat hyperlipidemia	Flushing, pruritus, hyperglycemia, hyperuricemia, increased liver enzymes
Pantothenic acid (vitamin B₅)	No deficiency state established			
Pyridoxine (vitamin B₆)	Inadequate intake or impaired absorption	Skin and mucous membrane lesions (seborrheic dermatitis, intertrigo, glossitis, stomatitis) Neurologic problems (convulsions, peripheral neuritis, mental depression)		
Riboflavin (vitamin B₂)	Inadequate intake or impaired absorption. Uncommon and usually occurs with deficiencies of other B-complex vitamins	Glossitis and stomatitis Seborrheic dermatitis Eye disorders (burning, itching, lacrimation, photophobia, vascularization of the cornea)		
Thiamine (vitamin B₁)	Inadequate diet, especially among pregnant women and infants; impaired absorption due to GI disorders Alcoholism	Mild deficiency—fatigue, anorexia, retarded growth, mental depression, irritability, apathy, lethargy Severe deficiency (beriberi)—peripheral neuritis, personality disturbances, heart failure, edema, Wernicke-Korsakoff syndrome in alcoholics		
Vitamin C (ascorbic acid)	Inadequate dietary intake (most likely in infants, older adults, indigent people, and alcoholics) Increased requirements (people who smoke cigarettes, take oral contraceptives, or have acute or chronic illness) Megadoses that are abruptly discontinued may cause a rebound deficiency. Deficiency also may occur in infants whose mothers took megadoses during pregnancy.	Mild deficiency—irritability, malaise, arthralgia, increased tendency to bleed Severe deficiency—scurvy and adverse effects on most body tissues (gingivitis; bleeding of gums, skin, joints, and other areas; disturbances of bone growth; anemia; and loosening of teeth). If not treated, coma and death may occur.	Megadoses may produce excessive amounts of oxalate in the urine.	Renal calculi

GI, gastrointestinal; RBCs, red blood cells.

TABLE 31-3 **Vitamin Drug Preparations**

Generic/Trade Name	Routes and Dosage Ranges
Fat-Soluble Vitamins	
Vitamin A (Aquasol A)	Adults with severe deficiency: PO, IM 100,000 IU daily for 3 d, then 50,000 IU daily for 2 wk, then 10,000–20,000 IU daily for another 2 mo.
	Children over 8 y with severe deficiency: PO, IM same as adults
	Infants and children under 8 y: PO 5000–10,000 IU daily for 2 mo; IM infants, 7500–15,000 IU daily for 10 d; children 1–8 y, 17,000–35,000 IU daily for 10 d
Vitamin E (Aquasol E)	Adults: PO 100–400 IU daily
	Children: PO 25–50 IU daily
Vitamin K	Adults and children: PO, IM 5–15 mg daily
Menadione sodium diphosphate (Synkayvite)	Adults: PO 5–10 mg daily; SC, IM, IV 5–15 mg daily
	Children: PO, SC, IM, IV 5–10 mg daily
Phytonadione (Mephyton, Aqua-Mephyton)	Adults and children: PO, SC, IM 2.5–25 mg daily
	Newborns: IV, IM 0.5–1 mg immediately after birth to *prevent* hemorrhagic disease of neonates; 1–2 mg daily to *treat* hemorrhagic disease
Water-Soluble Vitamins	
B-COMPLEX VITAMINS	
Calcium pantothenate (B$_5$)	Adults: PO 10–20 mg daily
Cyanocobalamin (B$_{12}$) (Rubramin)	Adults and children: PO 10–250 µg daily for 1 mo in an oral therapeutic multivitamin preparation when deficiency is due to increased requirements and gastrointestinal absorption is normal
	IM, SC, IV 30 µg daily for 5–10 d, then 100–200 µg monthly
Folic acid (Folvite)	Adults and children: PO, SC, IM, IV up to 1 mg daily until symptoms decrease and blood tests are normal, then maintenance dose of 0.1–0.25 mg daily
Niacin (nicotinic acid), **niacinamide** (nicotinamide)	Deficiency, PO, IM, IV 50–100 mg daily
	Pellagra, 500 mg daily
	Hyperlipidemia, PO 2–6 g daily
Pyridoxine (B$_6$)	Deficiency, PO, IM, IV 10–20 mg daily for 3 wk, then 2–5 mg daily
	Anemia, peripheral neuritis, 100–200 mg daily
	Pyridoxine dependency syndrome, up to 600 mg daily
Riboflavin	PO 5–25 mg daily
Thiamine (B$_1$)	PO 10–30 mg daily; IM 10–20 mg three times daily for 2 wk, supplemented with 5–10 mg orally; IV 100-200 mg
VITAMIN C	
Vitamin C (ascorbic acid)	Deficiency, PO, IM, IV 100–500 mg daily
	Scurvy, 300–1000 mg daily for at least 2 wk
	Infants receiving formula, 35–50 mg daily for first few weeks of life
	Urinary acidification, 4–12 g daily in divided doses every 4 h
	Prophylaxis, 50–100 mg daily

IM, intramuscular; IV, intravenous; PO, oral; SC, subcutaneous.

normally adequate may become inadequate in certain circumstances.
- Vitamin deficiencies are likely to occur in people who are poor, elderly, chronically or severely ill, or alcoholic.
- Vitamin excess states are rarely caused by excessive dietary intake but may occur with use of vitamin drug preparations, especially if megadoses are taken.

Nursing Diagnoses

- Altered Nutrition: Less Than Body Requirements related to vitamin deficiency
- Altered Nutrition: More Than Body Requirements related to vitamin excess with overuse of supplements
- Risk for Injury related to vitamin deficiency or overdose

- Knowledge Deficit: Importance of adequate vitamin intake in normal body functioning
- Knowledge Deficit: Dietary sources of various vitamins
- Knowledge Deficit: Selection of vitamin supplements
- Knowledge Deficit: Adverse effects of self-prescribed megadoses of vitamins

How Can You Avoid This Medication Error?

You receive an order for K 5 mg IM STAT for a patient. You see KCl in your stock supply that comes in 10 mEq/10 mL. You proceed to draw up and administer 5 mL of KCl IM to the patient.

Planning/Goals

The client will:

- Ingest appropriate amounts and sources of dietary vitamins
- Select and use vitamin supplements appropriately
- Avoid megadoses of vitamin supplements
- Avoid symptoms of vitamin deficiency or overdose

Interventions

Implement measures to prevent vitamin disorders; the safest and most effective way to prevent vitamin deficiencies is by increasing dietary intake of vitamins:

- A well-balanced, varied diet that is adequate in proteins and calories is adequate in vitamins for most people. Exceptions are those who have increased requirements or conditions that interfere with absorption or use of vitamins.
- Assist clients to increase dietary vitamin intake. Water-soluble vitamins are often destroyed by cooking or discarded in cooking water. Eating raw fruits and vegetables prevents loss of vitamins during cooking. When fruits and vegetables are cooked, vitamin losses can be minimized by using small amounts of water, steaming or microwave cooking for short periods, and keeping cooking utensils covered. In addition to cooking losses, vitamin C is lost with exposure of foods to air. Consequently, fruits and vegetables, including juices, should be kept covered during storage.
- When vitamin deficiency stems from inadequate dietary intake, correcting the diet is preferred over administering supplemental vitamins when feasible. Increasing fruit and vegetable intake to at least five servings daily is a recommended alternative to a vitamin supplement. For vitamin A deficiency, increasing daily intake of plant and animal sources may be sufficient. For vitamin C deficiency, citrus juices and fruits can be used therapeutically. When folic acid deficiency anemia stems from dietary lack, one fresh, uncooked fruit or vegetable or one glass of fruit juice added to the daily diet will probably correct the deficiency (except during pregnancy, when folate requirements are increased).
- Clients receiving only intravenous (IV) fluids or a clear liquid diet for more than 2 or 3 days need replacement vitamins.
- When requirements are increased or absorption is decreased, supplements may be needed to prevent deficiencies. Assist clients in choosing and using vitamin supplements, because they differ widely in the amount and type of vitamins contained. Recommendations should be based on RDAs and usual eating habits.
- Some oral multivitamin preparations considered appropriate for supplemental use are Poly-Vi-Sol, Tri-Vi-Sol, and Vi-Daylin for children and Dayalets for adults.

Evaluation

- Interview about and observe the amount and type of food intake.
- Interview about and observe for signs of vitamin deficiency or overdose.

CLIENT TEACHING GUIDELINES
Vitamins

General Considerations

✔ Vitamins are required for normal body metabolism and functioning. For the most part, they must be obtained from the diet or from vitamin supplements.

✔ The safest and most effective way to obtain needed vitamins is to eat a varied, well-balanced diet. A healthful diet supplies vitamins, minerals, protein, water, fiber, and probably other elements yet to be discovered. Thus, vitamin supplements cannot substitute for a healthy diet. Vitamin content of foods, especially B vitamins and vitamin C, can be increased by avoiding prolonged cooking.

✔ Although diseases caused by vitamin deficiencies are uncommon in the United States, studies indicate that less than 25% of adults meet the recommended dietary allowances (RDAs) for vitamins.

✔ An adequate vitamin intake, especially from the recommended minimum of five daily servings of fruits and vegetables, may help prevent heart disease and cancer.

✔ People who are healthy and who eat a well-balanced diet do not need to take a daily multivitamin supplement. However, a supplement is probably needed by pregnant women and people who smoke, ingest large amounts of alcohol, have impaired immune systems, or are elderly.

✔ Avoid large doses of vitamins. They will not promote health, strength, or youth. In addition, excessive amounts of B vitamins and vitamin C are eliminated in urine and some can cause adverse effects (eg, large doses of vitamin C can cause kidney stones; niacin can cause stomach upset, flushing, skin rashes, itching, and aggravation of asthma and gout; pyridoxine may cause numbness in

(continued)

limbs and difficulty in walking). Excessive amounts of vitamins A, D, E, and K are stored in the body and often lead to toxic effects. For example, high doses of vitamin A can result in headaches, diarrhea, nausea, loss of appetite, dry, itching skin, and elevated blood calcium. Excessive doses during pregnancy may cause birth defects.

✔ Although natural vitamins are advertised as being better than synthetic vitamins, there is no evidence to support this claim. The two types are chemically identical and used in the same way by the human body. Natural vitamins are usually much more expensive than synthetic vitamins.

✔ Sexually active women of childbearing potential need an adequate intake of folic acid to prevent severe birth defects in infants. To help prevent birth defects from folic acid deficiency, the Food and Drug Administration requires that folic acid be added to breads and cereal grain products.

✔ Vitamins from supplements exert the same physiologic effects as those obtained from foods.

✔ Multivitamin preparations often contain minerals as well, usually in smaller amounts than those recommended for daily intake. Large doses of minerals are toxic.

Self-administration

✔ If supplementary vitamins are taken, it is probably advisable to consult a health care provider. Available preparations differ widely in amounts and types of vitamin content. As a general rule, a multivitamin that contains no more than 100% of the recommended dietary allowance (RDA) for any vitamin is recommended because additional vitamins are obtained from food. In addition, the product should not contain more than rec-

ommended amounts of vitamin D, folic acid, and vitamin A because of possible adverse effects.

✔ When choosing a vitamin supplement, compare ingredients and costs. Store brands are usually effective and less expensive than name brands.

✔ Vitamin C supplements are available in tablet and powder forms of various dosages. Vitamin C is commonly included in multivitamin and other preparations sold as antioxidant supplements. The current RDA of 60 mg daily is being reviewed and some nutritionists are recommending an increase to 120 mg. A reasonable supplemental dose is approximately 100 to 200 mg daily. Large doses (eg, 1000 mg or more daily) may cause adverse effects and should be avoided. An adequate amount of vitamin C can also be obtained by eating at least five servings of fruit and vegetables daily.

✔ Take oral niacin preparations, except for timed-release forms, with or after meals or at bedtime to decrease stomach irritation. In addition, sit or lie down for approximately 30 minutes after taking a dose. Niacin causes blood vessels to dilate and may cause facial flushing, dizziness, and falls. Facial flushing can be decreased by aspirin 325 mg, taken 30 to 60 minutes before a dose of niacin. Itching, tingling, and headache may also occur. These effects usually subside with continued use of niacin.

✔ Swallow extended-release products whole; do not break, crush, or chew them. Breaking the product delivers the entire dose at once and may cause adverse effects

✔ Take prescribed vitamins as directed and for the appropriate time. In pernicious anemia, vitamin B_{12} injections must be taken for the remainder of life. In pregnancy and lactation, vitamin supplements are usually taken only during this period of increased need.

✔ Swallow vitamin E capsules whole; do not crush or chew.

PRINCIPLES OF THERAPY

Managing Vitamin Disorders

Vitamin disorders should be recognized as early as possible and appropriate treatment initiated. Early recognition and treatment can prevent a mild deficiency or excess from becoming severe. General guidelines include the following:

- For deficiency states, oral vitamin preparations are preferred when possible. They are usually effective (except in malabsorption syndromes), safe, convenient to administer, and relatively inexpensive. Multiple deficiencies are common and a multivitamin preparation used to treat them usually contains more

than 150% of the RDA. These products should be used only for therapeutic purposes and for limited periods. When fat-soluble vitamins are given to correct a deficiency, there is a risk of producing excess states. When water-soluble vitamins are given, excesses are less likely but may occur with large doses. These factors must be considered when determining vitamin dosage. Some oral preparations include Betalin Complex Elixir, Multicebrin, Natalins, Surbex, Tri-Vi-Sol, and Vi-Daylin. Some of these may be used for adults or children. Other preparations are available for use during pregnancy and lactation or for parenteral use.

- For excess states, the usual treatment is to stop administration of the vitamin preparation. There are no specific antidotes or antagonists.

Disorders of Fat-Soluble Vitamins A and K

- With vitamin A deficiency, increase intake of foods containing vitamin A or beta carotene when feasible. Use a single, pure form of vitamin A rather than a multivitamin unless multiple deficiencies are present. Give doses no larger than 25,000 U daily unless a severe deficiency is present. Give orally if not contraindicated; give intramuscularly if gastrointestinal (GI) absorption is severely impaired or ocular symptoms are severe. With vitamin A excess, immediately stop known sources of the vitamin.

- With vitamin K deficiency, bleeding may occur spontaneously or in response to trauma. Thus, administration of vitamin K and measures to prevent bleeding are indicated. If the deficiency is not severe, oral vitamin K may be given for a few days until serum prothrombin activity returns to a normal range. In obstructive jaundice, bile salts must be given at the same time as oral vitamin K, or vitamin K must be given parenterally. In malabsorption syndromes or diarrhea, parenteral administration is probably necessary. A single dose of vitamin K may be sufficient.

  With severe bleeding, vitamin K may be given IV. IV vitamin K must be given very slowly to decrease risks of hypotension and shock. Unfortunately, a therapeutic response does not occur for at least 4 hours. For more rapid control of bleeding, transfusions of plasma or whole blood are needed. When bleeding is caused by oral anticoagulant drugs, avoid overdoses of vitamin K. Oral anticoagulants are usually given for thromboembolic disorders. Giving vitamin K as an antidote to control bleeding reestablishes the risks of thrombi. Measures to prevent bleeding include avoiding trauma, injections, and drugs that may cause bleeding.

Disorders of B-Complex Vitamins

- Most deficiencies of B-complex vitamins are multiple rather than single. Also, many of these vitamins are obtained from the same foods. Treating deficiencies consists of increasing intake of foods containing B-complex vitamins or giving multivitamin preparations. Most preparations contain thiamine, riboflavin, niacin, pyridoxine, and cyanocobalamin; other vitamins may also be included.

- If a single deficiency seems predominant, that vitamin may be given alone or along with a multivitamin preparation. For example, folic acid deficiency is widespread. This is attributed to inadequate dietary intake, loss in cooking and food processing, and intestinal disorders that inhibit absorption. In addition, folic acid is depleted by alcohol and many medications, including analgesic and anti-inflammatory drugs (eg, ibuprofen, naproxen), antacids containing magnesium and aluminum (eg, Mylanta, Maalox, Amphojel), antibiotics containing trimethoprim (eg, Bac-trim, Septra, Proloprim), anticonvulsants (eg, phenytoin, carbamazepine, valproic acid), bile acid sequestrants (eg, cholestyramine), gastric acid suppressants (eg, cimetidine, ranitidine, famotidine, nizatidine), methotrexate, oral contraceptives, potassium-sparing diuretics (eg, Dyazide, Maxzide), and sustained-release potassium supplements (eg, K-Dur, Micro-K).

  Thiamine deficiency is common in alcoholics. Reasons include inadequate dietary intake and the use of large amounts of thiamine to metabolize ethanol.

- Some uncommon types of anemia occur with deficiencies of certain B vitamins. One type occurs with pyridoxine deficiency and is relieved by administration of pyridoxine. Megaloblastic anemias, characterized by abnormally large, immature red blood cells, occur with deficiency of folic acid or vitamin B_{12}. If megaloblastic anemia is severe, treatment is usually instituted with folic acid and vitamin B_{12}.

  - In pernicious anemia, vitamin B_{12} must be given by injection because oral forms are not absorbed from the GI tract. The injections must be continued for life. Vitamin B_{12} is also given to prevent pernicious anemia in clients who are strict vegetarians, who have had gastrectomy, or who have chronic small bowel disease. Although folic acid relieves hematologic disorders of pernicious anemia, giving folic acid alone allows continued neurologic deterioration. Thus, an accurate diagnosis is required.

  - In other types of megaloblastic anemias, vitamin B_{12} or folic acid is indicated. Although both of these are included in many multivitamin preparations, they usually must be given separately for therapeutic purposes. With vitamin B_{12}, doses in excess of 100 μg are rapidly excreted in urine. However, a single dose of 1000 μg is given when performing the Schilling test for pernicious anemia. With folic acid, oral administration is indicated for most clients. Daily doses in excess of 1 mg are excreted in the urine.

Disorders of Vitamin C

Treatment of vitamin C deficiency involves increased intake of vitamin C from dietary or pharmaceutical sources. Vitamin C is available alone for oral, intramuscular (IM),

---

Nursing Notes: Apply Your Knowledge

Jim Bagley, 40 years of age, was just diagnosed with pernicious anemia. Jim asks you why he must take shots rather than vitamin pills. You are assigned to provide his IM injection of vitamin B_{12} and provide patient teaching. Discuss how you will proceed.

or IV administration. It is also an ingredient in most multivitamin preparations for oral or parenteral use.

Since 1989, the RDA for vitamin C has been 60 mg daily. This is being revised by the Food and Nutrition Board of the National Academy of Sciences. Some nutritionists are recommending an increase to 120 mg/day. Others recommend an estimated intake of approximately 200 mg/day from five servings of fruits and vegetables or 100 mg/day of a vitamin C supplement. An additional recommendation is to limit intake to less than 1 g/day, which is considered the maximum amount that is unlikely to cause adverse effects.

Plasma levels of vitamin C are usually low in patients who are smokers, are postoperative, or have illnesses such as sepsis, human immunodeficiency virus infection, pancreatitis, adult respiratory distress syndrome, or other critical illnesses requiring intensive care. The significance of low plasma levels and whether increased levels would decrease smoking-related diseases or have beneficial effects in other illnesses is unknown. In addition, there are few data relating plasma levels to susceptibility to the common cold and other infections.

With excessive intake of vitamin C supplements (≥ 1 g daily), the main concern is formation of calcium oxalate kidney stones and potential obstruction or other renal damage. There is no known benefit of such large amounts, and their use should be discouraged.

Use in Children

Children need sufficient amounts of all required vitamins to support growth and normal body functioning. For healthy children consuming a well-balanced diet, vitamin supplements are probably not needed. However, if supplements are given, considerations include the following:

- Dosages should not exceed recommended amounts. There is a risk of overdosage by children and their parents. Because of manufacturers' marketing strategies, many supplements are available in flavors and shapes (eg, cartoon characters, animals) designed to appeal to children. Because younger children may think of these supplements as candy and take more than recommended, they should be stored out of reach and dispensed by an adult. Parents may lack knowledge of nutrition or be concerned about the adequacy of a child's diet. Their wish to promote health may lead them to give unneeded supplements or to give more than recommended amounts. Parents may need information about the potential hazards of acute and chronic vitamin overdoses.
- The content of supplements for infants and children younger than 4 years is regulated by the FDA; the content of preparations for older children is not regulated.
- Supplements given to children and adolescents should in general provide RDA levels of vitamins. Supplements containing 25% to 50% of the RDA minimize risks of deficiency states; those containing 100% of the RDA meet nutritional needs without producing excess states.
- Except for single supplements of vitamin K and vitamin E in infants, multivitamin products are commonly used. For infants, liquid formulations usually include vitamins A, D, C, and B complex. Folic acid is not included because it is unstable in liquid form. For older children, chewable tablets usually contain vitamins A, D, C, and B complex, including folic acid.
- A single IM dose of vitamin K is given to newborn infants to prevent hemorrhagic disease of newborns.
- Preterm infants need proportionately more vitamins than term infants because their growth rate is faster and their absorption of vitamins from the intestine is less complete. A multivitamin product containing the equivalent of RDAs for term infants is recommended.

Use in Older Adults

Vitamin requirements are the same as for younger adults. However, deficiencies are common in older adults, especially of vitamins A and D, folic acid, riboflavin, and thiamine. Numerous factors may contribute to deficiencies, including limited income, anorexia, lack of teeth or ill-fitting dentures, drugs that decrease absorption of dietary nutrients, and disease processes that interfere with the ability to obtain, prepare, or eat adequate amounts of a variety of foods.

Every older adult should be carefully assessed regarding nutritional status and use of drugs that interact with dietary nutrients. If an older adult cannot eat a varied, well-balanced diet for any reason, a vitamin supplement is probably desirable. In addition, requirements may be increased during illnesses, especially those affecting GI function. Overdoses, especially of the fat-soluble vitamins A and D, may cause toxicity and should be avoided.

Use in Cancer Prevention

Vitamin A, its precursor beta carotene, and vitamin C are the main vitamins associated with prevention of cancer. Anticancer effects are attributed to antioxidant activity. Vitamin A and beta carotene may reduce cancers of the lung, breast, oral mucosa, esophagus, and bladder. Although vitamin A supplements are not recommended, increasing dietary intake of fruits and vegetables is desirable. It is unknown whether anticancer effects stem from beta carotene or other components of fruits and vegetables.

With vitamin C, several studies indicate that diets with 200 mg or more from fruits and vegetables (five or more servings daily) are associated with reduced cancer risk, especially for cancers of the GI tract (eg, oral cavity, esophagus, stomach, and colon) and lung. However, in other studies, vitamin C supplements did not decrease the occurrence of stomach or colorectal cancer. Thus, the cancer-preventing effects of fruits and vegetables may be associated with factors other than vitamin C (eg, interactions between vitamin C and other components of these foods, food components other than vitamin C, or because people who eat fruits and vegetables also participate in other health-promoting activities).

Use in Preventing Cardiovascular Disease

Folic acid, vitamin C, and vitamin E are thought to have cardioprotective effects. Folic acid is important in the metabolism of homocysteine, a toxic amino acid and a major risk factor for heart disease. Homocysteine is normally produced during metabolism of methionine, another amino acid. Several B vitamins, including folic acid, are required for the metabolism of homocysteine to a nontoxic substance, and an increased blood level of homocysteine occurs with folic acid deficiency. Excessive homocysteine damages the endothelial lining of arteries and leads to plaque formation, arteriosclerosis, and thrombosis. Folic acid supplements can prevent or delay these effects by lowering blood levels of homocysteine. Although the recent FDA requirement that folic acid be added to cereal grain foods may be helpful, the folic acid intake that helps prevent cardiovascular disease is thought to be higher.

Vitamins C and E are thought to help prevent cardiovascular disease by their antioxidant effects. The atherogenic effects of blood lipids, especially low-density lipoprotein (LDL) cholesterol (see Chap. 58), are attributed to their chemical breakdown or oxidation. Vitamin C may be more effective in preventing oxidation of LDL cholesterol than vitamin E. Overall, however, the effects of vitamin C on prevention of coronary artery disease (CAD) are unclear. Some studies indicate an increased risk for CAD only with a severe vitamin C deficiency and that vitamin C has little effect on ischemic heart disease and stroke after adjustment for other risk factors. More research is needed before supplements of vitamins C and E are recommended for cardioprotective effects. However, fruits and vegetables are natural sources of antioxidants and increased intake may be beneficial.

Use in Renal Impairment

Patients with renal impairment usually have special needs in relation to vitamin intake because of difficulties in ingesting or using these nutrients. Considerations include:

* In patients with acute renal failure who are unable to eat an adequate diet, a vitamin supplement to meet RDAs is recommended. Large doses of vitamin C should be avoided because urinary excretion is impaired. In addition, oxalate (a product of vitamin C catabolism) may precipitate in renal tubules or form calcium oxalate stones, obstruct urine flow, and worsen renal function.

* In patients with chronic renal failure (CRF), deficiencies of water-soluble vitamins are common because many foods that contain these vitamins are restricted because of their potassium content. In addition, vitamin C is reabsorbed from renal tubules by a specific transport protein. When the transport protein becomes saturated, remaining vitamin C is excreted in urine. Vitamin C is removed by dialysis and patients receiving dialysis require vitamin C replacement. The optimal replacement dose is unknown but probably should not exceed 200 mg/day (to avoid increased oxalate and possible stones).

A multivitamin product with essential vitamins, including vitamin C 70 to 100 mg, pyridoxine 5 to 10 mg, and folic acid 1 mg, is recommended for daily use. Because patients with CRF often have increased vitamin A concentrations, vitamin A should be omitted or reduced in dosage for those requiring parenteral nutrition.

Use in Hepatic Impairment

Vitamin deficiencies commonly occur in patients with chronic liver disease because of poor intake and malabsorption. With hepatic failure, hepatic stores of vitamin A, pyridoxine, folic acid, riboflavin, pantothenic acid, vitamin B_{12}, and thiamine are depleted. Folic acid deficiency may lead to megaloblastic anemia. Thiamine deficiency may lead to Wernicke's encephalopathy. Therapeutic doses of vitamins should be given for documented deficiency states.

Niacin is contraindicated in liver disease because it may increase liver enzymes (alanine and aspartate aminotransferase, alkaline phosphatase) and bilirubin and cause further liver damage. Long-acting dosage forms may be more hepatotoxic than the fast-acting forms.

Use in Critical Illness

Patients with critical illnesses often experience vitamin deficiencies unless they are prevented by early supplementation.

Patients receiving enteral nutrition should usually be given RDA-equivalent amounts of all vitamins. Those with intestinal resections (short bowel syndrome) may be able to take most vitamins orally or by GI tube. However, they usually need injections of vitamin B_{12} because they are unable to absorb it from the GI tract. Those with fat malabsorption syndromes need supplements of the fat-soluble vitamins A, D, E, and K.

For patients receiving parenteral nutrition, guidelines for daily vitamin supplementation have been developed by the Nutrition Advisory Group of the American Medical

Association (NAG-AMA). These guidelines are based on the RDAs for healthy people; vitamin requirements for patients who are critically ill or have specific organ failures are unclear.

Several parenteral multivitamin formulations meet the NAG-AMA guidelines for adults and children. Those for adults do not contain vitamin K, which is usually injected weekly. The usual dose is 2 to 4 mg, but some clinicians give 5 to 10 mg. Vitamin K is included in pediatric parenteral nutrition solutions.

 Home Care

The home care nurse needs to assess household members and the home setting for indications of vitamin deficiencies or use of megadoses. If actual or potential difficulties are found, the nurse may need to counsel household members about dietary sources of vitamins and adverse effects of excessive vitamin intake.

(*text continues on page 467*)

NURSING ACTIONS	Vitamins

NURSING ACTIONS	RATIONALE/EXPLANATION
1. Administer accurately	
a. With fat-soluble vitamins:	
(1) Give as directed.	To increase therapeutic effects and avoid adverse reactions
(2) Do not give oral preparations at the same time as mineral oil.	Mineral oil absorbs the vitamins and thus prevents their systemic absorption.
(3) For subcutaneous or intramuscular administration of vitamin K, aspirate carefully to avoid intravenous injection, apply gentle pressure to the injection site, and inspect the site frequently. For intravenous injection, vitamin K may be given by direct injection or diluted in intravenous fluids (eg, 5% dextrose in water or saline).	Vitamin K is given to clients with hypoprothrombinemia, which causes a bleeding tendency. Thus, any injection may cause trauma and bleeding at the injection site.
(4) Administer intravenous vitamin K slowly, at a rate not to exceed 1 mg/min, whether diluted or undiluted.	Intravenous phytonadione may cause hypotension and shock from an anaphylactic type of reaction.
b. With B-complex vitamins:	
(1) Give parenteral cyanocobalamin (vitamin B$_{12}$) intramuscularly or deep subcutaneously.	
(2) Give oral niacin preparations, except for timed-release forms, with or after meals or at bedtime. Have the client sit or lie down for about ½ hour after administration.	To decrease anorexia, nausea, vomiting, diarrhea, and flatulence. Niacin causes vasodilation, which may result in dizziness, hypotension, and possibly injury from falls. Vasodilation occurs within a few minutes and may last 1 hour.
(3) Give intramuscular thiamine deeply into a large muscle mass. Avoid the intravenous route.	To decrease pain at the injection site. Hypotension and anaphylactic shock have occurred with rapid intravenous administration and large doses.
2. Observe for therapeutic effects (mainly decreased signs and symptoms of deficiency)	
a. With vitamin A, observe for improved vision, especially in dim light or at night, less dryness in eyes and conjunctiva (xerophthalmia), improvement in skin lesions.	Night blindness is usually relieved within a few days. Skin lesions may not completely disappear for several weeks.
b. With vitamin K, observe for decreased bleeding and more nearly normal blood coagulation tests (eg, prothrombin time).	Blood coagulation tests usually improve within 4 to 12 hours.

(*continued*)

NURSING ACTIONS	RATIONALE/EXPLANATION
c. With B-complex vitamins, observe for decreased or absent stomatitis, glossitis, cheilosis, seborrheic dermatitis, neurologic problems (neuritis, convulsions, mental deterioration, psychotic symptoms), cardiovascular problems (edema, heart failure), and eye problems (itching, burning, photophobia).	Deficiencies of B-complex vitamins commonly occur together and produce many similar manifestations.
d. With vitamin B_{12} and folic acid, observe for increased appetite, strength and feeling of well-being, increased reticulocyte counts, and increased numbers of normal red blood cells, hemoglobin, and hematocrit.	Therapeutic effects may be quite rapid and dramatic. The client usually feels better within 24 to 48 hours, and normal red blood cells begin to appear. Anemia is decreased within approximately 2 weeks, but 4 to 8 weeks may be needed for complete blood count to return to normal.
e. With vitamin C, observe for decreased or absent malaise, irritability, and bleeding tendencies (easy bruising of skin, bleeding gums, nosebleeds, and so on).	
3. Observe for adverse reactions	
a. With vitamin A, observe for signs of hypervitaminosis A (anorexia, vomiting, irritability, headache, skin changes [dryness, dermatitis, itching desquamation], fatigue, pain in muscles, bones, and joints, and other clinical manifestations, and serum levels of vitamin A above 1200 U/dL).	Severity of manifestations depends largely on dose and duration of excess vitamin A intake. Very severe states produce additional clinical signs, including enlargement of liver and spleen, altered liver function, increased intracranial pressure, and other neurologic manifestations.
b. With vitamin K, observe for hypotension and signs of anaphylactic shock with intravenous phytonadione.	Vitamin K rarely produces adverse reactions. Giving intravenous phytonadione slowly may prevent adverse reactions.
c. With B-complex vitamins, observe for hypotension and anaphylactic shock with parenteral niacin, thiamine, cyanocobalamin, and folic acid; anorexia, nausea, vomiting and diarrhea, and postural hypotension with oral niacin.	Adverse reactions are generally rare. They are unlikely with B-complex multivitamin preparations. They are most likely to occur with large intravenous doses and rapid administration.
d. With vitamin C megadoses, observe for diarrhea and rebound deficiency if stopped abruptly.	Adverse reactions are rare with usual doses and methods of administration.
4. Observe for drug interactions	
a. Fat-soluble vitamins:	
(1) Bile salts *increase* effects.	Increase intestinal absorption
(2) Laxatives, especially mineral oil, *decrease* effects.	Mineral oil combines with fat-soluble vitamins and prevents their absorption if both are taken at the same time. Excessive or chronic laxative use decreases intestinal absorption.
(3) Antibiotics may *decrease* effects.	With vitamin K, antibiotics decrease production by decreasing intestinal bacteria. With others, antibiotics may cause diarrhea and subsequent malabsorption.
b. B-complex vitamins:	
(1) Cycloserine (antituberculosis drug) *decreases* effects.	By increasing urinary excretion of vitamin B-complex

(continued)

NURSING ACTIONS	RATIONALE/EXPLANATION
(2) Isoniazid (INH) *decreases* effect.	Isoniazid has an antipyridoxine effect. When INH is given for prevention or treatment of tuberculosis, pyridoxine is usually given also.
(3) With folic acid: alcohol, methotrexate, oral contraceptives, phenytoin, and triamterene *decrease* effects.	Alcohol alters liver function and leads to poor hepatic storage of folic acid. Methotrexate and phenytoin act as antagonists to folic acid and may cause folic acid deficiency. Oral contraceptives decrease absorption of folic acid.

How Can You Avoid This Medication Error?

Answer: You need to clarify this order with the physician before you proceed, clarifying whether vitamin K or KCl is ordered. It is likely the intended drug is vitamin K because it is ordered in milligrams and given IM. KCl is usually ordered in mEq and never given IM or IV push. Also, 5 mL is a very large dose to administer IM.

Nursing Notes: *Apply Your Knowledge*

Answer: Explain to Jim that injections are required for pernicious anemia because the parietal cells in the lining of his stomach fail to secrete intrinsic factor, which is required for intestinal absorption of B_{12}. Monthly injection of B_{12} will be required for the rest of his life. Later, Jim may want to learn how to administer his own injections. Provide Jim with teaching pamphlets about pernicious anemia and encourage him to ask questions.

REVIEW AND APPLICATION EXERCISES

1. What roles do vitamins play in normal body functioning?

2. Identify client populations who are at risk for vitamin deficiencies and excesses.

3. How would you assess a client for vitamin imbalances?

4. Are fat-soluble or water-soluble vitamins more toxic in overdoses? Why?

5. For an outpatient or home care client who is likely to have vitamin deficiencies, what information can you provide to increase vitamin intake from food?

6. For a client who asks your advice about taking a multivitamin supplement daily, how would you reply? Justify your answer.

7. What evidence supports anticancer and cardioprotective effects of vitamins?

8. How do the vitamin requirements of children, older adults, and ill patients differ from those of healthy young and middle-aged adults?

SELECTED REFERENCES

Chessman, K.H. & Anderson, J.D. (1997). Pediatric and geriatric nutrition support. In J.T. DiPiro, R.L. Talbert, G.C. Yee, G.R. Matzke, B.G. Wells, & L.M. Posey (Eds.), *Pharmacotherapy: A pathophysiologic approach*, 3rd ed., pp. 2787–2804. Stamford, CT: Appleton & Lange.

Darby, M.K. & Loughead, J.L. (1996). Neonatal nutritional requirements and formula composition: A review. *Journal of Obstetrics, Gynecology, and Neonatal Nursing, 25,* 209–217.

Drug facts and comparisons. (Updated monthly). St. Louis: Facts and Comparisons.

Hillman, R.S. (1996). Hematopoietic agents: Growth factors, minerals, and vitamins. In J.G. Hardman, L.E. Limbird, P.B. Molinoff, & R.W. Ruddon (Eds.), *Goodman & Gilman's The pharmacological basis of therapeutics*, 9th ed., pp. 1311–1340. New York: McGraw-Hill.

Levine, M., Rumsey, S.C., Daruwala, R., Park, J.B., & Wang, Y. (1999). Criteria and recommendations for vitamin C intake. *Journal of the American Medical Association, 281,* 1415–1423.

Marcus, R. & Coulston, A.M. (1996). Water-soluble vitamins. In J.G. Hardman, L.E. Limbird, P.B. Molinoff, & R.W. Ruddon (Eds.), *Goodman & Gilman's The pharmacological basis of therapeutics*, 9th ed., pp. 1555–1572. New York: McGraw-Hill.

Marcus, R. & Coulston, A.M. (1996). Fat-soluble vitamins. In J.G. Hardman, L.E. Limbird, P.B. Molinoff, & R.W. Ruddon (Eds.), *Goodman & Gilman's The pharmacological basis of therapeutics*, 9th ed., pp. 1573–1590. New York: McGraw-Hill.

Pelton, R. (1999). Folic acid: Essential for cell division. *American Druggist, 216*(2), 60–62.

Pleuss, J. (1998). Alterations in nutritional status. In C.M. Porth (Ed.), *Pathophysiology: Concepts of altered health states*, 5th ed., pp. 1243–1263. Philadelphia: Lippincott Williams & Wilkins.

Spencer, A.P., Carson, D.S., & Crouch, M.A. (1999). Vitamin E and coronary artery disease. *Archives of Internal Medicine, 159,* 1313–1320.

Stenson, W.F. & Eisenberg, P. (1997). Parenteral and enteral nutrition. In W.N. Kelley (Ed.), *Textbook of internal medicine*, 3rd ed., pp. 890–902. Philadelphia: Lippincott-Raven.

Wallace, J.I. & Schwartz, R.S. (1997). Geriatric clinical nutrition including malnutrition and cachexia. In W.N. Kelley (Ed.), *Textbook of internal medicine*, 3rd ed., pp. 2554–2560. Philadelphia: Lippincott-Raven.

32

Minerals and Electrolytes

Objectives

After studying this chapter, the student will be able to:

1. Discuss functions and food sources of major minerals.

2. Identify clients at risk for development of selected mineral and electrolyte imbalances.

3. Describe signs, symptoms, and treatment of sodium, potassium, and magnesium imbalances.

4. Describe signs, symptoms, and treatment of iron deficiency anemia.

5. Discuss the chelating agents used to remove excessive copper, iron, and lead from body tissues.

6. Apply nursing process skills to prevent, recognize, or treat mineral or electrolyte imbalances.

Minnie Pearl, 62 years of age, has been started on a thiazide diuretic to remove excess fluid and decrease the workload on her heart. Potassium supplements have been ordered to prevent hypokalemia.

Reflect on:

▶ How diuretics might alter electrolyte balance.

▶ What laboratory values are important to monitor for Ms. Pearl (review normal values).

▶ Why potassium supplements are especially important for cardiac patients on diuretics that are not potassium sparing.

▶ Important dietary teaching to help ensure electrolyte balance.

DESCRIPTION AND USES

Minerals and electrolytes are essential constituents of bone, teeth, cell membranes, connective tissue, and many essential enzymes. They function to maintain fluid, electrolyte, and acid–base balance; maintain osmotic pressure; maintain nerve and muscle function; assist in transfer of compounds across cell membranes; and influence the growth process.

Minerals occur in the body and foods mainly in ionic form. Ions are electrically charged particles. Metals (eg, sodium, potassium, calcium, magnesium) form positive ions or cations; nonmetals (eg, chlorine, phosphorus, sulfur) form negative ions or anions. These cations and anions combine to form compounds that are physiologically inactive and electrically neutral. When placed in solution, such as a body fluid, the components separate into electrically charged particles called *electrolytes*. For example, sodium and chlorine combine to form sodium chloride ($NaCl$ or table salt). In a solution, $NaCl$ separates into Na^+ and Cl^- ions. (The plus sign after Na means that Na is a cation; the minus sign after Cl means that Cl is an anion.) At any given time, the body must maintain an equal number of positive and negative charges. Therefore, the ions are constantly combining and separating to maintain electrical neutrality or electrolyte balance.

These electrolytes also maintain the acid–base balance of body fluids, which is necessary for normal body functioning. When foods are digested in the body, they produce mineral residues that react chemically as acids or bases.

Acids are usually anions, such as chloride, bicarbonate, sulfate, and phosphate. Bases are usually cations, such as sodium, potassium, calcium, and magnesium. If approximately equal amounts of cations and anions are present in the mineral residue, the residue is essentially neutral, and the pH of body fluids does not require adjustment. If there is an excess of cations (base), the body must draw on its anions (acid) to combine with the cations, render them physiologically inactive, and restore the normal pH of the blood. Excess cations are excreted in the urine, mainly in combination with the anion phosphate. If there is an excess of anions (acid), usually sulfate or phosphate, they combine with hydrogen ions or other cations and are excreted in the urine.

Macronutrients

There are 22 minerals thought to be necessary for human nutrition. Some of these (calcium, phosphorus, sodium, potassium, magnesium, chlorine, sulfur) are required in relatively large amounts and thus are sometimes called *macronutrients*. Calcium and phosphorus are discussed in Chapter 26. Sulfur is a component of cellular protein molecules, several amino acids, B vitamins, insulin, and other essential body substances. No recommended dietary allowance (RDA) has been established; the dietary source is protein foods. The other macronutrients are described here in terms of characteristics, functions, RDAs, and food sources (Table 32-1). Imbalances of macronutrients

---

TABLE 32-1 **Minerals and Electrolytes**

Characteristics	Functions	Recommended Dietary Allowances (RDAs)	Food Sources
Sodium			
Major cation in extracellular body fluids (blood, lymph, tissue fluid)	Assists in regulating osmotic pressure, water balance, conduction of electrical impulses in nerves and muscles, electrolyte and acid–base balance	Approximately 2 g (estimated)	Present in most foods. Proteins contain relatively large amounts, vegetables and cereals contain moderate to small amounts, fruits contain little or no sodium.
Small amount in intracellular fluid	Influences permeability of cell membranes and assists in movement of substances across cell membranes		Major source in the diet is table salt added to food in cooking, processing, or seasoning. One teaspoon contains 2.3 g of sodium.
Large amounts in saliva, gastric secretions, bile, pancreatic and intestinal secretions	Participates in many intracellular chemical reactions		Water in some areas may contain significant amounts of sodium.
Potassium			
Major cation in intracellular body fluids	Within cells, helps to maintain osmotic pressure, fluid and electrolyte balance, and acid–base balance	Approximately 40 mEq	Present in most foods, including meat, whole-grain breads or cereals, bananas, citrus fruits, tomatoes, and broccoli
Present in all body fluids	In extracellular fluid, functions with sodium and calcium to regulate neuromuscular		
Eliminated primarily in urine. Normally functioning kidneys excrete excessive amounts of potassium, but they cannot			

(continued)

TABLE 32-1 **Minerals And Electrolytes** (*continued*)

Characteristics	Functions	Recommended Dietary Allowances (RDAs)	Food Sources
conserve potassium when intake is low or absent. The kidneys excrete 10 mEq or more daily in the absence of intake. Potassium excretion is influenced by acid–base balance and aldosterone secretion. A small amount is normally lost in feces and sweat.	excitability. Potassium is required for conduction of nerve impulses and contraction of skeletal and smooth muscle. It is especially important in activity of the myocardium. Participates in carbohydrate and protein metabolism. Helps transport glucose into cells and is required for glycogen formation and storage. Required for synthesis of muscle proteins		
Magnesium			
A cation occurring primarily in intracellular fluid Widely distributed in the body, approximately half in bone tissue and the remainder in soft tissue and body fluids Most dietary magnesium is not absorbed from the gastrointestinal tract and is excreted in feces.	Required for conduction of nerve impulses and contraction of muscle Especially important in functions of cardiac and skeletal muscles Serves as a component of many enzymes Essential for metabolism of carbohydrate and protein	Approximately 300 mg for adults. Increased amounts recommended for pregnant or lactating women and children.	Present in many foods; diet adequate in other respects contains adequate magnesium. Good food sources include nuts, cereal grains, dark green vegetables, and seafoods.
Chloride			
Ionized form of element chlorine The main anion of extracellular fluid Almost all chloride is normally excreted by the kidneys.	Functions with sodium to help maintain osmotic pressure and water balance Forms hydrochloric acid (HCl) in gastric mucosal cells Helps regulate electrolyte and acid–base balance by competing with bicarbonate ions for sodium Participates in a homeostatic buffering mechanism in which chloride shifts in and out of red blood cells in exchange for bicarbonate	80–110 mEq	Most dietary chloride is ingested as sodium chloride (NaCl), and foods high in sodium are also high in chloride.

are classified as deficiency states and excess states. Sodium imbalances (hyponatremia and hypernatremia) are described in Table 32-2, potassium imbalances (hypokalemia and hyperkalemia) in Table 32-3, magnesium imbalances (hypomagnesemia and hypermagnesemia) in Table 32-4, and chloride imbalances (hypochloremic metabolic alkalosis and hyperchloremic metabolic acidosis) in Table 32-5. Each imbalance is described in terms of causes, pathophysiology, and clinical signs and symptoms.

Micronutrients

The other 15 minerals are required in small amounts and are often called *micronutrients* or *trace elements*. Eight trace

elements (chromium, cobalt, copper, fluoride, iodine, iron, selenium, and zinc) have relatively well-defined roles in human nutrition (Table 32-6). Because of their clinical importance, iron imbalances are discussed separately in Table 32-7. Other trace elements (manganese, molybdenum, nickel, silicon, tin, and vanadium) are present in many body tissues. Some are components of enzymes and may be necessary for normal growth, structure, and function of connective tissue. For most of these, requirements are unknown, and states of deficiency or excess have not been identified in humans.

Several pharmacologic agents are used to prevent or treat mineral–electrolyte imbalances. Usually, neutral salts of minerals (eg, potassium chloride) are used in deficiency states, and nonmineral drug preparations are used in excess states.

TABLE 32-2 **Sodium Imbalances**

Causes	Pathophysiology	Signs and Symptoms
Hyponatremia 1. Inadequate intake. Unusual but may occur with sodium restricted diets and diuretic drug therapy or when water only is ingested after water and sodium are lost (eg, excessive sweating) 2. Excessive losses with vomiting, GI suction, diarrhea, excessive water enemas, excessive perspiration, burn wounds, and adrenal insufficiency states (eg, Addison's disease) 3. Excessive dilution of body fluids with water	1. Decreased serum sodium 2. Decreased plasma volume and cardiac output 3. Decreased blood flow to kidneys, decreased glomerular filtration rate, and decreased ability of kidneys to excrete water 4. Overhydration and swelling of brain cells (cerebral edema). Leads to impaired neurologic and muscular functions. 5. GI changes	1. Serum sodium <135 mEq/L 2. Hypotension and tachycardia 3. Oliguria and increased BUN 4. Headache, dizziness, weakness, lethargy, restlessness, confusion, delirium, muscle tremors, convulsions, ataxia, aphasia 5. Anorexia, nausea, and vomiting are common; abdominal cramps and paralytic ileus may develop.
Hypernatremia 1. Deficiency of water in proportion to the amount of sodium present. Water deficiency results from lack of intake or excessive losses (diarrhea, diuretic drugs, excessive sweating). 2. Excessive intake of sodium. An uncommon cause of hypernatremia because the thirst mechanism is normally activated, and water intake is increased. 3. Sodium retention due to hyperaldosteronism and Cushing's disease	1. Increased serum sodium 2. Hypernatremia due to water deficiency decreases fluid volume in extracellular fluid and intracellular fluid compartments (dehydration). 3. Hypernatremia due to sodium gain increases extracellular fluid volume and decreases intracellular fluid volume as water is pulled out of cells.	1. Serum sodium >145 mEq/L 2. Lethargy, disorientation, hyperactive reflexes, muscle rigidity, tremors and spasms, irritability, coma, cerebral hemorrhage, subdural hematoma 3. Hypotension 4. Fever, dry skin, and dry mucous membranes 5. Oliguria, concentrated urine with a high specific gravity, and increased BUN

BUN, blood urea nitrogen; GI, gastrointestinal.

INDIVIDUAL AGENTS USED IN MINERAL–ELECTROLYTE AND ACID–BASE IMBALANCES

Acidifying Agent

Ammonium chloride (NH_4Cl) is occasionally used in the treatment of hypochloremic metabolic alkalosis. As a general rule, chloride is preferably replaced with sodium chloride or potassium chloride rather than ammonium chloride. However, sodium chloride may be contraindicated in an edematous client, or the alkalosis may be unresponsive to sodium or potassium chloride. Ammonium chloride may also be used to acidify urine and facilitate the action or excretion of other drugs.

ROUTES AND DOSAGE RANGES

Adults: Oral (PO) 1–3 g two or four times daily
Intravenous (IV) 100–500 mL of a 2% solution, infused over a 3-h period; dosage depends on the client's status and on serum chloride concentration.

Alkalinizing Agents

Sodium bicarbonate has long been used to treat metabolic acidosis, which occurs with severe renal disease, diabetes mellitus, circulatory impairment due to hypotension, shock or fluid volume deficit, and cardiac arrest.

The drug dissociates into sodium and bicarbonate ions; the bicarbonate ions combine with free hydrogen ions to form carbonic acid. This action reduces the number of free hydrogen ions and thereby raises blood pH toward normal (7.35 to 7.45). However, the drug is not usually recommended now unless the acidosis is severe (eg, pH <7.1), or clinical shock is present. Even then, use must be based on frequent measurements of arterial blood gases and careful titration to avoid inducing alkalosis. Alkalosis makes the myocardium more sensitive to stimuli and increases the occurrence of arrhythmias. It also alters the oxyhemoglobin dissociation curve so less oxygen is released and hypoxemia becomes even more severe. Thus, drug administration may be more harmful than helpful. In most instances, treating the underlying cause of the acidosis is safer and more effective. For example, in diabetic ketoacidosis, fluid replacement and insulin may be effective. In cardiac arrest, interventions to maintain circulation and ventilation are more effective in alleviating acidosis.

Sodium bicarbonate also is used to alkalinize the urine. Alkalinization increases solubility of uric acid and sulfonamide drugs and increases excretion of some acidic drugs (eg, salicylates, phenobarbital) when taken in overdose.

ROUTES AND DOSAGE RANGES

Adults: PO 325 mg to 2 g, up to four times per day; maximum daily dose, 16 g for adults younger than 60 y, 8 g for adults older than 60 y

TABLE 32-3 Potassium Imbalances

Causes	Pathophysiology	Signs and Symptoms
Hypokalemia		
1. Inadequate intake. Uncommon in clients who can eat; may occur in those unable to eat or receiving only potassium-free intravenous fluids for several days.	1. Decreased serum potassium	1. Serum potassium <3.5 mEq/L
2. Excessive losses from the gastrointestinal tract (vomiting, gastric suction, diarrhea, overuse of laxatives and enemas) or urinary tract (polyuria from diuretic drugs, renal disease, excessive aldosterone)	2. Impaired cardiac conduction	2. Arrhythmias and ECG changes (depressed ST segment; flattened or inverted T wave; increased amplitude of P wave; prolonged P-R interval; prolonged QRS complex with normal shape and size). Premature atrial and ventricular beats or atrioventricular block may occur, usually in people taking digoxin. Death from cardiac arrest may occur.
3. Movement of potassium out of serum and into cells. This occurs with administration of insulin and glucose in treatment of diabetic ketoacidosis and in metabolic alkalosis.	3. Decreased strength of myocardial contraction and decreased cardiac output. Decreased response to catecholamines and other substances that normally raise blood pressure.	3. Postural hypotension
	4. Neurologic changes due to impaired conduction of nerve impulses	4. Confusion, memory impairment, lethargy, apathy, drowsiness, irritability, delirium
	5. Impaired function of skeletal, smooth, and cardiac muscle, most likely with serum potassium <2.5 mEq/L. Electrical impulses are slowed until muscle contraction cannot occur.	5. Muscle weakness and possibly paralysis. Weakness of leg muscles usually occurs first. Then weakness ascends to include respiratory muscles and cause respiratory insufficiency.
	6. Slowed gastric emptying and decreased intestinal motility, probably caused by muscle weakness	6. Abdominal distention, constipation, paralytic ileus
	7. Decreased ability of kidneys to concentrate urine and excrete acid. Decreased glomerular filtration rate with prolonged potassium deficiency.	7. Polyuria, polydipsia, nocturia. Prolonged deficiency may increase serum creatinine and blood urea nitrogen
	8. Impaired carbohydrate metabolism and decreased secretion of insulin	8. Hyperglycemia
Hyperkalemia		
1. Excess intake. Uncommon with normal kidney function.	1. Increased serum potassium	1. Serum potassium >5 mEq/L
2. Impaired excretion due to renal insufficiency, oliguria, potassium-saving diuretics, aldosterone deficiency, or adrenocortical deficiency	2. Impaired conduction of nerve impulses and muscle contraction	2. Muscle weakness, possibly paralysis and respiratory insufficiency
3. Combination of the above factors. Nonfood sources of potassium include potassium supplements, salt substitutes, transfusions of old blood, and potassium salts of penicillin (penicillin G potassium contains 1.7 mEq potassium per 1 million units).	3. Impaired cardiac conduction. Hyperkalemia "anesthetizes" nerve and muscle cells so electrical current cannot be built up to a sufficient level (repolarization) for an electrical impulse to be initiated and conducted.	3. Cardiotoxicity, with arrhythmias or cardiac arrest. Cardiac effects are not usually severe until serum levels are 7 mEq/L or above. ECG changes include a high, peaked T wave, prolonged P-R interval, absence of P waves, and prolonged QRS complex.
4. Movement of potassium from cells into serum with burns, crushing injuries, and acidosis		

ECG, electrocardiogram.

IV dosage individualized according to arterial blood gases

Children: IV dosage individualized according to arterial blood gases

Cation Exchange Resin

Sodium polystyrene sulfonate (Kayexalate) is a cation exchange resin used for treatment of hyperkalemia. Given orally or rectally, the resin acts in the colon to release sodium and combine with potassium. Potassium is then eliminated from the body in the feces. Each gram of resin removes approximately 1 mEq of potassium. Because the resin requires several hours to lower serum potassium levels, it is more likely to be used after other measures (eg, insulin and glucose infusions) have lowered serum levels. Insulin and glucose lower serum potassium levels by driving potassium into the cells. They do not remove potassium from the body.

ROUTES AND DOSAGE RANGES

Adults: PO 15 g in 100–200 mL of water and 70% sorbitol, one to four times daily

Rectally (retention enema) 30–50 g in 100–200 mL of water and 70% sorbitol q6h

TABLE 32-4) **Magnesium Imbalances**

Causes	Pathophysiology	Signs and Symptoms
Hypomagnesemia 1. Inadequate dietary intake or prolonged administration of magnesium-free intravenous fluids 2. Decreased absorption, as occurs with alcoholism 3. Excessive losses with diuretic drugs, diarrhea, or diabetic acidosis	1. Decreased serum magnesium 2. Impaired conduction of nerve impulses and muscle contraction	1. Serum magnesium <1.5 mEq/L 2. Confusion, restlessness, irritability, vertigo, ataxia, seizures 3. Muscle tremors, carpopedal spasm, nystagmus, generalized spasticity 4. Tachycardia, hypotension, premature atrial and ventricular beats
Hypermagnesemia 1. Renal failure 2. Impaired renal function accompanied by excessive intake of magnesium salts in antacids or cathartics 3. Overtreatment of magnesium deficiency	1. Increased serum magnesium 2. Depressant effects on central nervous and neuromuscular systems, which block transmission of electrical impulses	1. Serum magnesium >2.5 mEq/L 2. Skeletal muscle weakness and paralysis, cardiac arrhythmias, hypotension, respiratory insufficiency, drowsiness, lethargy, coma

TABLE 32-5) **Chloride Imbalances**

Causes	Pathophysiology	Signs and Symptoms
Hypochloremic Metabolic Alkalosis 1. Excessive losses of chloride from vomiting, gastric suctioning, diuretic drug therapy, diabetic ketoacidosis, excessive perspiration, or adrenocortical insufficiency 2. Excessive ingestion of bicarbonate or base	1. Decreased serum chloride 2. When chloride is lost, the body retains bicarbonate to maintain electroneutrality in extracellular fluids. The result is metabolic alkalosis, a relative deficiency of acid, and a relative excess of base. Hypokalemia is often present as well. 3. Hyperexcitability of the nervous system 4. Retention of carbon dioxide (acid) as a compensatory attempt to restore acid–base balance 5. Fluid loss and decreased plasma volume	1. Serum chloride <95 mEq/L; arterial blood pH >7.45 2. Paresthesias of face and extremities 3. Muscle spasms and tetany, which cannot be distinguished from the tetany produced by hypocalcemia 4. Slow, shallow respirations 5. Dehydration 6. Hypotension
Hyperchloremic Metabolic Acidosis 1. Most often caused by dehydration 2. Deficient bicarbonate 3. Hyperparathyroidism 4. Respiratory alkalosis 5. Excessive administration of sodium chloride or ammonium chloride	1. Increased serum chloride 2. In dehydration, the kidneys reabsorb water in an attempt to relieve the fluid deficit. Large amounts of chloride are reabsorbed along with the water. The result is metabolic acidosis, a relative excess of acid, and a relative deficiency of base. 3. Central nervous system depression 4. Increased exhalation of carbon dioxide as a compensatory attempt to restore acid–base balance	1. Serum chloride >103 mEq/L; arterial blood pH <7.35 2. Lethargy, stupor, disorientation, and coma if acidosis is not treated 3. Increased rate and depth of respiration

Chelating Agents (Metal Antagonists)

Deferoxamine (Desferal) is a chelating agent for iron and is the only drug available for removing excess iron from the body. When given orally within a few hours after oral ingestion of iron preparations, deferoxamine combines with the iron in the bowel lumen and prevents its absorption. When given parenterally, it removes iron from storage sites (eg, ferrin, hemosiderin) and combines with the iron to produce a water-soluble compound that can be excreted by the kidneys. The drug can remove approximately 10 to 50 mg of iron per day. The urine becomes reddish brown from the iron content.

(*text continues on page 476*)

TABLE 32-6	Selected Trace Elements		

Characteristics	Functions	Recommended Dietary Allowances (RDAs)	Food Sources
Chromium			
Deficiency produces impaired glucose tolerance (hyperglycemia, glycosuria), impaired growth and reproduction, and decreased life span.	Aids glucose use by increasing effectiveness of insulin and facilitating transport of glucose across cell membranes	Not established	Brewer's yeast and whole wheat products
Cobalt			
1. Stored in the liver, spleen, kidneys, and pancreas 2. Excreted mainly in urine 3. Deficiency of vitamin B_{12} produces pernicious anemia. 4. Excess state not established for humans. In animals, excess cobalt produces polycythemia, bone marrow hyperplasia, and increased blood volume.	A component of vitamin B_{12}, which is required for normal function of all body cells and for maturation of red blood cells	Approximately 1 mg in the form of vitamin B_{12}	Animal foods, including liver, muscle meats, and shellfish. Fruits, vegetables, and cereals contain no cobalt as vitamin B_{12}.
Copper			
1. Found in the brain, liver, heart, kidneys, bone, and muscle 2. Eliminated in urine, sweat, feces, and menstrual flow 3. Deficiency occurs with lack of food intake, malabsorption syndromes, and prolonged administration of copper-free IV hyperalimentation solutions 4. Signs and symptoms of deficiency include decreased serum levels of copper and ceruloplasmin (a plasma protein that transports copper); decreased iron absorption; anemia from impaired erythropoiesis; leukopenia. Death can occur. In infants, three deficiency syndromes have been identified. One is characterized by anemia, a second by chronic malnutrition and diarrhea, and a third (Menke's syndrome) by retarded growth and progressive mental deterioration. 5. Copper excess (hypercupremia) may occur in women who take oral contraceptives or who are pregnant and in clients with infections or liver disease. Wilson's disease is a rare hereditary disorder characterized by accumulation of copper in vital organs (brain, liver, kidneys). Signs and symptoms vary according to affected organs.	1. A component of many enzymes 2. Essential for correct functioning of the central nervous, cardiovascular, and skeletal systems 3. Important in formation of red blood cells, apparently by regulating storage and release of iron for hemoglobin	Not established; estimated at approximately 2 mg	Many foods, including liver, shellfish, nuts, cereals, poultry, dried fruits
Fluoride			
1. Present in water, soil, plants, and animals in small amounts. Often added to community supplies of drinking water. 2. Accumulates in the body until approximately 50–60 years of age	1. A component of tooth enamel 2. Strengthens bones, probably by promoting calcium retention in bones	Not established; average daily intake estimated at approximately 4 mg	Beef, canned salmon, eggs. Very little in milk, cereal grains, fruits, and vegetables. Fluoride content of foods depends on fluoride content of soil where they are grown.

(continued)

| TABLE 32-6 | Selected Trace Elements (*continued*) | | |

Characteristics	Functions	Recommended Dietary Allowances (RDAs)	Food Sources
3. Fluoride deficiency is indicated by dental caries and possibly a greater incidence of osteoporosis. 4. Fluoride excess results in mottling of teeth and osteosclerosis.	3. Adequate intake before ages 50–60 years may decrease osteoporosis and fractures during later years.		
Iodine 1. Iodine deficiency causes thyroid gland enlargement and may cause hypothyroidism 2. Iodine excess (iodism) produces edema, fever, conjunctivitis, lymphadenopathy, stomatitis, vomiting, and coryza. Iodism is unlikely with dietary intake but may occur with excessive intake of drugs containing iodine.	Essential component of thyroid hormones	150 mg for adults, larger amounts for children and pregnant or lactating women	Seafood is the best source. In vegetables, iodine content varies with the amount of iodine in soil where grown. In milk and eggs, content depends on the amount present in animal feed.

Iron
1. Nearly 75% of body iron is in hemoglobin in red blood cells; approximately 25% is stored in the liver, bone marrow, and spleen as ferritin and hemosiderin; the remaining small amount is in myoglobin and enzymes or bound to transferrin in plasma.
2. Absorption from foods is approximately 10%.
  A. Factors that *increase* absorption:
    (1) Presence of dietary ascorbic acid
    (2) Acidity of gastric fluids increases solubility of dietary iron.
    (3) Presence of calcium. Calcium combines with phosphate, oxalate, and phylate. If this reaction does not occur, iron combines with these substances and produces nonabsorbable compounds.
    (4) Physiologic states that increase iron absorption include periods of increased blood formation, such as pregnancy and growth. Also, more iron is absorbed when iron deficiency is present.
  B. Factors that *decrease* absorption:
    (1) Lack of hydrochloric acid in the stomach or administration of antacids, which produces an alkaline environment
    (2) Combination of iron with phosphates, oxalates, or phytates in the intestine. This results in nonabsorbable compounds.
	1. Essential component of hemoglobin, myoglobin, and several enzymes
	2. Hemoglobin is required for transport and use of oxygen by body cells; myoglobin aids oxygen transport and use by muscle cells; enzymes are important for cellular metabolism.
		10 mg for men and older women
		18 mg for women during childbearing years and children during periods of rapid growth
			Liver and other organ meats, lean meat, shellfish, dried beans and vegetables, egg yolks, dried fruits, molasses, whole grain and enriched breads. Milk and milk products contain essentially no iron.

(*continued*)

TABLE 32-6 **Selected Trace Elements (*continued*)**

Characteristics	Functions	Recommended Dietary Allowances (RDAs)	Food Sources
(3) Increased motility of the intestines, which decreases absorption of iron by decreasing contact time with the mucosa			
(4) Steatorrhea or any malabsorption disorder			
Selenium			
1. Has antioxidant properties similar to those of vitamin E	Important for function of myocardium and probably other muscles	70 µg for men; 55 µg for women, increased to 65 µg during pregnancy and 75 µg during lactation	Fish, meat, breads, and cereals
2. Deficiency most likely with long-term IV therapy. Signs and symptoms include myocardial abnormalities and other muscle discomfort and weakness.			
3. Highly toxic in excessive amounts. Signs and symptoms include fatigue, peripheral neuropathy, nausea, diarrhea, and alopecia.			
Zinc			
1. Deficiency may occur in liver cirrhosis, hepatitis, nephrosis, malabsorption syndromes, chronic infections, malignant diseases, myocardial infarction, hypothyroidism, and prolonged administration of zinc-free IV hyperalimentation solutions. Signs and symptoms are most evident in growing children and include impaired growth, hypogonadism in boys, anorexia, and sensory impairment (loss of taste and smell). Also, if the client has had surgery, wound healing may be delayed.	1. A component of many enzymes that are essential for normal metabolism (eg, carbonic anhydrase, lactic dehydrogenase, alkaline phosphatase).	15 mg for adolescents and adults	Animal proteins, such as meat, liver, eggs, and seafood. Wheat germ is also a good source.
	2. Necessary for normal cell growth, synthesis of nucleic acids (RNA and DNA), and synthesis of carbohydrates and proteins	10 mg for preadolescents	
	3. May be essential for use of vitamin A	25–30 mg for pregnant and lactating women	
2. Zinc excess is unlikely with dietary intake but may develop with excessive ingestion or inhalation of zinc. Ingestion may cause nausea, vomiting, and diarrhea; inhalation may cause vomiting, headache, and fever.			

IV, intravenous.

The major indication for use of deferoxamine is acute iron intoxication. It is also used in hemochromatosis due to blood transfusions or hemosiderosis due to certain hemolytic anemias. In these chronic conditions characterized by accumulation of iron in tissues, phlebotomy may be more effective in removing iron. Deferoxamine is more likely to be used in clients who are too anemic or hypoproteinemic to tolerate the blood loss.

ROUTES AND DOSAGE RANGES

Adults and children: PO 4–8 g, given within a few hours of oral ingestion of iron preparations

Intramuscular (IM) 1 g initially, then 500 mg q4h for two doses, then 500 mg q4–12h if needed; maximum dose, 6 g/24h

IV 1 g slowly (not to exceed 15 mg/kg/h), then 500 mg q4h for two doses, then 500 mg q4–12h if necessary; maximum dose, 6 g/24 h. This route is used only in the client in shock.

Penicillamine (Cuprimine) chelates copper, zinc, mercury, and lead to form soluble complexes that are excreted in the urine. The main therapeutic use is to remove excess copper in clients with Wilson's disease (see Table 32-6). It also can be used prophylactically, before clinical manifestations occur, in clients in whom this hereditary condition is likely to develop. Penicillamine may be used to treat cystinuria, a hereditary metabolic disorder characterized by large amounts of cystine in the urine and renal calculi. It may be used in lead poisoning and severe rheumatoid

TABLE 32-7) **Iron Imbalances**

Causes	Pathophysiology	Signs and Symptoms
Deficiency State		
1. Inadequate intake of iron in the diet 2. Faulty absorption of iron 3. Blood loss in gastrointestinal bleeding, heavy or prolonged menstrual flow, traumatic injury, and other conditions	1. Impaired erythropoiesis 2. Inadequate hemoglobin to transport sufficient oxygen to body tissues 3. Iron deficiency increases absorption of other minerals (eg, lead, cobalt, manganese) and may produce signs of excess.	1. Anemia (decrease in red blood cells, hemoglobin, and hematocrit) 2. With gradual development of anemia, minimal symptoms occur 3. With rapid development of anemia or severe anemia, dyspnea, fatigue, tachycardia, malaise, and drowsiness occur.
Acute Excess State		
Acute iron poisoning usually occurs in small children who take several tablets of an iron preparation.	Acute toxicity	Vomiting, diarrhea, melena, abdominal pain, shock, convulsions, and metabolic acidosis. Death may occur within 24 h if treatment is not prompt.
Chronic Excess State		
Chronic iron excess (hemochromatosis) is rare but may be caused by long-term ingestion of excessive iron salts (eg, ferrous sulfate), large numbers of blood transfusions, or a rare genetic trait that promotes iron absorption.	Excess iron is deposited in the heart, pancreas, kidney, liver, and other organs. It impairs cell function and eventually destroys cells.	Cardiac arrhythmias, heart failure, diabetes mellitus, bronze pigmentation of skin, liver enlargement, arthropathy, and others

arthritis that does not respond to conventional treatment measures.

ROUTE AND DOSAGE RANGES

Adults and older children: Wilson's disease, PO 250 mg four times per day, increased gradually, if necessary, up to 2 g/d
Lead poisoning, PO 250–500 mg twice a day
Rheumatoid arthritis, PO 125–250 mg/d for 4 wk, increased by 125–250 mg/d at 1- to 3-mo intervals, if necessary
Usual maintenance dose, 500–750 mg/d; maximum dose, 1000–1500 mg/d
Infants >6 mo and young children: Wilson's disease, PO 250 mg/d, dissolved in fruit juice
Lead poisoning, PO 125 mg three times per day

Succimer (Chemet) chelates lead to form water-soluble complexes that are excreted in the urine. The main therapeutic use is to treat lead poisoning in children with blood levels above 45 μg/100 mL. The most common adverse effects are anorexia, nausea, vomiting, and diarrhea.

ROUTE AND DOSAGE RANGES

Children: PO 10 mg/kg or 350 mg/m^2 q8h for 5 days, then q12h for 14 days (total of 19 days of drug administration). For young children who cannot swallow capsules, the capsule contents can be sprinkled on soft food or given with a spoon.

Iron Preparations

Ferrous gluconate (Fergon) is an oral preparation for treating iron deficiency anemia. It may be less irritating to gastrointestinal (GI) mucosa and therefore better tolerated than ferrous sulfate. Ferrous gluconate contains approximately 12% elemental iron, so each 320-mg tablet contains approximately 38 mg of iron. Indications for use, adverse reactions, and contraindications are the same as for ferrous sulfate.

ROUTE AND DOSAGE RANGES

Adults: PO 320–640 mg (40–80 mg elemental iron) three times per day
Children: PO 100–300 mg (12.5–37.5 mg elemental iron) three times per day
Infants: PO 100 mg or 30 drops of elixir initially, gradually increased to 300 mg or 5 mL of elixir daily (15–37.5 mg elemental iron) in divided doses

Ferrous sulfate (Feosol), which contains 20% elemental iron, is the prototype of oral iron preparations and the preparation of choice for prevention or treatment of iron deficiency anemia. It may be used as an iron supplement during periods of increased requirements (eg, childhood, pregnancy). Nausea and other GI symptoms may result from gastric irritation. Ferrous sulfate and other oral iron preparations discolor feces, producing a black-green color that may be mistaken for blood in the stool. Contraindications to oral iron preparations include peptic ulcer disease, inflammatory intestinal disorders, anemias other than iron deficiency anemia, multiple blood transfusions, hemochromatosis, and hemosiderosis.

ROUTE AND DOSAGE RANGES

Adults: PO 325 mg–1.2 g (60–240 mg elemental iron) daily in three or four divided doses
Children 6–12 y: PO 120–600 mg (24–120 mg elemental iron) daily in divided doses
Infants and children <6 y: 300 mg (60 mg elemental iron) daily in divided doses

Iron dextran injection (InFeD) is a parenteral form of iron useful in treating iron deficiency anemia when oral supplements are not feasible. One milliliter equals 50 mg of elemental iron. Reasons for using iron dextran injection include peptic ulcer or inflammatory bowel disease that is likely to be aggravated by oral iron preparations, the client's inability or unwillingness to take oral preparations, and a shortage of time for correcting the iron deficiency (eg, late pregnancy or preoperative status). A major advantage of parenteral iron is that body iron stores can be replenished rapidly. The drug is contraindicated in anemias not associated with iron deficiency and hypersensitivity to the drug (fatal anaphylactoid reactions have occurred).

Dosage is calculated for individual clients according to hemoglobin and weight (see manufacturer's literature).

Magnesium Preparations

Magnesium oxide or **hydroxide** may be given for mild hypomagnesemia in asymptomatic clients. **Magnesium sulfate** is given parenterally for moderate to severe hypomagnesemia, convulsions associated with pregnancy (eclampsia), and prevention of hypomagnesemia in total parenteral nutrition. Therapeutic effects in these conditions are attributed to the drug's depressant effects on the central nervous system and smooth, skeletal, and cardiac muscle. Oral magnesium salts may cause diarrhea; their uses as antacids and cathartics are discussed in Chapters 60 and 61, respectively. Magnesium preparations are contraindicated in clients who have impaired renal function or who are comatose.

ROUTES AND DOSAGE RANGES

Adults: Hypomagnesemia, PO magnesium oxide 250–500 mg three or four times daily, milk of magnesia 5 mL four times daily, or a magnesium-containing antacid 15 mL three times daily; IM 1–2 g (2–4 mL of 50% solution) once or twice daily based on serum magnesium levels

Eclampsia, IM 1–2 g (2–4 mL of 50% solution) initially, then 1 g every 30 min until seizures stop

Convulsive seizures, IM 1 g (2 mL of 50% solution) repeated PRN

IV, do not exceed 150 mg/min (1.5 mL/min of a 10% solution, 3 mL/min of a 5% solution)

Older children: IM, same dosage as adults

Potassium Preparations

Potassium chloride (KCl) is the drug of choice for preventing or treating hypokalemia because deficiencies of potassium and chloride often occur together. It is often prescribed for clients who are receiving potassium-losing diuretics (eg, hydrochlorothiazide, furosemide); those who are receiving digoxin (hypokalemia increases risks

of digoxin toxicity); and those who are receiving only IV fluids because of surgical procedures, GI disease, or other conditions. KCl also may be used to replace chloride in hypochloremic metabolic alkalosis. It is contraindicated in clients with renal failure and in those receiving potassium-saving diuretics, such as triamterene, spironolactone, or amiloride.

Potassium chloride can be given orally or IV. Oral preparations are recommended when feasible, but one disadvantage of oral liquids is an unpleasant taste. This has led to production of various flavored powders, liquids, and effervescent tablets (eg, Kay Ciel Elixir, K-Lor, Klorvess). Tablets containing a wax matrix (eg, Slow-K) are effective and better tolerated by most clients than liquid formulations. IV preparations of KCl must be diluted before administration to prevent hyperkalemia, cardiotoxicity, and severe pain at the injection site.

ROUTES AND DOSAGE RANGES

Adults: PO 15–20 mEq two to four times per day
IV (KCl injection) approximately 40–100 mEq/24 h. Dosage must be individualized and depends mainly on serum potassium levels. KCl must be diluted for IV administration. A generally safe dosage range is 20–60 mEq, diluted in 1000 mL of dextrose or sodium chloride IV solution and given no faster than 10–15 mEq/h or 60–120 mEq/24 h.

Sodium Preparations

Sodium chloride (NaCl) injection is available in several concentrations and sizes for IV use. Commonly used concentrations are 0.45% (hypotonic solution) and 0.9% (isotonic). NaCl is also available in combination with dextrose. Five percent dextrose in 0.22% NaCl and 5% dextrose in 0.45% NaCl are often used for IV fluid therapy. They contain 38.5 and 77 mEq/L, respectively, of sodium and chloride. Isotonic or 0.9% sodium chloride contains 154 mEq of both sodium and chloride. This solution may be used to treat hyponatremia.

ROUTE AND DOSAGE RANGE

Adults: IV 1500–3000 mL of 0.22%, 0.45% solution/24 h depending on the client's fluid needs; approximately 50 mL/h to keep IV lines open

---

How Can You Avoid This Medication Error?

Jean Watson, a postoperative patient, has a low serum potassium on her second postoperative day (2.1 mEq/L), and her physician orders an additional 20 mEq of KCl to be added to her IV bag. Currently, she has 1000 cc 5% D/.45% NaCl with 20 mEq KCl hanging with 200 cc left in the bag and infusing at 125 cc/hour. You draw up the 20 mEq of KCl and add it to the current infusion without changing the infusion rate.

Zinc Preparation

Zinc sulfate is available in tablets containing 110, 200, or 220 mg of zinc sulfate (equivalent to 25, 47, and 50 mg of elemental zinc, respectively) and in capsules containing 220 mg of zinc sulfate (equivalent to 50 mg of elemental zinc). It is also an ingredient in several vitamin–mineral combination products. Zinc sulfate is given orally as a dietary supplement to prevent or treat zinc deficiency.

> **ROUTE AND DOSAGE RANGE**
>
> *Adults:* PO 25–50 mg elemental zinc daily

Multiple Mineral–Electrolyte Preparations

There are numerous commercially prepared electrolyte solutions for IV use. One group provides *maintenance* amounts of fluids and electrolytes when oral intake of food and fluids is restricted or contraindicated. These solutions differ slightly in the number and amount of particular electrolytes. A second group provides *replacement* amounts of electrolytes (mainly sodium and chloride) when electrolytes are lost from the body in abnormal amounts. This group includes Normosol-R (Abbott), and Plasma-Lyte 148 (Travenol). These electrolyte preparations are available with dextrose 2.5% to 10%. Ringer's solution is another replacement fluid that is used often. It is manufactured by several different companies; health care agencies use one manufacturer's products for the most part.

Oral electrolyte solutions (eg, Lytren, Pedialyte) contain several electrolytes and a small amount of dextrose. They are used to supply maintenance amounts of fluids and electrolytes when oral intake is restricted. They are especially useful in children for treatment of diarrhea and may prevent severe fluid and electrolyte depletion. The amount given must be carefully prescribed and calculated to avoid excessive intake. They should not be used in severe circumstances in which IV fluid and electrolyte therapy is indicated. They must be cautiously used with impaired renal function. They should not be mixed with other electrolyte-containing fluids, such as milk or fruit juices.

> **ROUTES AND DOSAGE RANGES**
>
> *Adults:* IV 2000–3000 mL/24 h, depending on individual fluid and electrolyte needs
>
> *Children:* IV, PO, amount individualized according to fluid and electrolyte needs

NURSING PROCESS

Assessment

Assess each client for current or potential mineral–electrolyte or acid–base disorders. Specific assessment factors related to minerals and electrolytes include the following:

- Deficiency states are probably more common than excess states unless a mineral–electrolyte supplement is being taken. However, deficiencies and excesses may be equally harmful, and both must be assessed.
- Clients with other nutritional deficiencies are likely to have mineral–electrolyte deficiencies as well. Moreover, deficiencies are likely to be multiple, with overlapping signs and symptoms.
- Many drugs influence gains and losses of minerals and electrolytes, including diuretics and laxatives.
- Minerals and electrolytes are lost with gastric suction, polyuria, diarrhea, excessive perspiration, and other conditions.
- Assess laboratory reports when available.
  - Check the complete blood count for decreased red blood cells, hemoglobin, and hematocrit. Reduced values may indicate iron deficiency anemia, and further assessment is needed.
  - Check serum electrolyte reports for increases or decreases. All major minerals can be measured in clinical laboratories. The ones usually measured are sodium, chloride, and potassium; carbon dioxide content, a measure of bicarbonate, is also assessed. Normal values vary to some extent with the laboratory and the method of measurement, but a general range of normal values is sodium, 135 to 145 mEq/L; chloride, 95 to 105 mEq/L; potassium, 3.5 to 5 mEq/L; and carbon dioxide, 22 to 26 mEq/L.

Nursing Diagnoses

- Altered Nutrition: Less Than Body Requirements related to mineral–electrolyte deficiency
- Altered Nutrition: More Than Body Requirements related to excessive intake of drug preparations
- Risk for Injury related to mineral–electrolyte deficiency or overdose
- Knowledge Deficit: Importance of adequate mineral–electrolyte intake in normal body functioning
- Knowledge Deficit: Dietary sources of various mineral–electrolyte nutrients

Planning/Goals

The client will:

- Have an adequate dietary intake of minerals and electrolytes
- Avoid mineral–electrolyte supplements unless recommended by a health care provider
- Participate in follow-up procedures and laboratory tests as requested when mineral–electrolyte drugs are prescribed
- Take mineral–electrolyte drugs as prescribed
- Avoid adverse effects of drug preparations

Interventions

Implement measures to prevent mineral–electrolyte disorders:

- Promote a varied diet. A diet adequate in protein and calories usually provides adequate minerals and electrolytes. An exception is iron, which is often needed as a dietary supplement in women and children.
- If assessment data reveal potential development of a disorder, start preventive measures as soon as possible. For clients able to eat, foods high in iron may delay onset of iron deficiency anemia, foods high in potassium may prevent hypokalemia with diuretic therapy, and salty foods along with water help to prevent problems associated with excessive heat and perspiration. For people unable to eat, IV fluids and electrolytes are usually given. In general, oral food intake or tube feeding is preferable to IV therapy.
- Treat underlying disorders that contribute to the mineral–electrolyte deficiency or excess. Measures to relieve anorexia, nausea, vomiting, diarrhea, pain, and other symptoms help to increase intake or decrease output of certain minerals. Measures to increase urine output, such as forcing fluids, help to increase output of some minerals in the urine and therefore prevent excess states from developing.
- Mineral supplements are recommended only for current or potential deficiencies because all are toxic in excessive amounts. When deficiencies are identified, treat with foods when possible. Next, use oral mineral supplements. Use parenteral supplements only for clear-cut indications because they are potentially the most hazardous.
- For clients who have nasogastric tubes to suction, irrigate the tubes with isotonic sodium chloride solution. The use of tap water is contraindicated because it is hypotonic and would pull electrolytes into the stomach. Electrolytes are then lost in the aspirated and discarded stomach contents. For the same reason, only small amounts of ice chips or water are allowed per hour. Clients often request ice chips or water frequently and in larger amounts than desirable; the nurse must explain the reason for the restrictions.
- Assist clients to keep appointments for periodic blood tests and other follow-up procedures when mineral–electrolyte supplements are prescribed.

Evaluation

- Interview about and observe the amount and type of food intake in relation to required minerals and electrolytes.
- Interview and observe for signs of mineral–electrolyte deficiency or excess.

PRINCIPLES OF THERAPY

Diet Supplements

Many people take mineral preparations as dietary supplements, usually in a multivitamin preparation. Recommended doses should not be exceeded; minerals are toxic at high doses.

Prevention of an Excess State

When a mineral is given to correct a deficiency state, there is a risk of producing an excess state. Because both deficiency and excess states may be harmful, the amount of mineral supplement should be titrated closely to the amount needed by the body. Larger doses are needed to treat deficiency states than are needed to prevent deficiencies from developing. In addition to producing potential toxicity, large doses of one mineral may cause a relative deficiency of another mineral or nutrient.

Drug Selection

Oral drug preparations are preferred, when feasible, for preventing or treating mineral disorders. They are safer, less likely to produce toxicity, more convenient to administer, and less expensive than parenteral preparations.

Management of Sodium Disorders

Hyponatremia
Treatment of hyponatremia is aimed at restoring normal levels of serum sodium. This can be done with isotonic NaCl solution when hyponatremia is caused by sodium depletion, and with restriction of water when hyponatremia is caused by fluid volume excess (water intoxication).

Hypernatremia
Treatment of hypernatremia requires administration of sodium-free fluids, either orally or IV, until serum sodium levels return to normal. Milder states usually respond to increased water intake through the GI tract; more severe hypernatremia requires IV administration of 5% dextrose in water.

Management of Potassium Disorders

Hypokalemia
1. Assess for conditions contributing to hypokalemia, and attempt to eliminate them or reduce their impact. Such conditions are usually inadequate intake, excessive loss, or some combination of the two.

CLIENT TEACHING GUIDELINES
Mineral Supplements

General Considentations

✔ The best source of minerals and electrolytes is a well-balanced diet with a variety of foods. A well-balanced diet contains all the minerals needed for health in most people. An exception is iron, which is often needed as a dietary supplement in women and children.

✔ The safest course of action is to take mineral supplements only on a health care provider's advice, in the amounts and for the length of time prescribed. All minerals are toxic when taken in excess.

✔ Keep all mineral–electrolyte substances out of reach of children to prevent accidental overdose. Acute iron intoxication is a common problem among small children and can be fatal.

✔ Keep appointments with health care providers for periodic blood tests and other follow-up procedures when mineral–electrolyte supplements are prescribed (eg, potassium chloride). This helps prevent ingestion of excessive amounts.

✔ Minerals are often contained in multivitamin preparations, with percentages of the recommended dietary allowances supplied. These amounts differ in various preparations and should be included in estimations of daily intake.

Self- or Caregiver Administration

✔ Take iron preparations with or after meals, with approximately 8 oz of fluid, to prevent stomach upset. Do not crush or chew slow-release tablets or capsules. With liquid preparations, dilute with water, drink through a straw, and rinse the mouth afterward to avoid staining the teeth. Expect that stools will be dark green or black.

✔ With potassium preparations, mix oral solutions or effervescent tablets with at least 4 oz of water or juice to improve the taste, dilute the drug, and decrease gastric irritation. Do not crush or chew slow-release preparations. Take after meals initially to decrease gastric irritation. If no anorexia, nausea, vomiting, or other problems occur, the drug can be tried before meals because it is better absorbed from an empty stomach. Do *not* stop taking the medication without notifying the physician who prescribed it, especially if also taking digoxin or diuretics. Excessive amounts should also be avoided. Do not use salt substitutes unless they are recommended by a health care provider; they contain potassium chloride and may result in excessive intake. Serious problems may develop from either high or low levels of potassium in the blood.

---

2. Assess the severity of the hypokalemia. This is best done on the basis of serum potassium levels and clinical manifestations. Serum potassium levels alone are inadequate because they may not accurately reflect depletion of body potassium.

3. Potassium supplements are indicated in the following circumstances:
   a. When serum potassium level is below 3 mEq/L on repeated measurements, even if the client is asymptomatic
   b. When serum potassium is 3 to 3.5 mEq/L and clear-cut symptoms or electrocardiographic (ECG) changes indicate hypokalemia. Some clinicians advocate treatment in the absence of symptoms.
   c. In clients receiving digoxin, if necessary to maintain serum potassium levels above 3.5 mEq/L. This is indicated because hypokalemia increases digoxin toxicity.

4. When potassium supplements are necessary, oral administration is preferred when possible.

5. Potassium chloride is the drug of choice in most instances. Liquids, powders, and effervescent tablets for oral use must be diluted in at least 4 oz of water or juice to improve taste and decrease gastric irritation. Controlled-release tablets or capsules with KCl in a wax matrix or microencapsulated form are preferred by most clients.

6. Intravenous KCl is indicated when a client cannot take an oral preparation or has severe hypokalemia. The serum potassium level should be measured, total body deficit estimated, and adequate urine output established before IV potassium therapy begins.
   a. Intravenous KCl must be well diluted to prevent sudden hyperkalemia, cardiotoxic effects, and phlebitis at the venipuncture site. The usual dilution is KCl 20 to 60 mEq/1000 mL of IV fluid for maintenance and 10 mEq/50 mL or 20 mEq/100 mL for replacement.
   b. Dosage must be individualized. Clients receiving IV fluids only are usually given 40 to 60 mEq of KCl daily. This can be given safely with 20 mEq KCl/L of fluids and a flow rate of 100 to 125 mL/hour. In severe deficits, a higher concentration and a higher flow rate may be necessary. In these situations, an infusion pump to control flow rate accurately and continuous cardiac monitoring for detection of hyperkalemia are necessary. Also, serum potassium levels must be checked frequently and dosage adjusted if indicated. No more than 100 to 200 mEq KCl should be given within 24 hours, even if several days are required to replace the estimated deficit.
   c. Do not administer potassium-containing IV solutions into a central venous catheter. There is a

risk of hyperkalemia and cardiac arrhythmias or arrest because there is limited time for the solution to be diluted in the blood returning to the heart.

    d. In critical situations, KCl usually should be given in sodium chloride solutions rather than dextrose solutions. Administering dextrose solutions may increase hypokalemia by causing some potassium to leave the serum and enter cells.

Hyperkalemia

1. Eliminate any exogenous sources of potassium, such as potassium supplements, penicillin G potassium, salt substitutes, and blood transfusion with old blood.
2. Treat acidosis, if present, because potassium leaves cells and enters the serum with acidosis.
3. Use measures that antagonize the effects of potassium, that cause potassium to leave the serum and reenter cells, and that remove potassium from the body. Appropriate measures are determined mainly by serum potassium levels and ECG changes. Continuous cardiac monitoring is required.

    Severe hyperkalemia (serum potassium above 7 mEq/L and ECG changes indicating hyperkalemia) requires urgent treatment. Immediate IV administration of sodium bicarbonate 45 mEq, over a 5-minute period, causes rapid movement of potassium into cells. This can be repeated in a few minutes if ECG changes persist.

    Calcium gluconate 10%, 5 to 10 mL IV, is also given early in treatment to decrease the cardiotoxic effects of hyperkalemia. It is contraindicated if the client is receiving digoxin, and it cannot be added to fluids containing sodium bicarbonate because insoluble precipitates are formed.

    The next step is IV infusion of glucose and insulin. This also causes potassium to move into cells, although not as quickly as sodium bicarbonate.

4. When hyperkalemia is less severe or when it has been reduced by the aforementioned measures, sodium polystyrene sulfonate, a cation exchange resin, can be given orally or rectally to remove potassium from the body. Each gram of the resin combines with 1 mEq potassium, and both are excreted in feces. The resin is usually mixed with water and sorbitol, a poorly absorbed, osmotically active alcohol that has a laxative effect. The sorbitol offsets the constipating effect of the resin and aids in its expulsion. Oral administration is preferred, and several doses daily may be given until serum potassium is normal. When given as an enema, the solution must be retained from 1 to several hours, or repeated enemas must be given for therapeutic effect.
5. If the preceding measures fail to reduce hyperkalemia, peritoneal dialysis or hemodialysis may be used.

Management of Magnesium Disorders

Hypomagnesemia

1. Prevent hypomagnesemia, when possible, by giving parenteral fluids with magnesium when the fluids are the only source of nutrients. Multiple-electrolyte IV solutions contain magnesium chloride or acetate, and magnesium can be added to solutions for total parenteral nutrition.
2. For mild, asymptomatic hypomagnesemia, oral magnesium preparations may be given. For moderate to severe and symptomatic hypomagnesemia, parenteral (IV or IM) magnesium sulfate may be given daily as long as hypomagnesemia persists or continuing losses occur. Initial dosage may be larger, but the usual maintenance dose is approximately 8 mEq daily. A 10% solution is available in 10-mL vials that contain 8 mEq of magnesium sulfate for adding to IV solutions. A 50% solution is available in 2-mL vials (8 mEq) for IM administration.
3. Check serum magnesium levels daily.

Hypermagnesemia

1. Stop any source of exogenous magnesium, such as magnesium sulfate or magnesium-containing antacids, cathartics, or enemas.
2. Have calcium gluconate available for IV administration. It is an antidote for the sedative effects of magnesium excess.
3. Increase urine output by increasing fluid intake, if feasible. This increases removal of magnesium from the body in urine.
4. Clients with chronic renal failure are the most likely to become hypermagnesemic. They may require peritoneal dialysis or hemodialysis to lower serum magnesium levels.

Management of Iron Deficiency and Excess

Iron Deficiency Anemia

1. Anemia is a symptom, not a disease. Therefore, the underlying cause must be identified and eliminated, if possible.

Nursing Notes: Apply Your Knowledge

After surgery, George Lee will be taking ferrous sulfate, 300 mg tid with meals. The pharmacy supplies him with 300-mg tablets. Review important points to focus in your teaching plan before discharge.

2. Assess the client's intake of and attitude toward foods with high iron content. Encourage increased dietary intake of these foods.

3. Use oral iron preparations when possible. They are safe, effective, convenient to administer, and relatively inexpensive. Ferrous preparations (sulfate, gluconate, fumarate) are better absorbed than ferric preparations. Other iron salts do not differ significantly from ferrous sulfate, which is usually the drug of choice for oral iron therapy. Slow-release or enteric-coated products tend to decrease absorption of iron.

4. Dosage is calculated in terms of elemental iron. Iron preparations vary greatly in the amount of elemental iron they contain. Ferrous sulfate, for example, contains 20% iron; thus, each 325-mg tablet furnishes approximately 60 mg of elemental iron. With the usual regimen of one tablet three times daily, a daily dose of 180 mg of elemental iron is given. For most clients, probably half that amount (30 mg three times daily) would correct the deficiency. However, tablets are not manufactured in sizes to allow this regimen, and liquid preparations are not popular with clients. Thus, relatively large doses are usually given, but smaller doses may be just as effective, especially if GI symptoms become a problem with higher dosages. Whatever the dose, only about 10% to 15% of the iron is absorbed. Most of the remainder is excreted in feces, which turn dark green or black.

5. Oral iron preparations are better absorbed if taken on an empty stomach. However, because gastric irritation is a common adverse reaction, they are more often given with or immediately after meals.

6. Although normal hemoglobin levels return after approximately 2 months of oral iron therapy, an additional 6-month period of drug therapy is recommended to replenish the body's iron stores.

7. Reasons for failure to respond to iron therapy include continued blood loss, failure to take the drug as prescribed, or defective iron absorption. These factors must be reevaluated if no therapeutic response is evident within 3 to 4 weeks after drug therapy is begun.

8. Parenteral iron is indicated when oral preparations may further irritate a diseased GI tract, when the client is unable or unwilling to take the oral drugs, or when the anemia must be corrected rapidly.

9. For severe iron deficiency anemia, blood transfusions may be most effective.

Iron Excess

1. Acute iron overdosage requires treatment as soon as possible, even if overdosage is only suspected and the amount taken is unknown. It is unnecessary to wait until the serum iron level is measured.

   If treatment is begun shortly after oral ingestion of iron, induced vomiting or aspiration of stomach contents by nasogastric tube is helpful. This can be followed by lavage with 1% sodium bicarbonate solution to form insoluble iron carbonate compounds. The next step is to instill in the stomach 5 to 8 g of deferoxamine dissolved in 50 mL of distilled water to bind the iron remaining in the GI tract and prevent its absorption. Finally, deferoxamine is given IM or IV to bind with iron in tissues and allow its excretion in the urine. Throughout the treatment period, supportive measures may be needed for GI hemorrhage, acidosis, and shock.

2. For chronic iron overload or hemochromatosis, the first step in treatment is to stop the source of iron, if possible. Phlebotomy is the treatment of choice for most clients because withdrawal of 500 mL of blood removes approximately 250 mg of iron. Phlebotomy may be needed as often as weekly and for as long as 2 to 3 years. For clients resistant to or intolerant of phlebotomy, deferoxamine can be given. Approximately 10 to 50 mg of iron is excreted daily in the urine with deferoxamine administration.

Management of Acid–Base Disorders

Metabolic Acidosis

1. Assess the presence and severity of acidosis by measuring arterial blood gases. Results reflecting acidosis are decreased pH (<7.35) and decreased bicarbonate (<22 mEq/L).

2. Assess and treat the underlying condition, such as diabetic ketoacidosis.

3. If this does not relieve acidosis, or if acidosis is severe (arterial blood pH <7.2), sodium bicarbonate may be given parenterally to alkalinize the blood. It can be given by direct injection into a vein or as a continuous IV infusion. Ampules and prefilled syringes are available in 8.4% solution (50 mL contains 50 mEq) or 7.5% solution (50 mL contains 44.6 mEq). IV solutions of 5% and 1.4% sodium bicarbonate are also available in 500-mL bottles.

4. Monitor arterial blood gases and serum potassium levels frequently. Overtreatment of acidosis with sodium bicarbonate produces alkalosis. Serum potassium levels may change from high to normal levels initially (because acidosis causes potassium to be drawn into the bloodstream) to severely low levels as potassium reenters cells with treatment of acidosis. Thus, potassium replacement is likely to be needed during treatment of acidosis.

5. During severe acidosis, effective ventilation measures are needed along with sodium bicarbonate to remove carbon dioxide from the blood.

6. In lactic acidosis, larger doses of sodium bicarbonate may be required than in other types of acidosis. This is because of continued production of large amounts of lactic acid by body metabolism.

7. Chronic metabolic acidosis may occur with chronic renal failure. Sodium bicarbonate or citrate (which is converted to bicarbonate in the body) can be given orally in a dose sufficient to maintain a normal serum bicarbonate level.

Metabolic Alkalosis

1. Assess the presence and severity of the alkalosis by measuring arterial blood gases. Values indicating alkalosis are increased pH (>7.45) and increased bicarbonate (>26 mEq/L).
2. Assess and treat the underlying condition. Often, volume depletion and hypochloremia are present and can be corrected with isotonic 0.9% NaCl solution. If hypokalemia and hypochloremia are present, KCl will likely replace both deficits.
3. In severe alkalosis that does not respond to the preceding therapy, ammonium chloride can be given, but it must be given cautiously to avoid inducing acidosis.

Use in Children

Children need sufficient amounts of minerals and electrolytes to support growth and normal body functioning. In the healthy child, a varied, well-balanced diet is usually preferred over supplements. However, iron deficiency is common in young children and teenage girls, and an iron supplement is often needed. Guidelines include the following:

1. In children who eat poorly, a combined vitamin/mineral supplement every other day may be reasonable. In areas where water is not fluorinated, a combined vitamin/mineral supplement containing fluoride may be indicated for infants and children. Fluoride must be prescribed by a physician, dentist, or nurse practitioner.
2. If supplements are given, dosages should be discussed with a health care provider and usually should not exceed RDAs. All minerals and electrolytes are toxic in overdose and may cause life-threatening adverse effects. All such drugs should be kept out of reach of young children and should never be referred to as "candy."
3. If KCl and other electrolyte preparations are used to treat deficiency states in children, serum electrolyte levels must be monitored. In addition, doses must be carefully measured and given no more often than prescribed to avoid toxicity.
4. Accidental ingestion of iron-containing medications and dietary supplements is a common cause of poisoning death in children younger than 6 years of age. To help combat accidental poisoning, products containing iron must be labeled with a warning and prod-

ucts with 30 mg or more of iron (eg, prenatal iron products) must be packaged as individual doses. All iron-containing preparations should be stored in places that are inaccessible to young children.

Use in Older Adults

Mineral–electrolyte requirements are the same as for younger adults, but deficiencies of calcium and iron are common in older adults. Numerous factors may contribute to deficiencies, including limited income, anorexia, lack of teeth or ill-fitting dentures, drugs that decrease absorption of dietary nutrients, and disease processes that interfere with the ability to obtain, prepare, or eat adequate amounts of a variety of foods. Diuretic drugs, frequently prescribed for cardiovascular disorders in older adults, may cause potassium deficiency unless serum levels are carefully monitored and preventive measures taken.

Excess states also may occur in older adults. For example, decreased renal function promotes retention of magnesium and potassium. Hyperkalemia also may occur with the use of potassium supplements or salt substitutes. All minerals and electrolytes are toxic in overdose.

Every older adult should be assessed carefully regarding nutritional status and use of drugs that interact with dietary nutrients. Serum levels of minerals and electrolytes should be monitored carefully during illness, and measures taken to prevent either deficiency or excess states.

Use in Renal Impairment

Several mineral–electrolyte products are contraindicated in clients with renal impairment, including ammonium chloride, magnesium, and potassium chloride (severe impairment with oliguria or azotemia), because of potential accumulation and toxicity.

Frequent measurements of serum electrolyte levels may be indicated.

Use in Hepatic Impairment

Ammonium chloride is contraindicated in impaired hepatic function, and iron dextran must be used with extreme caution. Also, overdoses of chromium and copper are hepatotoxic and should be avoided.

Use in Critical Illness

Electrolyte and acid–base imbalances often occur in critically ill clients and are usually treated as in other clients, with very close monitoring of serum electrolyte levels and avoiding excessive amounts of replacement products.

Home Care

The home care nurse has the opportunity to assess household members and the environment for indications of mineral–electrolyte deficiency or excess. Depending on assessment data, teaching may be needed about dietary sources of these nutrients, when mineral supplements are indicated or should be avoided, and safety factors related to iron supplements in homes with small children.

(*text continues on page 489*)

NURSING ACTIONS	Mineral–Electrolyte Preparations

NURSING ACTIONS	RATIONALE/EXPLANATION
1. Administer accurately	
a. Give oral mineral–electrolyte preparations with food or immediately after meals.	To decrease gastric irritation. Iron and possibly some other agents are better absorbed when taken on an empty stomach. However, they are better tolerated when taken with food.
b. Given intravenous (IV) preparations slowly, as a general rule.	The primary danger of rapid IV injection or infusion is a transient excess in serum, which may cause cardiac arrhythmias or other serious problems.
c. Do not mix minerals and electrolytes with any other drug in a syringe.	High risk of physical incompatibility and precipitation of drugs
d. For IV infusion, most minerals and electrolytes are compatible with solutions of dextrose or sodium chloride. Do not mix with other solutions until compatibility is determined.	To avoid physical incompatibility and precipitation of contents
e. For IV sodium chloride (NaCl) solutions:	
(1) Give fluids at the prescribed flow rate.	Flow rates depend largely on reasons for use. For example, if a client is receiving no oral fluids (NPO) or only small amounts, the flow rate is often 100 to 125 mL/h or 2400 to 3000 mL/24 h. If used as a vehicle for IV antibiotics, the rate is often 50 mL/h or keep open rate (KOR). If the client is dehydrated, 150 to 200 mL/h may be given for a few hours or until a certain amount has been given. (Restrictions in time or amount are necessary to avoid circulatory overload or pulmonary edema.)
f. For potassium supplements:	
(1) Mix liquids, powders, and effervescent tablets in at least 4 oz of juice, water, or carbonated beverage.	To dilute, disguise the unpleasant taste, and decrease gastric irritation
(2) Give oral preparations with or after meals.	To decrease gastric irritation
(3) Never give undiluted potassium chloride (KCl) IV.	Transient hyperkalemia may cause life-threatening cardiotoxicity. Severe pain and vein sclerosis also may result.
(4) Dilute IV KCl 20 to 60 mEq in 1000 ml of IV solution, such as dextrose in water. Be sure that KCl is mixed well with the IV solution.	Dilution decreases risks of hyperkalemia and cardiotoxicity. It also prevents or decreases pain at the infusion site.
(5) Usually, give potassium-containing IV solutions at a rate that administers approximately 10 mEq/h or less.	This is the safest amount and rate of potassium administration. It is also usually effective.

(continued)

NURSING ACTIONS	RATIONALE/EXPLANATION
(6) For life-threatening arrhythmias caused by hypokalemia, potassium can be replaced with 20 to 40 mEq/h with appropriate cardiac monitoring.	Risks of hyperkalemia and life-threatening cardiotoxicity are greatly increased with high concentrations or rapid flow rates. Constant electrocardiogram monitoring is the best way to detect hyperkalemia.
g. For magnesium sulfate ($MgSO_4$):	
(1) Read the drug label carefully to be sure you have the correct preparation for the intended use.	$MgSO_4$ is available in concentrations of 10%, 25%, and 50% and in sizes of 2-, 10-, and 20-mL ampules, as well as a 30-mL multidose vial.
(2) For intramuscular administration, small amounts of 50% solution are usually used (1 g $MgSO_4$ = 2 mL of 50% solution).	
(3) For IV use, a 5% or 10% solution is used for direct injection, intermittent infusion, or continuous infusion. Whatever concentration is used, administer no more than 150 mg/min (1.5 mL/min of 10% solution; 3 mL/min of 5% solution).	
h. For sodium bicarbonate ($NaHCO_3$):	
(1) Read the label carefully to be sure you have the correct solution.	$NaHCO_3$ is available in several concentrations and sizes, such as 50-mL ampules or prefilled syringes with 50 mEq drug (8.4% solution) or 44.6 mEq drug (7.5% solution), or 500-mL bottles with 297.7 mEq drug (5% solution) or 83 mEq drug (1.4% solution).
(2) Inject directly into the vein or into the tubing of a flowing IV infusion solution in emergencies, such as cardiac arrest.	
(3) In nonemergency situations, titrate flow rate of infusions according to arterial blood gases.	To avoid iatrogenic alkalosis
(4) Flush IV lines before and after injecting and do not add any other medications to an IV containing $NaHCO_3$	$NaHCO_3$ is highly alkaline and may cause precipitation of other drugs.
(5) Monitor arterial blood gases for increased pH after each 50 to 100 mEq of $NaHCO_3$	To avoid overtreatment and metabolic alkalosis
i. For iron preparations:	
(1) Dilute liquid iron preparations, give with a straw, and have the client rinse the mouth afterward	To prevent temporary staining of teeth
(2) To give iron dextran intramuscularly, use a 2- to 3-inch needle and Z-track technique to inject the drug into the upper outer quadrant of the buttock.	To prevent discomfort and staining of subcutaneous tissue and skin
(3) To give iron dextran IV (either directly or diluted in sodium chloride solution and given over several hours), do not use the multidose vial.	The multidose vial contains phenol as a preservative and is not suitable for IV use. Ampules of 2 mL or 5 mL are available without preservative.
j. Refer to the individual drugs or package literature for instructions regarding administration of ammonium chloride, deferoxamine, penicillamine, and multiple electrolyte solutions.	*(continued)*

NURSING ACTIONS	RATIONALE/EXPLANATION

2. Observe for therapeutic effects

a. With NaCl, observe for decreased symptoms of hyponatremia and increased serum sodium level.

Therapeutic effects should be evident within a few hours.

b. With KCl or other potassium preparations, observe for decreased signs of hypokalemia and increased serum potassium levels.

c. With $MgSO_4$, observe for decreased signs of hypomagnesemia, increased serum magnesium levels, or control of convulsions.

d. With zinc sulfate ($ZnSO_4$), observe for improved wound healing.

e. With sodium bicarbonate ($NaHCO_3$), observe for decreased manifestations of acidosis and a rise in blood pH and bicarbonate levels.

f. With iron preparations, observe for:

(1) Increased vigor and feeling of well-being

(2) Improved appetite

(3) Less fatigue

(4) Increased red blood cells, hemoglobin, and hematocrit

(5) With parenteral iron, observe for an average increase in hemoglobin of 1 g/wk.

Therapeutic effects are usually evident within a month unless other problems are also present (eg, vitamin deficiency, achlorhydria, infection, malabsorption).

3. Observe for adverse effects

a. Mineral–electrolyte excess states:

These are likely to occur with excessive dosages of supplements. They can usually be prevented by using relatively low doses in nonemergency situations and by frequent monitoring of serum levels of electrolytes and iron.

(1) With NaCl injection, observe for hypernatremia and circulatory overload.

These are most likely to occur with rapid infusion of large amounts or with heart or kidney disease, which decreases water excretion and urine output. They also may occur with hypertonic solutions (eg, 3% NaCl), but these are infrequently used.

(2) With potassium preparations, observe for hyperkalemia.

This is most likely to occur with rapid IV administration, high dosages or concentrations, or in the presence of renal insufficiency and decreased urine output.

(3) With magnesium preparations, observe for hypermagnesemia.

See potassium preparations, above.

(4) With $NaHCO_3$, observe for metabolic alkalosis.

This is most likely to occur when large amounts of $NaHCO_3$ are given IV.

b. Gastrointestinal (GI) symptoms–anorexia, nausea, vomiting, diarrhea, and abdominal discomfort from gastric irritation

Most oral preparations of minerals and electrolytes are likely to cause gastric irritation. Taking the drugs with food or 8 oz of fluid may decrease symptoms.

c. Cardiovascular symptoms:

(1) Cardiac arrhythmias

Potentially fatal arrhythmias may occur with hyperkalemia or hypermagnesemia.

(continued)

NURSING ACTIONS	RATIONALE/EXPLANATION
(2) Hypotension, tachycardia, other symptoms of shock	May occur with deferoxamine and iron dextran injections
(3) Circulatory overload and possible pulmonary edema	Most likely to occur with large amounts of NaCl or NaHCO$_3$
d. With Kayexalate, observe for hypokalemia, hypocalcemia, hypomagnesemia, and edema.	Although this drug is used to treat hyperkalemia, it removes calcium and magnesium ions as well as potassium ions. Because it acts by trading sodium for potassium, the sodium retention may lead to edema.
4. Observe for drug interactions	
a. Drugs that *increase* effects of minerals and electrolytes and related drugs:	
(1) Acidifying agents (ammonium chloride): effects are increased by sodium chloride, potassium chloride, and ascorbic acid.	Systemic acidification by increased serum chloride; also increased urine acidity
(2) Alkalinizing agents (sodium bicarbonate): effects are increased by antacids, such as magnesium hydroxide, calcium carbonate, and aluminum hydroxide.	Small amounts of antacids may be absorbed to produce additive effects.
(3) Cation exchange resin (Kayexalate): diuretics increase potassium loss; other sources of sodium increase the likelihood of edema.	Additive effects
(4) Iron salts:	
(a) Allopurinol (Zyloprim)	This drug may increase the concentration of iron in the liver. It should not be given concurrently with any iron preparation.
(b) Ascorbic acid (vitamin C)	In large doses of 1 g or more, ascorbic acid increases absorption of iron by acidifying secretions.
(5) Potassium salts:	
(a) Spironolactone, triamterene, amiloride	These drugs are potassium-saving diuretics. They should *not* be given with a potassium supplement because of additive risks of producing life-threatening hyperkalemia.
(b) Salt substitutes (eg, Neo-Curtasol)	These contain potassium rather than sodium and may cause hyperkalemia if given with potassium supplements.
(c) Penicillin G potassium	This potassium salt of penicillin contains 1.7 mEq of potassium per 1 million units. It may produce hyperkalemia if given in combination with potassium supplements.
b. Drugs that *decrease* effects of minerals and electrolytes and related drugs:	
(1) Acidifying agents: effects are decreased by alkalinizing agents.	Alkalinizing agents neutralize the effects of acidifying agents.
(2) Alkalinizing agents: effects are decreased by acidifying drugs.	Acidifying drugs neutralize effects of alkalinizing agents.

(continued)

NURSING ACTIONS	RATIONALE/EXPLANATION
(3) Oral iron salts:	
(a) Antacids containing carbonate	The antacids decrease iron absorption by forming an insoluble, nonabsorbable compound of iron carbonate.
(b) Magnesium trisilicate	This antacid decreases absorption of iron.
(c) Pancreatic extracts	These inhibit iron absorption by increasing alkalinity of GI fluids.
(4) Potassium salts:	
(a) Calcium gluconate	Decreases cardiotoxic effects of hyperkalemia and is therefore useful in the treatment of hyperkalemia
(b) Sodium polystyrene sulfonate (Kayexalate)	Used in treatment of hyperkalemia because it removes potassium from the body

How Can You Avoid This Medication Error?

Answer: This could cause hyperkalemia that might be lethal for the patient. Adding KCl to an IV bag with only 200 cc remaining would create a solution too concentrated to administer IV. Also, adding KCl to an existing IV should be avoided whenever possible because if the potassium is not mixed adequately with the solution in the bag, a concentrated, potentially lethal dose could be infused. It would be prudent in this situation to waste the 200 cc of IV fluid in the bag that is hanging and hang a new 1000-cc bag with the additional 20 mEq of KCl added. This IV will have 40 mEq of KCL per 1000 cc, which can be safely given at 125 cc/hour. It would be safest to administer the IV through an infusion pump so sudden infusion of excess IV fluid can be avoided.

Nursing Notes: Apply Your Knowledge

Answer: Ferrous sulfate is an iron preparation that helps restore iron levels possibly depleted from blood loss during surgery. Take 1 tablet with meals to avoid gastric irritation, which can occur if taken on an empty stomach. Warn Mr. Lee that iron will turn his stool black or dark green and is very constipating. Because constipation may be a factor during the postoperative period because of other factors, a stool softener and laxatives may be needed to promote optimal bowel function.

REVIEW AND APPLICATION EXERCISES

1. What are the major roles of minerals and electrolytes in normal body functioning?

2. How would you assess a client for hypokalemia?

3. When a client is given potassium supplements for hypokalemia, how do you monitor for therapeutic and adverse drug effects?

4. Identify client populations at risk for development of hyperkalemia.

5. List interventions to decrease risks for development of hyperkalemia.

6. If severe hyperkalemia develops, how is it treated?

7. What are some causes of iron deficiency anemia?

8. In a client with iron deficiency anemia, what information could you provide about good food sources of iron?

9. What are advantages and disadvantages of iron supplements?

SELECTED REFERENCES

Chessman, K.H. & Anderson, J.D. (1997). Pediatric and geriatric nutrition support. In J.T. DiPiro, R.L. Talbert, G.C. Yee, G.R. Matzke, B.G. Wells, & L.M. Posey (Eds.), *Pharmacotherapy: A pathophysiologic approach*, 3rd ed., pp. 2787–2804. Stamford, CT: Appleton & Lange.

Darby, M.K. & Loughead, J.L. (1996). Neonatal nutritional requirements and formula composition: A review. *Journal of Obstetrics, Gynecology, and Neonatal Nursing, 25*, 209–217.

Drug facts and comparisons. (Updated monthly). St. Louis: Facts and Comparisons.

Food and Drug Administration. (1997). *Warnings required on iron-containing drugs and supplements*. FDA Press Release, January 15, 1997. Washington, D.C.: Author.

Helwick, C. (1999). Anemia is a symptom, not a disease. *Medical Tribune 40*(9), 3.

Hillman, R.S. (1996). Hematopoietic agents: Growth factors, minerals, and vitamins. In J.G. Hardman, L.E. Limbird, P.B. Molinoff, & R.W. Ruddon (Eds.), *Goodman & Gilman's The pharmacological basis of therapeutics*, 9th ed., pp. 1311–1340. New York: McGraw-Hill.

Martinez-Maldonado, M. (1997). Approach to the patient with hypokalemia. In W.N. Kelley (Ed.), *Textbook of internal medicine*, 3rd ed., pp. 959–963. Philadelphia: Lippincott-Raven.

Porth, C.M. (Ed.). (1998). *Pathophysiology: Concepts of altered health states*, 5th ed. Philadelphia: Lippincott Williams & Wilkins.

Schoolwerth, A.C., Feldman, G.M., & Culpepper, R.M. (1997). Approach to the patient with altered magnesium concentration. In W.N. Kelley (Ed.), *Textbook of internal medicine*, 3rd ed., pp. 967–970. Philadelphia: Lippincott-Raven.

Schultz, N.J. & Chitwood, K.K. (1997). Body electrolyte homeostasis. In J.T. DiPiro, R.L. Talbert, G.C. Yee, G.R. Matzke, B.G. Wells, & L.M. Posey (Eds.), *Pharmacotherapy: A pathophysiologic approach*, 3rd ed., pp. 1105–1137. Stamford, CT: Appleton & Lange.

Drugs Used to
Treat Infections

33

General Characteristics of Antimicrobial Drugs

Objectives

After studying this chapter, the student will be able to:

1. Identify populations who are at increased risk for development of infections.

2. Discuss common pathogens and methods of infection control.

3. Assess clients for local and systemic signs of infection.

4. Discuss common and potentially serious adverse effects of antimicrobial drugs.

5. Identify clients at increased risk for adverse drug reactions.

6. Discuss ways to increase benefits and decrease hazards of antimicrobial drug therapy.

7. Discuss ways to minimize emergence of drug-resistant microorganisms.

8. State appropriate nursing implications for a client receiving an antimicrobial drug.

9. Discuss important elements of using antimicrobial drugs in children, older adults, those with renal or hepatic impairment, and those with critical illness.

Antimicrobial drugs are used to prevent or treat infections caused by pathogenic (disease-producing) microorganisms. The human body and the environment contain many microorganisms, most of which live in a state of balance with the human host and do not cause disease. When the balance is upset and infection occurs, characteristics of the infecting microorganism(s) and the adequacy of host defense mechanisms are major factors in the severity of the infection and the person's ability to recover. Conditions that impair defense mechanisms increase the incidence and severity of infections and impede recovery. In addition, use of antimicrobial drugs may lead to serious infections caused by drug-resistant microorganisms. To help prevent infectious diseases and participate effectively in antimicrobial drug therapy, the nurse must be knowledgeable about microorganisms, host responses to microorganisms, and antimicrobial drugs.

MICROORGANISMS AND INFECTIONS

In an infection, microorganisms initially attach to host cell receptors (ie, proteins, carbohydrates, lipids). For example, some bacteria have hair-like structures that attach them to skin and mucous membranes. Most microorganisms preferentially attach themselves to particular body tissues. The microorganisms may then invade tissues, multiply, and produce infection. A major characteristic of microorganisms is their ability to survive in various environments. Bacteria, for example, may form mutant strains, alter their structures and functions, or become embedded in a layer of mucus. These adaptations may protect them from normal body defense mechanisms and antimicrobial drugs. Many bacteria produce drug-resistant strains in the presence of antimicrobial drugs. Classifications, normal microbial flora, and common pathogenic microorganisms are described in the following sections.

Classifications

Bacteria are subclassified according to whether they are aerobic (require oxygen) or anaerobic (cannot live in the presence of oxygen), their reaction to Gram's stain (gram positive or gram negative), and their shape (eg, cocci, bacilli).

Viruses are intracellular parasites that survive only in living tissues. They are officially classified according to their structures, but are more commonly described according to origin and the disorders or symptoms they produce. Human pathogens include adenoviruses, herpesviruses, and retroviruses (see Chap. 39).

Fungi are plant-like organisms that live as parasites on living tissue or as saprophytes on decaying organic matter. Approximately 50 species are pathogenic in humans (see Chap. 40).

Normal Microbial Flora

The human body normally has areas that are sterile and areas that are colonized with microorganisms. Sterile areas are body fluids and cavities, the lower respiratory tract (trachea, bronchi, lungs), much of the gastrointestinal (GI) and genitourinary tracts, and the musculoskeletal system. Colonized areas include the skin, upper respiratory tract, and colon.

Normal skin flora includes staphylococci, streptococci, diphtheroids, and transient environmental organisms. The upper respiratory tract contains staphylococci, streptococci, pneumococci, diphtheroids, and *Hemophilus influenzae*. The external genitalia contain skin organisms; the vagina contains lactobacilli, *Candida*, and *Bacteroides*. The colon contains *Escherichia coli*, *Klebsiella*, *Enterobacter*, *Proteus*, *Pseudomonas*, *Bacteroides*, clostridia, lactobacilli, streptococci, and staphylococci. Microorganisms that are part of the normal flora and nonpathogenic in one area of the body may be pathogenic in other parts of the body; for example, *E. coli* often cause urinary tract infections.

Normal flora protects the human host by occupying space and consuming nutrients. This interferes with the ability of potential pathogens to establish residence and proliferate. If the normal flora is suppressed by antimicrobial drug therapy, potential pathogens may thrive. For example, the yeast, *Candida albicans*, is a normal resident of the vagina and intestinal tract. An antibacterial drug may destroy the normal bacterial flora without affecting the fungal organism. As a result, *C. albicans* can proliferate and cause infection. Much of the normal flora can cause disease under certain conditions, especially in elderly, debilitated, or immunosuppressed people. Normal bowel flora also synthesizes vitamin K and vitamin B complex.

Infectious Diseases

Colonization involves the presence of normal microbial flora or transient environmental organisms that do not harm the host. Infectious disease involves the presence of a pathogen plus clinical signs and symptoms indicative of an infection. Accurate assessment and documentation of symptoms can aid diagnosis of infectious diseases.

Laboratory Identification of Pathogens

Laboratory tests of infected fluids or tissues can identify probable pathogens. *Culture* involves growing a microorganism in the laboratory. With bacteria, identification is based on microscopic appearance, Gram's stain reaction, shape, texture, and color of the colonies, and other characteristics of the organism. Identification of other microorganisms (eg, intracellular pathogens such as chlamydiae and viruses) may require different techniques. *Serology* identifies infectious agents indirectly by measuring the antibody level (titer) in the serum of a diseased host. A tentative diagnosis can be made if the antibody level against a specific pathogen rises during the acute phase of the disease and falls during convalescence. *Detection of antigens* uses features of culture and serology but reduces the time required for diagnosis.

Common Human Pathogens

Common human pathogens are viruses, gram-positive enterococci, streptococci and staphylococci, and gram-negative intestinal organisms (*E. coli, Bacteroides, Klebsiella, Proteus, Pseudomonas* species, and others; Box 33-1). These microorganisms are usually spread by air; direct contact with an infected person; or contaminated hands, food, water, or objects.

"Opportunistic" microorganisms are usually normal endogenous or environmental flora and nonpathogenic. They become pathogens, however, in hosts whose defense mechanisms are impaired. Opportunistic infections are likely to occur in people with severe burns, cancer, indwelling intravenous (IV) or urinary catheters, and antibiotic or corticosteroid drug therapy. Opportunistic bacterial infections, often caused by drug-resistant microorganisms, are usually serious and may be life threatening. Fungi of the *Candida* genus, especially *C. albicans*, may cause life-threatening bloodstream or deep tissue infections, such as

(*text continues on page 498*)

BOX 33–1 COMMON BACTERIAL PATHOGENS

Gram-Positive Bacteria

Staphylococci

Staphylococcus aureus organisms are part of the normal microbial flora of the skin and upper respiratory tract and also are common pathogens. Some people carry (are colonized with) the organism in the anterior nares. The organisms are spread mainly by direct contact with people who are infected or who are carriers. The hands of health care workers are considered a major source of indirect spread and nosocomial infections. The organisms also survive on inanimate surfaces for long periods of time.

S. aureus organisms cause boils, carbuncles, burn and surgical wound infections, and internal abscesses. Burns or surgical wounds often become infected from clients' own nasal carriage or from health care personnel. The organisms cannot penetrate intact skin or mucous membranes. However, they can penetrate damaged tissues and produce endotoxins that destroy erythrocytes, leukocytes, platelets, fibroblasts, and other human cells. Also, many strains produce enterotoxins that cause food poisoning when ingested. The enterotoxins survive heating at temperatures high enough to kill the organisms, so reheating foods does not prevent food poisoning.

High-risk groups for staphylococcal infections include newborns, the elderly, and those who are malnourished, diabetic, or obese. In children, staphylococcal infections of the respiratory tract are most common in those younger than 2 years of age. In adults, staphylococcal pneumonia often occurs in people with chronic lung disease or as a secondary bacterial infection after influenza. The influenza virus destroys the ciliated epithelium of the respiratory tract and thereby aids bacterial invasion.

Staphylococcus epidermidis organisms are also part of the normal microbial flora of the skin and mucosal surfaces and are increasingly common pathogens. Infections with these organisms are associated with the use of treatment devices such as intravascular catheters, prosthetic heart valves, cardiac pacemakers, orthopedic prostheses, cerebrospinal fluid shunts, and peritoneal catheters. *S. epidermidis* infections include endocarditis, bacteremia, and other serious infections and are especially hazardous to neutropenic and immunocompromised clients. Treatment usually requires removal of any infected medical device as well as appropriate antibiotic therapy.

Streptococci

S. viridans (alpha-hemolytic streptococcus) organisms are part of the normal microbial flora of the throat and nasopharynx in many healthy people. Infections are usually spread by inhalation of droplets from the upper respiratory tracts of carriers or people with infections. However, these organisms do not cause disease unless the mucosal barrier is damaged by trauma, previous infection, or surgical manipulation. Such damage allows the organisms to enter the bloodstream and gain access to other parts of the body. For example, the organisms may cause endocarditis if they reach damaged heart valves. Streptococcal endocarditis can usually be treated effectively by approximately 2 weeks of penicillin therapy.

S. pneumoniae organisms, often called pneumococci, are common bacterial pathogens. They cause pneumonia, sinusitis, otitis media, and meningitis. Pneumococcal pneumonia usually develops when the mechanisms that normally expel organisms inhaled into the lower airway (ie, the mucociliary blanket and cough reflex) are impaired by viral infection, smoking, immo-

(continued)

BOX 33–1 **COMMON BACTERIAL PATHOGENS** (*continued*)

bility, or other insults. When *S. pneumoniae* reach the alveoli, they proliferate, cause acute inflammation, and spread rapidly to involve one or more lobes. Alveoli fill with proteinaceous fluid, neutrophils, and bacteria. When the pneumonia resolves, there is usually no residual damage to the pulmonary parenchyma. Elderly adults have high rates of illness and death from pneumococcal pneumonia, which can often be prevented by pneumococcal vaccine. Pneumococcal vaccine (see Chap. 43) contains 23 strains of the pneumococci that cause most of the serious infections.

Pneumococcal sinusitis and otitis media usually follow a viral illness, such as the common cold. The viral infection injures the protective ciliated epithelium and fills the air spaces with nutrient-rich tissue fluid, in which the pneumococci thrive. *S. pneumoniae* cause approximately 35% of cases of bacterial sinusitis. In young children, upper respiratory tract infections may be complicated by acute sinusitis. With otitis media, most children have repeated episodes by 6 years of age and the pneumococcus causes approximately half of these cases. Recurrent otitis media during early childhood may result in reduced hearing acuity. Otitis media rarely occurs in adults.

Pneumococcal meningitis may develop from sinus or middle ear infections or an injury that allows organisms from the nasopharynx to enter the meninges. *S. pneumoniae* are a common cause of bacterial meningitis in adults. Other potential secondary complications include septicemia, endocarditis, pericarditis, and empyema.

Susceptible pneumococcal infections may be treated with penicillin G. For people who are allergic to penicillin, a first-generation cephalosporin or erythromycin may be effective for pneumonia, but pneumococcal meningitis should be treated with chloramphenicol.

S. pyogenes (beta-hemolytic streptococcus) are often part of the normal flora of the skin and oropharynx. The organisms spread from person to person by direct contact with oral or respiratory secretions. They cause severe pharyngitis ("strep throat"), scarlet fever, rheumatic fever, and endocarditis. With streptococcal pharyngitis, people remain infected with the organism for weeks after symptoms resolve and thus serve as a reservoir for infection.

Enterococci

Enterococci are normal flora in the human intestine but are also found in soil, food, water, and animals. Although the genus *Enterococcus* contains approximately 12 species, the main pathogens are *E. faecalis*, *E. faecium*, and *E. durans*. Most enterococcal infections occur in hospitalized patients, especially those in criti-

cal care units. Risk factors for nosocomial infections include serious underlying disease, prior surgery, renal impairment, and the presence of urinary or vascular catheters. These organisms, especially *E. faecalis*, are usually secondary invaders in urinary tract or wound infections. Enterococci may also cause endocarditis. This serious infection occurs most often in people with underlying heart disease, such as an injured valve. When the organisms reach a heart valve, they multiply and release emboli of foreign particles into the bloodstream. Symptoms of endocarditis include fever, heart murmurs, enlarged spleen, and anemia. This infection is diagnosed by isolating enterococci from blood cultures. If not treated promptly and appropriately, often with ampicillin and gentamicin, enterococcal endocarditis may be fatal.

Gram-Negative Bacteria

Bacteroides

Bacteroides are anaerobic bacteria normally found in the digestive, respiratory, and genital tracts. They are the most common bacteria in the colon, where they greatly outnumber *Escherichia coli*. *B. fragilis*, the major human pathogen, causes intra-abdominal and pelvic abscesses (eg, after surgery or trauma that allows fecal contamination of these tissues), brain abscesses (eg, from bacteremia or spread from a middle ear or sinus infection), and bacteremia, which may spread the organisms throughout the body.

Escherichia coli

E. coli inhabit the intestinal tract of humans and animals. They are normally nonpathogenic in the intestinal tract but common pathogens in other parts of the body. They may be beneficial by synthesizing vitamins and by competitively discouraging growth of potential pathogens.

E. coli cause most urinary tract infections. They also cause pneumonia and sepsis in immunocompromised hosts and meningitis and sepsis in newborns. *E. coli* pneumonia often occurs in debilitated patients after colonization of the oropharynx with organisms from their endogenous microbial flora. In healthy people, the normal gram-positive organisms of oral cavities attach to material that coats the surface of oral mucosa and prevents transient *E. coli* from establishing residence. Debilitated or severely ill people produce an enzyme that destroys the material that allows gram-positive flora to adhere to oral mucosa. This allows *E. coli* (and other gram-negative enteric bacteria) to compete successfully with the normal gram-positive flora and colonize the oropharynx. Then, droplets of

(*continued*)

BOX 33–1 COMMON BACTERIAL PATHOGENS (*continued*)

the oral flora are aspirated into the respiratory tract, where impaired protective mechanisms allow survival of the aspirated organisms.

E. coli also cause enteric gram-negative sepsis, which is acquired from the normal enteric bacterial flora. When *E. coli* and other enteric organisms reach the bloodstream of healthy people, host defenses eliminate the organisms. When the organisms reach the bloodstream of people with severe illnesses and conditions such as neutropenia, the host is unable to mount adequate defenses and sepsis occurs. In neonates, *E. coli* are the most common gram-negative organisms causing nosocomial septic shock and meningitis.

In addition, *E. coli* often cause diarrhea and dysentery. One strain, called 0157:H7, causes hemorrhagic colitis, a disease characterized by severe abdominal cramps, copious bloody diarrhea, and hemolytic-uremic syndrome (hemolytic anemia, thrombocytopenia, and acute renal failure). Hemolytic-uremic syndrome occurs most often in children. The main reservoir of this strain is the intestinal tract of animals, especially cattle, and several epidemics have been associated with ingestion of undercooked ground beef. Other sources include contaminated water and milk and person-to-person spread. Because it cannot survive in nature, the presence of *E. coli* in milk or water indicates fecal contamination.

Klebsiella

Klebsiella organisms, which are normal bowel flora, may infect the respiratory tract, urinary tract, bloodstream, burn wounds, and meninges, most often as opportunistic infections in debilitated persons. *K. pneumoniae* are a common cause of pneumonia, especially in people with pulmonary disease, bacteremia, and sepsis.

Proteus

Proteus organisms are normally found in the intestinal tract and in decaying matter. They most often cause urinary tract and wound infections but may infect any tissue, especially in debilitated people. Infection usually occurs with antibiotic therapy, which decreases drug-sensitive bacteria and allows drug-resistant bacteria to proliferate.

Pseudomonas

Pseudomonas organisms are found in water, soil, skin, and intestines. They are found in the stools of some healthy people and possibly 50% of hospital patients. *P. aeruginosa*, the species most often associated with human disease, can cause infections of the respiratory tract, urinary tract, wounds, burns, meninges, eyes, and ears. Because of its resistance to many antibiotics, it can

cause severe infections in people receiving antibiotic therapy for burns, wounds, and cystic fibrosis. *P. aeruginosa* colonizes the respiratory tract of most clients with cystic fibrosis and infects approximately 25% of burn patients. Infection is more likely to occur in hosts who are very young or very old or who have impaired immune systems. Sources of infection include catheterization of the urinary tract, trauma or procedures involving the brain or spinal cord, and contamination of respiratory ventilators.

P. cepacia infections are increasing, especially in patients with burns, cystic fibrosis, debilitation, or immunosuppression. These infections are especially difficult to treat because the organism is resistant to many of the antibiotics used to treat other gram-negative infections.

Serratia

S. marcescens organisms are found in infected people, water, milk, feces, and soil. They cause serious nosocomial infections of the urinary tract, respiratory tract, skin, burn wounds, and bloodstream. They also may cause hospital epidemics and produce drug-resistant strains. High-risk patients include newborns, the debilitated, and the immunosuppressed.

Salmonella

Approximately 1400 species have been identified; several are pathogenic to humans. The organisms cause gastroenteritis, typhoid fever, septicemia, and a severe, sometimes fatal type of food poisoning. The primary reservoir is the intestinal tract of many animals. Humans become infected through ingestion of contaminated water or food. Water becomes polluted by introduction of feces from any animal excreting salmonellae. Infection by food usually results from ingestion of contaminated meat or by hands transferring organisms from an infected source. In the United States, undercooked poultry and eggs are common sources.

Salmonella enterocolitis is a common cause of foodborne outbreaks of gastroenteritis. Diarrhea usually begins several hours after ingesting contaminated food and may continue for several days, along with nausea, vomiting, headache, and abdominal pain.

Shigella

Shigella species cause gastrointestinal problems ranging from mild diarrhea to severe bacillary dysentery. Humans, who seem to be the only natural hosts, become infected after ingestion of contaminated food or water. Effects of shigellosis are attributed to the loss of fluids, electrolytes, and nutrients and to the ulceration that occurs in the colon wall.

brain abscesses. Viral infections may cause fatal pneumonia in people with renal or cardiac disorders and in bone marrow transplant recipients.

Community-Acquired Versus Nosocomial Infections

Infections are often categorized as community acquired or hospital acquired (nosocomial). Because the microbial environments differ, the two types of infections often have different etiologies and require different antimicrobial drugs. As a general rule, community-acquired infections are less severe and easier to treat. Nosocomial infections may be more severe and difficult to manage because they often result from drug-resistant microorganisms and occur in people whose resistance to disease is impaired. Drug-resistant strains of staphylococci, *Pseudomonas*, and *Proteus* are common causes of nosocomial urinary tract and surgical wound infections.

Antibiotic-Resistant Microorganisms

The increasing prevalence of bacteria resistant to the effects of antibiotics, in both community-acquired and nosocomial infections, is a major public health concern. Antibiotic resistance occurs in most human pathogens. Infections caused by drug-resistant organisms often require more toxic and expensive drugs, lead to prolonged illness or hospitalization, and increase mortality rates.

Resistant microorganisms grow and multiply when susceptible organisms (eg, normal flora) are suppressed by antimicrobial drugs or when normal body defenses are impaired by immunosuppressive disorders or drugs. They may emerge during or after antimicrobial drug therapy. Contributing factors include:

1. **Widespread use of antimicrobial drugs, especially broad-spectrum agents**. Antibiotics affect the bacteria for which they are prescribed, transient organisms, other pathogens, and normal flora. When the normal flora is suppressed, space and nutrients become available to support the growth of organisms resistant to the effects of that antibiotic. The resistant organisms soon become the predominant strain. Once established, resistant bacteria can cause superinfection in the original host, spread to other hosts, and even spread their resistance properties for that antibiotic to other species of bacteria. In addition to resistance to the effects of one antibiotic, cross-resistance to similar antibiotics also occurs because most antibiotics are variations of a few basic types.

2. **Interrupted or inadequate antimicrobial treatment of infections**. Clients often stop taking a prescribed antibiotic when symptoms subside or they feel better. In such circumstances, only the most susceptible bacteria are affected and resistant organisms can become established residents.

3. **Type of bacteria**. Both gram-positive and gram-negative bacteria are producing more antibiotic-resistant strains. Gram-positive organisms include staphylococci, streptococci, and enterococci. Gram-negative bacteria associated with high rates of antibiotic resistance include *Pseudomonas aeruginosa* and *Serratia*, *Enterobacter*, and *Acinetobacter* species. These organisms are inherently resistant to penetration of antibiotics and acquire resistance by multiple mechanisms. One mechanism is an outer membrane with openings (porins) that regulate passage of antibiotics. Some gram-negative bacteria (eg, *E. coli*) have more permeable porins than others (eg, *P. aeruginosa*). Thus, *P. aeruginosa* organisms are generally resistant to many antibiotics.

4. **Type of infection**. Infections often associated with high rates of resistance include lower respiratory tract infections and those associated with cystic fibrosis or osteomyelitis. These infections are often difficult to treat because they tend to recur; involve multiple, gram-negative, or resistant organisms; and involve anatomic locations that antibiotics do not penetrate well.

5. **Condition of the host**. Clients who are malnourished, severely ill, immunosuppressed, or receiving mechanical ventilation are at high risk for infections, including those caused by antibiotic-resistant organisms.

6. **Location or setting**. Resistant organisms are especially likely to emerge in critical care units and large teaching hospitals, where seriously ill clients often require extensive antibiotic therapy. The constant presence of antibiotics provides strong pressures for selection and replication of resistant organisms.

Resistant organisms and the antibiotics to which they develop resistance vary in geographic areas, communities, and hospitals according to the use of particular antibiotics. Nationally, resistant bacterial strains of major concern include penicillin resistant *Streptococcus pneumoniae*, methicillin-resistant *Staphylococcus aureus* and *Staphylococcus epidermidis*, vancomycin-resistant enterococcus, and multidrug-resistant tuberculosis (MDR-TB). Actually, all of these organisms are resistant to multiple antibiotics. The first three are described in Box 33-2; MDR-TB is discussed in Chapter 38. Viruses and fungi also develop resistance to antimicrobial drugs, as discussed in Chapters 39 and 40.

Mechanisms of Resistance

Bacteria have developed numerous ways to acquire resistance to antimicrobial drugs, including:

- Production of enzymes that inactivate the drugs. For example, beta-lactamase enzymes change the chemical structure of penicillins and cephalosporins by

BOX 33–2   ANTIBIOTIC-RESISTANT STAPHYLOCOCCI, STREPTOCOCCI, AND ENTEROCOCCI

Methicillin-Resistant *Staphylococcus aureus*

Penicillin-resistant staphylococci developed in the early days of penicillin use because the organisms produced beta-lactamase enzymes (penicillinases) that destroyed penicillin. Methicillin was one of five drugs developed to resist the action of beta-lactamase enzymes and thus be effective in treating staphylococcal infections. Eventually, strains of *S. aureus* became resistant to these drugs as well. The mechanism of resistance in methicillin-resistant *S. aureus* (MRSA) is alteration of penicillin-binding proteins (PBPs). PBPs, the target sites of penicillins and other beta-lactam antibiotics, are enzymes required for synthesis of cell walls in *S. aureus* organisms. Susceptible *S. aureus* have five PBPs called 1, 2, 3, 3a or 3′, and 4. Beta-lactam antibiotics bind to these enzymes and produce defective bacterial cell walls, which kill the organisms. MRSA have an additional PBP called 2a or 2′. Methicillin cannot bind effectively to the PBPs and inhibit bacterial cell wall synthesis except with very high drug concentrations. Consequently, minimum inhibitory concentrations (MICs) of methicillin increased to high levels that were difficult to achieve.

The term MRSA is commonly used but misleading because the organisms are widely resistant to penicillins (including all of the antistaphylococcal penicillins, not just methicillin) and cephalosporins. Many strains of MRSA are also resistant to erythromycin, clindamycin, tetracycline, and the aminoglycosides. In addition, the incidence of methicillin-resistant *Staphylococcus epidermidis* (MRSE) isolates is increasing. MRSE frequently colonize nasal passages of health care workers and are increasing as a cause of nosocomial infections, especially in critical care units.

A major reason for concern about infections caused by MRSA and MRSE is that vancomycin is the drug of choice for treatment. However, vancomycin has been used extensively to treat infections caused by *S. epidermidis* and enterococci, and vancomycin resistance is increasing in those species. Because resistance genes from the other organisms can be transferred to *S. aureus*, vancomycin-resistant MRSA may develop. Vancomycin-resistant enterococci (VRE) are discussed later.

Penicillin-Resistant *Streptococcus pneumoniae* (Pneumococci)

Penicillin has long been the drug of choice for treating pneumococcal infections (eg, community-acquired pneumonia, bacteremia, meningitis, and otitis media in children). However, penicillin-resistant strains and multidrug-resistant strains are being identified with increasing frequency. Risk factors for the development of resistant strains include frequent antibiotic use and prophylactic antibiotics. Once developed, resistant strains spread to other people, especially in children's day care centers and in hospital settings. Children in day care centers are often colonized or infected with antibiotic-resistant *S. pneumoniae*. This is attributed to a high incidence of otitis media, which is often treated with a penicillin or cephalosporin. Resistant strains in adults and elderly clients are often associated with previous use of a penicillin or cephalosporin and hospitalization.

S. pneumoniae are thought to develop resistance to penicillin by decreasing the ability of their PBPs to bind with penicillin (and other beta-lactam antibiotics). In addition, some penicillin-resistant pneumococci are resistant to third-generation (extended-spectrum) cephalosporins. In pneumococcal infections resistant to penicillins and cephalosporins, vancomycin is the drug of choice. To decrease spread of resistant *S. pneumoniae*, the Centers for Disease Control and Prevention (CDC) have proposed:

- Improved surveillance to delineate prevalence by geographic area and assist clinicians in choosing appropriate antimicrobial therapy.
- Rational use of antimicrobials to reduce exposures to drug-resistant pneumococci. For example, prophylactic antibiotic therapy for otitis media may increase colonization and infection of young children with resistant organisms.
- Pneumococcal vaccination for people older than 2 years of age with increased risk of pneumococcal infection, and for all people older than 65 years of age.

Vancomycin-Resistant Enterococci

Enterococci have intrinsic and acquired resistance to many antibacterial drugs. For example, penicillins and cephalosporins inhibit rather than kill the organisms at achievable concentrations, and aminoglycosides are ineffective if used alone. As a result, standard treatment of an enterococcal infection outside of the urinary tract has involved a combination of a penicillin and an aminoglycoside. This combination is often successful because the penicillin damages the bacterial cell wall and allows the aminoglycoside to penetrate the bacterial cell. For penicillin-allergic clients, vancomycin is given with an aminoglycoside.

This treatment is becoming less effective because some strains of enterococci have developed resistance to penicillin, gentamicin, and vancomycin. The incidence of multidrug-resistant enterococci and VRE has

(continued)

increased in recent years. Two major types (Van A and Van B) of VRE have been described, with different patterns of antimicrobial susceptibility. Van B is susceptible to teicoplanin; Van A is resistant to teicoplanin but may be susceptible to minocycline, ciprofloxacin, or the newer agent quinupristin/dalfopristin (Synercid).

A major contributing factor to VRE is increased use of vancomycin to prevent or treat other infections such as staphylococcal (MRSA and MRSE) infections and antibiotic-associated (pseudomembranous) colitis (caused by toxins released by *Clostridium difficile* organisms). Therefore, to decrease the spread of VRE, the CDC recommends limiting the use of vancomycin. Specific recommendations include avoiding or minimizing use in routine surgical prophylaxis, empiric therapy for febrile patients with neutropenia (unless the prevalence of MRSA or MRSE is high), systemic or local prophylaxis for intravascular catheter infection or colonization, selective decontamination of the gastrointestinal tract, eradication of MRSA, primary treatment of antibiotic-associated colitis, and routine prophylaxis for very low birth weight infants or patients on continuous ambulatory peritoneal dialysis. Thorough hand washing and environmental cleaning are also important because VRE can survive for long periods on hands, gloves, stethoscopes, and environmental surfaces. Personnel should remove or change gloves after contact with clients known to be colonized or infected with VRE. Stethoscopes should be used only with an infected patient or cleaned thoroughly between patients if used for both VRE-infected and uninfected patients.

opening the beta-lactam ring and preventing the antibiotic from binding with its target site (enzymes called penicillin-binding proteins) in the bacterial cell wall.

- Genetic mutations that change target enzymes or change the genetic code to produce new enzymes. These changes decrease bacterial susceptibility to an antibiotic, largely by altering binding sites.
- Changing their metabolic pathways to bypass antibiotic activity.
- Changing their cell walls to produce porins that prevent penetration of the drug.
- Acquiring the ability to pump drug molecules out of the cell. Multiple, nonspecific efflux systems become activated to remove foreign chemicals.
- Transferring genetic material (deoxyribonucleic acid or plasmids) between microorganisms. Bacteria have efficient mechanisms for genetic exchange that allow them to spread antibiotic resistance from one bacterial strain to another, including different species or types of bacteria. Thus, when a new antibiotic is used, resistance may rapidly appear and be disseminated to multiple bacteria.

HOST DEFENSE MECHANISMS

Although the numbers and virulence of microorganisms help to determine whether a person acquires an infection, another major factor is the host's ability to defend itself against the would-be invaders.

Major defense mechanisms of the human body are intact skin and mucous membranes, various anti-infective secretions, mechanical movements, phagocytic cells, and the immune and inflammatory processes. The skin pre-

vents penetration of foreign particles, and its secretions and normal bacterial flora inhibit growth of pathogenic microorganisms. Secretions of the GI, respiratory, and genitourinary tracts (eg, gastric acid, mucus) kill, trap, or inhibit growth of microorganisms. Coughing, swallowing, and peristalsis help to remove foreign particles and pathogens trapped in mucus, as does the movement of cilia. Phagocytic cells in various organs and tissues engulf and digest pathogens and cellular debris. The immune system produces lymphocytes and antibodies (see Chap. 42). The inflammatory process (see Chap. 1) is the body's response to injury by microorganisms, foreign particles, chemical agents, or physical irritation of tissues. Inflammation localizes, destroys, dilutes, or removes the injurious agent so tissue healing can occur.

Many factors impair host defense mechanisms and predispose to infection by disease-producing microorganisms:

- Breaks in the skin and mucous membranes related to trauma, inflammation, open lesions, or insertion of prosthetic devices, tubes, and catheters for diagnostic or therapeutic purposes
- Impaired blood supply
- Neutropenia and other blood disorders
- Malnutrition
- Poor personal hygiene
- Suppression of normal bacterial flora by antimicrobial drugs
- Suppression of the immune system and the inflammatory response by immunosuppressive drugs, cytotoxic antineoplastic drugs, and adrenal corticosteroids
- Diabetes mellitus and other chronic diseases
- Advanced age

CHARACTERISTICS OF ANTI-INFECTIVE DRUGS

Terms and Concepts

Several terms are used to describe these drugs. *Anti-infective* and *antimicrobial* include antibacterial, antiviral, and antifungal drugs; *antibacterial* and *antibiotic* usually refer only to drugs used in bacterial infections. Most of the drugs in this section are antibacterials. Antiviral and antifungal drugs are discussed in Chapters 39 and 40, respectively.

Additional terms for antibacterial drugs include *broad spectrum*, for those effective against several groups of microorganisms, and *narrow spectrum*, for those effective against a few groups. The action of an antibacterial drug is usually described as *bactericidal* (kills the microorganism) or *bacteriostatic* (inhibits growth of the microorganism). Whether a drug is bactericidal or bacteriostatic often depends on its concentration at the infection site and the susceptibility of the microorganism to the drug. Successful treatment with bacteriostatic antibiotics depends on the ability of the host's immune system to eliminate the inhibited bacteria and an adequate duration of drug therapy. Stopping an antibiotic prematurely can result in rapid resumption of bacterial growth. Bactericidal drugs are preferred in serious infections, especially in people with impaired immune function.

Mechanisms of Action

Most antibiotics act on a specific target in the bacterial cell (Fig. 33-1). Almost any structure unique to bacteria, such as proteins or nucleic acids, can be a target for antibiotics. Specific mechanisms include the following:

1. Inhibition of bacterial cell wall synthesis or activation of enzymes that disrupt bacterial cell walls (eg, penicillins, cephalosporins, vancomycin)
2. Inhibition of protein synthesis by bacteria or production of abnormal bacterial proteins (eg, aminoglycosides, clindamycin, erythromycin, tetracyclines). These drugs bind irreversibly to bacterial ribosomes, intracellular structures that synthesize proteins. When antimicrobial drugs are bound to the ribosomes, bacteria cannot synthesize the proteins necessary for cell walls and other structures.
3. Disruption of microbial cell membranes (eg, antifungals)
4. Inhibition of organism reproduction by interfering with nucleic acid synthesis (eg, fluoroquinolones, rifampin, anti–acquired immunodeficiency syndrome antivirals)
5. Inhibition of cell metabolism and growth (eg, sulfonamides, trimethoprim)

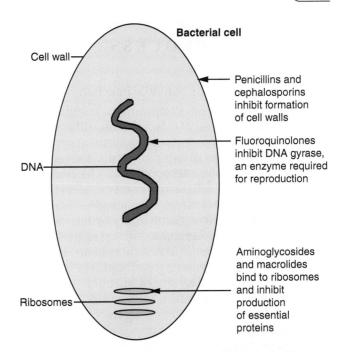

FIGURE 33–1   Actions of major antibacterials on bacterial cells.

Indications for Use

Antimicrobial drugs are used to treat and prevent infections. Because laboratory tests (except Gram's stain and a rapid test for group A streptococci) to identify causative organisms usually take 24 hours or longer, empiric therapy against the most likely pathogens is often begun. Once organisms are identified, more specific therapy is instituted. Prophylactic therapy is recommended to prevent:

1. Group A streptococcal infections and possibly rheumatic fever, rheumatic heart disease, and glomerulonephritis. Penicillin is commonly used.
2. Bacterial endocarditis in clients with cardiac valvular disease who are having dental, surgical or other invasive procedures
3. Tuberculosis. Isoniazid (see Chap. 38) is used.
4. Perioperative infections in high-risk clients (eg, those whose resistance to infection is lowered because of age, poor nutrition, disease, or drugs) and for high-risk surgical procedures (eg, cardiac or GI surgery, certain orthopedic procedures, organ transplants)
5. Sexually transmitted diseases (eg, gonorrhea, syphilis, chlamydial infections) after exposure has occurred
6. Recurrent urinary tract infections in premenopausal, sexually active women. A single dose of trimethoprim-sulfamethoxazole, cinoxacin, or cephalexin, taken after sexual intercourse, is often effective.

NURSING PROCESS

Assessment

Assess for current or potential infection:

- General signs and symptoms of infection are the same as those of inflammation, although the terms are not synonymous. Inflammation is the normal response to any injury; infection requires the presence of a microorganism. The two often occur together. Inflammation may weaken tissue, allowing microorganisms to invade and cause infection. Infection (tissue injury by microorganisms) arouses inflammation. Local signs include redness, heat, edema, and pain; systemic signs include fever and leukocytosis. Specific manifestations depend on the site of infection. Common sites are the respiratory tract, surgical or other wounds, and the genitourinary tract.
- Assess each client for the presence of factors that increase risks of infection (see the section on Host Defense Mechanisms, earlier).
- Assess culture reports for causative organisms.
- Assess susceptibility reports for appropriate antibacterial drug therapy.
- Assess clients for drug allergies. If present, ask about specific signs and symptoms.
- Assess baseline data about renal and hepatic function and other factors that aid monitoring for therapeutic and adverse drug effects.
- Assess for characteristics that increase risks of adverse drug effects.

Nursing Diagnoses

- Fatigue related to infection
- Self Care Deficit related to infection
- Activity Intolerance related to fatigue
- Diarrhea related to antimicrobial therapy
- Altered Nutrition: Less Than Body Requirements related to anorexia, nausea, and vomiting associated with antimicrobial therapy
- Risk for Injury related to infection or adverse drug effects
- Risk for Infection related to emergence of drug-resistant microorganisms
- Knowledge Deficit: Methods of preventing infections
- Knowledge Deficit: Appropriate use of antimicrobial drugs

Planning/Goals

The client will:

- Receive antimicrobial drugs accurately when given by health care providers or caregivers
- Take drugs as prescribed and for the length of time prescribed when self-administered as an outpatient

- Experience decreased fever, white blood cell (WBC) count, and other signs and symptoms of infection
- Be monitored regularly for therapeutic and adverse drug effects
- Receive prompt recognition and treatment of potentially serious adverse effects
- Verbalize and practice measures to prevent future infections
- Be safeguarded against nosocomial infections by health care providers

Interventions

- Use measures to prevent and minimize the spread of infection.
- Wash hands thoroughly and often. This is probably the most effective method of preventing infections.
- Support natural defense mechanisms by promoting general health measures (eg, nutrition, adequate fluid intake, rest, exercise).
- Keep the client's skin clean and dry, especially the hands, underarms, groin, and perineum, because these areas harbor large numbers of microorganisms. Also, take care to prevent trauma to the skin and mucous membrane. Damaged tissues are susceptible to infection.
- Treat all body fluids (eg, blood, aspirates from abdomen or chest) and body substances (eg, sputum, feces, urine, wound drainage) as infectious. Major elements of standard precautions to prevent transmission of hepatitis B, human immunodeficiency virus, and other pathogens include wearing gloves when likely to be exposed to any of these materials and thorough hand washing when the gloves are removed. Rigorous and consistent use of the recommended precautions helps to protect health care providers and clients.
- Implement isolation procedures appropriately.
- To prevent spread of respiratory infections, have clients wash hands after coughing, sneezing, or contact with infected people; cover mouth and nose with tissues when sneezing or coughing and dispose of tissues by placing them in a paper bag and burning it; expectorate sputum (swallowing may cause reinfection); avoid crowds when possible, especially during influenza season (approximately November through February); and recommend annual influenza vaccine to high-risk populations (eg, people with chronic diseases such as diabetes and heart, lung, or renal problems; older adults; and health care personnel who are likely to be exposed). Pneumococcal vaccine (see Chap. 43) is recommended as a single dose for the same populations.

- Assist or instruct clients at risk about pulmonary hygiene measures to prevent accumulation or promote removal of respiratory secretions. These measures include ambulating, turning, coughing and deep-breathing exercises, and incentive spirometry. Retained secretions are good culture media for bacterial growth.
- Use sterile technique when changing any dressing. If a wound is not infected, sterile technique helps prevent infection; if the wound is already infected, sterile technique avoids introducing new bacteria. For all but the smallest of dressings without drainage, remove the dressing with clean gloves, discard it in a moisture-proof bag, and wash hands before putting on sterile gloves to apply the new dressing.
- To minimize spread of staphylococcal infections, infected personnel with skin lesions should not work until lesions are healed; infected clients should be isolated. Personnel with skin lesions probably spread more staphylococci than clients because personnel are more mobile.
- For clients with infections, monitor temperature for increased or decreased fever, and monitor WBC count for decrease.

- For clients receiving antimicrobial therapy, maintain a total fluid intake of approximately 3000 mL/24 hours, if not contraindicated by the client's condition. An adequate intake and avoidance of fluid volume deficit may help to decrease drug toxicity, especially with aminoglycoside antibiotics. On the other hand, a client receiving IV antibiotics, with 50 to 100 mL of fluid per dose, may be at risk for development of fluid volume overload.
- Assist clients with hand washing, maintaining nutrition and fluid balance, getting adequate rest, and handling secretions correctly. These measures help the body to fight the infection, prevent further infection, and enhance the effectiveness of anti-infective drugs.
- Assist clients in using antimicrobial drugs safely and effectively.

Evaluation
- Interview and observe for compliance with instructions for using antimicrobial drugs.
- Observe for adverse drug effects.
- Interview and observe for practices to prevent infection.

CLIENT TEACHING GUIDELINES
Antimicrobial Drugs

General Considerations
- Wash hands often and thoroughly, especially before preparing food or eating and after exposure to any body secretions (eg, urine, feces, sputum, nasal secretions). This is probably the most effective way to prevent infection and to avoid spreading an infection to others.
- A balanced diet and adequate fluid intake, rest, and exercise also help the body to fight infection, prevent further infection, and increase the effectiveness of antimicrobial drugs.
- Take all prescribed doses of an antimicrobial; do not stop when symptoms are relieved. If medication is stopped too soon, symptoms of the current infection may recur and new infections that are caused by antibiotic-resistant organisms and harder to treat may develop.

- If problems occur with taking an antimicrobial drug, report them to a health care provider rather than stopping the drug.
- Do not take antimicrobials left over from a previous illness or prescribed for someone else. Even if infection is present, the likelihood of having the appropriate drug on hand, and in adequate amounts, is extremely small. Thus, taking drugs not prescribed for the particular illness tends to maximize risks and minimize benefits. Also, if the infection is viral, antibacterial drugs are ineffective and should not be used.
- Report any other drugs being taken to the prescribing physician. Drug interactions may occur, and changes in drug therapy may be indicated.
- Report any drug allergies to all health care providers and wear a medical identification emblem that lists allergens.

(continued)

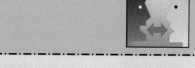
PRINCIPLES OF THERAPY

Treating Infection

The goal of treatment is to eradicate the causative microorganism and return the host to full physiologic functioning. This differs from the goal of most drug therapy, which is to relieve signs and symptoms rather than cure the underlying disorder.

Rational Use of Antimicrobial Drugs

Antimicrobials are among the most frequently used drugs worldwide. Their success in saving lives and decreasing severity and duration of infectious diseases has encouraged their extensive use. Some authorities believe that much antibiotic use involves overuse, misuse, or abuse of the drugs. That is, an antibiotic is not indicated at all or the wrong drug, dose, route, or duration is prescribed. Inappropriate use of antibiotics increases adverse drug effects, infections with drug-resistant microorganisms, and health care costs. In addition, it decreases the number of effective drugs for serious or antibiotic-resistant infections.

Guidelines to promote more appropriate use of the drugs include:

1. Avoid the use of broad-spectrum antibacterial drugs to treat trivial or viral infections; use narrow-spectrum agents when likely to be effective.

2. Give antibacterial drugs only when a significant bacterial infection is diagnosed or strongly suspected or when there is an established indication for prophylaxis. These drugs are ineffective and should not be used to treat viral infections.

3. Minimize antimicrobial drug therapy for fever unless other clinical manifestations or laboratory data indicate infection.

4. Use the drugs along with other interventions to decrease microbial proliferation, such as universal precautions, medical isolation techniques, frequent and thorough hand washing, and preoperative skin and bowel cleansing.

5. Follow recommendations of the Centers for Disease Control and Prevention for prevention and treatment of infections, especially those caused by drug-resistant organisms (eg, gonorrhea, penicillin-resistant streptococcal infections, methicillin-resistant staphylococcal infections, vancomycin-resistant enterococcal infections, and MDR-TB).

6. Consult infectious disease physicians and infection control nurses about local patterns of drug-resistant organisms and treatment of complicated infections.

Collection of Specimens

Collect specimens for culture and Gram's stain before giving the first dose of an antibiotic. For best results, specimens must be collected accurately and taken directly to the laboratory. If analysis is delayed, contaminants may overgrow pathogenic microorganisms.

Drug Selection

Once an infection requiring treatment is diagnosed, numerous factors influence the choice of an antimicrobial drug or combination of drugs.

Initial, empiric therapy. Because most laboratory tests to identify causative organisms require 48 to 72 hours, the physician usually prescribes for immediate administration a drug that is likely to be effective. This empiric therapy is based on an informed estimate of the most likely pathogen, given the client's signs and symptoms and apparent site of infection. A single broad-spectrum antibiotic or a combination of drugs is often chosen.

Culture and susceptibility studies allow the therapist to "match the drug to the bug." Culture identifies the causative organism; susceptibility tests determine which drugs are likely to be effective against the organism. Culture and susceptibility studies are especially important with suspected gram-negative infections because of the high incidence of drug-resistant microorganisms. However, drug-resistant gram-positive organisms are being identified with increasing frequency.

When a specific organism is identified by a laboratory culture, tests can be performed to measure the organism's susceptibility to particular antibiotics. Laboratory reports indicate whether the organism is susceptible (S) or resistant (R) to the tested drugs. One indication of susceptibility is the minimum inhibitory concentration (MIC). The MIC is the lowest concentration of an antibiotic that prevents visible growth of microorganisms. *Susceptible organisms* have low or moderate MICs that can be attained by giving usual doses of an antimicrobial agent. For the drug to be effective, serum and tissue concentrations should usually exceed the MIC of an organism for a period of time. How much and how long drug concentrations need to exceed the MIC depend on the drug class and the bacterial species. With beta-lactam agents (eg, penicillins, cephalosporins), the drug concentration usually needs to be maintained above the MIC of the infecting organism for the duration of antibiotic therapy. With the aminoglycosides (eg, gentamicin, others), the drug concentration does not need to be maintained above the MIC. Aminoglycosides have a postantibiotic effect, defined as a persistent effect of an antimicrobial on bacterial growth after brief exposure of the organisms to a drug. Some studies demonstrate that large doses of aminoglycosides, given once daily, are as effective as more frequent dosing and may cause less nephrotoxicity. *Resistant organisms* have high MICs and may require higher concentrations of drug than can be achieved, even with large doses. In some cases the minimum bactericidal concentration (MBC) is reported, indicating no growth of the organism in the presence of a particular antibiotic. The MBC is especially desirable for infected hosts with impaired immune functions.

Clients' responses to antimicrobial therapy cannot always be correlated with the MIC of an infecting pathogen. Thus, reports of drug susceptibility testing must be applied in the context of the site of infection, the characteristics of the drug, and the clinical status of the client.

Knowledge of antibiotic resistance patterns in the community and agency. Because these patterns change, continuing efforts must be made. *Pseudomonas aeruginosa* organisms are resistant to many antibiotics. Those strains resistant to gentamicin may be susceptible to amikacin, ceftazidime, imipenem, or aztreonam. Some gram-negative organisms have become increasingly resistant to aminoglycosides, third-generation cephalosporins, and aztreonam, but may be susceptible to imipenem.

Knowledge of the organisms most likely to infect particular body tissues. For example, urinary tract infections are often caused by *E. coli*, and a drug effective against this organism is indicated.

A drug's ability to penetrate infected tissues. Several antimicrobials are effective in urinary tract infections because they are excreted in the urine. However, the choice of an effective antimicrobial drug may be limited in infections of the brain, eyes, gallbladder, or prostate gland because many drugs are unable to reach therapeutic concentrations in these tissues.

A drug's toxicity and the risk-to-benefit ratio. In general, less toxic drugs should be used for mild infections and more toxic drugs should be reserved for serious infections.

Drug costs. If an older, less expensive drug meets the criteria for rational drug selection and is likely to be effective in a given infection, it should be used in preference to a more expensive agent. For hospitals and nursing homes, personnel costs in relation to preparation and administration should be considered as well as purchasing costs.

Antibiotic Combination Therapy

Antimicrobial drugs are often used in combination. Indications for combination therapy include:

* Infections caused by multiple microorganisms (eg, abdominal and pelvic infections)
* Nosocomial infections, which may be caused by many different organisms
* Serious infections in which a combination is synergistic (eg, an aminoglycoside and an antipseudomonal penicillin for pseudomonal infections)

- Likely emergence of drug-resistant organisms if a single drug is used (eg, tuberculosis). Although drug combinations to prevent resistance are widely used, the only clearly effective use is for treatment of tuberculosis.
- Fever or other signs of infection in clients whose immune systems are suppressed. Combinations of antibacterial plus antiviral or antifungal drugs may be needed.

Dosage

Dosage (amount and frequency of administration) should be individualized according to characteristics of the causative organism, the chosen drug, and the client's condition (eg, type and severity of infection, ability to use and excrete the chosen drug). For example, dosage may need to be increased for serious infections or reduced if the client has renal impairment or other disorders that delay drug elimination.

Route of Administration

Most antimicrobial drugs are given orally or IV for systemic infections. The route of administration depends on the client's condition (eg, location and severity of the infection, ability to take oral drugs) and the available drug dosage forms. In serious infections, the IV route is preferred for most drugs.

Duration of Therapy

Duration of therapy varies from a single dose to years, depending on the reason for use. For most acute infections, the average duration is approximately 7 to 10 days or until the recipient has been afebrile and asymptomatic for 48 to 72 hours.

Perioperative Use

When used to prevent infections associated with surgery, antimicrobials are usually given within 2 hours before the scheduled operation. This provides effective tissue concentration during the procedure, when contamination occurs. The choice of drug depends on the pathogens most likely to enter the operative area. A first-generation cephalosporin, such as cefazolin (Kefzol), is often used, usually in a single preoperative dose. An antistaphylococcal drug is often given before orthopedic procedures. Repeated doses may be given during surgery for procedures of long duration, procedures involving insertion of prosthetic materials, and contaminated or infected operative sites. Postoperative antimicrobials are indicated with dirty, traumatic wounds or ruptured viscera.

Use in Children

Antimicrobial drugs are commonly used in hospitals and ambulatory settings for respiratory infections, otitis media, and other infections. General principles of pediatric (see Chap. 4) and antimicrobial drug therapy apply. Other guidelines include the following:

1. **Penicillins and cephalosporins** are considered safe for most age groups. However, they are eliminated more slowly in neonates because of immature renal function and must be used cautiously. Carbenicillin, piperacillin, penicillin/beta-lactamase inhibitor combinations (eg, Augmentin), aztreonam, and intramuscular imipenem-cilastatin have not been established as safe and effective in children younger than 12 years of age. Intravenous imipenem and meropenem (Merrem) may be used.
2. **Erythromycin**, oral azithromycin (Zithromax), and clarithromycin (Biaxin) are considered safe. Dirithromycin (Dynabac) has not been established as safe and effective in children younger than 12 years of age.
3. **Aminoglycosides** (eg, gentamicin) may cause nephrotoxicity and ototoxicity in any client population. Neonates are at high risk because of immature renal function.
4. **Tetracyclines** are contraindicated in children younger than 8 years of age because of drug effects on teeth and bone (see Chap. 36).
5. When **clindamycin** (Cleocin) is given to neonates and infants, liver and kidney function should be monitored.
6. **Fluoroquinolones** (eg, ciprofloxacin [Cipro]) are contraindicated for use in children (<18 years of age) because weight-bearing joints have been impaired in young animals given the drugs.
7. **Trimethoprim** (often given in combination with sulfamethoxazole as Bactrim or Septra) has not been proven safe for children younger than 12 years of age.

Use in Older Adults

Antimicrobial drugs are commonly used in all health care settings for infections in older adults as in younger adults. General principles of geriatric (see Chap. 4) and antimicrobial drug therapy apply. Other guidelines include the following:

1. **Penicillins** are usually safe. However, hyperkalemia may occur with large IV doses of penicillin G potassium (1.7 mEq potassium per 1 million units), and hypernatremia may occur with ticarcillin (Ticar), which contains 5.6 mEq sodium per gram. Hyperkalemia and hypernatremia are more likely to occur with impaired renal function, a common condition in older adults.

2. **Cephalosporins** (eg, cefazolin) are considered safe but may cause or aggravate renal impairment, especially when other nephrotoxic drugs are used concurrently. Dosage of most cephalosporins should be reduced in the presence of renal impairment (see Chap. 34).

3. **Macrolides** (eg, erythromycin) are usually safe. Dosage of clarithromycin should be reduced with severe renal impairment.

4. **Aminoglycosides** (eg, gentamicin) are contraindicated in the presence of impaired renal function if less toxic drugs are effective against causative microorganisms. Older adults are at high risk of nephrotoxicity and ototoxicity from these drugs. Interventions to decrease adverse drug effects are described in Chapter 35.

5. **Clindamycin** may cause diarrhea and should be used with caution in the presence of GI disease, especially colitis.

6. **Trimethoprim-sulfamethoxazole** (Bactrim, Septra) may be associated with an increased risk of severe adverse effects in older adults, especially those with impaired liver or kidney function. Severe skin reactions and bone marrow depression are the most frequently reported severe reactions.

7. **Tetracyclines** (except doxycycline) and nitrofurantoin (Macrodantin) are contraindicated in the presence of impaired renal function if less toxic drugs are effective against causative organisms.

Use in Renal Impairment

Antimicrobial drug therapy requires extreme caution in clients with renal impairment. Many drugs are excreted primarily by the kidneys; some are nephrotoxic and may further damage the kidneys. In the presence of renal impairment, they may accumulate and produce toxic effects. Thus, dosage reductions are necessary for some drugs. Methods of calculating dosage are usually based on rates of creatinine clearance (CrCl).

The following formula may be used to estimate CrCl:

Male: Weight in kilograms × (140 − age), divided by 72 × serum creatinine (in milligrams per 100 mL)
Female: 0.85 × above value

Dosage may be reduced by giving smaller individual doses, by increasing the time interval between doses, or both. Anti-infective drugs can be categorized as follows in relation to renal impairment:

1. Drugs that are contraindicated in renal impairment (ie, CrCl <30 mL/minute) unless the infecting organism is sensitive only to a particular drug (eg, tetracyclines except doxycycline).

2. Drugs that are not used in renal impairment unless the infection is caused by organisms resistant to safer drugs. If used, dosage must be carefully adjusted, renal function must be closely monitored, and the client must be closely observed for adverse effects. These drugs include aminoglycosides, cephalexin, amphotericin B, ethambutol, flucytosine, and the fluoroquinolones. Serum drug levels are recommended for monitoring aminoglycoside antibiotics.

3. Drugs that require dosage reduction in severe renal impairment. These include penicillin G, ampicillin, most cephalosporins, and trimethoprim-sulfamethoxazole.

4. Drugs that require little or no dosage adjustment. These include chloramphenicol, clindamycin, dicloxacillin, doxycycline, erythromycin, isoniazid, nafcillin, and rifampin.

An additional factor is important in clients with acute or chronic renal failure who are receiving hemodialysis or peritoneal dialysis: some drugs are removed by dialysis, and an extra dose may be needed during or after dialysis.

Use in Hepatic Impairment

Antimicrobial therapy in clients with liver impairment is not well defined. Some drugs are excreted by the liver (eg, cefaperazone, chloramphenicol, clindamycin, erythromycin), and dosage must be reduced in clients with severe liver impairment. Some are associated with elevations of liver enzymes (eg, aztreonam, imipenem and meropenem, fluoroquinolones). Some are associated with hepatotoxicity (eg, fluoroquinolones, isoniazid, rifampin).

Penicillins and other beta-lactam drugs rarely cause jaundice, hepatitis, or liver failure. However, a large number of acute liver injuries have been reported with the combination of amoxicillin/clavulanate (Augmentin), and some cases of cholestatic jaundice have been reported with ticarcillin/clavulanate (Timentin). Hepatotoxicity is attributed to the clavulanate component. These drugs are contraindicated in clients who have had cholestatic jaundice or hepatic dysfunction associated with their use and must be used with caution in clients with hepatic impairment.

Fluoroquinolones may cause liver enzyme abnormalities and hepatotoxicity (eg, hepatitis, liver impairment or failure). The drugs should be used cautiously in clients with or at risk for development of impaired liver function. In addition, liver function tests should be monitored and the drug should probably be stopped if jaundice or any other symptoms of liver dysfunction develop. If trovafloxacin is used at all, the restrictions established by the Food and Drug Administration (see Chap. 35) should be strictly followed.

Use in Critical Illness

Antimicrobials are frequently given in critical care units. Many clients have multiple organ impairments or chronic diseases with a superimposed acute illness or injury (eg, surgery, trauma, burns). Thus, antimicrobial therapy is often more aggressive, complex, and expensive in critically ill clients than in other clients. In addition, measurement of plasma drug levels is often needed because there is a direct relationship between plasma levels and antimicrobial effectiveness or toxicity. Drug levels are usually measured after four or five doses are given so that steady-state concentrations have been reached.

Clients in critical care units are at high risk for acquiring nosocomial pneumonia because of the severity of their illness, duration of hospitalization, and antimicrobial drug therapy. The strongest predisposing factor is mechanical ventilation, which bypasses airway defenses against movement of microorganisms from the upper to the lower respiratory tract. Organisms often associated with nosocomial pneumonia are *S. aureus* and gram-negative bacilli. Bacterial pneumonia is usually treated with a broad-spectrum antibiotic until culture and susceptibility reports become available. Selection of antibacterial drugs may be difficult because of frequent changes in antibiotic resistance patterns.

Home Care

Infections are among the most common illnesses in all age groups, and they are often treated by antibiotic therapy at home, with medications administered by the client or a family member caregiver. If a home care nurse is involved, responsibilities may include teaching family members how to administer antibiotics (eg, teaching a parent how to store and measure a liquid antibiotic), care

for the person with an infection, and protect other people in the environment from the infection. General infection control practices include frequent and thorough hand washing, use of gloves when indicated, and appropriate handling and disposal of body substances (eg, blood, urine, feces, sputum, vomitus, wound drainage).

Increasingly, IV antibiotics are being given in the home. Any client who needs more than a few days of IV antibiotic therapy may be a candidate for home care. Some infections that require relatively long-term IV antibiotic therapy include endocarditis, osteomyelitis, pyelonephritis, and some surgical wound infections. Numerous people and agencies may be involved in providing this service. First, the client and family need to be able and willing to manage some aspects of therapy and to provide space for necessary supplies. Second, arrangements must be made for procuring equipment, supplies, and medication. In some areas, nurses employed by equipment companies help families prepare and use IV infusion pumps. Medication is usually obtained from a local pharmacy in a unit-dose package ready for administration.

The role of the home care nurse includes teaching the client and caregiver to store and administer the medication, monitor the IV site, monitor the infection, manage problems, and report client responses. Specific responsibilities may vary according to drug administration intermittently or by continuous infusion, whether the client has a peripheral or central IV line, and other factors. The family should be provided with detailed instructions and emergency telephone numbers of the home care nurse, the pharmacy, and the supply company.

(*text continues on page 511*)

NURSING ACTIONS	Antimicrobial Drugs

NURSING ACTIONS	RATIONALE/EXPLANATION
1. **Administer accurately**	
a. Schedule at evenly spaced intervals around the clock.	To maintain therapeutic blood levels
b. Give most oral antimicrobials on an empty stomach, approximately 1 h before or 2 h after meals.	To decrease binding to foods and inactivation by gastric acid.
c. For oral and parenteral solutions from powder forms, follow label instructions for mixing and storing. Check expiration dates.	Several antimicrobial drugs are marketed in powder forms because they are unstable in solution. When mixed, measured amounts of diluent must be added for drug dissolution and the appropriate concentration. Parenteral solutions are usually prepared in the pharmacy. Most solutions require refrigeration to prolong stability. None of the solutions should be used after the expiration date because drug decomposition is likely.

(*continued*)

NURSING ACTIONS	RATIONALE/EXPLANATION
d. Give parenteral antimicrobial solutions alone; do not mix with any other drug in a syringe or intravenous (IV) solution.	To avoid chemical and physical incompatibilities that may cause drug precipitation or inactivation
e. Give intramuscular (IM) antimicrobials deeply into large muscle masses (preferably gluteal muscles), and rotate injection sites.	To decrease tissue irritation
f. For IV administration, use dilute solutions, give direct injections slowly and intermittent infusions over 30 to 60 min. After infusions, flush the IV tubing with at least 10 mL of IV solution. For children, check references about individual drugs to avoid excessive concentrations and excessive fluids.	Most antimicrobials that are given IV can be given by intermittent infusion. Although instructions vary with specific drugs, most reconstituted drugs can be further diluted with 50 to 100 mL of IV fluid (D_5W, NS, D_5-¼% or D_5-½% NaCl). Dilution and slow administration minimize vascular irritation and phlebitis. Flushing ensures that the entire dose is given and prevents contact between drugs in the tubing.
2. Observe for therapeutic effects	
a. With local infections, observe for decreased redness, edema, heat, and pain.	Signs and symptoms of inflammation and infection usually subside within approximately 48 h after antimicrobial therapy is begun. Although systemic manifestations of infection are similar regardless of the cause, local manifestations vary with the type or location of the infection.
b. With systemic infections, observe for decreased fever and white blood cell count, increased appetite, and reports of feeling better.	
c. With wound infections, observe for decreased signs of local inflammation and decreased drainage. Drainage also may change from purulent to serous.	
d. With respiratory infections, observe for decreased dyspnea, coughing, and secretions. Secretions may change from thick and colored to thin and white.	
e. With urinary tract infections, observe for decreased urgency, frequency, and dysuria. If urinalysis is done, check the laboratory report for decreased bacteria and white blood cells.	
f. Absence of signs and symptoms of infection when given prophylactically.	
3. Observe for adverse effects	
a. Hypersensitivity	Reactions are more likely to occur in those with previous hypersensitivity reactions and those with a history of allergy, asthma, or hay fever.
(1) Anaphylaxis—hypotension, respiratory distress, urticaria, angioedema, vomiting, diarrhea	Hypersensitivity may occur with most antimicrobial drugs but is more common with penicillins. Anaphylaxis may occur with oral administration but is more likely with parenteral administration and may occur within 5 to 30 min of injection. Hypotension results from vasodilation and circulatory collapse. Respiratory distress results from bronchospasm or laryngeal edema.
(2) Serum sickness—chills, fever, vasculitis, generalized lymphadenopathy, joint edema and inflammation, bronchospasm, urticaria	This is a delayed allergic reaction, occurring 1 wk or more after the drug is started. Signs and symptoms are caused by inflammation.

(continued)

NURSING ACTIONS	RATIONALE/EXPLANATION
(3) Acute interstitial nephritis (AIN) hematuria, oliguria, proteinuria, pyuria	AIN is considered a hypersensitivity reaction that may occur with many antimicrobials, including penicillins, cephalosporins, aminoglycosides, sulfonamides, tetracyclines, and others. It is usually reversible if the causative agent is promptly stopped.
b. Superinfection	Superinfection is a new or secondary infection that occurs during antimicrobial therapy of a primary infection. Superinfections are common and potentially serious because responsible microorganisms are often drug-resistant staphylococci, gram-negative organisms (eg, *Pseudomonas aeruginosa*) or fungi (eg, *Candida*).
(1) Recurrence of systemic signs and symptoms (eg, fever, malaise)	
(2) New localized signs and symptoms—redness, heat, edema, pain, drainage, cough	
(3) Stomatitis or "thrush"—sore mouth, white patches on oral mucosa, black, furry tongue	From overgrowth of fungi
(4) Pseudomembranous colitis—severe diarrhea characterized by blood, pus, and mucus in stools	May occur with most antibiotics, but is most often associated with ampicillin, the cephalosporins, and clindamycin. These and other antibiotics suppress normal bacterial flora and allow the overgrowth of *Clostridium difficile*. The organism produces a toxin that kills mucosal cells and produces superficial ulcerations that are visible with sigmoidoscopy. Discontinuing the drug and giving metronidazole or oral vancomycin are curative measures. However, relapses may occur.
(5) Monilial vaginitis—rash in perineal area, itching, vaginal discharge	From overgrowth of yeast organisms
c. Phlebitis at IV sites; pain at IM sites	Many antimicrobial parenteral solutions are irritating to body tissues.
d. Nausea and vomiting	These often occur with oral antimicrobials, probably from irritation of gastric mucosa.
e. Diarrhea	Commonly occurs, caused by irritation of gastrointestinal mucosa and changes in intestinal bacterial flora; and may range from mild to severe. Pseudomembranous colitis (see earlier) is one type of severe diarrhea.
f. Nephrotoxicity	
(1) See AIN, earlier	More likely to occur in clients who are elderly or who have impaired renal function.
(2) Acute tubular necrosis (ATN)—increased blood urea nitrogen and serum creatinine, decreased creatinine clearance, fluid and electrolyte imbalances	Aminoglycosides are the antimicrobial agents most often associated with ATN.
g. Neurotoxicity—confusion, hallucinations, neuromuscular irritability, convulsive seizures	More likely with large IV doses of penicillins or cephalosporins, especially in clients with impaired renal function.

(continued)

NURSING ACTIONS	RATIONALE/EXPLANATION
h. Bleeding—hypoprothrombinemia, platelet dysfunction	Most often associated with penicillins and cephalosporins.
4. Observe for drug interactions	See following chapters. The most significant interactions are those that alter effectiveness or increase drug toxicity.

REVIEW AND APPLICATION EXERCISES

1. How does the body defend itself against infection?

2. When assessing a client, what signs and symptoms may indicate an infectious process?

3. Do all infections require antimicrobial drug therapy? Why or why not?

4. With antimicrobial drug therapy, what is meant by the terms *bacteriostatic, bactericidal, antimicrobial spectrum of activity*, and *minimum inhibitory concentration*?

5. Why is it important to identify the organism causing an infection?

6. Why are infections of the brain, eye, and prostate gland more difficult to treat than infections of the GI, respiratory, and urinary tracts?

7. What factors promote the development of drug-resistant microorganisms, and how can they be prevented or minimized?

8. What are common adverse effects associated with antimicrobial drug therapy?

9. When teaching a client about a prescribed antibiotic, a common instruction is to take all the medicine and not to stop prematurely. Why is this information important?

10. When a dose of an antibiotic is prescribed to prevent postoperative infection, should it be given before, during, or after surgery? Why?

11. What special precautions are needed for clients with renal or hepatic impairment or critical illness?

SELECTED REFERENCES

Barriere, S.L. (1997). Selection of antimicrobial regimens. In J.T. DiPiro, R.L. Talbert, P.E. Hayes, G.C. Yee, G.R. Matzke, B.G. Wells, & L.M. Posey (Eds.), *Pharmacotherapy: A pathophysiologic approach*, 3rd ed., pp. 1953–1969. Stamford, CT: Appleton & Lange.

Chambers, H.F. & Sande, M.A. (1996). Antimicrobial agents: General considerations. In J.G. Hardman, L.E. Limbird, P.B. Molinoff, & R.W. Ruddon (Eds.), *Goodman & Gilman's The pharmacological basis of therapeutics*, 9th ed., pp. 1029–1056. New York: McGraw-Hill.

Drug facts and comparisons. (Updated monthly). St. Louis: Facts and Comparisons.

Dudley, M.N. (1997). Use of laboratory tests in infectious diseases. In J.T DiPiro, R.L. Talbert, P.E. Hayes, G.C. Yee, G.R. Matzke, B.G. Wells, & L.M. Posey (Eds.), *Pharmacotherapy: A pathophysiologic approach*, 3rd ed., pp. 1931–1951. Stamford, CT: Appleton & Lange.

Dunne, W. M. (1998). Mechanisms of infectious disease. In C.M. Porth (Ed.), *Pathophysiology: Concepts of altered health states*, 5th ed., pp. 167–187. Philadelphia: Lippincott Williams & Wilkins.

Foxworth, J. (1997). Recognizing and preventing antibiotic-associated complications in the critical care setting. *Critical Care Nursing Quarterly, 20*(3), 1–11.

Goldmann, D.A., Weinstein, R.A., Wenzel, R.P., Tablan, O.C., Duma, R.J., Gaynes, R.P., Schlosser, J., & Martone, W.J. (1996). Strategies to prevent and control the emergence and spread of antimicrobial-resistant microorganisms in hospitals. *Journal of the American Medical Association, 275*, 234–240.

Holman, R.G. & Dellinger, E.P. (1996). Fever, infection, and antibiotics. In J.A. Weigelt and F.R. Lewis, Jr. (Eds.), *Surgical critical care*. Philadelphia: W.B. Saunders.

Jernigan, D.B., Cetron, M.S., & Breiman, R.F. (1996). Minimizing the impact of drug-resistant *Streptococcus pneumoniae* (DRSP). *Journal of the American Medical Association, 275*, 206–209.

Pinner, R.W., Teutsch, S.M., Simonsen, S., Klug, L.A. Graber, J.M., Clarke, M.J., & Berkelman, R.L. (1996). Trends in infectious diseases mortality in the United States. *Journal of the American Medical Association, 275*, 189–193.

Plouffe, J.F., Breiman, R.F., & Facklam, R.R. (1996). Bacteremia with *Streptococcus pneumoniae*: Implications for therapy and prevention. *Journal of the American Medical Association, 275*, 194–198.

Vial, T., Biour, M., Descotes, J., & Trepo, C. (1997). Antibiotic-associated hepatitis: Update from 1990. *Annals of Pharmacotherapy, 31*, 204–220.

Volk, W.A., Gebhardt, B.M., Hammarskjold, M.L., & Kadner, R.J. (1996). *Essentials of medical microbiology*, 5th ed. Philadelphia, Lippincott-Raven.

Zarama, M. & Abraham, P.A. (1997). Drug-induced renal disease. In J.T DiPiro, R.L. Talbert, P.E. Hayes, G.C. Yee, G.R. Matzke, B.G. Wells, & L.M. Posey (Eds.), *Pharmacotherapy: A pathophysiologic approach*, 3rd ed., pp. 1007–1031. Stamford, CT: Appleton & Lange.

34

Beta-Lactam Antibacterials: Penicillins, Cephalosporins, and Others

Objectives

After studying this chapter, the student will be able to:

1. Describe general characteristics of beta-lactam antibiotics.

2. Discuss penicillins in relation to effectiveness, safety, spectrum of antimicrobial activity, mechanism of action, indications for use, administration, observation of client response, and teaching of clients.

3. Differentiate among extended-spectrum penicillins.

4. Question clients about allergies before the initial dose of a penicillin.

5. Describe characteristics of beta-lactamase inhibitor drugs.

6. State the rationale for combining a penicillin and a beta-lactamase inhibitor drug.

7. Discuss similarities and differences between cephalosporins and penicillins.

8. Differentiate cephalosporins in relation to antimicrobial spectrum, indications for use, and adverse effects.

9. Apply principles of using beta-lactam antimicrobials in selected client situations.

Kurt, 5 months of age, is brought to the urgent care center at 4 AM. He has had a cold for 3 days and started to run a high temperature (over 39°C) last evening. His parents are visibly upset and worried. He has been crying continuously for the last 8 hours and appears to be in pain. The physician examines him and tells the parents he has a middle ear infection, for which he prescribes amoxicillin 200 mg q8h for 10 days.

Reflect on:

▶ Factors contributing to the increased incidence of ear infections in this age group.

▶ Why amoxicillin is a good choice for treatment. (Hint: think of the spectrum of coverage.)

▶ Important teaching to limit the potential for antimicrobial resistance.

▶ Factors in the situation that may make learning difficult for the parents, and how you will individualize teaching.

DESCRIPTION

Beta-lactam antibacterials derive their name from the beta-lactam ring that is part of their chemical structure. An intact beta-lactam ring is essential for antibacterial activity. Several gram-positive and gram-negative bacteria produce beta-lactamase enzymes that disrupt the beta-lactam ring and inactivate the drugs. This is a major mechanism by which microorganisms acquire resistance to beta-lactam antibiotics. Penicillinase and cephalosporinase are beta-lactamase enzymes that act on penicillins and cephalosporins, respectively.

Despite the common element of a beta-lactam ring, characteristics of beta-lactam antibiotics differ widely because of variations in their chemical structures. The drugs may differ in antimicrobial spectrum of activity, routes of administration, susceptibility to beta-lactamase enzymes, and adverse effects. Beta-lactam antibiotics include penicillins, cephalosporins, carbapenems, and monobactams, which are described in the following sections. Individual penicillins are listed in Table 34-1, oral cephalosporins are listed in Table 34-2, and parenteral cephalosporins are listed in Table 34-3.

Mechanism of Action

Beta-lactam antibacterial drugs inhibit synthesis of bacterial cell walls by binding to enzymes (penicillin-binding proteins) in bacterial cell membranes. This binding produces a defective cell wall that allows intracellular contents to leak out, destroying the microorganism. In subbactericidal concentrations, the drugs may inhibit growth, decrease viability, and alter the shape and structure of organisms. The latter characteristic may help to explain the development of mutant strains of microorganisms exposed to the drugs. Beta-lactam antibiotics are most effective when bacterial cells are dividing.

PENICILLINS

The penicillins are effective, safe, and widely used antimicrobial agents. The group includes natural extracts from the *Penicillium* mold and several semisynthetic derivatives. When penicillin G, the prototype, was introduced, it was effective against streptococci, staphylococci, gonococci, meningococci, *Treponema pallidum*, and other organisms. It had to be given parenterally because it was destroyed by gastric acid, and injections were very painful. With extensive use, strains of drug-resistant staphylococci appeared. Later penicillins were developed to increase gastric acid stability, beta-lactamase stability, and antimicrobial spectrum of activity, especially against gram-negative microorganisms. Semisynthetic derivatives are formed by adding side chains to the penicillin nucleus.

After absorption, penicillins are widely distributed and achieve therapeutic concentrations in most body fluids, including joint, pleural, and pericardial fluids and bile. Therapeutic levels are not usually obtained in intraocular and cerebrospinal fluids (CSF) unless inflammation is present because normal cell membranes act as barriers to drug penetration. Penicillins are rapidly excreted by the kidneys and produce high drug concentrations in the urine (an exception is nafcillin, which is excreted by the liver).

Indications for Use

Clinical indications for use of penicillins include bacterial infections caused by susceptible microorganisms. They usually are more effective in infections caused by gram-positive bacteria than those caused by gram-negative bacteria. However, their clinical uses vary according to the subgroup or individual drug and microbial patterns of resistance. The drugs are often useful in respiratory, gastrointestinal, and genitourinary infections. However, the incidence of resistance among streptococci, staphylococci, and other microorganisms continues to grow.

Contraindications to Use

Contraindications include hypersensitivity or allergic reactions to any penicillin preparation.

Subgroups and Individual Penicillins

Penicillins G and V

Penicillin G, the prototype, is widely used. Because of its effectiveness and minimal toxicity, it is recommended for treatment of infections caused by susceptible microorganisms. Although many strains of staphylococci and gonococci and some strains of streptococci have acquired resistance to penicillin G, the drug is still effective in many streptococcal infections. Thus, it is often the drug of choice for the treatment of streptococcal pharyngitis; for prevention of rheumatic fever, a complication of streptococcal pharyngitis; and for prevention of bacterial endocarditis in people with diseased heart valves who undergo dental or some surgical procedures.

Several preparations of penicillin G are available for intravenous (IV) and intramuscular (IM) administration (oral forms have been discontinued). They cannot be used interchangeably. Only aqueous preparations can be given IV. Preparations containing benzathine or procaine can be given only IM. Long-acting repository forms have additives that decrease their solubility in tissue fluids and delay their absorption.

Penicillin V is derived from penicillin G and has the same antibacterial spectrum. It is not destroyed by gastric acid and is given only by the oral route. It is well absorbed and produces therapeutic blood levels.

TABLE 34-1   **Penicillins**

Generic/Trade Name	Routes and Dosage Ranges	
	Adults	Children
Penicillins G and V		
Penicillin G potassium (Pfizerpen)	IM 300,000–8 million U daily IV 6–20 million U daily by continuous or intermittent infusion q2–4h. Up to 60 million U daily have been given in certain serious infections.	IM, IV 50,000–250,000 U/kg/d in divided doses q4h
Penicillin G benzathine (Bicillin)	IM 1.2–2.4 million U in a single dose Prophylaxis of rheumatic fever, IM 1.2 million U monthly or 600,000 U every 2 wk Treatment of syphilis, IM 2.4 million U (1.2 million U in each buttock) in a single dose	IM 50,000 U/kg in one dose Prophylaxis of rheumatic fever, IM 1.2 million U monthly or 600,000 U every 1–2 wk
Penicillin G procaine (Wycillin, others)	IM 600,000–1.2 million U daily in one or two doses	IM 25,000–50,000 U/kg/d in divided doses q12h
Penicillin V (V-Cillin K, PenVee K, others)	PO 125–500 mg four to six times daily	Same as adults Infants: PO 15–50 mg/kg/d in three to six divided doses
Penicillinase-Resistant (Antistaphylococcal) Penicillins		
Cloxacillin (Tegopen)	PO 250–500 mg q6h	Weight ≥ 20 kg: Same as adults Weight < 20 kg: PO 50–100 mg/kg/d in four divided doses q6h
Dicloxacillin (Dynapen)	PO, IM 125–250 mg q6h	Weight ≥ 40 kg: Same as adults Weight < 40 kg: 12.5–25 mg/kg/d in four divided doses q6h
Nafcillin (Unipen)	IM 500 mg q4–6h IV 500 mg–2 g in 15–30 mL sodium chloride injection, infused over 5–10 min, q4h; maximal daily dose, 12 g for serious infections	IM, IV 50–100 mg/kg/d in four to six divided doses q4–6h
Oxacillin (Prostaphlin)	PO, IM, IV 500 mg–1 g q4–6h. For direct IV injection, the dose should be well diluted and given over 10–15 min.	Weight > 40 kg: Same as adults Weight ≤ 40 kg: PO, IM, IV 50–100 mg/kg/d in four divided doses q6h
Ampicillins		
Ampicillin (Omnipen, Penbriten, others)	PO, IM, IV 250–500 mg q6h. In severe infections, doses up to 2 g q4h may be given IV.	Weight > 20 kg: Same as adults Weight ≤ 20 kg: PO, IM, IV 50–100 mg/kg/d in divided doses q6h
Amoxicillin (Amoxil, Larotid, others)	PO 250–500 mg q8h	Weight > 20 kg: Same as adults Weight ≤ 20 kg: 20–40 mg/kg/d in divided doses q8h
Bacampicillin (Spectrobid)	PO 400–800 mg q12h	Weight > 25 kg: Same as adults
Extended-Spectrum (Antipseudomonal) Penicillins		
Carbenicillin indanyl sodium (Geocillin)	PO 1–2 tablets (382 mg carbenicillin/tablet) four times daily	PO 30–50 mg/kg/d in divided doses q8h
Ticarcillin (Ticar)	IM, IV 1–3 g q6h. IM injections should not exceed 2 g/injection.	Weight < 40 kg: 100–300 mg/kg/d q6–8h
Mezlocillin (Mezlin)	IM, IV 200–300 mg/kg/d in four to six divided doses. Usual adult dosage, 3 g q4h or 4 g q6h	Age 1 mo–12 y: 300 mg/kg/d in six divided doses, q4h
Piperacillin (Pipracil)	IV, IM 200–300 mg/kg/d in divided doses q4–6h. Usual adult dosage, 3–4 g q4–6h; maximal daily dose, 24 g	Age < 12 y: Dosage not established
Penicillin/Beta-Lactamase Inhibitor Combinations		
Ampicillin/sulbactam (Unasyn)	IM, IV 1.5–3 g q6h	Age > 12 y, same as adults Age < 12 y, dosage not established
Amoxicillin clavulanate (Augmentin)	PO 250–500 mg q8h	Weight < 40 kg: 20–40 mg/kg/d in divided doses q8h
Piperacillin/tazobactam (Zosyn)	IV 3.375 g q6h	Dosage not established
Ticarcillin/clavulanate (Timentin)	IV 3.1 g q4-6h	Weight < 60 kg: 200–300 mg/kg/d in divided doses q4–6h

IM, intramuscular; IV, intravenous; PO, oral.

TABLE 34-2) **Oral Cephalosporins**

Generic/Trade Name	Characteristics	Routes and Dosage Ranges	
		Adults	Children
First Generation			
Cefadroxil (Duricef, Ultracef)	A derivative of cephalexin that has a longer half-life and can be given less often	PO 1–2 g twice daily	30 mg/kg/d in two doses q12h
Cephalexin (Keflex)	First oral cephalosporin; still used extensively	PO 250–500 mg q6h, increased to 4 g q6h if necessary in severe infections	PO 25–50 mg/kg/d in divided doses q6h
Cephradine (Anspor, Velosef)	Essentially the same as cephalexin, except it also can be given parenterally	PO 250–500 mg q6h, up to 4 g daily in severe infections	PO 25–50 mg/kg/d in divided doses q6h. In severe infections, up to 100 mg/kg/d may be given.
Second Generation			
Cefaclor (Ceclor)	More active against *H. influenzae* and *E. coli* than first-generation drugs	PO 250–500 mg q8h	PO 20–40 mg/kg/d in three divided doses q8h
Cefprozil (Cefzil)	Similar to cefaclor	PO 250–500 mg q12–24h	PO 15 mg/kg q12h
Cefuroxime (Ceftin)	1. Can also be given parenterally 2. Available only in tablet form 3. The tablet may be crushed and added to a food (eg, applesauce), but the crushed tablet leaves a strong, bitter, persistent aftertaste.	PO 250 mg q12h; severe infections, 500 mg q12h; urinary tract infection, 125 mg q12h	>12 y, same as adults; <12 y, 125 mg q12h Otitis media, >2 y, 250 mg q12h, <2 y, 125 mg q12h
Loracarbef (Lorabid)	A synthetic drug similar to cefaclor	PO 200–400 mg q12h	PO 15–30 mg/kg/d in divided doses q12h
Third Generation			
Cefdinir (Omnicef)	Indicated for bronchitis, pharyngitis, and otitis media caused by streptococci or *H. influenzae*	PO 300 mg q12h or 600 mg q24h for 10 d	≥13 y: PO Same as adults 6 mo–12 y: PO 7 mg/kg q12h or 14 mg/kg q24h for 10 d
Cefixime (Suprax)	First oral third-generation drug	PO 200 mg q12h or 400 mg q24h	PO 4 mg/kg q12h or 8 mg/kg q24h; give adult dose to children 50 kg of weight or ≥12 y
Cefpodoxime (Vantin)	Similar to cefixime except has some activity against staphylococci (except methicillin-resistant *S. aureus*)	PO 200–400 mg q12h	PO 5 mg/kg q12h Give 10 mg/kg (400 mg or adult dose) to children ≥13 y with skin and soft-tissue infections
Ceftibuten (Cedax)	1. Indicated for bronchitis, otitis media, pharyngitis, or tonsillitis caused by streptococci or *H. Influenzae.* 2. Can be given once daily 3. Available in a capsule for oral use and an oral pediatric suspension that comes in two concentrations (90 mg/5 mL and 180 mg/5 mL).	PO 400 mg daily for 10 d Renal impairment: CrCl 30–49 mL/min, 200 mg q24h CrCl 5–29 mL/min, 100 mg q24h	Oral suspension with 90 mg/mL *10 kg:* 5 mL daily *20 kg:* 10 mL daily *40 kg:* 20 mL daily *Above 45 kg:* Same as adults Oral suspension with 180 mg/ 5 mL *10 kg:* 2.5 mL daily *20 kg:* 5 mL daily *40 kg:* 10 mL daily *Above 45 kg:* Same as adults

CrCl, creatinine clearance; PO, oral.

Penicillinase-Resistant (Antistaphylococcal) Penicillins

Because methicillin is no longer marketed, this group now includes four drugs (**cloxacillin, dicloxacillin, nafcillin,** and **oxacillin**) that are effective in some infections caused by staphylococci resistant to penicillin G. The drugs are formulated to resist the penicillinases that inactivate other penicillins. These drugs are recommended for use in known or suspected staphylococcal infections, except for methicillin-resistant *Staphylococcus aureus* infections. Although called "methicillin-resistant," these staphylococcal microorganisms are also resistant to other

TABLE 34-3   **Parenteral Cephalosporins**

Generic/Trade Name	Characteristics	Routes and Dosage Ranges	
		Adults	Children
First Generation			
Cefazolin (Kefzol, Ancef)	Active against streptococci, staphylococci, *Neisseria*, *Salmonella*, *Shigella*, *Escherichia*, *Klebsiella*, *Listeria*, *Bacillus*, *Hemophilus influenzae*, *Corynebacterium diphtheriae*, *Proteus mirabilis*, and *Bacteroides* (except *B. fragilis*)	IM, IV 250 mg–1 g q6–8h	IM, IV 50–100 mg/kg/d in three to four divided doses
Cephapirin (Cefadyl)	No significant differences from cefazolin	IV, IM 500 mg–1 g q4–6h, up to 12 g daily, IV, in serious infections	IV, IM 40–80 mg/kg/d in four divided doses (q6h)
Cephradine (Anspor, Velosef)	No significant differences from cefazolin except it also can be given orally	IV, IM 500 mg–1 g two to four times daily, depending on severity of infection	IV, IM 75–125 mg/kg/d in divided doses q6h
Second Generation			
Cefmetazole (Zefazone)	Similar to cefoxitin in antibacterial spectrum and clinical use	IV 2 g q6–12h for 5–14 d Surgical prophylaxis, IV 1 or 2 g 30–90 min before surgery, repeated 8 and 16 h later (total of three doses)	
Cefonocid (Monocid)	1. Antimicrobial spectrum similar to other second-generation cephalosporins 2. Has a long half-life and can therefore be given once daily 3. Not approved for use in children	IV, IM 1 g daily (q24h) Surgical prophylaxis, IV, IM 1 g 1 h before procedure	
Cefotetan (Cefotan)	1. Effective against most organisms except *Pseudomonas* 2. Highly resistant to beta-lactamase enzymes	IV, IM 1–2 g q12h for 5–10 d; maximum dose, 3 g q12h in life-threatening infections Perioperative prophylaxis, IV 1–2 g 30–60 min before surgery	
Cefoxitin (Mefoxin)	1. The first cephamycin (derived from a different fungus than cephalosporins) 2. A major clinical use may stem from increased activity against *B. fragilis*, an organism resistant to most other antimicrobial drugs.	IV 1–2 g q4–6h	IV 80–160 mg/kg/d in divided doses q4–6h. Do not exceed 12 g/d.
Cefuroxime (Ceftin, Kefurox, Zinacef)	1. Similar to other second-generation cephalosporins 2. Penetrates cerebrospinal fluid in presence of inflamed meninges	IV, IM, 750 mg–1.5 g q8h Surgical prophylaxis, IV 1.5 g 30–60 min before initial skin incision, then 750 mg IV or IM q8h if procedure is prolonged	>3 mo: IV, IM 50–100 mg/kg/d in divided doses q6–8h Bacterial meningitis, IV 200–240 mg/kg/d in divided doses q6–8h, reduced to 100 mg/kg/d on clinical improvement
Third Generation			
Cefoperazone (Cefobid)	1. Active against gram-negative and gram-positive organisms, including gram-negative organisms resistant to earlier cephalosporins 2. Has increased activity against *Pseudomonas* organisms but cannot be used for single-agent treatment of systemic pseudomonal infections 3. Excreted primarily in bile; half-life prolonged in hepatic failure	IV, IM 2–4 g/d in divided doses q8–12h	Dosage not established

TABLE 34-3 **Parenteral Cephalosporins** (*continued*)

Generic/Trade Name	Characteristics	Routes and Dosage Ranges	
		Adults	Children
Cefotaxime (Claforan)	1. Antibacterial activity against most gram-positive and gram-negative bacteria, including several strains resistant to other antibiotics. It has activity against some strains of *Pseudomonas aeruginosa* resistant to first- and second-generation cephalosporins. 2. Recommended for serious infections caused by susceptible microorganisms	IV, IM 1 g q6–8h; maximum dose, 12 g/24h	Weight >50 kg: same as adults Weight <50 kg and age >1 mo: IV, IM 50–180 mg/kg/d, in divided doses q4–6h Neonates: ≤ 1 wk, IV 50 mg/kg q12h; 1–4 wk, IV 50 mg/kg q8h
Ceftazidime (Fortaz)	1. Active against gram-positive and gram-negative organisms 2. Especially effective against gram-negative organisms, including *P. aeruginosa* and other bacterial strains resistant to aminoglycosides 3. Indicated for serious infections caused by susceptible organisms	IV, IM 1 g q8–12h	1 mo to 12 y: IV 30–50 mg/kg q8h, not to exceed 6 g/d <1 mo: IV 30 mg/kg q12h
Ceftizoxime (Cefizox)	1. Broader gram-negative and anaerobic activity, especially against *B. fragilis* 2. More active against Enterobacteriaceae than cefoperazone 3. Dosage must be reduced with even mild renal insufficiency (CrCl <80 mL/min)	IV, IM 1–2 g q8–12h Gonorrhea, uncomplicated, IM 1 g as a single dose	>6 mo: IV, IM 50 mg/kg q6–8h, increased to a total daily dose of 200 mg/kg if necessary
Ceftriaxone (Rocephin)	First third-generation cephalosporin approved for once-daily dosing	IV, IM 1–2 g once daily (q24h) Surgical prophylaxis, IV, IM 1 g 0.5–2 h before the procedure	IV, IM 50–75 mg/kg/d, not to exceed 2 g daily, in divided doses q12h Meningitis, IV, IM 100 mg/kg/d, not to exceed 4 g daily, in divided doses q12h
Fourth Generation			
Cefepime (Maxipime)	1. Indicated for urinary tract infections caused by *Escherichia coli* or *Klebsiella pneumoniae*; skin and soft tissue infections caused by susceptible streptococci or staphylococci; and pneumonia caused by *Streptococcus pneumoniae* 2. Dosage must be reduced with renal impairment.	IV 0.5–2 g q12h for 10 d IM 0.5–1 g q12h for 7–10 d Renal impairment: CrCl 30–60 mL/min, 0.5–2 g q24h; CrCl 11–29 mL/min, 0.5–1 g q24h; CrCl ≤10 mL/min, 250–500 mg q24h	Dosage not established

CrCl, creatinine clearance; IM, intramuscular; IV, intravenous.

antistaphylococcal penicillins and antibacterial drugs except vancomycin.

Aminopenicillins

Ampicillin is a broad-spectrum, semisynthetic penicillin that is bactericidal for several types of gram-positive and gram-negative bacteria. It has been effective against *Proteus mirabilis, Salmonella, Shigella*, and most strains of *Escherichia coli*, but resistant forms of these organisms are increasing. Ampicillin is not used against gram-positive

cocci because penicillin G or V is more effective and less expensive. It is ineffective against penicillinase-producing staphylococci and gonococci. It is excreted mainly by the kidneys; thus, it is useful in urinary tract infections (UTI). Because some is excreted in bile, it is useful in biliary tract infections not caused by biliary obstruction. It is used in treatment of bronchitis, sinusitis, and otitis media.

Amoxicillin is similar to ampicillin but is better absorbed and produces therapeutic blood levels more rapidly. It also causes less gastrointestinal distress. **Bacam-**

picillin, which is converted to ampicillin in the body, has a long duration of action and can be given twice daily.

Extended-Spectrum (Antipseudomonal) Penicillins

The drugs in this group (**carbenicillin, ticarcillin, mezlocillin**, and **piperacillin**) have a broad spectrum of antimicrobial activity, especially against gram-negative organisms such as *Pseudomonas* and *Proteus* species and *E. coli*. For pseudomonal infections, one of these drugs is usually given concomitantly with an aminoglycoside (see Chap. 35). Carbenicillin is available as an oral formulation for UTI or prostatitis caused by susceptible pathogens. The other drugs are usually given by intermittent IV infusion, although most can be given IM.

Penicillin/Beta-Lactamase Inhibitor Combinations

Beta-lactamase inhibitors are drugs with a beta-lactam structure but little antibacterial activity. They bind irreversibly and inactivate the beta-lactamase enzymes produced by many bacteria (eg, *E. coli, Klebsiella, Enterobacter*, and *Bacteroides* species, and *S. aureus*). When combined with a penicillin, the beta-lactamase inhibitor protects the penicillin from destruction by the enzymes and extends the penicillin's spectrum of antimicrobial activity. Thus, the combination drug may be effective in infections caused by bacteria that are resistant to a beta-lactam antibiotic alone. Clavulanate, sulbactam, and tazobactam are the beta-lactamase inhibitors available in combinations with penicillins.

Unasyn is a combination of ampicillin and sulbactam available in vials with 1 g of ampicillin and 0.5 g of sulbactam or 2 g of ampicillin and 1 g of sulbactam. **Augmentin** contains amoxicillin and clavulanate. It is available in 250- and 500-mg tablets, each of which contains 125 mg of clavulanate. Thus, two 250-mg tablets are not equivalent to one 500-mg tablet. **Timentin** is a combination of ticarcillin and clavulanate available in an IV formulation containing 3 g ticarcillin and 100 mg clavulanate. **Zosyn** is a combination of piperacillin and tazobactam in an IV formulation. Three dosage strengths are available, with 2 g piperacillin and 0.25 g tazobactam, 3 g piperacillin and 0.375 g tazobactam, or 4 g piperacillin and 0.5 g tazobactam.

CEPHALOSPORINS

Cephalosporins are a widely used group of drugs that are derived from a fungus. Although technically cefoxitin and cefotetan (cephamycins derived from a different fungus) and loracarbef (a carbacephem) are not cephalosporins,

they are categorized with the cephalosporins because of their similarities to the group. Cephalosporins are broad-spectrum agents with activity against both gram-positive and gram-negative bacteria. Compared with penicillins, they are in general less active against gram-positive organisms but more active against gram-negative ones.

Once absorbed, cephalosporins are widely distributed into most body fluids and tissues, with maximum concentrations in the liver and kidneys. Many cephalosporins do not reach therapeutic levels in CSF; exceptions are cefuroxime, a second-generation drug, and the third-generation agents. These drugs reach therapeutic levels when meninges are inflamed. Cephalosporins are excreted through the kidneys (except for cefoperazone, which is excreted in bile).

First-Generation Cephalosporins

First-generation cephalosporins have essentially the same spectrum of antimicrobial activity and can be described as a group. They are effective against streptococci, staphylococci (except methicillin-resistant *S. aureus*), *Neisseria, Salmonella, Shigella, Escherichia, Klebsiella*, and *Bacillus* species, *Corynebacterium diphtheriae, Proteus mirabilis*, and *Bacteroides* species (except *Bacteroides fragilis*). They are not effective against *Enterobacter, Pseudomonas*, and *Serratia* species.

Second-Generation Cephalosporins

Second-generation cephalosporins are more active against some gram-negative organisms than older drugs. Thus, they may be effective in infections resistant to other antibiotics, including infections caused by *Hemophilus influenzae, Enterobacter* and *Klebsiella* species, *E. coli*, and some strains of *Proteus*. Because each of these drugs has a different antimicrobial spectrum, susceptibility tests must be performed for each drug rather than for the entire group, as was feasible with first-generation drugs. Cefoxitin (Mefoxin), for example, is active against *B. fragilis*, an anaerobic organism resistant to most drugs.

Third-Generation Cephalosporins

Third-generation cephalosporins further extend the spectrum of activity against gram-negative organisms. In addition to activity against the usual enteric pathogens (eg, *E. coli, Proteus* and *Klebsiella* species), they are also active against several strains resistant to other antibiotics and to first- and second-generation cephalosporins. Thus, they may be useful in infections caused by unusual strains of enteric organisms such as *Citrobacter, Serratia, Providencia*, and *Enterobacter*. Another difference is that third-generation cephalosporins penetrate inflamed meninges to reach therapeutic concentrations in CSF. Thus, they may be useful in meningeal infections caused by common pathogens, including *H. influenzae, Neisseria meningitidis*, and *Streptococcus pneumoniae*. Although some of the drugs are active against *Pseudomonas* organisms, drug-resistant strains emerge when a cephalosporin is used alone for treatment of pseudomonal infection.

Overall, cephalosporins gain gram-negative activity and lose gram-positive activity as they move from the first to the third generation. The second- and third-generation drugs are more active against gram-negative organisms because they are more resistant to the beta-lactamase enzymes (cephalosporinases) produced by some bacteria to inactivate cephalosporins.

Fourth-Generation Cephalosporins

Fourth-generation cephalosporins have a greater spectrum of antimicrobial activity and greater stability against breakdown by beta-lactamase enzymes compared with third-generation drugs. Cefepime is the first fourth-generation cephalosporin to be developed. It is active against both gram-positive and gram-negative organisms. With gram-positive organisms, it is active against streptococci and staphylococci (except for methicillin-resistant staphylococci). With gram-negative organisms, its activity against *Pseudomonas aeruginosa* is similar to that of ceftazidime and its activity against Enterobacteriaceae is greater than that of third-generation cephalosporins. Moreover, cefepime retains activity against strains of Enterobacteriaceae and *P. aeruginosa* that have acquired resistance to third-generation agents.

Indications for Use

Clinical indications include surgical prophylaxis and treatment of infections of the respiratory tract, skin and soft tissues, bones and joints, urinary tract, and bloodstream (septicemia). Cephalosporins are often used as alternative drugs in infections caused by organisms resistant to other drugs (eg, prevention or treatment of gonorrhea in areas with high rates of penicillin-resistant gonococci). They are most important clinically for gram-negative infections. In most infections with streptococci and staphylococci, penicillins are more effective and less expensive. In infections caused by methicillin-resistant *S. aureus*, cephalosporins are not clinically effective even if in vitro testing indicates susceptibility. The fourth-generation drug, cefepime, is indicated for use in severe infections of the lower respiratory and urinary tracts, skin and soft tissue, female reproductive tract, and in febrile neutropenic clients. It should be used as monotherapy for all infections caused by susceptible organisms except *P. aeruginosa*; a combi-

nation of drugs should be used for serious pseudomonal infections.

Contraindications to Use

A major contraindication to the use of cephalosporins is a previous severe anaphylactic reaction to penicillin. Because cephalosporins are chemically similar to penicillins, there is a risk of cross-sensitivity. However, incidence of cross-sensitivity is low, especially in clients who have had delayed reactions (eg, skin rash) to penicillins. Another contraindication is cephalosporin allergy. Immediate allergic reactions with anaphylaxis, bronchospasm, and urticaria occur less often than delayed reactions with skin rash, drug fever, and eosinophilia.

CARBAPENEMS

Carbapenems are broad-spectrum, bactericidal, beta-lactam antimicrobials. Like other beta-lactam drugs, they inhibit synthesis of bacterial cell walls by binding with penicillin-binding proteins. The group consists of two drugs.

Imipenem/cilastatin (Primaxin) is given parenterally and distributed in most body fluids. Imipenem is rapidly broken down by an enzyme (dehydropeptidase) in renal tubules and therefore reaches only low concentrations in urine. Cilastatin was synthesized to inhibit the enzyme and increase urine levels of the antibacterial agent. Recommended doses indicate the amount of imipenem; the solution contains an equivalent amount of cilastatin.

The drug is effective in infections caused by a wide range of bacteria, including penicillinase-producing staphylococci, *E. coli, Proteus* species, *Enterobacter-Klebsiella-Serratia* species, *P. aeruginosa*, and *Enterococcus faecalis*. Its main indication for use is treatment of infections caused by organisms resistant to other drugs. Adverse effects are the same as those occurring with other beta-lactam antibiotics. The solution for IM injection contains lidocaine, a local anesthetic to decrease pain. This solution is contraindicated in people allergic to this type of local anesthetic or who have severe shock or heart block.

How Can You Avoid This Medication Error?

Glen Rilley returns to your busy surgical unit with the following antibiotic order: Cefuroxime 1 g q12h. The antibiotic comes from the pharmacy labeled "ceftizoxime 1 g q12h (0900 & 2100). Infuse 50 cc over 30 minutes." You hook up the antibiotic and set the hour rate for 100 cc/hour.

ROUTE AND DOSAGE RANGES

Adults: IV 250–500 mg q6h; IM 500–750 mg q12h
Children below 40 kg weight: IV 60 mg/kg/d in divided
  doses: Children above 40 kg, use adult dosage

Meropenem (Merrem) is a newer carbapenem. It has a broad spectrum of antibacterial activity and may be used as a single drug for empiric therapy before causative microorganisms are identified. It is reportedly effective against penicillin-susceptible staphylococci and *S. pneumoniae*, most gram-negative aerobes (eg, *E. coli, H. influenzae, Klebsiella pneumoniae, P. aeruginosa*), and some anaerobes, including *B. fragilis*. It is indicated for use in intra-abdominal infections and bacterial meningitis caused by susceptible organisms. Compared with imipenem, meropenem costs more and seems to offer no clinical advantages.

ROUTE AND DOSAGE RANGES

Adults: IV 1 g q8h, as a bolus injection over 3 to 5 min
  or infusion over 15 to 30 min
Children ≥3 mo: IV 20–40 mg/kg q8h. Maximum dose
  2 g q8h.

MONOBACTAM

Aztreonam (Azactam) is active against gram-negative bacteria, including Enterobacteriaceae and *P. aeruginosa*, and many strains that are resistant to multiple antibiotics. Activity against gram-negative bacteria is similar to that of the aminoglycosides, but the drug does not cause kidney damage or hearing loss. Aztreonam is stable in the presence of beta-lactamase enzymes. Because gram-positive and anaerobic bacteria are resistant to aztreonam, the drug's ability to preserve normal gram-positive and anaerobic flora may be an advantage over most other antimicrobial agents.

Indications for use include UTI, lower respiratory tract infections, septicemia, and abdominal and gynecologic infections caused by susceptible organisms. Adverse effects are similar to those for penicillin.

ROUTES AND DOSAGE RANGES

Adults: UTI, IM, IV 0.5–1.0 g q8–12h
  Systemic infections, 1–2 g q6–12h
Children: Dosage not established

NURSING PROCESS

General aspects of the nursing process in antimicrobial drug therapy, as described in Chapter 33, apply to the client receiving penicillins, cephalosporins, aztreonam, imipenem/cilastatin, and meropenem. In this chapter, only those aspects related specifically to these drugs are included.

Assessment

With penicillins, ask clients whether they have ever taken a penicillin and, if so, whether they ever had a skin rash, hives, swelling, or difficulty breathing associated with the drug. With cephalosporins, ask clients if they have ever taken one of the drugs, as far as they know, and whether they ever had a severe reaction to penicillin. Naming a few cephalosporins (eg, Ceclor, Keflex, Rocephin, Suprax) may help the client identify previous usage.

Nursing Diagnoses

- Risk for Injury: Hypersensitivity reactions with penicillins or cephalosporins
- Risk for Injury: Renal impairment with cephalosporins
- Knowledge Deficit: Correct home care administration and usage of oral beta-lactams

Planning/Goals

The client will:

- Take oral beta-lactam antibacterials as directed
- Receive parenteral beta-lactam drugs by appropriate techniques to minimize tissue irritation
- Receive prompt and appropriate treatment if hypersensitivity reactions occur

Interventions

- After giving a penicillin parenterally in an outpatient setting, keep the client in the area for at least 30 minutes. Anaphylactic reactions are more likely to occur with parenteral than oral use and within a few minutes after injection.
- In any client care setting, keep emergency equipment and supplies readily available.
- Monitor client response to beta-lactam drugs.
- Monitor dosages of beta-lactam drugs for clients with impaired renal function.

Evaluation

- Observe for improvement in signs of infection.
- Interview and observe for adverse drug effects.

PRINCIPLES OF THERAPY

Guidelines Related to Hypersensitivity to Penicillins

1. Before giving the initial dose of any penicillin preparation, ask the client if he or she has ever taken penicillin and, if so, whether an allergic reaction occurred. Penicillin is the most common cause of drug-induced anaphylaxis, a life-threatening hyper-

CLIENT TEACHING GUIDELINES
Oral Penicillins

General Considerations

✔ Do not take any penicillin if you have ever had an allergic reaction to penicillin with which you had difficulty breathing, swelling, or skin rash. However, some people call a minor stomach upset an allergic reaction and are not given penicillin when that is the best antibiotic in a given situation.

✔ Complete the full course of drug treatment for greater effectiveness and prevention of secondary infection with drug-resistant bacteria.

✔ Follow instructions carefully about the dose and how often it is taken. Drug effectiveness depends on maintaining adequate blood levels.

✔ Penicillins often need more frequent administration than some other antibiotics, because they are rapidly excreted by the kidneys.

Self- or Caregiver Administration

✔ Take most penicillins on an empty stomach, 1 hour before or 2 hours after a meal. Penicillin V, amoxicillin, Augmentin, and bacampicillin can be taken without regard to meals.

✔ Take each dose with a full glass of water; do not take with orange juice or with other acidic fluids (they may destroy the drug).

✔ Take at even intervals, preferably around the clock.

✔ Shake liquid penicillins well, to mix thoroughly and measure the dose accurately.

✔ Discard liquid penicillin after 1 week if stored at room temperature or after 2 weeks if refrigerated. Liquid forms deteriorate and should not be taken after their expiration dates.

✔ Report skin rash, hives, itching, severe diarrhea, shortness of breath, fever, sore throat, black tongue, or any unusual bleeding. These symptoms may indicate a need to stop the penicillin.

---

sensitivity reaction, and a person known to be hypersensitive should be given another type of antibiotic.

2. In the rare instance in which penicillin is considered essential, a skin test may be helpful in assessing hypersensitivity. Benzylpenicilloyl polylysine (Pre-Pen) or a dilute solution of the penicillin to be administered (10,000 units/mL) may be applied topically to a skin scratch made with a sterile needle. If the scratch test is negative (no urticaria, erythema, or pruritus), the preparation may be injected intradermally. Allergic reactions, including fatal anaphylactic shock, have occurred with skin tests and after negative skin tests. If the scratch test is positive, desensitization can be accomplished by giving gradually increasing doses of penicillin.

Nursing Notes: Apply Your Knowledge

Ellen Driver is admitted to the emergency department with cellulitis in her left leg. Cefotetan (a second-generation cephalosporin) 1 g is given IV over 30 minutes. Before administering this medication, you note that she is allergic to penicillin, sulfa, and fish but she denies any allergies to other antibiotics. Ten minutes after the IV cefotetan starts to infuse, Ms. Driver complains that she feels odd. She appears flushed and her throat feels tight and itchy. Her respiratory rate is slightly elevated at 24 breaths per minute, but you do not see any rash. How should you proceed?

3. Because anaphylactic shock may occur with administration of the penicillins, especially by parenteral routes, emergency drugs and equipment must be readily available. Treatment may require parenteral epinephrine, oxygen, and insertion of an endotracheal or tracheostomy tube if laryngeal edema occurs.

Drug Selection

Choice of a beta-lactam antibacterial depends on the organism causing the infection, severity of the infection, and other factors. With penicillins, penicillin G is the drug of choice in many infections; ampicillin is useful in many gram-negative infections; an antipseudomonal penicillin is indicated in most *Pseudomonas* and *Proteus* infections; and an antistaphylococcal penicillin is indicated in staphylococcal infections. Antistaphylococcal drugs of choice are nafcillin for IV use and dicloxacillin for oral use.

With cephalosporins, *first-generation* drugs are often used for surgical prophylaxis, especially with prosthetic implants, because most postimplant infections are caused by gram-positive organisms such as staphylococci. They may also be used alone for treatment of infections caused by susceptible organisms in body sites where drug penetration and host defenses are adequate. Cefazolin (Kefzol) is a frequently used parenteral agent. It reaches a higher serum concentration, is more protein bound, and has a slower rate of elimination than other first-generation drugs. These factors prolong serum half-life, so cefazolin can be given in smaller doses or less frequently. Cefazolin is also

---

Oral Cephalosporins

General Considerations

✔ Inform your physician if you have ever had a severe allergic reaction to penicillin in which you had difficulty breathing, swelling, or skin rash. A small number of people are allergic to both penicillins and cephalosporins because the drugs are somewhat similar in their chemical structures.

✔ Also inform your physician if you have had a previous allergic reaction to a cephalosporin (eg, Ceclor, Keflex). If not sure whether a new prescription is a cephalosporin, ask the pharmacist before having the prescription filled.

✔ Complete the full course of drug treatment for greater effectiveness and prevention of secondary infection with drug-resistant bacteria.

✔ Follow instructions about dosing frequency; effectiveness depends on maintaining adequate blood levels.

Self- or Caregiver Administration

✔ Take most oral drugs with food or milk to prevent stomach upset.

✔ Take cefpodoxime (Vantin) and cefuroxime (Ceftin, Kefurox, Zinacef) with food to increase absorption

✔ Shake liquid preparations well to mix thoroughly and measure the dose accurately.

✔ Report the occurrence of diarrhea, especially if it is severe or contains blood, pus, or mucus. Cephalosporins can cause antibiotic-associated colitis and the drug may need to be stopped.

✔ Inform the prescribing physician if you are breastfeeding. These drugs enter breast milk.

---

preferred for IM administration because it is less irritating to body tissues.

Second-generation cephalosporins are also often used for surgical prophylaxis, especially for gynecologic and colorectal surgery. They are also used for treatment of intra-abdominal infections such as pelvic inflammatory disease, diverticulitis, penetrating wounds of the abdomen, and other infections caused by organisms inhabiting pelvic and colorectal areas.

Third-generation cephalosporins are recommended for serious infections caused by susceptible organisms that are resistant to first- and second-generation cephalosporins. They are often used in the treatment of infections caused by *E. coli, Proteus, Klebsiella*, and *Serratia* species, and other Enterobacteriaceae, especially when the infections occur in body sites not readily reached by other drugs (eg, CSF, bone) and in clients with immunosuppression. Although effective against many *Pseudomonas* strains, these drugs should not be used alone in treating pseudomonal infections because drug resistance develops.

Fourth-generation drugs are most useful in serious gram-negative infections, especially infections caused by organisms resistant to third-generation drugs. Cefepime has the same indications for use as ceftazidime, a third-generation drug.

Route of Administration and Dosage

Choice of route and dosage depends largely on the seriousness of the infection being treated. For serious infections, beta-lactam antibacterials are usually given IV in large doses. With penicillins, most must be given every 4 to 6 hours to maintain therapeutic blood levels because they are rapidly excreted by the kidneys. The oral route is often used, especially for less serious infections and for long-term prophylaxis of rheumatic fever; the IM route is rarely used in hospitalized clients but may be used in ambulatory settings. With cephalosporins, a few are sufficiently absorbed for oral administration; these are most often used in mild infections and UTI. Although some cephalosporins can be given IM, the injections cause pain and induration. Cefazolin is preferred for IM administration because it is less irritating to tissues.

Use of Penicillins in Specific Situations

Streptococcal Infections

Clinicians need to perform culture and susceptibility studies and know local patterns of streptococcal susceptibility or resistance before prescribing penicillins for streptococcal infections. When used, penicillins should be given for the full prescribed course to prevent complications such as rheumatic fever, endocarditis, and glomerulonephritis.

With Probenecid

Probenecid (Benemid) can be given concurrently with penicillins to increase serum drug levels. Probenecid acts by blocking renal excretion of the penicillins. This action may be useful when high serum levels are needed with oral penicillins or when a single large dose is given IM for prevention or treatment of syphilis.

With an Aminoglycoside

A penicillin is often given concomitantly with an aminoglycoside for serious infections, such as those caused by *P. aeruginosa*. The drugs should not be mixed in a syringe or an IV solution because that inactivates the aminoglycoside.

Perioperative Use of Cephalosporins

Many cephalosporins are used in surgical prophylaxis. The particular drug depends largely on the type of organism likely to be encountered in the operative area. First-generation drugs are often used for procedures associated with gram-positive postoperative infections, such as prosthetic implant surgery. Second-generation cephalosporins are often used for abdominal procedures, especially gynecologic and colorectal surgery, in which enteric gram-negative postoperative infections may occur. Third-generation drugs should not be used for surgical prophylaxis because they are less active against staphylococci than cefazolin, the gram-negative organisms they are most useful against are rarely encountered in elective surgery, widespread usage for prophylaxis promotes emergence of drug-resistant organisms, and they are very expensive.

When used perioperatively, a cephalosporin should be given approximately 30 to 60 minutes before the first skin incision is made so the drug has time to reach therapeutic serum and tissue concentrations. A single dose is usually sufficient. With prosthetic implants and open heart surgery, the drug may be continued for 3 to 5 days.

Use in Children

Penicillins and cephalosporins are widely used to treat infections in children and are generally safe. They should be used cautiously in neonates because immature kidney function slows their elimination. Dosages should be based on age, weight, severity of the infection being treated, and renal function. Although no children's dosage has been established for aztreonam, the drug has been given to children with various infections in doses of 30 mg/kg every 6 to 8 hours and in doses of 50 mg/kg every 4 to 6 hours for infections caused by *P. aeruginosa.*

Use in Older Adults

Beta-lactam antibacterials are relatively safe, although decreased renal function, other disease processes, and concurrent drug therapies increase the risks of adverse effects in older adults. With penicillins, hyperkalemia may occur with large IV doses of penicillin G potassium and hypernatremia may occur with ticarcillin (Ticar). Hypernatremia is less likely with other antipseudomonal penicillins such as mezlocillin and piperacillin. Cephalosporins may aggravate renal impairment, especially when other nephrotoxic drugs are used concurrently. Dosage of most cephalosporins must be reduced in the presence of renal impairment, depending on creatinine clearance.

With aztreonam, dosage is determined by renal status as indicated by creatinine clearance. No guidelines have been established for the use of imipenem/cilastatin or meropenem in older adults.

Use in Renal Impairment

Beta-lactam antimicrobials are excreted mainly by the kidneys and may accumulate in the presence of renal impairment. Dosage of many beta-lactams must be decreased according to creatinine clearance (CrCl) levels. In addition, some of the drugs are nephrotoxic. Non-nephrologist prescribers should consult a nephrologist or drug literature about dosages recommended for various levels of creatinine clearance. Additional considerations are included in the following sections.

Penicillins
- Dosage of penicillin G, bacampicillin, carbenicillin, mezlocillin, piperacillin, piperacillin/tazobactam, and ticarcillin should be reduced.
- Clients on hemodialysis usually need an additional dose after treatment because hemodialysis removes substantial amounts and produces subtherapeutic serum drug levels.
- Carbenicillin, which is used to treat UTIs, does not reach therapeutic levels in urine in clients with severe renal impairment (CrCl <10 mL/minute).
- Nephropathy, such as interstitial nephritis, although infrequent, has occurred with all penicillins. It is most often associated with high doses of parenteral penicillins and is attributed to hypersensitivity reactions. Manifestations include fever, skin rash, eosinophilia, and possibly increased levels of blood urea nitrogen and serum creatinine.
- Electrolyte imbalances, mainly hypernatremia and hyperkalemia, may occur. Hypernatremia is most likely to occur when ticarcillin (5.6 mEq sodium/g) is given to clients with renal impairment or congestive heart failure. Hypokalemic metabolic acidosis may also occur with ticarcillin because potassium loss is enhanced by high sodium intake. Hyperkalemia may occur with large IV doses of penicillin G potassium (1.7 mEq/1 million units).

Cephalosporins
- May be nephrotoxic. Use with caution in clients with severe renal impairment (CrCl <50 mL/minute). Monitor clients' renal status carefully during therapy.
- Reduce dosage because usual doses may produce high and prolonged serum drug levels. In renal failure (CrCl <20 to 30 mL/minute), dosage of all cephalosporins except cefoperazone should be reduced by 50%. Cefoperazone is excreted primarily through the bile and therefore does not accumulate with renal failure.
- Cefotaxime is converted to active metabolites that are normally eliminated by the kidneys. These metabolites accumulate and may cause toxicity in clients with renal impairment.

Aztreonam

- May increase serum drug levels and serum creatinine levels. Thus, after an initial loading dose, reduce dosage by 50% or more in clients with CrCl levels of 30 mL/minute or less. Give at the usual intervals of 6, 8, or 12 hours.
- For serious or life-threatening infections in clients on hemodialysis, give 12.5% of the initial dose after each hemodialysis session, in addition to maintenance doses.

Carbapenems

- Dosage of imipenem should be reduced in most clients with renal impairment and the drug is contraindicated in clients with severe renal impairment (CrCl ≤5 mL/minute) unless hemodialysis is started within 48 hours. For clients already on hemodialysis, the drug may cause seizures and should be used very cautiously, if at all.
- Dosage of meropenem should be reduced with renal impairment (CrCl <50 mL/minute). In addition, meropenem may cause renal failure.

Use in Hepatic Impairment

A few beta-lactam antibiotics may cause or aggravate hepatic impairment. Amoxicillin/clavulanate (Augmentin) should be used with caution in clients with hepatic impairment. It is contraindicated in clients who have had cholestatic jaundice and hepatic dysfunction with previous use of the drug. Cholestatic liver impairment usually subsides when the drug is stopped. Hepatotoxicity is attributed to the clavulanate component and has also occurred with ticarcillin/clavulanate (Timentin).

Cefoperazone is excreted mainly in bile and its serum half-life increases in clients with hepatic impairment or biliary obstruction. Adverse effects include cholestasis, jaundice, and hepatitis. Serum drug levels should be monitored if high doses are given (>4 g).

Aztreonam, imipenem, and meropenem may cause abnormalities in liver function test results (ie, elevated aspartate and alanine aminotransferase and alkaline phosphatase), but hepatitis and jaundice rarely occur.

Use in Critical Illness

Beta-lactam antimicrobials are commonly used in critical care units to treat pneumonia, wound infections, and other infections.

Because clients often have multiorganism or nosocomial infections, the beta-lactam drugs are often given concomitantly with other antimicrobial drugs. Because clients are seriously ill, renal, hepatic, and other organ functions should be monitored and drug dosages should be reduced when indicated.

With penicillins, the extended-spectrum drugs (eg, piperacillin) and penicillin–beta-lactamase inhibitor combinations (eg, Unasyn) are most likely to be used. With cephalosporins, third-generation drugs are commonly used and usually given by intermittent bolus IV infusions every 8 or 12 hours. Currently, possible advantages of continuous infusion are being discussed. Like other beta-lactam antibacterials, blood levels of cephalosporins need to be maintained above the minimum inhibitory concentration for microorganisms causing the infection being treated. Thus, continuous infusions may be of benefit with serious infections, especially those caused by relatively resistant organisms such as *Pseudomonas*.

 Home Care

Many beta-lactam antibiotics are given in the home setting. With oral agents, the role of the home care nurse is mainly to teach accurate administration and observation for therapeutic and adverse effects. With liquid suspensions for children, shaking to resuspend medication and measuring with a measuring spoon or calibrated device are required for safe dosing. Household spoons should *not* be used because they vary widely in capacity. General guidelines for IV therapy are discussed in Chapter 33; specific guidelines depend on the drug being given.

(*text continues on page 527*)

NURSING ACTIONS	**Beta-Lactam Antibacterials**

NURSING ACTIONS	RATIONALE/EXPLANATION

1. **Administer accurately**
  a. With penicillins:
    (1) Give most oral penicillins on an empty stomach, approximately 1 h before or 2 h after a meal. Penicillin V, amoxicillin, amoxicillin/clavulanate, and bacampicillin may be given without regard to meals.
	To decrease binding to foods and inactivation by gastric acid. The latter four drugs are not significantly affected by food.

(*continued*)

NURSING ACTIONS	RATIONALE/EXPLANATION
(2) Give oral drugs with a full glass of water, preferably; do not give with orange juice or other acidic fluids.	To promote absorption and decrease inactivation, which may occur in an acidic environment
(3) Give intramuscular (IM) penicillins deeply into a large muscle mass.	To decrease tissue irritation
(4) For intravenous (IV) administration, usually dilute reconstituted penicillins in 50 to 100 mL of 5% dextrose or 0.9% sodium chloride injection and infuse over 30 to 60 min.	To minimize vascular irritation and phlebitis
(5) Give reconstituted ampicillin IV or IM within 1 h.	The drug is stable in solution for a limited time, after which effectiveness is lost.
b. With cephalosporins:	
(1) Give most oral drugs with food or milk.	To decrease nausea and vomiting. Food delays absorption but does not affect the amount of drug absorbed. An exception is the pediatric suspension of ceftibuten, which must be given at least 2 h before or 1 h after a meal.
(2) Give IM drugs deeply into a large muscle mass.	The drugs are irritating to tissues and cause pain, induration, and possibly sterile abscess. The IM route is rarely used.
(3) For IV administration, usually dilute reconstituted drugs in 50 to 100 mL of 5% dextrose or 0.9% sodium chloride injection and infuse over 30 min.	These drugs are irritating to veins and cause thrombophlebitis. This can be minimized by using small IV catheters, large veins, adequate dilution, slow infusion rates, and changing venipuncture sites. Thrombophlebitis is more likely to occur with doses of more than 6 g/d for longer than 3 d.
c. With aztreonam:	
(1) For IM administration, add 3 mL diluent per gram of drug, and inject into a large muscle mass.	
(2) For IV injection, add 6 to 10 mL sterile water, and inject into vein or IV tubing over 3 to 5 min.	
(3) For IV infusion, mix in at least 50 mL of 0.9% NaCl or 5% dextrose injection per gram of drug and give over 20 to 60 min.	
d. With imipenem/cilastatin: IV: Mix reconstituted solution in 100 mL of 0.9% NaCl or 5% dextrose injection. Give 250- to 500-mg doses over 20 to 30 min; give 1-g doses over 40 to 60 min. IM: Inject deeply into a large muscle mass with a 21-gauge, 2-inch needle	
2. Observe for therapeutic effects	See Chapter 33.
a. Decreased signs of local and systemic infection	
b. Decreased signs and symptoms of the infection for which the drug is given	
c. Absence of signs and symptoms of infection when given prophylactically	

(continued)

NURSING ACTIONS	RATIONALE/EXPLANATION
3. Observe for adverse effects	
a. Hypersensitivity—anaphylaxis, serum sickness, skin rash, urticaria	See Nursing Actions in Chapter 33 for signs and symptoms. Reactions are more likely to occur in those with previous hypersensitivity reactions and those with a history of allergy, asthma, or hay fever. Anaphylaxis is more likely with parenteral administration and may occur within 5 to 30 min of injection.
b. Phlebitis at IV sites and pain at IM sites	Parenteral solutions are irritating to body tissue.
c. Superinfection	See Chapter 33 for signs and symptoms.
d. Nausea and vomiting	May occur with all beta-lactam drugs, especially with high oral doses
e. Diarrhea, colitis, pseudomembranous colitis	Diarrhea commonly occurs with beta-lactam drugs and may range from mild to severe. The most severe form is pseudomembranous colitis, which is more often associated with ampicillin and the cephalosporins than other beta-lactams.
f. Nephrotoxicity	
(1) Acute interstitial nephritis (AIN)—hematuria, oliguria, proteinuria, pyuria	AIN may occur with any of the beta-lactams, especially with high parenteral doses of penicillins.
(2) Increased blood urea nitrogen and serum creatinine; casts in urine	More likely with cephalosporins, especially in clients who are elderly or have impaired renal function, unless dosage is reduced
g. Neurotoxicity—confusion, hallucinations, neuromuscular irritability, convulsive seizures	More likely with large IV doses of penicillins or cephalosporins, especially in clients with impaired renal function
h. Bleeding—hypoprothrombinemia, platelet dysfunction	Ticarcillin may cause decreased platelet aggregation. Cefoperazone, cefotetan, and ceftriaxone may cause hypoprothrombinemia (by killing intestinal bacteria that normally produce vitamin K or a chemical structure that prevents activation of prothrombin) or platelet dysfunction. Hypoprothrombinemia can be treated by giving vitamin K. Vitamin K does not restore normal platelet function or normal bacterial flora in the intestines.
4. Observe for drug interactions	
a. Drugs that *increase* effects of penicillins:	
(1) Gentamicin and other aminoglycosides	Synergistic activity against *Pseudomonas* organisms when given concomitantly with extended-spectrum (antipseudomonal) penicillins
	Synergistic activity against enterococci that cause subacute bacterial endocarditis, brain abscess, meningitis, or urinary tract infection
	Synergistic activity against *S. aureus* when used with nafcillin
(2) Probenecid (Benemid)	Decreases renal excretion of penicillins, thus elevates and prolongs penicillin blood levels
b. Drugs that *decrease* effects of penicillins:	
(1) Acidifying agents (ammonium chloride, ascorbic acid, cranberry juice, methenamine, methionine, orange juice)	Most oral penicillins are destroyed by acids, including gastric acid. Amoxicillin and penicillin V are acid stable.

(continued)

NURSING ACTIONS	RATIONALE/EXPLANATION
(2) Erythromycin	Erythromycin inhibits the bactericidal activity of penicillins against most organisms but potentiates activity against resistant strains of *S. aureus*.
(3) Tetracyclines	These bacteriostatic antibiotics slow multiplication of bacteria and thereby inhibit the penicillins, which act against rapidly multiplying bacteria.
c. Drugs that *increase* effects of cephalosporins:	
(1) Loop diuretics (furosemide, ethacrynic acid)	Increased renal toxicity
(2) Gentamicin and other aminoglycoside antibiotics	Additive renal toxicity especially in older clients, those with renal impairment, those receiving high dosages, and those receiving probenecid
(3) Probenecid	Increases blood levels by decreasing renal excretion of the cephalosporins. This may be a desirable interaction to increase blood levels and therapeutic effectiveness or allow smaller doses.
d. Drugs that *decrease* effects of cephalosporins:	
(1) Tetracyclines	Tetracyclines are bacteriostatic and slow the rate of bacterial reproduction. Cephalosporins are bactericidal and are most effective against rapidly multiplying bacteria. Thus, tetracyclines should not be given concurrently with cephalosporins.
e. Drugs that *increase* or *decrease* effects of aztreonam and imipenem/cilastatin	Although few interactions have been reported with these drugs, potential interactions are those that occur with other beta-lactam antibiotics.

How Can You Avoid This Medication Error?

Answer: You have just administered the wrong medication to this patient. Although the names are similar (many cephalosporin names sound and look alike), these are two different drugs. Cefuroxime is a second-generation cephalosporin and ceftizoxime is a third-generation cephalosporin, meaning their bacterial coverage and pharmacokinetics are different. When the dispensed medication is not identical to the prescribed medication, check with the pharmacist to see if the substitution is appropriate or if it is a mistake.

Nursing Notes: Apply Your Knowledge

Answer: Ms. Driver may be experiencing anaphylaxis. Although she did not state an allergy to cephalosporin antibiotics, 5% to 10% of people allergic to penicillin may have a cross-sensitivity to cephalosporins because structurally all beta-lactams are similar. Stop the infusing cefotetan but keep the IV line open because you may need to give emergency drugs IV if her condition worsens. Take her vital signs, administer oxygen, and have someone stay with her while you contact the physician. Make sure that you have epinephrine on hand.

 REVIEW AND APPLICATION EXERCISES

1. How do beta-lactam drugs act against bacteria?
2. What adverse effects are associated with beta-lactam drugs, and how may they be prevented or minimized?
3. What are beta-lactamase enzymes, and what do they do to beta-lactam antibacterial drugs?
4. How are penicillins and other beta-lactam drugs excreted?
5. What are the main differences between penicillin G or V and antistaphylococcal and antipseudomonal penicillins?
6. What is the reason for combining clavulanate, sulbactam, or tazobactam with a penicillin?
7. When giving injections of penicillin in an outpatient setting, it is recommended to keep clients in the area and observe them for at least 30 minutes. Why?
8. When probenecid is given concurrently with a penicillin, what is its purpose?
9. What are the signs and symptoms of anaphylaxis?z
10. For clients with renal impairment, which drugs in this chapter require reduced dosages?

11. Which drugs from this chapter may cause pseudo-membranous (antibiotic-associated) colitis?

12. What are the signs, symptoms, and treatment of pseudomembranous colitis?

SELECTED REFERENCES

Drug facts and comparisons. (Updated monthly). St. Louis: Facts and Comparisons.

Dunne, W.M., Jr. (1998). Mechanisms of infectious disease. In C.M. Porth (Ed.), *Pathophysiology: Concepts of altered health states*, 5th ed., pp. 167–187. Philadelphia: Lippincott Williams & Wilkins.

Limauro, D.L., Chan-Tompkins, N.H., Carter, R.W., Brodmerkel, G.J., Jr., & Agrawal, R.M. (1999). Amoxicillin/clavulanate associated hepatic failure with progression to Stevens-Johnson syndrome. *Annals of Pharmacotherapy, 33*, 560–564.

Mandell, G.L. & Petri, W.A., Jr. (1996). Antimicrobial agents: Penicillins, cephalosporins, and other beta-lactam antibiotics. In J.G. Hardman, L.E. Limbird, P.B. Molinoff, & R.W. Ruddon (Eds.), *Goodman & Gilman's The pharmacological basis of therapeutics*, 9th ed., pp. 1073–1101. New York: McGraw-Hill.

Sheff, B. (1999). Minimizing the threat of *C. difficile*. *Nursing, 29*(2), 33–38.

35

Aminoglycosides and Fluoroquinolones

Objectives

After studying this chapter, the student will be able to:

1. Describe characteristics of aminoglycosides in relation to effectiveness, safety, spectrum of antimicrobial activity, indications for use, administration, and observation of client responses.

2. Discuss factors influencing selection and dosage of aminoglycosides.

3. State the rationale for the increasing use of single daily doses.

4. Discuss the importance of serum drug levels during aminoglycoside therapy.

5. Describe measures to decrease nephrotoxicity and ototoxicity with aminoglycosides.

6. Describe characteristics, uses, adverse effects, and nursing process implications of fluoroquinolones.

7. Discuss principles of using aminoglycosides in renal impairment and critical illness.

8. Discuss principles of using fluoroquinolones in renal and hepatic impairment.

George Masury, accompanied by his wife Jennie, visits his primary care provider complaining of upper respiratory symptoms. George and Jennie have been married for 52 years and Jennie has always cared for George when he was sick and helped make decisions for him. George is hard of hearing, has some "forgetfulness," and does not talk very much. His physician prescribes ciprofloxacin (Cipro) 250 mg bid for 10 days.

Reflect on:

- ▶ How you will include George and Jennie in the teaching session.
- ▶ Essential information to teach about Cipro.
- ▶ Teaching strategies to individualize for hearing deficits and memory deficits.
- ▶ How you will evaluate George and Jennie's learning and their ability to comply with the newly prescribed medication.

The aminoglycosides have been widely used to treat serious gram-negative infections for many years. The quinolones are older drugs originally used only for treatment of urinary tract infections (see Chap. 36). The fluoroquinolones are synthesized by adding a fluorine molecule to the quinolone structure. This addition increases drug activity against gram-negative microorganisms, broadens the antimicrobial spectrum to include several other microorganisms, and allows use of the drugs in treating some systemic infections. General characteristics, mechanisms of action, indications for and contraindications to use, nursing process implications, and principles of therapy for these drugs are described in this chapter. Individual drugs, with routes of administration and dosage ranges, are listed in Tables 35-1 and 35-2.

AMINOGLYCOSIDES

Aminoglycosides are bactericidal agents with similar pharmacologic, antimicrobial, and toxicologic characteristics. They are used to treat infections caused by gram-negative microorganisms such as *Pseudomonas* and *Proteus* species, *Escherichia coli*, and *Klebsiella*, *Enterobacter*, and *Serratia* species.

These drugs are poorly absorbed from the gastrointestinal (GI) tract. Thus, when given orally, they exert local effects in the GI tract. They are well absorbed from intramuscular injection sites and reach peak effects in 30 to 90 minutes if circulatory status is good. After intravenous (IV) administration, peak effects occur within 30 to 60 minutes. Plasma half-life is 2 to 4 hours with normal renal function.

After parenteral administration, aminoglycosides are widely distributed in extracellular fluid and reach therapeutic levels in blood, urine, bone, inflamed joints, and pleural and ascitic fluids. They accumulate in high concentrations in the kidney and inner ear. They are poorly distributed to the central nervous system, intraocular fluids, and respiratory tract secretions.

Injected drugs are not metabolized; they are excreted unchanged in the urine, primarily by glomerular filtration. Oral drugs are excreted in feces.

Mechanism of Action

Aminoglycosides penetrate the cell walls of susceptible bacteria and bind irreversibly to 30S ribosomes, intracellular structures that synthesize proteins. As a result, the bacteria cannot synthesize the proteins necessary for their function and replication.

Indications for Use

The major clinical use of parenteral aminoglycosides is to treat serious systemic infections caused by susceptible aerobic gram-negative organisms. Many hospital-acquired infections are caused by gram-negative organisms. These infections have become more common with control of other types of infections, widespread use of antimicrobial drugs, and diseases (eg, acquired immunodeficiency syndrome [AIDS]) or treatments (eg, radical surgery and therapy with antineoplastic or immunosuppressive drugs) that lower host resistance. The infections occur in the respiratory and genitourinary tracts, skin, wounds, bowel, and bloodstream. Any infection with gram-negative organisms may be serious and potentially life threatening. Management is difficult because the organisms are in general less susceptible to antibacterial drugs, and drug-resistant strains develop rapidly. The few drugs that are effective against them are relatively toxic. In pseudomonal infections, an aminoglycoside is often given concurrently with an antipseudomonal penicillin (eg, piperacillin) for synergistic therapeutic effects. The penicillin-induced breakdown of the bacterial cell wall makes it easier for the aminoglycoside to reach its site of action inside the bacterial cell. However, the drugs are chemically and physically incompatible. Therefore, they should not be mixed in a syringe or an IV fluid because the aminoglycoside will be deactivated.

A second clinical use is for treatment of tuberculosis. Streptomycin was often used before the development of isoniazid and rifampin. Now, it may be used for treatment of tuberculosis resistant to other antitubercular drugs. Multidrug-resistant strains of the tuberculosis organism, including strains resistant to both isoniazid and rifampin, are being identified with increasing frequency. This development is leading some authorities to recommend an aminoglycoside as part of a four- to six-drug regimen.

A third clinical use is oral administration to suppress intestinal bacteria. Neomycin and kanamycin may be given before bowel surgery and to treat hepatic coma. In hepatic coma, intestinal bacteria produce ammonia, which enters the bloodstream and causes encephalopathy. Drug therapy to suppress intestinal bacteria decreases ammonia production. Paromomycin is used mainly in the treatment of intestinal amebiasis.

A few aminoglycosides are administered topically to the eye or to the skin. These are discussed in Chapters 65 and 66, respectively.

Contraindications to Use

Aminoglycosides are contraindicated in infections for which less toxic drugs are effective. The drugs are nephrotoxic and ototoxic and must be used very cautiously in the presence of renal impairment. Dosages are adjusted according to serum drug levels and creatinine clearance. The drugs must also be used cautiously in clients with myasthenia gravis and other neuromuscular disorders because muscle weakness may be increased.

(text continues on page 533)

TABLE 35-1 **Aminoglycosides**

Generic/Trade Name	Characteristics	Routes and Dosage Ranges	
		Adults	**Children**
Amikacin (Amikin)	Has a broader spectrum of antibacterial activity than other aminoglycosides because it resists degradation by most enzymes that inactivate gentamicin and tobramycin Major clinical use is in infections caused by organisms resistant to other aminoglycosides (eg, *Pseudomonas, Proteus, Escherichia coli, Klebsiella, Enterobacter, Serratia*), whether community or hospital acquired	IM, IV 15 mg/kg q24h, 7.5 mg/kg q12h, or 5 mg/kg q8h	*Older children:* Same as adults *Neonates:* IM, IV 10 mg/kg initially, then 7.5 mg/kg q12h
Gentamicin (Garamycin)	Effective against several gram-negative organisms, although some strains have become resistant Acts synergistically with antipseudomona penicillins against *Pseudomonas aeruginosa.* The combination also inhibits the emergence of resistant bacteria that may occur when either drug is used alone.	IV, IM 3–5 mg/kg q24h, 1.5–2.5 mg/kg q12h, or 1–1.7 mg/kg q8h	*Children:* IV, IM 6–7.5 mg/kg/d in three divided doses, q8h *Infants and neonates:* IV, IM 7.5 mg/kg/d in three divided doses, q8h *Premature infants and neonates <1 wk:* IV, IM 5 mg/kg/d in two divided doses, q12h
Kanamycin (Kantrex)	Occasionally used to decrease bowel organisms before surgery, treat hepatic coma, or to treat multidrug-resistant tuberculosis	IV, IM 15 mg/kg/d, in two or three divided doses Suppression of intestinal bacteria PO 1 g every hour for four doses, then 1 g q6h for 36 to 72 h Hepatic coma PO 8–12 g daily in divided doses	IV, IM same as adults
Neomycin	Given orally or topically only because too toxic for systemic use Although poorly absorbed from GI tract, toxic levels may accumulate in presence of renal failure. Used topically, often in combination with other drugs, to treat infections of the eye, ear, and skin (burns, wounds, ulcers, dermatoses) When used for wound or bladder irrigations, systemic absorption may occur if the area is large or if drug concentration exceeds 0.1%.	Suppression of intestinal bacteria (with erythromycin 1 g) PO 1 g at 19, 18, and 9 h before surgery (three doses) Hepatic coma PO 4–12 g daily in divided doses	
Netilmicin (Netromycin)	Similar to gentamicin in antimicrobial spectrum, but is reportedly less active against *P. aeruginosa*	IM, IV 4–6.5 mg/kg/d in two or three divided doses, q8–12h	*Infants and children (6 wk to 12 y):* 5.5 to 8 mg/kg/d in 2 or 3 divided doses, q8–12h *Neonates (<6 wk):* 4–6.5 mg/kg/d, in two divided doses, q12h
Paromomycin (Humatin)	Acts against bacteria and amebae in the intestinal lumen Used to treat hepatic coma and intestinal amebiasis. It is not effective in amebic infections outside the intestine.	Intestinal amebiasis PO 25–35 mg/kg/d, in three divided doses, with meals, for 5–10 d. Repeat after 2 wk, if necessary. Hepatic coma PO 4 g/d in divided doses for 5–6 d	Intestinal amebiasis, same as adults

(continued)

TABLE 35-1   Aminoglycosides (continued)

Generic/Trade Name	Characteristics	Routes and Dosage Ranges	
		Adults	Children
	Usually not absorbed from GI tract and unlikely to cause ototoxicity and nephrotoxicity associated with systemically absorbed aminoglycosides. However, systemic absorption may occur in the presence of inflammatory or ulcerative bowel disease.		
Streptomycin	May be used in a four- to six-drug regimen for treatment of multidrug-resistant tuberculosis	IM 15 mg/kg/d (maximum 1 g) or 25–30 mg/kg two or three times weekly (maximum 1.5 g per dose)	IM 20–40 mg/kg/d in two divided doses, q12h (maximum dose, 1 g/d)
Tobramycin (Nebcin)	Similar to gentamicin in antibacterial spectrum, but may be more active against Pseudomonas organisms May be indicated in serious staphylococcal infections when penicillins or other less toxic drugs are contraindicated or ineffective Often used with other antibiotics for septicemia and infections of burn wounds, other soft tissues, bone, the urinary tract and the central nervous system	IV, IM 3–5 mg/kg q24h, 1.5–2.5 mg/kg q12h, or 1–1.7 mg/kg q8h	Same as adults Neonates (≤1 wk): IM, IV up to 4 mg/kg/d in two divided doses, q12h

GI, gastrointestinal; IM, intramuscular; IV, intravenous.

TABLE 35-2	Fluoroquinolones	
Generic/Trade Name	Characteristics	Routes and Dosage Ranges
Cinoxacin (Cinobac)	1. Used only for UTI 2. Effective against most gram-negative bacteria that commonly cause UTI (*Escherichia coli, Klebsiella, Enterobacter, Proteus*)	PO 1 g daily in two to four divided doses for 7-14 d
Ciprofloxacin (Cipro)	1. Effective in respiratory, urinary tract, gastrointestinal tract, and skin and soft tissue infections as well as sexually transmitted diseases caused by chlamydiae and gonorrhea organisms 2. Used as one of four to six drugs in treatment of multidrug-resistant tuberculosis	UTI, PO 250 mg q12h Systemic infections, PO 500–750 mg q12h
Enoxacin (Penetrex)	Used only for UTI and uncomplicated gonorrhea	UTI, PO 200–400 mg q12h for 7–14 d Gonorrhea, PO 400 mg as a single dose
Gatifloxacin (Tequin)	Indicated for pneumonia, bronchitis, skin and soft tissue infections, urinary infections, gonorrhea	PO, IV infusion 400 mg once daily Give IV dose after 60 minutes; avoid rapid administration
Levofloxacin (Levaquin)	A broad-spectrum agent effective for treatment of bronchitis, cystitis, pneumonia, and sinusitis	PO, IV 250–500 mg once daily. Infuse IV dose slowly, over 60 min
Lomefloxacin (Maxaquin)	1. See ciprofloxacin, above 2. Also approved for prophylactic therapy before transurethral surgical procedures	PO 400 mg once daily Preoperatively, PO 400 mg as a single dose, 2-6 h before surgery
Moxifloxacin (Avelox)	Indicated for pneumonia and skin and soft tissue infections	PO 400 mg once daily
Norfloxacin (Noroxin)	Used only for UTI and uncomplicated gonorrhea	PO 400 mg twice daily
Ofloxacin (Floxin)	See ciprofloxacin, above	PO, IV 200–400 mg q12h for 3–10 d Gonorrhea, PO 400 mg as a single dose
Sparfloxacin (Zagam)	Indicated for community-acquired pneumonia caused by *Chlamydia pneumoniae, Streptococcus pneumoniae*, or *Hemophilus influenzae* and acute bacterial exacerbations of chronic bronchitis caused by above organisms, *Klebsiella pneumoniae*, or *Staphylococcus aureus*	PO 400 mg as loading dose, then 200 mg once daily for 10 d Renal impairment (creatinine clearance <50 mL/min), PO 400 mg as loading dose, then 200 mg q48h for a total of 9 d of therapy (6 tablets)

IV, intravenous; PO, oral; UTI, urinary tract infection.

FLUOROQUINOLONES

Fluoroquinolones are synthetic bactericidal drugs with activity against gram-negative and gram-positive organisms. They may allow oral ambulatory treatment of infections that previously required parenteral therapy and hospitalization. Most are given orally, after which they are well absorbed, achieve therapeutic concentrations in most body fluids, and are metabolized to some extent in the liver. The kidneys are the main route of elimination, with approximately 30% to 60% of an oral dose excreted unchanged in the urine. Dosage should be reduced in renal impairment.

Mechanism of Action

The drugs act by interfering with deoxyribonucleic acid (DNA) gyrase, an enzyme required for synthesis of bacterial DNA and therefore required for bacterial growth and replication.

Indications for Use

Fluoroquinolones are indicated for various infections caused by aerobic gram-negative and other microorganisms. Thus, they may be used to treat infections of the respiratory, genitourinary, and GI tracts as well as infections of bones, joints, skin, and soft tissues. Additional uses include treatment of gonorrhea, multidrug-resistant tuberculosis (see Chap. 38), *Mycobacterium avium* complex (MAC) infections in clients with AIDS, and fever in neutropenic cancer clients. Indications vary with individual drugs and are listed in Table 35-2.

Contraindications to Use

Fluoroquinolones are contraindicated in children younger than 18 years of age, in pregnant or lactating women, and in those who have experienced a hypersensitivity reaction.

NURSING PROCESS

General aspects of the nursing process as described in Chapter 33 apply to the client receiving aminoglycosides and fluoroquinolones. In this chapter, only those aspects related specifically to these drugs are included.

Assessment

With aminoglycosides, assess for the presence of factors that predispose to nephrotoxicity or ototoxicity:

- Check laboratory reports of renal function (eg, serum creatinine, creatinine clearance, blood urea nitrogen [BUN]) for abnormal values.
- Assess for impairment of balance or hearing, including audiometry reports if available.
- Analyze current medications for drugs that interact with aminoglycosides to increase risks of nephrotoxicity or ototoxicity.

With fluoroquinolones, assess for the presence of factors that increase risks of adverse drug effects (eg, impaired renal function, inadequate fluid intake, frequent or prolonged exposure to sunlight in usual activities of daily living):

- Assess laboratory tests (eg, complete blood counts and tests of renal and hepatic function) for abnormal values.

Planning/Goals

The client will:

- Receive aminoglycoside dosages that are individualized by age, weight, renal function, and serum drug levels

- Have serum aminoglycoside levels monitored when indicated
- Have renal function tests performed regularly during aminoglycoside and fluoroquinolone therapy
- Be well hydrated during aminoglycoside and fluoroquinolone therapy
- Be observed regularly for adverse drug effects

Interventions

- With aminoglycosides, weigh clients accurately (dosage is based on weight), monitor laboratory reports of BUN, serum creatinine, serum drug levels, and urinalysis for abnormal values.
- Force fluids to at least 2000 to 3000 mL daily if not contraindicated. Keeping the client well hydrated reduces risks of nephrotoxicity with aminoglycosides and crystalluria with fluoroquinolones.
- Avoid concurrent use of other nephrotoxic drugs when possible.

Evaluation

- Interview and observe for improvement in the infection being treated.
- Interview and observe for adverse drug effects.

PRINCIPLES OF THERAPY

Choice of Drug

Of the aminoglycosides, gentamicin is often given for systemic infections if resistant microorganisms have not developed in the clinical setting. If gentamicin-resistant organisms have developed, amikacin or tobramycin may

CLIENT TEACHING GUIDELINES
Oral Fluoroquinolones

General Considerations

✔ Avoid exposure to sunlight during and for several days after taking one of these drugs. Stop taking the drug and notify the prescribing physician if skin burning, redness, swelling, rash, or itching occurs. Sunscreen lotions do not prevent photosensitivity reactions.

✔ Be very careful if driving or doing other tasks requiring alertness or physical coordination. These drugs may cause dizziness or light-headedness.

Self-administration

✔ Take norfloxacin (Noroxin) and enoxacin (Penetrex) 1 hour before or 2 hours after meals. Do not take ofloxacin with

food. Ciprofloxacin (Cipro), gatifloxacin (Tequin), lomefloxacin (Maxaquin), and sparfloxacin (Zagam) can be taken without regard to meals.

✔ Drink 2 to 3 quarts of fluid daily if able. This helps to prevent kidney problems.

✔ Do not take antacids containing magnesium or aluminum (eg, Mylanta or Maalox) or any products containing iron or zinc at the same time, within 4 hours before, or within 2 hours after a dose of the antibiotic.

be given because they are less susceptible to drug-destroying enzymes. In terms of toxicity, the drugs cause similar effects, except that tobramycin may cause less nephrotoxicity and netilmicin may cause less ototoxicity. When fluoroquinolones are prescribed, ciprofloxacin or a newer drug is often used.

Dosage of Aminoglycosides

Dosage of aminoglycosides must be carefully regulated because therapeutic doses are close to toxic doses. Two major dosing schedules are used, one involving multiple daily doses and one involving a single daily dose. The multiple-dose regimen has been used for many years, and guidelines are well defined. The single-dose regimen is being used increasingly, and guidelines are still evolving as studies and clinical experience accumulate. These two regimens are described in the following sections.

Multiple Daily Dosing

1. An *initial loading dose*, based on weight and the desired peak serum level, is given to achieve therapeutic serum levels rapidly. If the client is obese, lean or ideal body weight should be used because aminoglycosides are not significantly distributed in body fat. In clients with normal renal function, the recommended loading dose for gentamicin, tobramycin, and netilmicin is 1.5 to 2 mg/kg of body weight; for amikacin the loading dose is 5 to 7.5 mg/kg.
2. *Maintenance doses* are based on serum drug levels. Peak serum levels should be assessed 30 to 60 minutes after drug administration (5 to 8 µg/mL for gentamicin and tobramycin, 20 to 30 µg/mL for amikacin, 4 to 12 µg/mL for netilmicin). Measurement of both peak and trough levels helps to maintain therapeutic serum levels without excessive toxicity. For gentamicin and tobramycin, peak levels above 10 to 12 µg/mL and trough levels above 2 µg/mL for prolonged periods have been associated with nephrotoxicity. For accuracy, blood samples must be drawn at the correct times.
3. *With impaired renal function*, dosage of aminoglycosides must be reduced. Methods of reducing dosage

include measuring serum drug levels or lengthening the time between doses according to creatinine clearance levels. For specific instructions, consult the manufacturers' literature.

4. *In urinary tract infections*, smaller doses can be used than in systemic infections because the aminoglycosides reach high concentrations in the urine. Also, alkalinizing the urine increases the activity and effectiveness of aminoglycoside therapy.

Single Daily Dosing

The use of once-daily (q24h) aminoglycoside dosing is increasing. This practice evolved from increased knowledge about the concentration-dependent bactericidal effects and postantibiotic effects of aminoglycosides. Concentration-dependent bactericidal effects mean that the drugs kill more microorganisms with a large dose and high peak serum concentrations. Postantibiotic effects mean that aminoglycosides continue killing microorganisms even with low serum concentrations. These characteristics allow administration of high doses to achieve high peak serum concentrations and optimal killing of microorganisms. The 24-hour interval until the next dose allows the client to eliminate the drug to very low serum levels for approximately 6 hours. During this low-drug period, the postantibiotic effect is active and there is minimal drug accumulation in body tissues. Reported advantages of this regimen include increased bactericidal effects, less nephrotoxicity, reduced need for serum drug levels, and reduced nursing time for administration.

Dosage of Fluoroquinolones

Recommended dosages of fluoroquinolones should not be exceeded in any clients, and dosages should be reduced in the presence of renal impairment.

Guidelines for Reducing Toxicity of Aminoglycosides

In addition to the preceding recommendations, guidelines to decrease the incidence and severity of adverse effects include the following:

1. Identify clients at high risk for adverse effects (eg, neonates, older adults, clients with renal impairment, clients with disease processes or drug therapies that impair blood circulation and renal function).
2. Keep clients well hydrated to decrease drug concentration in serum and body tissues. The drugs reach higher concentrations in the kidneys and inner ears than in other body tissues. This is a major factor in nephrotoxicity and ototoxicity. The goal of an adequate fluid intake is to decrease the incidence and severity of these adverse effects.
3. Avoid concurrent administration of diuretics. Diuretics may increase nephrotoxicity by decreasing fluid volume, thereby increasing drug concentration in serum and tissues. Dehydration is most likely to occur with loop diuretics such as furosemide.
4. Give the drug for no longer than 10 days. Clients are most at risk when high doses are given for prolonged periods.
5. Detect adverse effects early and reduce dosage or discontinue the drug. Changes in renal function tests that indicate nephrotoxicity may not occur until the client has received an aminoglycoside for approximately 5 days. If nephrotoxicity occurs, it is usually reversible if the drug is stopped. Early ototoxicity is detectable only with audiometry.

Use in Children

Aminoglycosides must be used cautiously in children as with adults. Dosage must be accurately calculated according to weight and renal function. Serum drug levels must be monitored and dosage adjusted as indicated to avoid toxicity. Neonates may have increased risk of nephrotoxicity and ototoxicity because of their immature renal function. Neomycin is not recommended for use in infants and children. Fluoroquinolones are not recommended for use in children because they have been associated with permanent damage in cartilage and joints.

Use in Older Adults

With aminoglycosides, advanced age is considered a major risk factor for development of toxicity. However, the drugs are commonly used in older adults because of intolerance to other antibacterials and infections caused by organisms resistant to other antibacterials. Aminoglycosides should not be given to older adults with impaired renal function if less toxic drugs are effective against causative organisms. When the drugs are given, extreme caution is required. Because of impaired renal function, other disease processes, and multiple-drug therapy, older adults are at high risk for development of nephrotoxicity and ototoxicity. Interventions to decrease the incidence and severity of adverse drug effects are listed in the section on Guidelines for Reducing Toxicity of Aminoglycosides.

These interventions are important with any client receiving an aminoglycoside, but are especially important with older adults. In addition, prolonged therapy (>1 week) increases toxicity and should be avoided when possible.

Fluoroquinolones are commonly used in older adults for the same indications as in younger adults. In older adults with normal renal function, the drugs should be accompanied by an adequate fluid intake and urine output to prevent drug crystals from forming in the urinary tract. In addition, urinary alkalinizing agents, such as calcium-containing antacids, should be avoided because drug crystals form more readily in alkaline urine. In those with impaired renal function, a common condition in older adults, the drugs should be used cautiously and in reduced dosages.

Use in Renal Impairment

Aminoglycosides and fluoroquinolones are nephrotoxic and must be used very cautiously in clients with renal impairment. Dosage guidelines have been established according to creatinine clearance and often involve lower dosages and prolonged intervals between doses (eg, 36 to 72 hours). Guidelines for reducing nephrotoxicity of aminoglycosides are as listed previously.

With fluoroquinolones, reported renal effects include azotemia, crystalluria, hematuria, interstitial nephritis, nephropathy, and renal failure. Nephrotoxicity occurs less often than with aminoglycosides, and most cases of acute renal failure have occurred in older adults. It is unknown whether renal failure is caused by hypersensitivity or a direct toxic effect. Crystalluria rarely occurs in acidic urine but may occur in alkaline urine. Guidelines for reducing nephrotoxicity include lower dosages, longer intervals between doses, adequate hydration, and avoiding substances that alkalinize the urine.

Use in Hepatic Impairment

With aminoglycosides, hepatic impairment is not a significant factor because the drugs are excreted through the kidneys. With fluoroquinolones, however, hepatotoxicity has been observed with most of the drugs. Clinical manifestations range from abnormalities in liver enzyme test results to hepatitis, liver necrosis, or hepatic failure. Because of serious hepatotoxicity with trovafloxacin, the Food and Drug Administration issued a public health advisory to use the drug only for serious infections, give initial doses in an inpatient setting, administer no longer than 14 days, and discontinue the drug if liver dysfunction occurs.

Use in Critical Illness

Aminoglycosides and fluoroquinolones are often used in critically ill clients because this population has a high incidence of serious infections. Aminoglycosides are usually given with other antimicrobials to provide broad-spectrum activity. In critical care units, as in other settings, there is increased use of once-daily dosing. Because critically ill clients are at high risk for development of nephrotoxicity and ototoxicity with aminoglycosides, guidelines for safe drug usage should be strictly followed.

Because fluoroquinolones may be nephrotoxic and hepatotoxic, renal and hepatic function should be monitored during therapy. Ciprofloxacin, a commonly used fluoroquinolone, is usually infused IV in critically ill clients. However, administration orally or by GI tube (eg, nasogastric, gastrostomy, or jejunostomy) may be feasible in some clients. Concomitant administration of antacids or enteral feedings decreases absorption.

 Home Care

Parenteral aminoglycosides are usually given in a hospital setting. Oral fluoroquinolones are often self-administered at home. The role of the home care nurse is primarily to teach clients or caregivers how to take the drugs effectively and to observe for adverse drug effects.

(*text continues on page 539*)

NURSING ACTIONS	Aminoglycosides and Fluoroquinolones

NURSING ACTIONS	RATIONALE/EXPLANATION
1. Administer accurately	
a. With aminoglycosides:	
(1) For intravenous (IV) administration, dilute the drug in 50 to 100 mL of 5% dextrose or 0.9% sodium chloride injection and infuse over 30 to 60 min. The concentration of gentamicin solution should not exceed 1 mg/mL.	To achieve therapeutic blood levels
(2) Give intramuscular aminoglycosides in a large muscle mass, and rotate sites.	To avoid local tissue irritation. This is less likely to occur with aminoglycosides than with most other antibiotics.
b. With fluoroquinolones:	
(1) Give norfloxacin and enoxacin 1 h before or 2 h after a meal. Do not give ofloxacin with food. Ciprofloxacin, lomefloxacin, and sparfloxacin may be given without regard to food intake.	To promote therapeutic plasma drug levels. Food in the gastrointestinal (GI) tract interferes with absorption of most oral fluoroquinolones.
(2) Give IV infusions over 60 min.	To decrease vein irritation and phlebitis
(3) When giving ciprofloxacin IV into a primary IV line (eg, using piggyback or Y connector), stop the primary solution until ciprofloxacin is infused.	To avoid physical or chemical incompatibilities
2. Observe for therapeutic effects	
a. Decreased signs and symptoms of the infection for which the drug is being given	See Chapter 33
3. Observe for adverse effects	
a. With aminoglycosides, observe for:	Adverse effects are more likely to occur with parenteral administration of large doses for prolonged periods. However, they may occur with oral administration in the presence of renal impairment and with usual therapeutic doses.
(1) Nephrotoxicity—casts, albumin, red or white blood cells in urine, decreased creatinine clearance, increased serum creatinine, increased blood urea nitrogen.	Renal damage is most likely to occur in clients who are elderly, receive high doses or prolonged therapy, have prior renal damage, or receive other nephrotoxic drugs. This is the most serious adverse

(*continued*)

NURSING ACTIONS	RATIONALE/EXPLANATION
	reaction. Risks of kidney damage can be minimized by using the drugs appropriately, detecting early signs of renal impairment, and keeping clients well hydrated.
(2) Ototoxicity—deafness or decreased hearing, tinnitus, dizziness, ataxia	This results from damage to the eighth cranial nerve. Incidence of ototoxicity is increased in older clients and those with previous auditory damage, high doses or prolonged duration, and concurrent use of other ototoxic drugs.
(3) Neurotoxicity—respiratory paralysis and apnea	This is caused by neuromuscular blockade and is more likely to occur after rapid IV injection, administration to a client with myasthenia gravis, or concomitant administration of general anesthetics or neuromuscular blocking agents (eg, succinylcholine, tubocurarine). This effect also may occur if an aminoglycoside is administered shortly after surgery, owing to the residual effects of anesthetics or neuromuscular blockers. Neostigmine or calcium may be given to counteract apnea.
(4) Hypersensitivity—skin rash, urticaria	This is an uncommon reaction except with topical neomycin, which may cause sensitization in as many as 10% of recipients.
(5) Nausea, vomiting, diarrhea, peripheral neuritis, paresthesias	Uncommon with parenteral aminoglycosides. Diarrhea often occurs with oral administration.
b. With fluoroquinolones, observe for:	The drugs are usually well tolerated.
(1) Hepatotoxicity (abnormal liver enzyme tests, hepatitis, hepatic failure)	Hepatotoxicity has been observed with most of the drugs. Trovafloxacin use is restricted because of liver damage and failure.
(2) Allergic reactions (anaphylaxis, urticaria)	Uncommon, but some fatalities have been reported.
(3) Nausea, vomiting, diarrhea, pseudo-membranous colitis	Nausea is the most common GI symptom.
(4) Headache, dizziness	
(5) Crystalluria	Uncommon, but may occur with an inadequate fluid intake
(6) Photosensitivity (skin redness, rash, itching)	May occur with most fluoroquinolones with exposure to sunlight
(7) Other	Adverse effects involving most body systems have been reported with one or more of the fluoroquinolones. Most have a low incidence (<1%) of occurrence.
4. Observe for drug interactions	
a. Drugs that *increase* effects of aminoglycosides:	The listed drugs increase toxicity.
(1) Loop diuretics (furosemide, ethacrynic acid, bumetanide)	Increased nephrotoxicity apparently caused by increased drug concentration in serum and tissues when the client is relatively "dehydrated" by potent diuretics

(continued)

NURSING ACTIONS	RATIONALE/EXPLANATION
(2) Methoxyflurane (Penthrane) and nephrotoxic antimicrobial agents (amphotericin B, cephalosporins)	Increased nephrotoxicity
(3) Drugs with neuromuscular blocking activity (methoxyflurane, procainamide, promethazine, quinidine, sodium citrate, succinylcholine, tubocurarine)	Increased neuromuscular blockade with possible paralysis of respiratory muscles and apnea. This is most likely to occur with succinylcholine and tubocurarine.
b. Drugs that *increase* effects of fluoroquinolones: Cimetidine, probenecid	These drugs inhibit elimination of fluoroquinolones and may increase serum drug levels.
c. Drugs that *decrease* effects of fluoroquinolones:	
(1) Antacids, iron preparations, sucralfate, zinc preparations	These drugs interfere with absorption of fluoroquinolones from the GI tract.
(2) Antineoplastic drugs	These drugs may decrease serum levels of fluoroquinolones.
(3) Bismuth subsalicylate (eg, Pepto-Bismol) decreases enoxacin absorption if given with or within 1 h after enoxacin.	These drugs should not be taken together or within 1 h of each other.
(4) Nitrofurantoin may decrease the antibacterial effect of norfloxacin in the urinary tract.	

Nursing Notes: Apply Your Knowledge

Answer: Peak and trough gentamicin levels are obtained to assess whether the proper dosage is being administered and to avoid toxicity that can cause permanent damage to renal function and hearing. Peak (highest) blood levels should be drawn 30 to 60 minutes after administering the drug and trough (lowest) blood level should be drawn just before the dose is administered. The laboratory results indicate that the peak level is normal but the trough level is high (4 µg/mL rather than less than 2 µg/mL). Dosage will need to be decreased to avoid renal damage. Considering Mr. Howles' age, he may have some renal impairment already that has decreased the rate of gentamicin excretion. Check to see if Mr. Howles' creatinine and blood urea nitrogen levels are elevated, which would indicate renal insufficiency. Notify the physician with the test result so that the gentamicin dose can be adjusted.

How Can You Avoid This Medication Error?

Answer: A nurse may change the dose of a medication only if she has prescriptive authority (eg, ARNP). This is not indicated in this situation. Your concerns are valid regarding aminoglycoside toxicity for this patient. It would be prudent to place another call to the physician and hold the gentamicin until you hear from her or him.

REVIEW AND APPLICATION EXERCISES

1. How do aminoglycosides exert bactericidal effects?

2. Why must aminoglycosides be given parenterally for systemic infections?

3. How are aminoglycosides excreted?

4. What are risk factors for aminoglycoside-induced nephrotoxicity and ototoxicity?

5. How would you assess a client for nephrotoxicity or ototoxicity?

6. What is the reason for giving an aminoglycoside and an antipseudomonal penicillin in the treatment of serious infections caused by *Pseudomonas aeruginosa*?

7. Why should an aminoglycoside and an antipseudomonal penicillin *not* be combined in a syringe or IV fluid for administration?

8. Which laboratory tests need to be monitored regularly for a client receiving a systemic aminoglycoside?

9. What is the rationale for giving an oral aminoglycoside to treat hepatic coma?

10. How do fluoroquinolones exert their antibacterial effects?

11. What are the main clinical uses of fluoroquinolones?

12. What are adverse effects of fluoroquinolones, and how may they be prevented or minimized?

13. Why is it important to maintain an adequate fluid intake and urine output with the fluoroquinolones?

14. Why are fluoroquinolones not given to children?

SELECTED REFERENCES

Chambers, H.F. & Sande, M.A. (1996). Antimicrobial agents: The aminoglycosides. In J.G. Hardman, L.E. Limbird, P.B. Molinoff, & R.W. Ruddon (Eds.), *Goodman & Gilman's The pharmacological basis of therapeutics*, 9th ed., pp. 1103–1121. New York: McGraw-Hill.

Craig, W.A. (1997). Antimicrobial therapeutic agents. In W.N. Kelley (Ed.), *Textbook of internal medicine*, 3rd ed., pp. 1843–1852. Philadelphia: Lippincott-Raven.

Drug facts and comparisons. (Updated monthly). St. Louis: Facts and Comparisons.

Food and Drug Administration. (1999). *Public health advisory: Trovan (trovafloxacin)*. Washington, D.C.: Author.

Foxworth, J. (1997). Recognizing and preventing antibiotic-associated complications in the critical care setting. *Critical Care Nursing Quarterly, 20*(3), 1–11.

Hooper, D.C. (1998). Expanding uses of fluoroquinolones: Opportunities and challenges. *Annals of Internal Medicine, 129*, 908–911.

Lipsky, B.A. & Baker, C.A. (1999). Fluoroquinolone toxicity profiles: A review focusing on newer agents. *Clinical Infectious Diseases, 28*, 352–364.

Maljanian, R. & Quintiliani, R. (1999). When once is enough: Administering aminoglycosides effectively. *Nursing, 29*(5), 41–44.

Mandell, G.L. & Petri, W.A., Jr. (1996). Antimicrobial agents: Sulfonamides, trimethoprim-sulfamethoxazole, quinolones, and agents for urinary tract infections. In J.G. Hardman, L.E. Limbird, P.B. Molinoff, & R.W. Ruddon (Eds.), *Goodman & Gilman's The pharmacological basis of therapeutics*, 9th ed., pp. 1057–1072. New York: McGraw-Hill.

Paterson, D.L., Robson, J.M.B., & Wagener, M.M. (1998). Risk factors for toxicity in elderly patients given aminoglycosides once daily. *Journal of General Internal Medicine, 13*, 735–739.

36

Tetracyclines, Sulfonamides, and Urinary Agents

Objectives

After studying this chapter, the student will be able to:

1. Discuss major characteristics and clinical uses of tetracyclines.

2. Recognize doxycycline as the tetracycline of choice for use in clients with renal failure.

3. Discuss characteristics, clinical uses, adverse effects, and nursing implications of selected sulfonamides.

4. Recognize trimethoprim-sulfamethoxazole as a combination drug that is commonly used for urinary tract and systemic infections.

5. Describe the use of urinary antiseptics in the treatment of urinary tract infections.

6. Teach clients strategies for preventing, recognizing, and treating urinary tract infections.

Faye Sullivan, 15 years of age, comes to the walk-in clinic with symptoms of urgency, frequency, and dysuria. A routine urinalysis indicates the presence of infection. The urinary tract infection (UTI) is treated with Bactrim for 10 days.

Reflect on:

▶ Factors that increase the incidence of UTI for adolescent girls.

▶ Important information to include when teaching Faye about Bactrim therapy.

▶ Strategies to prevent future UTIs.

▶ Data to collect to determine if Faye's UTI is responding to treatment.

DESCRIPTION

Tetracyclines and sulfonamides are older, broad-spectrum, bacteriostatic drugs that are rarely used for systemic infections because of microbial resistance and the development of more effective or less toxic drugs. However, the drugs are useful in selected infections. Urinary antiseptics are used only in urinary tract infections (UTI). These drugs are described later in this chapter and listed in Tables 36-1, 36-2, and 36-3.

The tetracyclines are similar in pharmacologic properties and antimicrobial activity. They are effective against a wide range of gram-positive and gram-negative organisms as well as rickettsiae, mycoplasma, some protozoa, spirochetes, and others. They are widely distributed into most body tissues and fluids. The older tetracyclines are excreted mainly in urine, the newer ones (doxycycline and minocycline) mainly in feces.

Sulfonamides are bacteriostatic against a wide range of bacteria, including pneumococci; *Neisseria* species; *Escherichia coli*; *Klebsiella*, *Proteus*, and *Enterobacter* species; and *Hemophilus influenzae*. Individual drugs vary in extent of systemic absorption and clinical indications.

(*text continues on page 547*)

TABLE 36-1 Tetracyclines

Generic/Trade Name	Characteristics	Routes and Dosage Ranges	
		Adults	Children
Tetracycline (Achromycin, others)	1. Prototype drug 2. Marketed under generic and numerous trade names	PO 250–500 mg q6h	PO 22–44 mg/kg/d in four divided doses
Demeclocycline (Declomycin)	1. Has a longer half-life than tetracycline, and smaller doses produce therapeutic serum levels 2. The tetracycline most likely to cause photosensitivity 3. May be used to promote diuresis when fluid retention is caused by inappropriate secretion of antidiuretic hormone	PO 150 mg q6h or 300 mg q12h Gonorrhea in penicillin-sensitive clients, PO 600 mg initially, followed by 300 mg q12h for 4 d	Age>8 y: PO 3–6 mg/kg/d in two to four divided doses
Doxycycline (Vibramycin)	1. Well absorbed from the gastrointestinal tract. Oral administration yields serum drug levels equivalent to those obtained by parenteral administration. 2. Highly lipid soluble; therefore, reaches therapeutic levels in CSF, the eye, and the prostate gland 3. Can be given in smaller doses and less frequently than other tetracyclines because of long serum half-life (approximately 18 h) 4. Excreted by kidneys to a lesser extent than other tetracyclines and is considered safe for clients with impaired renal function	PO 100 mg q12h for two doses, then once daily or in divided doses; severe infections, 100 mg q12h IV 200 mg the first day, then 100–200 mg daily in one or two doses	PO, IV same as adults for children weighing ≥45 kg Those weighing <45 kg: PO 4.4 mg/kg (2 mg/lb) q12h for two doses, then 1 mg/kg/d in a single dose; severe infections, 2 mg/kg q12h IV 4.4 mg/kg/d in one or two doses, then 1–2 mg/kg/d, depending on severity of infection
Minocycline (Minocin)	1. Well absorbed after oral administration 2. Like doxycycline, readily penetrates CSF, the eye, and the prostate 3. Metabolized more than other tetracyclines, and smaller amounts are excreted in urine and feces	PO, IV 200 mg initially, then 100 mg q12h	>12 y: PO, IV same as adults <12 y: PO, IV 4 mg/kg initially, then 2 mg/kg q12h

CSF, cerebrospinal fluid; IV, intravenous; PO, oral.

TABLE 36-2 **Sulfonamide Preparations**

Generic/Trade Name	Characteristics	Clinical Indications	Routes and Dosage Ranges	
			Adults	Children
Single Agents				
Sulfadiazine	1. A short-acting, rapidly absorbed, rapidly excreted agent for systemic infections 2. Low solubility 3. Therapeutic blood levels are 10–15 mg/100 mL.	1. Urinary tract infections 2. Prophylaxis of rheumatic fever in clients allergic to penicillin 3. Nocardiosis 4. Meningococcal meningitis 5. Toxoplasmosis	PO 2–4 g initially, then 2–4 g daily in three to six divided doses	>2 mo: PO 75 mg/kg initially, then 150 mg/kg/d in four to six divided doses: maximal daily dose, 6 g Prophylaxis of rheumatic fever, PO 500 mg once daily for children weighing <30 kg; 1 g daily for children weighing >30 kg
Sulfamethizole (Thiosulfil)	A highly soluble, rapidly absorbed, and rapidly excreted agent that is similar to sulfisoxazole in actions and uses	Urinary tract infections	PO 500 mg–1 g three or four times daily	>2 mo: PO 30–45 mg/kg/d in four divided doses
Sulfamethoxazole (Gantanol)	1. Similar to sulfisoxazole in therapeutic effects but absorbed and excreted more slowly. More likely to produce excessive blood levels and crystalluria than sulfisoxazole. 2. An ingredient in mixtures with trimethoprim (see Combination Agent, below)	1. Systemic infections 2. Urinary tract infections	PO 2 g initially, then 1–2 g two or three times daily	>2 mo: PO 50–60 mg/kg initially, then 30 mg/kg q12h; maximal daily dose, 75 mg/kg
Sulfasalazine (Azulfidine)	1. Poorly absorbed 2. Does not alter normal bacterial flora in the intestine. Effectiveness in ulcerative colitis may be due to antibacterial (sulfapyridine) and antiinflammatory (aminosalicylic acid) metabolites.	1. Ulcerative colitis 2. Rheumatoid arthritis	Ulcerative colitis, PO 3–4 g daily in divided doses initially; 2 g daily in four doses for maintenance; maximal daily dose, 8 g Rheumatoid arthritis, PO 2 g daily in divided doses	PO 40–60 mg/kg/d in three to six divided doses initially, followed by 30 mg/kg/d in four divided doses
Sulfisoxazole	1. Rapidly absorbed, rapidly excreted: 2. Highly soluble and less likely to cause crystalluria than most other sulfonamides	1. Urinary tract infections 2. Vaginitis 3. Ocular infections	PO 2–4 g initially, then 4–8 g daily in three to six divided doses Intravaginally, 2.5–5 g of vaginal cream (10%) twice daily	>2 mo: PO 75 mg/kg of body weight initially, then 150 mg/kg/d in four to six divided doses; maximal daily dose, 6 g
Combination Agent				
Trimethoprim-sulfamethoxazole (Bactrim, Septra, others)	1. Synergistic effectiveness against many organisms, including streptococci (*S. pneumoniae, S. viridans*); staphylococci (*S.epidermidis, S. aureus*): *Escherichia coli; Proteus; Enterobacter; Salmonella; Shigella;*	1. Acute and chronic urinary tract infections 2. Acute exacerbations of chronic bronchitis 3. Acute otitis media caused by susceptible strains of *Hemophilus influenzae* and *S. pneumoniae* 4. Shigellosis	Urinary tract infections, trimethoprim 160 mg and sulfamethoxazole 800 mg PO q12h for 10–14 d Shigellosis, same dose as above for 5 d Severe urinary tract infections, PO 8–10 mg (trimethoprim component) per kg/d in two	Urinary tract infections, otitis media, and shigellosis, PO 8 mg/kg trimethoprim and 40 mg/kg sulfamethoxazole in two divided doses q12h for 10 d Severe urinary tract infections, IV 8–10 mg (trimethoprim compo-

(continued)

TABLE 36-2	Sulfonamide Preparations (*continued*)			

			Routes and Dosage Ranges	
Generic/Trade Name	**Characteristics**	**Clinical Indications**	**Adults**	**Children**

	Serratia; Klebsiella, Nocardia: and others. Most strains of *Pseudomonas* are resistant.
	 2. The two drugs have additive antibacterial effects because they interfere with different steps in bacterial synthesis and activation of folic acid, an essential nutrient.
	 3. The combination is less likely to produce resistant bacteria than either agent alone.
	 4. Oral preparations contain different amounts of the two drugs, as follows:
	   a. "Regular" tablets contain trimethoprim 80 mg and sulfamethoxazole 400 mg.
	   b. Double-strength tablets (eg, Bactrim D.S., Septra D.S.) contain trimethoprim 160 mg and sulfamethoxazole 800 mg.
	   c. The oral suspension contains trimethoprim 40 mg and sulfamethoxazole 200 mg in each 5 mL.
	 5. The IV preparation contains trimethoprim 80 mg and sulfamethoxazole 400 mg in 5 mL.
	 6. Dosage must be reduced in renal insufficiency.
	 7. The preparation is contraindicated if creatinine clearance is less than 15 mL/min.
		5. Infection by *Pneumocystis carinii* (prevention and treatment)
		 6. Intravenous preparation indicated for *P. carinii* pneumonia, severe urinary tract infections, and shigellosis
			to four divided doses, up to 14 d
			 P. carinii pneumonia, IV 15–20 mg (trimethoprim component) per kg/d in three or four divided doses, q6–8h up to 14 d
				nent)/kg in two to four divided doses q6–8h or q12h up to 14 d
				 P. carinii pneumonia, IV 15–20 mg (trimethoprim component) per kg/d in three or four divided doses, q6–8h up to 14 d

(*continued*)

TABLE 36-2 **Sulfonamide Preparations** (*continued*)

Generic/Trade Name	Characteristics	Clinical Indications	Routes and Dosage Ranges	
			Adults	Children
Topical Sulfonamides				
Mafenide (Sulfamylon)	1. Effective against most gram-negative and gram-positive organisms, especially *Pseudomonas* 2. Application causes pain and burning. 3. Mafenide is absorbed systemically and may produce metabolic acidosis.	Prevention of bacterial colonization and infection of severe burn wounds	Topical application to burned area, once or twice daily, in a thin layer	Same as adults
Silver sulfadiazine (Silvadene)	1. Effective against most *Pseudomonas* species, the most common pathogen in severe burn sepsis, *E. coli, Klebsiella, Proteus,* staphylococci, and streptococci 2. Application is painless. 3. Does not cause electrolyte or acid–base imbalances 4. Significant amounts may be absorbed systemically with large burned areas and prolonged use.	Same as mafenide. Usually the preferred drug.	Same as mafenide	Same as mafenide

IV, intravenous; PO, oral.

TABLE 36-3 **Miscellaneous Drugs for Urinary Tract Infections**

Generic/Trade Name	Characteristics	Routes and Dosage Ranges	
		Adults	Children
Fosfomycin (Monurol)	1. Broad-spectrum, long-acting agent 2. Most common adverse effects are diarrhea and headache.	PO 3 g in a single dose, taken with or without food. Powder should be mixed with one-half cup of water and drunk immediately.	Dosage not established
Methenamine mandelate (Mandelamine)	1. Antibacterial activity only at a urine pH <5.5. In acidic urine, the drug forms formaldehyde, which is the antibacterial component. Acidification of urine (eg, with ascorbic acid) is usually needed. 2. Formaldehyde is active against several gram-positive and gram-negative organisms, including *Escherichia coli*. It is most useful for long-term suppression of bacteria in chronic, recurrent infections.	PO 1 g four times daily	Age 6–12 y: PO 500 mg four times daily Age <6 y: PO 50 mg/kg/d, in three divided doses

(*continued*)

TABLE 36-3   **Miscellaneous Drugs for Urinary Tract Infections** (*continued*)

Generic/Trade Name	Characteristics	Routes and Dosage Ranges	
		Adults	Children
	3. It is not indicated in acute infections. 4. Contraindicated in renal failure		
Methanamine-hippurate (Hiprex)	See methenamine mandelate, above	PO 1 g twice daily	PO 500 mg–1 g twice daily
Nalidixic acid (NegGram)	1. Prototype of quinolones 2. Active against most gram-negative organisms that cause UTI, but rarely used because organisms develop resistance rapidly and other effective drugs are available.	PO 4 g daily in four divided doses for 1–2 wk, then 2 g/d if long-term treatment is required	PO 55 mg/kg/d in four divided doses, reduced to 33 mg/kg/d for long-term use in children <12 y. Contraindicated in infants <3 mo.
Nitrofurantoin (Furadantin, Macrodantin)	1. Antibacterial activity against *E. coli* and most other organisms that cause UTI. 2. Used for short-term treatment of UTI or long-term suppression of bacteria in chronic, recurrent UTI. 3. Bacterial resistance develops slowly and to a limited degree. 4. Contraindicated in severe renal disease	PO 50–100 mg four times daily Prophylaxis of recurrent UTI in women, PO 50–100 mg at bedtime	>3 mo: PO 5–7 mg/kg/d, in four divided doses
Phenazopyridine (Pyridium)	1. An azo dye that acts as a urinary tract analgesic and relieves symptoms of dysuria, burning, and frequency and urgency of urination, which occur with UTI. 2. It has no anti-infective action. 3. It turns urine orange-red, which may be mistaken for blood. 4. It is contraindicated in renal insufficiency and severe hepatitis.	PO 200 mg three times daily after meals	6–12 y: PO 12 mg/kg/d, in three divided doses
Trimethoprim (Proloprim, Trimpex)	1. A folate antagonist drug with antibacterial effects 2. Available as a single agent for treatment of UTI caused by susceptible strains of *E. coli,* and other gram-negative organisms 3. Most often used in a fixed-dose combination with sulfamethoxazole (Bactrim, Septra) 4. Contraindicated in clients with hypersensitivity to trimethoprim or megaloblastic anemia due to folate deficiency. 5. Rash and pruritus are the most common adverse effects. Nausea, vomiting, glossitis, thrombocytopenia, leukopenia, and methemoglobinemia occasionally occur.	PO 100 mg q12h for 10 d	

PO, oral; UTI, urinary tract infection.

Some are well absorbed and can be used in systemic infections; others are poorly absorbed and exert more local effects.

Urinary antiseptics may be bactericidal for sensitive organisms in the urinary tract because they are concentrated in renal tubules and reach high levels in urine. They are not used in systemic infections because they do not attain therapeutic plasma levels. An additional drug, phenazopyridine, is given to relieve pain associated with UTI. It has no antibacterial activity.

Mechanisms of Action

Tetracyclines penetrate microbial cells by passive diffusion and an active transport system. Intracellularly, they bind to 30S ribosomes, like the aminoglycosides, and inhibit microbial protein synthesis. Sulfonamides act as antimetabolites of para-aminobenzoic acid (PABA), which microorganisms require to produce folic acid; folic acid, in turn, is required for the production of bacterial intracellular proteins. Sulfonamides enter into the reaction instead of PABA, compete for the enzyme involved, and cause formation of nonfunctional derivatives of folic acid. Thus, sulfonamides halt multiplication of new bacteria but do not kill mature, fully formed bacteria. With the exception of the topical sulfonamides used in burn therapy, the presence of pus, serum, or necrotic tissue interferes with sulfonamide action because these materials contain PABA. Some bacteria can change their metabolic pathways to use precursors or other forms of folic acid and thereby develop resistance to the antibacterial action of sulfonamides. Once resistance to one sulfonamide develops, cross-resistance to others is common.

Indications for Use

A tetracycline is the drug of choice in a few infections (eg, cholera, granuloma inguinale, chancroid, Rocky Mountain spotted fever, psittacosis, typhus, trachoma). Other drugs (eg, penicillins) are usually preferred in gram-positive infections, and most gram-negative organisms are resistant to tetracyclines. However, a tetracycline may be used if bacterial susceptibility is confirmed. Specific clinical indications for tetracyclines include:

1. Treatment of uncomplicated urethral, endocervical, or rectal infections caused by *Chlamydia* organisms.
2. Adjunctive treatment, with other antimicrobials, in the treatment of pelvic inflammatory disease and sexually transmitted diseases.
3. Long-term treatment of acne. Tetracyclines interfere with the production of free fatty acids and decrease *Corynebacterium* in sebum. These actions decrease the inflammatory, pustular lesions associated with severe acne.

4. As a substitute for penicillin in penicillin-allergic clients. Tetracyclines may be effective in treating gonorrhea and syphilis when penicillin cannot be given. They should not be substituted for penicillin in treating streptococcal pharyngitis because microbial resistance is common, and tetracyclines do not prevent rheumatic fever. In addition, they should not be substituted for penicillin in any serious staphylococcal infection because microbial resistance commonly occurs.
5. Doxycycline may be used to prevent traveler's diarrhea due to enterotoxic strains of *E. coli.*
6. Demeclocycline may be used to inhibit antidiuretic hormone in the management of chronic inappropriate antidiuretic hormone secretion.

Sulfonamides are commonly used to treat UTI (eg, acute and chronic cystitis, asymptomatic bacteriuria) caused by *E. coli* and *Proteus* or *Klebsiella* organisms. In acute pyelonephritis, other agents are preferred. Additional uses include ulcerative colitis and uncommon infections such as chancroid, lymphogranuloma venereum, nocardiosis, toxoplasmosis, and trachoma. Topical sulfonamides are used in prevention of burn wound infections and in treatment of ocular, vaginal, and other soft tissue infections. For specific clinical indications of individual drugs, see Table 36-2.

Urinary antiseptics are used only for UTI.

Contraindications to Use

Both tetracyclines and sulfonamides are contraindicated in renal failure. Tetracyclines are also contraindicated in pregnant women and in children up to 8 years of age. In the fetus and young child, tetracyclines are deposited in bones and teeth along with calcium. If given during active mineralization of these tissues, tetracyclines can cause permanent brown coloring (mottling) of tooth enamel and can depress bone growth. Sulfonamides are also contraindicated in late pregnancy, lactation, children younger than 2 months of age (except for treatment of congenital toxoplasmosis), and people who have had hypersensitivity reactions to them or to chemically related drugs (eg, thiazide diuretics or antidiabetic sulfonylureas). Sulfasalazine (Azulfidine) is contraindicated in people who are allergic to salicylates and people with intestinal or urinary tract obstruction.

How Can You Avoid This Medication Error?

Trimethoprim-sulfamethoxazole (Bactrim) DS bid is ordered for a client after urologic surgery. He takes no medications and reports an allergy to eggs, nuts, sulfa, and morphine. The unit dose provided from the pharmacy is a tablet containing 160 mg of trimethoprim and 800 mg of sulfamethoxazole. You give him one tablet at 0900 for his morning dose.

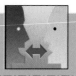

CLIENT TEACHING GUIDELINES
Oral Tetracyclines

General Considerations

✔ Because tetracyclines inhibit rather than kill bacteria, they must be taken correctly to achieve desired effects.

✔ These drugs increase sensitivity to sunlight and risks of sunburn. Avoid sunlamps, tanning beds, and intense or prolonged exposure to sunlight; if unable to avoid exposure, wear protective clothing and a sunblock preparation.

✔ Report severe nausea, vomiting, diarrhea, skin rash, or perineal itching. These symptoms may indicate a need for changing or stopping the tetracycline.

Self-administration

✔ Take most tetracyclines on an empty stomach, at least 1 hour before or 2 hours after meals. Doxycycline and minocycline may be taken with food (except dairy products).

✔ Do not take with or within 2 hours of dairy products, antacids, or iron supplements. If an antacid must be taken, take at least 2 hours before or after tetracycline.

✔ Take each dose with a full glass of water (240 mL).

NURSING PROCESS

General aspects of the nursing process in antimicrobial drug therapy, as described in Chapter 33, apply to the client receiving tetracyclines, sulfonamides, and urinary antiseptics. In this chapter, only those aspects related specifically to these drugs are included.

Assessment

With tetracyclines, assess for conditions in which the drugs must be used cautiously or are contraindicated, such as impaired renal or hepatic function.

With sulfonamides, assess for signs and symptoms of disorders for which the drugs are used:

- For *UTI*, assess urinalysis reports for white blood cells and bacteria, urine culture reports for type of bacteria, and symptoms of dysuria, frequency, and urgency of urination.
- For *burns*, assess the size of the wound, amount and type of drainage, presence of edema, and amount of eschar.
- Ask clients specifically if they have ever taken a sulfonamide and, if so, whether they had an allergic reaction.

With urinary antiseptics, assess for signs and symptoms of UTI.

Nursing Diagnoses

- Risk for Injury: Hypersensitivity reaction, kidney, liver, or blood disorders with sulfonamides
- Knowledge Deficit: Correct administration and use of tetracyclines, sulfonamides, and urinary antiseptics

Planning/Goals

The client will:

- Receive or self-administer the drugs as directed
- Receive prompt and appropriate treatment if adverse effects occur

Interventions

- During tetracycline therapy for systemic infections, monitor laboratory tests of renal function for abnormal values.
- During sulfonamide therapy, encourage sufficient fluids to produce a urine output of at least 1200 to 1500 mL daily. A high fluid intake decreases the risk of crystalluria (precipitation of drug crystals in the urine).
- Avoid urinary catheterization when possible. If catheterization is necessary, use sterile technique. The urinary tract is normally sterile except for the lower third of the urethra. Introduction of any bacteria into the bladder may cause infection.
- A single catheterization may cause infection. With indwelling catheters, bacteria colonize the bladder and produce infection within 2 to 3 weeks, even with meticulous care.
- When indwelling catheters must be used, measures to decrease UTI include using a closed drainage system; keeping the perineal area clean; forcing fluids, if not contraindicated, to maintain a dilute urine; and removing the catheter as soon as possible. Do not disconnect the system and irrigate the catheter unless obstruction is suspected. *Never* raise the urinary drainage bag above bladder level.
- Force fluids in anyone with a UTI unless contraindicated. Bacteria do not multiply as rapidly in

dilute urine. In addition, emptying the bladder frequently allows it to refill with uninfected urine. This decreases the bacterial population of the bladder.

- Teach women to cleanse themselves from the urethral area toward the rectum after voiding or defecating to avoid contamination of the urethral area with bacteria from the vagina and rectum. Also, voiding after sexual intercourse helps cleanse the lower urethra and prevent UTI.

Evaluation

- Observe for improvement in signs of the infection for which drug therapy was given.
- Interview and observe for adverse drug effects.

PRINCIPLES OF THERAPY

Tetracyclines

1. Culture and sensitivity studies are needed before tetracycline therapy is started because many strains of organisms are either resistant or vary greatly in drug susceptibility. Cross-sensitivity and cross-resistance are common among tetracyclines.
2. The oral route of administration is usually effective and preferred. Intravenous therapy is used when oral administration is contraindicated or for initial treatment of severe infections.
3. Tetracyclines decompose with age, exposure to light, and extreme heat and humidity. Because the breakdown products may be toxic, it is very important to store these drugs correctly. Also, the manu-

facturer's expiration dates on containers should be noted and outdated drugs should be discarded.

Sulfonamides and Urinary Antiseptics

1. With systemically absorbed sulfonamides, an initial loading dose may be given to produce therapeutic blood levels (12 to 15 mg/100 mL) more rapidly. The amount is usually twice the maintenance dose.
2. Urine pH is important in drug therapy with sulfonamides and urinary antiseptics.
   a. With sulfonamide therapy, alkaline urine increases drug solubility and helps prevent crystalluria. It also increases the rate of sulfonamide excretion and the concentration of sulfonamide in the urine. The urine can be alkalinized by giving sodium bicarbonate. Alkalinization is not needed with sulfisoxazole (because the drug is highly soluble) or sulfonamides used to treat intestinal infections or burn wounds (because there is little systemic absorption).
   b. With mandelamine therapy, urine pH must be acidic (<5.5) for the drug to be effective. At a higher pH, mandelamine does not hydrolyze to formaldehyde, the antibacterial component. Urine can be acidified by concomitant administration of ascorbic acid.
3. Urine cultures and sensitivity tests are indicated in suspected UTI because of wide variability in possible pathogens and their susceptibility to antibacterial drugs. The best results are obtained with drug therapy indicated by the microorganisms isolated from each client.

CLIENT TEACHING GUIDELINES
Oral Sulfonamides

General Considerations

✔ Sulfonamides inhibit rather than kill bacteria. Thus, it is especially important to take them as prescribed, for the length of time prescribed.

✔ These drugs increase sensitivity to sunlight and risks of sunburn. Avoid sunlamps, tanning beds, and intense or prolonged exposure to sunlight; if unable to avoid exposure, wear protective clothing and a sunblock preparation.

✔ Notify the prescribing physician if you have blood in urine, skin rash, difficulty in breathing, fever, or sore throat. These symptoms may indicate adverse drug effects and the need to change or stop the drug.

Self-administration

✔ Take oral sulfonamides on an empty stomach with a full glass of water.

✔ With oral suspensions, shake well, refrigerate after opening, and discard the unused portion after 14 days.

✔ Drink 2 to 3 quarts of fluid daily, if able. A good fluid intake helps the drugs to be more effective, especially in urinary tract infections, and decreases the likelihood of damaging the kidneys.

Use in Children

Tetracyclines should not be used in children younger than 8 years of age because of their effects on teeth and bones. In teeth, the drugs interfere with enamel development and may cause a permanent yellow, gray, or brown discoloration. In bone, the drugs form a stable compound in bone-forming tissue and may interfere with bone growth.

Systemic sulfonamides are contraindicated during late pregnancy, lactation, and in children younger than 2 months. If a fetus or young infant receives a sulfonamide by placental transfer, in breast milk, or by direct administration, the drug displaces bilirubin from binding sites on albumin. As a result, bilirubin may accumulate in the bloodstream (hyperbilirubinemia) and central nervous system (kernicterus) and cause life-threatening toxicity.

Sulfonamides are often used to treat UTI in children older than 2 months. Few data are available regarding the effects of long-term or recurrent use of sulfamethoxazole (Gantanol) in children younger than 6 years of age with chronic renal disease. Sulfamethoxazole is often given in combination with trimethoprim (Bactrim, Septra), although trimethoprim has not been established as safe and effective in children younger than 12 years of age.

Some clinicians recommend that asymptomatic bacteriuria be treated in children younger than 5 years of age to decrease risks of long-term renal damage. Treatment is the same as for symptomatic UTI.

Use in Older Adults

A major concern with the use of tetracyclines and sulfonamides in older adults is renal impairment, which commonly occurs in this population. Except for doxycycline and minocycline, tetracyclines are contraindicated in clients with renal impairment. Sulfonamides may cause additional renal impairment. As with younger adults, a fluid intake of about 2 L daily is needed to reduce formation of crystals and stones in the urinary tract.

With the combination of sulfamethoxazole and trimethoprim (Bactrim, Septra), older adults are at increased risk for severe adverse effects. Severe skin reactions and bone marrow depression are most often reported. Folic acid deficiency may also occur because both of the drugs interfere with folic acid metabolism.

Use in Renal Impairment

As discussed previously, most tetracyclines are contraindicated in clients with renal impairment. High concentrations of tetracyclines inhibit protein synthesis in human cells. This antianabolic effect increases tissue breakdown (catabolism) and the amount of waste products to be excreted by the kidneys. The increased workload can be

---

> ### Nursing Notes: Apply Your Knowledge
>
> You are working in a nursing home, caring for an elderly, incontinent client who has an indwelling urinary catheter. You notice her urine is cloudy with lots of sediment and it has a strong, foul odor. The client is afebrile and is not complaining of any pain. Analyze these data and discuss how you will proceed.

---

handled by normally functioning kidneys, but waste products are retained when renal function is impaired. This leads to azotemia, increased blood urea nitrogen, hyperphosphatemia, hyperkalemia, and acidosis. If a tetracycline is necessary because of an organism's sensitivity or the host's inability to take other antimicrobial drugs, doxycycline or minocycline may be given.

Systemic sulfonamides should probably be avoided in clients with renal impairment, if other effective drugs are available. Acute renal failure (ARF) has occurred when the drugs or their metabolites precipitated in renal tubules and caused obstruction. ARF is rarely associated with newer sulfonamides, which are more soluble than older ones, but has increased with the use of sulfadiazine to treat toxoplasmosis in clients with acquired immunodeficiency syndrome (AIDS). Preventive measures include a fluid intake of 2 to 3 L daily.

Use in Hepatic Impairment

Tetracyclines are contraindicated in pregnant women because they may cause fatal hepatic necrosis in the mother. They must be used cautiously in the presence of liver or kidney impairment. Because tetracyclines are metabolized in the liver, hepatic impairment or biliary obstruction slows drug elimination. In clients with renal impairment, high intravenous (IV) doses (>2 g/day) have been associated with death from liver failure. If necessary in clients with known or suspected renal and hepatic impairment, renal and liver function test results should be monitored. In addition, serum tetracycline levels should not exceed 15 µg/mL, and other hepatotoxic drugs should be avoided.

Sulfonamides cause cholestatic jaundice in a small percentage of clients and should be used with caution in clients with hepatic impairment.

Use in Critical Illness

Tetracyclines may be used to treat sepsis caused by rickettsial, chlamydial, or mycoplasma infection and pulmonary infection caused by *Mycoplasma pneumoniae* or *Legionella pneumophila*.

When necessary, doxycycline is the drug of choice because it can be given to clients with renal impairment, a common problem in critical care settings.

Sulfonamides are rarely used in critical care settings except for the combination of trimethoprim and sulfamethoxazole (eg, Bactrim) and the topical silver sulfa-

diazine (Silvadene) used to treat burn wounds. Bactrim may be used to treat *Pneumocystis carinii* pneumonia. Although often given IV in critical care settings, oral or nasogastric tube administration may be used in selected clients (eg, clients with AIDS and respiratory failure).

(*text continues on page 553*)

NURSING ACTIONS — Tetracyclines, Sulfonamides, and Urinary Agents

NURSING ACTIONS	RATIONALE/EXPLANATION
1. Administer accurately	
a. With tetracyclines:	
(1) Give oral drugs with food that does not contain dairy products; do not give with or within 2 h of dairy products, antacids, or iron supplements.	To decrease nausea and other gastrointestinal (GI) symptoms. Tetracyclines combine with metallic ions (eg, aluminum, calcium, iron, magnesium) and are not absorbed.
(2) For intravenous (IV) administration, dilute with an appropriate type and amount of IV solution, and infuse over 1–4 h.	Rapid administration should be avoided. IV doses are usually mixed in hospital pharmacies.
b. With sulfonamides:	
(1) Give oral drugs before or after meals, with a full glass of water.	Absorption is better when taken on an empty stomach; however, taking with food decreases GI upset.
(2) Infuse IV trimethoprim-sulfamethoxazole (diluted in 125 mL of 5% dextrose in water) over 60–90 min. Do not mix with other drugs or solutions and flush IV lines to remove any residual drug.	Manufacturer's recommendations
(3) For topical sulfonamides to burn wounds, apply a thin layer with a sterile gloved hand after the surface has been cleansed of previously applied medication.	Burn wounds may be cleansed by whirlpool, shower, or spot cleansing with sterile saline, gauze pads, and gloves.
c. Give nitrofurantoin with or after meals.	Food decreases nausea, vomiting and diarrhea.
2. Observe for therapeutic effects	Therapeutic effects depend on the reason for use.
a. With tetracyclines, observe for decreased signs and symptoms of the infection for which the drug is being given.	
b. With sulfonamides, observe for decreased symptoms of urinary tract infection (UTI), decreased diarrhea when given for ulcerative colitis or bacillary dysentery, lack of fever and wound drainage and evidence of healing in burn wounds.	Topical sulfonamides for burns are used to prevent rather than treat infection.
c. With urinary antiseptics, observe for decreased symptoms of UTI.	
3. Observe for adverse effects	
a. Nausea, vomiting, diarrhea	Commonly occur with tetracyclines, sulfonamides, and urinary antiseptics, probably from local irritation of GI mucosa. After several days of an oral

(*continued*)

NURSING ACTIONS	RATIONALE/EXPLANATION
	tetracycline, diarrhea may be caused by superinfection.
b. Hematologic disorders—anemia, neutropenia, thrombocytopenia	
c. Hypersensitivity—anaphylaxis, skin rash, urticaria, serum sickness	
d. Photosensitivity—sunburn reaction	This can be prevented or minimized by avoiding exposure to sunlight or other sources of ultraviolet light, wearing protective clothing and using sunscreen lotions.
e. Thrombophlebitis at IV infusion sites	These drugs are irritating to tissues. Irritation can be decreased by diluting the drugs and infusing them at the recommended rates.
f. Nephrotoxicity—increased blood urea nitrogen and serum creatinine, hematuria, proteinuria, crystalluria	Nephrotoxicity is more likely to occur in people who already have impaired renal function. Keeping clients well hydrated may help prevent renal damage.
g. Hepatotoxicity—elevated aspartate aminotransferase and other enzymes	Hepatitis, cholestasis, and other serious liver disorders rarely occur with these drugs.
h. Superinfection—sore mouth, white patches on oral mucosa, black, furry tongue, diarrhea, skin rash, itching in the perineal area, pseudomembranous colitis	Superinfection may occur with tetracyclines because of their broad spectrum of antimicrobial activity. Signs and symptoms usually indicate monilial infection.
	Meticulous oral and perineal hygiene helps prevent these problems. The drug should be stopped if severe diarrhea occurs, with blood, mucus, or pus in stools.
4. Observe for drug interactions	
a. Drugs that *decrease* effects of tetracyclines:	
(1) Aluminum, calcium, iron, or magnesium preparations (eg, antacids, ferrous sulfate)	These metals combine with oral tetracyclines to produce insoluble, nonabsorbable compounds that are excreted in feces.
(2) Cathartics	Decrease absorption
(3) Barbiturates, carbamazepine, phenytoin, rifampin	These drugs induce drug-metabolizing enzymes in the liver and may speed up metabolism of doxycycline.
b. Drugs that *increase* effects of sulfonamides:	
(1) Alkalinizing agents (eg, sodium bicarbonate)	Increase rate of urinary excretion, thereby raising levels of sulfonamides in the urinary tract and increasing effectiveness in UTIs
(2) Methenamine compounds, urinary acidifiers (eg, ascorbic acid)	These drugs increase the risk of nephrotoxicity and should not be used with sulfonamides. They may cause precipitation of sulfonamide with resultant blockage of renal tubules.
(3) Salicylates (eg, aspirin), nonsteroidal anti-inflammatory drugs (eg, ibuprofen), oral anticoagulants, phenytoin, methotrexate	Increase toxicity by displacing sulfonamides from plasma protein-binding sites, thereby increasing plasma levels of free drug

(continued)

NURSING ACTIONS	RATIONALE/EXPLANATION
c. Drugs that alter effects of nitrofurantoin:	
(1) Antacids	May decrease absorption
(2) Acidifying agents	Increase antibacterial activity of nitrofurantoin by decreasing renal excretion. Nitrofurantoin is most active against organisms causing UTI when urine pH is 5.5 or less.

How Can You Avoid This Medication Error?

Answer: Bactrim should not be given to this client because he has an allergy to sulfa, and the sulfamethoxazole component is a sulfonamide. You might want to ask him what type of reaction he experienced when he previously took sulfa. If he reports nausea, this is an adverse side effect rather than an allergic response. An allergic response is a histamine-mediated reaction with symptoms such as hives, rash, pruritus, or, in severe cases, bronchospasm and cardiovascular collapse. If any allergic symptoms occurred, hold the medication and call the physician. If the client is not allergic to sulfa, giving one tablet would provide an accurate double-strength (DS) dose.

Nursing Notes: Apply Your Knowledge

Answer: An indwelling catheter significantly increases the incidence of urinary tract infection (UTI). Cloudy, foul-smelling urine with lots of sediment also supports the presence of a UTI. Because of their depressed immune function, elderly clients do not always experience common symptoms of UTI such as fever or pain. Obtain an order for a urine culture and sensitivity so appropriate antibiotics can be prescribed. Encourage fluids, at least 8 glasses per day unless contraindicated. Work on a long-term plan for bladder retraining or intermittent catheterization to decrease risk of chronic, recurrent UTIs.

 REVIEW AND APPLICATION EXERCISES

1. What foods and drugs interfere with absorption of oral tetracyclines? How can interference be prevented or minimized?

2. What are potentially serious adverse effects of tetracyclines?

3. What is the rationale for long-term, low-dose administration of a tetracycline for acne?

4. Which tetracyclines may be given to clients with renal impairment?

5. Why are sulfonamides often effective in UTI?

6. What are major adverse effects of sulfonamides, and how may they be prevented or minimized?

7. What is the rationale for combining sulfamethoxazole and trimethoprim?

8. What are important characteristics of urinary antiseptics?

SELECTED REFERENCES

Drug facts and comparisons. (Updated monthly). St. Louis: Facts and Comparisons.

Kapusnik-Uner, J.E., Sande, M.A., & Chambers, H.F. (1996). Antimicrobial agents: Tetracyclines, chloramphenicol, erythromycin, and miscellaneous antibacterial agents. In J.G. Hardman, L.E. Limbird, P.B. Molinoff, & R.W. Ruddon (Eds.), *Goodman & Gilman's The pharmacological basis of therapeutics*, 9th ed., pp. 1123–1153. New York: McGraw-Hill.

Mandell, G.L. & Petri, W.A. Jr., (1996). Antimicrobial agents: Sulfonamides, trimethoprim-sulfamethoxazole, quinolones, and agents for urinary tract infections. In J.G. Hardman, L.E. Limbird, P.B. Molinoff, & R.W. Ruddon (Eds.), *Goodman & Gilman's The pharmacological basis of therapeutics*, 9th ed., pp. 1057–1072. New York: McGraw-Hill.

Marchiondo, K. (1998). A new look at urinary tract infection. *American Journal of Nursing* 98(3), 34–38.

37

Macrolides and Miscellaneous Antibacterials

Objectives

After studying this chapter, the student will be able to:

1. Discuss characteristics and specific uses of erythromycin and other macrolides.

2. Compare and contrast macrolides with other commonly used antibacterial drugs.

3. Describe the interference of erythromycin with the metabolism of other drugs.

4. Apply principles of using macrolides in selected client situations.

5. Discuss characteristics, indications for use, and precautions for using chloramphenicol, clindamycin, metronidazole, teicoplanin, and vancomycin.

6. Discuss the roles of metronidazole and oral vancomycin in the treatment of pseudomembranous colitis.

You are an infection control nurse who will be providing long-term care nurses with an update on methicillin-resistant *Staphylococcus aureus* (MRSA). Because MRSA has been a significant problem over the last decade, especially in long-term care facilities, your goal is to increase knowledge about the development of drug resistance and appropriate measures to prevent spread of this organism.

Reflect on:

▶ Factors that promote resistance to antibiotics.

▶ Why vancomycin may be the drug of choice for MRSA.

▶ What risks are involved when vancomycin is used consistently to treat MRSA.

▶ What infection control practices are necessary to limit the spread of MRSA and other resistant organisms.

The drugs described in this chapter are heterogeneous in their antimicrobial spectra, characteristics, and clinical uses. Some are used often; some are used only in specific circumstances. The macrolides and other drugs are described in the following sections.

MACROLIDES

The macrolides, which include erythromycin, azithromycin (Zithromax), clarithromycin (Biaxin), and dirithromycin (Dynabac), have similar antibacterial spectra and mechanisms of action. They are widely distributed into body tissues and fluids and may be bacteriostatic or bactericidal, depending on drug concentration in infected tissues. They are effective against gram-positive cocci, including group A streptococci, pneumococci, and most staphylococci. They are also effective against species of *Corynebacterium*, *Treponema*, *Neisseria*, and *Mycoplasma* and against some anaerobic organisms such as *Bacteroides* and *Clostridia*. Azithromycin and clarithromycin also are active against the atypical mycobacteria that cause *Mycobacterium avium* complex (MAC) disease. MAC is an opportunistic infection that occurs mainly in people with advanced human immunodeficiency virus infection.

Erythromycin, the prototype, is now used less often because of microbial resistance, numerous drug interactions, and the development of newer macrolides. Erythromycin is metabolized in the liver and excreted mainly in bile; approximately 20% is excreted in urine. Compared with erythromycin, the newer drugs require less frequent administration and cause less nausea, vomiting, and diarrhea. Azithromycin and dirithromycin are excreted mainly in bile, and clarithromycin is metabolized to an active metabolite in the liver, which is then excreted in urine.

Erythromycin is available in several preparations. Topical and ophthalmic preparations are discussed in Chapters 65 and 66; individual erythromycin formulations and other macrolides are listed in Table 37-1.

Mechanism of Action

The macrolides enter microbial cells and attach to 50S ribosomes, thereby inhibiting microbial protein synthesis.

Indications for Use

The macrolides are widely used for treatment of respiratory tract and skin/soft tissue infections caused by streptococci and staphylococci. Erythromycin is also used as a penicillin substitute in clients who are allergic to penicillin; for prevention of rheumatic fever, gonorrhea, syphilis, pertussis, and chlamydial conjunctivitis in newborns (ophthalmic ointment); and to treat other infections (eg, Legionnaire's disease, genitourinary infections caused by *Chlamydia trachomatis*, intestinal amebiasis caused by *Entamoeba histolytica*).

In addition, azithromycin is approved for treatment of urethritis and cervicitis caused by *C. trachomatis* organisms, and is being used for the prevention and treatment of MAC disease, although it is not yet approved by the Food and Drug Administration for this indication. Clarithromycin is approved for prevention and treatment of MAC disease. For prevention, clarithromycin may be used alone; for treatment, it is combined with one or two other drugs (eg, ethambutol or rifabutin) to prevent the emergence of drug-resistant organisms. Clarithromycin is also used to treat *Helicobacter pylori* infections associated with peptic ulcer disease.

Contraindications to Use

The drugs are contraindicated in people who have hypersensitivity reactions to macrolides. They are also contraindicated or must be used with caution in clients with pre-existing liver disease.

MISCELLANEOUS ANTIBACTERIAL DRUGS

Chloramphenicol

Chloramphenicol is a broad-spectrum, bacteriostatic antibiotic that is active against most gram-positive and gram-negative bacteria, rickettsiae, chlamydiae, and treponemes. It acts by interfering with microbial protein synthesis. It is well absorbed and diffuses well into body tissues and fluids, including cerebrospinal fluid (CSF), but low drug levels are obtained in urine. It is metabolized in the liver and excreted in the urine.

Chloramphenicol is rarely used in infections caused by gram-positive organisms because of the effectiveness and low toxicity of penicillins, cephalosporins, and macrolides. It is the drug of choice only in typhoid fever. Otherwise, it is indicated for use in serious infections for which no adequate substitute drug is available. Specific infections include meningococcal, pneumococcal, or *Hemophilus* meningitis in penicillin-allergic clients; anaerobic brain abscess; *Bacteroides fragilis* infections; rickettsial infections and brucellosis when tetracyclines are contraindicated; and *Klebsiella* and *Hemophilus* infections that are resistant to other drugs.

ROUTES AND DOSAGE RANGES

Adults: Oral (PO), intravenous (IV) 50–100 mg/kg/d, in four divided doses, q6h

Children and full-term infants >2 wk: PO 50 mg/kg/d, in three or four divided doses, q6–8h

TABLE 37-1 **Macrolides**

Generic/Trade Name	Usual Routes and Dosage Ranges	
	Adults	Children
Azithromycin (Zithromax)	Respiratory and skin infections, PO 500 mg as a single dose on the first day, then 250 mg once daily for 4 d. Nongonococcal urethritis and cervicitis caused by *Chlamydia trachomatis,* give 1 g as a single dose.	6 mo and older: Acute otitis media PO, 10 mg/kg as a single dose (not to exceed 500 mg) on the first day, then 5 mg/kg (not to exceed 250 mg) once daily for 4 d 2 y and older: Pharyngitis/tonsillitis, PO 12 mg/kg (not to exceed 500 mg) once daily for 5 d
Clarithromycin (Biaxin)	PO 250–500 mg q12h for 7 to 14 d. Prevention or treatment of MAC, PO 500 mg q12h	PO 7.5 mg/kg q12h, not to exceed 500 mg q12h Prevention or treatment of MAC: same as above
Dirithromycin (Dynabac)	Bronchitis caused by *Streptococcus pneumoniae* or *Moraxella catarrhalis* and skin infections caused by methicillin-susceptible *Staphylococcus aureus*, PO 500 mg once daily for 7 d Pharyngitis/tonsillitis caused by *Streptococcus pyogenes,* PO 500 mg once daily for 10 d Community-acquired pneumonia caused by *Legionella pneumophila, Mycoplasma pneumoniae* or *S. pneumoniae* PO 500 mg once daily for 14 d	Dosage not established
Erythromycin base (E-mycin)	PO 250–500 mg q6h; severe infections, up to 4 g or more daily in divided doses	PO 30–50 mg/kg/d in divided doses q6–12h, severe infections, 100 mg/kg/d in divided doses
Erythromycin estolate (Ilosone)	PO 250 mg q6h; maximal daily dose, 4 g	Weight >25 kg, PO same as adults Weight 10–25 kg, PO 30–50 mg/kg/d in divided doses Weight <10 kg, PO 10 mg/kg/d in divided doses q6–12h Dosages may be doubled in severe infections.
Erythromycin ethylsuccinate (E.E.S.)	PO 400 mg four times daily; severe infections, up to 4 g or more daily in divided doses	PO 30–50 mg/kg/d in four divided doses q6h. Severe infections, 60–100 mg/kg/d in divided doses
Erythromycin lactobionate	IV 15–20 mg/kg/d in divided doses; severe infections, up to 4 g daily	IV same as adults
Erthromycin stearate (Erythrocin stearate)	PO 250 mg q6h or 500 mg q12h; severe infections, up to 4 g daily	PO 30–50 mg/kg/d in four divided doses q6h; severe infections, 60–100 mg/kg/d

IV, intravenous; PO, oral.

Clindamycin

Clindamycin is similar to the macrolides in its mechanism of action and antimicrobial spectrum. It is bacteriostatic in usual doses. It is effective against gram-positive cocci, including group A streptococci, pneumococci, most staphylococci, and some anaerobes such as *Bacteroides* and *Clostridia.* Clindamycin enters microbial cells and attaches to 50S ribosomes, thereby inhibiting microbial protein synthesis.

Clindamycin is often used to treat infections caused by *B. fragilis.* Because these bacteria are usually mixed with gram-negative organisms from the gynecologic or gastrointestinal (GI) tracts, clindamycin is usually given with another drug, such as gentamicin, to treat mixed infections. The drug may be useful as a penicillin substitute in clients who are allergic to penicillin and who have serious streptococcal, staphylococcal, or pneumococcal infections in which the causative organism is sensitive to clindamycin. A topical solution is used in the treatment of acne, and a vaginal cream is available. Despite its effectiveness in infections caused by gram-positive microorganisms, clindamycin should be used only in infections in which it is clearly more effective than other drugs (eg, anaerobic infections) because of the diarrhea and pseudomembranous colitis associated with its use. Clindamycin does not reach therapeutic concentrations in the central nervous system (CNS) and should not be used for treating meningitis.

Clindamycin is well absorbed with oral administration and reaches peak plasma levels within 1 hour after a dose. It is widely distributed in body tissues and fluids, except

CSF, and crosses the placenta. It is highly bound (≥90%) to plasma proteins. It is metabolized in the liver, and the metabolites are excreted in bile and urine. Dosage may need to be reduced in clients with severe hepatic failure to prevent accumulation and toxic effects.

Clindamycin Hydrochloride

ROUTE AND DOSAGE RANGES

Adults: PO 150–300 mg q6h; up to 450 mg q6h for severe infections

Children: PO 8–16 mg/kg/d in three or four divided doses, q6–8h; up to 20 mg/kg/d in severe infections

Clindamycin Phosphate

ROUTES AND DOSAGE RANGES

Adults: Intramuscular (IM) 600 mg—2.7 g/d in two to four divided doses, q6–12h

IV 600 mg—2.7 g/d in two to four divided doses; up to 4.8 g/d in life-threatening infections

Children: IM, IV 15–40 mg/kg/d in three or four divided doses, q6–8h; up to 40 mg/kg/d in severe infections

Clindamycin Palmitate Hydrochloride (Cleocin Pediatric—75 mg/mL)

ROUTE AND DOSAGE RANGES

Children: PO 8–12 mg/kg/d in three or four divided doses; up to 25 mg/kg/d in very severe infections. For children weighing 10 kg or less, the minimum dose is 37.5 mg, three times per day.

Metronidazole

Metronidazole (Flagyl) is effective against anaerobic bacteria, including gram-negative bacilli such as *Bacteroides*, gram-positive bacilli such as *Clostridium*, and some gram-positive cocci. It is also effective against protozoa that cause amebiasis, giardiasis, and trichomoniasis (see Chap. 41).

Clinical indications for use include prevention or treatment of anaerobic bacterial infections (eg, in colorectal surgery and intra-abdominal infections) and treatment of *Clostridium difficile* infections associated with pseudomembranous colitis. It is contraindicated during the first trimester of pregnancy and must be used with caution in clients with CNS or blood disorders.

Metronidazole is carcinogenic in rodents, if given in high doses for prolonged periods, but there is no evidence that people treated with therapeutic doses have increased risks for development of cancer. Metronidazole is widely distributed in body fluids and tissues, metabolized in the liver, and excreted mostly (60% to 80%) in urine, with a small amount excreted in feces.

ROUTES AND DOSAGE RANGES

Adults: Anaerobic bacterial infection, IV 15 mg/kg (approximately 1 g for a 70-kg adult) as a loading dose, infused over 1 h, followed by 7.5 mg/kg (approximately 500 mg for a 70-kg adult) q6h as a maintenance dose, infused over 1 h; duration usually 7–10 d; maximum dose 4 g/24 h.

Surgical prophylaxis, colorectal surgery, IV 15 mg/kg, infused over 30–60 min, infusion to be completed approximately 1 h before surgery, followed by 7.5 mg/kg, infused over 30–60 min, at 6 h and 12 h after the initial dose

C. difficile colitis, PO 1–2 g daily for 7–10 d

Spectinomycin

Spectinomycin is used for treatment of gonococcal exposure or infection in people who are allergic to or unable to take preferred drugs (the cephalosporins ceftriaxone or cefixime, or the fluoroquinolones ciprofloxacin or ofloxacin). It may be used during pregnancy when clients cannot tolerate cephalosporins and when fluoroquinolones are contraindicated. Spectinomycin has no activity against infections caused by *Chlamydia* organisms, which often accompany gonorrhea.

ROUTE AND DOSAGE RANGE

Adults: IM 2 g in a single dose

Vancomycin and Teicoplanin

Vancomycin and **teicoplanin** (Targocid) are active only against gram-positive microorganisms. They act by inhibiting cell wall synthesis. Vancomycin is indicated only for the treatment of severe infections. Parenteral vancomycin has been used extensively to treat infections caused by methicillin-resistant *Staphylococcus aureus* (MRSA) and *Staphylococcus epidermidis* (MRSE) and endocarditis caused by *Streptococcus viridans* (in clients allergic to or with infections resistant to penicillins and cephalosporins) or *Enterococcus faecalis* (with an aminoglycoside). The drug has also been widely used for prophylaxis of gram-positive infections in clients requiring long-term use of intravascular catheters and other invasive treatment or monitoring devices and to treat infections caused by penicillin-resistant *Streptococcus pneumoniae*. Oral vancomycin has been used extensively to treat staphylococcal enterocolitis and pseudomembranous colitis caused by *C. difficile*.

Partly because of this widespread use, vancomycin-resistant enterococci (VRE) are being encountered more often, especially in critical care units, and treatment options for infections caused by these organisms are very limited. To decrease the spread of VRE, the Centers for Disease Control and Prevention recommends limiting the use of vancomycin. Specific recommendations include avoiding or minimizing use in empiric treatment of febrile clients with neutropenia (unless the prevalence of MRSA or MRSE is high); initial treatment for *C. difficile* colitis (metronidazole is preferred); and prophylaxis for surgery, low-birthweight infants, intravascular catheter colonization or infection, and peritoneal dialysis.

For systemic infections, vancomycin is given IV and reaches therapeutic plasma levels within 1 hour after infusion. It is very important to give IV infusions slowly, over 1 to 2 hours, to avoid an adverse reaction characterized by hypotension and flushing and skin rash. This reaction, sometimes called *red man syndrome*, is attributed to histamine release. Vancomycin is excreted through the kidneys; dosage should be reduced in the presence of renal impairment. For bacterial colitis, vancomycin is given orally because it is not absorbed from the GI tract and acts within the bowel lumen. Large amounts of vancomycin are excreted in the feces after oral administration.

Teicoplanin is a newer drug that is similar to vancomycin and reportedly as effective as vancomycin in the treatment of streptococcal and staphylococcal infections. It also may be effective in some enterococcal infections that are resistant to vancomycin. It is excreted almost entirely by the kidneys, and dosage should be reduced with renal impairment. Teicoplanin differs from vancomycin in that it can be given IM as well as IV for systemic infections, it does not cause red man syndrome, and it can be given once daily for most infections because it has a long serum half-life.

Vancomycin

ROUTES AND DOSAGE RANGES

Adults: PO 500 mg q6h or 1 g q12h; maximum dose, 4 g/d
IV 2 g/d in two to four divided doses, q6–12h
Children: PO, IV 40 mg/kg/d in divided doses
Infants and Neonates: IV 15 mg/kg initially, then 10 mg/kg q12h for neonates up to 7 d of age, then q8h up to 1 mo of age

Teicoplanin

ROUTES AND DOSAGE RANGES

Adults: IV, IM 6 mg/kg/d, up to 30 mg/kg/d for serious staphylococcal infections

---

NURSING PROCESS

Assessment

- Assess for infections that macrolides and the designated miscellaneous drugs are used to prevent or treat.
- Assess each client for signs and symptoms of the specific current infection.

- Assess culture and susceptibility reports when available.
- Assess each client for risk factors that increase risks of infection (eg, immunosuppression) or risks of adverse drug reactions (eg, impaired renal or hepatic function).

Nursing Diagnoses

- Knowledge Deficit related to type of infection
- Knowledge Deficit related to appropriate use of prescribed antimicrobial drugs
- Risk for Injury related to adverse drug effects
- Risk for Injury related to infection with antibiotic-resistant microorganisms

Planning/Goals

The client will:

- Take or receive macrolides and miscellaneous antimicrobials accurately, for the prescribed length of time
- Experience decreased signs and symptoms of the infection being treated
- Be monitored regularly for therapeutic and adverse drug effects
- Verbalize and practice measures to prevent recurrent infection

Interventions

- Use measures to prevent and minimize the spread of infection (see Chap. 33).
- Monitor for fever and other signs and symptoms of infection.
- Monitor laboratory reports for indications of the client's response to drug therapy (eg, white blood cells [WBC], tests of renal function).
- Encourage fluid intake to decrease fever and maintain good urinary tract function.
- Provide foods and fluids with adequate nutrients to maintain or improve nutritional status, especially if febrile and hypermetabolic.
- Assist clients to prevent or minimize infections with streptococci, staphylococci, and other gram-positive organisms

CLIENT TEACHING GUIDELINES
Macrolides

General Considerations

✔ Complete the full course of drug therapy. The fastest and most complete relief of infections occurs with accurate usage of antibiotics. Moreover, inaccurate use may cause other, potentially more severe infections.

✔ These drugs are often given for infections of the respiratory tract or skin (eg, bronchitis, pneumonia, cellulitis). Good hand washing can help prevent the development and spread of these infections.

✔ Report symptoms of infection that recur or develop during antibiotic therapy. Such symptoms can indicate recurrence of the original infection (ie, the antibiotic is not effective because it is the wrong drug or wrong dosage for the infection or it is not being taken accurately) or a new infection with antibiotic-resistant bacteria or fungi.

✔ Report nausea, vomiting, diarrhea, abdominal cramping or pain, yellow discoloration of the skin or eyes (jaundice), dark urine, pale stools, or unusual tiredness. These symptoms may indicate liver damage, which sometimes occurs with these drugs.

Self-administration

✔ Take each dose with 6 to 8 oz of water, at evenly spaced time intervals, preferably around the clock.

✔ With erythromycin, ask a health care provider if not instructed when to take the drug in relation to food. Erythromycin is available in several preparations. Some should be taken on an empty stomach (at least 1 hour before or 2 hours after meals) or may be taken with a small amount of food if gastrointestinal upset occurs. Some preparations may be taken without regard to meals.

✔ Take azithromycin (Zithromax) oral solution on an empty stomach, 1 h before or 2 h after a meal; take tablets without regard to meals. Do not take with an antacid.

✔ Take clarithromycin (Biaxin) without regard to meals. With the oral suspension, do not refrigerate, and shake well before measuring the dose.

✔ Take dirithromycin (Dynabac) with food or within 1 hour of having eaten. Do not cut, chew, or crush the tablets.

PRINCIPLES OF THERAPY

Culture and Susceptibility Studies

Specimens for culture and sensitivity studies should be obtained before the first dose of macrolides and clindamycin because these drugs have a narrow spectrum of antibacterial activity and some organisms are resistant. Drug therapy is often started before results are available, especially with serious infections.

Effects of Erythromycin on Other Drugs

Erythromycin interferes with the elimination of several drugs, especially those metabolized by the cytochrome P450 enzymes in the liver. As a result, the affected drugs are eliminated more slowly, their serum levels are increased, and they are more likely to cause adverse effects and toxicity unless dosage is reduced. Interacting drugs include alfentanil (Alfenta), bromocriptine (Parlodel), carbamazepine (Tegretol), cyclosporine (Sandimmune), digoxin (Lanoxin), disopyramide (Norpace), methylprednisolone (Medrol), theophylline (Theo-Dur), triazolam (Halcion), and warfarin (Coumadin). These drugs represent a variety of drug classes. Erythromycin is contraindicated in clients who are receiving fluoro-quinolone antibacterials (eg, ciprofloxacin) because serious ventricular arrhythmias and fatalities have been reported.

Preventing Toxicity With Chloramphenicol

Clients taking chloramphenicol need a complete blood count, platelet count, reticulocyte count, and serum iron every 3 days. These tests are necessary because chloramphenicol may lead to serious bone marrow depression, including aplastic anemia. In addition, periodic measurements of serum drug levels are recommended. Therapeutic levels are 10 to 20 μg/mL.

Preventing Toxicity With Clindamycin

If diarrhea develops in a client receiving clindamycin, stools should be checked for WBC, blood, and mucus, and proctoscopy should be done to determine whether the client has pseudomembranous colitis, a potentially fatal adverse reaction. If lesions are seen on proctoscopy, the drug should be stopped immediately. Although pseudomembranous colitis may occur with any antibiotic, it has often been associated with clindamycin therapy.

After gynecologic surgery, Susan Miller contracts a serious wound infection. She is treated with IV clindamycin and IV gentamicin. After 5 days of treatment, Ms. Miller develops severe diarrhea (12 watery, bloody stools per day) and feels dizzy and weak, especially when getting out of bed. She is afebrile. Based on these assessment data, how should you proceed?

Use in Children

Erythromycin is in general considered safe for treatment of infections caused by susceptible organisms. Oral azithromycin is used in young children for some infections, but safety and effectiveness of the IV formulation have not been established for children younger than 16 years of age. Clarithromycin has been used in young children; safety and effectiveness of dirithromycin have not been established for children younger than 12 years of age.

Dosage of chloramphenicol must be reduced in premature infants and in full-term infants less than 2 weeks of age because impaired metabolism may lead to accumulation and adverse effects. Clindamycin should be given to neonates and infants only if clearly indicated, and then liver and kidney function must be monitored. Diarrhea and pseudomembranous colitis may occur with topical clindamycin for treatment of acne. The safety and efficacy of metronidazole have been established in children only for the treatment of amebiasis. Vancomycin is often used in children, including preterm and full-term neonates, for the same indications as in adults. Monitoring serum drug levels is recommended with IV vancomycin.

Use in Older Adults

Erythromycin is in general considered safe. Because it is metabolized in the liver and excreted in bile, it may be useful in clients with impaired renal function. Dosage reductions are not indicated with azithromycin and dirithromycin, but may be needed if clarithromycin is given to older adults with severe renal impairment. The miscellaneous drugs are used in older adults for the same indications as in younger adults. Dosage of vancomycin should be reduced when renal function is impaired, a common condition in older adults.

Use in Renal Impairment

With the macrolides, dosage of erythromycin does not need reduction because it is excreted mainly by the liver. With the newer drugs, there are no data about azithromycin dosage in renal impairment and no dosage reduc-

tion is recommended for dirithromycin. However, clarithromycin dosage should be halved or the dosing interval doubled in clients with severe renal impairment (creatinine clearance [CrCl] <30 mL/minute). In addition, the combination of clarithromycin and ranitidine bismuth citrate therapy (Tritec; used to treat peptic ulcers associated with *H. pylori* infection) is not recommended in clients with severe renal impairment (CrCl <25 mL/minute)

Dosage of clindamycin does not need reduction in renal impairment because it is excreted primarily by the liver. Dosage of vancomycin and teicoplanin should be reduced because they are excreted mainly by the kidneys and accumulate in renal impairment. In addition, vancomycin may be nephrotoxic with IV administration, high serum concentrations, prolonged therapy, use in elderly or neonates, and concomitant use of other nephrotoxic drugs. Thus, in addition to reduced dosage, renal function and serum drug levels should be monitored (therapeutic levels are 10 to 25 µg/mL).

Use in Hepatic Impairment

Erythromycin should be used cautiously, if at all, in clients with hepatic impairment. It is metabolized in the liver to an active metabolite that is excreted in the bile. Avoiding the drug or dosage reduction may be needed in liver failure. It has also been associated with cholestatic hepatitis, most often with the estolate formulation (eg, Ilosone). Symptoms, which may include nausea, vomiting, fever, and jaundice, usually occur after 1 to 2 weeks of drug administration and subside when the drug is stopped.

Other macrolides vary in their hepatic effects. Azithromycin is mainly eliminated unchanged in bile and could accumulate with impaired liver function. It should be used with caution. Clarithromycin is metabolized in the liver to an active metabolite that is then excreted through the kidneys. Dosage reduction is not recommended for clients with hepatic impairment and normal renal function but is required with severe renal impairment (see above). Dirithromycin is metabolized in the liver to an active metabolite that is then excreted in bile and feces. No dosage reduction is recommended for mild hepatic impairment. Because effects in moderate to severe hepatic impairment have not been studied, the drug should be used only if absolutely necessary.

Clindamycin, chloramphenicol, and metronidazole should be used cautiously, if at all, in the presence of liver disease. Because these drugs are eliminated through the liver, they may accumulate and cause toxic effects. When feasible, other drugs should be substituted. If no effective substitutes are available, dosage should be reduced.

Use in Critical Illness

Erythromycin is seldom used in critical care settings, partly because broader-spectrum bactericidal drugs are usually needed in critically ill clients, and partly because it inhibits liver metabolism and slows elimination of several other drugs. For a critically ill client who needs a macrolide antibiotic, one of the newer drugs is preferred because they have broader spectrums of antibacterial activity and apparently do not alter metabolism of other drugs.

Clindamycin should be used only when necessary (ie, for serious infections caused by susceptible anaerobes) because critically ill clients may develop hepatic impairment and pseudomembranous colitis (also called antibiotic-associated colitis). These clients are at high risk for development of pseudomembranous colitis because they often receive aggressive antibiotic therapy with multiple or broad-spectrum antibacterial drugs that destroy normal bowel microorganisms. Metronidazole is often used in critically ill clients with mixed infections. These clients are at risk for drug toxicity from accumulation of active metabolites. Vancomycin penetrates tissues well in critically ill clients and achieves therapeutic levels well

above the minimum inhibitory concentration for most staphylococci and enterococci. Plasma drug levels and renal function should be monitored. Although usually given by IV infusion, vancomycin is given orally to treat pseudomembranous colitis.

 Home Care

Most of the macrolides and miscellaneous drugs may be taken in the home setting. The role of the home care nurse is generally the same as with other antibiotic therapy; that is, the nurse may need to teach clients or caregivers about drug administration and expected effects. For clients taking oral metronidazole or vancomycin for pseudomembranous colitis, stool specimens may need to be collected and tested in the laboratory for *C. difficile* organisms or toxins.

(*text continues on page 564*)

NURSING ACTIONS	Macrolides and Miscellaneous Antibacterials

NURSING ACTIONS	RATIONALE/EXPLANATION
1. Administer accurately	
a. Give oral erythromycin preparations according to manufacturers' instructions, with 6 to 8 oz of water, at evenly spaced intervals, around the clock.	Some should be taken on an empty stomach; some can be taken without regard to meals. Adequate water aids absorption; regular intervals help to maintain therapeutic blood levels.
b. With azithromycin, give the oral suspension on an empty stomach, 1 h before or 2 h after a meal. Give tablets without regard to meals. Do not give oral azithromycin with aluminum- or magnesium-containing antacids.	Food decreases absorption of the suspension; antacids decrease absorption of tablets and the suspension
c. With clarithromycin, give with or without food. Shake the suspension well before measuring the dose.	All suspensions should be mixed well to measure accurately.
d. With dirithromycin, give with food or within 1 h after a meal.	
e. For intravenous (IV) erythromycin, consult the manufacturer's instructions for dissolving, diluting, and administering the drug. Infuse continuously or intermittently (eg, q6h over 30–60 min).	The IV formulation has limited stability in solution, and instructions must be followed carefully to achieve therapeutic effects. Also, instructions differ for intermittent and continuous infusions. IV erythromycin is the treatment of choice for Legionnaire's disease. Otherwise, it is rarely used.
f. With chloramphenicol:	
(1) Give oral drug 1 h before or 2 h after meals, q6h around the clock. If gastrointestinal (GI) upset occurs, give with food.	To increase absorption and maintain therapeutic blood levels

(continued)

NURSING ACTIONS	RATIONALE/EXPLANATION
(2) Mix IV chloramphenicol in 50–100 mL of 5% dextrose in water and infuse over 15–30 min.	
g. With clindamycin:	
(1) Give capsules with a full glass of water.	To avoid esophageal irritation
(2) Do not refrigerate reconstituted oral solution.	Refrigeration is not required for drug stability and may thicken the solution, making it difficult to measure and pour accurately.
(3) Give intramuscular injections deeply, and rotate sites. Do not give more than 600 mg in a single injection.	To decrease pain, induration, and abscess formation
(4) For IV administration, dilute 300 mg in 50 mL of IV fluid and give over 10 min, or dilute 600 mg in 100 mL and give over 20 min. *Do not* give clindamycin undiluted or by direct injection.	Dilution decreases risks of phlebitis. Cardiac arrest has been reported with bolus injections of clindamycin.
h. With IV metronidazole, check the manufacturer's instructions.	The drug requires specific techniques for preparation and administration.
i. With vancomycin, dilute 500-mg doses in 100 mL and 1-g doses in 200 mL of 0.9% NaCl or 5% dextrose injection and infuse over at least 60 min.	To decrease hypotension and flushing (ie, "red man syndrome") that may occur with more rapid IV administration. This reaction is attributed to histamine release and may be prevented by prior administration of diphenhydramine, an antihistamine. Dilution also decreases pain and phlebitis at the injection site.
2. Observe for therapeutic effects	
a. Decreased local and systemic signs of infection	See Chapter 33.
b. Decreased signs and symptoms of the specific infection for which the drug is being given	
3. Observe for adverse effects	
a. With macrolides:	
(1) Nausea, vomiting, diarrhea	These are the most frequent adverse reactions, reportedly less common with azithromycin and clarithromycin than with erythromycin.
(2) With IV erythromycin, phlebitis at the IV infusion site	The drug is very irritating to body tissues. Phlebitis can be minimized by diluting the drug well, infusing it slowly, and not using the same vein more than 48–72 h, if possible.
(3) Hepatotoxicity—nausea, vomiting, abdominal cramps, fever, leukocytosis, abnormal liver function, and possibly jaundice	More likely to occur with the estolate formulation of erythromycin, but has been reported with other preparations as well
(4) Allergic reactions (anaphylaxis, skin rash, urticaria)	Potentially serious but infrequent
b. With chloramphenicol:	
(1) Anemia, leukopenia, thrombocytopenia	Blood dyscrasias are the most serious adverse reaction to chloramphenicol. They are caused by bone marrow depression.

(continued)

NURSING ACTIONS	RATIONALE/EXPLANATION

(2) Clinical signs of infection or bleeding

c. With clindamycin:

(1) Nausea, vomiting, diarrhea

These are the most frequent adverse effects and may be severe enough to require stopping the drug.

(2) Pseudomembranous colitis (also called antibiotic-associated colitis)—severe diarrhea, fever, stools containing neutrophils and shreds of mucous membrane

May occur with most antibiotics but is more common with oral clindamycin. It is caused by *Clostridium difficile*. The organism produces a toxin that kills mucosal cells and produces superficial ulcerations that are visible with sigmoidoscopy. Discontinuing the drug and giving oral metronidazole are curative measures.

d. With metronidazole:

(1) Central nervous system effects—convulsive seizures, peripheral paresthesias, ataxia, confusion, dizziness, headache

Convulsions and peripheral neuropathy may be serious effects; GI effects are most common.

(2) GI effects—nausea, vomiting, diarrhea

(3) Dermatologic effects—skin rash, pruritus, thrombophlebitis at infusion site

e. With vancomycin:

(1) Nephrotoxicity—oliguria, increased blood urea nitrogen and serum creatinine

Uncommon. Most likely to occur with large doses, concomitant administration of an aminoglycoside antibiotic, or pre-existing renal impairment. Usually resolves when vancomycin is discontinued.

(2) Ototoxicity—hearing loss, tinnitus

Most likely to occur in people with renal impairment or a preexisting hearing loss

(3) Red man syndrome—hypotension, skin flushing

Occurs with rapid infusion of IV vancomycin. Can be prevented by adequate dilution and infusing over 1–2 h or premedicating with diphenhydramine (an antihistamine). This reaction does not occur with teicoplanin.

4. Observe for drug interactions

a. Drugs that *decrease* effects of azithromycin:

(1) Antacids

Antacids decrease peak serum levels

b. Drug that *increases* effects of clarithromycin:

(1) Fluconazole

c. Drugs that *increase* effects of dirithyromycin:

(1) Antacids, histamine-2 (H₂) receptor antagonists

These agents raise gastric pH and slightly increase absorption of dirithromycin.

d. Drugs that *increase* effects of erythromycin:

(1) Chloramphenicol

The combination is effective against some strains of resistant *Staphylococcus aureus*.

(2) Streptomycin

The combination is effective against the enterococcus in bacteremia, brain abscess, endocarditis, meningitis, and urinary tract infection

e. Drugs that *decrease* effects of chloramphenicol:

(continued)

NURSING ACTIONS	RATIONALE/EXPLANATION
(1) Barbiturates, rifampin	Reduce serum levels, probably by accelerating liver metabolism of chloramphenicol
f. Drugs that *decrease* effects of clindamycin: (1) Erythromycin (2) Kaolin-pectin	 Delays absorption
g. Drug that *increases* effects of metronidazole: (1) Cimetidine	 Inhibits hepatic metabolism
h. Drugs that *decrease* effects of metronidazole: (1) Phenobarbital, phenytoin, prednisone, rifampin	 These drugs induce hepatic enzymes and decrease effects of metronidazole by accelerating its rate of hepatic metabolism.

How Can You Avoid This Medication Error?

Answer: This error occurred because the drug infused too rapidly. Although the IV rate was calculated correctly, the IV could have been positional, which could have caused the sudden infusing of medication. When giving a medication such as this, it is best to use an IV controller pump to regulate the infusion rate. The rapid infusion of vancomycin caused the flushing, which is sometimes referred to as the "red man effect." This is not an allergic reaction, but is caused by histamine release and vasodilation when infusion is too fast. This reaction can be limited by slowing the infusion or premedication with an antihistamine.

Nursing Notes: Apply Your Knowledge

Answer: Diarrhea is a side effect of many antibiotics. When diarrhea is severe, it is important to determine if the cause is pseudomembranous colitis, which is caused when antibiotics suppress the growth of normal flora and allow the overgrowth of *Clostridium difficile*. This organism produces a toxin that kills mucosal cells and creates ulcerations. Pseudomembranous colitis is often associated with the use of clindamycin. Contact the physician for an order for a stool culture for *C. difficile* (C-diff). Treatment includes metronidazole (Flagyl) or oral vancomycin. Ms. Miller's dizziness may be caused by volume depletion. Adequate fluids must be restored to prevent shock.

REVIEW AND APPLICATION EXERCISES

1. Why is erythromycin called a penicillin substitute?
2. What are adverse effects with erythromycin, and how may they be prevented or minimized?

3. How do the newer macrolides differ from erythromycin?
4. How would you recognize pseudomembranous colitis in a client? What would you do if you thought a client might have it? Why?
5. Why is metronidazole preferred over vancomycin for initial treatment of pseudomembranous colitis?
6. Which antibacterial drug is considered the drug of choice for MRSA and MRSE?
7. What is "red man syndrome," and how can it be prevented or minimized?

SELECTED REFERENCES

Belliveau, R.P., Rothman, A.L., & Maday, C.E. (1996). Limiting vancomycin use to combat vancomycin-resistant *Enterococcus faecium*. *American Journal of Health-System Pharmacy, 53*, 1570–1575.

Drug facts and comparisons. (Updated monthly). St. Louis: Facts and Comparisons.

Horsburgh, C.R., Jr. (1996). Advances in the prevention and treatment of *Mycobacterium avium* disease (editorial). *New England Journal of Medicine, 335*, 428–429.

Kapusnik-Uner, J.E., Sande, M.A., & Chambers, H.F. (1996). Antimicrobial agents: Tetracyclines, chloramphenicol, erythromycin, and miscellaneous antibacterial agents. In J.G. Hardman, L.E. Limbird, P.B. Molinoff, & R.W. Ruddon (Eds.), *Goodman & Gilman's The pharmacological basis of therapeutics*, 9th ed., pp. 1123–1153. New York: McGraw-Hill.

Pierce, M., Crampton, S., Henry, D., et al. (1996). A randomized trial of clarithromycin as prophylaxis against disseminated *Mycobacterium avium* complex infection in patients with advanced acquired immunodeficiency syndrome. *New England Journal of Medicine, 335*, 384–391.

Woeltje, K.F. & Ritchie, D.J. (1998). Antimicrobials. In C.F. Carey, H.H. Lee, & K.F. Woeltje (Eds.), *The Washington manual of medical therapeutics*, 29th ed., pp. 244–259. Philadelphia: Lippincott Williams & Wilkins.

38

Drugs for Tuberculosis and Mycobacterium avium Complex (MAC) Disease

Objectives

After studying this chapter, the student will be able to:

1. Describe unique characteristics of tuberculosis infection.

2. Discuss the increased incidence of tuberculosis, especially multidrug-resistant tuberculosis (MDR-TB).

3. Identify populations at high risk for contracting tuberculosis.

4. List characteristics, uses, effects, and nursing implications of using isoniazid, rifampin, and pyrazinamide.

5. Describe the rationale for multiple drug therapy in treatment of tuberculosis.

6. Discuss common problems associated with drug therapy of drug-susceptible and MDR-TB.

7. Discuss the use of aminoglycosides and fluoroquinolones in the treatment of MDR-TB.

8. Describe *Mycobacterium avium* complex disease and the drugs used to prevent or treat it.

John Phillips, a homeless person with a history of drug and alcohol abuse, comes to the emergency department with a productive cough, complaints of night sweats, and fatigue. The physician suspects tuberculosis (TB) and orders a purified protein derivative (PPD), chest x-ray, and sputum for acid-fast bacillus.

Reflect on:

▶ The necessary infection control measures to use before TB is confirmed or ruled out.

▶ Why multidrug treatment would be important if TB is confirmed.

▶ Factors that affect compliance with drug treatment for John Phillips and a plan to improve and monitor compliance.

▶ How long Mr. Phillips will require drug treatment, and how you can evaluate when the TB is cured.

TUBERCULOSIS

Tuberculosis is an infectious disease that usually affects the lungs but may involve the kidneys, meninges, bone, adrenal glands, and gastrointestinal (GI) tract. It commonly occurs in many parts of the world and has increased in the United States in recent years. This increase is largely attributed to a high incidence in people with acquired immunodeficiency syndrome (AIDS) and in immigrants from countries where the disease is common. There is also an increase in drug-resistant tuberculosis.

Tuberculosis is caused by *Mycobacterium tuberculosis*, the tubercle bacillus. These organisms multiply slowly; they may lie dormant in the body for many years, encapsulated in calcified tubercles; they resist phagocytosis and survive in phagocytic cells; and they develop resistance to antitubercular drugs.

MULTIDRUG-RESISTANT TUBERCULOSIS

Drug-resistant mutants of *M. tuberculosis* microorganisms are present in any infected person. When infected people receive antitubercular drugs, drug-resistant mutants continue to appear and reproduce in the presence of the drugs. These strains may become predominant as the drugs eliminate susceptible strains and provide more space and nutrients for resistant strains. Most drug-resistant strains develop when previously infected clients do not take the drugs and doses prescribed for the length of time prescribed. However, drug-resistant strains can be spread from one person to another and cause new infections, especially in people whose immune systems are suppressed by disease (eg, advanced human immunodeficiency virus [HIV] infection) or drugs (eg, antineoplastic drugs and those used to prevent rejection of organ transplants). Multidrug-resistant tuberculosis (MDR-TB) indicates organisms that are resistant to two or more antitubercular drugs, often including both isoniazid (INH) and rifampin, the most effective drugs available.

CHEMOPROPHYLAXIS OF TUBERCULOSIS

Adequate drug therapy of infected people is an effective method for prevention of tuberculosis. If effective preventive therapy is implemented, active tuberculosis does not occur. For many years, INH was the only drug prescribed for chemoprophylaxis of tuberculosis (usually for 6 to 12 months), and it is still the drug of choice when INH-susceptible organisms predominate in the client's community. With the increasing prevalence of INH-resistant tuberculosis and MDR-TB, optimal drug therapy for chemoprophylaxis has not been established, and various regimens are being tried. For people with positive tuberculin

reactions who have been exposed to someone with INH-resistant tuberculosis, rifampin may be given alone or in combination with ethambutol or pyrazinamide for 12 months. For people with exposure to someone with documented MDR-TB, a combination of pyrazinamide (25 to 30 mg/kg/day) and ofloxacin (400 mg twice daily) may be given.

TREATMENT OF TUBERCULOSIS

Adequate drug therapy of clients with active disease usually produces improvement within 2 to 3 weeks, with decreased fever and cough, weight gain and improved well-being, and improved chest x-rays. Most clients have negative sputum cultures within 3 to 6 months. If the client is symptomatic or the culture is positive after 3 months, noncompliance or drug resistance must be considered. Cultures that are positive after 6 months often include drug-resistant organisms, and an alternative drug therapy regimen is probably needed.

For several years, initial treatment of new cases of active tuberculosis involved a three-drug regimen (INH, rifampin, and pyrazinamide daily for 2 months, followed by continued INH and rifampin for 4 additional months, daily or twice weekly). Organism susceptibility to INH and rifampin was assumed and usually validated by effectiveness of treatment. This regimen may still be used in communities with rare isolates of drug-resistant organisms. In the twice-weekly schedule, health care providers either administer the drugs or observe the client taking them (called directly observed therapy, or DOT). This method was developed for clients unable or unwilling to self-administer the drugs independently.

With the increasing prevalence of MDR-TB, guidelines for treatment have changed and continue to evolve in the attempt to promote client adherence to treatment and to manage MDR-TB, two of the major problems in drug therapy of tuberculosis. Some of the current regimens are described below:

- The Centers for Disease Control and Prevention recommend performing culture and susceptibility tests with all cases; prescribing four antitubercular drugs (INH, rifampin, pyrazinamide, and either ethambutol or streptomycin) until susceptibility reports become available (usually several weeks); directly observing therapy to ensure that the client actually takes the drugs; and continuing treatment at least 6 months, or 3 months after cultures become negative. This regimen is indicated for clients in areas where drug-resistant organisms have been isolated, and for clients who require intensive treatment (eg, those with advanced HIV infection). (A five- or six-drug regimen, including two or three drugs not taken before, is recommended for clients who have received several courses of drug therapy and are therefore at high risk of having MDR-TB.)

- This four-drug regimen is evaluated when culture and susceptibility reports become available. If the causative strain of *M. tuberculosis* is susceptible to INH, rifampin, and pyrazinamide, the regimen is continued as with the three-drug regimen described previously and the fourth drug (ethambutol or streptomycin) is discontinued.

- If the causative organism is resistant to INH, rifampin and ethambutol are given for 12 months. Opinions differ about adding INH, with some clinicians believing INH should be a component of all treatment regimens.

- If the causative organism is resistant to rifampin, INH and ethambutol are given for 18 months, with pyrazinamide also being given during the first 2 months.

- When culture reports identify MDR-TB, a five- or six-drug regimen, individualized according to susceptibility reports and containing at least three drugs to which the organism is susceptible, should be instituted. Such regimens include second-line antitubercular drugs and other drugs with activity against *M. tuberculosis*, such as amikacin, ciprofloxacin, or ofloxacin. Some clinicians include at least one injectable agent. The drugs should be given for 1 to 2 years after cultures become negative, preferably with direct observation. Intermittent administration is not recommended for MDR-TB.

- For clients who are unable to tolerate pyrazinamide, INH and rifampin may be given for 9 months.

- During pregnancy, a three-drug regimen of INH, rifampin, and ethambutol is considered safe.

CHARACTERISTICS OF ANTITUBERCULAR DRUGS

Antitubercular drugs are divided into primary and secondary agents. Primary drugs (eg, INH, rifampin, pyrazinamide) are used in the initial treatment of tuberculosis. Secondary drugs, used when organisms develop resistance to primary drugs, are less effective, more toxic, or both. Amikacin, ciprofloxacin, levofloxacin, and ofloxacin (see Chap. 35) are not usually considered antitubercular drugs, but they are used in prevention and treatment of MDR-TB.

Mechanisms of Action

INH inhibits formation of cell walls in mycobacteria. The drug is actively transported into the bacterium, where it kills actively growing organisms and inhibits the growth of dormant organisms in macrophages and tuberculous lesions. Its exact mechanism of action is unknown, but it is thought to combine with an enzyme needed by INH-susceptible tuberculosis organisms. Rifampin inhibits synthesis of ribonucleic acid (RNA) in mycobacterial cells, thereby causing defective, nonfunctional proteins to be

produced. It also penetrates intact cells and kills intracellular bacteria. This ability contributes to its effectiveness in treating tuberculosis because mycobacteria are harbored in host cells. Thus, it acts synergistically with INH. Pyrazinamide is bactericidal against actively growing mycobacteria in macrophages, but its exact mechanism of action is unknown. Ethambutol probably inhibits bacterial synthesis of RNA. Streptomycin acts only against extracellular organisms; it does not penetrate macrophages and tuberculous lesions.

Indications for Use

INH is used to prevent and treat tuberculosis. Because the drug may cause hepatotoxicity, there is some controversy about who should receive prophylaxis. In general, however, candidates include the following groups who are at high risk for development of active disease:

1. Household and other close contacts of clients with recently diagnosed tuberculosis. These people should receive INH for 3 months. Then, if a skin test and chest x-ray are negative, the drug may be stopped. If the tests are positive, INH should be continued for 9 additional months.
2. People who are newly infected (ie, recent converters from negative to positive skin tests)
3. People with positive skin tests and additional risk factors (lung lesions on chest x-ray; diseases such as diabetes mellitus, silicosis, AIDS, leukemia, or lymphoma; alcoholism; postgastrectomy status; on chronic hemodialysis; on corticosteroid or other immunosuppressive drugs; immigrants from Southeast Asia or Mexico)
4. Children and adults younger than 35 years of age with positive skin tests

In chemotherapy of active tuberculosis, INH is included in most drug regimens. It is always used in conjunction with one or two other primary antitubercular drugs to inhibit emergence of drug-resistant organisms. Rifampin, pyrazinamide, and ethambutol were formerly used only for treatment of active disease. Now, they are being used for chemoprophylaxis with drug-resistant tuberculosis. (Rifampin is also used for prophylaxis of meningitis in close contacts of clients with meningitis.) Streptomycin is used in the treatment of active tuberculosis.

Contraindications to Use

Chemoprophylaxis with INH is contraindicated in clients with hepatic disease, in those who have had reactions to the drug, in pregnant women, and possibly older adults. Rifampin is contraindicated in people who have had hypersensitivity reactions and must be used with caution in the presence of liver disease. Pyrazinamide should be used in the presence of liver disease only if necessary.

INDIVIDUAL ANTITUBERCULAR DRUGS

Primary and secondary drugs are described in the following sections; dosages of selected drugs are listed in Table 38-1.

Primary Drugs

INH is the prototype and most commonly used antitubercular drug. It penetrates body cells and is effective against bacilli growing in cells. Although it can be used alone for chemoprophylaxis of tuberculosis, it must be used with one or two other antitubercular drugs for treatment of active disease.

INH is well absorbed from the GI tract and widely distributed in body tissues and fluids, including cerebrospinal fluid. It is acetylated in the liver to acetylisoniazid, which is excreted by the kidneys. Metabolism of INH is genetically determined; some people are "slow acetylators" and others are "rapid acetylators." A person's rate of acetylation may be significant in determining response to INH. Slow acetylators have less N-acetyltransferase, the acetylating enzyme,

in their livers. In these clients, INH is more likely to accumulate to toxic concentrations, and the development of peripheral neuropathy is more likely. However, there is no significant difference in the clinical effectiveness of INH. Rapid acetylators may require unusually high doses of INH. They also may be more susceptible to serious liver injury related to the formation of hepatotoxic metabolites.

Potentially serious adverse effects include hepatotoxicity and peripheral neuropathy. Hepatotoxicity may be manifested by symptoms of hepatitis (eg, anorexia, nausea, fatigue, malaise, and jaundice) or elevated liver enzymes. The drug should be stopped if hepatitis develops or liver enzymes (eg, alanine [ALT] and aspartate aminotransferases [AST]) are more than five times the normal values. Hepatitis is more likely to occur during the first 8 weeks of INH therapy. Clients receiving INH should be monitored monthly for signs and symptoms of hepatitis. Some clinicians also monitor liver enzymes monthly. Because of the risk of hepatotoxicity, INH should not be used for prophylaxis and should be used very cautiously for treatment of clients with preexisting liver disease. Peripheral neuropathy may be manifested by numbness

TABLE 38-1 **Selected Antitubercular Drugs**

| Generic/Trade Name | Routes and Dosage Ranges | |
	Adults	Children
Single Drugs		
Isoniazid	Treatment of active disease, PO, IM 4–5 mg/kg/d in a single dose (maximum dose, 300 mg/d), for at least 6 mo or daily for 2 mo, then 15 mg/kg twice weekly for 4 mo Chemoprophylaxis, PO, IM 300 mg/d in a single dose for 3–12 mo Disseminated tuberculosis or pulmonary disease resulting from atypical mycobacteria, PO, IM 10–20 mg/kg/d, perhaps for years	Treatment of active disease, PO, IM 10–15 mg/kg/d or 20–30 mg/kg twice weekly for at least 6 mo; maximum dose, 300 mg/d or 900 mg twice weekly Chemoprophylaxis, 10 mg/kg/d in a single dose (maximum dose, 300 mg/d), for 3–12 mo
Rifampin	Treatment of tuberculosis, PO 600 mg or 10–20 mg/kg/d in a single dose for at least 6 mo or daily for 2 mo, then 10 mg/kg twice weekly for 4 mo	Treatment of tuberculosis, PO 10–20 mg/kg once daily or twice weekly for at least 6 mo; maximum dose, 600 mg/d
Ethambutol	Initial treatment, PO 15 mg/kg/d in a single dose Retreatment, 25 mg/kg/d for 2 months, then 15 mg/kg/d	*>13 y:* Initial treatment, PO 15 mg/kg/d in a single dose Retreatment, 25 mg/kg/d for 2 months, then 15 mg/kg/d *6–12 y:* PO 10–15 mg/kg/d
Pyrazinamide	PO 15–30 mg/kg/d, in a single dose, to a maximum dose of 3 g/d or 50–70 mg/kg twice weekly to a maximum dose of 4 g, for the initial 2 mo of antitubercular drug therapy	PO 20–40 mg/kg/d or 50 mg/kg twice weekly; maximum dose 2 g/d
Rifapentine (Priftin)	PO 150 mg twice weekly for 2 mo, with at least 3 d between doses, then once weekly for 4 mo	Dosage not established
Combination Drugs		
Rifamate	PO 2 tablets daily for 6 mo	
Rifater	First 2 mo of a 6-mo treatment regimen, PO 4 tablets daily for patients weighing ≤44 kg, 5 tablets daily for those weighing 45 to 54 kg, and 6 tablets daily for those weighing ≥55 kg.	

IM, intramuscular; PO, oral.

and tingling in the hands and feet. It is most likely to occur in clients who are malnourished or elderly, or who have alcoholism, diabetes mellitus, or uremia. Pyridoxine 25 to 50 mg daily is usually given with INH to minimize peripheral neuropathy.

Rifampin is bactericidal for both intracellular and extracellular tuberculosis organisms. It is always used with other drugs to minimize the occurrence of drug-resistant organisms. Rifampin and INH in combination eliminate tuberculosis bacilli from sputum and produce clinical improvement faster than any other drug regimen, unless organisms resistant to one or both drugs are causing the disease.

Rifampin is well absorbed with oral administration and diffuses well into body tissues and fluids, with highest concentrations in the liver, lungs, gallbladder, and kidneys. It is metabolized in the liver and excreted primarily in bile; a small amount is excreted in urine. The drug causes a harmless red-orange discoloration of body secretions, including urine, tears, saliva, sputum, perspiration, and feces. It may stain contact lenses.

Rifampin induces hepatic microsomal enzymes and accelerates the metabolism of numerous other drugs, thereby decreasing their half-lives and therapeutic effects. Affected drugs include acetaminophen, anti-AIDS drugs, benzodiazepines, oral contraceptives, corticosteroids, cyclosporine, estrogens, fluconazole, ketoconazole, mexilitene, methadone, metoprolol, phenytoin, propranolol, quinidine, oral sulfonylureas, theophylline, verapamil, and warfarin. With warfarin, decreased anticoagulant effect occurs approximately 5 to 8 days after rifampin is started and lasts for 5 to 7 days after rifampin is stopped. With methadone, concurrent administration with rifampin may precipitate signs and symptoms of opiate withdrawal.

Rifapentine (Priftin) is a newer drug that is similar to rifampin in effectiveness, adverse effects, and enzyme induction activity. It is indicated for use in the treatment of pulmonary tuberculosis and must be used with at least one other drug to which the causative organisms are susceptible. The main advantage over rifampin is less frequent administration (once or twice weekly rather than daily).

Ethambutol is a tuberculostatic drug that inhibits synthesis of ribonucleic acid and thus interferes with mycobacterial protein metabolism. It is well absorbed from the GI tract, even when given with food. It is excreted primarily by the kidneys, either unchanged or as metabolites. Mycobacterial resistance to ethambutol develops slowly. Ethambutol may be a component in a four-drug regimen for initial treatment of tuberculosis that may be caused by multidrug-resistant organisms.

Dosage is determined by body weight because no practical method of measuring serum drug levels is available. Also, dosage is changed during treatment if significant changes in body weight occur. Dosage must be reduced with impaired renal function. To obtain therapeutic serum levels, the total daily dose is given at one time. Ethambutol is not recommended for young children (eg, <5 years

of age) whose visual acuity cannot be monitored, but may be considered for children of any age when organisms are susceptible to ethambutol and resistant to other drugs.

A major adverse effect is optic neuritis, which decreases visual acuity and ability to differentiate red from green. Tests of visual acuity and red-green discrimination are recommended before starting ethambutol and periodically during therapy. If optic neuritis develops, the drug should be promptly stopped. Recovery usually occurs when ethambutol is discontinued.

Pyrazinamide is used for the first 2 months of tuberculosis treatment, along with INH and rifampin. It is well absorbed with oral administration, widely distributed through the body, and excreted mainly through the kidneys.

A major adverse effect is hepatotoxicity, and the drug should not be given to a client with preexisting liver impairment unless it is considered essential. For clients without liver impairment, liver function studies should be done before starting pyrazinamide and periodically during treatment. Increased plasma levels of ALT and AST are usually the first clinical signs of liver damage. If significant liver damage is indicated, pyrazinamide should be stopped.

Pyrazinamide inhibits urate excretion. This characteristic causes hyperuricemia in most clients and may cause acute attacks of gout.

Streptomycin, an aminoglycoside (see Chap. 35), is mainly used in a regimen of four to six drugs in the treatment of tuberculosis suspected or known to be resistant to INH, rifampin, or both. It may be discontinued when cultures become negative or after a few months of therapy.

Secondary Drugs

Para-aminosalicylic acid (PAS), **capreomycin** (Capastat), **cycloserine** (Seromycin), and **ethionamide** (Trecator SC) are diverse drugs that share tuberculostatic properties. These drugs are in general less effective or more toxic than primary drugs. They are indicated for use only when other agents are contraindicated or in disease caused by drug-resistant organisms. They must be given concurrently with other tuberculostatic drugs to inhibit emergence of resistant mycobacteria. PAS is available only on special order from the manufacturer.

Other Drugs Used in Multidrug-Resistant Tuberculosis

Amikacin and kanamycin are aminoglycoside antibiotics with activity against mycobacteria. Although they are not usually considered antitubercular drugs, one may be a component of a four- to six-drug regimen to treat suspected or known MDR-TB. Similarly, the fluoroquinolones ciprofloxacin, levofloxacin, and ofloxacin have antimycobacterial activity and may be used to prevent or treat MDR-TB.

Combination Antitubercular Drugs

Rifamate and **Rifater** are combination products developed to increase convenience to clients and promote adherence to the prescribed drug therapy regimen (for drug-susceptible tuberculosis). Each Rifamate tablet contains INH 150 mg and rifampin 300 mg, and two tablets daily provide the recommended doses for a 6-month, short-course treatment regimen. Rifater contains INH 50 mg, rifampin 120 mg, and pyrazinamide 300 mg and is approved for the first 2 months of a 6-month, short-course treatment regimen. Dosage depends on weight, with four tablets daily for clients weighing 44 kg or less, five tablets daily for those weighing 45 to 54 kg, and six tablets daily for those weighing 55 kg or more.

MYCOBACTERIUM AVIUM COMPLEX DISEASE

Mycobacterium avium and *Mycobacterium intracellulare* are different types of mycobacteria that resemble each other so closely they are usually grouped together as MAC. These atypical mycobacteria are found in water and soil throughout the United States. The organisms are thought to be transmitted by inhalation of droplets of contaminated water; there is no evidence of spread to humans from animals or other humans.

M. avium complex rarely causes significant disease in immunocompetent people but causes an opportunistic pulmonary infection in approximately 50% of clients with advanced HIV infection. Symptoms include a productive cough, weight loss, hemoptysis, and fever. As the disease becomes disseminated through the body, chronic lung disease develops and the organism is found in the blood, bone marrow, liver, lymph nodes, and other body tissues.

MAC disease was formerly treated with a combination of antitubercular drugs. However, these drugs are not very effective because of high rates of drug resistance and relapse. Newer drugs used in prevention and treatment of MAC disease are the macrolides, azithromycin and clarithromycin (see Chap. 37), and rifabutin. Prophylactic drug therapy is recommended to be lifelong, and azithromycin or clarithromycin should be included in any treatment regimen.

Rifabutin

Rifabutin (Mycobutin) is an antimycobacterial drug that is chemically related to rifampin, an antituberculosis drug. It is approved for prevention of MAC disease in clients with advanced HIV infection. Although opinions differ, rifabutin may be started when CD4+ cell counts are below 100 cells/mm^3. Rifabutin has no advantage over rifampin in treatment of tuberculosis but may be given concur-

rently with INH to clients who need prophylaxis against both *M. tuberculosis* and *M. avium*.

Rifabutin is absorbed from the GI tract, metabolized in the liver, and eliminated in urine and bile. The drug and its metabolites may cause a brownish-orange discoloration of urine, feces, saliva, sputum, perspiration, tears, and skin. Soft contact lenses may be permanently discolored. Like rifampin, rifabutin induces drug-metabolizing enzymes in the liver and accelerates metabolism of several drugs, including ketoconazole, phenytoin, prednisone, propranolol, quinidine, warfarin, and zidovudine. The drug is usually well tolerated. Adverse effects include skin rash, nausea, vomiting, diarrhea, neutropenia, and uveitis (an eye disorder characterized by inflammation, pain, and impaired vision). Safety and effectiveness in children have not been established.

ROUTE AND DOSAGE RANGE

Adults: PO 300 mg once daily

NURSING PROCESS

Assessment

Assess for current or potential tuberculosis:

- For potential tuberculosis, identify high-risk clients (ie, people who are close contacts of someone with active tuberculosis; are elderly or undernourished; have diabetes mellitus, silicosis, Hodgkin's disease, leukemia, or AIDS; are alcoholics; are receiving immunosuppressive drugs; or are immigrants from Southeast Asia and other parts of the world where the disease is endemic).
- For current disease, clinical manifestations include fatigue, weight loss, anorexia, malaise, fever, and a productive cough. In early phases, however, there may be no symptoms. If available, check diagnostic test reports for indications of tuberculosis (chest x-ray, tuberculin skin test, and sputum smear and culture).
- In children, initial signs and symptoms often occur within 1 to 2 months after exposure (before skin tests become positive, which usually takes approximately 3 months) and resemble those of bacterial pneumonia. In addition, indications of disease in lymph nodes, GI and urinary tracts, bone marrow, and meninges may be present.
- In older adults, signs and symptoms of tuberculosis are often less prominent than in younger adults, or similar to those in other respiratory disorders. Thus, an older adult is less likely to have fever, positive skin test, significant sputum production, hemoptysis, or night sweats. However, mental status changes and mortality rates are higher in older than in younger adults.

- In clients with HIV infection, skin tests showing 5 mm of induration are considered positive. In addition, disease manifestations in clients with AIDS differ from those of people with undamaged immune systems. For example, malaise, weight loss, weakness, and fever are prominent. Others often resemble those of bacterial pneumonia, involve multiple lobes of the lungs, and involve extrapulmonary sites.
- Assess for signs and symptoms of MAC disease, especially in clients with advanced HIV infection who have a CD4+ cell count of 100/mm³ or less.

Nursing Diagnoses

- Anxiety or Fear related to chronic illness and long-term drug therapy
- Knowledge Deficit: Disease process and need for treatment
- Noncompliance related to adverse drug effects and need for long-term treatment
- Knowledge Deficit: Consequences of noncompliance with the drug therapy regimen
- Risk for Injury: Adverse drug effects

Planning/Goals

The client will:

- Take drugs as prescribed
- Keep appointments for follow-up care
- Report adverse drug effects
- Act to prevent spread of tuberculosis

Interventions

Assist clients to understand the disease process and the necessity for long-term treatment and follow-up. This is extremely important for the client and the community, because lack of knowledge and

---

CLIENT TEACHING GUIDELINES
Isoniazid, Rifampin, and Pyrazinamide

✔ Isoniazid (INH) is one of the most commonly used medications for tuberculosis infection. It is given to people with positive skin tests to prevent development of active disease, usually for 1 year. Vitamin B₆ (pyridoxine) is usually given along with the INH to prevent leg numbness and tingling. Take INH and pyridoxine in a single dose once daily. Take on an empty stomach if possible; if stomach upset occurs, the drugs may be taken with food.

✔ For treatment of active disease, INH, rifampin, and pyrazinamide are usually given daily or twice weekly for 2 months, then the pyrazinamide is stopped and the others are continued for an additional 4 months.

✔ All three of these drugs can cause liver damage. As a result, you should avoid alcoholic beverages, have periodic blood tests of liver function, and report signs or symptoms of hepatitis (eg, nausea, yellowing of skin or eyes, dark urine, light-colored stools).

✔ Rifampin should be taken in a single dose, once daily or twice weekly, on an empty stomach, 1 hour before or 2 hours after a meal.

✔ Rifampin causes a reddish discoloration of urine, tears, saliva, and other body secretions. This is harmless, except that soft contact lenses may be permanently stained.

✔ Use all available resources to learn about tuberculosis and the medications used to prevent or treat the infection. This is extremely important because the information can help you understand the reasons long-term treatment and follow-up care are needed. In addition to personal benefit, taking medications as prescribed can help your family and community by helping to prevent spread of tuberculosis. The American Lung Association publishes many helpful pamphlets that are available from local

health departments and health care providers. Additional information is available on the Internet. Some sites that provide reliable information include the Centers for Disease Control and Prevention (CDC) Division of Tuberculosis Elimination (DTBE) at http://www.cdc.gov/nchstp/tb/dtbe/html; and the National Tuberculosis Center at http://www.nationaltbcenter.edu/resource.html.

✔ Learn how to prevent spread of tuberculosis:
  ✔ Cover mouth and nose when coughing or sneezing. This prevents expelling tuberculosis germs into the surrounding air, where they can be inhaled by and infect others.
  ✔ Cough and expectorate sputum into at least two layers of tissue. Place the used tissues in a waterproof bag, and dispose of the bag, preferably by burning.
  ✔ Wash hands after coughing or sneezing.

✔ A nourishing diet and adequate rest help healing of infection.

✔ Periodic visits to a health care provider are needed for follow-up care and to monitor medications.

✔ The importance of taking medications as prescribed cannot be overemphasized. If not taken in the doses and for the length of time needed, there is a high likelihood for development of tuberculosis infection that is resistant to the most effective antituberculosis drugs. If this happens, treatment is much longer, very expensive, and requires strong drugs that cause more adverse effects. In addition, this very serious infection can be spread to family members and other close contacts. Thus, avoiding drug-resistant tuberculosis should be a strong incentive to complete the full course of treatment.

failure to comply with the therapeutic regimen lead to disease progression and spread. The American Lung Association publishes many helpful pamphlets, written for the general public, that can be obtained from a local chapter and given to clients and their families. Do not use these as a substitute for personal contact, however.

Use measures to prevent the spread of tuberculosis:

- Isolate suspected or newly diagnosed hospitalized clients in a private room for 2 or 3 weeks, until drug therapy has rendered them noninfectious.
- Wear masks with close contact, and wash hands thoroughly afterward.
- Have clients wear masks when out of the room for diagnostic tests.
- Assist clients to take antitubercular drugs as prescribed, for the length of time prescribed.

Evaluation

- Observe for improvement in signs and symptoms of tuberculosis and MAC disease.
- Interview and observe for adverse drug effects; check laboratory reports of hepatic and renal function, when available.
- Question regarding compliance with instructions for taking antitubercular and anti-MAC drugs.

PRINCIPLES OF THERAPY

Drug-Susceptible Tuberculosis

1. Sputum culture and susceptibility reports require 6 to 8 weeks because the tubercle bacillus multiplies slowly. Consequently, initial drug therapy is based on other factors, such as the extent of disease, whether the client has previously received antitubercular drugs, and whether multidrug-resistant strains are being isolated in the particular community.
2. Multiple drugs are required to inhibit emergence of drug-resistant organisms.
3. Duration of drug therapy varies with the purpose, extent of disease, and clinical response. INH for positive tuberculin reactors is given for 6 to 12 months. Treatment of active disease with multiple drugs ranges from 6 months to 1 year or more, depending on clinical response and culture reports.

Multidrug-Resistant Tuberculosis

1. Multidrug-resistant strains may occur anywhere. However, in the United States, they have been most evident in populations with AIDS, in closed environments (eg, hospitals, prisons), and in large urban areas.

2. Drug therapy regimens for people exposed to someone with MDR-TB or suspected of having MDR-TB should be designed in consultation with infectious disease specialists.
3. Prevention or treatment of MDR-TB requires concurrent administration of more drugs, for a longer period of time, than for drug-susceptible tuberculosis, and may require 2 years or longer.
4. All drug therapy for suspected or known MDR-TB should involve daily administration and directly observed therapy (DOT).
5. The fluoroquinolones are not recommended for use in children.

Increasing Compliance With Antituberculosis Drug Therapy

1. Close supervision by a health care provider is needed during chemoprophylaxis and treatment regimens to monitor the client's response and compliance. In addition, continued contact is needed during the year after completion of drug therapy because most relapses occur during that time.
2. Intermittent dosing (eg, twice weekly rather than daily) and DOT (ie, a health care provider watching a person take a drug dose) are two strategies designed to increase compliance with drug therapy and decrease drug-resistant tuberculosis. All intermittent regimens should be administered under direct observation. In addition, alcoholics, drug abusers, homeless people, and others at high risk for noncompliance should be treated under DOT.
3. Combinations of drugs may reduce the number of pills to be taken per dose and promote compliance. However, they are more expensive than purchasing each drug separately.

Use in Human Immunodeficiency Virus Infection

Tuberculosis is a common opportunistic infection in people with advanced HIV infection and may develop from an initial infection or reactivation of an old infection. For chemoprophylaxis in clients with positive skin tests, 1 year

Nursing Notes: Apply Your Knowledge

Christine Sommers, during chemotherapy for breast cancer, experienced symptoms of tuberculosis (TB) and had an abnormal chest x-ray. Sputum results are not yet available but treatment with isoniazid and rifampin is started. Ms. Sommers voices anxiety about taking medications that are "toxic" and have so many side effects. How can you individualize your teaching for Ms. Sommers?

Nursing Notes: Ethical/Legal Dilemma

Hong Pham was recently diagnosed with active tuberculosis (TB). His physician is discussing treatment options through a translator. Mr. Pham is against taking medications (isoniazid, rifampin, and ethambutol) that the doctor is prescribing, requesting that he be allowed to cure the TB with herbal remedies.

Reflect on:

- Mr. Pham's right to refuse treatment.
- The role culture may play in Mr. Pham's decision.
- The rights of the general public to be protected from infectious disease.
- How to work with Mr. Pham to resolve this conflict.

of INH (300 mg) daily has been used for several years. Recent studies indicate that a 2-month regimen of rifampin (450 to 600 mg) and pyrazinamide (1500 to 2500) daily or twice weekly is equally effective and promotes greater compliance than 6- or 12-month regimens.

Treatment of active disease is difficult and long term (2 to 3 years) because of the damaged immune system. Clients with AIDS do not absorb most antitubercular drugs very well, and this may lead to treatment failures and drug-resistant organisms. These clients are also at high risk for development of primary infection with multidrug-resistant organisms. An additional complication is that INH, rifampin, and related drugs may decrease the effectiveness of several anti-AIDS drugs.

Use in Children

Tuberculosis occurs in children of all ages. Infants and preschool children are especially in need of early recognition and treatment because they can rapidly progress from primary infection to active pulmonary disease and perhaps to extrapulmonary involvement. Tuberculosis is usually discovered during examination of a sick child or investigation of the contacts of someone with newly diagnosed active tuberculosis. Children in close contact with a case of tuberculosis should receive skin testing, a physical examination, and a chest x-ray.

When children require antitubercular drugs for prevention or treatment, treatment is mainly empiric. For example, some drugs are not established as safe or effective or are not recommended for use in children. For drugs that are used, dosage ranges are not well defined because few data are available about the pharmacokinetics of antitubercular drugs in children. In addition, most of the drugs are not available in pediatric dosage forms and are given as crushed portions of adult dosage forms. INH is available as a solution, but it contains sorbitol and may cause diarrhea.

As with adults, drug therapy regimens vary with particular circumstances and continue to evolve. Health care providers need to follow current recommendations of pediatric infectious disease specialists. Children with exposure to tuberculosis but negative skin tests should be given INH for 3 months. If exposure stops and the skin test and examination remain negative, the INH can be stopped. For older children and adolescents with negative skin tests and no symptoms, chemoprophylaxis may be omitted or delayed until skin tests become positive or other signs and symptoms develop.

Children who are infected but without disease (ie, have positive skin tests) should receive preventive therapy. If the infection to which the child was exposed was drug susceptible, INH should be given daily for approximately 9 months (≥12 months for children with HIV infection or immunosuppression). If the causative strain in the index case was INH resistant, rifampin may be given empirically. Children with suspected disease should receive multidrug treatment until infection can be ruled out.

If the drug-susceptibility patterns of the *M. tuberculosis* strain causing the index case are known, the child is treated with those drugs; if this information is not available, the pattern of drug resistance in the community where the child likely became infected should be the guide for selecting the drug therapy regimen. As in adults, drug-susceptible tuberculosis is treated with INH, rifampin, and pyrazinamide for 2 months. Then, pyrazinamide is stopped and the INH and rifampin are continued for 4 more months. If drug-resistant organisms have been identified in the community, a fourth drug, ethambutol or streptomycin, should be given until the client's culture and susceptibility data become available. If pyrazinamide is not given, INH and rifampin are recommended for 9 months. When INH or rifampin cannot be used, therapy should continue for 12 to 24 months.

Drug-resistant tuberculosis in children is usually acquired from an adult family member or other close contact with active, drug-resistant disease. For children exposed to MDR-TB, there is no proven preventive therapy. Several regimens are used empirically, including ethambutol and pyrazinamide or ethionamide and cycloserine. When INH and rifampin cannot be given because of MDR-TB, drug therapy should continue for 24 months after sputum smears or cultures become negative. Ciprofloxacin, levofloxacin, and ofloxacin are used for prevention and treatment of MDR-TB in adults, but are not recommended for use in children because of possible cartilage damage, especially in weight-bearing joints. If they are used, children must be monitored often for joint pain or swelling. Clients with MDR-TB may require months of treatment before sputum smears become negative, and they are infectious during this period. To guide dosage and minimize adverse drug effects, serum drug levels should be measured periodically, especially in clients with GI, renal or hepatic disease, or with advanced HIV infection.

In children with HIV infection, the American Academy of Pediatrics recommends three drugs for at least 12 months. If drug resistant or extrapulmonary disease is suspected, four drugs are indicated.

Use in Older Adults

Although INH is the drug of choice for chemoprophylaxis, its use is controversial in older adults. Because risks of drug-induced hepatotoxicity are higher in this population, some clinicians believe those with positive skin tests should have additional risk factors (eg, recent skin test conversion, immunosuppression, or previous gastrectomy) before receiving INH. When INH is given, people who drink alcoholic beverages daily are most likely to sustain serious liver impairment.

For treatment of active disease caused by drug-susceptible organisms, INH, rifampin, and pyrazinamide are given, as in younger adults. Because all three drugs may cause hepatotoxicity, liver function tests should be monitored and the drugs discontinued if signs and symptoms of hepatotoxicity occur. For treatment of suspected or known MDR-TB, four to six drugs are used.

Use in Renal Impairment

Rifampin is mainly eliminated by the liver. However, up to 30% of a dose is excreted by the kidneys and dose reduction may be needed in clients with renal impairment. In addition, dosage of amikacin, capreomycin, cycloserine, ethambutol, fluoroquinolones, and streptomycin should be reduced in clients with impaired renal function. Cycloserine is contraindicated in severe renal impairment.

Use in Hepatic Impairment

Most antitubercular drugs are metabolized in the liver and several (eg, INH, rifampin, and pyrazinamide) are hepatotoxic. To detect hepatotoxicity as early as possible, plasma ALT and AST should be measured before starting and periodically during drug therapy. If hepatitis develops, these enzymes usually increase before other signs and symptoms develop.

With INH, mild increases in AST and ALT occur in approximately 10% to 20% of clients but are not considered significant and usually resolve without stopping the drug. Hepatitis and liver damage are more likely to occur during the first 8 weeks of INH therapy and in middle-aged and older adults.

Clients should be assessed monthly for symptoms of hepatitis (anorexia, nausea, fatigue, malaise, and jaundice). If symptoms occur or if AST and ALT increase significantly (more than five times the normal values), INH should be discontinued. Because of the risk of hepatotoxicity, INH should not be used for prophylaxis and should be used very cautiously for treatment of clients with preexisting liver disease.

With rifampin, liver damage is most likely to occur with preexisting liver disease or concurrent use of other hepatotoxic drugs. AST and ALT should be measured before starting rifampin and every 2 to 4 weeks during rifampin therapy. The drug should be stopped if signs of liver damage occur.

With pyrazinamide, the drug should not be given to a client with preexisting liver impairment unless it is considered absolutely essential. For clients without liver impairment, liver function studies should be done before and during treatment. Increased ALT and AST values are early signs of liver injury. If significant elevations occur or if other evidence of liver damage becomes apparent, the drug must be stopped.

 Home Care

The home care nurse has major roles to play in the health care of clients, families, and communities. With individual clients receiving preventive or therapeutic antitubercular drugs, the home care nurse needs to assist in taking the drugs as directed. Specific interventions vary widely and may include administering the drugs (DOT); teaching about the importance of taking the drugs and the possible consequences of not taking them (ie, more severe disease, longer treatment regimens with more toxic drugs, spreading the disease to others); monitoring for adverse drug effects and assisting the client to manage them or reporting them to the drug prescriber; assisting in obtaining the drugs; and keeping follow-up appointments for blood tests and chest x-rays; and others. Family members may also need teaching related to preventing spread of the disease and assisting the client to obtain adequate treatment. In relation to community needs, the nurse needs to be active in identifying cases, investigating contacts of newly diagnosed cases, and promoting efforts to manage tuberculosis effectively.

NURSING ACTIONS Antitubercular Drugs	
NURSING ACTIONS	**RATIONALE/EXPLANATION**
1. **Administer accurately** **a.** Give isoniazid (INH), ethambutol, and rifampin in a single dose once daily.	A single dose with the resulting higher blood levels is more effective. Also, fewer doses may increase client compliance with drug therapy.

(*continued*)

NURSING ACTIONS	RATIONALE/EXPLANATION
b. Give ethionamide with food.	To minimize nausea, vomiting, and diarrhea
c. Give rifampin 1 h before or 2 h after a meal.	Food delays absorption.
d. Give capreomycin and parenteral INH by deep intramuscular injection into a large muscle mass, and rotate injection sites.	To decrease local pain and tissue irritation
2. Observe for therapeutic effects	
a. Clinical improvement	Therapeutic effects are usually apparent within the first 2 or 3 weeks of drug therapy.
(1) Decreased cough, sputum, fever, night sweats, and fatigue	
(2) Increased appetite, weight, and feeling of well-being.	
b. Negative sputum smear and culture	
c. Improvement in chest x-ray studies	
3. Observe for adverse effects	
a. Nausea, vomiting, diarrhea	These symptoms are likely to occur with any of the oral antitubercular drugs and are usually most severe with para-aminosalicylic acid.
b. Neurotoxicity:	
(1) Eighth cranial nerve damage—vertigo, tinnitus, hearing loss	A major adverse reaction to aminoglycoside antibiotics
(2) Optic nerve damage—decreased vision and color discrimination	The major adverse reaction to ethambutol
(3) Peripheral neuritis—tingling, numbness, paresthesias	Often occurs with INH but can be prevented by administering pyridoxine (vitamin B$_6$). Also may occur with ethambutol.
(4) Central nervous system changes—confusion, convulsions, depression	More often associated with INH, but similar changes may occur with ethambutol
c. Hepatotoxicity—increased serum aspartate aminotransferase, alanine aminotransferase, and serum bilirubin; jaundice; and other symptoms of hepatitis	May occur with INH, rifampin, and pyrazinamide, especially if the client already has liver damage
d. Nephrotoxicity—increased blood urea nitrogen and serum creatinine, cells in urine, oliguria	A major adverse reaction to aminoglycosides
e. Hypersensitivity—fever, tachycardia, anorexia, and malaise are early symptoms. If the drug is not discontinued, exfoliative dermatitis, hepatitis, renal abnormalities, and blood dyscrasias may occur.	Hypersensitivity reactions are more likely to occur between the third and eighth weeks of drug therapy. Early detection and drug discontinuation are necessary to prevent progressive worsening of the client's condition. Severe reactions can be fatal.
4. Observe for drug interactions	
a. Drugs that *increase* effects of antitubercular drugs: Other antitubercular drugs	Potentiate antitubercular effects. These drugs are always used in combinations of two or more for treatment of tuberculosis. For chemoprophylaxis, INH is used alone.
b. Drugs that *alter* the effects of INH:	
(1) Alcohol and oral antacids decrease effects.	Alcohol induces hepatic enzymes, which accelerate the rate of isoniazid metabolism and may increase the likelihood of toxicity. Oral antacids may decrease absorption of oral INH.

(continued)

NURSING ACTIONS	RATIONALE/EXPLANATION
(2) Disulfiram	May cause behavioral changes and impairments in coordination
(3) Pyridoxine (vitamin B$_6$)	Pyridoxine decreases peripheral neuritis, a common adverse effect of INH, and is usually combined with INH for this purpose.
(4) Sympathomimetics	May result in increased blood pressure owing to the monoamine oxidase inhibitory activity of INH
c. Drugs that *alter* effects of rifampin: Halothane and INH *increase* effects.	Additive risk of hepatotoxicity
d. Drugs that *alter* effects of aminoglycosides	See Chapter 35.

Nursing Notes: Apply Your Knowledge

Answer: First, it is important that you hear Ms. Sommers' concerns and acknowledge them. To comply with treatment, Ms. Sommers needs to see that the benefits are greater than the risks. Provide Ms. Sommers with specific information concerning side effects and how they will be monitored. Peripheral neuropathy and hepatotoxicity are significant side effects. Tell Ms. Summers to alert you about tingling in her feet or hands. Vitamin B$_6$ tablets can be given to decrease this side effect. Liver function is monitored by watching for symptoms such as jaundice and fatigue and by assessing laboratory results (liver enzymes, bilirubin levels). Warn Ms. Sommers that her urine and other body fluids may turn red, but this is not harmful in any way. Ms. Sommers should also check with her doctor before taking over-the-counter medications because drug interactions with TB medications are common. Provide Ms. Sommers with written material and encourage her to call if she has any questions.

 ## REVIEW AND APPLICATION EXERCISES

1. How do tuberculosis infections differ from other bacterial infections?

2. Why are clients with AIDS at high risk for development of tuberculosis?

3. What are the main risk factors for development of drug-resistant tuberculosis?

4. Who should receive INH to prevent tuberculosis? Who should not be given INH? Why?

5. When INH is given alone for prophylaxis, how long should it be taken?

6. If you worked in a health department with clients on INH prophylaxis, what are some interventions to promote client adherence to the drug regimen?

7. Why is active, symptomatic tuberculosis always treated with multiple drugs?

8. In a client with tuberculosis newly started on drug therapy, how could you explain the emergence of drug-resistant organisms and the importance of preventing this problem?

9. What are advantages and disadvantages of short-course (6 to 9 months) treatment programs?

10. For which clients would intermittent, direct administration of antitubercular drugs be preferred?

11. What adverse effects are associated with INH, rifampin, pyrazinamide, and ethambutol, and how may they be prevented or minimized?

12. In a client with MDR-TB, what are nursing implications?

SELECTED REFERENCES

Boutotte, J.M. (1999). Keeping TB in check. *Nursing, 29*(3), 34–39.

Carter, M. (1998). TB prevention and treatment. *Infections in Medicine 15*(1), 32–34, 37. [Online: Available http://www.medscape.com. Accessed July 9, 1999.]

Chaisson, R.E. & Bishai, W. (1998). Short course preventive therapy for tuberculosis in HIV-infected patients. *Medscape HIV/AIDS 4*(1) 1998. [Online: Available http://www.medscape.com. Accessed July 9, 1999.]

Ebert, S.C. (1997). Tuberculosis. In J.T. DiPiro, R.L. Talbert, G.C. Yee, G.R. Matzke, B.G. Wells, & L.M. Posey (Eds.), *Pharmacotherapy: A pathophysiologic approach*, 3rd ed., pp. 2101–2124. Stamford, CT: Appleton & Lange.

Field, K.W. & Vezeau, T.M. (1998). Nursing interventions for MDR-TB. *American Journal of Nursing, 98*(6), 16E, 16H, 16J.

Horsburgh, C.R. (1996). Advances in the prevention and treatment of *Mycobacterium avium* complex disease (Editorial). *New England Journal of Medicine, 335,* 428–429.

Humma, L.M. (1996). Prevention and treatment of drug-resistant tuberculosis. *American Journal of Health-System Pharmacy, 53,* 2291–2298.

Jackson, M.M. & McLeod, R.P. (1998). Tuberculosis in infants, children, and adolescents: An update with case studies. *Pediatric Nursing, 23,* 411–420.

Mandell, G.L. & Petri, W.A., Jr. (1996). Drugs used in the chemotherapy of tuberculosis, *Mycobacterium avium* complex disease, and leprosy. In J.G. Hardman, L.E. Limbird, P.B. Molinoff, & R.W. Ruddon (Eds.), *Goodman & Gilman's The pharmacological basis of therapeutics,* 9th ed., pp. 1155–1174. New York: McGraw-Hill.

Mundy, L.M. & L'Ecuyer, P.B. (1998). Treatment of infectious diseases: Tuberculosis. In C.F. Carey, H.H. Lee, & K.F. Woeltje (Eds.), *The Washington manual of medical therapeutics,* 29th ed., pp. 279–281. Philadelphia: Lippincott Williams & Wilkins.

Porth, C.M. (Ed.). (1998). *Pathophysiology: Concepts of altered health states,* 5th ed., pp. 510–513. Philadelphia: Lippincott Williams & Wilkins.

Portyansky, E. (1998). New anti-TB agent offers more convenient dosing schedule. *Drug Topics, 142*(14), 22.

Toossi, Z. & Ellner, J.J. (1997). Tuberculosis. In W.N. Kelley (Ed.), *Textbook of internal medicine,* 3rd ed., pp. 1687–1696. Philadelphia: Lippincott-Raven.

39

Antiviral Drugs

Objectives

After studying this chapter, the student will be able to:

1. Describe characteristics of viruses and common viral infections.

2. Discuss difficulties in developing and using antiviral drugs.

3. Identify clients at risk for development of systemic viral infections.

4. Differentiate types of antiviral drugs used for herpes infections, human immunodeficiency virus (HIV) infections, influenza A, and respiratory syncytial virus infections.

5. Describe commonly used antiviral drugs in terms of indications for use, adverse effects, and nursing process implications.

6. Discuss the rationale for using combinations of drugs in treating HIV infection.

7. Discuss guidelines for using antiviral drugs in special populations.

8. Teach clients techniques to prevent viral infections.

Mark, a 32-year-old bisexual man, was recently diagnosed with human immunodeficiency virus (HIV) infection with a CD4+ cell count of less than 200. He is started on aggressive drug therapy including didanosine (ddI), a reverse transcriptase inhibitor, and ritonavir, a protease inhibitor. Each day he takes 22 pills at a cost of $400/week.

Reflect on:

▶ What is the expected outcome of antiviral therapy in a person infected with HIV?

▶ Is the HIV-infected person still able to spread the infection to others while on antiviral treatment?

▶ Who should be responsible for the cost of treatment if private insurance lapses when Mark is no longer able to work?

▶ Ethical issues concerning possible effects when these drugs are used for a long period of time.

GENERAL CHARACTERISTICS OF VIRUSES AND VIRAL INFECTIONS

Viruses produce many diseases, including acquired immunodeficiency syndrome (AIDS), hepatitis, pneumonia, and other disorders that affect almost every body system. Many potentially pathogenic viral strains exist. For example, more than 150 viruses infect the human respiratory tract, including approximately 100 types of rhinovirus that cause the common cold. Viruses are spread by secretions from infected people, ingestion of contaminated food or water, breaks in skin or mucous membrane, blood transfusions, sexual contact, pregnancy, breastfeeding, and organ transplantation. Viral infections vary from mild, localized disease with few symptoms to severe systemic illness and death. Severe infections are more common when host defense mechanisms are impaired by disease or drugs. Additional characteristics of viruses and viral infections are described in the following; selected infections are described in Box 39-1.

1. Viruses are intracellular parasites that can live and reproduce only while inside other living cells. They gain entry to human host cells by binding to receptors on cell membranes. All human cells do not have receptors for all viruses; cells that lack receptors for a particular virus are resistant to infection by that virus. Thus, the locations and numbers of the receptors determine which host cells can be infected by a virus. For example, the mucous membranes lining the tracheobronchial tree have receptors for the influenza A virus, and certain white blood cells (eg, helper T lymphocytes) have CD4 molecules, which are the receptors for the human immunodeficiency virus (HIV).

2. Once inside host cells, viruses use cellular metabolic activities for their own survival and replication. Viral replication involves dissolution of the protein coating and exposure of the genetic material (deoxyribonucleic acid [DNA] or ribonucleic acid [RNA]). With DNA viruses, the viral DNA enters the host cell's

---

BOX 39–1 SELECTED VIRAL INFECTIONS

Herpesvirus Infections

Cytomegalovirus Disease and Retinitis

Cytomegalovirus (CMV) infection is extremely common, and most people become infected by adulthood. Infection is usually asymptomatic in healthy, immunocompetent adults. Like other herpesviruses, CMV can cause a primary infection, then remain latent in body tissues, probably for life. This means the virus can be shed in secretions of an asymptomatic host and spread to others by contact with infected saliva, blood, urine, semen, breast milk, and cervical secretions. It also means the virus is ready to cause an opportunistic infection when the host becomes immunosuppressed. During pregnancy, CMV is transmitted to the fetus across the placenta and may cause infection in the brain, inner ears, eyes, liver, and bone marrow. Learning disabilities and mental retardation may result from congenital CMV infection. Children spread the virus to each other in saliva or urine; adolescents and adults transmit the virus mainly through sexual contact.

Major populations at risk for development of CMV infection are clients with cancer who receive immunosuppressant drugs; organ transplant recipients, who must receive immunosuppressant drugs to prevent their body's rejection of the transplanted organ; and those with advanced human immunodeficiency virus (HIV) infection. Systemic CMV infection occurs mainly from reactivation of endogenous virus, although it may occur from an exogenous source, and it may cause cellular necrosis and inflammation in various body tissues. Common disorders are pneumonitis, hepatitis, encephalitis, adrenal insufficiency, and gastrointestinal inflammation and ulcers.

In the eye, CMV infection produces retinitis, usually characterized by blurred vision and decreased visual acuity. Visual impairment is progressive and irreversible, if untreated, and causes blindness in one or both eyes. CMV retinitis may also indicate systemic CMV disease, or it may be asymptomatic or discovered at autopsy.

Genital Herpes Infection

Genital herpes infection is caused by the herpes simplex virus (HSV) and produces recurrent, painful, blister-like eruptions of the skin and mucous membranes. The virus is usually transmitted from person to person by direct contact with open lesions or secretions, including genital secretions. Primary infection occurs at a site of viral entry, where the virus infects epithelial cells, produces progeny viruses, and destroys the infected cells. Recovery from the primary infection leaves latent infection in sensory nerve cells. In response to various stimuli, such as intense sunlight, emotional stress, febrile illness, or menstruation, the latent infection is reactivated periodically, with viral reproduction and shedding.

In the fetus, HSV may be transmitted from an infected birth canal, and neonatal herpes is a serious complication of maternal genital herpes. Neonatal herpes usually becomes evident within the first week of life and may be manifested by the typical clusters of blister-like lesions on skin or mucous membranes. Irritability,

(continued)

BOX 39–1 **SELECTED VIRAL INFECTIONS** *(continued)*

lethargy, jaundice, bleeding problems, respiratory distress, seizures, or coma may also occur. The lesions heal in 1 to 2 weeks, but neonatal herpes still carries a high mortality rate. In immunosuppressed people, HSV infection may result in severe, systemic disease.

Herpes Zoster

Herpes zoster is caused by the varicella-zoster virus, which is highly contagious and present worldwide. Most children in the United States are infected by early school age. The virus produces chickenpox on first exposure and is spread from person to person by the respiratory route or by contact with secretions from the skin lesions. Recovery from the primary infection leaves latent infection in nerve cells. Reactivation of the latent infection causes herpes zoster (commonly called shingles), a localized cluster of painful, blister-like skin eruptions. The skin lesions have the same appearance as those of chickenpox and genital herpes. Over several days, the vesicles become pustules, then rupture and heal. Because the virus remains in sensory nerve cells, pain can persist for months after the skin lesions heal. Most cases of herpes zoster infection occur among the elderly and the immunocompromised.

Human Immunodeficiency Virus Infection

Human immunodeficiency virus (HIV) infection is caused by a retrovirus that attacks the immune system. Two types of HIV virus have been identified. Most infections are caused by HIV-1; HIV-2 infections occur mainly in Africa. HIV-1 binds to a receptor protein (CD4 molecule) on the surface of susceptible cells, primarily T lymphocytes (also called helper T cells and CD4+ cells) and monocyte/macrophages. The infection and destruction of CD4+ cells lead to the severe impairment of the immune system.

Progression of HIV-1 infection to acquired immunodeficiency syndrome (AIDS) occurs during phases of disease development. One phase is characterized by the primary infection, during which influenza-like symptoms (eg, fever, chills, muscle aches) may last several weeks. During this time, the virus is rapidly growing and spreading to lymphoid and other body tissues. The next phase is characterized by a dramatic decline in the rate of viral replication, attributed to a partially effective immune system response, and no visible manifestations of HIV infection. However, there is continued replication of HIV in body tissues, destruction of lymphoid tissues, and the presence of HIV antibodies in the blood (called seroconversion). During this period, which may last 10 years, the person is seropositive (HIV+) and infectious but asymptomatic. Eventually, the immune system

is substantially damaged and the rate of viral reproduction accelerates. When the viral load and immunodeficiency reach significant levels, the illness is called advanced HIV infection or AIDS. This phase is characterized by decreased CD4+ cell counts, loss of immune responses, and clinical disease most often manifested by opportunistic infections such as *Pneumocystis carinii* pneumonia.

HIV can spread to a new host during any phase of infection and is spread by sexual intercourse, injection of intravenous drugs with contaminated needles, mucous membrane contact with blood or body fluids containing HIV, and perinatally, from mother to fetus. Although the virus has been found in most body fluids, blood, semen, or vaginal secretions have been associated with most infections. Health care workers have been infected by needlestick injuries. The virus is not spread through casual contact.

Respiratory Syncytial Virus Infection

The respiratory syncytial virus (RSV) is present worldwide, is highly contagious, and infects most children by school age. Epidemics of RSV infection may occur in nurseries, day care centers, and pediatric hospital units during winter months. This virus infects and destroys respiratory epithelium in the bronchi, bronchioles, and alveoli. It is spread by respiratory droplets and secretions, direct contact with an infected person, and contact with fomites, including the hands of caregivers.

RSV is the most common cause of bronchiolitis and pneumonia in infants and causes the most severe illness in those younger than 6 months of age. These infants usually have wheezing, cough, and respiratory distress, and may have fever. The infection is usually self-limited and resolves in 1 to 2 weeks. Antiviral therapy with ribavirin is used in some cases. The mortality rate from RSV infection is low in children who are generally healthy but increases substantially in those with congenital heart disease or immunosuppression. Recurrent infection occurs but is usually less severe than the primary infection. In older children, RSV infection produces much milder disease but may be associated with acute exacerbations of asthma.

In adults, RSV infection causes colds and bronchitis, with symptoms of fever, cough, and nasal congestion. Infection occurs most often in those with household or other close contact with children, including pediatric health care workers. In elderly adults, RSV infection may cause pneumonia and require hospitalization. In immunocompromised patients, RSV infection may cause severe and potentially fatal pneumonia.

nucleus, where it becomes incorporated into the host cell's chromosomal DNA. Then, host cell genes are coded to produce new viruses. In addition, the viral DNA incorporated with host DNA is transmitted to the host's daughter cells during host cell mitosis and becomes part of the inherited genetic information of the host cell and its progeny. With RNA viruses (eg, HIV), the viral RNA must be converted to DNA by an enzyme called reverse transcriptase before replication can occur.

Once new viruses are formed, they are released from the infected cell by budding out and breaking off from the cell membrane (leaving the host cell intact) or by causing lysis of the cell. When the cell is destroyed, the viruses are released into the blood and surrounding tissues, from which they can transmit the viral infection to other host cells.

3. Viruses induce antibodies and immunity. Antibodies are proteins that defend against microbial or viral invasion. They are very specific (ie, an antibody protects only against a specific virus or other antigen). For instance, in a person who has had measles, antibody protection (immunity) develops against future infection by the measles virus, but immunity does not develop against other viral infections, such as chickenpox or hepatitis.

The protein coat of the virus allows the immune system of the host to recognize the virus as a "foreign invader" and to produce antibodies against it. This system works well for most viruses but does not work for the influenza A virus, which can alter its protein covering so much and so often that the immune system does not recognize it as foreign to the body. Thus, last year's antibody cannot recognize and neutralize this year's virus.

Antibodies against infecting viruses can prevent the viruses from reaching the bloodstream or, if they are already in the bloodstream, prevent their invasion of host cells. Once the virus has penetrated the cell, it is protected from antibody action, and the host depends on cell-mediated immunity (lymphocytes and macrophages) to eradicate the virus along with the cell harboring it.

4. Viral infection may occur without signs and symptoms of illness. If illness does occur, the clinical course is usually short and self-limited. Recovery occurs as the virus is eliminated from the body. Some viruses (eg, herpesviruses) can survive in host cells for many years and cause a chronic, latent infection that periodically becomes reactivated. Also, autoimmune diseases may be caused by viral alteration of host cells so lymphocytes are fooled into thinking the host's own tissues are foreign.

5. Symptoms usually associated with acute viral infections include fever, headache, cough, malaise, mus-

cle pain, nausea and vomiting, diarrhea, insomnia, and photophobia. White blood cell count is usually normal. Other signs and symptoms vary with the type of virus and the body organs involved.

Antiviral Drugs

Few antiviral drugs were available before the AIDS epidemic. Since then, numerous drugs have been developed to treat HIV infection and opportunistic viral infections that occur in hosts whose immune systems are suppressed by AIDS or immunosuppressant drugs given to organ transplant recipients. Drug therapy for viral infections is still limited, however, because drug development is difficult. Viruses use the metabolic and reproductive mechanisms of host cells for their own vital functions, and few drugs inhibit viruses without being excessively toxic to host tissues. The drugs inhibit viral reproduction but do not eliminate viruses from tissues. Available drugs are expensive, relatively toxic, and effective in a limited number of infections. Some may be useful in treating an established infection if given promptly and in chemoprophylaxis if given before or soon after exposure. Protection conferred by chemoprophylaxis is immediate but lasts only while the drug is being taken. Subgroups of antiviral drugs are described in the following sections; additional characteristics and dosage ranges are listed in Tables 39-1 and 39-2.

Drugs for Herpesvirus Infections

Acyclovir, famciclovir, and **valacyclovir** penetrate virus-infected cells, become activated by an enzyme, and inhibit viral DNA reproduction. They are used in the treatment of herpes simplex and herpes zoster infections. Acyclovir is used to treat genital herpes, in which it decreases viral shedding and the duration of skin lesions and pain. It does not eliminate inactive virus in the body and thus does not prevent recurrence of the disease unless oral drug therapy is continued. Acyclovir is also used for treatment of herpes simplex infections in immunocompromised clients. Prolonged or repeated courses of acyclovir therapy may result in the emergence of acyclovir-resistant viral strains, especially in immunocompromised clients. Acyclovir can be given orally or intravenously (IV), or applied topically to lesions. IV use is recommended for severe genital herpes in nonimmunocompromised clients and any herpes infections in immunocompromised clients. Oral and IV acyclovir is excreted mainly in urine, and dosage should be decreased in clients who are elderly or have renal impairment.

Famciclovir and valacyclovir are oral drugs for herpes zoster and recurrent genital herpes. Famciclovir is metabolized to penciclovir, its active form, and excreted mainly

TABLE 39-1   Drugs for Prevention or Treatment of Selected Viral Infections

Generic/Trade Name	Indications for Use	Routes and Dosage Ranges	
		Adults	Children
Herpes Virus Infections			
Acyclovir (Zovirax)	Oral mucocutaneous lesions (eg, cold sores, fever blisters) Genital herpes Herpes simplex encephalitis Varicella (chickenpox) in immunocompromised hosts Herpes zoster (shingles) in normal and immuno-compromised hosts	Genital herpes, PO 200 mg q4h, five times daily for 10 d for initial infection; 400 mg two times daily to prevent recurrence of chronic infection; 200 mg q4h five times daily for 5 d to treat recurrence Herpes zoster, PO 800 mg q4h five times daily for 7–10 d Chickenpox, PO 20 mg/kg (maximum dose 800 mg) four times daily for 5 d Mucosal and cutaneous herpes simplex virus (HSV) infections in immunocompromised hosts (ICH), IV 5 mg/kg infused at constant rate over 1 h, q8h for 7 d Varicella-zoster infections in ICH, IV 10 mg/kg, infused as above, q8h for 7 d HSV encephalitis, IV 10 mg/kg infused as above, q8h for 10 d Topically to lesions q3h, six times daily for 7 d	Children <12 y: IV 250 mg/m² q8h for 7 d
Cidofovir (Vistide)	Treatment of CMV retinitis in persons with AIDS	IV infusion, 5 mg/kg over 1 h, every 2 wk	Dosage not established
Famciclovir (Famvir)	Acute herpes zoster Genital herpes, recurrent episodes	*Herpes zoster*, PO 500 mg q8h for 7 d *Genital herpes*, PO 125 mg twice daily for 5 d	Dosage not established
Foscarnet (Foscavir)	Treatment of CMV retinitis in persons with AIDS Treatment of acyclovir-resistant mucocutaneous HSV infections in immunocompromised clients	CMV retinitis, IV 60 mg/kg q8h for 2–3 wk, depending on clinical response, then 90–120 mg/kg/d for maintenance HSV infections, IV 40 mg/kg q8–12h for 2–3 wk or until lesions are healed Reduce dosage with impaired renal function	
Ganciclovir (Cytovene)	CMV retinitis in immuno-compromised clients Prevention of CMV disease in clients with organ transplants or advanced HIV infection	CMV retinitis, IV 5 mg/kg q12h for 14–21 d, then 5 mg/kg once daily for 7 d/wk or 6 mg/kg once daily for 5 d/wk or PO 1000 mg three times daily for maintenance Prevention in transplant recipients, IV 5 mg/kg once daily 7 d/wk or 6 mg/kg once daily 5 d/wk Prevention in clients with HIV infection, PO 1000 mg three times daily	
Trifluridine (Viroptic)	Keratoconjunctivitis caused by herpes viruses	Topically to eye, 1% ophthalmic solution, 1 drop q2h while awake (maximum 9 drops/d) until re-epithelialization of corneal ulcer occurs; then 1 drop q4h (maximum 5 drops/d) for 7 d	

TABLE 39-1 **Drugs for Prevention or Treatment of Selected Viral Infections** (*continued*)

Generic/Trade Name	Indications for Use	Routes and Dosage Ranges	
		Adults	Children
Valacyclovir (Valtrex)	Herpes zoster and recurrent genital herpes in immuno-competent clients	Herpes zoster, PO 1 g q8h for 7 d Recurrent genital herpes, PO 500 mg q12h daily for 5 d Reduce dosage with renal impairment (creatinine clearance <50 mL/min)	
Vidarabine (Vira-A)	Keratoconjunctivitis caused by herpes viruses	IV 15 mg/kg/d dissolved in 2500 mL of fluid and given over 12–24 h daily for 10 d Topically to eye, 3% ophthalmic ointment, applied q3h until re-epithelialization, then twice daily for 7 d	
Influenza Virus Infection			
Amantadine (Symmetrel)	Prevention or treatment of influenza A infection	PO 200 mg once daily or 100 mg twice daily Reduce dosage with renal impairment (creatinine clearance <50 mL/min)	9 to 12 y: PO 100 mg twice daily 1 to 9 y: PO 4.4 to 8.8 mg/kg/d given in one single dose or two divided doses, not to exceed 150 mg/d
Oseltamivir (Tamiflu)	Treatment of influenza	PO 75 mg twice daily for 5 d	Dosage not established
Rimantadine (Flumadine)	Prevention or treatment of influenza A infection in adults Prophylaxis of influenza A in children	PO 100 mg twice daily	<10 y: 5 mg/kg once daily, not exceeding 150 mg >10 y: Same as adults
Zanamivir (Relenza)	Treatment of influenza A or B infection	Oral inhalation, 1 Rotadisk twice daily for 5 days	≥12 y: Same as adults
Respiratory Syncytial Virus Infection			
Ribavirin (Virazole)	Treatment of hospitalized infants and young children with severe lower respiratory tract infections		Inhalation; diluted to a concentration of 20 mg/mL for 12 to 18 h/d for 3 to 7 d

AIDS, acquired immunodeficiency syndrome; CMV, cytomegalovirus; IV, intravenous; PO, oral.

in the urine. Valacyclovir is metabolized to acyclovir by enzymes in the liver or intestine or both, and excreted in the urine. As with acyclovir, dosage of these drugs must be reduced in the presence of renal impairment.

Cidofovir, foscarnet, and **ganciclovir** also inhibit viral reproduction after activation by a viral enzyme found in virus-infected cells. The drugs are used to treat cytomegalovirus (CMV) retinitis in clients with AIDS. In addition, foscarnet is used to treat acyclovir-resistant mucocutaneous herpes simplex infections in people with impaired immune functions and ganciclovir is used to prevent CMV disease, mainly in clients with organ transplants or HIV infection. Dosage of these drugs must be reduced with renal impairment. Ganciclovir causes granulocytopenia and thrombocytopenia in approximately 20% to 40% of recipients. These hematologic effects often occur during the first 2 weeks of therapy but may occur at any time. If severe bone marrow depression occurs, ganciclovir should be discontinued. Recovery usually occurs within a week of stopping the drug.

Trifluridine and **vidarabine** are applied topically to treat keratoconjunctivitis and corneal ulcers caused by the herpes simplex virus (herpetic keratitis). Trifluridine should not be used longer than 21 days because of possible ocular toxicity. Vidarabine also is given IV to treat herpes zoster infections in clients whose immune systems are impaired and encephalitis caused by herpes simplex viruses. IV dosage must be reduced with impaired renal function.

Drugs for HIV Infection and AIDS (Antiretrovirals)

The three types of drugs used for HIV infections are nucleoside reverse transcriptase inhibitors (NRTIs), nonnucleoside reverse transcriptase inhibitors (NNRTIs), and protease inhibitors. The drugs inhibit enzymes required for viral replication in human host cells (Fig. 39-1). To (*text continues on page 586*)

TABLE 39-2 **Drugs for Human Immunodeficiency Virus Infection and Acquired Immunodeficiency Syndrome**

Generic/Trade Name	Characteristics	Routes and Dosage Ranges	
		Adults	Children
Nucleoside Reverse Transcriptase Inhibitors (NRTIs)			
Zidovudine (AZT, ZVD, Retrovir)	Prototype NRTI Well absorbed with oral administration Metabolized in the liver to an inactive metabolite, which is excreted in urine Often causes severe anemia and granulocytopenia, which may require reducing dosage, stopping the drug, giving blood transfusions, or giving filgrastim or sargramostim to hasten bone marrow recovery May also cause peripheral neuropathy and pancreatitis	Symptomatic HIV infection, PO 100 mg q4h (total daily dose 600 mg), IV 1–2 mg/kg q4h around the clock Asymptomatic HIV infection, PO 100 mg q4h while awake (total daily dose 500 mg) Maternal dose after 14 wk of pregnancy, PO 100 mg 5 times daily until labor begins. During labor and delivery, IV 2 mg/kg over 1 h, then IV 1 mg/kg/h until umbilical cord clamped	3 mo to 12 y: 180 mg/m² q6h (not to exceed 200 mg q6h) Neonate born of HIV-infected mother who took the drug during pregnancy, labor, and delivery, PO 2 mg/kg q6h starting within 12 h of birth and continuing until 6 wk of age. If unable to take oral drug, give 1.5 mg/kg IV q6h, infused over 30 min.
Abacavir (Ziagen)	Well absorbed with oral administration Approximately 50% bound to plasma proteins Metabolized to inactive metabolites that are excreted in urine and feces May cause serious hypersensitivity reactions	PO 300 mg twice daily	>3 mo: PO 8 mg/kg twice daily (maximum dose, 300 mg twice daily)
Didanosine (ddI, Videx)	Used for patients who do not respond to or cannot tolerate zidovudine	35–49 kg: PO 125 mg q12h 50–74 kg: PO 200 mg q12h ≥75 kg: PO 300 mg q12h	<0.4 m² BSA: PO 25 mg q12h 0.5–0.7 m² BSA: PO 50 mg q12h 0.8–1 m² BSA: PO 75 mg q12h 1.1–1.4 m² BSA: PO 100 mg q12h
Lamivudine (Epivir)	Used to treat advanced HIV infection and chronic hepatitis B Well absorbed with oral administration and mainly eliminated unchanged in urine Dosage should be reduced with renal impairment	PO 150 mg twice daily Weight <50 kg (110 lbs): PO 2 mg/kg twice daily	3 mo to 12 y: PO 4 mg/kg twice daily 12–16 y: PO same as adults
Stavudine (Zerit)	Used to treat adults who do not improve with or do not tolerate other anti-HIV medications May be useful against zidovudine-resistant strains of HIV Approximately 40% is eliminated through the kidneys, and dosage should be reduced with renal impairment May cause peripheral neuropathy	Weight ≥60 kg, PO 40 mg q12h Weight <60 kg, PO 30 mg q12h	Dosage not established
Zalcitabine (Hivid)	Used with zidovudine to treat advanced HIV infection in adults whose condition continues to deteriorate while receiving zidovudine May cause peripheral neuropathy	PO 0.75 mg q8h (2.25 mg/d) with zidovudine 200 mg q8h (600 mg/d)	Dosage not established
Non-nucleoside Reverse Transcriptase Inhibitors (NNRTIs)			
Delavirdine (Rescriptor)	Used with NRTIs and protease inhibitors Well absorbed with oral administration and metabolized in the liver	PO 400 mg (four 100 mg tablets) three times daily	Dosage not established

TABLE 39-2 **Drugs for Human Immunodeficiency Virus Infection and Acquired Immunodeficiency Syndrome** (*continued*)

Generic/Trade Name	Characteristics	Routes and Dosage Ranges	
		Adults	Children
Efavirenz (Sustiva)	Induces drug-metabolizing enzymes in the liver and increases metabolism of itself and other drugs Common adverse effects are nausea and skin rash. May be as effective with two NRTIs as a protease inhibitor plus two NRTIs	PO 600 mg once daily	≥3 y and weight 10–40 kg (22–88 lbs): PO 200–400 mg, depending on weight Weight >40 kg: PO same as adults
Nevirapine (Viramune)	Well absorbed with oral administration and metabolized in the liver Induces drug-metabolizing enzymes in the liver and increases metabolism of itself and other drugs Adverse effects include severe skin reactions and hepatotoxicity.	PO 200 mg once daily for 2 wk, then 200 mg twice daily	Dosage not established
Protease Inhibitors			
Amprenavir (Agenerase)	Well absorbed after oral administration Oral solution less bioavailable than capsules, thus the two dosage forms are not equivalent on a milligram basis Highly bound to plasma proteins Metabolized in liver; small amount of unchanged drug excreted in urine and feces May cause serious skin reactions	PO 1200 mg (eight 150-mg capsules) twice daily	13–16 y and weight ≥50 kg: PO same as adults 4–12 y, or 13–16 y and weight <50 kg: PO 20/mg/kg twice daily or 15 mg/kg three times daily (maximum daily dose, 2400 mg); Oral solution, 22.5 mg/kg twice daily or 17 mg/kg three times daily (maximum daily dose, 2800 mg)
Indinavir (Crixivan)	Well absorbed and approximately 60% bound to plasma proteins. Metabolized in the liver and excreted mainly in feces May cause GI upset and kidney stones	PO 800 mg (two 400 mg capsules) q8h	Dosage not established
Nelfinavir (Viracept)	Metabolized in the liver and excreted mainly in feces The most common adverse effect is diarrhea, which can usually be controlled with over-the-counter drugs such as loperamide.	PO 750 mg (three 250-mg tablets) three times daily	2–13 y: PO 20–30 mg/kg/dose, three times daily
Ritonavir (Norvir)	Metabolized in the liver and excreted mainly in feces Usually well tolerated but may cause GI upset	PO 600 mg twice daily	Dosage not established
Saquinavir (Fortovase)	Not well absorbed, undergoes first-pass metabolism in the liver, and is highly bound to plasma proteins Metabolized in the liver and excreted mainly in feces May cause GI upset May produce fewer drug interactions than indinavir and ritonavir	PO 1200 mg (six 200-mg tablets) three times daily, with an NRTI	Dosage not established

BSA, body surface area; GI, gastrointestinal; HIV, human immunodeficiency virus; IV, intravenous; PO, oral.

increase effectiveness and decrease viral mutations and emergence of drug-resistant viral strains, the drugs are used in combination. All of the drugs can cause serious adverse effects.

Nucleoside Reverse Transcriptase Inhibitors

The NRTIs are similar to a component of DNA (adenosine, cytosine, guanosine, or thymidine) and thus are able to enter human cells and viruses in human cells. For example, zidovudine, the prototype, is able to substitute for thymidine. In the infected cell, these drugs inhibit reverse transcriptase, an enzyme required by retroviruses to convert RNA to DNA and allow replication. The drugs are more active in preventing acute infection than in treating chronically infected cells. Thus, they slow progression but do not cure HIV infection or prevent transmission of the virus through sexual contact or blood contamination.

Zidovudine, the first NRTI, is still widely used. However, zidovudine-resistant viral strains are increasing. Other NRTIs are usually given with zidovudine or as a substitute for zidovudine in clients who are unable to take or do not respond to zidovudine.

Non-nucleoside Reverse Transcriptase Inhibitors

The NNRTIs inhibit viral replication in infected cells by directly binding to reverse transcriptase and preventing its function. They are used in combination with NRTIs to treat clients with advanced HIV infection. Because the two types of drugs inhibit reverse transcriptase by different mechanisms, they have synergistic antiviral effects. NNRTIs are also used with other antiretroviral drugs because drug-resistant strains emerge rapidly when the drugs are used alone.

Protease Inhibitors

Protease inhibitors attack the HIV at a different phase of its life cycle than reverse transcriptase inhibitors. Protease is an enzyme in HIV-infected cells that is required to process protein precursors into mature viral particles capable of infecting other cells. The drugs inhibit the enzyme by binding to the protease-active site. This inhibition causes the production of immature, noninfectious viral particles. These drugs are active in both acutely and chronically infected cells because they block viral maturation.

The protease inhibitors are metabolized in the liver by the cytochrome P450 enzyme system and should be used cautiously in clients with impaired liver function. They should be used only if necessary in pregnant women because no studies have been done. It is unknown whether the drugs are excreted in breast milk. However, the Cen-

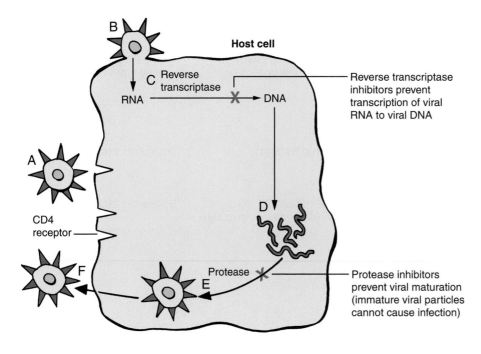

FIGURE 39–1 HIV replication and actions of anti-HIV drugs. (**A**) The virus attaches to receptors (eg, CD4 molecules) on the host cell membrane and fuses to the cell membrane. (**B**) The virus becomes uncoated and releases its RNA into the host cell. (**C**) The enzyme reverse transcriptase converts RNA to DNA, which is necessary for viral replication. (**D**) The DNA codes for protein synthesis, which produces immature viral particles. (**E**) The enzyme protease assembles the immature viral particles into mature viruses. (**F**) Mature viruses are released from the host cell.

ters for Disease Control and Prevention (CDC) advises women with HIV infection to avoid breastfeeding because HIV may be transmitted to an uninfected infant. Safety and efficacy of protease inhibitors in children have not been established.

Indinavir, ritonavir, and saquinavir are the oldest and best-known protease inhibitors, but their long-term effects are unknown. Two major concerns are viral resistance and drug interactions. Viral resistance develops fairly rapidly, with resistant strains developing in approximately half of the recipients within a year of drug therapy. In relation to drug interactions, protease inhibitors interfere with metabolism, increase plasma concentrations, and increase risks of toxicity of numerous other drugs metabolized by the cytochrome P450 enzymes in the liver.

The most interactions occur with ritonavir, which increases plasma concentrations of amiodarone, bepridil, bupropion, clozapine, flecainide, meperidine, piroxicam, propafenone, propoxyphene, quinidine, and rifabutin. None of these drugs should be given concomitantly with ritonavir because high plasma concentrations may cause cardiac arrhythmias, hematologic abnormalities, seizures, and other potentially serious adverse effects. In addition, ritonavir may increase sedation and respiratory depression with benzodiazepines (eg, alprazolam, diazepam) and zolpidem, and should not be given concomitantly with these drugs.

Indinavir increases plasma concentrations of several of the same drugs listed previously and should not be given concomitantly with them because of potential cardiac arrhythmias or prolonged sedation. Saquinavir may produce fewer interactions because it inhibits the cytochrome P450 enzyme system to a lesser extent than indinavir and ritonavir. However, if saquinavir is given with clindamycin, quinidine, triazolam, or a calcium channel blocker, clients should be monitored closely for increased plasma levels and adverse drug effects.

Amprenavir is a sulfonamide and should be used with caution in clients known to be allergic to sulfonamides. The likelihood of cross-sensitivity reactions between amprenavir and other sulfonamides is unknown. The drug formulation contains vitamin E and clients taking it should be cautioned against taking additional vitamin E supplements. Amprenavir should be discontinued with the occurrence of severe skin rashes or moderate rashes with systemic symptoms.

Drugs for Influenza A

Amantadine and **rimantadine** inhibit replication of the influenza A virus and are used to prevent or treat influenza A infections. Postexposure prophylaxis with either drug protects contacts of people with influenza A infections. Seasonal prophylaxis may be used in high-risk clients if the influenza vaccine cannot be given or may be ineffective.

In epidemics, one of the drugs is recommended for clients at high risk who have not been vaccinated. The high-risk population includes older adults, those who have chronic lung disease, and those who have immunodeficiency disorders. During an epidemic, amantadine or rimantadine may be given approximately 2 weeks if the client is vaccinated at the beginning of drug therapy or approximately 4 to 8 weeks if the client is not vaccinated. Protection is lost within a few days after drug therapy is stopped. For treatment of influenza A infection, either drug may shorten the illness if started soon after onset and continued for 5 days. The drugs may also decrease viral shedding and spread of the disease.

Amantadine and rimantadine are well absorbed after oral administration. Amantadine is excreted in the urine unchanged. It accumulates in the body of elderly adults and others with impaired renal function, and dosage therefore should be reduced in these groups. Rimantadine is extensively metabolized, with small amounts excreted in the urine. The most common adverse effects of the drugs are gastrointestinal (anorexia, nausea) and central nervous system (CNS) (nervousness, lightheadedness, difficulty concentrating) symptoms. CNS effects are more likely to occur with amantadine than rimantadine, and high plasma levels of amantadine have been associated with delirium, hallucinations, seizures, coma, and cardiac arrhythmias. Amantadine has also been associated with exacerbations of preexisting seizure disorders and psychiatric symptoms. Amantadine is teratogenic in animals, and neither drug has been established as safe for pregnant women.

Amantadine is also used in the treatment of Parkinson's disease and extrapyramidal symptoms associated with the use of some antipsychotic drugs (see Chap. 12).

Oseltamivir (Tamiflu) and **zanamivir** (Relenza) are approved for treatment of influenza A or B in clients with symptoms for 2 days or less. They are used for 5 days. Oseltamivir is an oral drug; zanamivir is a powder form for oral inhalation with a device called a Diskhaler. Zanamivir may cause bronchospasm in clients with asthma or chronic obstructive pulmonary disease.

Drug for Respiratory Syncytial Virus Respiratory Tract Infections

Ribavirin is used for the treatment of bronchiolitis or pneumonia caused by the respiratory syncytial virus (RSV). It is used in hospitalized infants and young children and given by inhalation with the Viratek Small Particle Aerosol Generator. The drug is not recommended for clients on ventilators because it precipitates and blocks tubes, including endotracheal tubes. Deterioration of pulmonary function is a common adverse effect. The drug is absorbed systemically after administration by aerosol. Most infants and children with RSV infections have mild, self-limited disease that does not involve the lower respiratory tract and does not require hospitalization or ribavirin therapy.

NURSING PROCESS

Assessment

- Assessment varies with the type of viral infection and may include signs and symptoms of influenza or other viral infections of the respiratory tract, genital herpes, viral infections of the eye, or other conditions.
- Assess renal function and adequacy of fluid intake.
- With HIV infection, assess baseline data to assist in monitoring response to drug therapy. Baseline data may include vital signs, weight and nutritional status, signs and symptoms of the disease, signs and symptoms of opportunistic infections associated with the disease and immunosuppression, and available reports of laboratory tests (eg, complete blood count, CD4+ lymphocyte counts, plasma levels of viral RNA, blood urea nitrogen and serum creatinine, liver function tests).

Nursing Diagnoses

- Self Care Deficit related to systemic infection
- Anxiety related to a medical diagnosis of HIV infection, genital herpes, or CMV retinitis

- Altered Sexuality Patterns related to sexually transmitted viral infections (HIV infection, genital herpes)
- Body Image Disturbance related to sexually transmitted infection
- Social Isolation related to a medical diagnosis of HIV infection or genital herpes
- Knowledge Deficit: Disease process and methods of spread
- Knowledge Deficit: Availability of vaccines and other prophylactic interventions
- Risk for Injury: Recurrent infection
- Risk for Injury: Adverse drug effects or interactions
- Risk for Injury: Infections and other problems associated with compromised immune systems in HIV infection

Planning/Goals

The client will:

- Receive or take antiviral drugs as prescribed
- Be safeguarded against new or recurrent infection
- Act to prevent spread of viral infection to others and recurrence in self
- Avoid preventable adverse drug effects
- Receive emotional support and counseling to assist in coping with HIV infection or genital herpes

Interventions

- Follow recommended policies and procedures for preventing spread of viral infections.

(*text continues on page 590*)

CLIENT TEACHING GUIDELINES
Miscellaneous Antiviral Drugs

General Considerations

✔ Prevention is better than treatment, partly because medications to treat viral infections may cause serious adverse effects. Thus, you need to use techniques to prevent viral infections, when possible.
  ✔ Frequent and thorough hand washing helps prevent most infections.
  ✔ Maintain immunizations against viral infections as indicated.
  ✔ With genital herpes, avoid sexual intercourse when visible lesions are present and always wash hands after touching any lesion.

✔ Drugs may relieve symptoms but do not cure viral infections. For example, treatment of genital herpes does not

prevent transmission to others and treatment of cytomegalovirus (CMV) retinitis does not prevent disease progression.

✔ Ask a health care provider for information about managing adverse drug effects.

✔ If taking foscarnet or ganciclovir for CMV retinitis, have eye examinations approximately every 6 weeks.

Self-administration

✔ With acyclovir, famciclovir, and valacyclovir for genital herpes, start oral drugs for recurrent lesions as soon as signs and symptoms begin.

✔ Use gloves to apply acyclovir ointment to lesions.

CLIENT TEACHING GUIDELINES
Anti-Human Immunodeficiency Virus Drugs

General Considerations

✔ Prevention is better than treatment, partly because medications to treat viral infections may cause serious adverse effects. Thus, you need to use techniques to prevent viral infections, when possible.
  ✔ Frequent and thorough hand washing helps prevent most infections.
  ✔ Maintain immunizations against viral infections as indicated.
  ✔ With human immunodeficiency virus (HIV) infection, use a condom with sexual activity and avoid sharing intravenous needles with anyone.

✔ Drugs may relieve symptoms but do not cure HIV infection, prevent transmission of the virus, or prevent other illnesses associated with advanced HIV infection.

✔ Effective treatment of HIV infection requires close adherence to a drug therapy regimen of several drugs and several doses daily. Missing a dose or two can cause the blood level of the drug to fall and allow HIV to mutate. With each mutation, the virus becomes more drug resistant, and after three or four mutations, it might become completely resistant.

✔ Request information about adverse effects associated with the specific drugs you are taking and what you should do if they occur. Adverse effects vary among the drugs; some are potentially serious.

✔ Have regular blood tests of viral load, CD4+ cell count, complete blood count, and others as indicated (eg, tests of kidney and liver function, because some of the medications cause adverse effects in these organs and medication changes may be needed).

✔ Keep your physician and other health care providers informed about all medications being taken; do not take any other drugs (including drugs of abuse, herbal preparations, vitamin/mineral supplements, nonprescription drugs) without consulting a health care provider. These preparations may make anti-HIV medications less effective or more toxic.

✔ If amprenavir is prescribed:
  ✔ Tell the prescriber if you are allergic to sulfa drugs (eg, Bactrim). Amprenavir is a sulfonamide; it is unknown whether people allergic to sulfa drugs are allergic to amprenavir.
  ✔ Women who take hormonal contraceptives need to use other methods of contraception.

✔ Do not take vitamin E supplements because amprenavir capsules and oral solution contain more than the recommended daily amount of vitamin E.

✔ With nelfinavir, women taking oral contraceptives need to use alternate or additional contraceptive methods.

Self-administration

✔ Take the medications exactly as prescribed. Do not change doses or stop the medications without consulting a health care provider. If a dose is missed, do not double the next dose. The drugs must be taken consistently to suppress HIV infection and minimize adverse drug effects.

✔ These medications vary in their interactions with food and should be taken appropriately for optimal benefit. Unless otherwise instructed, take the drugs as follows:
  ✔ **Abacavir, amprenavir, delavirdine, efavirenz, famciclovir, lamivudine, nevirapine, stavudine,** and **valacyclovir** may be taken with or without food. However, do not take abacavir, amprenavir, or efavirenz with a high-fat meal. Also, if taking an antacid or didanosine, take **amprenavir** at least 1 hour before or after a dose of antacid or didanosine.
  ✔ Take **didanosine** and **indinavir** on an empty stomach. This usually means 1 hour before or 2 hours after a meal. Although indinavir is best absorbed if taken on an empty stomach, with water, it may also be taken with skim milk, juice, coffee, tea, or a light meal (eg, toast, cereal). If you are taking indinavir and didanosine, the drugs should be taken at least 1 hour apart on an empty stomach.
  ✔ Take **ganciclovir, nelfinavir,** and **ritonavir** with food. The oral solution of ritonavir may be mixed with chocolate milk or Ensure to improve the taste.
  ✔ Take **saquinavir** within 2 hours after a meal.

✔ **Delavirdine** tablets may be mixed in water by adding four tablets to at least 3 oz of water, waiting a few minutes, and then stirring. Drink the mixture promptly, rinse the glass, and swallow the rinse to be sure the entire dose is taken.

✔ To give **nelfinavir** to infants and young children, the oral powder can be mixed with a small amount of water, milk, or formula. Once mixed, the entire amount must be taken to obtain the full dose. Acidic foods or juices (eg, apple sauce, orange juice, apple juice) should not be used because they produce a bitter taste.

- Assist clients in learning ways to control spread and recurrence of viral infection.
- Assist clients to maintain immunizations against viral infections.
- For clients receiving systemic antiviral drugs, monitor serum creatinine and other tests of renal function, complete blood count, and fluid balance.
- Spend time with the client when indicated to reduce anxiety and support usual coping mechanisms.
- For clients with HIV infection, monitor for changes in baseline data during each contact; prevent opportunistic infections (eg, CMV retinitis, herpes infections) when possible; and manage signs and symptoms, disease complications, and adverse effects of drug therapy to promote quality of life.

Evaluation

- Observe for improvement in signs and symptoms of the viral infection for which a drug is given.
- Interview outpatients regarding their compliance with instructions for taking antiviral drugs.
- Interview and observe for use of infection control measures.
- Interview and observe for adverse drug effects.
- Observe the extent and severity of any symptoms in clients with HIV infection.

PRINCIPLES OF THERAPY

Prevention of Viral Infections

General preventive measures include vaccination, hand washing, teaching infected clients to cover their mouth and nose when coughing or sneezing, treatment of symptoms, and recognition and treatment of complications. Of the sexually transmitted viral infections, genital herpes can be prevented by avoiding sex when skin lesions are present and using condoms; HIV infection can be prevented by the consistent use of condoms and not sharing needles among drug users.

Viral Vaccines

Viral vaccines are used for active immunization of clients before exposure or to control epidemics of viral disease in a community. Vaccines for prevention of poliomyelitis, measles, rubella, mumps, smallpox, and yellow fever and for protection against influenza and rabies are available (see Chap. 43). Live attenuated viral vaccines are in general safe and nontoxic. However, they probably should not be used in clients who are pregnant, immunodeficient, or receiving corticosteroids, antineoplastic or immunosuppressive drugs, or irradiation. Influenza vaccines prevent infection in most clients. If infection does occur, less virus is shed in respiratory secretions. Thus, vaccination reduces transmission of influenza by decreasing the number of susceptible people and by decreasing transmission by immunized people who still become infected. The multiplicity of rhinoviruses (common cold), enteroviruses, and respiratory viruses hinders development of practical vaccines for these common diseases.

Use of Antibacterial Drugs in Viral Infections

Antibacterial drugs should not be used in viral infections in the hope of preventing complications. They do have a role, however, in treating bacterial complications of viral infections. For example, bacterial pneumonia may develop as a complication of influenza.

Use of Antiretroviral Drugs in HIV Infection

1. The goals of drug therapy include prolonging and improving the quality of life, decreasing the viral load to undetectable levels in plasma as long as possible, stopping disease progression, and restoring immune function.
2. Treatment of HIV infection is complex and recommendations change often as new drugs and research reports become available. Thus, when possible, a physician with expertise in the care of HIV-infected clients should prescribe or supervise drug therapy. When this is not possible, primary physicians should consult specialists and other sources for current treatment recommendations.
3. Drug therapy requires substantial commitment of time and energy by therapists and their clients. Therapists must keep abreast of new developments and monitor clients' responses; clients must be willing to adhere to a complex regimen and manage or tolerate adverse drug effects. Nonadherence may lead to a lack of effectiveness or emergence of drug-resistant viral strains. Thus, therapists and clients need to discuss benefits and risks and participate in decision making.
4. Drug therapy is usually started early in the course of the infection. The initial infection is manifested by an illness similar to influenza, with fever, chills, and muscle aches that may last for several weeks. This period is usually followed by a quiescent phase, which may last up to 10 years, during which there may be no clinical manifestations. This phase was once thought to indicate viral latency and inactiv-

ity. However, research has shown that the initial infection is characterized by explosive viral growth and spread to body tissues, especially the lymphoid system. The period after the initial infection is characterized by a partially effective immune system response, which decreases viral replication. However, some viral replication and destruction of lymphoid tissue continue during this period. Early treatment that reduces the number of HIV (viral load) may delay progression of the disease and development of clinical signs and symptoms.

5. Guidelines for drug therapy in adults and adolescents, as developed by the Panel on Clinical Practices for Treatment of HIV Infection (convened by the Department of Health and Human Services and the Henry J. Kaiser Family Foundation), include the following:

    a. Treatment is recommended for clients with the acute HIV syndrome, those within 6 months of seroconversion, and those with symptoms attributed to HIV infection. For asymptomatic clients, treatment is usually recommended with fewer than 500 CD4+ T cells/mm^3 or a high viral load (plasma HIV RNA levels above 10,000 or 20,000 copies/mL, depending on the type of test).

    b. A combination of antiretroviral drugs should be used. A commonly used three-drug regimen includes two NRTIs and a protease inhibitor. Other options include two NRTIs and the NNRTI efavirenz or two protease inhibitors plus one or two NRTIs. The choice of specific drugs must consider client health status, adverse drug effects, and potential drug interactions. For example, anorexia may prevent clients from following dietary recommendations to promote absorption of some protease inhibitors; bone marrow suppression induced by zidovudine may make the drug intolerable; combinations of NRTIs may increase neuropathy; and multiple drug interactions occur, especially between protease inhibitors and many other drugs. Because of the high risk of drug interactions, clients considering new drugs (including over-the-counter, herbal, or other preparations) should discuss the potential effects on their anti-HIV drug regimen with a health care provider.

    A single anti-HIV medication should not be used except in pregnancy, to reduce perinatal transmission, and when there are no other options.

    c. When starting drug therapy, most drugs should be started at the same time and in full therapeutic doses. Starting at smaller doses and increasing them gradually are recommended for ritonavir and nevirapine.

    d. Potentially serious drug interactions, especially between protease inhibitors and other agents, are

extensive and often require changes in drugs or doses to avoid toxicity. Clients should be assessed for signs and symptoms of adverse drug effects at least twice during the first month of treatment, when new signs and symptoms develop, and approximately every 3 months during therapy.

    e. Effective drug therapy usually produces significantly reduced plasma HIV RNA levels by 2 months and undetectable levels (<500 copies/mL) by 4 to 6 months. Failure to obtain these results may result from nonadherence, inadequate drugs or doses, drug-resistant viral strains, and other factors.

    f. Laboratory tests are used to determine when to start drug therapy and to assess adherence and response to therapy. The preferred test (called HIV RNA levels or copies) measures the number of HIV in the blood; it does not measure viral levels in tissues, where viral reproduction may be continuing. Measurement is recommended at the time of diagnosis and every 3 to 4 months in untreated clients. In treated clients, HIV RNA levels should be done before and 2 to 8 weeks after starting drug therapy, then every 3 to 4 months. Serial measurements should be done in the same laboratory because there are differences among tests and techniques.

    CD4+ cell counts may also be used and are expected to increase with effective drug therapy. They should be measured at the time of diagnosis and approximately every 3 to 6 months thereafter.

    Complete blood counts, tests of renal and hepatic function, and other tests are also needed.

    g. Clients receiving drug therapy for advanced HIV infection should continue medications during an opportunistic infection or malignancy, unless there are significant drug intolerances, toxicities, or interactions.

    h. Reasons for temporary interruption of therapy include intolerable adverse effects, drug interactions, and unavailability of drug. Although interruptions increase the risk of drug resistance, the time interval between stopping drug therapy and the development of drug resistance is unknown. If one antiretroviral drug must be stopped for a prolonged period, it may be better to stop all of them. Continuing one or two drugs may be more likely to cause drug-resistant viral strains.

    i. The Panel plans to update these guidelines regularly on the HIV/AIDS Treatment Information Service website (*http://www.hivatis.org*).

Use in Children

The use of systemic antiviral drugs may be difficult in children because several of the available agents have not been established as safe and effective, are not available in pediatric formulations, or do not have pediatric dosages.

Amantadine is given to prevent or treat influenza A in children 1 year of age or older, and rimantadine is given only for prevention in children. The optimal dose and duration of amantadine or rimantadine therapy have not been established.

Cidofovir should probably not be used in children because of long-term risks of carcinogenicity and reproductive toxicity. It is also nephrotoxic.

There are few guidelines for the use of anti-HIV drugs in children. Most HIV infections in children result from perinatal transmission. Thus, pregnant women with possible exposure to HIV should be tested and, if HIV positive, should receive zidovudine to prevent perinatal transmission. After delivery, zidovudine is given to the infant for the first 6 weeks of life. If perinatal infection occurs, the infant usually has symptoms (eg, an opportunistic infection or failure to thrive) within the first 3 to 8 months of life and the disease continues to progress rapidly. Zidovudine is approved for treatment of HIV infection in children and is usually the drug of choice. As in adults, anemia and neutropenia are common adverse effects of zidovudine.

Abacavir can be used in clients 3 months to 13 years of age; amprenavir can be used in children 4 to 16 years of age; didanosine may be given to children who do not respond to zidovudine; nelfinavir may be used in children 2 years of age and older; and delavirdine and zalcitabine may be used in adolescents. Safety and effectiveness of several drugs have not been established (eg, famciclovir, indinavir, and stavudine for any age group; ritonavir for those younger than 12 years of age; and saquinavir for those younger than 16 years).

Use in Older Adults

Antiviral drug selection and dosage should be done very cautiously because older adults often have impaired organ function, concomitant disease, or other drug therapy. For example, most systemic antiviral drugs are excreted by the kidneys. Because renal impairment is common in older adults, there are greater risks of toxicity. These risks may be minimized by reducing drug dosage when indicated by decreased creatinine clearance (CrCl), close monitoring of renal function, and maintaining adequate fluid intake. When amantadine is given to prevent or treat influenza A, dosage should be reduced with renal impairment, and older adults must be monitored closely for CNS effects (eg, hallucinations, depression, confusion) and cardiovascular effects (eg, congestive heart failure, orthostatic hypotension). Rimantadine reportedly causes fewer CNS effects.

There is little information about the effects of anti-HIV medications in older adults. However, as in other populations, dosage may need to be decreased with renal impairment, and protease inhibitors may be contraindicated with hepatic impairment.

Use in Renal Impairment

Antiviral drugs must be used very cautiously in clients with impaired renal function because some are nephrotoxic, most are eliminated by the kidneys, and many require dosage reductions because their elimination may be decreased. All clients with renal impairment should be monitored closely for abnormal renal function tests and drug-related toxicity. Renal effects and guidelines for usage of selected drugs are described in the following sections.

Nephrotoxic Drugs

* **Acyclovir** may precipitate in renal tubules and cause renal impairment with high doses of oral drug or IV administration (eg, to treat acute herpes zoster). This is most likely to occur in clients who are dehydrated and may be minimized by maintaining a high urine output. Although clients on hemodialysis usually need reduced doses, an additional dose is needed after dialysis because the treatment removes approximately 51% of acyclovir in the body.
* **Cidofovir** is nephrotoxic in approximately 50% of clients. It is contraindicated in clients who are taking other nephrotoxic drugs or who have abnormal renal function tests (eg, baseline serum creatinine >1.5 mg/dL, CrCl ≤55 mL/minute, or proteinuria 2+ or above). Acute renal failure has occurred and renal function may not return to baseline after the drug is stopped.

Guidelines to minimize nephrotoxicity include avoiding higher-than-recommended doses, rates of infusion, and frequencies of administration; prehydration with IV 0.9% sodium chloride injection; giving probenecid with each infusion; and monitoring serum creatinine and urine protein within 48 hours before each dose, and decreasing the dose when indicated. The drug should be decreased in dosage or stopped with evidence of deteriorating renal function.

- **Foscarnet** may cause or worsen renal impairment and should be used with caution in all clients. Nephrotoxicity occurs to some extent in most clients. Manifestations of renal impairment are most likely to occur during the second week of induction therapy but may occur any time during treatment. Renal impairment may be minimized by monitoring renal function (eg, at baseline, two to three times weekly during induction, and at least every 1 to 2 weeks during maintenance therapy) and reducing dosage accordingly. The drug should be stopped if CrCl drops below 0.4 mL/minute/kg. Adequate hydration should also be maintained throughout the course of drug therapy.
- **Indinavir** may cause nephrolithiasis, flank pain, and hematuria. Symptoms usually subside with increased hydration and stopping the drug for 1 to 3 days. A fluid intake of at least 1500 mL daily is recommended during indinavir therapy.

Drugs That Require Dosage Reduction

- **Amantadine, famciclovir, ganciclovir, lamivudine, stavudine, valacyclovir**, and **zalcitabine** are eliminated mainly through the kidneys. In clients with renal impairment, they may accumulate, produce higher blood levels, have longer half-lives, and cause toxicity. For all the drugs except famciclovir, dosage should be reduced with CrCl levels below 50 mL/minute. With famciclovir, dosage should be decreased with CrCl below 60 mL/minute. For clients receiving hemodialysis, dosages should be calculated according to CrCl, with daily doses given after dialysis. Prescribers should consult manufacturers' recommendations for dosages in relation to CrCl.
- **Zidovudine** dosage should be decreased with severe renal impairment. It is mainly metabolized in the liver to an inactive metabolite that is then eliminated renally (approximately 60% to 75% of a dose); another 20% is excreted as unchanged drug in the urine. Thus, mild to moderate renal impairment does not lead to drug accumulation or a need for reduced dosage. With severe impairment, however, drug half-life is prolonged, possibly because some metabolism occurs in the kidneys as well as the liver. Also, clients with

renal impairment may be more likely to experience zidovudine-induced hematologic adverse effects because of decreased production of erythropoietin. Because of these factors, it is recommended that the daily dosage be reduced by approximately 50% in clients with severe renal impairment (CrCl <25 mL/minute) and clients on hemodialysis. In addition, clients should be carefully monitored for adverse drug effects.

- **Didanosine** doses are approximately 60% excreted in the urine as unchanged drug. The remainder is metabolized in the liver to several metabolites, including one with antiviral activity similar to that of the parent drug. In clients with severe renal impairment, didanosine is eliminated slowly and has a longer half-life. Thus, dosage reduction is indicated to prevent drug accumulation and toxic effects. In addition, because didanosine tablets contain sodium and magnesium, dosage reductions help to prevent edema and hypermagnesemia.

Other Drugs

Delavirdine, nelfinavir, nevirapine, ritonavir, and **saquinavir** are primarily metabolized by the liver and are unlikely to need dosage reductions with impaired renal function.

Use in Hepatic Impairment

The antiviral drugs of most concern in hepatic impairment are the anti-HIV agents, especially the protease inhibitors. Although most antiretroviral drugs have not been studied in clients with hepatic impairment, several are primarily metabolized in the liver and may produce high blood levels and cause adverse effects in the presence of liver dysfunction. In addition, clients with HIV infection may have concomitant liver disease that further impairs hepatic metabolism and elimination of the drugs. Although few guidelines are available, dosages should be individualized according to the severity of hepatic impairment and HIV infection, other drug therapies (for HIV infection, opportunistic infections, or other conditions), additional risk factors for drug toxicity, and the potential for drug interactions. In addition, all clients with hepatic impairment should be monitored closely for abnormal liver function tests (LFTs) and drug-related toxicity. Hepatic effects and considerations for usage of selected drugs are as follows:

- **Amprenavir, delavirdine, didanosine, nelfinavir, nevirapine, ritonavir**, and **saquinavir** may need dosage reductions with impaired hepatic function.
- **Nevirapine** may cause abnormal LFTs, and a few cases of fatal hepatitis have been reported. If moderate or severe LFT abnormalities occur, nevirapine administration should be stopped until LFTs return

to baseline values. If liver dysfunction recurs when the drug is resumed, nevirapine should be discontinued permanently.

- **Zidovudine** is eliminated more slowly and has a longer half-life in clients with moderate to severe liver disease. Thus, it is recommended that daily doses be reduced by 50% in clients with hepatic impairment.

 Home Care

Most antiviral drugs are self-administered by clients or given by caregivers in the home setting. Precautions to prevent viral infections from occurring or spreading are especially important because of the close contacts among members of a household. The home care nurse may need to teach infection control precautions and to assess the immunization status of all household members. If immunizations are indicated, the nurse may need to teach, encourage, provide, or somehow facilitate their accomplishment.

Home care of clients with HIV infection may include a variety of activities such as assisting with drug therapy for HIV or opportunistic infections, coordinating medical and social services, managing symptoms of the disease or adverse drug effects, preventing or minimizing opportunistic infections, teaching clients and others that HIV infection is a chronic illness that progresses differently among individuals, and making referrals for hospitalization or hospice care when indicated.

(*text continues on page 598*)

| NURSING ACTIONS | Antiviral Drugs |

NURSING ACTIONS	RATIONALE/EXPLANATION
1. Administer accurately **a.** Give oral drugs as recommended in relation to meals:	Manufacturers' recommendations to promote absorption and bioavailability
(1) Give abacavir, amprenavir, delavirdine, efavirenz, famciclovir, lamivudine, nevirapine, stavudine, and valacyclovir with or without food. However, do not give abacavir, amprenavir, or efavirenz with a high-fat meal. Also, if the patient is taking an antacid or didanosine, give amprenavir at least 1 h before or after a dose of antacid or didanosine.	
(2) Give didanosine and indinavir on an empty stomach, 1 h before or 2 h after a meal. Although indinavir is best absorbed if taken on an empty stomach, with water, it may also be taken with skim milk, juice, coffee, tea or a light meal (eg, toast, cereal). If the patient is taking indinavir and didanosine, the drugs should be given at least 1 h apart on an empty stomach.	
(3) Give ganciclovir, nelfinavir, and ritonavir with food. The oral solution of ritonavir may be mixed with chocolate milk or Ensure to improve the taste.	
(4) Give saquinavir within 2 h after a meal.	
b. Delavirdine tablets may be mixed in water by adding four tablets to at least 3 oz of water, waiting a few minutes, and then stirring. Have the client drink the mixture promptly, rinse the glass, and swallow the rinse to be sure the entire dose is taken.	

(*continued*)

NURSING ACTIONS	RATIONALE/EXPLANATION
c. To give nelfinavir to infants and young children, the oral powder can be mixed with a small amount of water, milk, or formula. Once mixed, the entire amount must be taken to obtain the full dose.	Acidic foods or juices (eg, orange juice, apple juice, apple sauce) should not be used because they produce a bitter taste.
d. Give intravenous (IV) acyclovir, cidofovir, foscarnet, and ganciclovir over 1 h.	To decrease tissue irritation and increased toxicity from high plasma levels
e. With cidofovir therapy, give probenecid 2 g 3 h before cidofovir, 1 g 2 h before cidofovir, and 1 g 8 h after completion of the cidofovir infusion	To slow renal excretion of cidofovir and decrease nephrotoxic effects
f. With topical acyclovir, wear a glove to apply.	To prevent spread of infection because lesions contain herpesvirus
g. With ribavirin, follow the manufacturer's instructions.	Specific techniques are required for accurate usage
2. Observe for therapeutic effects	
a. With acyclovir for genital herpes, observe for fewer recurrences when given for prophylaxis; observe for healing of lesions and decreased pain and itching when given for treatment.	
b. With amantadine, observe for absence of symptoms when given for prophylaxis of influenza A and decreased fever, cough, muscle aches, and malaise when given for treatment.	
c. With cidofovir, ganciclovir or foscarnet for cytomegalovirus retinitis, observe for improved vision.	
d. With ophthalmic drugs, observe for decreased signs of eye infection.	
e. With anti–human immunodeficiency virus (HIV) drugs, observe for improved clinical status (fewer signs and symptoms) and improved laboratory markers (eg, decreased viral load, increased CD4+ cell count)	
3. Observe for adverse effects	
a. General effects—anorexia, nausea, vomiting, diarrhea, fever, headache	These effects occur with most systemic antiviral drugs and may range from mild to severe.
b. With IV acyclovir—phlebitis at injection site, skin rash, urticaria, increased blood urea nitrogen or serum creatinine, encephalopathy manifested by confusion, coma, lethargy, seizures, tremors	Encephalopathy is rare but potentially serious; other effects commonly occur.
c. With topical acyclovir—burning or stinging and pruritus	These effects are usually transient.
d. With amantadine and rimantadine—central nervous system (CNS) effects with anxiety, ataxia, dizziness, hyperexcitability, insomnia, mental confusion, hallucinations, slurred speech	CNS symptoms are reportedly more likely with amantadine than with rimantadine and may be similar to those caused by atropine and CNS stimulants. Adverse reactions are more likely to occur in older adults and those with renal impairment.

(continued)

NURSING ACTIONS	RATIONALE/EXPLANATION
e. With didanosine, zalcitabine, and zidovudine—peripheral neuropathy (numbness, burning, pain in hands and feet), pancreatitis (abdominal pain, severe nausea and vomiting, elevated serum amylase)	Peripheral neuropathy may be more likely with zalcitabine, and the drug should be stopped promptly if symptoms appear, to avoid irreversible neuropathy. Pancreatitis may be more likely with didanosine, especially in those with previous episodes, alcohol consumption, elevated serum triglycerides, or advanced HIV infection. Didanosine should be stopped promptly if symptoms of pancreatitis occur.
f. With ganciclovir and foscarnet—bone marrow depression (anemia, leukopenia, neutropenia, thrombocytopenia), renal impairment (increased serum creatinine and decreased creatinine clearance), neuropathy	Renal impairment may be more likely to occur with foscarnet.
g. With indinavir, ritonavir, and saquinavir—circumoral and peripheral paresthesias, debilitation, fatigue	The most frequent adverse effects are the general ones listed above. Most are relatively mild.
h. With lamivudine and stavudine—peripheral neuropathy, flu-like syndrome (fever, malaise, muscle and joint aches or pain), dizziness, insomnia, depression	
i. With ribavirin—increased respiratory distress	Pulmonary function may deteriorate.
j. With zidovudine—bone marrow depression (BMD; anemia, leukopenia, granulocytopenia, thrombocytopenia); anemia and neutropenia in newborn infants	Anemia may occur within 2–4 wk of starting the drug; granulocytopenia is more likely after 6–8 wk. A complete blood count should be done every 2 wk. Dosage should be reduced with moderate BMD, and the drug should be stopped with severe BMD (hemoglobin <7.5 g/dL; granulocyte count <750 mm^3), until the bone marrow recovers. Colony-stimulating factors (filgrastim or sargramostim) may be given to aid recovery of bone marrow function. Blood transfusions may be given for anemia.
	The hematologic effects on newborn infants may occur when the mothers received zidovudine during pregnancy.
k. With ophthalmic antiviral drugs—pain, itching, edema, or inflammation of the eyelids	These symptoms result from tissue irritation or hypersensitivity reactions.
4. Observe for drug interactions	Antiviral drugs are often given concomitantly with each other and with many other drugs, especially those used to treat opportunistic infections and other illnesses associated with HIV infection and organ transplantation. In general, combinations of drugs that cause similar, potentially serious adverse effects (eg, bone marrow depression, peripheral neuropathy) should be avoided, when possible.
a. Drugs that *increase* effects of acyclovir:	
(1) Probenecid	May increase blood levels of acyclovir by slowing its renal excretion
(2) Zidovudine	Severe drowsiness and lethargy may occur.

(continued)

NURSING ACTIONS	RATIONALE/EXPLANATION
b. Drugs that *increase* effects of amantadine and rimantadine:	
(1) Anticholinergics—atropine, first-generation antihistamines, antipsychotics, tricyclic antidepressants	These drugs add to the anticholinergic effects (eg, blurred vision, mouth dryness, urine retention, constipation, tachycardia) of the antiviral agents.
(2) CNS stimulants	These drugs add to the CNS-stimulating effects (eg, confusion, insomnia, nervousness, hyperexcitability) of the antiviral agents.
c. Drugs that *increase* effects of cidofovir and foscarnet:	
(1) Aminoglycoside antibiotics, amphotericin B, didanosine, IV pentamidine	These drugs are nephrotoxic and increase risks of nephrotoxicity.
d. Drugs that *increase* effects of ganciclovir:	
(1) Imipenem/cilastatin	Increased risk of seizures; avoid the combination if possible.
(2) Nephrotoxic drugs (eg, amphotericin B, cyclosporine)	Increased serum creatinine and potential nephrotoxicity
(3) Probenecid	May increase blood levels of ganciclovir by decreasing its renal excretion
e. Drugs that *increase* effects of indinavir:	
(1) Clarithromycin, ketoconazole, quinidine, zidovudine.	Increase blood levels of indinavir, probably by decreasing its metabolism and elimination
f. Drugs that *decrease* effects of indinavir:	
(1) Didanosine	Didanosine increases gastric pH and decreases absorption of indinavir. If the two drugs are given concurrently, give at least 1 h apart, on an empty stomach.
(2) Fluconazole	Decreases blood levels of indinavir
(3) Rifampin, rifabutin	These drugs speed up metabolism of indinavir by inducing hepatic drug-metabolizing enzymes.
g. Drug that *increases* the effects of lamivudine:	
(1) Trimethoprim/sulfamethoxazole	Decreases elimination of lamivudine
h. Drugs that *increase* the effects of ritonavir:	
(1) Clarithromycin, fluconazole, fluoxetine:	Increase blood levels, probably by slowing metabolism of ritonavir
i. Drug that *decreases* the effects of ritonavir:	
(1) Rifampin	Accelerates metabolism of ritonavir by inducing drug-metabolizing enzymes in the liver
j. Drug that *increases* the effects of saquinavir:	
(1) Ketoconazole	Increases blood levels of saquinavir
k. Drugs that *decrease* the effects of saquinavir:	
(1) Rifampin, rifabutin	Accelerate metabolism of ritonavir by inducing drug-metabolizing enzymes in the liver

(continued)

NURSING ACTIONS	RATIONALE/EXPLANATION
l. Drugs that *increase* the effects of zalcitabine:	
(1) Chloramphenicol, cisplatin, didanosine, ethionamide, isoniazid, metronidazole, nitrofurantoin, phenytoin, ribavirin, vincristine	Zalcitabine and these drugs are associated with peripheral neuropathy; concomitant use increases risks of this adverse effect. Didanosine and zalcitabine should not be used concomitantly.
(2) Cimetidine, probenecid	Increase blood levels of zalcitabine by decreasing its elimination
(3) Pentamidine (IV)	Increased risk of pancreatitis. If IV pentamidine is used to treat *Pneumocystis carinii* pneumonia, zalcitabine should be interrupted.
m. Drugs that *decrease* effects of zalcitabine:	
(1) Antacids, metoclopramide	Decrease absorption. Do not give antacids at the same time as zalcitabine.
n. Drugs that *increase* effects of zidovudine:	
(1) Doxorubicin, vincristine, vinblastine	Increased bone marrow depression, including neutropenia
(2) Amphotericin B, flucytosine	Increased nephrotoxicity
(3) Ganciclovir and pentamidine	Increased neutropenia
(4) Probenecid, trimethoprim	May increase blood levels of zidovudine, probably by decreasing renal excretion
o. Drugs that *decrease* effects of zidovudine:	
(1) Rifampin, rifabutin	Accelerate metabolism of zidovudine

Nursing Notes: Apply Your Knowledge

Answer: Nick may feel embarrassed or ashamed about this diagnosis and reluctant to ask questions. If his stress level is high, he may not hear and remember everything that is said. Provide written information for his future reference. Stress that genital herpes is a sexually transmitted disease that will be controlled but not cured with the acyclovir. He should complete the entire 10-day prescription, then take 400 mg bid for recurrences. Factors such as illness, emotional stress, or intense sunlight can increase recurrence. Because genital herpes is not cured, it is important to use a condom to prevent transmission of herpes to a sexual partner. The diagnosis of herpes is stressful and affects future life decisions. Listen to Nick's concerns and offer counseling.

 REVIEW AND APPLICATION EXERCISES

1. What is the major effect of antiviral drugs on susceptible viruses?

2. Which viral infections may be prevented by administration of an antiviral drug?

3. What are the major adverse effects associated with commonly used antiviral drugs? How would you assess for each of the adverse effects?

4. Why is it important to monitor renal function in any client receiving a systemic antiviral drug?

5. What is the advantage of combination drug therapy for HIV infection?

6. List nursing interventions to prevent or minimize adverse effects of anti-HIV drugs.

SELECTED REFERENCES

Andrist, L.C. (1997). Genital herpes: Overcoming barriers to diagnosis and treatment. *American Journal of Nursing, 97*(10), 16AAA–16DDD.

Balfour, H.H. (1999). Antiviral drugs. *New England Journal of Medicine, 340*, 1255–1268.

Bartlett, J.G. (1999). *The Johns Hopkins Hospital guide to medical care of patients with HIV infection*, 8th ed. Baltimore: Williams & Wilkins.

Bjorgen, S. (1998). Herpes zoster. *American Journal of Nursing, 98*(2), 46.

Carpenter, C.C., Fischl, M.A., Hammer, S.M., et al. (1996). Antiretroviral therapy for HIV infection in 1996: Recommendations of an international panel. *Journal of the American Medical Association, 276*, 146–154.

Collier, A.C. (1996). Efficacy of combination antiretroviral therapy. In J. Mills, P.A. Volberding, & L. Corey (Eds.), *Antiviral chemotherapy*, pp. 355–372. New York: Plenum Press.

Deitz, S.E. (1998). Acquired immunodeficiency syndrome. In C.M. Porth (Ed.), *Pathophysiology: Concepts of altered health states*, 5th ed., pp. 235–248. Philadelphia: Lippincott Williams & Wilkins.

Drug facts and comparisons. (Updated monthly). St. Louis: Facts and Comparisons.

Fletcher, C.V. & Collier, A.C. (1997). Principles and management of the acquired immunodeficiency syndrome. In J.T. DiPiro, R.L. Talbert, P.E. Hayes, G.C. Yee, G.R. Matzke, B.G. Wells, & L.M. Posey (Eds.). *Pharmacotherapy: A pathophysiologic approach*, 3rd ed., pp. 2353–2386. Stamford, CT: Appleton & Lange.

Goldschmidt, R.H. & Moy, A. (1996). Antiretroviral drug treatment for HIV/AIDS. *American Family Physician, 54*, 574–580.

Hayden, F.G. (1996). Antiviral agents. In J.G. Hardman, L.E. Limbird, P.B. Molinoff, & R.W. Ruddon (Eds.), *Goodman & Gilman's The pharmacological basis of therapeutics*, 9th ed., pp. 1191–1223. New York: McGraw-Hill.

Hilts, A.E. & Fish, D.N. (1998). Dosage adjustment of antiretroviral agents in patients with organ dysfunction. *American Journal of Health-System Pharmacy, 55*, 2528–2533.

Holtzer, C.D. & Roland, M. (1999). The use of combination antiretroviral therapy in HIV-infected patients. *Annals of Pharmacotherapy, 33*, 198–209.

Kaul, D.R., Cinti, S.K., Carver, P.L., & Kazanjian, P.H. (1999). HIV Protease inhibitors: Advances in therapy and adverse reactions, including metabolic complications. *Pharmacotherapy, 19*, 281–298.

Kirsten, V.L. & Whipple, B. (1998). Treating HIV disease: Hope on the horizon. *Nursing 28*(11), 33–39.

Lisanti, P. & Zwolski, K. (1997). Understanding the devastation of AIDS. *American Journal of Nursing, 97*(7), 26–34.

Pai, V.B. & Nahata, M.C. (1999). Nelfinavir mesylate: A protease inhibitor. *Annals of Pharmacotherapy, 33*, 325–339.

Panel on Clinical Practices for Treatment of HIV Infection. (1999). Guidelines for the use of antiretroviral agents in HIV-infected adults and adolescents. [Online: Available HIV/AIDS Treatment Information Service website: *http://www.hivatis.org*, accessed July 17, 1999.]

Portyansky, E. (1999, January 18). A powerful antiretroviral joins the nucleoside analog class in the fight against HIV-1 infection. *Drug Topics*, 23.

Rana, K.Z. & Dudley, M.N. (1999). Human immunodeficiency virus protease inhibitors. *Pharmacotherapy 19*, 35–49.

Varav, H. & Holtzer, C.D. (1999). Simultaneous use of two protease inhibitors in HIV infection. *American Journal of Health-System Pharmacy, 56*, 273–276.

Volk, W.A., Gebhardt, B.M., Hammarskjold, M.L., & Kadner, R.J. (1996). *Essentials of medical microbiology*, 5th ed. Philadelphia: Lippincott-Raven.

40

Antifungal Drugs

Objectives

After studying this chapter, the student will be able to:

1. Describe characteristics of fungi and fungal infections.

2. Discuss antibacterial drug therapy and immunosuppression as risk factors for development of fungal infections.

3. Describe commonly used antifungal drugs in terms of indications for use, adverse effects, and nursing process implications.

4. Differentiate between adverse effects associated with systemic and topical antifungal drugs.

5. Differentiate among formulations of amphotericin B.

6. Teach clients about prevention and treatment of fungal infections.

John Morgan, 79 years of age, is diagnosed with prostate cancer. He has been receiving chemotherapy for the last 3 months. After his third course of treatment, he becomes neutropenic and an infection develops that is treated with two broad-spectrum antibiotics.

Reflect on:

▶ Why John is at risk for a fungal infection.

▶ Why a fungal infection in John is likely to be serious and systemic.

▶ What assessments you will make to detect a fungal infection.

FUNGI AND FUNGAL INFECTIONS

Fungi are molds and yeasts that are widely dispersed in the environment. Fungal infections (mycoses) may be mild and superficial or life threatening and systemic. For example, *Candida albicans* is part of the indigenous microbial flora of the skin, mouth, intestine, and vagina. It is an opportunistic organism that often causes superficial mucosal infections (eg, oral, intestinal, or vaginal candidiasis) with antibiotic, antineoplastic, corticosteroid, and immunosuppressant drug therapy. Other fungi that cause superficial infections of the skin, hair, and nails are called *dermatophytes*. They obtain nourishment from keratin, a protein in skin, hair, and nails. Dermatophytic infections, which are of concern primarily because of their cosmetic appearance, include tinea pedis (athlete's foot) and tinea capitis (ringworm of the scalp) (see Chap. 66).

Systemic infections caused by opportunistic fungi (eg, *C. albicans* and *Aspergillus* species) usually occur only in immunocompromised hosts. Fungi that cause other serious infections are not part of the body's normal flora; they grow in soil and decaying organic matter. Most invasive fungal infections are acquired by inhalation of airborne spores from contaminated soil. Severity of disease increases with intensity of exposure.

Infections such as histoplasmosis, coccidioidomycosis, and blastomycosis usually occur as pulmonary disease but may be systemic. Other serious, systemic infections include cryptococcosis and sporotrichosis. These infections can occur in both healthy and immunocompromised people but are more likely to be severe and widespread in immunocompromised hosts.

Serious systemic fungal infections commonly occur, largely because of acquired immunodeficiency syndrome (AIDS), the use of immunosuppressant drugs to treat clients with cancer or organ transplants, the use of indwelling intravenous (IV) catheters for prolonged drug therapy or parenteral nutrition, implantation of prosthetic devices, and widespread use of broad-spectrum antibacterial drugs. Characteristics of selected fungal infections are described in Box 40-1.

(*text continues on page 603*)

BOX 40-1   SELECTED FUNGAL INFECTIONS

Aspergillosis is caused by an opportunistic mold that mainly causes infection in debilitated and immunocompromised people, including those with leukemia, lymphoma, or acquired immunodeficiency syndrome (AIDS) and those with neutropenia from a disease process or drug therapy. *Aspergillus* infection is characterized by inflammatory granulomatous lesions, which may develop in the bronchi, lungs, ear canal, skin, or mucous membranes of the eye, nose, or urethra. It may extend into blood vessels, lungs, liver, kidneys, and other organs. Invasive aspergillosis is a serious illness associated with thrombosis, ischemic infarction of involved tissues, and progressive disease.

For people with asthma in whom aspergillosis develops, an allergic reaction may occur and produce permanent fibrotic damage.

Blastomycosis is usually initiated by inhalation of spores from a fungus that grows in soil and decaying organic matter. The organism is endemic in the southeastern United States, Minnesota, Wisconsin, Michigan, and New York. The infection may be asymptomatic or produce pulmonary symptoms resembling pneumonia or tuberculosis. It may also be systemic and involve other organs, especially the skin and bone. Skin lesions, which may include pustules, ulcerations, and abscesses, may progress over a period of years and eventually involve large areas of the body. Bone invasion, with arthritis and bone destruction, occurs in 25% to 50% of clients.

Blastomycosis can occur in healthy people with sufficient exposure but is usually more severe and more likely to be systemic in immunocompromised clients.

Candidiasis is a yeast infection that often occurs in clients with malignant lymphomas, diabetes mellitus, or AIDS and in clients receiving antibiotic, antineoplastic, corticosteroid, and immunosuppressant drug therapy. Most candidal infections are caused by *Candida albicans*, which is part of the normal body flora and causes infection in certain circumstances. Oral, intestinal, vaginal, and systemic candidiasis can occur. Early recognition and treatment of local infections may prevent systemic candidiasis.

- **Oral candidiasis** (thrush) is characterized by painless white plaques on oral and pharyngeal mucosa. It often occurs in newborn infants, who become infected during passage through an infected or colonized vagina. In older children and adults, thrush may occur as a complication of diabetes mellitus, as a result of poor oral hygiene, or after taking antibiotics or corticosteroids. It may also occur as an early manifestation of AIDS.
- **Gastrointestinal candidiasis** most often occurs after prolonged broad-spectrum antibacterial therapy, which destroys a large part of the normal flora of the intestine. The main symptom is diarrhea.
- **Vaginal candidiasis** commonly occurs in women who are pregnant, have diabetes mellitus, or take

(continued)

BOX 40–1   SELECTED FUNGAL INFECTIONS (*continued*)

oral contraceptives or antibacterial drugs. The main symptom is a yellowish vaginal discharge. The infection may produce inflammation of the perineal area and spread to the buttocks and thighs. The organism is difficult to eradicate, and many women have recurrent infections.

- **Skin candidiasis** usually occurs in people with metabolic disorders that cause obesity, which results in continuously moist folds of skin, or with moist surgical dressings. The organism also may cause diaper rash and perineal rashes. Skin lesions are red and macerated.
- **Systemic** or **invasive candidiasis** occurs when the organism gets into the bloodstream and is circulated throughout the body. It often occurs as a nosocomial infection in clients with serious illnesses or drug therapies that suppress their immune systems. Invasive infections may be present in any organ and may produce such disorders as urinary tract infection, endocarditis, and meningitis. It is usually diagnosed by positive cultures of blood or tissue. Signs and symptoms depend on the severity of the infection and the organs affected.

Coccidioidomycosis is caused by an organism that grows in soil and decaying organic matter and is commonly found in the southwestern United States and northern Mexico. Infection results from inhalation of spores and often causes asymptomatic or mild respiratory infection. However, it may cause acute pulmonary infection with fever, chest pain, cough, headache, and loss of appetite. X-rays may show small nodules in the lung like those seen in tuberculosis. In some cases, chronic disease develops in which the organisms remain localized and cause large, organism-filled cavities in the lung. These cavities may become fibrotic and eventually require surgical excision. In a few cases, severe, disseminated disease occurs, either soon after the primary infection or after years of chronic pulmonary disease. Disseminated coccidioidomycosis may produce an acute or chronic meningitis or a generalized disease with lesions in many internal organs. Skin lesions appear as granulomas that may eventually heal or become ulcerations. Most clients with primary infection recover without treatment; clients with disseminated disease require prolonged chemotherapy.

Coccidioidomycosis may occur in healthy or immunocompromised people but is more severe and more likely to become systemic in immunocompromised clients. For example, clients with AIDS who live in endemic areas are highly susceptible to this infection. The severity of the disease also increases with intensity of exposure.

Cryptococcosis is caused by inhalation of *Cryptococcus neoformans*, an organism found worldwide. Primary infection occurs in the lungs; it is usually asymptomatic and heals without treatment. However, pneumonia may occur and lead to spread of the organisms by the bloodstream. Cryptococcosis may occur in both healthy and immunocompromised people, but is likely to be more severe and to become disseminated in immunocompromised clients. People with AIDS are highly susceptible.

Although the infection may involve the lungs, skin, and other body organs, it often attacks the meninges and produces abscesses in the brain. Clinical manifestations include headache, dizziness, and neck stiffness and the condition is often mistaken for brain tumor. Later symptoms include coma, respiratory failure, and death if the meningitis is not treated effectively.

Histoplasmosis is a common fungal infection that occurs worldwide, especially in the central and mideastern United States. The causative fungus is found in soil and organic debris around chicken houses, bird roosts, and caves inhabited by bats. Histoplasmosis develops when the organisms are inhaled into the lungs, where they develop into yeast cells that reach the bloodstream and become distributed throughout the body. In most cases, the organisms are destroyed or encapsulated by the host's immune system. The lung lesions heal by fibrosis and calcification and resemble the lesions of tuberculosis.

Clinical manifestations may vary widely. In people with normal immune responses, manifestations can be correlated with the extent of exposure. Most infections are asymptomatic or produce minimal symptoms for which treatment is not sought. When symptoms occur, they usually resemble an acute, influenza-like respiratory infection. However, people exposed to large amounts of spores may have a high fever and severe pneumonia, which usually resolves with a low mortality rate. Some people, most often adult men with underlying emphysema or other lung disease, develop chronic pulmonary histoplasmosis with recurrent episodes of cough, fever, and weakness. Histoplasmosis may also develop years after the primary infection, probably from reactivation of a latent lesion. This is likely to occur in clients with AIDS.

In addition, histoplasmosis occasionally infects the liver, spleen, and other organs and is rapidly fatal if not treated effectively. As with many other infections, the severe, disseminated form usually occurs in patients whose immune systems are suppressed by diseases or drugs.

Sporotrichosis occurs when contaminated soil or plant material is inoculated into the skin through small wounds (eg, splinters, thorn pricks) on the fin-

(*continued*)

BOX 40–1   SELECTED FUNGAL INFECTIONS (*continued*)

gers, hands, or arms. It is most likely to occur among people who handle sphagnum moss, roses, or baled hay. Thus, infection is an occupational hazard for gardeners and greenhouse workers. It can occur in both healthy and immunocompromised people, but is usually more severe and disseminated in the immuno-compromised host.

Initial lesions, usually small, painless bumps resembling insect bites, occur 1 week to 6 months after in-

oculation. The subcutaneous nodule develops into a necrotic ulcer, which heals slowly as new ulcers appear in adjacent areas. Local lymphatic channels and lymph nodes also develop abscesses, nodules, and ulcers that may persist for months or years if the disease is not treated effectively.

In immunocompromised people, sporotrichosis may enter the bloodstream and spread to various tissues, including the meninges.

ANTIFUNGAL DRUGS

Drugs for superficial fungal infections of skin and mucous membranes are usually applied topically. Numerous preparations are available, many without a prescription. Drugs for systemic infections are given IV or orally. Amphotericin B, which is active against most types of pathogenic fungi, is considered the drug of choice for most serious fungal infections. It must be given IV and produces numerous adverse effects in most recipients. The lipid formulations cause less nephrotoxicity than the older deoxycholate formulation. The various preparations cannot be used interchangeably and instructions for administration differ. Amphotericin B is usually given for 6 to 12 weeks.

The azole antifungal agents (eg, fluconazole, itraconazole, ketoconazole) are widely used drugs that cause fewer adverse effects than amphotericin B. Fluconazole is effective for candidiasis, cryptococcosis, and coccidioidomycosis. It is also used for long-term maintenance therapy of cryptococcal meningitis in clients with AIDS, after initial use of amphotericin B. Itraconazole is the drug of choice for blastomycosis, histoplasmosis, and sporotrichosis and is useful in treating aspergillosis.

Fluconazole can be given orally or IV; the others are given orally. Fluconazole and itraconazole increase serum levels, prolong half-lives, or decrease the clearance of numerous drugs. These drug interactions increase the risks of adverse effects with cyclosporine, phenytoin, sulfonylureas, theophylline, warfarin, and zidovudine. Indications for use and dosages of individual antifungal drugs are listed in Table 40-1.

Mechanism of Action

Most antifungal drugs bind with essential components in fungal cell membranes. This binding increases permeability of the cell membrane and allows intracellular contents to leak out.

NURSING PROCESS

Assessment

Assess for fungal infections. Specific signs and symptoms vary with location and type of infection.

- Superficial lesions of skin, hair, and nails are usually characterized by pain, burning, and itching. Some lesions are moist; others are dry and scaling. They also may appear inflamed or discolored.
- Candidiasis occurs in warm, moist areas of the body. Skin lesions are likely to occur in perineal and intertriginous areas. They are usually moist, inflamed, pruritic areas with papules, vesicles, and pustules. Oral lesions are white patches that adhere to the buccal mucosa. Vaginal infection causes a cheesy vaginal discharge, burning, and itching. Intestinal infection causes diarrhea. Systemic infection causes chills and fever, myalgia, arthralgia, and prostration.
- Blastomycosis, coccidioidomycosis, and histoplasmosis may be asymptomatic or simulate influenza, pneumonia, or tuberculosis, with cough, fever, malaise, and other pulmonary manifestations. Severe histoplasmosis may also cause fever, anemia, enlarged spleen and liver, leukopenia, and gastrointestinal tract ulcers.
- Cryptococcosis may involve the lungs, skin, and other body organs. In clients with AIDS or other immunosuppressant disorders, it often involves the central nervous system (CNS) and produces mental status changes, headache, dizziness, and neck stiffness.
- Sporotrichosis involves the skin and lymph nodes. It usually produces small nodules that look like insect bites initially and ulcerations later. Nodules and ulcers also may develop in local lymphatic channels and nodes. The infection can

(*text continues on page 606*)

TABLE 40-1   **Selected Antifungal Drugs**

Generic/Trade Name	Clinical Indications	Routes and Dosage Ranges	
		Adults	**Children**
Amphotericin B deoxycholate (Fungizone)	Serious, systemic fungal infections (eg, candidiasis, histoplasmosis) Cutaneous candidiasis Oral candidiasis	IV, individualized according to disease severity and client tolerance. Initial dose often 0.25 mg/kg/d, gradually increased to 0.5–1 mg/kg/d, infused over 2–6 h. Topically to skin lesions two to four times daily for 1–4 wk Oral suspension (100 mg/mL), 1 mL "swish and swallow" four times daily	Same as for adults for IV, skin preparations, and oral suspension
Amphotericin B lipid complex (Abelcet)	Systemic infections in clients who do not tolerate Fungizone	IV 5 mg/kg/d	Same as adults
Liposomal amphotericin B (AmBisome)	Systemic infections in clients who do not tolerate Fungizone Empirical treatment of presumed fungal infections in febrile, neutropenic clients	Immunocompetent clients, IV 3–5 mg/d on days 1 through 5, 14, and 21; course of therapy may be repeated if necessary. Immunosuppressed clients, IV 4 mg/kg/d on days 1 through 5, 10, 17, 24, 31, and 38 Febrile, neutropenic clients, IV 3 mg/kg/d by infusion pump, over approximately 2 h, depending on client tolerance	Same as adults
Amphotericin B cholesteryl (Amphotec)	Systemic infections in clients who do not tolerate Fungizone	IV, 3–4 mg/kg/d	Same as adults
Butoconazole (Femstat)	Vaginal candidiasis	Intravaginally, once daily for 3 d	
Ciclopirox (Loprox)	Tinea infections, cutaneous candidiasis	Topically to skin lesions, twice daily for 2–4 wk	
Clotrimazole (Lotrimin, Mycelex, Gyne-Lotrimin)	Cutaneous dermatophytosis; oral, cutaneous, and vaginal candidiasis	Orally, 1 troche dissolved in mouth five times daily Topically to skin twice daily Intravaginally, once daily	Same as for adults Dosage not established
Econazole (Spectazole)	Tinea infections, cutaneous candidiasis	Topically to skin lesions, once or twice daily for 2–4 wk	
Fluconazole (Diflucan)	Oropharyngeal, esophageal, vaginal, and systemic candidiasis Prevention of candidiasis after bone marrow transplantation Cryptococcal meningitis	Oropharyngeal candidiasis, PO, IV 200 mg first day, then 100 mg daily for 2 wk Esophageal candidiasis, PO, IV, 200 mg first day, then 100 mg daily for at least 3 wk Vaginal candidiasis, PO 150 mg as a single dose Systemic candidiasis, PO, IV 50–400 mg/d Prophylaxis, PO, IV 400 mg once daily Cryptococcal meningitis, PO, IV, 400 mg first day, then 200 mg/d	Oropharyngeal candidiasis, PO, IV 6 mg/kg first day, then 3 mg/kg/d for at least 2 wk Esophageal candidiasis, PO, IV, 6 mg/kg first day, then 3 mg/kg/d for at least 3 wk Systemic candidiasis, PO, IV 6–12 mg/kg/d Cryptococcal meningitis, PO, IV 12 mg/kg first day, then 6 mg/kg/d
Flucytosine (Ancobon)	Systemic mycoses due to *Candida* species or *Cryptococcus neoformans*	PO 50–150 mg/kg/d in divided doses q6h. Dosage must be decreased with impaired liver function	Same as for adults

| TABLE 40-1 | Selected Antifungal Drugs (*continued*) | | |

		Routes and Dosage Ranges	
Generic/Trade Name	Clinical Indications	Adults	Children
Griseofulvin (Fulvicin)	Dermatophytosis (skin, hair, nails)	Microsize, PO 500 mg–1 g daily in divided doses q6h Ultramicrosize, PO 250–500 mg daily	Microsize, PO 10 mg/kg in divided doses q6h Ultramicrosize, PO 5–7 mg/kg/d
Haloprogin (Halotex)	Dermatophytosis, mainly tinea pedis (athlete's foot), cutaneous candidiasis	Topically to skin, 1% cream or solution twice daily for 2–4 wk	Dosage not established
Itraconazole (Sporanox)	Systemic fungal infections, including aspergillosis, in neutropenic and immuno-compromised hosts Onychomycosis	Systemic infection, PO 200 mg once or twice daily Onchomycosis, PO 200 mg once daily for 12 wk	
Ketoconazole (Nizoral)	Candidiasis, histoplasmosis, coccidioidomycosis Cutaneous candidiasis Tinea infections	PO 200 mg once daily, increased to 400 mg once daily if necessary in severe infections Topically to skin, once daily for 2–6 wk	≥2 y: PO 3.3–6.6 mg/kg/d as a single dose
Miconazole (Monistat)	Dermatophytosis, cutaneous and vulvo-vaginal candidiasis	Topically to skin, once or twice daily for 4 wk Intravaginally, once daily for 1–2 wk	
Naftifine (Naftin)	Tinea infections (athlete's foot, jock itch, ringworm)	Topically to skin, once daily (cream) or twice daily (gel)	Safety and efficacy not established
Natamycin (Natacyn)	Fungal infections of the eye	Topically to eye, 1 drop q1–2h for 3–4 d, then 1 drop six to eight times daily for 14–24 d	
Nystatin (Mycostatin)	Candidiasis of skin, mucous membrane, and intestinal tract	Oral or intestinal infection, PO 400,000–600,000 U four times daily Topically to skin lesions, two or three times daily, continued for 1 wk after cure Intravaginally, 1 vaginal tablet once daily for 14 d	Oral infection, PO 100,000 U three or four times daily
Oxiconazole (Oxistat)	Tinea infections	Topically to skin lesions, once daily in evening for 2–4 wk	
Sulconazole (Exelderm)	Tinea infections	Topically to skin lesions once or twice daily for 3 to 4 wk	Safety and efficacy not established
Terconazole (Terazol)	Vaginal candidiasis	Intravaginally, 1 applicator once daily at bedtime for 7 doses	
Terbinafine (Lamisil)	Tinea infections Onychomycosis of fingernails or toenails	Tinea infections, topically to skin, once or twice daily for at least 1 wk and no longer than 4 wk Fingernail infections, PO 250 mg daily for 6 wk Toenail infections, PO 250 mg daily for 12 wk	Same as for adults Dosage not established
Tioconazole (Vagistat)	Vaginal candidiasis	Intravaginally, 1 applicator at bedtime	
Tolnaftate (Tinactin)	Cutaneous mycoses (dermatophytosis)	Topically to skin lesions, twice daily for 2–6 wk	Same as for adults
Triacetin (Fungoid)	Dermatophytosis (eg, athlete's foot), cutaneous candidiasis	Topically to skin lesions, twice daily until 1 wk after symptoms are relieved	Same as for adults
Zinc undecylenate (Desenex)	Dermatophytosis	Topically to skin twice daily for 2–4 wk	Same as for adults

IV, intravenous; PO, oral.

spread to other parts of the body in immuno-compromised clients.

- Systemic mycoses are confirmed by recovery of organisms from specimens of body tissues or fluids.

Nursing Diagnoses

- Self Care Deficit related to systemic infection
- Knowledge Deficit: Prevention and treatment of fungal infection
- Knowledge Deficit: Accurate drug usage
- Noncompliance related to the need for long-term therapy
- Risk for Injury: Adverse drug effects with systemic antifungal drugs

Planning/Goals

The client will:

- Receive systemic antifungal drugs as prescribed
- Apply topical drugs accurately
- Act to prevent recurrence of fungal infection
- Avoid preventable adverse effects from systemic drugs

Interventions

- Use measures to prevent spread of fungal infections:
  - Observe universal precautions while assessing or providing care to clients with skin lesions. Superficial infections (eg, ringworm) are highly contagious and can be spread by sharing towels and hairbrushes. Systemic mycoses are not contagious.
  - Decrease client exposure to environmental fungi. For inpatients who are neutropenic or otherwise immunocompromised, do not allow soil-containing plants in the room and request regular cleaning and inspection of air-conditioning systems. Aspergillosis has occurred after inhalation of airborne mold spores from air-conditioning units. For outpatients, assist to identify and avoid areas of potential exposure (eg, soil contaminated by chicken, other bird, or bat droppings). If exposure is unavoidable, instruct to spray areas with water to minimize airborne spores and to wear disposable clothing and a face mask. For clients at risk of exposure to sporotrichosis (eg, those who garden or work in plant nurseries), assist to identify risk factors and preventive measures (eg, wearing gloves and long sleeves).
- For obese clients with skin candidiasis, apply dry padding to intertriginous areas to help prevent irritation and candidal growth.

- For clients with oropharyngeal ulcerations, provide soothing oral hygiene, nonacidic fluids, and soft, bland foods.
- For clients with systemic fungal infections, monitor respiratory, cardiovascular, and neurologic status at least every 8 hours. Provide comfort measures and medications (eg, analgesics, antihistamines, antipyretics, antiemetics) for clients receiving IV amphotericin B.

Evaluation

- Observe for relief of symptoms for which an antifungal drug was prescribed.
- Interview outpatients regarding their compliance with instructions for using antifungal drugs.
- Interview and observe for adverse drug effects with systemic antifungal agents.

Nursing Notes: Apply Your Knowledge

Harold Johnson has oral candidiasis and is being treated with nystatin 5 cc, S & S, after meals and at bedtime. What nursing considerations are important to ensure therapeutic effect?

PRINCIPLES OF THERAPY

General Considerations

- Some fungal infections are asymptomatic or resolve spontaneously without treatment. In addition, candidal infections of blood or urine often respond to the removal of predisposing factors, such as antibacterial drugs, corticosteroids or other immunosuppressive drugs, and indwelling IV or bladder catheters.
- When antifungal drug therapy is required, it is usually long term, over many weeks to months. In some cases, it may be lifelong. If drug therapy is stopped too soon, relapse of the infection commonly occurs. However, in clients with AIDS, who often require long-term antifungal drug therapy, drug-resistant infections may develop. Fluconazole-resistant candidiasis is being increasingly recognized in this population.
- The selection of antifungal drugs is determined mainly by the type of fungal infection. For example, drugs that are effective in candidiasis are not usually effective in dermatophytic infections, and vice versa. For serious, systemic infections, amphotericin B is often the first drug of choice.
- Routes of administration are determined mainly by locations and severity of the infections. For example,

local infections can often be treated by topical applications, whereas more serious or systemic infections require oral or IV routes.

- Dosages depend on illness severity, with high amounts required for systemic infections, especially in immunocompromised hosts.

- Clients with impaired immune responses often become reinfected after effective antifungal drug therapy.

Drugs Used in Specific Infections

- **Aspergillosis.** Itraconazole for approximately 1 year may be effective in mild to moderate infection. Amphotericin B is indicated for serious invasive disease, and large doses are required.

- **Blastomycosis.** Amphotericin B is the drug of first choice for seriously ill clients. Itraconazole may also be used, alone for at least 6 months or after a course of amphotericin B.

- **Candidiasis. Oral candidiasis** is often treated with nystatin suspension, which is swished in the mouth to

allow medication contact with the mucosa and then swallowed. Other options include nystatin or clotrimazole troches, dissolved slowly in the mouth; oral fluconazole or ketoconazole; and low-dose amphotericin B IV for 1 to 2 weeks. **Vaginal candidiasis** may be treated with vaginal tablets, creams, or suppositories containing clotrimazole, miconazole, nystatin, tioconazole, or terconazole. Some of these preparations are available over the counter. A concern with self-treatment with nonprescription products is an incorrect diagnosis. Antifungal preparations do not help a bacterial vaginal infection. Pregnant clients should consult their obstetrician before using these drugs. **Gastrointestinal candidiasis** is usually treated with oral nystatin or fluconazole. **Systemic candidiasis** is usually treated with amphotericin B. If the CNS is involved, flucytosine is used in conjunction with amphotericin B, although some strains of *C. albicans* are resistant to flucytosine. Oral or IV fluconazole may also be used for non-neutropenic clients who cannot tolerate amphotericin B.

- **Coccidioidomycosis.** Amphotericin B is preferred for severe or disseminated disease and is usually given for 1 to 3 months. For milder infections, an oral azole (eg, fluconazole) may be given. Azole therapy is usually continued for more than 6 months after the disease becomes inactive. Some clients may require long-term therapy with itraconazole.

- **Cryptococcosis.** A combination of amphotericin B and flucytosine for 2 to 6 weeks is the initial treatment of first choice. This may be followed by 6 months of oral fluconazole for treatment of meningitis.
- **Histoplasmosis.** Amphotericin B is the drug of choice for treating moderate to severe disease in immunocompromised hosts. Itraconazole may be given, usually for 6 to 12 months, for mild disease in immunocompetent hosts. Ketoconazole may also be used. Relapses have occurred with each drug.
- **Sporotrichosis.** Itraconazole, for 3 to 6 months, is probably the drug of choice for localized lymphocutaneous infection. Amphotericin B is used to treat pulmonary, disseminated, and relapsing infections.

Characteristics and Usage of Amphotericin B

Amphotericin B has long been the gold standard of drug therapy for serious fungal infections. However, its use is problematic because of different preparations, special requirements for administration, and toxicity. These aspects are summarized below:

- **Preparations.** The deoxycholate preparation (Fungizone), often called conventional amphotericin B, is the oldest, most widely used form. Lipid preparations were developed to decrease the toxicity of the deoxycholate form, and three are currently available. These preparations have similar antifungal spectra, but they differ from the deoxycholate formulation and from each other in other respects. The cholesteryl form (Amphotec) and the lipid complex form (Abelcet) have longer half-lives than the liposomal form (AmBisome).

  The lipid formulations are indicated for clients who are unable to tolerate, or do not respond to, conventional amphotericin B. For example, these formulations may be useful for clients with renal impairment.
- **Administration.** These drugs should be reconstituted and prepared for IV administration in a pharmacy. If not prepared in a pharmacy, the manufacturer's instructions should be followed for each preparation. Additional factors include the following:
  - A test dose is usually recommended to assess the client's tolerance of the drug.
  - Maintenance doses can be doubled and infused on alternate days. However, a single daily dose should not exceed 1.5 mg/kg; overdoses can result in cardiorespiratory arrest.

  - Small initial doses (eg, 5 to 10 mg/day) are recommended for clients with impaired cardiovascular or renal function or a severe reaction to the test dose.
  - Larger doses of lipid preparations are needed to achieve therapeutic effects similar to those of the deoxycholate preparation.
  - An in-line filter may be used with Fungizone and AmBisome but should not be used with Abelcet or Amphotec.
  - Although manufacturers recommend covering containers during administration, to protect from light, this is probably not necessary if the solution is infused within 8 hours of reconstitution.
- **Decreasing adverse effects.** Several recommendations for reducing toxicity of IV amphotericin B have evolved, but most of them have not been tested in controlled studies. Recommendations to decrease nephrotoxicity are listed in the section on Use in Renal Impairment; those to decrease fever and chills include premedication with acetaminophen, diphenhydramine, IV corticosteroid, and meperidine; and those to decrease phlebitis at injection sites include administering on alternate days, adding 500 to 2000 units of heparin to the infusion, rotating infusion sites, administering through a large central vein, removing the needle after infusion, and using a pediatric scalp vein needle. A test dose is often given, but this does not reliably predict or rule out anaphylaxis, which is a rare adverse effect of both conventional and lipid formulations.

  Supplemental potassium may be used to treat hypokalemia, and recombinant erythropoietin may be used to treat anemia if the client has a low plasma level of erythropoietin.

Use in Children

Guidelines for the use of topical antifungal drugs in children are the same as those for adults. With most oral and

---

How Can You Avoid This Medication Error?

Amphotericin B is ordered for Harry Little, who has aspergillosis. You collect the following information before administering the medication: blood pressure 110/68, pulse 92, respiratory rate 18, temperature 37.8°C. Laboratory test results include K^+ 3.2 mEq/L, Na^+ 140 mEq/L, hemoglobin 14 g/dL, hematocrit 43%, blood urea nitrogen (BUN) 48 mg/dL, and creatinine 3.5 mg/dL. You have an order to premedicate Mr. Little with meperidine and diphenhydramine IV, which you do. He has a central line and the IV amphotericin is diluted in 500 cc, to run over 2 hours. You set the IV infusion pump for 250 cc/hour after you check the site and see that there is no redness.

parenteral agents, safety, effectiveness, and guidelines for use have not been established. In addition, some agents have no established dosages and others have age restrictions. Despite these limitations, most oral and parenteral drugs have been used successfully to treat children with serious fungal infections, without unusual or severe adverse effects. These include conventional and lipid formulations of amphotericin B, fluconazole, itraconazole, and ketoconazole. As in other populations receiving these drugs, children should receive the lowest effective dosage and be monitored closely for adverse effects.

Use in Older Adults

No geriatric guidelines have been established for antifungal drugs. The main concern is with oral or parenteral drugs because topical agents produce few adverse effects.

Virtually all adults receiving IV amphotericin B experience adverse effects. With the impaired renal and cardiovascular functions that usually accompany aging, older adults are especially vulnerable to serious adverse effects. They must be monitored closely to reduce the incidence and severity of nephrotoxicity, hypokalemia, and other adverse drug reactions. Lipid formulations are less nephrotoxic than the conventional deoxycholate formulation and may be preferred for older adults.

Use in Clients With Cancer

Clients with cancer are at high risk for development of serious, systemic fungal infections. In clients receiving cytotoxic anticancer drugs, antifungal therapy is often used to prevent or treat infections caused by *Candida* and *Aspergillus* organisms. For prophylaxis, topical, oral, or IV agents are given before and during the period of drug-induced neutropenia, often to prevent recurrence of infection that occurred during previous neutropenic episodes. For treatment, oral or IV drugs may be given at the onset of fever and neutropenia, when fever persists or recurs in a neutropenic client despite appropriate antimicrobial therapy, or when maintenance therapy is needed after acute treatment of coccidioidomycosis, cryptococcosis, or histoplasmosis. These infections often relapse if antifungal drugs are discontinued. Clients must be closely monitored for adverse effects of antifungal drugs.

Use in Renal Impairment

Amphotericin B deoxycholate (Fungizone), the conventional formulation, is nephrotoxic. Renal impairment occurs in most clients (up to 80%) within the first 2 weeks of therapy, but usually subsides with dosage reduction or drug discontinuation. Permanent impairment occurs in a few clients. Recommendations to decrease nephrotoxic-ity include hydrating clients with a liter of 0.9% sodium chloride solution IV and monitoring serum creatinine and blood urea nitrogen (BUN) at least weekly. If the BUN exceeds 40 mg/dL or the serum creatinine exceeds 3 mg/dL, the drug should be stopped or dosage should be reduced until renal function recovers. A newer strategy is to give a lipid formulation (eg, Abelcet, AmBisome, or Amphotec), which is less nephrotoxic. For clients who already have renal impairment or other risk factors for development of renal impairment, a lipid formulation seems indicated. Renal function should still be monitored frequently.

Fluconazole is mainly excreted in the urine as unchanged drug. Dosage may need to be reduced in clients with renal impairment. However, for clients receiving hemodialysis, an extra dose may be needed because 3 hours of hemodialysis lowers plasma drug levels by approximately 50%.

Flucytosine is excreted renally and may accumulate in renal impairment. Accumulation may increase BUN and serum creatinine and lead to renal failure unless dosage is reduced. Plasma drug levels should be monitored and dosage should be adjusted to maintain blood levels below 100 μg/mL.

Use in Hepatic Impairment

The azole antifungals may cause hepatotoxicity. With fluconazole, hepatic dysfunction has ranged from mild, transient elevations in transaminases to clinical hepatitis, cholestasis, hepatic failure, and death. Fatal hepatic damage occurred primarily in clients with serious underlying conditions, such as AIDS or malignancy, and with multiple concomitant medications. Liver function tests should be monitored during fluconazole therapy. If abnormalities develop, clients should be closely monitored for signs of hepatic injury. If clinical manifestations of liver disease occur, fluconazole should be discontinued. Hepatotoxicity may be reversible if the drug is discontinued.

Ketoconazole may cause serious hepatic impairment, including toxic hepatitis. When used for long periods in immunocompromised clients, liver function tests should be monitored. Asymptomatic, reversible elevations in hepatic aminotransferases occur with ketoconazole and itraconazole. Hepatic injury may be reversible if recognized promptly and the drug is discontinued.

Liver function tests should also be monitored when clients are receiving amphotericin B.

Use in Critical Illness

Amphotericin B and fluconazole are the drugs most often used for serious fungal infections. Amphotericin B penetrates tissues well, except for cerebrospinal fluid (CSF), and only small amounts are excreted in urine. With prolonged administration, the half-life increases from 1 to 15 days. Hemodialysis does not remove the drug. Lipid formulations may be preferred in critically ill clients because of less nephrotoxicity.

Fluconazole penetrates tissues well, including CSF. Although IV administration may be necessary in many critically ill clients, the drug is well absorbed when administered orally or by nasogastric tube, with bioavailability greater than 90%. Impaired renal function may require reduced dose.

When itraconazole is used in critically ill clients, a loading dose of 200 mg three times daily (600 mg/day) may be given for the first 3 days. Treatment should be continued for at least 3 months; inadequate treatment may lead to recurrent infection.

 Home Care

Antifungal drugs may be taken at home by a variety of routes. For topical and oral routes, the role of the home care nurse may be teaching correct usage and encouraging clients to persist with the long-term treatment usually required. With IV antifungal drugs for serious infections, the home care nurse may need to assist in administration and monitoring for adverse reactions.

(*text continues on page 612*)

NURSING ACTIONS	Antifungal Drugs

NURSING ACTIONS	RATIONALE/EXPLANATION
1. Administer accurately	
a. Give amphotericin B according to manufacturers' recommendations for each product:	Test doses and all other solutions should be prepared in the pharmacy.
(1) Follow manufacturers' recommendations for administration of test doses.	Concentrations and administration times vary among formulations.
(2) Use an infusion pump.	To regulate flow accurately
(3) Use a separate intravenous (IV) line if possible; if necessary to use an existing line, flush with 5% dextrose in water before and after each infusion.	
(4) Fungizone IV—give in 5% dextrose in water, over 2–6 h; use an in-line filter and an infusion pump; do not mix with other IV medications; cover the container if the solution is not infused within 8 h after reconstitution.	Administration times can vary according to patient tolerance.
(5) Abelcet—give IV over approximately 2 h; if infusion time exceeds 2 h, shake the container q2h to mix contents; do not use an in-line filter.	
(6) AmBisome—infuse over 2 h or longer; may use an in-line filter.	
(7) Amphotec—refrigerate after reconstitution and use within 24 h; infuse over at least 2 h; do not use an in-line filter.	
(8) Apply cream or lotion liberally to skin lesions and rub in gently.	
b. With IV fluconazole, follow instructions for preparation carefully; give as a continuous infusion at a maximum rate of 200 mg/h.	
c. With flucytosine, give one to two capsules at a time over 15 min.	To decrease nausea and vomiting

(*continued*)

NURSING ACTIONS	RATIONALE/EXPLANATION
d. Give itraconazole capsules after a full meal; give the oral solution on an empty stomach and ask the client to swish the medication around in the mouth for a few minutes, then swallow the medication.	To decrease gastrointestinal (GI) upset and increase absorption. The oral solution is effective only for oropharyngeal candidiasis, and correct administration enhances contact with mucosal lesions.
e. Give oral ketoconazole with food. However, do not give with antacids or other gastric acid suppressants. If such drugs are required, give them approximately 2 h after a dose of ketoconazole.	Food decreases GI upset. Antacids and antiulcer drugs that suppress gastric acid decrease absorption because the drug is dissolved and absorbed only in an acidic environment.
f. With nystatin suspension for mouth lesions (thrush), ask the client to swish the medication around in the mouth for a few minutes, then swallow the medication.	To increase drug contact with the lesions. Nystatin is not absorbed from the GI tract.
2. Observe for therapeutic effects	
a. Decreased fever and malaise with systemic mycoses	
b. Healing of lesions on skin and mucous membranes	
c. Diminished diarrhea with intestinal candidiasis	
d. Decreased vaginal discharge and discomfort with vaginal candidiasis	
3. Observe for adverse effects	
a. With amphotericin B, observe for fever, chills, anorexia, nausea, vomiting, renal damage (elevated blood urea nitrogen and serum creatinine), hypokalemia, hypomagnesemia, headache, stupor, coma, convulsions, anemia from bone marrow depression, phlebitis at venipuncture sites, anaphylaxis.	Amphotericin B is a highly toxic drug and most recipients develop some adverse reactions, including some degree of renal damage. Antipyretic and antiemetic drugs may be given to help minimize adverse reactions and promote patient comfort. Adequate hydration and lipid formulations may decrease renal damage.
b. With fluconazole, itraconazole, or ketoconazole, observe for unusual fatigue, loss of appetite, nausea, vomiting, jaundice, dark urine, pale stools, fever, abdominal pain, or diarrhea.	These may be signs of liver damage or other adverse drug effects. Drug therapy may need to be discontinued.
c. With flucytosine, observe for nausea, vomiting, and diarrhea.	These are common effects. Hepatic, renal, and hematologic functions also may be affected.
d. With ketoconazole, observe for nausea, vomiting, pruritus, and abdominal pain.	Gastrointestinal upset occurs in approximately 20% of clients taking 200 mg daily and in 50% or more of clients taking 400 mg daily.
e. With griseofulvin, observe for GI symptoms, hypersensitivity (urticaria, photosensitivity, skin rashes, angioedema), headache, mental confusion, fatigue, dizziness, peripheral neuritis, and blood dyscrasias (leukopenia, neutropenia, granulocytopenia).	Incidence of serious reactions is very low.
f. With oral terbinafine, observe for diarrhea, dyspepsia, headache, skin rash or itching, liver enzyme abnormalities.	

(continued)

NURSING ACTIONS	RATIONALE/EXPLANATION
g. With topical drugs, observe for skin rash and irritation.	Adverse reactions are usually minimal with topical drugs, although hypersensitivity may occur.
4. Observe for drug interactions	
a. Drugs that *increase* effects of amphotericin B:	
(1) Antineoplastic drugs	May increase risks of nephrotoxicity, hypotension, and bronchospasm
(2) Corticosteroids	May potentiate hypokalemia and precipitate cardiac dysfunction.
(3) Zidovudine	Increases renal and hematologic adverse effects of the liposomal formulation of amphotericin B. Renal and hematologic functions should be monitored closely.
b. Drug that *increases* effects of fluconazole:	
(1) Hydrochlorothiazide	Increased serum level of fluconazole, attributed to decreased renal excretion
c. Drugs that *decrease* effects of fluconazole:	
(1) Cimetidine, rifampin	Decrease serum levels
d. Drugs that *decrease* effects of griseofulvin: Barbiturates and other drugs that induce liver enzymes	Enzyme inducers inhibit effects of griseofulvin by increasing its rate of metabolism.
e. Drugs that *decrease* effects of itraconazole:	
(1) Histamine H$_2$ antagonists, phenytoin, rifampin	Decrease serum levels
f. Drugs that *decrease* effects of ketoconazole:	
(1) Antacids, histamine H$_2$ antagonists	These drugs increase gastric pH; this may inhibit absorption of ketoconazole.
(2) Isoniazid, rifampin	Decrease serum levels
g. Drug that *decreases* effects of terbinafine:	
(1) Rifampin	Causes rapid clearance of terbinafine

Nursing Notes: Apply Your Knowledge

Answer: Nystatin works topically to treat fungal infestation in the oral cavity. "S & S" means "swish and swallow." To ensure that nystatin remains in contact with the oral mucosa for as long as possible, it should be administered after meals and all other medications. Instruct the patient not to drink anything for 30 minutes.

How Can You Avoid This Medication Error?

Answer: Amphotericin B is very nephrotoxic. You should not administer it to Mr. Little when his BUN is 48 mg/dL and his creatinine is 3.5 mg/dL because both values indicate renal impairment. Notify his physician of this laboratory data to see if he or she would like to decrease the dose.

REVIEW AND APPLICATION EXERCISES

1. What environmental factors predispose clients to development of fungal infections?

2. What signs and symptoms occur with candidiasis, and how would you assess for these?

3. Which fungal infections often mimic other respiratory infections?

4. What are the clinical indications for use of IV amphotericin B?

5. What are nursing interventions to decrease adverse effects of IV amphotericin B?

6. What are the differences between amphotericin B deoxycholate and the lipid formulations?

7. What are the clinical indications for use of oral antifungal drugs?

SELECTED REFERENCES

Bennett, J.E. (1996). Antifungal agents. In J.G. Hardman, L.E. Limbird, P.B. Molinoff, & R.W. Ruddon (Eds.), *Goodman & Gilman's The pharmacological basis of therapeutics*, 9th ed., pp. 1175–1190. New York: McGraw-Hill.

Carver, P.L. (1997). Invasive fungal infections. In J.T. DiPiro, R.L. Talbert, G.C. Yee, G.R. Matzke, B.G. Wells, & L.M. Posey (Eds.), *Pharmacotherapy: A pathophysiologic approach*, 3rd ed., pp. 2251–2279. Stamford, CT: Appleton & Lange.

Drug facts and comparisons. (Updated monthly.) St. Louis: Facts and Comparisons.

Lewis, R.E. & Klepser, M.E. (1999). The changing face of nosocomial candidemia: Epidemiology, resistance, and drug therapy. *American Journal of Health-System Pharmacy, 56*, 525–536.

Rex, J.H. (1997). Approach to the treatment of systemic fungal infections. In W.N. Kelley (Ed.), *Textbook of internal medicine*, 3rd ed., pp. 1853–1854. Philadelphia: Lippincott-Raven.

Warnock, D.W. (1998). Treatment of invasive fungal infections (Editorial). *Hospital Medicine, 59*, 266–267.

Volk, W.A., Gebhardt, B.M., Hammarskjold, M.L., & Kadner, R.J. (1996). *Essentials of medical microbiology*, 5th ed. Philadelphia: Lippincott-Raven.

41

Antiparasitics

Objectives

After studying this chapter, the student will be able to:

1. Describe environmental and other major factors in prevention and recognition of selected parasitic diseases.

2. Discuss assessment and treatment of pinworm infestations and pediculosis in school-age children.

3. Discuss the drugs used to treat *Pneumocystis carinii* pneumonia in clients with acquired immunodeficiency syndrome.

4. Teach preventive interventions to clients planning travel to a malarious area.

You are the school nurse in an elementary school. There is an outbreak of head lice in one of the fourth grade classrooms. Four girls are affected. You are responsible for identifying infested students and developing prevention programs.

Reflect on:

▶ How the infested child feels.

▶ How the parents feel when they find out their child has head lice.

▶ Appropriate infection control measures to prevent the spread of head lice to other children in the classroom or family members.

▶ Teaching about the safe use of topical agents such as Nix.

A parasite is a living organism that survives at the expense of another organism, called the *host*. Parasitic infestations are common human ailments worldwide. The effects of parasitic diseases on human hosts vary from minor and annoying to major and life threatening. Parasitic diseases in this chapter are those caused by protozoa, helminths (worms), the itch mite, and pediculi (lice). Protozoa and helminths can infect the digestive tract and other body tissues; the itch mite and pediculi affect the skin.

PROTOZOAL INFECTIONS

Amebiasis

Amebiasis is a common disease in Africa, Asia, and Latin America, but it can occur in any geographic region. In the United States it is most likely to occur in residents of institutions for the mentally retarded, homosexual and bisexual men, and residents or travelers in countries with poor sanitation.

Amebiasis is caused by the pathogenic protozoan *Entamoeba histolytica*, which exists in two forms. The cystic form is inactive and resistant to drugs, heat, cold, and drying and can live outside the body for long periods. Amebiasis is transmitted by the fecal–oral route, such as ingesting food or water contaminated with human feces containing amebic cysts. Once ingested, some cysts break open in the ileum to release amebae, which produce trophozoites. Other cysts remain intact to be expelled in feces and continue the chain of infection. Trophozoites are active amebae that feed, multiply, move about, and produce clinical manifestations of amebiasis. Trophozoites produce an enzyme that allows them to invade body tissues. They may form erosions and ulcerations in the intestinal wall and cause diarrhea (this form of the disease is called *intestinal amebiasis* or *amebic dysentery*), or they may penetrate blood vessels and be carried to other organs, where they form abscesses. These abscesses are usually found in the liver (hepatic amebiasis), but they also may occur in the lungs or brain.

Drugs used to treat amebiasis (amebicides) are classified according to their site of action. For example, iodoquinol is an *intestinal amebicide* because it acts within the lumen of the bowel; chloroquine is a *tissue* or *extraintestinal amebicide* because it acts in the bowel wall, liver, and other tissues. Metronidazole (Flagyl) is effective in both intestinal and extraintestinal amebiasis. No available amebicides are recommended for prophylaxis of amebiasis.

Giardiasis

Giardiasis is caused by *Giardia lamblia*, a common intestinal parasite. It is spread by food or water contaminated with human feces containing encysted forms of the organism or by contact with infected people or animals. Person-to-person spread often occurs among children in day care centers, institutionalized people, and homosexual men. The organism is also found in people who camp or hike in wilderness areas or who drink untreated well water in areas where sanitation is poor. Giardiasis may affect children more than adults, and it has caused community outbreaks of diarrhea.

Giardial infections occur 1 to 2 weeks after ingestion of the cysts and may be asymptomatic or produce diarrhea and abdominal cramping and distention. If untreated, giardiasis may resolve spontaneously or progress to a chronic disease with anorexia, nausea, malaise, weight loss, and continued diarrhea with large, foul-smelling, light-colored, fatty stools. Deficiencies of vitamin B_{12} and fat-soluble vitamins may occur. Adults and children older than 8 years with symptomatic giardiasis should be treated with oral metronidazole.

Malaria

Malaria is a common cause of morbidity and mortality in many parts of the world, especially in tropical regions. In the United States, malaria is rare and affects travelers or immigrants from malarious areas.

Malaria is caused by four species of protozoa of the genus *Plasmodium*. The human being is the only natural reservoir of these parasites. All types of malaria are transmitted only by *Anopheles* mosquitoes. *Plasmodium vivax*, *Plasmodium malariae*, and *Plasmodium ovale* cause recurrent malaria by forming reservoirs in the human host. In these types of malaria, signs and symptoms may occur months or years after the initial attack. *Plasmodium falciparum* causes the most life-threatening type of malaria but does not form a reservoir. This type of malaria may be cured and prevented from recurring.

Plasmodia have a life cycle in which one stage of development occurs within the human body. When a mosquito bites a person with malaria, it ingests blood that contains gametocytes (male and female forms of the protozoan parasite). From these forms, sporozoites are produced and transported to the mosquito's salivary glands. When the mosquito bites the next person, the sporozoites are injected into that person's bloodstream. From the bloodstream, the organisms lodge in the liver and other tissues, where they reproduce and form merozoites. The liver cells containing the parasite eventually rupture and release the merozoites into the bloodstream, where they invade red blood cells. After a period of growth and reproduction, merozoites rupture red blood cells, invade other erythrocytes, form gametocytes, and continue the cycle. After several cycles, clinical manifestations of malaria occur because of the large numbers of parasites. The characteristic cycles of chills and fever correspond to the release of merozoites from erythrocytes.

Antimalarial drugs act at different stages in the life cycle of plasmodial parasites. Some drugs (eg, chloroquine) are effective against erythrocytic forms and are therefore useful in preventing or treating acute attacks of malaria. These drugs do not prevent infection with the parasite, but they do prevent clinical manifestations. Other drugs (eg, primaquine) act against exoerythrocytic or tissue forms of the parasite to prevent initial infection and recurrent attacks or to cure some types of malaria. Combination drug therapy, administered concomitantly or consecutively, is common with antimalarial drugs.

Pneumocystosis

Pneumocystosis is caused by *Pneumocystis carinii*, a parasitic organism once considered a protozoan but now considered a fungus. Sources and routes of spread have not been clearly delineated. It is apparently widespread in the environment, and most people are exposed at an early age. Infections are mild or asymptomatic in immunocompetent people. However, the organism can form cysts in the lungs, persist for long periods, and become activated in immunocompromised hosts. Activation produces *P. carinii* pneumonia (PCP), an acute, life-threatening respiratory infection characterized by cough, fever, dyspnea, and presence of the organism in sputum. Groups at risk include those with acquired immunodeficiency syndrome (AIDS); those receiving corticosteroids, antineoplastics, and other immunosuppressive drugs; and probably caregivers of infected people. PCP is often the cause of death in people with AIDS. PCP is discussed in this chapter because antiprotozoan drugs are used to treat the condition.

Toxoplasmosis

Toxoplasmosis is caused by *Toxoplasma gondii*, a parasite spread by ingesting undercooked meat or other food containing encysted forms of the organism, by contact with feces from infected cats, and by congenital spread from mothers with acute infection. Once infected, the organism may persist in tissue cysts for the life of the host. However, symptoms rarely occur unless the immune system is impaired or becomes impaired at a later time. Although symptomatic infection may occur in anyone with immunosuppression (eg, people with cancer or organ transplants), it is especially common and serious in people with AIDS, in whom it often causes encephalitis and death.

Trichomoniasis

The most common form of trichomoniasis is a vaginal infection caused by *Trichomonas vaginalis*. The disease is usually spread by sexual intercourse. Antitrichomonal drugs may be administered systemically (ie, metronidazole) or applied locally as douche solutions or vaginal creams.

HELMINTHIASIS

Helminthiasis, an infestation with parasitic worms, is a major disease in many parts of the world. Helminths are most often found in the gastrointestinal (GI) tract. However, several types of parasitic worms penetrate body tissues or produce larvae that migrate to the blood, lymph channels, lungs, liver, and other body tissues. Helminthic infections are described in Box 41-1.

Drugs used for treatment of helminthiasis are called *anthelmintics*. Most anthelmintics act locally to kill or cause expulsion of parasitic worms from the intestines; some anthelmintics act systemically against parasites that have penetrated various body tissues. The goal of anthelmintic therapy may be to eradicate the parasite completely or to decrease the magnitude of infestation ("worm burden").

SCABIES AND PEDICULOSIS

Scabies and pediculosis are parasitic infestations of the skin. Scabies is caused by the itch mite (*Sarcoptes scabiei*), which burrows into the skin and lays eggs that hatch in 4 to 8 days. The burrows may produce visible skin lesions, most often between the fingers and on the wrists.

Pediculosis is caused by three types of lice, which are blood-sucking insects. Pediculosis capitis (head lice) is the most common type of pediculosis in the United States. It is diagnosed by finding louse eggs (nits) attached to hair shafts close to the scalp. Pediculosis corporis (body lice) is diagnosed by finding lice in clothing, especially in seams. Body lice can transmit typhus and other diseases. Pediculosis pubis (pubic or crab lice) is diagnosed by finding lice in the pubic and genital areas. Occasionally, these lice infest the axillae, mustache, or eyelashes. Pediculosis is usually associated with poor personal hygiene and spread by social and sexual contact.

Although scabies and pediculosis are caused by different parasites, the conditions have several characteristics in common:

- They are more likely to occur in areas of poverty, overcrowding, and poor sanitation. However, they may occur in any geographic area and socioeconomic group.
- They are highly communicable and transmitted by direct contact with an infected person or the person's personal effects (eg, clothing, combs and hairbrushes, bed linens).
- Pruritus is usually the major symptom. It results from an allergic reaction to parasite secretions and excrement. In addition to the intense discomfort associated with pruritus, scratching is likely to cause skin excoriation with secondary bacterial infection and formation of vesicles, pustules, and crusts.
- They are treated with some of the same topical medications.

Hookworm infections are caused by *Necator americanus*, a species found in the United States, and *Ancylostoma duodenale*, a species found in Europe, the Middle East, and North Africa. Hookworm is spread by ova-containing feces from infected people. Ova develop into larvae when deposited on the soil. Larvae burrow through the skin (eg, if the person walks on the soil with bare feet), enter blood vessels, and migrate through the lungs to the pharynx, where they are swallowed. Larvae develop into adult hookworms in the small intestine and attach themselves to the intestinal mucosa.

Pinworm infections (enterobiasis), caused by *Enterobius vermicularis*, are the most common parasitic worm infections in the United States. They are highly communicable and often involve school children and household contacts. Infection occurs from contact with ova in food or water or on bed linens. The female pinworm migrates from the bowel to the perianal area to deposit eggs, especially at night. Touching or scratching the perianal area deposits ova on hands and any objects touched by the contaminated hands.

Roundworm infections (ascariasis), caused by *Ascaris lumbricoides*, are the most common parasitic worm infections in the world. They occur most often in tropical regions but may occur wherever sanitation is poor. The infection is transmitted by ingesting food or water contaminated with feces from infected people. Ova are swallowed and hatch into larvae in the intestine. The larvae penetrate blood vessels and migrate through the lungs before returning to the intestines, where they develop into adult worms.

Tapeworms attach themselves to the intestinal wall and may grow as long as several yards. Segments called proglottids, which contain tapeworm eggs, are expelled in feces. Tapeworms are transmitted by ingestion of contaminated, raw, or improperly cooked beef, pork, or fish. Beef and fish tapeworm infections are not usually considered serious illnesses. Pork tapeworm, which is uncommon in the United States, is more serious because it produces larvae that enter the bloodstream and migrate to other body tissues (ie, muscles, liver, lungs, and brain).

Threadworm infections (strongyloidiasis), caused by *Strongyloides stercoralis*, are potentially serious infections. This worm burrows into the mucosa of the small intestine, where the female lays eggs. The eggs hatch into larvae that can penetrate all body tissues.

Trichinosis, a parasitic worm infection caused by *Trichinella spiralis*, occurs worldwide. It is caused by ingestion of inadequately cooked meat, especially pork. Encysted larvae are ingested in infected pork. In the intestine, the larvae excyst, mature, and produce eggs that hatch into new larvae. The larvae enter blood and lymphatic vessels and are transported throughout the body. They penetrate various body tissues (eg, muscles and brain) and evoke inflammatory reactions. Eventually, the larvae are re-encysted or walled off in the tissues and may remain for 10 years or longer.

Whipworm infections (trichuriasis) are caused by *Trichuris trichiura*. Whipworms attach themselves to the wall of the colon.

ANTIPARASITIC DRUGS

Antiparasitic drugs include amebicides, antimalarials, other antiprotozoal agents, anthelmintics, scabicides, and pediculocides. These are described below and listed in Table 41-1.

Amebicides

Chloroquine (Aralen) is used primarily for its antimalarial effects. When used as an amebicide, the drug is effective in extraintestinal amebiasis (ie, hepatic amebiasis) but usually ineffective in intestinal amebiasis. The phosphate salt is given orally. When the oral route is contraindicated, severe nausea and vomiting occur, or the infection is severe, the hydrochloride salt can be given intramuscularly. Treatment is usually combined with an intestinal amebicide.

Iodoquinol (Yodoxin) is an iodine compound that acts against active amebae (trophozoites) in the intestinal lumen. It may be used alone in asymptomatic intestinal amebiasis to decrease the number of amebic cysts passed in the feces. When given for symptomatic intestinal amebiasis (eg, amebic dysentery), it is usually given with other amebicides in concurrent or alternating courses. Iodoquinol is ineffective in amebic hepatitis and abscess formation. Its use is contraindicated with iodine allergy and liver disease.

Metronidazole (Flagyl) is effective against protozoa that cause amebiasis, giardiasis, and trichomoniasis and against anaerobic bacilli, such as *Bacteroides* and *Clostridia* (see Chap. 37). In amebiasis, metronidazole is amebicidal at intestinal and extraintestinal sites of infection. It is a drug of choice for all forms of amebiasis except asymptomatic intestinal amebiasis (in which amebic cysts are expelled in the feces). In trichomoniasis, metronidazole is the only systemic trichomonacide available, and it is more effec-
(*text continues on page 621*)

TABLE 41-1 **Antiparasitic Drugs**

		Routes and Dosage Ranges	
Generic/Trade Name	**Indications for Use**	**Adults**	**Children**
Amebicides			
Chloroquine (Aralen)	Extraintestinal amebiasis	Phosphate, PO 1 g/d for 2 d, then 500 mg/d for 2 to 3 wk Hydrochloride, IM 200 to 250 mg/d for 10 to 12 d	Phosphate, PO 20 mg/kg/d, in two divided doses, for 2 d, then 10 mg/kg/d for 2 to 3 wk Hydrochloride, IM 15 mg/kg/d for 2 d, then 7.5 mg/kg/d for 2 to 3 wk
Iodoquinol (Yodoxin)	Intestinal amebiasis	Asymptomatic carriers, PO 650 mg/d Symptomatic intestinal amebiasis, PO 650 mg three times daily after meals for 20 d; repeat after 2 to 3 wk if necessary	PO 40 mg/kg/d in three divided doses for 20 d (maximum dose, 2 g/d); repeat after 2 to 3 wk if necessary
Metronidazole (Flagyl)	Intestinal and extraintestinal amebiasis Giardiasis Trichomoniasis	Amebiasis, PO 500 to 750 mg three times daily for 5–10 d Giardiasis, PO 250 mg three times daily for 7 d Trichomoniasis, PO 250 mg three times daily for 7 d, 1 g twice daily for 1 d, or 2 g in a single dose. Repeat after 4 to 6 wk, if necessary. *Gardnerella vaginalis* vaginitis, PO 500 mg twice daily for 7 d	Amebiasis, PO 35 to 50 mg/kg/d in three divided doses, for 10 d Giardiasis, PO 15 mg/kg/d in three divided doses, for 7 d
Tetracycline (Sumycin) and doxycycline (Vibramycin)	Intestinal amebiasis	PO 250–500 mg q6h, up to 14 d	PO 25 to 50 mg/kg/d in four divided doses for 7–10 d
Antimalarial Agents			
Chloroquine phosphate and chloroquine hydrochloride (Aralen)	Prevention and treatment of malaria	Prophylaxis, PO 5 mg/kg (chloroquine base) weekly (maximum of 300 mg weekly), starting 2 wk before entering a malarious area and continuing for 8 wk after return Treatment, PO 1 g (600 mg of base) initially, then 500 mg (300 mg of base) after 6 to 8 h, then 500 mg daily for 2 d (total of 2.5 g in four doses)	Treatment, PO 10 mg/kg (chloroquine base) initially, then 5 mg/kg after 6 h, then 5 mg/kg/d for 2 d (total of four doses)
		Treatment of malarial attacks, (hydrochloride) IM 250 mg (equivalent to 200 mg of chloroquine base) initially, repeated q6h if necessary, to a maximal dose of 800 mg of chloroquine base in 24 h	Treatment of malarial attacks, (hydrochloride) IM 5 mg/kg chloroquine base initially, repeated after 6 h if necessary; maximal dose, 10 mg/kg/24 h
Hydroxychloroquine (Plaquenil)	Erythrocytic malaria	Prophylaxis, PO 5 mg/kg, not to exceed 310 mg (of hydroxychloroquine base), once weekly for 2 wk before entry to and 8 wk after return from malarious areas Treatment of acute malarial attacks, PO 620 mg initially, then 310 mg 6 h later, and 310 mg/d for 2 d (total of four doses)	Prophylaxis, PO 5 mg/kg (of hydroxychloroquine base) once weekly for 2 wk before entry to and 8 wk after return from malarious areas Treatment of acute malarial attacks, PO 10 mg/kg initially, then 5 mg/kg 6 h later, and 5 mg/kg/d for two doses (total of four doses)
Chloroquine with primaquine	Prophylaxis of malaria	PO 1 tablet weekly for 2 wk before entering and 8 wk after leaving malarious areas	PO same as adults for children weighing >45 kg; 1/2 tablet for children weighing 25–45 kg.

TABLE 41-1 **Antiparasitic Drugs** (*continued*)

Generic/Trade Name	Indications for Use	Routes and Dosage Ranges	
		Adults	Children
			For younger children, a suspension is prepared (eg, 40 mg of chloroquine and 6 mg of primaquine in 5 mL). Dosages are then 2.5 mL for children weighing 5 to 7 kg, 5 mL for 8 to 11 kg, 7.5 mL for 12 to 15 kg, 10 mL for 16 to 20 kg, and 12.5 mL for 21 to 24 kg. Dosages are given weekly for 2 wk before entering and 8 wk after leaving malarious areas.
Halofantrine (Halfan)	Treatment of malaria, including chloroquine- or multidrug-resistant strains.	PO 500 mg q6h for three doses, repeat in 1 wk for clients without previous exposure to malaria (eg, travelers)	<40 kg: PO 8 mg/kg according to the schedule for adults
Mefloquine (Lariam)	Prevention and treatment of malaria	Prophylaxis, PO 250 mg 1 wk before travel, then 250 mg weekly during travel and for 4 wk after leaving a malarious area Treatment, 1250 mg (5 tablets) as a single dose	Prophylaxis, PO 1/4 tablet for 15–19 kg weight; 1/2 tablet for 20–30 kg; 3/4 tablet for 31–45 kg; and 1 tablet for >45 kg, according to the schedule for adults
Primaquine	Prevention of malaria	PO 26.3 mg (equivalent to 15 mg of primaquine base) daily for 14 d, beginning immediately after leaving a malarious area, or 79 mg (45 mg of base) once a week for 8 wk. To prevent relapse, the same dose is given with chloroquine or a related drug daily for 14 d.	PO 0.3 mg of base/kg/d for 14 d, according to the schedule for adults, or 0.9 mg of base/kg/wk for 8 wk
Pyrimethamine (Daraprim)	Prevention of malaria	PO 25 mg once weekly, starting 2 wk before entering and continuing for 8 wk after returning from malarious areas	PO 25 mg once weekly, as for adults, for children >10 y; 6.25–12.5 mg once weekly for children <10 y
Quinine (Quinamm)	Treatment of malaria	PO 650 mg q8h for 10–14 d	PO 25 mg/kg/d in divided doses q8h for 10–14 d
*Anti–*Pneumocystis carinii *Agents*			
Trimethoprim–sulfamethoxazole or **TMP-SMX** (Bactrim, others)	Prevention and treatment of PCP	Prophylaxis, PO 1 double-strength tablet (160 mg TMP and 800 mg SMX) q24h Treatment, IV 15–20 mg/kg/d (based on trimethoprim) q6–8 h, for up to 14 d; PO 15–20 mg/kg TMP/ 100 mg/kg SMX per day, in divided doses, q6h, for 14–21 d	Prophylaxis, PO 150 mg/m² TMP/750 mg/m² SMX per day, in divided doses q12h, on 3 consecutive days per week. Maximum daily dose, 320 mg TMP/1600 mg SMX. Treatment, IV 15–20 mg/kg/d (based on trimethoprim) q6–8 h, for up to 14 d; PO 15–20 mg/kg TMP/100 mg/kg SMX per day, in divided doses, q6h, for 14–21 d
Atovaquone (Mepron)	Prevention and treatment of PCP in people who are unable to take TMP-SMX	Prevention, PO 1500 mg once daily with a meal Treatment, PO 750 mg twice daily with food for 21 d	Adolescents 13–16 y: Same as adults Children <13 y: Dosage not established
Pentamidine (Pentam 300, NebuPent)	Prevention and treatment of PCP	Treatment, IM, IV 4 mg/kg once daily for 14 d Prophylaxis, inhalation, 300 mg every 4 wk	IM, IV same as adults Inhalation, dosage not established

(continued)

TABLE 41-1) **Antiparasitic Drugs** (*continued*)

		Routes and Dosage Ranges	
Generic/Trade Name	Indications for Use	Adults	Children
Trimetrexate (Neutrexin)	Treatment of PCP in immuno-compromised clients who are unable to take TMP-SMX	IV infusion 45 mg/m² daily, over 60–90 min, for 21 d (with leucovorin, PO, IV 20 mg/m² q6h for 24 d; give IV doses over 5–10 min)	Dosage not established
Anthelmintics			
Mebendazole (Vermox)	Treatment of hookworm, pinworm, roundworm, whipworm, and tapeworm infections	Most infections, PO 100 mg morning and evening for 3 consecutive d. For pinworms, a single 100-mg dose may be sufficient. A second course may be given in 3 wk, if necessary.	Same as adults
Pyrantel (Antiminth)	Treatment of roundworm, pinworm, and hookworm infections	Roundworms and pinworms, PO 11 mg/kg (maximal dose, 1 g) as a single dose; for hookworms, the same dose is given daily for 3 consecutive days. The course of therapy may be repeated in 1 mo, if necessary.	Same as adults
Thiabendazole (Mintezol)	Treatment of threadworm, pinworm, hookworm, roundworm, and whipworm infections	PO 22 mg/kg (maximal single dose, 3 g) twice daily after meals; 1 d for pinworms, repeated after 1–2 wk; 2 d for other infections, except trichinosis, which requires approximately 5 d	Same as adults
Scabicides and Pediculicides			
Permethrin (Nix, Elimite)	Pediculosis Scabies	Scabies, massage Elmite into the skin over the entire body except the face, leave on for 8–14 h, wash off. Pediculosis, apply Nix after shampooing, rinsing, and towel drying hair. Saturate hair and scalp, leave on for 10 min, rinse off with water.	Same as adults
Gamma benzene hexachloride (Kwell, Lindane)	Pediculosis Scabies	Scabies, apply topically to entire skin except the face, neck, and scalp, leave in place for 24 h, then remove by shower Pediculosis, rub cream or lotion into affected area, leave in place for 12 h, then wash or shampoo (rub into the affected area for 4 min and rinse thoroughly)	Same as adults
Malathion (Ovide)	Pediculosis (head lice)	Applied to hair, rubbed in well to wet hair, then hair dried without covering or using a hair dryer. After 8–12 h, shampoo, rinse, and comb hair with a fine-toothed comb to remove dead lice and eggs. If necessary, treatment can be repeated in 7–9 d.	Same as adults for children >2 y Safety and effectiveness not established for children <2 y

IM, intramuscular; IV, intravenous; PCP, *Pneumocystis carinii* pneumonia; PO, oral.

tive than any locally active agent. Because trichomoniasis is transmitted by sexual intercourse, partners should be treated simultaneously to prevent reinfection.

Metronidazole is usually contraindicated during the first trimester of pregnancy and must be used with caution in clients with central nervous system (CNS) or blood disorders.

Tetracycline and **doxycycline** are antibacterial drugs (see Chap. 36) that act against amebae in the intestinal lumen by altering the bacterial flora required for amebic viability. One of these drugs may be used with other amebicides in the treatment of all forms of amebiasis except asymptomatic intestinal amebiasis.

Antimalarial Agents

Chloroquine is a widely used antimalarial agent. It acts against erythrocytic forms of plasmodial parasites to prevent or treat malarial attacks. When used for prophylaxis, it is given before, during, and after travel or residence in endemic areas. When used for treatment of malaria caused by *P. vivax*, *P. malariae*, or *P. ovale*, chloroquine relieves symptoms of the acute attack. However, the drug does not prevent recurrence of malarial attacks because it does not act against the tissue (exoerythrocytic) forms of the parasite. When used for treatment of malaria caused by *P. falciparum*, chloroquine relieves symptoms of the acute attack and eliminates the parasite from the body because *P. falciparum* does not have tissue reservoirs. However, chloroquine-resistant strains of *P. falciparum* have developed in some geographic areas.

Chloroquine also is used in protozoal infections other than malaria, including extraintestinal amebiasis and giardiasis. It should be used with caution in clients with hepatic disease or severe neurologic, GI, or blood disorders.

Hydroxychloroquine (Plaquenil) is a derivative of chloroquine with essentially the same actions, uses, and adverse effects as chloroquine. It is also used to treat rheumatoid arthritis and lupus erythematosus.

Chloroquine with **primaquine** is a mixture available in tablets containing chloroquine phosphate 500 mg (equivalent to 300 mg of chloroquine base) and primaquine phosphate 79 mg (equivalent to 45 mg of primaquine base). This combination is effective for prophylaxis of malaria and may be more acceptable to clients. It also may be more convenient for use in children because no pediatric formulation of primaquine is available.

Halofantrine (Halfan) is indicated for treatment of malaria caused by *P. falciparum* or *P. vivax*, including chloroquine- or multidrug-resistant strains.

Mefloquine (Lariam) is used to prevent *P. falciparum* malaria, including chloroquine-resistant strains, and to treat acute malaria caused by *P. falciparum* or *P. vivax*.

Primaquine is used to prevent the initial occurrence of malaria; to prevent recurrent attacks of malaria caused by *P. vivax*, *P. malariae*, and *P. ovale*; and to achieve "radical cure" of these three types of malaria. (Radical cure involves eradicating the exoerythrocytic forms of the plasmodium and preventing the survival of the blood forms.) The clinical usefulness of primaquine stems primarily from its ability to destroy tissue (exoerythrocytic) forms of the malarial parasite. Primaquine is especially effective in *P. vivax* malaria. Thus far, plasmodial strains causing the three relapsing types of malaria have not developed resistance to primaquine. When used to prevent initial occurrence of malaria (causal prophylaxis), primaquine is given concurrently with a suppressive agent (eg, chloroquine or hydroxychloroquine) after the client has returned from a malarious area. Primaquine is not effective for treatment of acute attacks of malaria.

Pyrimethamine (Daraprim) is a folic acid antagonist used to prevent malaria caused by susceptible strains of plasmodia. It is sometimes used with a sulfonamide and quinine to treat chloroquine-resistant strains of *P. falciparum*. Folic acid antagonists and sulfonamides act synergistically against plasmodia because they block different steps in the synthesis of folic acid, a nutrient required by the parasites.

Quinine (Quinamm) is derived from the bark of the cinchona tree. Quinine was the primary antimalarial drug for many years but has been largely replaced by synthetic agents that cause fewer adverse reactions. However, it may still be used in the treatment of chloroquine-resistant *P. falciparum* malaria, usually in conjunction with pyrimethamine and a sulfonamide. Quinine also relaxes skeletal muscles and is used for prevention and treatment of nocturnal leg cramps.

Anti-*Pneumocystis carinii* Agents

Trimethoprim-sulfamethoxazole (TMP-SMX, Bactrim, others) (see Chap. 36) is the drug of choice for prevention and treatment of PCP. Prophylaxis is indicated for adults and adolescents with human immunodeficiency virus (HIV) infection and a low CD4+ T-helper cell count (<200); children with HIV; newborns whose mothers have HIV; organ transplant recipients; clients with leukemia or lymphoma who are receiving cytotoxic chemotherapy; and for clients receiving high doses of corticosteroids (equivalent to 20 mg or more daily of prednisone), including the tapering period, and for 1 month after the corticosteroid is stopped.

Adverse effects include nausea, fever, skin rash, and others, with some attributed to hypersensitivity reactions to the sulfamethoxazole. These effects seem to be more severe in clients with HIV infection.

Atovaquone (Mepron) is used for treatment of PCP in people who are unable to take TMP-SMX. Adverse effects include nausea, vomiting, diarrhea, fever, insomnia, and elevated hepatic enzymes.

Trimetrexate (Neutrexin) is a folate antagonist (which must be used with leucovorin rescue) approved only for treatment of moderate to severe PCP in immunocompromised clients, including those with advanced HIV infection, who are unable to take TMP-SMX. Hematologic toxicity is the main dose-limiting adverse effect. Leucovorin must be given daily during trimetrexate therapy and for 72 hours after the last trimetrexate dose. Dosage of trimetrexate must be reduced and dosage of leucovorin must be increased with significant neutropenia or thrombocytopenia.

Pentamidine (Pentam 300, NebuPent) is used to prevent or treat PCP. Pentamidine interferes with production of ribonucleic acid and deoxyribonucleic acid by the organism. The drug is given parenterally for treatment of PCP and by inhalation for prophylaxis. It is excreted by the kidneys and accumulates in the presence of renal failure, so dosage should be reduced with renal failure. With parenteral pentamidine, appropriate tests should be performed before, during, and after treatment (eg, complete blood count, platelet count, serum creatinine, blood urea nitrogen, blood glucose, serum calcium, and electrocardiogram).

Anthelmintics

Mebendazole (Vermox) is a broad-spectrum anthelmintic used in the treatment of parasitic infections by hookworms, pinworms, roundworms, and whipworms. It is also useful but less effective in tapeworm infection. Mebendazole kills helminths by preventing uptake of the glucose necessary for parasitic metabolism. The helminths become immobilized and die slowly, so they may be expelled from the GI tract up to 3 days after drug therapy is completed. Mebendazole acts locally in the GI tract, and less than 10% of the drug is absorbed systemically.

Mebendazole is usually the drug of choice for single or mixed infections caused by the aforementioned parasitic worms. The drug is contraindicated during pregnancy because of teratogenic effects in rats; it is relatively contraindicated in children younger than 2 years of age because it has not been extensively investigated for use in this age group.

Pyrantel (Antiminth) is effective in infestations of roundworms, pinworms, and hookworms. The drug acts locally to paralyze worms in the intestinal tract. Pyrantel is poorly absorbed from the GI tract, and most of an administered dose may be recovered in feces. Pyrantel is contraindicated in pregnancy and is not recommended for children younger than 1 year of age.

Thiabendazole (Mintezol) is most effective against threadworms and pinworms. It is useful but less effective against hookworms, roundworms, and whipworms. Because of the broad spectrum of anthelmintic activity, thiabendazole may be especially useful in mixed parasitic infestations. In trichinosis, thiabendazole decreases symptoms and eosinophilia but does not eliminate larvae from muscle tissues. The mechanism of anthelmintic action is uncertain but probably involves interference with parasitic metabolism. The drug is relatively toxic compared with other anthelmintic agents.

Thiabendazole is a drug of choice for threadworm infestations. For other types of helminthiasis, it is usually considered an alternative drug. It is rapidly absorbed after oral administration and most of the drug is excreted in urine within 24 hours. It should be used with caution in clients with liver or kidney disease.

Scabicides and Pediculicides

Permethrin is the drug of choice for both pediculosis and scabies. A single application eliminates parasites and ova and is usually curative. For pediculosis, permethrin is used in a 1% liquid (Nix), a nonprescription drug. For scabies, it is used in a 5% cream (Elimite), which requires a prescription. Permethrin is safer than other scabicides and pediculicides, especially for infants and children.

Permethrin is derived from a chrysanthemum plant, and people with a history of allergy to ragweed or chrysanthemum flowers should use it cautiously. The most frequent adverse effect is pruritus.

To avoid reinfection, close contacts should be treated simultaneously. With pediculosis, clothing and bedding should be sterilized by boiling or steaming and seams of clothes should be examined to verify that all lice are eliminated.

Gamma benzene hexachloride (Kwell, Lindane) is a second-line drug for scabies and pediculosis. It may be used for people who have hypersensitivity reactions to permethrin. It is applied topically, and substantial amounts are absorbed through intact skin. CNS toxicity has been reported with excessive use, especially in infants and children. The drug is available in a 1% concentration in a cream, lotion, and shampoo.

Malathion (Ovide) is a pediculicide used in the treatment of head lice, and **Pyrethrin** preparations (eg, Barc, RID) are available over the counter as gels, shampoos, and liquid suspensions for treatment of pediculosis. **Crotamiton** (Eurax) is used as a 10% cream or lotion for scabies.

NURSING PROCESS

Assessment

Assess for conditions in which antiparasitic drugs are used.

- Assess for exposure to parasites. Although exposure is influenced by many variables (eg, geographic location, personal hygiene, environmental sanitation), some useful questions may include the following:
  - Does the person live in an institution, an area of poor sanitation, an underdeveloped country, a tropical region, or an area of overcrowded housing? These conditions predispose to para-

sitic infestations with lice, the itch mite, proto-zoa, and worms.

○ Are parasitic diseases present in the person's environment? For example, head lice, scabies, and pinworm infestations often affect school children and their families.

○ Has the person recently traveled (within the previous 1 to 3 weeks) in malarious regions? If so, were prophylactic measures used appropriately?

○ With vaginal trichomoniasis, assess in relation to sexual activity. The disease is spread by sexual intercourse, and sexual partners need simultaneous treatment to prevent reinfection.

○ With pubic (crab) lice, assess sexual activity. Lice may be transmitted by sexual and other close contact and by contact with infested bed linens.

• Assess for signs and symptoms. These vary greatly, depending on the type and extent of parasitic infestation.

○ **Amebiasis.** The person may be asymptomatic, have nausea, vomiting, diarrhea, abdominal cramping, and weakness, or experience symptoms from ulcerations of the colon or abscesses of the liver (amebic hepatitis) if the disease is severe, prolonged, and untreated. Amebiasis is diagnosed by identifying cysts or trophozoites of *E. histolytica* in stool specimens.

○ **Malaria.** Initial symptoms may resemble those produced by influenza (eg, headache, myalgia). Characteristic paroxysms of chills, fever, and copious perspiration may not be present in early malaria. During acute malarial attacks, the cycles occur every 36 to 72 hours. Additional symptoms include nausea and vomiting, splenomegaly, hepatomegaly, anemia, leukopenia, thrombocytopenia, and hyperbilirubinemia. Malaria is diagnosed by identifying the plasmodial parasite in peripheral blood smears (by microscopic examination).

○ **Trichomoniasis.** Women usually have vaginal burning, itching, and yellowish discharge; men may be asymptomatic or have symptoms of urethritis. The condition is diagnosed by finding *T. vaginalis* organisms in a wet smear of vaginal exudate, semen, prostatic fluid, or urinary sediment (by microscopic examination). Cultures may be necessary.

○ **Helminthiasis.** Light infestations may be asymptomatic. Heavy infestations produce symptoms according to the particular parasitic worm. Hookworm, roundworm, and threadworm larvae migrate through the lungs and may cause symptoms of pulmonary congestion. The hookworm may cause anemia by sucking blood from the intestinal mucosa; the fish tapeworm may cause megaloblastic or pernicious anemia by absorbing folic acid and vitamin B_{12}. Large masses of roundworms or tape-worms may cause intestinal obstruction. The major symptom usually associated with pinworms is intense itching in the perianal area (pruritus ani). Helminthiasis is diagnosed by microscopic identification of parasites or ova in stool specimens. Pinworm infestation is diagnosed by identifying ova on anal swabs, obtained by touching the sticky side of cellophane tape to the anal area. (Early-morning swabs are best because the female pinworm deposits eggs during sleeping hours.)

○ **Scabies and pediculosis.** Pruritus is usually the primary symptom. Secondary symptoms result from scratching and often include skin excoriation and infection (ie, vesicles, pustules, and crusts). Pediculosis is diagnosed by visual identification of lice or ova (nits) on the client's body or clothing.

Nursing Diagnoses

• Knowledge Deficit: Management of disease process and prevention of recurrence
• Knowledge Deficit: Accurate drug administration
• Altered Nutrition: Less Than Body Requirements related to parasitic disease or drug therapy
• Self-Esteem Disturbance related to a medical diagnosis of parasitic infestation
• Noncompliance related to need for hygienic and other measures to prevent and treat parasitic infestations

Planning/Goals

The client will:

• Experience relief of symptoms for which antiparasitic drugs were taken
• Self-administer drugs accurately
• Avoid preventable adverse effects
• Act to prevent recurrent infestation
• Keep appointments for follow-up care

Nursing Notes: Apply Your Knowledge

You are a nurse in a travel clinic. Sally and Bill, college students, plan to spend part of their summer vacation traveling in Africa. You update their immunizations and then talk with them about malaria prevention. The physician has written a prescription for chloroquine phosphate and primaquine, 1 tablet every week. What information would you include in your teaching?

CLIENT TEACHING GUIDELINES
Antiparasitic Drugs

General Considerations

✔ Use measures to prevent parasitic infection or reinfection:
  ✔ Support public health measures to maintain a clean environment (ie, sanitary sewers, clean water, regulation of food-handling establishments and food-handling personnel).
  ✔ When traveling to wilderness areas or to tropical or underdeveloped countries, check with the local health department about precautions needed to avoid parasitic infections.
  ✔ Practice good hand washing and other personal hygienic practices.
  ✔ When a family member or other close contact contracts a parasitic infection, be sure appropriate treatment and follow-up care are completed.
  ✔ Avoid raw fish and undercooked meat.
  ✔ With vaginal infections, avoid sexual intercourse, or have the male partner use a condom.

Self- or Caregiver Administration

✔ Use antiparasitic drugs as prescribed; their effectiveness depends on accurate use.

✔ Take atovaquone, chloroquine and related drugs, iodoquinol, and oral metronidazole with or after meals. Food increases absorption of atovaquone and decreases gastrointestinal irritation of the other drugs.

✔ To use pentamidine by inhalation, dissolve the contents of one vial in 6 mL of sterile water, place the solution in the nebulizer chamber of a Respirgard II device, and deliver by way of oxygen or compressed air flow until the nebulizer chamber is empty (approximately 30 to 45 minutes).

✔ Take or give most anthelmintics without regard to mealtimes or food ingestion. Mebendazole tablets should be chewed or crushed and mixed with food; thiabendazole should be taken with food to decrease stomach upset. Chew chewable tablets thoroughly before swallowing.

✔ Use pediculicides and scabicides as directed on the label or product insert. Instructions vary among preparations.

Interventions

Use measures to avoid exposure to or prevent transmission of parasitic diseases.

- Environmental health measures include the following:
  ○ Sanitary sewers to prevent deposition of feces on surface soil and the resultant exposure to helminths
  ○ Monitoring of community water supplies, food-handling establishments, and food-handling personnel
  ○ Follow-up examination and possibly treatment of household and other close contacts of people with helminthiasis, amebiasis, trichomoniasis, scabies, and pediculosis
  ○ Mosquito control in malarious areas and prophylactic drug therapy for travelers to malarious areas. In addition, teach travelers to decrease exposure to mosquito bites (eg, wear long-sleeved, dark clothing; use an effective insect repellent such as DEET; and sleep in well-screened rooms or under mosquito netting). These measures are especially needed at dusk and dawn, the maximal feeding times for mosquitoes.
- Personal and other health measures include the following:
  ○ Maintain personal hygiene (ie, regular bathing and shampooing, handwashing before eating or handling food and after defecation or urination).
  ○ Avoid raw fish and undercooked meat. This is especially important for anyone with immunosuppression.
  ○ Avoid contaminating streams or other water sources with feces.
  ○ Control flies and avoid foods exposed to flies.
  ○ With scabies and pediculosis infestations, drug therapy must be accompanied by adjunctive measures to avoid reinfection or transmission to others. For example, close contacts should be examined carefully and treated if indicated. Clothes, bed linens, and towels should be washed and dried on hot cycles. Clothes that cannot be washed should be dry cleaned. With head lice, combs and brushes should be cleaned and disinfected; carpets and upholstered furniture should be vacuumed.
  ○ With pinworms, clothing, bed linens, and towels should be washed daily on hot cycles. Toilet seats should be disinfected daily.
  ○ Ensure follow-up measures, such as stool specimens, vaginal examinations, anal swabs, smears, and cultures.
  ○ With vaginal infections, avoid sexual intercourse, or have the male partner use a condom.

Evaluation

- Interview and observe for relief of symptoms.
- Interview outpatients regarding compliance with instructions for taking antiparasitic drugs and measures to prevent recurrence of infestation.
- Interview and observe for adverse drug effects.
- Interview and observe regarding food intake or changes in weight.

PRINCIPLES OF THERAPY

1. Antiparasitic drugs should be used along with personal and public health control measures to prevent spread of parasitic infestations. Specific measures vary according to the type of organism, the environment, and the host.
2. Many of the drugs described in this chapter are quite toxic; they should be used only when clearly indicated (ie, laboratory documentation of parasitic infection).

Use in Children

Children often receive an antiparasitic drug for head lice or worm infestations. These should be used exactly as directed and with appropriate precautions to prevent reinfection. Malaria is usually more severe in children than in adults, and children should be protected from exposure when possible. When chemoprophylaxis or treatment for malaria is indicated, the same drugs are used for children as for adults, with appropriate dosage adjustments. An exception is that tetracyclines should not be given to children younger than 8 years of age. Giardiasis seems to be more common in children than adults.

Use in Older Adults

Older adults are more likely to experience adverse effects of antiparasitic drugs because they often have impaired renal and hepatic function.

 Home Care

Most antiparasitic drugs are given primarily in the home setting. The home care nurse may need to examine close contacts of the infected person and assess their need for treatment, assist parents and clients to use the drugs appropriately, and teach personal and environmental hygiene measures to prevent reinfection. When children have parasitic infestations, the home care nurse may need to collaborate with day care centers and schools to prevent or control outbreaks.

(*text continues on page 628*)

NURSING ACTIONS | **Antiparasitics**

NURSING ACTIONS	RATIONALE/EXPLANATION
1. Administer accurately	
a. Give atovaquone, chloroquine and related drugs, iodoquinol, and oral metronidazole with or after meals.	Food improves absorption of atovaquone and decreases gastrointestinal (GI) irritation of the other drugs.
b. With pentamidine:	
(1) For intramuscular (IM) administration, dissolve the drug in 3 mL of sterile water for injection and inject deeply in a large muscle mass.	IM administration is painful and may cause sterile abscesses.
(2) For intravenous administration, dissolve the calculated dose in 3–5 mL of sterile water or 5% dextrose in water. Dilute further with 50–250 mL of 5% dextrose solution and infuse over 60 min.	
(3) For aerosol use, dissolve the contents of one vial in 6 mL of sterile water, place the solution in the nebulizer chamber of a Respirgard II device, and deliver by way of oxygen or compressed air flow until the nebulizer chamber is empty (approximately 30–45 min).	

(continued)

NURSING ACTIONS	RATIONALE/EXPLANATION
c. Give anthelmintics without regard to mealtimes or food ingestion. Mebendazole tablets may be chewed, swallowed, or crushed and mixed with food.	Food in the GI tract does not decrease effectiveness of most anthelmintics.
d. For pediculicides and scabicides, follow the label or manufacturer's instructions.	Instructions vary among preparations.
2. Observe for therapeutic effects	
a. With chloroquine for acute malaria, observe for relief of symptoms and negative blood smears.	Fever and chills usually subside within 24–48 h, and blood smears are negative for plasmodia within 48–72 h.
b. With amebicides, observe for relief of symptoms and negative stool examinations.	Relief of symptoms does not indicate cure of amebiasis; laboratory evidence is required. Stool specimens should be examined for amebic cysts and trophozoites periodically for approximately 6 mo.
c. With anti–*Pneumocystis carinii* agents for prophylaxis, observe for absence of symptoms; when used for treatment, observe for decreased fever, cough, and respiratory distress.	
d. With anthelmintics, observe for relief of symptoms, absence of the parasite in blood or stool for three consecutive examinations, or a reduction in the number of parasitic ova in the feces.	The goal of anthelmintic drug therapy may be complete eradication of the parasite or reduction of the "worm burden."
e. With pediculicides, inspect affected areas for lice or nits.	For most clients, one treatment is effective. For others, a second treatment may be necessary.
3. Observe for adverse effects	
a. With amebicides, observe for anorexia, nausea, vomiting, epigastric burning, diarrhea.	GI effects may occur with all amebicides.
(1) With iodoquinol, observe for agitation, amnesia, peripheral neuropathy, and optic neuropathy.	These effects are most likely to occur with large doses or long-term drug administration.
b. With antimalarial agents, observe for nausea, vomiting, diarrhea, pruritus, skin rash, headache, central nervous system (CNS) stimulation.	These effects may occur with most antimalarial agents. However, adverse effects are usually mild because small doses are used for prophylaxis, and the larger doses required for treatment of acute malarial attacks are given only for short periods. When chloroquine and related drugs are used for long-term treatment of rheumatoid arthritis or lupus erythematosus, adverse effects increase (eg, blood dyscrasias, retinal damage).
(1) With pyrimethamine, observe for anemia, thrombocytopenia, and leukopenia.	This drug interferes with folic acid metabolism.
(2) With quinine, observe for signs of cinchonism (headache, tinnitus, decreased auditory acuity, blurred vision).	These effects occur with usual therapeutic doses of quinine. They do not usually necessitate discontinuance of quinine therapy.
c. With metronidazole, observe for convulsions, peripheral paresthesias, nausea, diarrhea, unpleasant taste, vertigo, headache, and vaginal and urethral burning sensation.	CNS effects are most serious: GI effects are most common.

(continued)

NURSING ACTIONS	RATIONALE/EXPLANATION
d. With parenteral pentamidine, observe for leukopenia, thrombocytopenia, hypoglycemia, hypocalcemia, hypotension, acute renal failure, ventricular tachycardia, and Stevens-Johnson syndrome.	Severe hypotension may occur after a single parenteral dose. Deaths from hypotension, hypoglycemia, and cardiac arrhythmias have been reported.
e. With aerosol pentamidine, observe for fatigue, shortness of breath, bronchospasm, cough, dizziness, rash, anorexia, nausea, vomiting, chest pain.	These are the most common adverse effects.
f. With atovaquone, observe for nausea, vomiting, diarrhea, fever, headache, skin rash.	
g. With trimetrexate, observe for anemia, neutropenia, thrombocytopenia, increased bilirubin and liver enzymes (aspartate and alanine aminotransferases, alkaline phosphatase), fever, skin rash, pruritus, nausea, vomiting, hyponatremia, hypocalcemia.	
h. With topical antitrichomonal agents, observe for hypersensitivity reactions (eg, rash, inflammation), burning, and pruritus.	Hypersensitivity reactions are the major adverse effects. Other effects are minor and rarely require that drug therapy be discontinued.
i. With permethrin, observe for pruritus, burning, or tingling; with Lindane, observe for CNS stimulation (nervousness, tremors, insomnia, convulsions).	Antihistamines or topical corticosteroids may be used to decrease itching. CNS toxicity is more likely to occur with excessive use of Lindane (ie, increased amounts, leaving in place longer than prescribed, or applying more frequently than prescribed).
4. Observe for drug interactions	Few clinically significant drug interactions occur because many antiparasitic agents are administered for local effects in the GI tract or on the skin. Most of the drugs also are given for short periods.
a. Drugs that alter effects of chloroquine:	
(1) Acidifying agents (eg, ascorbic acid)	Inhibit chloroquine by increasing the rate of urinary excretion
(2) Alkalinizing agents (eg, sodium bicarbonate)	Potentiate chloroquine by decreasing the rate of urinary excretion
(3) Monoamine oxidase inhibitors	Increase risk of toxicity and retinal damage by inhibiting hepatic enzymes.
b. Drugs that alter effects of metronidazole:	
(1) Phenobarbital, phenytoin	These drugs induce hepatic enzymes and decrease effects of metronidazole by accelerating its rate of hepatic metabolism.
(2) Cimetidine	May increase effects by inhibiting hepatic metabolism of metronidazole.
c. Drugs that *decrease* effects of atovaquone and trimetrexate: Rifampin and other drugs that induce P450 drug-metabolizing enzymes in the liver	Although few interactions have been reported, any enzyme-inducing drug can potentially decrease effects of atovaquone and trimetrexate by accelerating their metabolism in the liver.

Nursing Notes: Apply Your Knowledge

Answer: Explain that malaria is transmitted by mosquito bites, and thus it is important to limit exposure to mosquitoes (by using insect repellent, wearing long pants and long-sleeve shirts, sleeping in screened or well-netted areas). Mosquitoes are most active at dusk and dawn, so prevention is especially important at these times. Prophylactic medications must be started 2 weeks before entering infested areas and continued for 8 weeks after return. The medication should be taken on the same day of the week at approximately the same time. If acute symptoms appear (headache, malaise, fever, chills), additional medication can be taken to treat the infection. Clear, written instructions regarding the dosage should be provided.

REVIEW AND APPLICATION EXERCISES

1. What groups are at risk for development of parasitic infections (eg, amebiasis, malaria, pediculosis, helminthiasis)?

2. What interventions are needed to prevent parasitic infections?

3. How would you assess for a parasitic infection in a client who has been in an environment associated with a particular infestation?

4. How can you assess a client's personal hygiene practices and environmental sanitation facilities?

5. How would you instruct a mother about treatment and prevention of reinfection with head lice or pinworms?

6. What are adverse effects of commonly used antiparasitic drugs, and how may they be prevented or minimized?

SELECTED REFERENCES

Anandan, J.V. (1997). Parasitic diseases. In J.T. DiPiro, R.L. Talbert, G.C Yee, G.R. Matzke, B.G. Wells, & L.M. Posey (Eds.), *Pharmacotherapy: A pathophysiologic approach*, 3rd ed., pp. 2161–2170. Stamford, CT: Appleton & Lange.

Drug facts and comparisons. (Updated monthly). St. Louis: Facts and Comparisons.

Grubman, S. & Simonds, R.J. (1996). Preventing *Pneumocystis carinii* pneumonia in human immunodeficiency virus-infected children: New guidelines for prophylaxis. *Pediatric Infectious Disease Journal, 15*, 165–168.

Kelley, W.N. (1997). *Textbook of internal medicine*, 3rd ed. Philadelphia: Lippincott-Raven.

Peterson, C.M. & Eichenfield, L.F. (1996). Scabies. *Pediatric Annals, 25*, 97–100.

Smeltzer, S.C. & Bare, B.G. (1996). *Brunner and Suddarth's Textbook of medical-surgical nursing*, 8th ed. Philadelphia: Lippincott-Raven.

Tracy, J.W. & Webster, L.T., Jr. (1996). Chemotherapy of parasitic infections. In J.G. Hardman, L.E. Limbird, P.B. Molinoff, & R.W. Ruddon (Eds.), *Goodman & Gilman's The pharmacological basis of therapeutics*, 9th ed., pp. 955–1026. New York: McGraw-Hill.

Drugs Affecting Hematopoiesis and the Immune System

42

Physiology of the Hematopoietic and Immune Systems

Objectives

After studying this chapter, the student will be able to:

1. Review hematopoiesis and body defense mechanisms.

2. Differentiate between cellular and humoral types of immunity.

3. Describe the antigen–antibody reaction.

4. Discuss similarities and differences between inflammation and the immune response.

5. Discuss roles of various white blood cells in the immune response.

6. Describe the functions and roles of cytokines and hematopoietic growth factors.

7. Discuss therapeutic uses of selected cytokines.

HEMATOPOIESIS

All blood cells originate in bone marrow in stem cells that are capable of becoming different types of blood cells. As these pluripotential stem cells reproduce during the life of the host, some reproduced cells are exactly like the original multipotential cells and are retained in bone marrow to maintain a continuing supply. However, most reproduced stem cells differentiate to form other types of cells. The early offspring are committed to become a particular type of cell, and a committed stem cell that will produce a cell type is called a colony-forming unit (CFU), such as CFU-erythrocyte or CFU-granulocyte. Hematopoietic growth factors control the reproduction, growth, and differentiation of the CFU. They also initiate the processes required to produce fully mature cells.

HEMATOPOIETIC CYTOKINES

Cytokines (Table 42-1) are substances produced by blood cells and other body cells that regulate many cellular activities by acting as chemical messengers among cells. Some cytokines are growth factors that induce proliferation and differentiation of blood cells. These cytokine hematopoietic growth factors comprise a large group of proteins that are structurally and functionally diverse. They were initially

TABLE 42-1 Cytokines

Type	Name	Main Source	Main Functions
Colony-stimulating factors (CSF)	G-CSF	Leukocytes	Stimulates growth of bone marrow
			Generates neutrophils
	M-CSF		Generates macrophages
			Stimulates growth of macrophages
	GM-CSF		Stimulates growth of monocyte–macrophages
	Erythropoietin	Kidneys	Stimulates bone marrow production of red blood cells
	Thrombopoietin	Liver and kidneys	Stimulates bone marrow production of platelets
Interferons (IFN)	IFN-alpha	Leukocytes	Antiviral, antiproliferative, and immunomodulating effects
			Stimulates macrophages and NK cells
	IFN-beta	Fibroblasts	Antiviral and immunoregulatory effects
	IFN-gamma	Circulating T cells and NK cells	Induces cell membrane antigens (eg, major histocompatibility complex)
			Influences functions of basophils and mast cells by increasing their ability to release histamine and decreasing their capacity for growth
Interleukins (IL)	IL-1	Monocytes	Interacts with tumor necrosis factor to induce other growth factors
			Stimulates growth of blood cells, especially B and T lymphocytes
			Enhances interactions between monocytes and lymphocytes
			Causes inflammation
			Causes fever
	IL-2	T lymphocytes	Promotes growth of T cells
			Activates T and B cells and NK cells
			Augments production of other lymphokines, such as interferon-gamma
			Influences the expression of histocompatibility antigens
			May inhibit granulocyte–macrophage colony formation and erythropoiesis
	IL-3 (multi-CSF)	T lymphocytes	Stimulates bone marrow; growth factor for all blood cells
			Stimulates growth of macrophages, eosinophils, and mast cells
	IL-4	Helper T cells	Stimulates growth of T and B cells and mast cells
			Promotes immunoglobulin synthesis and reactions
			Interacts with other cytokines to stimulate granulocytes, macrophages, mast cells, and other cells

TABLE 42-1   Cytokines (*continued*)

Type	Name	Main Source	Main Functions
	IL-5	Helper T cells	Stimulates B-cell growth, differentiation, and antibody secretion Stimulates eosinophils; promotes eosinophilia Stimulates T-cell replacement
	IL-6	Fibroblasts and others	Interacts with other growth factors to stimulate growth and differentiation of B and T cells and production of antibodies Augments inflammatory and Immune responses Augments colony formation induced by other growth factors Stimulates granulocyte–macrophage and megakaryocyte colony formation
	IL-7 (lymphopoietin-1)	Stromal cells of bone marrow	Generates pre–B and pre–T cells Stimulates lymphocyte growth Activates B and T cells
	IL-8	Macrophages and others	Regulates growth and movement of neutrophils and lymphocytes Induces immediate inflammatory responses
	IL-9	T lymphocytes	Stimulates production of red blood cells and platelets
	IL-10	T and B lymphocytes, macrophages	Inhibits cytokine synthesis
	IL-11	Stromal cells of bone marrow	Stimulates growth of megakaryocytes, B cells, and blast cells
	IL-12	Lymphocytes	Activates T lymphocytes and NK cells
	IL-13	Activated T lymphocytes	Induces proliferation of B lymphocytes Suppresses inflammatory cytokines
	TNF-alpha	T lymphocytes, macrophages	Inflammatory, immunoenhancing
	TNF-beta	T lymphocytes	Tumoricidal
T-lymphocyte growth factor (TGF)	TGF-beta	Platelets, bone, other tissue	Fibroplasia and immunosuppression Wound healing and bone remodeling

NK, natural killer; TNF, tumor necrosis factor.

named and defined by their action on one type of blood cell, but some of them act on multiple types of blood cells. They are primarily categorized as colony-stimulating factors (CSF), interleukins, and interferons.

Colony-Stimulating Factors

As their name indicates, CSF stimulate the production of red blood cells (erythropoietin), platelets (thrombopoietin), granulocytes (G-CSF), granulocyte–macrophages (GM-CSF), and monocyte–macrophages (M-CSF). In addition to granulocytes (neutrophils, basophils, and eosinophils), G-CSF also affects other blood cells (eg, erythrocytes, platelet precursors, and macrophages). In addition, interleukin-3 (IL-3) is sometimes called multi-CSF because it stimulates the production of all types of blood cells.

Interleukins

Interleukins (ILs) were named because they were thought to be produced by and to act only on leukocytes and lym-phocytes. However, they can be produced by body cells other than leukocytes and they can act on nonhematopoietic cells. Important interleukins include IL-3 (stimulates growth of stem cell precursors of all blood cells), IL-2 (stimulates T and B lymphocytes), IL-12 (stimulates hematopoietic cells and lymphocytes), and IL-11 (stimulates platelets and other cells). Interleukin action may occur only when combined with another factor, may be suppressive rather than stimulatory (eg, IL-10), or may involve a specific function (eg, IL-8 mainly promotes movement of leukocytes into injured tissues as part of the inflammatory response).

Interferons

Interferons "interfere" with the ability of viruses in infected cells to replicate and spread to uninfected cells. They also inhibit reproduction and growth of other cells, including tumor cells, and activate natural killer cells. These antiproliferative and immunomodulatory activities play important roles in normal host defense mechanisms.

OVERVIEW OF BODY DEFENSE MECHANISMS

The immune system is one of several mechanisms that protect the body from potentially harmful substances, including pathogenic microorganisms. The body's primary external defense mechanism is intact skin, which prevents entry of foreign substances and produces secretions that inhibit microbial growth. The mucous membranes lining the gastrointestinal (GI) and respiratory tracts are internal defense mechanisms that act as physical barriers and produce mucus that traps foreign substances so they may be expelled from the body. Mucous membranes also produce other secretions (eg, gastric acid) that kill ingested microorganisms. Additional internal mechanisms include the normal microbial population, which is usually nonpathogenic and controls potential pathogens, and secretions (eg, perspiration, tears, and saliva) that contain lysozyme, an enzyme that destroys the cell walls of gram-positive bacteria.

If a foreign substance gets through the aforementioned defenses and penetrates body tissues, an inflammatory response begins immediately. Inflammation is a generalized reaction to cellular injury from any cause. It involves phagocytic leukocytes and chemical substances that destroy the foreign invader.

The final defense mechanism is the immune response, which stimulates production of antibodies and activated lymphocytes to destroy foreign invaders and mutant body cells. Immune responses occur more slowly than inflammatory responses. Inflammatory and immune responses interact in complex ways and share a number of processes, including phagocytosis. As a result, understanding inflammation promotes understanding of immunity and vice versa. Cellular physiology and inflammation as a response to cellular injury are discussed in Chapter 1.

IMMUNITY

Immunity indicates protection from a disease, and the major function of the immune system is to detect and eliminate foreign substances that may cause tissue injury or disease. To perform this function, the immune system must be able to differentiate body tissues (self) from foreign substances (nonself). Self tissues are recognized by distinctive protein molecules on the surface membranes of body cells. These molecules or markers (also called autoantigens) are encoded by a group of genes called the major histocompatibility complex (MHC). MHC markers are essential to immune system function because they regulate the antigens to which a person responds and allow immune cells (eg, lymphocytes and macrophages) to recognize and communicate with each other. Nonself or foreign antigens are also recognized by distinctive molecules, called epitopes, on their surfaces. Epitopes vary widely in type, number, and ability to elicit an immune response.

A normally functioning immune system does not attack body tissues labeled as self, but attacks nonself substances. In most instances, a normally functioning immune system is highly desirable. With organ or tissue transplants, however, the system responds appropriately but undesirably when it attacks the nonself grafts. An abnormally functioning immune system causes numerous diseases. When the system is hypoactive, immunodeficiency disorders develop in which the person is highly susceptible to infectious and neoplastic diseases. When the system is hyperactive, it perceives ordinarily harmless environmental substances (eg, foods, plant pollens) as harmful and induces allergic reactions. When the system is inappropriately activated (it loses its ability to distinguish between self and nonself, so an immune response is aroused against the host's own body tissues), the result is autoimmune disorders, such as systemic lupus erythematosus and rheumatoid arthritis. Many other disorders, including diabetes mellitus, myasthenia gravis, and inflammatory bowel diseases are thought to involve autoimmune mechanisms. To aid understanding of the immune response and drugs used to alter immune response, more specific characteristics, processes, and functions of the immune system are described.

Types of Immunity

Innate immunity, which includes the general protective mechanisms described previously, is not produced by the immune system. It is often described as species dependent. Thus, humans have an inborn resistance to many infectious diseases that affect other species because human tissues do not provide a suitable environment for growth of the causative microorganisms.

Acquired immunity develops during gestation or after birth and may be active or passive. *Active immunity* is produced by the person's own immune system in response to a disease caused by a specific antigen or administration of an antigen (eg, a vaccine) from a source outside the body, usually by injection. The immune response stimulated by the antigen produces activated lymphocytes and antibodies against the antigen. When an antigen is present for the first time, production of antibodies requires several days. As a result, the serum concentration of antibodies does not reach protective levels for approximately 7 to 10 days, and the disease develops in the host. When the antigen is eliminated, the antibody concentration gradually decreases over several weeks.

The duration of active immunity may be brief (eg, to influenza viruses), or it may last for years or a lifetime. Long-term active immunity has a unique characteristic called *memory*. When the host is re-exposed to the antigen, lymphocytes are activated and antibodies are produced rapidly, and the host does not contract the disease.

This characteristic allows "booster" doses of antigen to increase antibody levels and maintain active immunity against some diseases.

Passive immunity occurs when antibodies are formed by the immune system of another person or animal and transferred to the host. For example, an infant is normally protected for several months by maternal antibodies received through the placenta during gestation. Also, antibodies previously formed by a donor can be transferred to the host by an injection of immune serum. These antibodies act against antigens immediately. Passive immunity is short term, lasting only a few weeks or months.

Types of acquired immunity have traditionally been separated into cellular immunity (mainly involving activated T lymphocytes in body tissues) and humoral immunity (mainly involving B lymphocytes and antibodies in the blood). However, it is now known that the two types are closely connected, that virtually all antigens elicit both cellular and humoral responses, and that most humoral (B cell) responses require cellular (T cell) stimulation.

Although most humoral immune responses occur when antibodies or B cells encounter antigens in blood, some occur when antibodies or B cells encounter antigens in other body fluids (eg, tears, sweat, saliva, mucus, and breast milk). The antibodies in body fluids other than blood are produced by a part of humoral immunity sometimes called the secretory or mucosal immune system. The B cells of the mucosal system migrate through lymphoid tissues of tear ducts, salivary glands, breasts, bronchi, intestines, and genitourinary structures. The antibodies (mostly immunoglobulin A [IgA], some IgM and IgG) secreted at these sites act locally rather than systemically. This local protection combats foreign substances, especially pathogenic microorganisms, that are inhaled, swallowed, or otherwise come in contact with external body surfaces. When the foreign substances bind to local antibodies, they are unable to attach to and invade mucosal tissue.

Antigens

Antigens are the foreign (nonself) substances, usually microorganisms, other proteins, or polysaccharides, that initiate immune responses. Antigens have specific sites that interact with immune cells to induce the immune response. The number of antigenic sites on a molecule depends largely on its molecular weight. Large protein and polysaccharide molecules are complete antigens because of their complex chemical structures and multiple antigenic sites. Smaller molecules (eg, animal danders, plant pollens, and most drugs) are incomplete antigens (called haptens) and cannot act as antigens by themselves. However, they have antigenic sites and can combine with carrier substances to become antigenic. Antigens also may be called *immunogens*. In discussions of allergic conditions, antigens are often called *allergens*.

Immune Responses to Antigens

The immune response involves antigens that induce the formation of antibodies or sensitized T lymphocytes. The initial response occurs when an antigen is first introduced into the body. B lymphocytes recognize the antigen as foreign and develop antibodies against it. Antibodies are proteins called immunoglobulins that interact with specific antigens. *Antigen–antibody interactions* may result in formation of antigen–antibody complexes, agglutination or clumping of cells, neutralization of bacterial toxins, destruction of pathogens or cells, attachment of antigen to immune cells, activation of complement (a group of plasma proteins essential to normal inflammatory and immunologic responses), and coating of the antigen so that it is more readily phagocytized (opsonization). With a later exposure to the antigen, antibody is rapidly produced. The number of exposures required to produce enough antibodies to bind a significant amount of antigen is unknown. Thus, an allergic reaction may occur with the second exposure or after several exposures, when sufficient antibodies have been produced.

Antigen–T lymphocyte interactions stimulate production and function of other T lymphocytes and help to regulate antibody production by B lymphocytes. T cells are involved in delayed hypersensitivity reactions, rejection of tissue or organ transplants, and response to neoplasms and some infections.

IMMUNE CELLS

Immune cells (Fig. 42-1) are white blood cells (WBCs) found throughout the body in lymphoid tissues (bone marrow, spleen, thymus, tonsils and adenoids, Peyer's patches in the small intestine, lymph nodes, and blood and lymphatic vessels that transport the cells). When exposure to an antigen occurs and an immune response is aroused, WBCs move toward the antigen in a process called *chemotaxis*. Once WBCs reach the area, they phagocytize the antigen. Specific WBCs are granulocytes (neutrophils, eosinophils, basophils), monocytes, and lymphocytes. Although all WBCs play a role, neutrophils, monocytes, and lymphocytes are especially important in phagocytic and immune processes.

Neutrophils arrive first and start phagocytosis; *monocytes* arrive several hours later. Compared with neutrophils, monocytes are larger, can ingest larger amounts of antigen, and have a much longer lifespan. In addition to their activity in the bloodstream, monocytes can enter tissue spaces (and are then called tissue macrophages). Tissue macrophages are widely distributed throughout the body and form the mononuclear phagocyte system. Both mobile monocytes and fixed monocyte–macrophages can initiate the immune response by activating lymphocytes. They perform this function as part of phagocytosis, in which they engulf a circulating antigen, break it into frag-

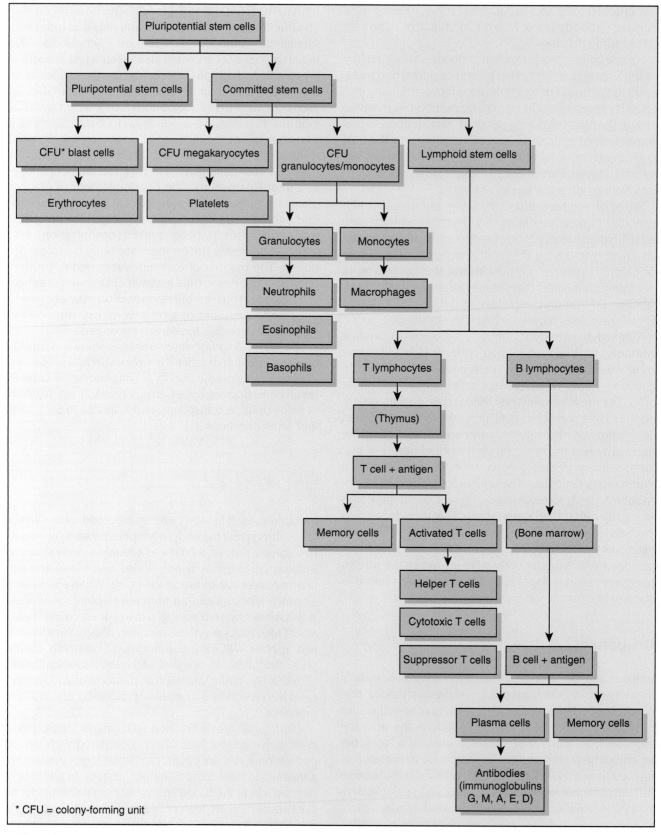

FIGURE 42–1 Hematopoiesis and formation of immune cells.

ments, and return antigenic fragments to the cell surface. The antigenic fragments are recognized as foreign material by circulating T and B lymphocytes, and an immune response is initiated. Because the monocytes prepare the antigen to interact with T and B lymphocytes, they are called antigen-processing and antigen-presenting cells.

Lymphocytes are the main immunocytes, and those in tissues are in dynamic equilibrium with those in circulating blood. These cells continuously travel through blood and lymph vessels from one lymphoid organ to another. The three types of lymphocytes are natural killer cells, T cells, and B cells.

Natural killer cells, so called because they do not need to interact with a specific antigen to become activated, destroy infectious microorganisms and malignant cells by releasing powerful chemicals. T lymphocytes are especially able to combat intracellular infections (eg, virus-infected cells), whereas B lymphocytes secrete antibodies that can neutralize pathogens before their entry into host cells. Both T and B cells must be activated by antigens before they can fulfill their immune functions, and both have proteins on their cell membrane surfaces that act as receptors for antigens.

Each T or B lymphocyte reacts only with a specific type of antigen and is capable of forming only one type of antibody or one type of T cell. When a specific antigen attaches to cell membrane receptors to form an antigen–antibody complex, the complex activates the lymphocyte to form tremendous numbers of duplicate lymphocytes (clones) that are exactly like the parent cell. Clones of a B lymphocyte eventually secrete antibodies that circulate throughout the body. Clones of a T lymphocyte are sensitized T cells that are released into lymphatic ducts, carried to the blood, circulated through all tissue fluids, then returned to lymphatic ducts and recirculated. Additional participants in the activation process are phagocytic macrophages and helper T cells, which secrete cytokines that regulate the growth, reproduction, and function of lymphocytes.

T Lymphocytes

T lymphocytes are the primary regulators of immune responses because they direct the activities of B cells and macrophages. They originate in pluripotential stem cells in the bone marrow and differentiate into immune cells in the thymus gland. The thymus produces a substance called thymosin, which is necessary for T cell maturation. When T cells bind with an antigen, specific genes are activated to produce substances that direct T cell proliferation and differentiation. One such substance is IL-2, which stimulates T cell deoxyribonucleic acid replication and mitosis. Cell division is necessary for production of large numbers of antigen-reactive cells and for cellular changes associated with the different subgroups of T cells. Specific types and functions of T cells include the following:

- *Helper T cells* (also called CD4 cells), the largest subgroup, regulate virtually all immune functions by producing protein substances called lymphokines (cytokines produced by lymphocytes). Lymphokines stimulate the growth of bone marrow and other cells of the immune system (eg, cytotoxic and suppressor T cells and B cells). They also activate macrophages and facilitate phagocytosis. Important lymphokines include IL-2, -3, -4, -5, and -6, GM-CSF, and interferon gamma. The devastating effects of acquired immunodeficiency syndrome (AIDS) result primarily from the ability of the human immunodeficiency virus to destroy helper T cells.
- *Cytotoxic T cells* (also called killer T cells) are recruited and activated by helper T cells. More specifically, helper T cells secrete IL-2, which is necessary for activation and proliferation (clonal expansion) of cytotoxic T cells. Once activated by antigen and IL-2, cytotoxic T cells bind to antigens on surfaces of target cells and release substances that form large holes in the target cell membrane. The damaged cell membrane allows water, electrolytes, and other molecules to enter the cell, resulting in cellular edema and death. Once these cytotoxic cells have damaged the target cells, they can detach themselves and attack other target cells.

  Cytotoxic T cells are especially lethal to virus-infected cells because virus particles become entrapped in the membranes of the cells and act as strong antigens that attract the T cells. These cells persist in tissues for months, even after destruction of all the invaders that elicited the original cytotoxic activity. Thus, T cells are especially important in killing body cells that have been invaded by foreign microorganisms or cells that have become malignant. Cytotoxic T cells also play a role in the destruction of transplanted organs and delayed hypersensitivity reactions.
- *Suppressor T cells* (also called CD8 cells) stop the immune response when an antigen has been destroyed by decreasing the activities of B cells and other T cells. This function is important in preventing further tissue damage. In autoimmune disorders, suppressor T-cell function is impaired, and extensive tissue damage may result.

B Lymphocytes

B lymphocytes originate in stem cells in the bone marrow, differentiate into cells capable of forming antibodies (also in the bone marrow), and migrate to the spleen, lymph nodes, or other lymphoid tissue. In lymphoid tissue, the cells may be dormant until exposed to an antigen. In response to an antigen and IL-2 from helper T cells, B cells multiply rapidly, enlarge, and differentiate into plasma cells, which then produce antibodies (immunoglobulins

[IGs]) to oppose the antigen. Immunoglobulins are secreted into lymph and transported to the bloodstream for circulation throughout the body. There are five main classes of immunoglobulins:

- *IgG* is the most abundant immunoglobulin, constituting approximately 80% of the antibodies in human serum. Molecules of IgG combine with molecules of antigen, and the antigen–antibody complex activates complement. Activated complement causes an inflammatory reaction, promotes phagocytosis, and inactivates or destroys the antigen. IgG also crosses the placenta to provide maternally acquired antibodies (passive immunity) to the infant.
- *IgA* is located primarily in secretions of the respiratory and GI tracts, where it acts against antigens entering those areas.
- *IgM* constitutes approximately 10% of serum antibodies and reacts with antigens in the bloodstream because its large molecular size prevents transport through capillary walls. It activates complement to destroy microorganisms.
- *IgE* is located mainly in tissues and is thought to be responsible for allergic reactions, including anaphylaxis. IgE sensitizes mast cells, which then release histamine and other chemical mediators that cause bronchoconstriction, edema, urticaria, and other manifestations of allergic reactions. IgE does not activate complement. The production of IgE is stimulated by T lymphocytes and lymphokines (mainly IL-4, -5, and -6) and inhibited by the interferons. Small amounts of IgE are present in the serum of nonallergic people; larger amounts are produced by people with allergies.
- *IgD* is present in serum in trace amounts and probably functions in recognition of antigens.

Immune System Cytokines

Although the hematopoietic cytokines described previously include the immune system cytokines, the emphasis here is on those that regulate growth, mobility, and differentiation of immune cells. It is thought that cytokines formed by activated macrophages enter the bone marrow, where they induce the synthesis and release of other cytokines that activate resting stem cells to produce more granulocytes and monocyte–macrophages. Newly formed granulocytes and monocytes leave the bone marrow and enter the circulating blood in approximately 3 days. Cytokines produced by monocyte–macrophages are called *monokines* and those produced by lymphocytes are called *lymphokines*.

Lymphokines enhance macrophage activity by two main mechanisms. First, they cause macrophages to accumulate in damaged tissues by delaying or stopping macrophage migration from the area. Second, they increase the capacity and effectiveness of phagocytosis. Some lymphokines, especially IL-2, directly stimulate helper T cells and enhance their antiantigenic activity. They also enhance the antiantigenic activity of the entire immune system. Interleukins 4, 5, and 6 are especially important in B-cell activities.

Tumor necrosis factors (TNF) are produced by activated macrophages and other cells and act on many immune and nonimmune target cells. They participate in the inflammatory response and cause hemorrhagic necrosis in several types of tumor cells. TNF-alpha is structurally the same as cachectin, a substance associated with debilitation and weight loss in patients with cancer. TNF-beta is also called lymphotoxin.

PATIENT-RELATED FACTORS THAT INFLUENCE IMMUNE FUNCTION

Age

Immune Function During Fetal and Neonatal Periods

During the first few months of gestation, the fetal immune system is deficient in antibody production and phagocytic activity. During the last trimester, the fetal immune system may be able to respond to infectious antigens, such as cytomegalovirus, rubella virus, and *Toxoplasma*. However, most fetal protection against infectious microorganisms is by maternal antibodies that reach the fetal circulation through the placenta. In the placenta, maternal blood and fetal blood are separated only by a layer of specialized cells called trophoblasts. Because antibodies are too large to diffuse across the trophoblastic layer, they are actively transported from the maternal to the fetal circulation by the trophoblastic cells.

At birth, the neonatal immune system is still immature, but IgG levels (from maternal blood) are near adult levels in umbilical cord blood. However, the source of maternal antibodies is severed at birth. Antibody titers in infants decrease over approximately 6 months as maternal antibodies are catabolized. Although the infant does start producing IgG, the rate of production is lower than the rate of breakdown of maternal antibodies. Cell-mediated immunity is probably completely functional at birth.

Immune Function in Older Adults

Both humoral and cell-mediated immune functions decline with aging, and this decline is probably a major factor in the older adult's increased susceptibility to infections and tumors. The regulation of immunologic functions also declines with age, which may account for the greater frequency of autoimmune diseases in this age group. Lymphocytes are less able to proliferate in response to antigenic stimulation, and a relative state of immunodeficiency prevails. With T lymphocytes, function is impaired, and the numbers in peripheral blood may be decreased. The functional impairment includes decreased activity of helper

T cells and increased activity of suppressor T cells. With B lymphocytes, the numbers probably do not decrease, but the cells are less able to form antibodies in response to antigens. Abnormal antibody production results from impaired function of B cells and helper T cells. In addition, older adults have increased blood levels of antibodies against their own tissues (autoantibodies).

Impaired immune mechanisms have several implications for clinicians who care for elderly patients, including the following:

- Older adults are more likely to contract infections and less able to recover from them. Therefore, older adults need protective measures, such as rigorous personal hygiene; good nutrition; adequate exercise, rest, and sleep; minimal exposure to potential pathogens, when possible; and appropriate immunizations (eg, influenza, pneumonia, tetanus). When an infection develops in older adults, signs and symptoms (eg, fever and drainage) may be absent or less pronounced than in younger adults.
- Older adults have impaired immune responses to antigens. Thus, achieving protective antibody titers may require higher doses of immunizing antigens in older adults than in younger adults.
- Older adults often exhibit a less intense positive reaction in skin tests for tuberculosis (indicating a decreased delayed hypersensitivity response).

Nutritional Status

Nutritional status can have profound effects on immune function. Adequate nutrient intake contributes to immunocompetence (ability of the immune system to function effectively). Malnutrition contributes to immunodeficiency. A severe lack of calories or protein decreases numbers and functions of T cells, complement activity, neutrophil chemotaxis, and phagocytosis. An inadequate zinc intake can depress the functions of T and B cells. Zinc is a cofactor for many enzymes, some of which are found in lymphocytes and are required for lymphocyte function. Zinc deficiency also may result from inadequate absorption in the GI tract or excessive losses in urine, feces, or through the skin with such disorders as chronic renal disease, chronic diarrhea, burns, or severe psoriasis. Vitamin deficiencies may also depress T- and B-cell function because several (eg, A, E, folic acid, pantothenic acid, and pyridoxine) also are enzyme cofactors in lymphocytes.

Stress

There is evidence that stress depresses immune function and therefore increases risks for development of infection and cancer. The connection between the stress response and the immune response is thought to involve neuroendocrine mechanisms. The stress response is character-ized by increased activity of catecholamine neurotransmitters in the central and autonomic nervous systems (eg, norepinephrine, epinephrine) and increased secretion of cortisol from the adrenal cortex. Cortisol and other corticosteroids are well known to suppress immune function and are used therapeutically for that purpose. The immune response is affected by these neuroendocrine influences on lymphoid organs and lymphocyte functions because lymphocytes have receptors for many neurotransmitters and hormones.

IMMUNE DISORDERS

Dysfunction of the immune system is related to many different disease processes, including allergic, autoimmune, immunodeficiency, and neoplastic disorders. Each of these is described in the following list to assist in understanding the use of drugs to alter immune functions:

- In *allergic disorders,* the body erroneously perceives normally harmless substances (eg, foods, pollens) as antigens and mounts an immune response. More specifically, IgE binds to antigen on the surface of mast cells and causes the release of chemical mediators (eg, histamine) that produce the allergic manifestations. This reaction may cause tissue damage ranging from mild skin rashes to life-threatening anaphylaxis.
- In *autoimmune disorders,* the body erroneously perceives its own tissues as antigens and elicits an immune response, often inflammatory in nature. Rheumatoid arthritis and systemic lupus erythematosus have long been considered autoimmune disorders. More recently, type 1 diabetes mellitus, myasthenia gravis, and several other disorders have been added to the list. Autoimmune processes may damage virtually every body tissue.
- In *immunodeficiency disorders,* the body is especially susceptible to infections and neoplastic diseases. AIDS is a major immunodeficiency disorder that decreases the numbers and almost all functions of T lymphocytes and several functions of B lymphocytes and monocytes. Immunodeficiency also is induced by severe malnutrition, cancer, and immunosuppressant drugs.
- In *neoplastic disease,* immune cells lose their ability to destroy mutant cells or early malignant cells. This effect could result from immunodeficiency states or from cancer cells that are overwhelming in number or highly malignant. Mutant cells constantly occur during cell division, but few survive or lead to cancer. Most mutant cells simply die; some survive but retain the normal controls that prevent excessive growth; and some are destroyed by immune processes activated by abnormal proteins found in most mutant cells.

DRUGS THAT ALTER HEMATOPOIETIC AND IMMUNE RESPONSES

Several hematopoietic and immune cytokines have been synthesized for therapeutic purposes. Hematopoietic agents are used to prevent or treat symptoms (eg, anemia, neutropenia) caused by disease processes or their treatments.

Drugs that modify the immune system are used to prevent or treat infections, treat immunodeficiency disorders and cancer, and to prevent or treat rejection of transplanted tissues or organs.

Methods include administering exogenous antigens (eg, immunizations and desensitization procedures), strengthening antigens (eg, an antigen that is too weak to elicit an immune response), or suppressing the normal response to an antigen. In desensitization procedures, weak extracts of antigenic substances (eg, foods, plant pollens, penicillin) are prepared as drugs and administered in small, increasing amounts so the patient develops a tolerance for the substances and avoids serious allergic reactions.

Overall, drugs can be given to stimulate immune responses (immunizing agents [see Chap. 43]; stimulate hematopoiesis and immune responses [see Chap. 44]); or suppress normal immune responses (immunosuppressants [see Chap. 45]).

REVIEW AND APPLICATION EXERCISES

1. What is the difference between innate and acquired immunity?

2. What are methods of producing active acquired immunity?

3. Which WBCs are phagocytes?

4. Describe phagocytosis.

5. Where are T lymphocytes formed, and what are their functions?

6. Where are B lymphocytes formed, and what are their functions?

7. What are antigens, and how do they elicit an immune response?

8. What are cytokines, and how do they function in the immune response?

9. What is complement, and how does it function in the immune response?

10. What are the main consequences of immunodeficiency states?

SELECTED REFERENCES

Guyton, A.C. & Hall, J.E. (1996). *Textbook of medical physiology,* 9th ed. Philadelphia: W.B. Saunders.

Hall, P.D. & Tami, J.A. (1997). Function and evaluation of the immune system. In J.T. DiPiro, R.L. Talbert, G.C. Yee, G.R. Matzke, B.G. Wells, & L.M. Posey (Eds.), *Pharmacotherapy: A pathophysiologic approach,* 3rd ed., pp. 1647–1660. Stamford, CT: Appleton & Lange.

Porth, C.M. (Ed.). (1998). *Pathophysiology: Concepts of altered health states,* 5th ed. Philadelphia: Lippincott Williams & Wilkins.

Rich, R.R., Fleisher, T.A., Schwartz, B.D., Shearer, W.T., & Strober, W. (Eds.). (1996). *Clinical immunology: Principles and practice.* St. Louis: C.V. Mosby.

Winchester, R. (1997). Principles of the immune response. In W.N. Kelley (Ed.), *Textbook of internal medicine,* 3rd ed., pp. 18–24. Philadelphia: Lippincott-Raven.

43

Immunizing Agents

Objectives

After studying this chapter, the student will be able to:

1. Discuss common characteristics of immunizations.

2. Discuss the importance of immunizations in promoting health and preventing disease.

3. Identify immunizations recommended for adults.

4. Identify immunizations recommended for children.

5. Discuss ways to promote immunization of children.

6. Teach parents about recommended immunizations and record keeping.

A young couple brings their 6-week-old infant to the clinic for a well-baby check and her required "shots." First, you examine the baby and talk with the couple about how new parenthood is going. Both seem very motivated to be good parents. They have lots of questions and ask whether all those shots are really necessary. The mother admits that she has always been afraid of shots and just can't watch her baby be hurt.

Reflect on:

▶ How you can acknowledge the mother's concerns without minimizing her feelings.

▶ Basic information regarding immunizations that every new parent should have.

▶ Teaching regarding what the parents may expect for 2 to 3 days after the injection and appropriate symptom management.

▶ The importance of keeping up-to-date immunization records.

Immune responses and types of immunity are described in Chapter 42. Many antigens that activate the immune response are microorganisms that cause infectious diseases. Early scientists observed that people who contracted certain diseases were thereafter protected despite repeated exposure to the disease. As knowledge evolved, it was discovered that protection stemmed from body substances called antibodies, and that antibodies could also be induced by deliberate, controlled exposure to the antigen. Subsequently, immunization techniques were developed.

IMMUNIZATION

Immunization or vaccination involves administration of an antigen to induce antibody formation (for active immunity) or serum from immune people or animals (for passive immunity). Preparations used for immunization are biologic products prepared by pharmaceutical companies and regulated by the Food and Drug Administration.

AGENTS FOR ACTIVE IMMUNITY

The biologic products used for active immunity are vaccines and toxoids. *Vaccines* are suspensions of microorganisms that have been killed or attenuated (weakened or reduced in virulence) so that they can induce antibody formation while preventing or causing very mild forms of the disease. *Toxoids* are bacterial toxins that have been modified to destroy toxicity while retaining antigenic properties (ie, ability to induce antibody formation). For maximum effectiveness, vaccines and toxoids must be given before exposure to the pathogenic microorganism.

Indications for Use

Clinical indications for use of vaccines and toxoids include the following:

1. Routine immunization of all children against diphtheria, hepatitis B, tetanus, pertussis (whooping cough), rubeola (red measles), rubella (German measles), mumps, and poliomyelitis
2. Immunization of adults against tetanus
3. Immunization of prepubertal girls or women of childbearing age against rubella. Rubella during the first trimester of pregnancy is associated with a high incidence of birth defects in the newborn.
4. Immunization of people at high risk of serious morbidity or mortality from a particular disease. For example, hepatitis B, influenza, and pneumococcal vaccines are recommended for selected groups of people (Table 43-1).
5. Immunization of adults and children at high risk of exposure to a particular disease. For example, several diseases (eg, yellow fever, cholera) rarely occur in most parts of the world. Thus, immunization is recommended only for people who live in or travel to geographic areas where the disease can be contracted.

(*text continues on page 649*)

TABLE 43-1   **Vaccines and Toxoids for Active Immunity**

Generic/Trade Name	Characteristics	Clinical Indications	Routes and Dosage Ranges Adults	Routes and Dosage Ranges Children
Cholera vaccine	Sterile suspension of killed cholera organisms Protects approximately 50% of recipients for 3–6 mo. Does not prevent transmission of cholera. Protection begins approximately 1 wk after the initial dose.	Travel to endemic areas (Asia, Africa, Middle East) Living in endemic areas	IM, SC 0.5 mL initially, 0.5 mL 4 wk later, then 0.5 mL every 6 mo if indicated	Age >10 y, same as adults Age 5–10 y, IM, SC 0.3 mL initially, 0.3 mL 4 wk later, then 0.3 mL every 6 mo if indicated Age 6 mo–4 y, IM, SC 0.2 mL initially, 0.2 mL 4 wk later, then 0.2 mL every 6 mo if indicated
Hemophilus influenzae b (Hib) **conjugate vaccine** (HibTITER, PedvaxHIB, ProHIBIT)	Formed by conjugating a derivative of the organism with a protein	To prevent infection with Hib, a common cause of serious bacterial infections, including meningitis, in children younger than 5 y of age		HibTITER age 2–5 mo, IM 0.5 mL every 2 mo for 3 doses; age 15 mo, 0.5 mL as a single booster dose Age 7–11 mo, IM 0.5 mL every 2 mo for two doses; age 15 mo, 0.5 mL as a single booster dose

| TABLE 43-1 | Vaccines and Toxoids for Active Immunity (*continued*) |

| | | | Routes and Dosage Ranges | |
Generic/Trade Name	Characteristics	Clinical Indications	Adults	Children
				Age 12–14 mo, IM 0.5 mL as single dose; age 15 mo, 0.5 mL as a single booster dose, at least 2 mo after the first dose
				Age 15–59 mo, IM 0.5 mL as a single dose (no additional booster dose)
				Pedvax HIB age 2–6 mo, IM 0.5 mL every 2 mo for two doses; age 12 mo, 0.5 mL as a booster dose
				Age 7–11 mo, IM 0.5 mL every 2 mo for two doses; age 15 mo, 0.5 mL as booster dose
				Age 12–14 mo, IM 0.5 mL as single dose; age 15 mo, 0.5 mL as a single booster dose, at least 2 mo after the first dose
				Age 15–59 mo, IM 0.5 mL as a single dose (no additional booster dose)
				ProHIBit Age 15–59 mo, IM 0.5 mL as a single dose (no additional booster dose)
Hepatitis A vaccine (Havrix)	Inactivated whole virus More than 90% effective Duration of protection unknown Contraindicated during febrile illness, immuno-suppression The adult formulation contains 1440 units in 1 mL; the pediatric formulation contains 360 units in 0.5 mL	Workers in day care centers, laboratories, food-handling establishments; homosexual men; intravenous drug users; military personnel; travelers to areas where hepatitis A is endemic; community residents during an outbreak	IM one dose of 1440 units Booster dose 6–12 mo after initial dose	2–18 y, IM, two doses of 360 units each, given 1 mo apart Booster dose 6–12 mo after initial dose
Hepatitis B vaccine (recombinant) (Recombivax HB, Engerix-B)	Prepared by recombinant DNA techniques of inserting the gene coding for production of hepatitis B surface antigen (HBsAG) into yeast cells Contains no blood or blood products Approximately 96% effective in children and young adults;	Pre-exposure immunization of high-risk groups, such as health care providers (nurses, physicians, dentists, laboratory workers); clients with cancer, organ transplants, hemodialysis, immunosuppressant drug therapy, or multiple infusions of blood or	Engerix, IM 20 μg (1 mL) × three doses, initially and at 1 mo and 6 mo after the first dose Booster, IM 20 μg × one dose Dialysis clients, IM 40 μg (2 mL) × four doses, initially and at 1, 2, and 6 mo after the first dose	Engerix, neonates to 10 y, IM 10 μg (0.5 mL) × three doses, initially and at 1 mo and 6 mo after first dose Booster, IM 10 μg × one dose >10 y, IM 20 μg (1 mL) × three doses, same schedule as above Booster, IM 20 μg × one dose

(*continued*)

TABLE 43-1 **Vaccines and Toxoids for Active Immunity** (*continued*)

Generic/Trade Name	Characteristics	Clinical Indications	Routes and Dosage Ranges	
			Adults	Children
	approximately 88% effective in adults >40 y Duration of protection unknown; can measure serum antibody levels periodically (protective levels approximately 10 million U/mL)	blood products; male homosexuals; intravenous drug abusers; residents and staff of institutions for mentally handicapped people	Recombivax, IM 10 µg (1 mL) × three doses, initially and at 1 mo and 6 mo after the first dose Booster 10 µg × one dose Dialysis formulation, IM 40 µg (1 mL) × three doses, initially and at 1 mo and 6 mo after the first dose Booster 40 µg × one dose if antibody level <10 million U/mL 1–2 mo after third dose of above schedule	Recombivax, birth to 10 years, IM 2.5 µg (0.25 mL) × three doses, initially and at 1 mo and 6 mo after the first dose 11–19 y, IM 5 µg (0.5 mL) × three doses, same schedule as above
Influenza vaccine (Fluogen)	Inactivated strains of A and B influenza viruses, reformulated annually to include current strains Protects 60%–75% of recipients for a few months. Maximal antibody production occurs the second week after vaccination; the titer remains constant for approximately 1 mo, then gradually declines Grown in chick embryos; therefore, contraindicated in clients who are highly allergic to eggs	Recommended annually for health care providers; older adults; and people chronically ill with pulmonary, cardiovascular, or renal disorders, diabetes mellitus, or adrenocortical insufficiency	IM 0.5 mL as single dose	<3 y, IM 0.25 mL as single dose >3 y, IM 0.5 mL as single dose Note: Children <9 y not previously immunized need two doses, at least 1 mo apart
Lyme disease vaccine (LYMErix)	A non-infectious recombinant vaccine Contains no substances of animal origin All three doses required for optimal protection	Immunization of people 15–70 y of age who live, work, or travel in wooded areas (potential exposure to disease-carrying ticks)	IM 30 µg/0.5 mL at 0, 1, and 12 mo	Adolescents ≥15 y, same as adults
Measles vaccine (Attenuvax)	Sterile preparation of live, attenuated measles (rubeola) virus Protects approximately 95% of recipients for several years or lifetime Usually given with mumps and rubella vaccines. A combination product con-	Routine immunization of children ≥1 y Immunization of adults not previously immunized	SC 0.5 mL in a single dose	SC, same as adults

TABLE 43-1) **Vaccines and Toxoids for Active Immunity** (*continued*)

Generic/Trade Name	Characteristics	Clinical Indications	Routes and Dosage Ranges Adults	Children
	taining all three antigens is available and preferred. Measles vaccine should not be given for 3 mo after administration of immune serum globulin, plasma, or whole blood			
Measles and rubella vaccine (M-R-Vax II)	Mixture of live attenuated rubeola virus (Attenuvax) and rubella (German measles) virus	Immunization of 15-mo-old children against rubeola and rubella		SC, total volume of reconstituted vial
Measles, mumps, and rubella vaccine (M-M-R II)	Mixture of three vaccines (rubeola, rubella, mumps) Usually preferred over single immunizing agents	Immunization from age 15 mo to puberty		SC, total volume of reconstituted vial
Meningitis vaccine (Menomune-A/C Menomune-A/C/Y/W-135)	Suspension prepared from groups A and C or A, C, Y, and W-135 of *Neisseria meningitidis*	Immunization of people at risk in epidemic or endemic areas Type A only should be given to infants and children <2 y	SC 0.5 mL	
Mumps vaccine (Mumpsvax)	Sterile suspension of live, attenuated mumps virus Provides active immunity in about 97% of children and 93% of adults for at least 10 y Most often given in combination with measles and rubella vaccines	Routine immunization of children (≥1 y) and adults	SC 0.5 mL in a single dose of reconstituted vaccine. (Reconstituted vaccine retains potency for 8 h if refrigerated. Discard if not used within 8 h.)	>1 y, same as adults (vaccination not indicated in children <1 y)
Plague vaccine	Sterile suspension of killed plague bacilli	Immunization of high-risk people (eg, laboratory workers, people in disaster areas)	IM 1.0 mL initially, then 0.2 mL after 1–3 mo and 3–6 mo (total of three doses) Booster doses of 0.1–0.2 mL every 6 mo during active exposure	5–10 y, 3/5 adult dose 1–4 y, 2/5 adult dose <1 y, 1/5 adult dose
Pneumococcal vaccine, polyvalent (Pneumovax 23, Pnu-Imune 23)	Consists of 23 strains of pneumococci, which cause approximately 85%–90% of the serious pneumococcal infections in the United States Protection begins approximately the third week after vaccination and lasts years.	Adults with chronic cardiovascular or pulmonary diseases Adults with chronic disease associated with increased risk of pneumococcal infection (eg, splenic dysfunction, Hodgkin's disease, multiple myeloma, cirrhosis, alcohol dependence, renal	SC IM 0.5 mL as a single dose	Same as adults

(continued)

TABLE 43-1 **Vaccines and Toxoids for Active Immunity** (*continued*)

Generic/Trade Name	Characteristics	Clinical Indications	Routes and Dosage Ranges	
			Adults	Children
	Not recommended for children <2 y because they may be unable to produce adequate antibody levels	failure, immunosuppression) Adults ≥65 y who are otherwise healthy Children ≥2 y with chronic disease associated with increased risk of pneumococcal infection (eg, asplenia, nephrotic syndrome, immunosuppression)		
Poliomyelitis vaccine, inactivated (IPOL)	A suspension of inactivated poliovirus types I, II, and III	Routine immunization of infants. May be used for all four doses or for the first two doses, followed by two doses of the oral vaccine Immunization of adults not previously immunized and at risk of exposure (eg, health care or laboratory workers)	SC 0.5 mL monthly for two doses, then a third dose 6–12 mo later	SC 0.5 mL at 2, 4, 6–18 mo, and 4–6 y of age (four doses) or at 2 and 4 mo (two doses)
Poliovirus vaccine trivalent, oral (Sabin) (Orimune)	A suspension of live, attenuated poliovirus types I, II, and III Effective in >90% of recipients	Infants for third and fourth doses of primary immunization (after two doses of injected vaccine) Infants whose parents refuse injected vaccine Mass immunizations during outbreaks of poliovirus infection	Not recommended for routine immunization of adults	PO 0.5 mL at 6–18 mo and 4–6 y of age (two doses) or at 2, 4, 6–18 mo, and 4–6 y of age (four doses)
Rabies vaccine (human diploid cell rabies vaccine [HDCV]) (Imovax)	An inactivated virus vaccine Immunity develops in 7–10 d and lasts 1 y or longer	Preexposure immunization in people at high risk of exposure (veterinarians, animal handlers, laboratory personnel who work with rabies virus) Postexposure prophylaxis in people who have been bitten by potentially rabid animals or who have skin scratches or abrasions exposed to animal saliva (eg, animal licking of wound), urine, or blood	Preexposure prophylaxis, IM 1.0 mL for three doses. The second dose is given 1 wk after the first; the third dose is given 4 wk after the first. Thereafter, booster doses (1 mL) are given every 2 y in high-risk people. Postexposure, IM 1 mL for five doses. After the initial dose, remaining doses are given 3, 7, 14, and 28 d later. Rabies immunoglobulin is administered at the same time as the initial dose of HDVC vaccine	

TABLE 43-1   Vaccines and Toxoids for Active Immunity (*continued*)

Generic/Trade Name	Characteristics	Clinical Indications	Routes and Dosage Ranges	
			Adults	Children
Rubella vaccine (Meruvax II)	Sterile suspension of live, attenuated rubella virus Protects approximately 95% of recipients at least 15 y, probably for lifetime Should not be given for 3 mo after receiving immune serum globulin, plasma, or whole blood Usually given with measles and mumps vaccines. A combination product containing all three antigens is available and preferred.	Routine immunization of children ≥1 y Initial or repeat immunization of adolescent girls or women of childbearing age *if* serum antibody levels are low	SC 0.5 mL in a single dose	SC same as adults
Rubella and mumps vaccine (Biavax II)	A mixture of mumps and rubella virus strains Less frequently used than measles, mumps, and rubella vaccine	Immunization of children		≥1 y, SC, total volume of reconstituted vial
Tuberculosis vaccine (Bacillus Calmette-Guérin) (TICE BCG)	Suspension of attenuated tubercle bacillus Converts negative tuberculin reactors to positive reactors. Therefore, precludes use of the tuberculin skin test for screening or early diagnosis of tuberculosis. Contraindicated in clients who have not had a (negative) tuberculin skin test within the preceding 2 wk; who are actually ill or suspected of having respiratory tract, skin, or other infection; who have dysgammaglobulinemia; and who have a positive tuberculin skin test	People at high risk for exposure, including newborns of women with tuberculosis	Percutaneous, by multiple puncture disk, 0.2–0.3 mL	Newborns, percutaneous, by multiple puncture disk, 0.1 mL >1 mo, same as adults

(*continued*)

TABLE 43–1   **Vaccines and Toxoids for Active Immunity** (*continued*)

Generic/Trade Name	Characteristics	Clinical Indications	Routes and Dosage Ranges	
			Adults	Children
Typhoid vaccine (Vivotif Berna)	Sterile suspension of attenuated or killed typhoid bacilli Protects >70% of recipients	High-risk people (household contacts of typhoid carriers or people whose occupation or travel predisposes to exposure)	SC 0.5 mL for two doses at least 4 wk apart, then a booster dose of 0.5 mL (or 0.1 mL intradermal) at least every 3 y for repeated or continued exposure PO 1 capsule every other day × four doses; repeat every 4 y as a booster dose with repeated or continued exposure	>10 y, SC 0.5 mL for two doses at least 4 wk apart, then a booster dose of 0.5 mL at least every 3 y for repeated or continued exposure Age 6 mo–10 y, SC 0.25 mL for two doses, at least 4 wk apart, then a booster dose of 0.25 mL (or 0.1 mL intradermal) every 3 y if indicated >6 y, PO same as adults
Varicella virus vaccine (Varivax)	Vaccine contains live, attenuated varicella virus Contraindicated in people with hematologic or lymphatic malignancy, immunosuppression, febrile illness, or pregnancy	Children ≥12 mo Adults who have frequent contact with children and have not had chickenpox (eg, health care personnel, teachers, day care center staff, others)	SC 0.5 mL, followed by a second dose of 0.5 mL 4–8 wk after the first dose	1–12 y, SC one dose of 0.5 mL Adolescents, ≥13 y, SC 0.5 mL, followed by a second dose of 0.5 mL 4–8 wk after the first dose
Yellow fever vaccine (YF-Vax)	Suspension of live, attenuated yellow fever virus Protects approximately 95% of recipients for 10 y or longer	Laboratory personnel at risk of exposure Travel to endemic areas (Africa, South America)	SC 0.5 mL; booster dose of 0.5 mL every 10 y if in endemic areas	>6 mo, SC same as adults
Diphtheria and tetanus toxoids and whole-cell pertussis vaccine (DTwP) (Tri-Immunol)	Diphtheria component is a preparation of detoxified growth products of *Corynebacterium diphtheriae* Pertussis component is killed, whole bacterial cells	Routine immunization of infants and children ≤6 y		IM 0.5 mL for three doses at 4- to 6-wk intervals, beginning at 2 mo of age, followed by a reinforcing dose 7–12 mo later and a booster dose when the child is 5–6 y of age
Diphtheria and tetanus toxoids and acellular pertussis vaccine (DTaP) (Acel-Imune, Tripedia)	Differs from Tri-Immunol in that the pertussis component is acellular bacterial particles, formulated to decrease serious adverse reactions associated with the whole-cell vaccine	As fourth or fifth dose, after initial immunization with whole cell vaccine, in children at least 15 mo of age		IM 0.5 mL at approximately 18 mo of age: repeat at 4–6 y of age
Diphtheria and tetanus toxoids and whole-cell pertussis and *Hemophilus influenzae* type B conjugate vaccines (DTwP-HibTITER) (Tetramune)	A mixture of DTwP (Tri-Immunol) and Hib vaccine (HibTITER)	Immunization of children 2 mo to 5 y of age when indications for diphtheria, tetanus, pertussis (DTP) and *H. influenzae* b conjugate vaccine coincide (usually at 2, 4, 6, and 15 mo of age)		IM 0.5 mL at age 2, 4, 6, and 15 mo (total of four doses)

TABLE 43-1 Vaccines and Toxoids for Active Immunity (*continued*)

Generic/Trade Name	Characteristics	Clinical Indications	Routes and Dosage Ranges Adults	Children
Diphtheria and tetanus toxoids adsorbed (pediatric type)	Also called DT Contains a larger amount of diphtheria antigen than tetanus and diphtheria toxoids, adult type (Td)	Routine immunization of infants and children ≤6 y of age in whom pertussis vaccine is contraindicated (ie, those who have adverse reactions to initial doses of DTP)		Infants and children ≤6 y. IM 0.5 mL for two doses at least 4 wk apart, followed by a reinforcing dose 1 y later and at the time the child starts school
Tetanus toxoid, adsorbed	Preparation of detoxified growth products of *Clostridium tetani* Protects approximately 100% of recipients for 10 y or more Usually given in combination with DTP or diphtheria toxoid (DT) for primary immunization of infants and children ≤6 y of age Usually given alone or combined with diphtheria toxoid (Td adult type) for primary immunization of adults	Routine immunization of infants and young children Primary immunization of adults Prevention of tetanus in previously immunized people who sustain a potentially contaminated wound	Primary immunization in adults not previously immunized IM 0.5 mL initially, followed by 0.5 mL in 4–8 wk, followed by 0.5 mL 6–12 mo later (total of three doses). Then, 0.5 mL booster dose every 10 y. Prophylaxis, IM 0.5 mL if wound severely contaminated and no booster dose received for 5 y; 0.5 mL if wound clean and no booster dose received for 10 y	Primary immunization and prophylaxis, same as adults
Tetanus and diphtheria toxoids, adsorbed (adult type)	Also called Td Contains a smaller amount of diphtheria antigen than diphtheria and tetanus toxoids, pediatric type	Primary immunization or booster doses in adults and children >6 y of age	IM 0.5 mL for two doses, at least 4 wk apart, followed by a reinforcing dose 6–12 mo later and every 10 y thereafter	>6 y, same as adults

IM, intramuscular; SC, subcutaneous.

Contraindications to Use

Vaccines and toxoids are usually contraindicated during febrile illnesses; immunosuppressive drug therapy (see Chap. 45); immunodeficiency states; leukemia, lymphoma, or generalized malignancy; and pregnancy.

AGENTS FOR PASSIVE IMMUNITY

The biologic products used for passive immunity are immune serums and antitoxins. These substances may be obtained from human or animal sources, and they may consist of whole serum or the immunoglobulin portion of serum in which the specific antibodies are concentrated. When possible, human serum is preferred to animal serum because risks of severe allergic reactions are reduced. Also, immunoglobulin fractions are preferred over whole serum because they are more likely to be effective. Human immunoglobulins are available for measles, hepatitis, rabies, respiratory syncytial virus, rubella, tetanus, and varicella-zoster infections.

To obtain antitoxins or animal immune serums, an animal such as a horse is injected with a purified toxin or toxoid. After antibodies have had time to develop, blood is withdrawn from the animal and prepared for clinical use. Antitoxins are available for rabies, botulism, diphtheria, gas gangrene, and tetanus. A major disadvantage of antitoxins is that a relatively high number of people are allergic to horse serum.

Immune serums and antitoxins are used to provide temporary immunity in people exposed to or experiencing a particular disease. The goal of therapy is to prevent or modify the disease process (ie, decrease incidence and severity of symptoms). Antitoxins are contraindicated in clients allergic to horse serum.

INDIVIDUAL IMMUNIZING AGENTS

Vaccines and toxoids are listed in Table 43-1; immune serums and antitoxins are listed in Table 43-2.

NURSING PROCESS

Assessment

Assess the client's immunization status by obtaining the following information:

- Determine the client's previous history of diseases for which immunizing agents are available (eg, measles, influenza).

- Ask if the client has had previous immunizations.
  - For which diseases were immunizations received?
  - Which immunizing agent was received?
  - Were any adverse effects experienced? If so, what symptoms occurred, and how long did they last?
  - Was tetanus toxoid given for any cuts or wounds?
  - Did any foreign travel require immunizations?
- Determine whether the client has any conditions that contraindicate administration of immunizing agents (eg, malignancy, pregnancy, immunosuppressive drug therapy).

(*text continues on page 652*)

TABLE 43-2	Immune Serums and Antitoxins for Passive Immunity		
Generic/Trade Name	**Characteristics**	**Clinical Indications**	**Routes and Dosage Ranges**
Immune Serums			
Cytomegalovirus immune globulin, IV, human (CMV-IGIV) (CytoGam)	Contains antibodies against CMV	Treat CMV infection in renal transplant recipients	IV infusion, 150 mg/kg within 72 h of transplantation; 100 mg/kg 2–8 wk after transplantation: 50 mg/kg 12–16 wk after transplantation
Hepatitis B immune globulin, human (H-BIG, Hyper-Hep, Hep-B-Gammagee)	A solution of immunoglobulins that contains antibodies to hepatitis B surface antigen	To prevent hepatitis after exposure	Adults and children: IM 0.06 mL/kg as soon as possible after exposure. Repeat dose in 1 mo.
Immune serum globulin (human) (ISG) (Gammar)	Commonly called gamma globulin Obtained from pooled plasma of normal donors Consists primarily of IgG, which contains concentrated antibodies Produces adequate serum levels of IgG in 2–5 d	To decrease the severity of hepatitis A, measles, and varicella after exposure To treat immunoglobulin deficiency Adjunct to antibiotics in severe bacterial infections and burns To lessen possibility of fetal damage in pregnant women exposed to rubella virus (however, routine use in early pregnancy is not recommended)	Adults and children: Exposure to hepatitis A, IM 0.02–0.04 mL/kg Exposure to measles, IM 0.25 mL/kg given within 6 d of exposure Exposure to varicella, IM 0.6–1.2 mL/kg Exposure to rubella (pregnant women only), IM 0.55 mL/kg Immunoglobulin deficiency, IM 1.3 mL/kg initially, then 0.6 mL/kg every 3–4 wk Bacterial infections, IM 0.5–3.5 mL/kg
Immune serum globulin IV (IGIV) (Gamimune, Sandoglobulin)	Given IV only Provides immediate antibodies Half-life approximately 3 wk Mechanism of action in idiopathic thrombocytopenic purpura (ITP) unknown	Immunodeficiency syndrome ITP	Gamimune: IV infusion 100–200 mg/kg once a month. May be given more often or increased to 400 mg/kg if clinical response or serum level of IgG is insufficient. ITP, IV infusion, 400 mg/kg daily for 5 consecutive days Sandoglobulin: IV infusion, 200 mg/kg once a month. May be given more often or increased to 300 mg/kg if clinical response or level of IgG is inadequate. ITP, IV infusion, 400 mg/kg daily for 5 consecutive days

TABLE 43-2 Immune Serums and Antitoxins for Passive Immunity (*continued*)

Generic/Trade Name	Characteristics	Clinical Indications	Routes and Dosage Ranges
Rabies immune globulin (human) (Hyperab, Imogam)	Gamma globulin obtained from plasma of people hyperimmunized with rabies vaccine Not useful in treatment of clinical rabies infection	Postexposure prevention of rabies, in conjunction with rabies vaccine	Adults and children: IM 20 U/kg (half the dose may be infiltrated around the wound) as soon as possible after possible exposure (eg, animal bite)
Respiratory syncytial virus immune globulin intravenous (human) (RSV-IGIV) (Hypermune RSV, RespiGam)	Reduces severity of RSV illness and the incidence and duration of hospitalization in high-risk infants	Prevention of serious RSV infections in high-risk children <2 y (ie, those with bronchopulmonary dysplasia or history of premature birth [gestation of ≤35 wk]) Treatment of RSV lower respiratory tract infections in hospitalized infants and young children	Children: IV infusion via infusion pump, 1.5 mL/kg/h for 15 min; then 3 mL/kg/h for 15 min, then 6 mL/kg/h until the infusion is completed, once monthly, if tolerated. Maximum monthly dose, 750 mg/kg
Rh₀(D) immune globulin (human) (Gamulin Rh, HypRho-D, RhoGAM)	Prepared from fractionated human plasma A sterile concentrated solution of specific immunoglobulin (IgG) containing anti-Rh₀(D) For IM use only	To prevent sensitization in a subsequent pregnancy to the Rh₀(D) factor in an Rh-negative mother who has given birth to an Rh-positive infant by an Rh-positive father To prevent Rh₀(D) sensitization in Rh-negative clients accidently transfused with Rh-positive blood Also available in microdose form (MICRhoGAM) for the prevention of maternal Rh immunization after abortion or miscarriage up to 12 wk gestation	Obstetric use: Inject contents of 1 vial IM for every 15 mL fetal packed red cell volume within 72 h after delivery, miscarriage, or abortion Transfusion accidents: Inject contents of 1 vial IM for every 15 mL of Rh-positive packed red cell volume Consult package instructions for blood typing and drug administration procedures.
Tetanus immune globulin (human) (Hyper-Tet)	Solution of globulins from plasma of people hyperimmunized with tetanus toxoid Tetanus toxoid should be given at the same time (in a different syringe and injection site) to initiate active immunization.	To prevent tetanus in clients with wounds possibly contaminated with *Clostridium tetani* and whose immunization history is uncertain or included less than two immunizing doses of tetanus toxoid Treatment of tetanus	Adults and children: Prophylaxis, IM 250 U as a single dose Treatment of clinical disease IM 3000–6000 U
Varicella-zoster immune globulin (human) (VZIG) (Varicella-zoster immune globulin)	The globulin fraction of human plasma Antibodies last 1 mo or longer.	To prevent or decrease severity of varicella infections (chickenpox, shingles) in children <15 y of age who are immunodeficient because of illness (eg, leukemia, lymphoma) or drug therapy (eg, corticosteroids, antineoplastics) and who have had significant exposure to chickenpox or herpes zoster (ie, playmate, household or hospital contact) May be used in other children <15 y and adults on an individualized basis	IM 125 U/10 kg up to a maximum of 625 U as soon as possible after exposure, up to 96 h after exposure. Minimal dose, 125 U

Animals Serums (Antitoxins)

Antirabies serum, equine	A hyperimmune horse serum used only if human rabies immune globulin is not available	To prevent rabies after severe exposure (eg, multiple, deep animal bites, especially	Adults and children: IM 55 U/kg (half the dose may be infiltrated around the wound) as

(*continued*)

TABLE 43-2 **Immune Serums and Antitoxins for Passive Immunity** (*continued*)

Generic/Trade Name	Characteristics	Clinical Indications	Routes and Dosage Ranges
		around the head). Used in conjunction with rabies vaccine.	soon as possible. A test for hypersensitivity to horse serum should precede administration.
Botulism antitoxin	Obtained from blood of horses immunized against toxins of *Clostridium botulinum* The only specific agent available for treatment of botulism. Prompt use markedly decreases mortality May be obtained from the Centers for Disease Control and Prevention	For treatment of suspected botulism (a severe form of food poisoning that develops from raw or improperly preserved foods, such as home-canned vegetables). Botulism has a 20% to 35% mortality rate.	Adults and children: Consult the manufacturer's instructions regarding dosages and routes of administration. Testing for hypersensitivity to horse serum should precede administration of the antitoxin.
Diphtheria antitoxin	Obtained from blood of horses hyperimmunized against diphtheria toxin Used in conjunction with antibiotics (eg, penicillin, tetracycline, erythromycin), which eliminate bacteria but do not eliminate bacterial toxins	To prevent diphtheria in exposed, nonimmunized clients For treatment of diphtheria infection (based on clinical diagnosis, without waiting for bacteriologic confirmation of *Corynebacterium diphtheriae*)	Adults and children: Prophylaxis, IM 10,000 U Treatment, IV 20,000–120,000 U

CMV, cytomegalovirus; IgG, immunoglobulin G; IM, intramuscular; IV, intravenous; RSV, respiratory syncytial virus.

- For pregnant women not known to be immunized against rubella, serum antibody titer should be measured to determine resistance or susceptibility to the disease.
- For clients with wounds, assess the type of wound and determine how, when, and where it was sustained. Such information may reveal whether tetanus immunization is needed.
- For clients exposed to infectious diseases, try to determine the extent of exposure (eg, household or brief, casual contact) and when it occurred.

Nursing Diagnoses

- Knowledge Deficit: Importance of maintaining immunizations for both children and adults
- Knowledge Deficit: Risk of disease development versus risk of immunization
- Risk for Fluid Volume Deficit related to inadequate intake and febrile reactions to immunizing agent
- Noncompliance in obtaining recommended immunizations related to fear of adverse effects
- Risk for Injury related to disease development
- Risk for Injury related to hypersensitivity, fever, and other adverse drug effects

Planning/Goals

The client will:

- Avoid diseases for which immunizations are given

- Obtain recommended immunizations for children and self
- Keep appointments for immunizations

Interventions

Use measures to prevent infectious diseases, and provide information about the availability of immunizing agents. General measures include those to promote health and resistance to disease (eg, nutrition, rest, and exercise). Additional measures include the following:

- Education of the public, especially parents of young children, regarding the importance of immunizations to personal and public health. Include information about the diseases that can be prevented and where immunizations can be obtained.
- Assisting clients in developing a system to maintain immunization records for themselves and their children. This is important because immunizations are often obtained at different places and over a period of years. Written, accurate, up-to-date records help to prevent diseases and unnecessary immunizations.
- Prevention of disease transmission. The following are helpful measures:
  ○ Hand washing (probably the most effective method)

CLIENT TEACHING GUIDELINES
Vaccinations

✔ Appropriate vaccinations should be maintained for adults as well as for children. Consult a health care provider periodically because recommendations and personal needs change fairly often.

✔ Maintain immunization records for yourself and your children. This is important because immunizations are often obtained at different places and over a period of years. Written, accurate, up-to-date records help to prevent diseases and unnecessary immunizations.

✔ If a physician recommends an immunization and you do not know whether you have had the immunization or the disease, it is probably safer to take the immunization than to risk having the disease. Immunization after a previous immunization or after having the disease usually is not harmful.

✔ To avoid rubella-induced abnormalities in fetal development, women of childbearing age who receive a rubella immunization must avoid becoming pregnant (ie, must use effective contraceptive methods) for 3 months.

✔ Women of childbearing age who receive a varicella immunization must avoid becoming pregnant (ie, must use effective contraceptive methods) for 3 months.

✔ Some vaccines cause fever and soreness at the site of injection. Acetaminophen (Tylenol) can be taken two to three times daily for 24 to 48 hours (by adults and children) to decrease fever and discomfort.

✔ After receiving varicella vaccine (to prevent chickenpox), avoid close contact with newborns, pregnant women, and anyone whose immune system is impaired. Also, use effective methods of contraception to avoid pregnancy for at least 3 months after immunization. Vaccinated people may transmit the vaccine virus to susceptible close contacts. Effects of the vaccine on the fetus are unknown, but fetal harm has occurred with natural varicella infection during pregnancy.

✔ After receiving a vaccine, stay in the area for approximately 30 minutes. If an allergic reaction is going to occur, it will usually do so within that time.

○ Avoiding contact with people who have known or suspected infectious diseases, when possible
○ Using isolation techniques when appropriate
○ Using medical and surgical aseptic techniques

• For someone exposed to rubeola, administration of measles vaccine within 48 hours to prevent the disease

• For someone with a puncture wound or a dirty wound, administration of tetanus immune globulin to prevent tetanus, a life-threatening disease

• For someone with an animal bite, washing the wound immediately with large amounts of soap and water. Health care should then be sought. Administration of rabies vaccine may be needed to prevent rabies, a life-threatening disease.

• Explaining to the client that contracting rubella or undergoing rubella immunization during pregnancy, especially during the first trimester, may cause severe birth defects in the infant. The goal of immunization is to prevent congenital rubella syndrome. Current recommendations are to immunize children against rubella at 12 to 15 months of age.

It is recommended that previously unimmunized girls 11 to 13 years of age be immunized. Further, nonpregnant women of childbearing age should have rubella antibody tests. If antibody concentrations are low, the women should be immunized. Pregnancy should be avoided for 3 months after immunization.

Evaluation

• Interview and observe for symptoms.
• Interview and observe for adverse drug effects.
• Check immunization records when indicated.

PRINCIPLES OF THERAPY

Sources of Information

Recommendations regarding immunizations change periodically as additional information and new immunizing agents become available. Consequently, health care personnel should update their knowledge at least annually. The best sources of information regarding current recommendations are the local health department and the Centers for Disease Control and Prevention, U.S. Public Health Service, Department of Health and Human Services, Atlanta, Georgia (Internet address: http://www.cdc.gov). Local health departments can be consulted on routine immunizations and those required for foreign travel.

Nursing Notes: Apply Your Knowledge

You are working in an urgent care clinic. A 53-year-old housewife sustains a laceration and puncture wound on a rusty nail while gardening. Prioritize what immunization history to obtain from this patient, and why.

Storage of Vaccines

To maintain effectiveness of vaccines and other biologic preparations, the products must be stored properly. Most products require refrigeration at 2°C to 8°C (35.6°F to 46.4°F); some (eg, measles-mumps-rubella [MMR]) require protection from light. Follow manufacturers' instructions for storage.

Use in Children

Routine immunization of children has greatly reduced the prevalence of many common childhood diseases. However, many children are not being immunized appropriately, and diseases for which vaccines are available still occur. Standards of practice, aimed toward increasing immunizations, have been established and are supported by most pediatric provider groups (Box 43-1).

Guidelines for children whose immunizations begin in early infancy are given in the following list. Different schedules are recommended for children 1 to 5 years of age and for those older than 6 years of age who are being immunized for the first time.

1. Hepatitis B vaccine to all newborns or infants
2. DTP (diphtheria and tetanus toxoids, pertussis vaccine) at 2 months, 4 months, 6 months, 18 months, and 4 to 6 years of age
3. *Hemophilus influenzae* type b vaccine (Hib) at 2, 4, 6, and 12 to 15 months of age
4. Inactivated poliovirus vaccine (IPV) injection at 2 and 4 months of age, then either the IPV or oral poliovirus vaccine (OPV) for the third dose at 6 to 18 months and the fourth dose at 4 to 6 years of age. IPV may also be given for the entire four-dose schedule and for immunocompromised people and their household contacts. OPV may be given when a parent refuses IPV and remains the vaccine of choice for outbreaks of poliovirus infection.
5. MMR at 12 to 15 months of age, usually as a combined vaccine. These vaccines are given later than DTP and IPV because sufficient antibodies may not be produced until passive immunity acquired from the mother dissipates (at 12 to 15 months of age).
6. Tetanus-diphtheria (adult type) at 14 to 16 years of age and every 10 years thereafter

---

BOX 43–1   STANDARDS FOR PEDIATRIC IMMUNIZATION PRACTICES

The following standards are recommended for use by all health professionals in the public and private sector who administer vaccines to or manage immunization services for infants and children.

Standard 1. …Immunization services are *readily* available.

Standard 2. …There are no barriers or unnecessary prerequisites to the receipt of vaccines.

Standard 3. …Immunization services are available free or for a minimal fee.

Standard 4. …Providers use all clinical encounters to screen and, when indicated, immunize children.

Standard 5. … Providers educate parents and guardians about pediatric immunizations in general terms.

Standard 6. … Providers question parents or guardians about contraindications and, before immunizing a child, inform them in specific terms about the risks and benefits of the immunizations their child is to receive.

Standard 7. … Providers follow only true contraindications.

Standard 8. … Providers administer simultaneously all vaccine doses for which a child is eligible at the time of each visit.

Standard 9. …Providers use accurate and complete recording procedures.

Standard 10. … Providers coschedule immunization appointments in conjunction with appointments for other child health services.

Standard 11. …Providers report adverse events after immunization promptly, accurately, and completely.

Standard 12. … Providers operate a tracking system.

Standard 13. … Providers adhere to appropriate procedures for vaccine management.

Standard 14. … Providers conduct semiannual audits to assess immunization coverage levels and to review immunization records in the patient population they serve.

Standard 15. … Providers maintain up-to-date, easily retrievable medical protocols at all locations where vaccines are administered.

Standard 16. …Providers operate with patient-oriented and community-based approaches.

Standard 17. … Vaccines are administered by properly trained individuals.

Standard 18. … Providers receive ongoing education and training on current immunization recommendations.

7. Varicella at 12 to 18 months and again at approximately 12 years of age

8. For children with acquired immunodeficiency syndrome (AIDS), live viral and bacterial vaccines (MMR, OPV, varicella, bacillus Calmette-Guérin) are contraindicated because they may cause the disease rather than prevent it. However, immunizations with DTP, IPV, and Hib are recommended even though they may be less effective than in children with competent immune systems. Also recommended are annual administration of inactivated influenza vaccine for children over 6 months of age and one-time administration of pneumococcal vaccine for children older than 2 years of age.

Use in Healthy Adolescents, Young Adults, and Middle-Aged Adults

Adolescents who completed all primary immunizations as younger children should have hepatitis B vaccine (if not received earlier) and a tetanus-diphtheria booster. Young adults who are health care workers, are sexually active, or belong to high-risk groups should have hepatitis B vaccine if not previously received; a tetanus-diphtheria booster every 10 years; MMR if not pregnant and rubella titer is inadequate or proof of immunization is unavailable; and varicella. In addition, young adults who are health care providers should have influenza vaccine annually.

Middle-aged adults should maintain immunizations against tetanus; high-risk groups (eg, those with chronic illness) and health care providers should receive hepatitis B once (if not previously taken) and influenza vaccine annually.

Use in Older Adults

Annual influenza vaccine and one-time administration of pneumococcal vaccine are recommended for healthy older adults and those with chronic respiratory, cardiovascular, and other diseases. As with younger adults,

Nursing Notes: Ethical/Legal Dilemma

Jim and Sue bring in their newborn for a well-child examination. When you bring up the immunization schedule for infants, they voice concerns about the safety of some immunizations. They further explain that they read an article outlining several cases that involved serious complications (deaths and life-long disabilities) after infant immunizations.

Reflect on:

• Additional information you might want to collect from the parents.

• How you feel as a health care provider when people select not to participate in widely accepted health practices.

• How you can help these parents make an informed decision.

• How you can support these parents in their decision, even if it is different from what you personally would choose.

immunization for most other diseases is recommended for older adults at high risk of exposure.

Use in Immunosuppression

Live, attenuated viral vaccines (MMR, oral polio, varicella) should not be given to people with AIDS, other immune diseases, or impaired immune systems due to leukemia, lymphoma, corticosteroid or anticancer drugs, or radiation therapy. The virus may be able to reproduce and cause infection in these people. If a person is exposed to measles or varicella, immune globulin or varicella-zoster immune globulin may be given for passive immunization. With hepatitis A and B vaccines, additional or larger doses may be required in immunosuppressed people.

(*text continues on page 658*)

NURSING ACTIONS — Immunizing Agents

NURSING ACTIONS	RATIONALE/EXPLANATION
1. Administer accurately **a.** Read the package insert, and check the expiration date on all biologic products (eg, vaccines, toxoids, human immune serums, and antitoxins).	Concentration, dosage, and administration of biologic products often vary with the products. Fresh products are preferred; avoid administration of expired products. Also, use reconstituted products within designated time limits because they are usually stable for only a few hours.

(continued)

NURSING ACTIONS	RATIONALE/EXPLANATION
b. Give trivalent oral poliovirus vaccine (TOPV) into the side of an infant's mouth with a dropper, by placing on a child's tongue or a sugar cube or by mixing with milk, distilled water, or chlorine-free water.	Several methods of administration are effective and can be varied to meet the needs of individual infants or children. Avoid administering TOPV to a crying child because the dose may be lost or aspirated into the lungs.
c. Check the child's temperature before giving diphtheria, tetanus, pertussis (DTP) vaccine.	If the temperature is elevated, do not give the vaccine.
d. Give DTP in the lateral thigh muscle of the infant.	The vastus lateralis is the largest skeletal muscle mass in the infant and the preferred site for all intramuscular (IM) injections.
e. With measles, mumps, rubella (MMR) vaccine, use only the diluent provided by the manufacturer, and administer the vaccine subcutaneously (SC) within 8 h after reconstitution.	The reconstituted preparation is stable for approximately 8 h. If not used within 8 h, discard the solution.
f. Give hepatitis B vaccine IM in the anterolateral thigh of infants and young children and in the deltoid of older children and adults. Although the IM route is preferred, the drug can be given SC in people at high risk of bleeding from IM injections (eg, clients with hemophilia).	Higher blood levels of protective antibodies are produced when the vaccine is given in the thigh or deltoid than when it is given in the buttocks, probably because of injection into fatty tissue rather than gluteal muscles.
g. Give IM human immune serum globulin with an 18- to 20-gauge needle, preferably in gluteal muscles. If the dose is 5 mL or more, divide it and inject it into two or more IM sites. Follow manufacturer's instruction for preparation and administration of IV formulations.	To promote absorption and minimize tissue irritation and other adverse reactions
h. Test for sensitivity to horse serum before administering any antitoxin (eg, botulism, diphtheria). This test is preferably performed by the physician. If done by the nurse, a physician should be in close proximity. Also, a syringe with 1 mL of epinephrine 1:1000 should be prepared *before* testing.	Anaphylactic shock may occur. Epinephrine aqueous solution 1:1000 is used for emergency treatment of anaphylaxis. Epinephrine is injected subcutaneously in a dose of 0.5 mL for adults and 0.01 mL/kg for children.
(1) For the intradermal test, inject 0.1 to 0.2 mL of a 1:1000 dilution of horse serum into the forearm. The test is positive (ie, indicates allergy to horse serum) if a wheal appears at the injection site within 30 min.	If sensitivity tests are positive and antitoxins are deemed necessary, special desensitization procedures may be performed. Follow the manufacturer's recommendations for desensitization.
(2) For the conjunctival test, 1 drop of a 1:10 dilution of horse serum in isotonic saline solution is instilled in one eye. The test is positive if lacrimation and conjunctivitis appear within 30 min.	
i. Aspirate carefully before IM or SC injection of any immunizing agent.	To avoid inadvertent intravenous administration and greatly increased risks of severe adverse effects
j. Have aqueous epinephrine 1:1000 readily available before administering any vaccine.	For immediate treatment of allergic reactions
k. After administration of an immunizing agent in a clinic or office setting, have the client stay in the area for at least 30 min.	To be observed for allergic reactions, which usually occur within 30 min

(continued)

NURSING ACTIONS	**RATIONALE/EXPLANATION**
2. Observe for therapeutic effects	
a. Absence of diseases for which immunized	
b. Decreased incidence and severity of symptoms when given to modify disease processes	
3. Observe for adverse effects	Immunizing agents may cause adverse, life-threatening reactions. The risk of serious adverse effects from immunization is usually much smaller than the risk of the disease immunized against. Adverse effects may be caused by the immunizing agent or by foreign protein incorporated with the immunizing agent (eg, egg protein in viral vaccines grown in chick embryos).
a. Pain, tenderness, redness at injection sites	Local tissue irritation may occur with an injected immunizing agent. It is especially likely to occur with adsorbed DTP or tetanus toxoid. With DTP, a nodule or lump may persist for months but eventually resolves.
b. Fever, malaise, myalgia	These adverse effects are relatively common with vaccines and toxoids. They rarely occur with human immune serums given for passive immunity.
c. Severe fever, shock, somnolence, convulsions, encephalopathy	These are rare adverse reactions to DTP. If they occur, they are thought to be caused by the pertussis antigen, and further administration of pertussis vaccine or DTP is contraindicated.
d. Paralysis (Guillain-Barré syndrome)	This is a rare reaction to oral poliovirus vaccine.
e. Anaphylaxis (cardiovascular collapse, shock, laryngeal edema, urticaria, angioneurotic edema, severe respiratory distress)	Anaphylaxis is most likely to occur with injections of antitoxins (horse serum) but may occasionally occur with other immunizing agents. Anaphylaxis is a medical emergency that requires immediate treatment with SC epinephrine (0.5 mL for adults; 0.01 mL/kg for children). Anaphylaxis is most likely to occur within 30 min after immunizing agents are injected.
f. Serum sickness (urticaria, fever, arthralgia, enlarged lymph nodes)	Serum sickness is a delayed hypersensitivity reaction that occurs several days or weeks after an injection of serum. It is most likely to occur with antitoxins (horse serum). Treatment is symptomatic. Symptoms are usually relieved by aspirin, antihistamines, and corticosteroids.
4. Observe for drug interactions	
a. Drugs that alter effects of vaccines: Immunosuppressant agents (eg, corticosteroids, antineoplastic drugs, phenytoin [Dilantin])	Vaccines may be contraindicated in clients receiving immunosuppressive drugs. These clients cannot produce sufficient amounts of antibodies for immunity and may develop the illness produced by the particular organism contained in the vaccine. The disease is most likely to occur with the live virus vaccines (measles, mumps, rubella). Similar effects occur when the client is receiving irradiation and phenytoin, an anticonvulsant drug that suppresses both cellular and humoral immune responses.

(continued)

NURSING ACTIONS	RATIONALE/EXPLANATION
b. With varicella vaccine, salicylates may increase risk of Reye's syndrome.	Aspirin and other salicylates should be avoided for 6 wk after vaccine administration because of potential Reye's syndrome, which has been reported with salicylate use after natural varicella infection.

Nursing Notes: *Apply Your Knowledge*

Answer: Ask the patient how long ago she received a tetanus booster. Life-long immunity is not provided for tetanus, necessitating booster injections every 10 years. Adults often do not keep good immunization records. If the patient is not absolutely sure she has had a recent booster injection, a tetanus immunization should be given. Tetanus is common with puncture wounds and can be lethal.

REVIEW AND APPLICATION EXERCISES

1. What is the difference between active immunity and passive immunity?

2. How do vaccines act to produce active immunity?

3. What are the sources and functions of immune serums?

4. List common childhood diseases for which immunizing agents are available.

5. Which immunizations are recommended for adults?

6. What are advantages of administering a combination of immunizing agents rather than single agents?

7. What are common adverse reactions to immunizing agents, and how may they be prevented or minimized?

8. Why should live vaccines not be given to people whose immune systems are suppressed by drugs or diseases?

SELECTED REFERENCES

Ad Hoc Working Group for the Development of Standards for Pediatric Immunization Practices. (1993). Standards for pediatric immunization practices. *Journal of the American Medical Association, 269,* 1817–1822.

American Academy of Pediatrics Committee on Infectious Diseases. (1999). Recommended childhood immunization schedule—United States, January–December 1999. *Pediatrics, 103,* 182–183.

American Academy of Pediatrics Committee on Infectious Diseases. (1999). Poliomyelitis prevention: Revised recommendations for use of inactivated and live oral poliovirus vaccines. *Pediatrics, 103,* 171–172.

Association for Professionals in Infection Control and Epidemiology, Inc. (APIC) Guidelines Committee. (1999). APIC position paper: Immunization. *American Journal of Infection Control, 27,* 52–53.

Bertino, J.S. & Casto, D.T. (1997). Vaccines, toxoids, and other immunobiologics. In J.T. DiPiro, R.L. Talbert, G.C. Yee, G.R. Matzke, B.G. Wells, & L.M. Posey (Eds.), *Pharmacotherapy: A pathophysiologic approach,* 3rd ed., pp. 2319–2350. Stamford, CT: Appleton & Lange.

Drug facts and comparisons. (Updated monthly). St. Louis: Facts and Comparisons.

Eickhoff, T.C. (1997). Immunizations. In W.N. Kelley (Ed.), *Textbook of internal medicine,* 3rd ed., pp. 151–155. Philadelphia: Lippincott-Raven.

Kraisinger, M. (1998). Update on childhood immunization. *American Journal of Health-System Pharmacy, 55,* 563–569.

Porth, C.M. (Ed.). (1998). *Pathophysiology: Concepts of altered health states,* 5th ed. Philadelphia: Lippincott Williams & Wilkins.

Selekman, J. (1999). Recommended immunization schedule for 1999: Update on the changes. *Pediatric Nursing, 25,* 217–218.

44

Hematopoietic and Immunostimulant Drugs

Objectives

After studying this chapter, the student will be able to:

1. Describe the goals and methods of enhancing hematopoietic and immune functions.

2. Discuss the use of hematopoietic agents in the treatment of anemia and thrombocytopenia.

3. Discuss the use of filgrastim and sargramostim in neutropenia and bone marrow transplantation.

4. Describe the adverse effects and nursing process implications of administering filgrastim and sargramostim.

5. Discuss interferons and aldesleukin in terms of clinical uses, adverse effects, and nursing process implications.

Mrs. Reynolds, a 67-year-old who has had chronic renal failure for the last 7 years, is severely anemic. Her physician prescribes epoetin alfa (Epogen) to stimulate red blood cell production. You are responsible for teaching her about the drug, including subcutaneous administration.

Reflect on:

▶ Review why renal failure causes anemia and how Epogen works to increase red blood cell counts.

▶ What assessment data should you collect before teaching Mrs. Reynolds self-injection technique?

▶ How will you evaluate whether the Epogen is working? Consider decreased symptoms of anemia and expected changes in laboratory values.

OVERVIEW

Enhancing a person's own body systems to fight infection and cancer is an evolving concept. Hematopoietic and immunostimulant drugs (also called biologic response modifiers) are given to restore normal function or increase the ability of the immune system to eliminate potentially harmful invaders. Those available for therapeutic use include colony-stimulating factors (CSF; eg, epoetin alfa, filgrastim, sargramostim), several interferons, and two interleukins. These drugs, which are the primary focus of this chapter, are described in the following sections and in Table 44-1.

Bacillus Calmette-Guérin (BCG) vaccine, used in the treatment of bladder cancer, is also discussed. Other drugs with immunostimulant properties are discussed in other chapters. These include traditional immunizing agents (see Chap. 43); levamisole (Ergamisol), which restores functions of macrophages and T cells and is used with fluorouracil in the treatment of intestinal cancer (see Chap. 64); and antiviral drugs used in the treatment of acquired immunodeficiency syndrome (AIDS) (see Chap. 39). Levamisole and antiviral drugs are more accurately called immunorestoratives because they help a compromised immune system regain normal function rather than stimulating "supranormal" function. In AIDS, the human immunodeficiency

TABLE 44-1	Hematopoietic and Immunostimulant Agents		
Generic/Trade Name	**Indication for Use**	**Routes and Dosage Ranges**	**Comments**
Hematopoietic Agent			
Epoetin alfa (Epogen, Procrit)	Prevention and treatment of anemia associated with chronic renal failure (CRF), zidovudine therapy, or anticancer chemotherapy Reduction of blood transfusions in anemic clients undergoing elective noncardiac, nonvascular surgery	CRF IV, SC 50–100 U/kg three times weekly to achieve or maintain a hematocrit of approximately 30%–36% Zidovudine therapy IV, SC 100 U/kg three times weekly Cancer chemotherapy SC 150 U/kg three times weekly initially, increased up to 300 U/kg three times weekly if necessary Surgery SC 300 U/kg/d for 10 d before surgery, on the day of surgery and for 4 d after surgery	All patients should receive iron supplementation throughout epoetin alfa therapy.
Colony-Stimulating Factors (CSF)			
Filgrastim (G-CSF) (Neupogen)	To prevent infection in patients with neutropenia induced by cancer chemotherapy or bone marrow transplantation To mobilize stem cells from bone marrow to peripheral blood, where they can be collected and reinfused after chemotherapy that depresses bone marrow function To treat severe chronic neutropenia	Myelosuppressive chemotherapy, 5 µg/kg/d, up to 2 wk until ANC reaches 10,000/mm³ Bone marrow transplantation, IV or SC infusion, 10 µg/kg/d initially, then titrated according to neutrophil count (5 µg/kg/d if ANC >1000/mm³ for 3 consecutive days; stop drug if >1000/mm³ for 6 d. If ANC drops below 1000/mm³, restart filgrastim at 5 µg/kg/d). Collection of peripheral stem cells, SC 10 µg/kg/d, by bolus injection or by continuous infusion, for 6–7 d, with collection on the last 3 days of drug administration Severe, chronic neutropenia, SC 5 or 6 µg/kg, once or twice daily, depending on clinical response and ANC	Do not give 24 h before or after a dose of cytotoxic chemotherapy. Dosage may be increased if indicated by neutrophil count. Stop the drug if the ANC exceeds 10,000/mm³
Sargramostim (GM-CSF) (Leukine)	After bone marrow transplantation to promote bone marrow function or to treat graft failure or delayed function	Bone marrow reconstitution, IV infusion over 2 h, 250 µg/m²/d, starting 2–4 h after bone marrow infusion, and continuing for 21 d	

TABLE 44-1) **Hematopoietic and Immunostimulant Agents (*continued*)**

Generic/Trade Name	Indication for Use	Routes and Dosage Ranges	Comments
	Mobilization of stem cells in peripheral blood so they can be collected.	Graft failure or delay, IV infusion over 2 h, 250 µg/m²/d, for 14 d. Course of treatment may be repeated after 7 d off therapy if engraftment has not occurred. Mobilization of stem cells, SC or IV over 24 h, 250 µg/m²/d	
Interleukins			
Aldesleukin (interleukin-2) (Proleukin)	Metastatic renal cell carcinoma in adults*	IV infusion over 15 min 600,000 IU or 0.037 mg/kg q8h for 14 doses: after 9d, repeat q8h for 14 doses	Adverse reactions are common and may be serious or fatal. Drug administration must be interrupted or stopped for serious toxicity.
Oprelvekin (Neumega)	Prevention of severe thrombo-cytopenia with antineoplastic chemotherapy that depresses bone marrow function, in clients with nonmyeloid malignancies	SC 50 µg/kg once daily	Start 6–24 h after completion of chemotherapy and continue until postnadir platelet count is ≥50,000 cells/mm³, usually 10–21 d. Discontinue oprelvekin at least 2 d before the next cycle of chemotherapy.
Interferons			
Interferon alfa-2a (Roferon-A)	Hairy cell leukemia in adults* AIDS-related Kaposi's sarcoma in adults* Chronic myelogenous leukemia	Hairy cell leukemia SC, IM Induction, 3 million IU daily for 16–24 wk Maintenance, 3 million IU three times weekly Kaposi's sarcoma SC, IM Induction, 36 million IU daily for 10–12 wk Maintenance, 36 million IU three times weekly Chronic myelogenous leukemia (CML) SC, IM 9 million IU daily	SC recommended for patients with platelet counts <50,000/mm³ or who are at risk for bleeding Omit single doses or reduce dosage by 50% if severe adverse reactions occur. May be better tolerated if started with 3 million IU for 3 d, then given 6 million IU for 3 d before giving the full dose of 9 million IU daily for CML
Interferon alfa-2b (Intron A)	Hairy cell leukemia in adults* AIDS-related Kaposi's sarcoma in adults* Condylomata (genital warts) Chronic hepatitis (B and C) Malignant melanoma, after surgical excision, to delay recurrence and prolong survival	Hairy cell leukemia SC, IM Induction and maintenance, 2 million IU/m² three times weekly Kaposi's sarcoma SC, IM Induction and maintenance, 30 million IU/m² three times weekly Chronic hepatitis B SC, IM 5 million IU daily or 10 million IU three times weekly (total of 30–35 million IU per wk) for 16 wk Chronic hepatitis C SC, IM 3 million IU three times weekly Malignant melanoma induction, IV 20 million IU/m² on 5 consecutive days per week for 4 wk; maintenance, SC 10 million IU/m² three times per week for 48 wk, unless disease progression occurs Condylomata intralesionally 1 million IU/lesion (maximum of five lesions) three times weekly for 3 wk	Omit single doses or reduce dosage by 50% if severe adverse reactions occur.

(continued)

TABLE 44-1 **Hematopoietic and Immunostimulant Agents** (*continued*)

Generic/Trade Name	Indication for Use	Routes and Dosage Ranges	Comments
Interferon alfa-2b (Intron A) and **ribavirin** (Rebetron)	Chronic hepatitis C in patients who have relapsed after interferon therapy	Interferon alfa-2b SC 3 million IU 3 times weekly Ribavirin PO 400–600 mg bid	
Interferon alfacon-1 (Infergen)	Chronic hepatitis C in adults*	SC 9 µg three times weekly for 24 wk, with at least 48 h between doses	
Interferon alfa-n1 lymphoblastoid (Wellferon)	Chronic hepatitis C in adults*	SC, IM 3 million IU three times weekly for 48 wk	
Interferon beta-1a (Avonex)	Multiple sclerosis, to reduce frequency of exacerbations	IM, 30 µg once per week	
Interferon beta-1b (Betaseron)	Same as Interferon beta-1a, above	SC 0.25 mg every other day	
Interferon gamma-1b (Actimmune)	Reducing frequency and severity of serious infections associated with chronic granulomatous disease	SC 50 µg/m^2 if body surface area (BSA) is >0.5 m^2; 1.5 µg/kg if BSA <0.5 m^2 three times weekly (eg, Mon., Wed., Fri.)	
Vaccine			
Bacillus Calmette-Guérin (TICE BCG, TheraCys)	Bladder cancer	Intravesical instillation by urinary catheter, three vials, reconstituted according to manufacturer's instructions, then diluted further in 50 mL of sterile, preservative-free saline solution (total volume per dose, 53 mL). Repeat once weekly for 6 wk, then give one dose monthly for 6–12 mo (TICE BCG) or one dose at 3, 6, 12, 18, and 24 mo (TheraCys).	Start 7–14 d after bladder biopsy or transurethral resection

AIDS, acquired immunodeficiency syndrome; ANC, absolute neutrophil count; IM, intramuscular; IV, intravenous; SC, subcutaneous.
* 18 years of age and older.

virus causes immune system malfunction, so the antiviral drugs indirectly improve immunologic function.

CHARACTERISTICS OF HEMATOPOIETIC AND IMMUNOSTIMULANT DRUGS

1. Most are facsimiles of natural endogenous protein substances (see Chap. 42). Techniques of molecular biology are used to delineate the type and sequence of amino acids and to identify the genes responsible for producing the substances. These genes are then inserted into bacteria (usually *Escherichia coli*) or yeasts capable of producing the substances exogenously. Some (eg, interferon beta-1b) are synthetic versions of deoxyribonucleic acid (DNA) recombinant products.

2. Exogenous drug preparations have the same mechanisms of action as the endogenous products described in Chapter 42. Thus, CSF bind to receptors on the cell surfaces of immature blood cells in the bone marrow and increase the number, maturity, and functional ability of the cells. Interferons also bind to specific cell surface receptors and, in viral infections, induce enzymes that inhibit protein synthesis and degrade viral ribonucleic acid. As a result, viruses are less able to enter uninfected cells, reproduce, and release new viruses. In multiple sclerosis, the action of interferon beta is unknown.

In cancer, the exact mechanisms by which interferons and interleukins exert antineoplastic effects are unknown. However, their immunostimulant effects are thought to enhance activities of immune cells (ie, natural killer cells, T cells, B cells, and macrophages), induce tumor cell antigens (which make tumor cells more easily recognized by immune cells), or alter the expression of oncogenes (genes that can cause a normal cell to change to a cancer cell). BCG vaccine is thought to act against cancer of the urinary bladder by stimulating the immune system and eliciting a local inflammatory response, but its exact mechanism of action is unknown.

3. They are given by subcutaneous or intravenous (IV) injection because they are proteins that would be destroyed by digestive enzymes if given orally. Epoetin alfa (Epogen), filgrastim (Neupogen), oprelvekin (Neumega), and the interferons are often self- or caregiver-administered to ambulatory clients.

4. They may produce adverse effects so that clients do not feel better when taking one of these drugs.

5. The combination of injections and adverse effects may lead to noncompliance in taking the drugs as prescribed.

6. *Epoetin alfa* is a recombinant DNA version of erythropoietin, a hormone from the kidney that stimulates bone marrow production of red blood cells. It is used to prevent or treat anemia.

7. *Aldesleukin* is a recombinant DNA version of interleukin-2 (IL-2). It differs from native IL-2, but has the same biologic activity (eg, activates cellular immunity; produces tumor necrosis factor, IL-1, and interferon gamma; and inhibits tumor growth). It is used to treat metastatic renal cell carcinoma and is being investigated for use in malignant melanoma and other types of cancer. The drug is given by IV infusion, after which it is rapidly distributed to extravascular, extracellular spaces and eliminated by metabolism in the kidneys.

Aldesleukin is contraindicated for initial use in clients who have had organ transplantation or those with serious cardiovascular disease (eg, an abnormal thallium stress test, which reflects coronary artery disease) or serious pulmonary disease (eg, abnormal pulmonary function tests). It is contraindicated for repeated courses of therapy in clients who had serious toxicity during earlier courses, including the following:
Cardiac—arrhythmias unresponsive to treatment or ventricular tachycardia lasting for five beats or more, recurrent episodes of chest pain with electrocardiographic evidence of angina or myocardial infarction, pericardial tamponade
Renal—impairment requiring dialysis for longer than 72 hours
Gastrointestinal (GI)—bleeding requiring surgery, bowel ischemia or perforation
Respiratory—intubation required longer than 72 hours
Central nervous system—coma or toxic psychosis lasting longer than 72 hours, repetitive or hard to control seizures

8. *Oprelvekin* is recombinant IL-11, which stimulates platelet production. It is used to prevent severe thrombocytopenia and reduce the need for plate-

let transfusions in clients with cancer who are receiving chemotherapy that depresses the bone marrow.

9. Interferons have antiviral, antiproliferative, and immunoregulatory activities and are used mainly to treat viral infections and some specific cancers. They are designated as alfa, beta, or gamma according to specific characteristics. *Interferons alfa-2a* and *alfa-2b*, structurally the same except for one amino acid, are used to treat hairy cell leukemia and Kaposi's sarcoma associated with AIDS. Interferon alfa-2b is also approved for the treatment of viral infections, such as chronic hepatitis and condylomata acuminata (genital warts associated with infection by human papillomavirus). *Interferon alfa-n1* and *alfacon-1* are newer drugs approved for treatment of chronic hepatitis C. *Interferon gamma* is used to treat chronic granulomatous disease, and *interferon beta* is used for multiple sclerosis, in which it reduces progression of neurologic dysfunction.

Interferons are being investigated for additional uses, especially in cancer and viral infections, including AIDS. In cancer, for example, interferon alfa has demonstrated antitumor effects in non-Hodgkin's lymphoma, chronic myelogenous leukemia, multiple myeloma, malignant melanoma, and renal cell carcinoma. Common solid tumors of the breast, lung, and colon are unresponsive. In chronic hepatitis C, interferon improves liver function in approximately 50% of clients, but relapse often occurs when drug therapy is stopped. Interferon alfa-2b is being combined with ribavirin, another antiviral drug, in efforts to increase effectiveness in chronic hepatitis C. In condylomata, interferon alfa-2b is injected directly into the lesions for several weeks, and most of the lesions disappear completely.

Systemic interferons are usually well absorbed, widely distributed, and eliminated primarily by the kidneys.

10. *Bacillus Calmette-Guérin* vaccine is a suspension of attenuated *Mycobacterium bovis*, long used as an immunizing agent against tuberculosis. The drug's immunostimulant properties stem from its ability to stimulate cell-mediated immunity. It is used as a topical agent to treat superficial cancers of the urinary bladder, in which approximately 80% of clients achieve a therapeutic response. BCG is contraindicated in immunosuppressed clients because the live tubercular organisms may cause tuberculosis in this high-risk population.

11. All of the drugs are contraindicated for use in clients who have previously experienced hypersensitivity reactions to any component of the pharmaceutical preparations.

NURSING PROCESS

Assessment

- Assess the client's status in relation to infection or cancer.
- Assess nutritional status, including appetite and weight.
- Assess functional abilities in relation to activities of daily living (ADLs).
- Assess adequacy of support systems for outpatients (eg, transportation for clinic visits).
- Assess ability and attitude toward planned drug therapy and associated monitoring and follow-up.
- Assess coping mechanisms of client and significant others in stressful situations.
- Assess client for factors predisposing to infection (eg, skin integrity, invasive devices, cigarette smoking).
- Assess environment for factors predisposing to infection (eg, family or health care providers with infections).
- Assess baseline values of laboratory and other diagnostic test reports to aid monitoring of responses to hematopoietic and immunostimulant drug therapy.

Nursing Diagnoses

- Risk for Injury: Infection related to drug-induced neutropenia, immunosuppression, malnutrition, chronic disease
- Risk for Injury: Bleeding related to anemia or thrombocytopenia
- Risk for Injury: Adverse drug effects
- Altered Nutrition: Less Than Body Requirements related to disease process or drug therapy
- Activity Intolerance related to weakness, fatigue from debilitating disease, or drug therapy
- Anxiety related to the diagnosis of cancer or AIDS, disease progression, and treatment
- Self Care Deficit related to debilitation from disease process or drug therapy
- Self-Esteem Disturbance related to illness, inability to perform usual ADLs
- Knowledge Deficit: Disease process
- Knowledge Deficit: Hematopoietic and immunostimulant drug therapy
- Ineffective Individual Coping related to a medical diagnosis of life-threatening illness
- Ineffective Family Coping related to illness and treatment of a family member

Planning/Goals

The client will:

- Participate in interventions to prevent or decrease infection

- Remain afebrile during immunostimulant therapy
- Experience increased immunocompetence as indicated by increased white blood cell (WBC) count (if initially leukopenic) or tumor regression
- Avoid preventable infections
- Experience relief or reduction of disease symptoms
- Maintain independence in ADLs when able; be assisted appropriately when unable
- Maintain adequate levels of nutrition and fluids, rest and sleep, and exercise
- Maintain or increase appetite and weight if initially anorexic and underweight
- Be assisted to cope with stresses of the disease process and drug therapy
- Learn to self-administer medications accurately when indicated

Interventions

- Practice and promote good hand washing techniques by clients and all others in contact with the client.
- Use sterile technique for all injections, IV site care, wound dressing changes, and any other invasive diagnostic or therapeutic measures.
- Allow clients to perform hygienic care when able, or provide assistance when unable.
- Screen staff and visitors for signs and symptoms of infection; if infection is noted, do not allow contact with the client.
- Allow clients to participate in self-care and decision making when possible and appropriate.
- Use isolation procedures when indicated, usually when the neutrophil count is below 500/mm^3.
- Promote adequate nutrition, with nutritious fluids, supplements, and snacks when indicated.
- Promote adequate rest, sleep, and exercise (eg, schedule frequent rest periods, avoid interrupting sleep when possible, individualize exercise or activity according to the client's condition).
- Inform clients about diagnostic test results, planned changes in therapeutic regimens, and evidence of progress.
- Allow family members or significant others to visit clients when feasible.
- Monitor complete blood count (CBC) and other diagnostic test reports for normal or abnormal values.
- Schedule and coordinate drug administration, diagnostic tests, and other elements of care to conserve clients' energy and decrease stress.
- Consult other health care providers (eg, physician, dietitian, social worker) on the client's behalf when indicated.
- Assist clients to learns ways to prevent or reduce the incidence of infections (eg, meticulous per-

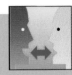

CLIENT TEACHING GUIDELINES
Blood Cell and Immune System Stimulants

General Considerations

✔ Help your body maintain immune mechanisms and other defenses by healthy lifestyle habits, such as a nutritious diet, adequate rest and sleep, and avoidance of tobacco and alcohol.

✔ Practice meticulous personal hygiene and avoid people and circumstances in which you are exposed to infection.

✔ Keep appointments with health care providers for follow-up care, blood tests, and so forth.

✔ Inform any other physician, dentist, or health care provider about your condition and the medications you are taking.

✔ Several of these medications can be taken at home, even though they are taken by injection. If you are going to self-inject a medication at home, allow sufficient time to learn and practice the techniques under the supervision of a health care provider. Correct preparation and injection are necessary to increase beneficial effects and decrease adverse effects.

✔ With oprelvekin, report the occurrence of ankle edema, shortness of breath, or dizzy spells. Edema and breathing difficulty may be caused by fluid retention, a common adverse effect, and dizziness may result from an irregular heartbeat, which is most likely to occur in older adults.

✔ With interferons, report the occurrence of depression or thoughts of suicide, dizziness, hives, itching, chest tightness, cough, difficulty breathing or wheezing, or visual problems. These symptoms may require that the drug be stopped or the dosage reduced. In addition, avoid pregnancy (use effective contraceptive methods) and avoid prolonged exposure to sunlight, wear protective clothing, and use sunscreens.

Self- or Caregiver Administration

✔ Take the drugs as prescribed. Although this is important with all medications, it is especially important with these. Obtaining beneficial effects and decreasing adverse effects depend to a great extent on how the drugs are taken.

✔ Use correct techniques to prepare and inject the medications. Instructions for mixing the drugs should be followed exactly.

✔ With interferons:
  ✔ Store in the refrigerator.
  ✔ Do not freeze or shake the drug vial.
  ✔ Do not change brands (changes in dosage may result).
  ✔ Take at bedtime to reduce some common adverse effects (eg, flu-like symptoms such as fever, headache, fatigue, anorexia, nausea and vomiting).
  ✔ Take acetaminophen (eg, Tylenol, others), if desired, to prevent or decrease fever and headache.
  ✔ Maintain a good fluid intake (eg, 2 to 3 quarts daily).

---

sonal hygiene, avoiding contact with infected people)

• Assist clients to learn ways to enhance immune mechanisms and other body defenses by healthy lifestyle habits, such as a nutritious diet, adequate rest and sleep, and avoidance of tobacco and alcohol

• Assist clients or caregivers in learning how to prepare and inject epoetin alfa, filgrastim, an interferon, or oprelvekin, when indicated.

Evaluation

• Determine the number and type of infections that have occurred in neutropenic clients.

• Compare current CBC reports with baseline values for changes toward normal levels (eg, WBC count 5000 to 10,000/mm³).

• Compare weight and nutritional status with baseline values for maintenance or improvement.

• Observe and interview for decreased numbers or severity of disease symptoms.

• Observe for increased energy and ability to participate in ADLs.

• Observe and interview outpatients regarding compliance with follow-up care.

• Observe and interview regarding the mental and emotional status of the client and family members.

PRINCIPLES OF THERAPY

Inpatient Versus Outpatient Settings for Drug Administration

Choosing inpatient or outpatient administration of hematopoietic and immunostimulant therapy depends on many factors, including the condition of the client, route of drug administration, expected duration of therapy, and potential severity of adverse drug reactions. Most of these drugs are proteins, and anaphylactic or other allergic reactions may occur, especially with parenteral administration. Thus, initial doses should be given where appropriate supplies and personnel are available to treat allergic reactions.

Epoetin alfa, filgrastim, interferons, and oprelvekin may be taken at home if the client or a caregiver can prepare and inject the medication. Because severe, life-threatening adverse effects may occur with high-dose aldesleukin, this drug should be given only in a hospital with intensive care facilities, under the supervision of health care providers experienced in critical care.

Dosage

Optimal dosages for interferons and aldesleukin have not been established. For clients who experience severe adverse reactions with interferon alfa, dosage should be reduced by 50% or administration stopped until the reaction subsides. For clients who experience severe reactions to aldesleukin, dosage reduction is not recommended. Instead, one or more doses should be withheld, or the drug should be discontinued. Withhold the dose for cardiac arrhythmias, hypotension, chest pain, agitation or confusion, sepsis, renal impairment (oliguria, increased serum creatinine), hepatic impairment (encephalopathy, increasing ascites), positive stool guaiac test, or severe dermatitis until the condition is resolved. The drug should be discontinued for the occurrence of any of the conditions listed as contraindications for repeat courses of aldesleukin therapy (eg, sustained ventricular tachycardia, angina, myocardial infarction, pulmonary intubation, renal dialysis, coma, and GI bleeding).

Laboratory Monitoring

A CBC with WBC differential and platelet count should be done before and during hematopoietic and immunostimulant drug therapy to monitor response and prevent avoidable adverse drug reactions. With CSF, these tests are recommended twice weekly during drug administration. With aldesleukin, these tests plus electrolytes and renal and liver function tests are recommended daily during drug administration. With interferons alfacon-1 and alfa-n1, tests of platelet and neutrophil counts, hemoglobin, serum creatinine or creatinine clearance, serum albumin, and thyroid-stimulating hormone are recommended for all clients before starting therapy, 2 weeks later, and periodically thereafter during the 24 weeks of therapy.

Uses in Clients With Cancer

Colony-Stimulating Factors

Filgrastim and *sargramostim* are used to restore, promote, or accelerate bone marrow function in clients with cancer who are undergoing chemotherapy or bone marrow

transplantation. In cancer chemotherapy, many therapeutic drugs cause bone marrow depression and result in anemia and neutropenia. Neutropenic clients are at high risk for development of infections, often from the normal microbial flora of the client's body or environmental microorganisms, and they may involve bacteria, fungi, and viruses. The client is most vulnerable to infection when the neutrophil count falls below 500/mm^3. Filgrastim helps to prevent infection by reducing the incidence, severity, and duration of neutropenia associated with several chemotherapy regimens. Most clients taking filgrastim have fewer days of fever, infection, and antimicrobial drug therapy. In addition, by promoting bone marrow recovery after a course of cytotoxic antineoplastic drugs, filgrastim also may allow higher doses or more timely administration of subsequent antitumor drugs.

When filgrastim is given to prevent infection in neutropenic clients with cancer, the drug should be started at least 24 hours after the last dose of the antineoplastic agent. It should then be continued during the period of maximum bone marrow suppression and the lowest neutrophil count (nadir) and during bone marrow recovery. CBC and platelet counts should be performed twice weekly during therapy, and the drug should be stopped if the neutrophil count exceeds 10,000/mm^3. When sargramostim is given to clients with cancer who have had bone marrow transplantation, the drug should be started 2 to 4 hours after the bone marrow infusion and at least 24 hours after the last dose of antineoplastic chemotherapy or 12 hours after the last radiotherapy treatment. CBC should be done twice weekly during therapy, and the neutrophil count should not exceed approximately 20,000/mm^3.

Epoetin alfa may be used to prevent or treat anemia in clients with cancer. An adequate intake of iron is required for drug effectiveness. In addition to dietary sources, a supplement is usually necessary.

Interleukins

Aldesleukin is a highly toxic drug and contraindicated in clients with preexisting serious cardiovascular or pulmonary impairment. Therefore, when it is used to treat metastatic renal cell carcinoma, clients must be carefully selected, evaluated, and monitored. The drug is most effective in clients with prior nephrectomy and low tumor

---

Nursing Notes: Apply Your Knowledge

John Miller is receiving monthly chemotherapy. The nadir is expected 10 days after treatment. Last month, the nadir lasted for 6 days, during which his neutrophil count was less than 1000/mm^3. This month he is given filgrastim (granulocyte colony-stimulating factor [G-CSF]). Why is the G-CSF given, and how will you evaluate its effectiveness?

burden. Still, only about 15% to 25% of clients experience therapeutic responses.

Measures to decrease toxicity are also needed. One strategy is to give the drug by continuous infusion rather than bolus injection. Another is to use cancer-fighting T cells found within tumors. These T cells, called tumor-infiltrating lymphocytes, can be removed from the tumors, incubated in vitro with aldesleukin, and reinjected into the client. Tumor-infiltrating lymphocytes return to the tumor and are more active in killing malignant cells than untreated T cells. This technique allows lower and therefore less toxic doses of aldesleukin. Corticosteroids can also decrease toxicity, but their use is not recommended because they also decrease the antineoplastic effects of aldesleukin.

In addition, any preexisting infection should be treated and resolved before initiating aldesleukin therapy because the drug may impair neutrophil function and increase the risk of infections, including septicemia and bacterial endocarditis. Clients with indwelling central IV devices should be given prophylactic antibacterials that are effective against *Staphylococcus aureus* (eg, nafcillin, vancomycin).

Oprelvekin may be used to prevent or treat thrombocytopenia and risks of bleeding in clients with cancer.

Interferons

In hairy cell leukemia, interferons normalize WBC counts in 70% to 90% of clients, with or without prior splenectomy. Drug therapy must be continued indefinitely to avoid relapse, which usually develops rapidly after the drug is discontinued. In AIDS-related Kaposi's sarcoma, larger doses are required than in other clinical uses, with resultant increases in toxicity. Interferon alfa is recommended for clients with CD4 cell counts higher than 200/mL (CD4 cells are the helper T cells attacked by the AIDS virus), who have no systemic symptoms, and who have had no opportunistic infections. Approximately 40% of these clients achieve a therapeutic response that lasts approximately 1 to 2 years. In addition to antineoplastic effects, data indicate that viral replication is suppressed in responding clients. Research studies suggest that a combination of interferon alfa and zidovudine, an antiviral drug used in the treatment of AIDS, may have synergistic antineoplastic and antiviral effects. Lower doses of interferon must be used when the drug is combined with zidovudine to minimize neutropenia.

Bacillus Calmette-Guérin

Bacillus Calmette-Guérin, when instilled into the urinary bladder of clients with superficial bladder cancer, causes remission in up to 82% of clients for an average of 4 years. Early, successful treatment of carcinoma in situ also prevents development of invasive bladder cancer. A specific protocol has been developed for administration of BCG solution, and it should be followed accurately.

Use in Bone Marrow and Stem Cell Transplantation

Filgrastim and *sargramostim* are used to treat clients who undergo bone marrow transplantation for Hodgkin's disease, non-Hodgkin's lymphoma, or acute lymphoblastic leukemia. Before receiving a bone marrow transplant, the client's immune system is suppressed by anticancer drugs or irradiation. After transplantation, it takes 2 to 4 weeks for the engrafted bone marrow cells to mature and begin producing blood cells. During this time, the client has virtually no functioning granulocytes and is at high risk for infection. Sargramostim promotes engraftment and function of the transplanted bone marrow, thereby decreasing risks of infection. If the graft is successful, the granulocyte count starts to rise in approximately 2 weeks. Sargramostim also is used to treat graft failure.

In stem cell transplantation, filgrastim or sargramostim is used to stimulate the movement of hematopoietic stem cells from the bone marrow to circulating blood, where they can be readily collected (in a process called peripheral blood progenitor cell collection). Transplantation of large numbers of stem cells can lead to more rapid engraftment and recovery, with less risk of transplant failure and complications.

Use in Children

There has been limited experience with hematopoietic and immunostimulant drugs in children (younger than 18 years of age), and the drugs' safety and effectiveness have not been established. *Filgrastim* and *sargramostim* have been used in children with therapeutic and adverse effects similar to those in adults. In clinical trials, filgrastim produced a greater incidence of subclinical spleen enlargement in children than in adults, but whether this affects growth and development or has other long-term consequences is unknown. *Oprelvekin* has been given to a few children with adverse effects similar to those observed in adults. Reports indicate that tachycardia occurs more often in children and that larger doses are needed (eg, a dose of 75 to 100 µg/kg in children produces similar plasma levels to a dose of 50 µg/kg in adults). Long-term effects on growth and development are unknown.

Little information is available about the use of interferons in children. *Interferon alfacon-1* (Infergen) is not recommended for use in children.

Use in Older Adults

In general, hematopoietic and immunostimulant agents have the same uses and responses in older adults as in younger adults. As with many other drugs, older adults may be at greater risk of adverse effects, especially if large doses are used. *Oprelvekin* should be used with caution in clients with a history of or risk factors for atrial fibrillation or flutter; these arrhythmias occurred in approximately 10% of clients during clinical trials. In addition, older adults are more likely to have fluid retention, with resultant symptoms of peripheral edema, dyspnea on exertion, and dilutional anemia.

Use in Renal Impairment

Except for epoetin alfa, which is used to treat anemia in clients with chronic renal failure, little information is available about the use of hematopoietic and immunostimulant drugs in clients with renal impairment. In some clients with preexisting renal impairment, sargramostim increased serum creatinine. Values declined to baseline levels when the drug was stopped or its dosage reduced. Renal function tests are recommended approximately every 2 weeks in clients with preexisting impairment.

With aldesleukin, renal impairment occurs during therapy. This impairment may be increased if other nephrotoxic drugs are taken concomitantly. In addition, drug-induced renal impairment may delay elimination of other medications and increase risks of adverse effects.

Use in Hepatic Impairment

In some clients with preexisting hepatic impairment, sargramostim increased serum bilirubin and liver enzymes. Values declined to baseline levels when the drug was stopped or its dosage reduced. Hepatic function tests are recommended approximately every 2 weeks in clients with preexisting impairment.

With aldesleukin, hepatic impairment occurs during therapy. This impairment may be increased if other hepatotoxic drugs are taken concomitantly. In addition, drug-

induced hepatic impairment may delay metabolism and elimination of other medications and increase risks of adverse effects.

Interferons may aggravate hepatic impairment. Interferons alfa-2b, alfacon-1, and alfa-n1 are contraindicated in clients with decompensated liver disease (ie, signs and symptoms such as jaundice, ascites, bleeding disorders, or decreased serum albumin), autoimmune hepatitis, a history of autoimmune disease, or post-transplantation immunosuppression. Worsening of liver disease, with jaundice, hepatic encephalopathy, hepatic failure, and death, has occurred in these clients. The drugs should be discontinued in clients with signs and symptoms of liver failure.

 Home Care

Epoetin alfa (Epogen), filgrastim (Neupogen), oprelvekin (Neumega), and the interferons are often self-administered or given by a caregiver to chronically ill clients. The home care nurse may need to teach clients or caregivers accurate drug preparation and injection techniques, as well as proper disposal of needles and syringes. Assistance may also be needed in obtaining appropriate laboratory tests (eg, CBC, platelet count, tests of renal or hepatic function) to monitor clients' responses to the medications. Other interventions depend on the drug being taken. For example, epoetin alfa is not effective unless sufficient iron is present, and most clients need an iron supplement. When an iron preparation is prescribed, the home care nurse may need to emphasize the importance of taking it. With filgrastim, the nurse may need to help the client and family with techniques to reduce exposure to infection.

(*text continues on page 671*)

NURSING ACTIONS	Hematopoietic and Immunostimulant Agents
NURSING ACTIONS	**RATIONALE/EXPLANATION**
1. Administer accurately	For hospitalized clients, the drugs may be prepared for administration in a pharmacy. When nurses prepare the drugs, they should consult the manufacturer's instructions. Outpatients may be taught self-administration techniques.
a. Give epoetin alfa intravenously (IV) or subcutaneously (SC); do not shake the vial; and discard any remainder of multidose vials 21 d after opening.	For clients with chronic renal failure on hemodialysis, epoetin alfa can be given by bolus injection at the end of dialysis. For other patients with an IV line, the drug can be given IV. For patients without an IV line or who are ambulatory, the drug is injected SC. Shaking can inactivate the medication; the manufacturer does not ensure sterility or stability of multidose vials after 21 days. *(continued)*

NURSING ACTIONS	RATIONALE/EXPLANATION
b. Give filgrastim according to indication for use:	
(1) With cancer chemotherapy, give by SC bolus injection, IV infusion over 15–30 min, or continuous SC or IV infusion	
(2) For bone marrow transplantation, give by IV infusion over 4 h or by continuous IV or SC infusion	
(3) For collection of stem cells, give as a bolus or a continuous infusion	
(4) For chronic neutropenia, give SC	
c. Give sargramostim by IV infusion over 2 h, after reconstitution with 1 mL sterile water for injection and addition to 0.9% sodium chloride.	
d. With aldesleukin, review institutional protocols or the manufacturer's instructions for administration.	This drug has limited uses and is rarely given. Thus, most nurses will need to review instructions each time.
e. Inject interferon for condylomata intralesionally into the base of each wart with a small-gauge needle. For large warts, inject at several points.	Manufacturer's recommendation
f. With intravesical *Bacillus Calmette-Guérin (BCG):*	
(1) Reconstitute solution (see Table 44-1).	Reconstituted solution should be used immediately or refrigerated. Discard if not used within 2 h.
(2) Wear gown and gloves.	
(3) Insert a sterile urethral catheter and drain bladder.	
(4) Instill medication slowly by gravity.	
(5) Remove catheter.	
(6) Have the patient lie on abdomen, back, and alternate sides for 15 min in each position. Then, allow to ambulate but ask to retain solution for a total of 2 h before urinating, if able.	
(7) Dispose of all equipment in contact with BCG solution appropriately.	BCG contains live mycobacterial organisms and is therefore infectious material.
(8) Do not give if catheterization causes trauma (eg, bleeding), and wait 1 wk before a repeat attempt.	
2. Observe for therapeutic effects	
a. With epoetin alfa, observe for increased red blood cells, hemoglobin, and hematocrit.	Therapeutic effects depend on the dose and the client's underlying condition. The goal is usually to achieve and maintain a hematocrit between 30% and 36%.
b. With oprelvekin, observe for maintenance of a normal or near-normal platelet count when used to prevent thrombocytopenia and an increased platelet count or fewer platelet transfusions when used to treat thrombocytopenia.	Platelet counts usually increase in approximately 1 wk and continue to increase for approximately 1 wk after the drug is stopped. Then, counts decrease toward baseline during the next 2 wk.

(continued)

NURSING ACTIONS	RATIONALE/EXPLANATION
c. With aldesleukin, observe for tumor regression (improvement in signs and symptoms).	Tumor regression may occur as early as 4 wk after the first course of therapy and may continue up to 12 mo.
d. With parenteral interferons, observe for improvement in signs and symptoms.	With hairy cell leukemia, hematologic tests may improve within 2 mo, but optimal effects may require 6 mo of drug therapy. With acquired immunodeficiency syndrome (AIDS)–related Kaposi's sarcoma, skin lesions may resolve or stabilize over several weeks. With chronic hepatitis, liver function tests may improve within a few weeks.
e. With intralesional interferons, observe for disappearance of genital warts.	Lesions usually disappear after several weeks of treatment.

3. Observe for adverse effects

a. With epoetin alfa, observe for nausea, vomiting, diarrhea, arthralgias, and hypertension.	The drug is usually well tolerated, with adverse effects similar to those of placebo and which may result from the underlying disease processes.
b. With oprelvekin, observe for atrial fibrillation or flutter, dyspnea, edema, fever, mucositis, nausea, neutropenia, tachycardia, vomiting	In clinical trials, most adverse events were mild or moderate in severity and reversible after stopping drug administration. Atrial arrhythmias are more likely to occur in older adults. Dyspnea and edema are attributed to fluid retention.
c. With filgrastim, observe for bone pain, erythema at SC injection sites, and increased serum lactate dehydrogenase, alkaline phosphatase, and uric acid levels.	Bone pain reportedly occurs in 20% to 25% of patients and can be treated with acetaminophen or a nonsteroidal anti-inflammatory drug (NSAID).
d. With sargramostim, observe for bone pain, fever, headache, myalgias, generalized maculopapular skin rash, and fluid retention (peripheral edema, pleural effusion, pericardial effusion).	Pleural and pericardial effusions are more likely at doses greater than 20 μg/kg/d. Adverse effects occur more often with sargramostim than filgrastim.
e. With interferons, observe for acute flu-like symptoms (eg, fever, chills, fatigue, muscle aches, headache), chronic fatigue, depression, leukopenia, and increased liver enzymes.	Acute effects occur in most patients, increasing with higher doses and decreasing with continued drug administration. Symptoms can be relieved by acetaminophen. Fatigue and depression occur with long-term administration and are dose-limiting effects.
f. With aldesleukin, observe for capillary leak syndrome (hypotension, shock, angina, myocardial infarction, arrhythmias, edema, respiratory distress, gastrointestinal bleeding, renal insufficiency, mental status changes). Other effects may involve most body systems, such as chills and fever, blood (anemia, thrombocytopenia, eosinophilia), and central nervous system (CNS) (seizures, psychiatric symptoms), skin (erythema, burning, pruritus), hepatic (cholestasis), endocrine (hypothyroidism), and bacterial infections. In addition, drug-induced tumor breakdown may cause hypocalcemia, hyperkalemia, hyperphosphatemia, hyperuricemia, renal failure, and electrocardiogram changes.	Adverse effects are frequent, often serious, and sometimes fatal. Most subside within 2 to 3 d after stopping the drug. Capillary leak syndrome, which may begin soon after treatment starts, is characterized by a loss of plasma proteins and fluids into extravascular space. Signs and symptoms result from decreased organ perfusion, and most patients can be treated with vasopressor drugs, cautious fluid replacement, diuretics, and supplemental oxygen.

(continued)

NURSING ACTIONS	RATIONALE/EXPLANATION
g. With intravesical BCG, assess for symptoms of bladder irritation (eg, frequency, urgency, dysuria, hematuria) and systemic symptoms of fever, chills, and malaise.	These effects occur in more than 50% of patients, usually starting a few hours after administration and lasting 2 to 3 d. They can be decreased by phenazopyridine (Pyridium), an analgesic, propantheline (Pro-Banthine) or oxybutynin (Ditropan), antispasmodics; and acetaminophen (Tylenol) or ibuprofen (Motrin), analgesic–antipyretic agents.
4. Observe for drug interactions	
a. Drugs that *increase* effects of sargramostim:	
(1) Corticosteroids, lithium	These drugs have myeloproliferative (bone marrow stimulating) effects of their own, which may add to those of sargramostim.
b. Drugs that *alter* effects of interferons:	
(1) Other antineoplastic agents	Additive therapeutic and myelosuppressive effects
c. Drugs that *increase* effects of aldesleukin:	All of the listed drug groups may potentiate adverse effects of aldesleukin.
(1) Aminoglycoside antibiotics (eg, gentamicin, others)	Increased nephrotoxicity
(2) Antihypertensives	Increased hypotension
(3) Antineoplastics (eg, asparaginase, doxorubicin, methotrexate)	Increased toxic effects on bone marrow, heart, and liver. Aldesleukin is usually given as a single antineoplastic agent; its use in combination with other antineoplastic drugs is being evaluated.
(4) Opioid analgesics	Increased CNS adverse effects
(5) NSAIDs (eg, ibuprofen)	Increased nephrotoxicity
(6) Sedative-hypnotics	Increased CNS adverse effects
d. Drugs that *decrease* effects of aldesleukin:	
(1) Corticosteroids	These drugs should not be given concurrently with aldesleukin. Although they decrease some adverse effects, such as fever, renal impairment, confusion, and others, they also decrease the drug's therapeutic antineoplastic effects.

Nursing Notes: Apply Your Knowledge

Answer: G-CSF is given to decrease the length and severity of bone marrow suppression after chemotherapy. Laboratory values (white blood cell count and differential) evaluate the degree of bone marrow suppression and whether G-CSF is effective. In this situation, nadir (lowest neutrophil count) should be above 1000/mm³ and should last for less than 6 days. Although bone marrow suppression can affect red blood cells and platelets, white blood cells (neutrophils) are most significant because a low neutrophil count increases infection risk. Infection in a neutropenic patient can be life threatening.

REVIEW AND APPLICATION EXERCISES

1. What are the hematopoietic, colony-stimulating cytokines, and how do they function in the body?

2. What are adverse effects of filgrastim and sargramostim, and how may they be prevented or minimized?

3. What are the clinical uses of pharmaceutical interleukins and interferons?

4. What are the adverse effects of interleukins and interferons, and how can they be prevented or minimized?

5. Describe the clinical uses of hematopoietic and immunostimulant drugs in the treatment of anemia,

neutropenia, thrombocytopenia, cancer, and bone marrow transplantation.

SELECTED REFERENCES

Balmer, C. & Valley, A.W. (1997). Basic principles of cancer treatment and cancer chemotherapy. In J.T. DiPiro, R.L. Talbert, G.C. Yee, G.R. Matzke, B.G. Wells, & L. M. Posey (Eds.), *Pharmacotherapy: A pathophysiologic approach*, 3rd ed., pp. 1879–1929. Stamford, CT: Appleton & Lange.

Diasio, R.B. & LoBuglio, A.F. (1996). Immunomodulators: Immunosuppressive agents and immunostimulants. In J.G. Hardman, L.E. Limbird, P.B. Molinoff, & R.W. Ruddon (Eds.), *Goodman & Gilman's The pharmacological basis of therapeutics*, 9th ed., pp. 2403–2465. New York: McGraw-Hill.

Drug facts and comparisons. (Updated monthly). St. Louis: Facts and Comparisons.

Hillman, R.S. (1996). Hematopoietic agents: Growth factors, minerals, and vitamins. In J.G. Hardman, L.E. Limbird, P.B. Molinoff, & R.W. Ruddon (Eds.), *Goodman & Gilman's The pharmacological basis of therapeutics*, 9th ed., pp. 1311–1340. New York: McGraw-Hill.

Moore, M. (1997). Hematopoietic growth factors. In W.N. Kelley (Ed.), *Textbook of internal medicine*, 3rd ed., pp. 1522–1525. Philadelphia: Lippincott-Raven.

Urba, W.J. & Chabner, B.A. (1997). Principles of biologic therapy. In W.N. Kelley (Ed.), *Textbook of internal medicine*, 3rd ed., pp. 1519–1522. Philadelphia: Lippincott-Raven.

Immunosuppressants

Objectives

After studying this chapter, the student will be able to:

1. Describe characteristics and consequences of immunosuppression.

2. Discuss characteristics and uses of major immunosuppressant drugs in autoimmune disorders and organ transplantation.

3. Identify adverse effects of immunosuppressant drugs.

4. Discuss nursing interventions to decrease adverse effects of immunosuppressant drugs.

5. Teach clients, family members, and caregivers about safe and effective immunosuppressant drug therapy.

6. Assist clients and family members to identify potential sources of infection in the home care environment.

Jane Reily, 46 years of age, is scheduled to have a kidney transplant this week. After transplantation, she will be on a regimen of immunosuppressive drugs, including corticosteroids and cyclosporine. You are responsible for Ms. Reily's teaching.

Reflect on:

▶ Why lifelong immunosuppression is necessary after an organ transplant.

▶ What symptoms Ms. Reily might experience if she rejected her transplanted kidney.

▶ How you will teach Ms. Reily to reduce her risk of infection.

▶ What lifelong measures for medical follow-up and management are necessary for a transplant recipient.

DESCRIPTION

Immunosuppressant drugs interfere with the production or function of immune cells. The drugs are used to decrease an inappropriate or undesirable immune response. The immune response is normally a protective mechanism (see Chap. 42) that helps the body defend itself against potentially harmful external (eg, microorganisms) and internal agents (eg, cancer cells). However, numerous disease processes are thought to be caused or aggravated when the immune system perceives the person's own body tissues as harmful invaders and tries to eliminate them. This inappropriate activation of the immune response is a major factor in a growing list of serious diseases believed to involve autoimmune processes, including rheumatoid arthritis, systemic lupus erythematosus, inflammatory bowel disease, and others.

An appropriate but undesirable immune response is elicited when foreign tissue is transplanted into the body. If the immune response is not sufficiently suppressed, the body reacts as with other antigens and attempts to destroy (reject) the foreign organ or tissue. Although numerous advances have been made in transplantation technology, the immune response remains a major factor in determining the success or failure of transplantation.

Most of the available immunosuppressant drugs inhibit the immune response in a general or nonspecific manner. However, the number of drugs that suppress the immune response to specific antigens is increasing. Drugs used therapeutically as immunosuppressants comprise a diverse group, several of which also are used for other purposes. These include corticosteroids (see Chap. 24) and certain cytotoxic antineoplastic drugs (see Chap. 64). These drugs are discussed here primarily in relation to their effects on the immune response. The drugs used to treat autoimmune disorders or to prevent or treat transplant rejection reactions are the main focus of this chapter (Fig. 45-1). These drugs are described in the following sections and in Table 45-1. To aid understanding of immunosuppressive drug therapy, autoimmune disorders, tissue and organ transplantation, and rejection reactions are described.

AUTOIMMUNE DISORDERS

Autoimmune disorders occur when a person's immune system loses its ability to differentiate between antigens on its own cells (called self-antigens or autoantigens) and antigens on foreign cells. As a result, an undesirable immune response is aroused against host tissues. In most instances, the autoantigen is a protein. Thus, in rheumatoid arthritis, the antigen is a protein found in joint tissue.

The mechanisms by which autoantigens are altered to elicit an immune response are unclear. Genetic susceptibility and possible "triggering" events such as damage by microorganisms or trauma, similarity in appearance between autoantigens and foreign antigens, or a linkage between a foreign antigen and an autoantigen may be involved. Once an autoantigen is changed and perceived as foreign or "nonself," the immune response may involve T lymphocytes in direct destruction of tissue, production of proinflammatory cytokines that recruit and activate phagocytes, and stimulation of B lymphocytes to produce autoantibodies that produce inflammation and tissue damage.

In addition to the factors that activate an immune response, there are also factors that prevent the immune system from "turning off" the abnormal immune or inflammatory process. The most prominent factor noted thus far is a deficient number of suppressor T cells.

TISSUE AND ORGAN TRANSPLANTATION

Tissue and organ transplantation usually involves replacing diseased host tissue with healthy donor tissue. The goal of such treatment is to save or enhance the quality of the host's life. Skin and renal grafts are commonly and successfully performed; heart, liver, lung, pancreas, and bone marrow transplantations are increasing. Although numerous factors affect graft survival, including the degree of matching between donor tissues and recipient tissues, drug-induced immunosuppression is a major part of transplantation technology. The goal is to provide adequate, but not excessive, immunosuppression. If immunosuppression is inadequate, graft rejection reactions occur with solid organ transplantation, and graft-versus-host disease (GVHD) occurs with bone marrow transplantation. If immunosuppression is excessive, serious infections and other adverse effects from immunosuppressant drugs develop in the client.

Rejection Reactions With Solid Organ Transplantation (Host-Versus-Graft Disease)

A rejection reaction occurs when the host's immune system is stimulated to destroy the transplanted organ. The immune cells of the transplant recipient attach to the donor cells of the transplanted organ and react against the antigens of the donor organ. The rejection process involves T and B lymphocytes, antibodies, multiple cytokines, and inflammatory mediators. In general, T-cell activation and proliferation are more important in the rejection reaction than B-cell activation and formation of antibodies. Cytotoxic and helper T cells are activated; activated helper T cells stimulate B cells to produce antibodies and lead to a delayed hypersensitivity reaction. The initial target of the recipient antibodies is the blood vessels of the transplanted organ. The antibodies can injure the transplanted organ by

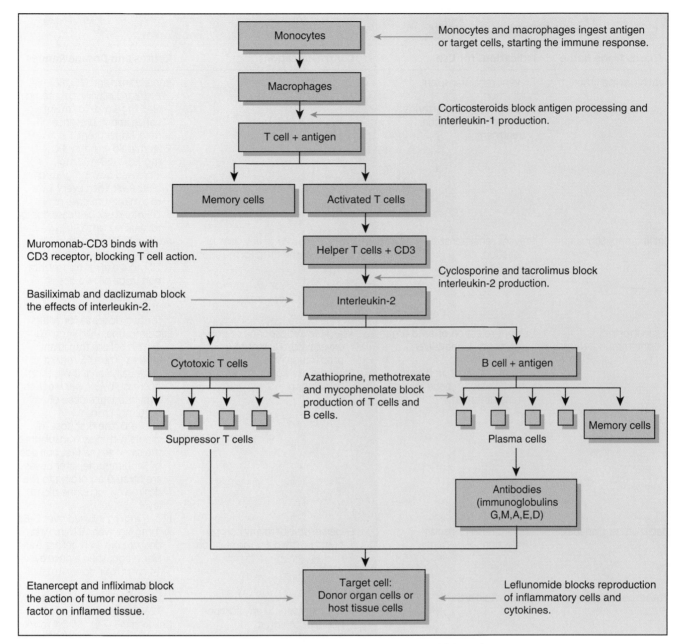

FIGURE 45–1   Sites of action of immunosuppressants. Available immunosuppressants inhibit the immune response by blocking that response at various sites.

activating complement, producing antigen–antibody complexes, or causing antibody-mediated tissue breakdown. This reaction can destroy the solid organ graft within 2 weeks unless the recipient's immune system is adequately suppressed by immunosuppressant drugs.

Rejection reactions are designated as hyperacute, acute, or chronic, depending on the time elapsed between transplantation and rejection. *Hyperacute* reactions occur as soon as blood from the recipient perfuses the grafted organ. This type of reaction is rare and usually occurs in recipients who have previously formed antibodies against antigens in the graft. The antibodies bind to the graft and induce inflammation. *Acute* reactions, which may occur approximately 2 weeks to a few months after transplanta-

tion, often involve humoral and cell-mediated immune responses. Characteristics include signs of organ failure and vasculitis lesions that often lead to arterial narrowing or obliteration. *Chronic* reactions may occur after months or years of normal function and are characterized by fibrosis of blood vessels and progressive failure of the transplanted organ.

Rejection reactions produce general manifestations of inflammation and specific manifestations depending on the organ involved. With renal transplantation, for example, acute rejection reactions produce fever, flank tenderness over the graft organ site, and symptoms of renal failure (eg, increased serum creatinine, decreased urine output, edema and weight gain, hypertension). Chronic rejection

TABLE 45-1 **Immunosuppressants**

Generic/Trade Name	Indications for Use	Contraindications	Routes and Dosage Ranges
Azathioprine (Imuran)	Prevent renal transplant rejection Severe rheumatoid arthritis unresponsive to other treatment	Pregnancy Allergy to azathioprine	Renal transplant: PO, IV 3–5 mg/kg/d initially, decreased (1–3 mg/kg/d) for maintenance and in presence of renal impairment Rheumatoid arthritis: PO 1 mg/kg/d (50–100 mg), increased by 0.5 mg/kg/d after 8 wk, then every 5 wk to a maximum dose of 2.5 mg/kg/d. Decrease dosage for maintenance.
Basiliximab (Simulect)	Prevent renal transplant rejection	Hypersensitivity to any components of the drug formulation	Adults: IV 20 mg within 2 h before transplantation and 20 mg 4 d after transplantation (total of two doses) Children (2–15 y): IV 12 mg/m² up to a maximum of 20 mg for two doses as for adults
Cyclosporine (Sandimmune, Neoral)	Prevent rejection of solid organ (eg, heart, kidney, liver) transplant Prevent and treat graft-versus-host disease in bone marrow transplantation	Allergy to cyclosporine or poly-oxyethylated castor oil (in IV preparation only) Cautious use during pregnancy or lactation	Sandimmune, PO 15 mg/kg 4–12 h before transplant surgery, then 15 mg/kg once daily for 1–2 wk, then decrease by 5% per week to a maintenance dose of 5–10 mg/kg/d Neoral, PO, the first dose in clients with new transplants is the same as the first oral dose of Sandimmune; later doses are titrated according to the desired cyclosporine blood level IV 5–6 mg/kg infused over 2–6 h
Daclizumab (Zenapax)	Prevent renal transplant rejection	Hypersensitivity to any components of the drug formulation	IV 1 mg/kg over 15 min. First dose within 24 h before transplantation, then a dose every 14 d for four doses (total of five doses)
Etanercept (Enbrel)	Rheumatoid arthritis	Sepsis Hypersensitivity to any components of the drug formulation	Adults: SC 25 mg twice weekly, 72–96 h apart Children (4–17 y): SC 0.4 mg/kg up to a maximum of 25 mg per dose, twice weekly, 72–96 h apart
Infliximab (Remicade)	Crohn's disease, moderate to severe or fistulizing	Hypersensitivity to mouse proteins or any other components of the formulation	Crohn's disease, moderate to severe: IV infusion 5 mg/kg as a single dose Crohn's disease, fistulizing: IV infusion 5 mg/kg initially and 2 and 6 wk later (total of three doses)
Leflunomide (Arava)	Rheumatoid arthritis	Hypersensitivity to any components of the drug formulation Pregnancy	PO 100 mg once daily for 3 d, then 20 mg once daily
Lymphocyte immune globulin, antithymocyte globulin (Equine) (Atgam)	Prevent or treat renal transplant rejection Treat aplastic anemia	Allergy to horse serum or prior allergic reaction to Atgam	IV 15 mg/kg/d for 14 d, then every other day for 14 d (21 doses)
Methotrexate (MTX) (Rheumatrex)	Severe rheumatoid arthritis unresponsive to other therapy	Allergy to methotrexate Pregnancy, lactation Liver disease Blood dyscrasias	PO 7.5 mg/wk as single dose, or 2.5 mg q12h for three doses once weekly

TABLE 45-1	Immunosuppressants (*continued*)		
Generic/Trade Name	**Indications for Use**	**Contraindications**	**Routes and Dosage Ranges**
Muromonab-CD3 (Orthoclone OKT3)	Treatment of renal transplant rejection	Allergy to muromonab-CD3 Signs of fluid overload (eg, heart failure, weight gain during week before starting drug therapy) Cautious use during pregnancy	IV 5 mg bolus injection once daily for 10–14 d
Mycophenolate mefetil (CellCept)	Prevent renal transplant rejection	Hypersensitivity to the drug or any component of the product	Renal transplantation: PO, IV 1 g twice daily Cardiac transplantation: PO, IV 1.5 g twice daily
Tacrolimus (Prograf)	Prevent liver, kidney, and heart transplant rejection	Hypersensitivity to the drug or the castor oil used in the IV formulation	Adults: IV infusion, 25–50 µg/kg/d, starting no sooner than 6 h after transplantation, until the patient can tolerate oral administration, usually 2–3 d PO 150–200 µg/kg/d, in two divided doses q12h, with the first dose 8–12 h after stopping the IV infusion Children: IV 50–100 µg/kg/d PO 200–300 µg/kg/d

IV, intravenous; PO, oral; SC, subcutaneous.

reactions are characterized by a gradual increase in serum creatinine levels over approximately 4 to 6 months.

Bone Marrow Transplantation and Graft-Versus-Host Disease

With bone marrow transplantation, the donor bone marrow mounts an immune response (mainly by stimulating T lymphocytes) against antigens on the host's tissues, producing GVHD. Tissue damage is produced directly by the action of cytotoxic T cells or indirectly through the release of inflammatory mediators such as complement and cytokines such as tumor necrosis factor (TNF)-alpha and interleukins.

Acute GVHD occurs in approximately 30% to 50% of clients, usually within 6 weeks. Signs and symptoms include delayed recovery of bone marrow production of blood cells, skin rash, liver dysfunction (indicated by increased alkaline phosphatase, aminotransferases, and bilirubin), and diarrhea. The skin reaction is usually a pruritic maculopapular rash that begins on the palms and soles and may extend over the entire body. Liver involvement can lead to bleeding disorders and coma.

Chronic GVHD occurs when symptoms persist or occur 100 days or more after transplantation. It is characterized by abnormal humoral and cellular immunity, severe skin disorders, and liver disease. Chronic GVHD appears to be an autoimmune disorder in which activated T cells perceive autoantigens as foreign antigens.

IMMUNOSUPPRESSANT DRUGS

Drugs used as immunosuppressants are diverse agents with often overlapping mechanisms of actions and effects. Older drugs generally depress the immune system. Two major adverse effects of immunosuppression are infection and malignancy. Infections may occur with any bacteria, viruses, fungi, or protozoa, at any time during the immunosuppressed state. Lymphoma is most likely to occur with the long-term immunosuppression required in autoimmune disorders and organ transplantation.

For many reasons, including adverse effects of older drugs and the efforts to develop more effective agents, extensive research has been done to develop drugs that modify the immune response (often called immunomodulators or biologic response modifiers). As a result, several drugs with more specific immunosuppressive actions have been approved in recent years. Most are used in combination with older immunosuppressants for synergistic effects.

Immunosuppressants are discussed here as corticosteroids, cytotoxic antiproliferative agents, conventional antirejection agents, antibody preparations, and miscellaneous drugs. This grouping is rather arbitrary because most of the drugs could also fit in one or more other categories (eg, the cytotoxic drugs and most of the antibody preparations are also antirejection drugs; some of the drugs can also be called anticytokines because they block the actions of cytokines such as interleukin-2 [IL-2] and TNF). It is hoped that the chosen groupings will assist the reader in differentiating drug sources, effects, and clinical uses.

Corticosteroids

Corticosteroids have long been used to suppress inflammation and immune reactions. In many disorders, they relieve signs and symptoms by decreasing the accumulation of lymphocytes and macrophages and the production of cell-damaging cytokines at sites of inflammatory reactions. Because inflammation is a common response to chemical mediators or antigens that cause tissue injury, the anti-inflammatory and immunosuppressive actions of corticosteroids often overlap and are indistinguishable. Despite this somewhat arbitrary separation, corticosteroid effects on the immune response are emphasized here. In general, the drugs suppress growth of all lymphoid tissue and therefore decrease formation and function of antibodies and T cells. Specific effects include the following:

- Increased numbers of circulating neutrophils (more are released from bone marrow and fewer leave the circulation to enter inflammatory exudates). In terms of neutrophil functions, corticosteroids increase chemotaxis and release of lysosomal enzymes but decrease the release of nonlysosomal proteolytic enzymes, such as collagenase and plasminogen activator.
- Decreased numbers of circulating basophils, eosinophils, and monocytes. The reduced availability of monocytes is thought to be a major factor in the anti-inflammatory activity of corticosteroids. Functions of monocyte–macrophages are also impaired. Corticosteroids suppress phagocytosis and initial antigen processing (necessary to initiate an immune response), impair migration to areas of tissue injury, and block the differentiation of monocytes to macrophages.
- Decreased numbers of circulating lymphocytes (immune cells), resulting from impaired production (ie, inhibition of deoxyribonucleic acid [DNA], ribonucleic acid [RNA], and protein synthesis), sequestration in lymphoid tissues, or lysis of the cells. T cells are markedly reduced; B cells are moderately reduced.
- Impaired function of cellular (mainly T-cell) and humoral (B-cell) immunity. Corticosteroids inhibit the production of immunostimulant cytokines (eg, IL-1 and IL-2) required for activation and clonal expansion of lymphocytes and cytotoxic cytokines, such as TNF and interferons. When administered for 2 to 3 weeks, the drugs also inhibit immune reactions to antigenic skin tests and reduce serum concentrations of some antibodies (immunoglobulins [Ig] G and A but not IgM).

Cytotoxic, Antiproliferative Agents

Cytotoxic, antiproliferative drugs damage or kill cells that are able to reproduce, such as immunologically competent lymphocytes. These drugs are used primarily in cancer chemotherapy. However, in small doses, some also exhibit immunosuppressive activities and are used to treat autoimmune disorders (eg, methotrexate) and to prevent rejection reactions in organ transplantation (azathioprine). These drugs cause generalized suppression of the immune system and can kill lymphocytes and nonlymphoid proliferating cells (eg, bone marrow blood cells, gastrointestinal mucosal cells, and germ cells in gonads).

Azathioprine
Azathioprine is an antimetabolite that interferes with production of DNA and RNA and thus blocks cellular reproduction, growth, and development. Once ingested, azathioprine is metabolized by the liver to 6-mercaptopurine, a purine analog. The purine analog is then incorporated into the DNA of proliferating cells in place of the natural purine bases, leading to the production of abnormal DNA. Rapidly proliferating cells are most affected, including T and B lymphocytes, which normally reproduce rapidly in response to stimulation by an antigen. The drug acts especially on T cells to block cell division, clonal proliferation, and differentiation. Azathioprine is well absorbed after oral administration, with peak serum concentrations in 1 to 2 hours and a half-life of less than 5 hours. The mercaptopurine resulting from initial biotransformation is inactivated mainly by the enzyme xanthine oxidase. Impaired liver function may decrease metabolism of azathioprine to its active metabolite and therefore decrease pharmacologic effects. Azathioprine is used mainly to prevent organ graft rejection and has little effect on acute rejection reactions. It is also used to treat severe rheumatoid arthritis not responsive to conventional treatment. When used to prevent graft rejection, azathioprine is used lifelong. Dosage varies among transplantation centers and types of transplants, but depends largely on white blood cell (WBC) and platelet counts.

Methotrexate
Methotrexate is a folate antagonist. It inhibits dihydrofolate reductase, the enzyme that converts dihydrofolate to the tetrahydrofolate required for biosynthesis of DNA and cell reproduction. The resultant DNA impairment inhibits production and function of immune cells, especially T cells. Methotrexate has long been used in the treatment of cancer. Other uses have evolved from its immunosuppressive effects, including treatment of autoimmune or inflammatory disorders, such as severe arthritis and psoriasis, that do not respond to other treatment measures. It is also used (with cyclosporine) to prevent GVHD associated with bone marrow transplantation, but it is not approved by the Food and Drug Administration for this purpose. Lower doses are

given for these conditions than for cancers, and adverse drug effects are fewer and less severe.

Conventional Antirejection Agents

Cyclosporine

Cyclosporine is used to prevent rejection reactions (destruction of the transplanted tissues by the body's immune system) after solid organ transplantation (eg, kidney, liver), or to treat chronic rejection in clients previously treated with other immunosuppressive agents. The drug inhibits both cellular and humoral immunity but affects T lymphocytes more than B lymphocytes. With T cells, cyclosporine reduces proliferation of helper and cytotoxic T cells and synthesis of several lymphokines (eg, IL-2, interferons). Suppressor T cells seem to be less affected by cyclosporine. With B cells, cyclosporine reduces production and function to some extent, but considerable activity is retained.

Transplant rejection reactions mainly involve cellular immunity or T cells. With cyclosporine-induced deprivation of IL-2, T cells stimulated by the graft antigen do not undergo clonal expansion and differentiation, and graft destruction is inhibited. In addition to its use in solid organ transplantation, cyclosporine is used to prevent and treat GVHD, a potential complication of bone marrow transplantation. In GVHD, T lymphocytes from the transplanted marrow of the donor mount an immune response against the tissues of the recipient.

Absorption of cyclosporine is slow and incomplete with oral administration. The drug is highly bound to plasma proteins (90%), and approximately 50% is distributed in erythrocytes, so drug levels in whole blood are significantly higher than those in plasma. Peak plasma levels occur 4 to 5 hours after a dose, and the elimination half-life is approximately 10 to 27 hours. Cyclosporine is metabolized in the liver and excreted in bile; less than 10% is excreted unchanged in urine. Because the drug is insoluble in water, other solvents are used in commercial formulations. Thus, it is prepared in alcohol and olive oil for oral administration and in alcohol and polyoxyethylated castor oil for intravenous (IV) administration. Anaphylactic reactions, attributed to the castor oil, have occurred with the IV formulation. Neoral is a microemulsion formulation of cyclosporine that is better absorbed than oral Sandimmune. The two formulations are not equivalent and cannot be used interchangeably. Neoral is available in capsules and an oral solution; Sandimmune is available in capsules, oral solution, and an IV solution.

Mycophenolate

Mycophenolate is similar to azathioprine. It is used for prevention and treatment of rejection reactions with renal and cardiac transplantation. It inhibits proliferation and function of T and B lymphocytes. It has synergistic effects with corticosteroids and cyclosporine and is used in combination with these drugs.

After oral or IV administration, the drug is rapidly broken down to mycophenolic acid, the active component. Mycophenolic acid is further metabolized to inactive metabolites that are eliminated in bile and urine. Neutropenia and thrombocytopenia may occur but are less common and less severe than with azathioprine. Infections with mycophenolate occur at approximately the same rate as with other immunosuppressant drugs. Because of its lesser toxicity, mycophenolate may be preferred over azathioprine, at least in clients who are unable to tolerate azathioprine.

Tacrolimus

Tacrolimus (formerly FK506) is similar to cyclosporine in its mechanisms of action, pharmacokinetic characteristics, and adverse effects. It prevents rejection of transplanted organs by inhibiting growth and proliferation of T lymphocytes. Although survival of clients and grafts is approximately the same as with cyclosporine, potential advantages of tacrolimus include less corticosteroid therapy and shorter, less costly hospitalizations. Tacrolimus is not well absorbed orally, so higher oral doses than IV doses must be given to obtain similar blood levels. It is well distributed through the body and reaches higher concentrations in erythrocytes than in plasma. It is metabolized in the liver and intestine to several metabolites. Impaired liver function may slow its metabolism and elimination.

Dosage ranges of tacrolimus vary according to clinical response, adverse effects, and blood concentrations. Serum drug levels are routinely monitored, with therapeutic ranges approximately 10 to 20 ng/mL for 6 months after transplantation, then 5 to 15 ng/mL. Children with transplants metabolize tacrolimus more rapidly than adults with transplants, on a body weight basis. Thus, children require higher doses, based on milligrams per kilogram, to maintain similar plasma drug levels. Dosage does not need to be reduced in renal insufficiency because there is little renal elimination of the drug.

There are numerous potential drug interactions that increase or decrease blood levels and effects of tacrolimus. Because tacrolimus is metabolized mainly by the cytochrome P450 enzymes that metabolize cyclosporine, drug interactions known to alter cyclosporine effects are likely to alter tacrolimus effects. In addition, tacrolimus is a macrolide and may have drug interactions similar to those occurring with erythromycin. Erythromycin is known to increase blood levels and risks of toxicity of several drugs, including oral anticoagulants, digoxin, and theophylline.

The role of tacrolimus in transplantation immunosuppression is not well defined. Because successful liver and intestinal transplantations have been attributed to the drug, some people suggest that tacrolimus may replace cyclosporine as the immunosuppressant of choice for new clients. It may also be useful for clients who do not respond to cyclosporine. In renal transplantation, its role is less clear because high success rates have been achieved with cyclosporine. However, cyclosporine is given with corticosteroids and tacrolimus may allow corticosteroids to be reduced or stopped, thereby decreasing the adverse effects of long-term corticosteroid therapy. Nephrotoxicity occurs at an approximately equal rate with both drugs.

Antibody Preparations

Antibody preparations are derived from animals injected with human lymphoid tissue to stimulate an immune response. The antibodies may be nonspecific polyclonal or specific monoclonal. Polyclonal preparations are a mixture of antibodies (eg, IgA, IgD, IgE, IgG, or IgM) produced by several clones of B lymphocytes. Each clone produces a structurally and functionally different antibody, even though the humoral immune response was induced by a single antigen.

Monoclonal antibodies are produced in the laboratory by procedures that isolate and clone individual B lymphocytes, resulting in the production of completely identical antibody molecules. It is easiest to make monoclonal antibodies in mice, and most are derived from murine (mouse) B-lymphocyte cells. A mouse is injected with an antigen from the tissue targeted for destruction and mounts an immune response to the antigen. Then, the B lymphocytes are removed from the mouse's spleen and manipulated so that they grow in a culture medium. As they grow, they secrete antibodies that can be isolated from the culture and prepared for clinical use. Because the antibodies are proteins and would be destroyed if taken orally, they must be given by injection.

Older murine antibodies (see LIG, ATG and muromonab-CD3, later) are themselves antigenic; they usually elicit human antibodies against the "foreign" mouse cells within 2 weeks. Newer murine antibodies (eg, basiliximab) have had human antibodies added by recombinant DNA technology and are less likely to elicit an immune response. However, because the products are proteins, there is some risk of hypersensitivity reactions.

Because they are derived from one cell line or clone, monoclonal antibodies can be designed to suppress the specific components of the immune system that are causing tissue damage in particular disorders. Note that the generic names of monoclonal antibodies used as drugs end in *mab* and thus identify their origin.

Polyclonal Antibody
Lymphocyte Immune Globulin, Antithymocyte Globulin

Lymphocyte immune globulin, antithymocyte globulin (LIG, ATG) is a nonspecific antibody with activity against all blood cells, although it acts mainly against T lymphocytes. LIG, ATG is obtained from the serum of horses immunized with human thymus tissue or T lymphocytes. It contains antibodies that destroy lymphoid

tissues and decrease the number of circulating T cells, thereby suppressing cellular and humoral immune responses. In addition to its high concentration of antibodies against T lymphocytes, the preparation contains low concentrations of antibodies against other blood cells. A skin test is recommended before administration to determine whether the client is allergic to horse serum. Because there is a high risk of anaphylactic reactions in recipients previously sensitized to horse serum, clients with positive skin tests should be desensitized before drug therapy is begun. LIG, ATG may be given for a few weeks to treat rejection reactions after solid organ transplantation, and it may be used to treat aplastic anemia.

Monoclonal Antibodies
Basiliximab and Daclizumab

Basiliximab (Simulect) and daclizumab (Zenapax) are very similar drugs. They are humanized IgE (ie, a combination of human and murine antibody sequences). They are called IL-2 receptor antagonists because they bind to IL-2 receptors on the surface of activated lymphocytes. This action inhibits the ability of IL-2 to stimulate proliferation and cytokine production of lymphocytes, a critical component of the cellular immune response involved in allograft rejection. The drugs are used to prevent organ rejection in clients receiving renal transplants and are given in combination with cyclosporine and a corticosteroid. In clinical trials, adverse effects were consistent with those of transplant status, underlying disease, and concomitant immunosuppressive and other drug therapy. They were also similar to those reported with placebo (ie, basiliximab or daclizumab + cyclosporine and a corticosteroid vs. placebo + cyclosporine and a corticosteroid).

Infliximab

Infliximab (Remicade) is a humanized IgG monoclonal antibody approved for treatment of Crohn's disease and being investigated for use in rheumatoid arthritis. It inhibits a cytokine, TNF-alpha, from binding to its receptors and thus neutralizes its actions. Biologic activities attributed to TNF-alpha include induction of other proinflammatory cytokines (eg, IL-1 and IL-6), increasing leukocyte migration into sites of injury or inflammation, and stimulating neutrophil and eosinophil activity. Infliximab's ability to neutralize TNF-alpha accounts for its anti-inflammatory effects. (It does not neutralize TNF-beta [lymphotoxin], a related cytokine that uses the same receptors.)

In Crohn's disease, elevated concentrations of TNF-alpha have been found in clients' stools and correlate with episodes of increased disease activity. Infliximab reduces infiltration of inflammatory cells, production of TNF-alpha in inflamed areas of the intestine, and the number of cells that can produce TNF-alpha. It is indicated for clients with moderate to severe disease who do not respond adequately to conventional treatment measures, and for those with draining enterocutaneous fistulas.

Infliximab therapy (ie, anti-TNF therapy) may lead to the formation of autoimmune antibodies and hypersensitivity reactions. Dyspnea, hypotension, and urticaria have occurred. The drug should be administered in settings in which personnel and supplies (eg, epinephrine, antihistamines, corticosteroids) are available for treatment of hypersensitivity reactions, and should be discontinued if severe reactions occur. In addition, infections developed in approximately 21% of clients in clinical trials.

Muromonab-CD3

Muromonab-CD3 (Orthoclone OKT3) is a monoclonal antibody that acts against an antigenic receptor called CD3, which is found on the surface membrane of most T cells in blood and body tissues. *CD* indicates *clusters of differentiation*, or groups of cells with the same surface markers (antigenic receptors). The CD3 molecule is associated with the antigen recognition structure of T cells and is essential for T-cell activation. Muromonab-CD3 binds with its antigen (CD3) and therefore blocks all known functions of T cells containing the CD3 molecule. Because rejection reactions are mainly T-cell–mediated immune responses against antigenic (nonself) tissues, the drug's ability to suppress such reactions accounts for its therapeutic effects in treating renal transplant rejection. It is usually given for 10 to 14 days. After treatment, CD3-positive T cells reappear rapidly and reach pretreatment levels within 1 week. The drug's name is derived from its source (murine or mouse cells) and its action (monoclonal antibody against the CD3 antigen). Because the drug is a protein and induces antibodies in most clients, decreased effectiveness and serious allergic reactions may occur if it is readministered later. Second courses of treatment must be undertaken cautiously.

Miscellaneous Immunosuppressants

Etanercept

Etanercept (Enbrel) is a manufactured TNF receptor that binds with TNF and prevents it from binding with its "normal" receptors on cell surfaces. This action inhibits TNF activity in inflammatory and immune responses.

Tumor necrosis factor is a naturally occurring cytokine that enhances leukocyte migration into areas of tissue injury and induces the production of other cytokines, such as IL-6. In rheumatoid arthritis, TNF is increased in joint synovial fluid and considered important in joint inflammation and destruction.

The biologic activity of TNF requires its binding to TNF-alpha or TNF-beta receptors on cell surfaces. Etanercept inhibits binding of both TNF-alpha and TNF-beta to cell surface TNF receptors and thereby inactivates TNF.

Etanercept is indicated for the treatment of moderate to severe rheumatoid arthritis in adults and children who have not received adequate relief of symptoms with other treatments. It can be used in combination with methotrexate in clients who do not respond adequately to methotrexate alone.

Leflunomide

Leflunomide (Arava) has antiproliferative and anti-inflammatory activities that are attributed to its effects on the immune system. The drug inhibits the synthesis of pyrimidines, which are components of DNA and RNA and therefore important in cell reproduction and growth. Leflunomide is used to treat rheumatoid arthritis in adults. In addition to relieving signs and symptoms, it also slows the progressive destruction of joint tissues.

After oral administration, leflunomide is metabolized to an active metabolite (called M1) that exerts almost all of the drug's effects. M1 has a half-life of approximately 2 weeks, and a loading dose is usually given for 3 days to achieve therapeutic blood levels more rapidly. It is highly bound to serum albumin and eventually eliminated by further metabolism and renal or biliary excretion. Some of the M1 excreted in bile is reabsorbed, and this contributes to its long half-life.

NURSING PROCESS

Assessment

- Assess clients receiving or anticipating immunosuppressant drug therapy for signs and symptoms of current infection.
- Assess clients receiving or anticipating immunosuppressant drug therapy for factors predisposing them to potential infection (eg, impaired skin integrity, invasive devices, cigarette smoking).
- Assess the environment for factors predisposing to infection (eg, family or health care providers with infections, contact with young children, and potential exposure to childhood infectious diseases).
- Assess nutritional status, including appetite and weight.
- Assess response to planned drug therapy and associated monitoring and follow-up.
- Assess baseline values of laboratory and other diagnostic test results to aid monitoring of responses to immunosuppressant drug therapy. With pretransplantation clients, this includes assessing for impaired function of the diseased organ and for abnormalities that need treatment before surgery.
- Assess adequacy of support systems for transplantation recipients.
- Assess post-transplantation clients for surgical wound healing, manifestations of organ rejection, and adverse effects of immunosuppressant drugs.

- Assess clients with autoimmune disorders (eg, rheumatoid arthritis, Crohn's disease) for manifestations of the disease process and responses to drug therapy.

Nursing Diagnoses

- Risk for Injury: Infection related to immunosuppression and increased susceptibility
- Risk for Injury: Cancer related to immunosuppression and increased susceptibility
- Risk for Injury: Adverse drug effects
- Knowledge Deficit: Disease process or planned treatment
- Knowledge Deficit: Immunosuppressant therapy
- Anxiety related to the diagnosis of serious disease or need for organ transplantation
- Body Image Disturbance: Cushingoid changes with long-term corticosteroid therapy; alopecia with azathioprine
- Ineffective Individual Coping related to chronic illness and long-term treatment
- Ineffective Family Coping related to illness and treatment of a family member
- Fear related to potential transplantation complications, disease progression, or death
- Social Isolation related to activities to reduce exposure to infection

Planning/Goals

The client will:

- Participate in decision making about the treatment plan

Nursing Notes: *Ethical/Legal Dilemma*

Anne Robins, a chronic alcoholic for many years, has just received a liver transplant. She will have to be on very expensive immunosuppressive medications for the rest of her life. She has private insurance, but there is some question whether it will cover the cost of her medications.

Reflect on:

- Do you think medical insurance companies should include expensive medications, which must be taken for life, in their benefit package?
- Explore the impact on Ms. Robins and her family if this benefit is denied.
- Explore the impact on insurance rates for other plan members who are healthy and require no long-term management if this benefit is included.
- Should Ms. Robins' history of alcoholism affect any decision that is made?

- Receive or take immunosuppressant drugs correctly
- Verbalize or demonstrate essential drug information
- Participate in interventions to prevent infection (eg, maintain good hygiene, avoid known sources of infection) while immunosuppressed
- Experience relief or reduction of disease symptoms
- Maintain adequate levels of nutrition and fluids, rest and sleep, and exercise
- Be assisted to cope with anxiety and fear related to the disease process and drug therapy
- Keep appointments for follow-up care
- Have adverse drug effects prevented or recognized and treated promptly
- Maintain diagnostic test values within acceptable limits
- Maintain family and other emotional or social support systems
- Receive optimal instructions and information about the treatment plan, self-care in activities of daily living, reporting adverse drug effects, and other concerns
- Before and after tissue or organ transplantation, receive appropriate care, including prevention or early recognition and treatment of rejection reactions

Interventions

- Practice and emphasize good personal hygiene and hand washing techniques by clients and all others in contact with clients.
- Use sterile technique for all injections, IV site care, wound dressing changes, and any other invasive diagnostic or therapeutic measures.
- Screen staff and visitors for signs and symptoms of infection; if infection is noted, do not allow contact with the client.
- Report fever and other manifestations of infection *immediately.*
- Allow clients to participate in decision making when possible and appropriate.
- Use isolation techniques according to institutional policies, usually after transplantation or when the neutrophil count is below 500/mm^3.
- Assist clients to maintain adequate nutrition, rest and sleep, and exercise.
- Inform clients about diagnostic test results, planned changes in therapeutic regimens, and evidence of progress.
- Allow family members or significant others to visit clients when feasible.
- Monitor complete blood count (CBC) and other diagnostic test results related to blood, liver, and kidney function throughout drug therapy. Spe-

cific tests vary with the client's health or illness status and the immunosuppressant drugs being taken.
- Schedule and coordinate drug administration to maximize therapeutic effects and minimize adverse effects.
- Consult other health care providers (eg, physician, dietitian, social worker) on the client's behalf when indicated. Multidisciplinary consultation is essential for transplantation clients and desirable for clients with autoimmune disorders.
- Assist clients in learning strategies to manage day-to-day activities during long-term immunosuppression.

Evaluation

- Interview and observe for accurate drug administration.
- Interview and observe for personal hygiene practices and infection-avoiding maneuvers.
- Interview and observe for therapeutic and adverse drug effects with each client contact.
- Interview regarding knowledge and attitude toward the drug therapy regimen, including follow-up care and symptoms to report to health care providers.
- Determine the number and types of infections that have occurred in the neutropenic client.
- Compare current CBC and other reports with baseline values for acceptable levels, according to the client's condition.
- Observe and interview outpatients regarding compliance with follow-up care.
- Observe and interview regarding the mental and emotional status of clients and family members or significant others.
- Interview and observe for organ function and absence of rejection reactions in post-transplantation clients.

PRINCIPLES OF THERAPY

Risk–Benefit Factors

Immunosuppression is a serious, life-threatening condition that may result from disease processes or drug therapy. At the same time, immunosuppressant drugs are used to treat serious illnesses, and their use may be required. Rational use of these drugs requires thorough assessment of a client's health or illness status, clear-cut indications for use, a lack of more effective and safer alternative treatments, analysis of potential risks versus potential benefits, cautious administration, and vigilant monitoring of the client's response. If a decision is then made that immuno-

suppressant drug therapy is indicated and benefits outweigh risks, the therapeutic plan must be discussed with the client (ie, reasons, expected benefits, consequences for the client's health, behavior, and lifestyle).

In addition to the specific risks or adverse effects of individual immunosuppressant drugs, general risks of immunosuppression include infection and cancer. Infection is a major cause of morbidity and mortality, especially in clients who are neutropenic (neutrophil count <1000/mm^3) from cytotoxic immunosuppressant drugs or who have had bone marrow or solid organ transplantation. For the latter group, who must continue lifelong immunosuppression to avoid graft rejection, serious infection is a constant hazard. Extensive efforts are made to prevent infections; if these efforts are unsuccessful and infections occur, they may be fatal unless recognized promptly and treated vigorously. Common infections are bacterial (gram-positive, such as *Staphylococcus aureus* or *S. epidermidis*, and gram-negative, such as *Escherichia coli, Klebsiella*, and *Pseudomonas* species), fungal (candidiasis, aspergillosis, pneumocystosis), or viral (cytomegalovirus, herpes simplex, or herpes zoster).

Cancer, most commonly lymphoma or skin cancer, may result from immunosuppression. The normal immune system is thought to recognize and destroy malignant cells as they develop, as long as they can be differentiated from normal cells. With immunosuppression, the malignant cells are no longer destroyed and thus are allowed to proliferate.

The consequences of immunosuppression may be lessened by newer drugs that target specific components of the immune response rather than causing general suppression of multiple components. However, there is apparently still some risk of infection and malignancy.

Use in Transplantation

The use of immunosuppressant drugs in transplantation continues to evolve as new drugs, combinations of drugs, and other aspects are developed and tested. Specific protocols vary among transplantation centers and types of transplants. As a general rule, immunosuppressant drugs used in transplantation are often used in highly technical, complex circumstances to manage life-threatening illness. Consequently, except for corticosteroids, the drugs should be used only by specialist physicians who are adept in their management. In addition, all health care providers need to review research studies and other current literature regularly for ways to maximize safety and effectiveness and minimize adverse effects of immunosuppression.

Combinations of Immunosuppressant Drugs

Most immunosuppressant drugs are used to prevent rejection of transplanted tissues. The rejection reaction involves

CLIENT TEACHING GUIDELINES
Immunosuppressant Drugs

General Considerations

✔ People taking medications that suppress the immune system are at high risk for development of infections. As a result, clients, caregivers, and others in the client's environment need to wash their hands often and thoroughly, practice meticulous personal hygiene, avoid contact with infected people, and practice other methods of preventing infection.

✔ Report adverse drug effects (eg, signs or symptoms of infection such as sore throat or fever, decreased urine output if taking cyclosporine, easy bruising or bleeding if taking azathioprine or methotrexate) to a health care provider.

✔ Try to maintain healthy lifestyle habits, such as a nutritious diet, adequate rest and sleep, and avoiding tobacco and alcohol. These measures enhance immune mechanisms and other body defenses.

✔ Carry identification that lists the drugs being taken; the dosage; the physician's name, address, and telephone number; and instructions for emergency treatment. This information is needed if an accident or emergency situation occurs.

✔ Inform all health care providers that you are taking these drugs.

✔ Maintain regular medical supervision. This is extremely important for detecting adverse reactions, evaluating disease status, evaluating drug responses and indications for dosage change, and having blood tests or other monitoring tests when needed.

✔ Take no other drugs, prescription or nonprescription, without notifying the physician who is managing immunosuppressant therapy. Immunosuppressant drugs may influence reactions to other drugs, and other drugs may influence reactions to the immunosuppressants. Thus, taking other drugs may decrease therapeutic effects or increase adverse effects. In addition, vaccinations may be less effective, and some should be avoided while taking immunosuppressant drugs.

✔ People of reproductive capability who are sexually active should practice effective contraceptive techniques during immunosuppressive drug therapy. With methotrexate, use contraception during and for at least 3 months (men) or one ovulatory cycle (women) after stopping the drug. With mycophenolate, effective contraception should be continued for 6 weeks after the drug is stopped.

✔ Wear protective clothing and use sunscreens to decrease exposure of skin to sunlight and risks of skin cancers. Also, methotrexate increases sensitivity to sunlight and may increase sunburn.

Self-administration

✔ Follow instructions about taking the drugs. This is vital to achieving beneficial effects and decreasing adverse effects. If unable to take a medication, report to the prescribing physician or other health care provider; do not stop unless advised to do so. For transplant recipients, missed doses may lead to transplant rejection; for clients with autoimmune diseases, missed doses may lead to acute flare-ups of symptoms. In addition, take at approximately the same time each day to maintain consistent drug levels in the blood.

✔ Take oral azathioprine in divided doses, after meals, to decrease stomach upset.

✔ With cyclosporine, use the same oral solution consistently. The two available solutions (Neoral and Sandimmune) are not equivalent and cannot be used interchangeably. If a change in formulation is necessary, it should be made cautiously and only under supervision of the prescribing physician.

  Measure oral cyclosporine solution with the dosing syringe provided; add to orange or apple juice that is at room temperature (avoid grapefruit juice); stir well and drink at once (do not allow diluted solution to stand before drinking). Use a glass container, not plastic. Rinse the glass with more diluent to ensure the total dose is taken. Do not rinse the dosing syringe with water or other cleaning agents. Take on a consistent schedule with regard to time of day and meals.

  These are the manufacturer's recommendations. Mixing with orange or apple juice improves taste; grapefruit juice should not be used because it affects metabolism of cyclosporine. The amount of fluid should be large enough to increase palatability, especially for children, but small enough to be consumed quickly. Rinsing ensures the entire dose is taken.

✔ Take mycophenolate on an empty stomach; food decreases the amount of active drug by 40%. Do not crush mycophenolate tablets and do not open or crush the capsules.

✔ Take tacrolimus with food to decrease stomach upset.

✔ If giving or taking an injected drug (eg, etanercept), be sure you understand how to mix and inject the medication correctly. For example, with etanercept, rotate injection sites, give a new injection at least 1 inch from a previous injection site, and do not inject the medication into areas where the skin is tender, bruised, red, or hard. When possible, practice the required techniques and perform the first injection under supervision of a qualified health care professional.

T and B lymphocytes, multiple cytokines, and inflammatory mediators. Thus, drug combinations are rational because they act on different components of the immune response and often have overlapping and synergistic effects. They may also allow lower doses of individual drugs, which usually cause fewer or less severe adverse effects. For example, most organ transplantation centers use a combination regimen for prevention and treatment of rejection reactions. Once the transplanted tissue is functioning and rejection has been successfully prevented or treated, it often is possible to maintain the graft with fewer drugs or lower drug dosages. Some recommendations to increase safety or effectiveness of drug combinations include the following:

- *Lymphocyte immune globulin, antithymocyte globulin* is usually given concomitantly with azathioprine and a corticosteroid.
- *Azathioprine* is usually given with cyclosporine and prednisone.
- *Basiliximab* and *daclizumab* are given with cyclosporine and a corticosteroid.
- *Corticosteroids* may be given alone or included in multidrug regimens with cyclosporine and muromonab-CD3. A corticosteroid should always accompany cyclosporine administration to enhance immunosuppression. In prophylaxis of organ transplant rejection, the combination seems more effective than azathioprine alone or azathioprine and a corticosteroid. A corticosteroid may not be required, at least long-term, with tacrolimus.
- *Cyclosporine* should be used cautiously with immunosuppressants other than corticosteroids to decrease risks of excessive immunosuppression and its complications.
- *Methotrexate* may be used alone or with cyclosporine for prophylaxis of GVHD after bone marrow transplantation.
- *Muromonab-CD3* may be given cautiously with reduced numbers or dosages of other immunosuppressants. When coadministered with prednisone and azathioprine, the maximum daily dose of prednisone is 0.5 mg/kg, and the maximum for azathioprine is 25 mg. When muromonab-CD3 is coadministered with cyclosporine, cyclosporine dosage should be reduced or the drug temporarily discontinued. If discontinued, cyclosporine is restarted 3 days before completing the course of muromonab-CD3 therapy, to resume a maintenance level of immunosuppression.
- *Mycophenolate* is used with cyclosporine and a corticosteroid. It may be used instead of azathioprine.
- *Tacrolimus* is being substituted for cyclosporine in some long-term immunosuppressant regimens. An advantage of tacrolimus is that corticosteroid therapy can often be discontinued, with the concomitant elimination of the adverse effects associated with the long-term use of corticosteroids.

Dosage Factors

Immunosuppressant drugs are relatively toxic, and adverse effects occur more often and are more severe with higher doses. Thus, the general principle of using the smallest effective dose for the shortest period of time is especially important with immunosuppressant drug therapy. Dosage must be individualized according to the client's clinical response (ie, improvement in signs and symptoms or occurrence of adverse effects). Factors to be considered in drug dosage decisions include the following:

- *Azathioprine* dosage should be reduced or the drug discontinued if severe bone marrow depression occurs (eg, reduced red blood cells, WBCs, and platelets on CBC). If it is necessary to stop the drug, administration may be resumed at a smaller dosage once the bone marrow has recovered. With renal transplant recipients, the dosage required to prevent rejection and minimize toxicity varies. When given long-term for maintenance of immunosuppression, the lowest effective dose is recommended. If given concomitantly with muromonab-CD3, the dosage is reduced to 25 mg/day.
- *Corticosteroid* dosages vary among transplantation centers. The highest doses are usually given immediately after transplantation and during treatment of acute graft rejection reactions. Doses are usually tapered by 6 months after the transplantation, and long-term maintenance doses of prednisone are usually under 10 mg/day. Doses of corticosteroids may also be reduced when the drugs are given in combination with other immunosuppressants. For some clients, the drugs may be discontinued.
- *Cyclosporine* dosage should be individualized according to drug concentration in blood, serum creatinine, and the client's clinical status. Higher doses are usually given for approximately 3 months posttransplantation and may be given IV for a few days after surgery (at one-third the oral dosage). Higher doses are also given if cyclosporine is used with one other drug than if used with two other drugs. After a few months, the dose is reduced for long-term maintenance of immunosuppression after solid organ transplantation.

  When a client receiving cyclosporine is given muromonab-CD3, cyclosporine is stopped temporarily or given in reduced doses.
- *Muromonab-CD3* dosage should follow established amounts and protocols.
- Optimal dosage regimens of *mycophenolate* and *tacrolimus* have not been established.

Drug Administration Schedules

The effectiveness of immunosuppressant therapy may be enhanced by appropriate timing of drug administration.

For example, corticosteroids are most effective when given just before exposure to the antigen, whereas the cytotoxic agents (eg, azathioprine, methotrexate) are most effective when given soon after exposure (ie, during the interval between exposure to the antigen and the production of sensitized T cells or antibodies). The newer drugs, basiliximab and daclizumab, are started a few hours before transplantation and continued for a few doses afterward.

Type of Transplant

Cardiac transplant recipients are usually given azathioprine, cyclosporine, and prednisone. Tacrolimus may be used instead of cyclosporine. Because rejection reactions are more likely to occur during the first 6 months after transplantation, transvenous endomyocardial biopsies are performed at regular intervals up to a year, then as needed according to the client's clinical status.

Renal transplant recipients receive variable immunosuppressive drug therapy, depending on the time interval since the transplant surgery. For several days posttransplantation, high doses of IV methylprednisolone are usually given. The dose is tapered and discontinued as oral prednisone is initiated.

Cyclosporine may not be used because of its unpredictable absorption and its nephrotoxicity. If used, it is given in very low doses. If not used, adequate immunosuppression must be maintained with other agents. Whichever drugs are used in the immediate postoperative period and up to 3 months post-transplantation, high doses are required to prevent organ rejection. These high doses may result in serious complications, such as infection and corticosteroid-induced diabetes. Doses are usually reduced if clients have serious adverse effects (eg, opportunistic infections, nephrotoxicity, or hepatotoxicity).

After approximately 3 months, maintenance immunosuppressant therapy usually consists of azathioprine and prednisone alone or with cyclosporine or tacrolimus. Doses are gradually decreased over 6 to 12 months, and some drugs may be discontinued (eg, prednisone, when tacrolimus is given). In addition, cyclosporine may be discontinued if chronic nephrotoxicity or severe hypertension occurs.

Liver transplant recipients may be given various drugs. There are several effective regimens and no clear indications that one is significantly better than another. Most regimens use methylprednisolone initially, with cyclosporine or tacrolimus; some include azathioprine or mycophenolate. At some centers, corticosteroids are eventually discontinued and clients are maintained on tacrolimus alone. Treatment of rejection reactions also varies among liver transplantation centers and may include the addition of high-dose corticosteroids and muromonab-CD3 or LIG, ATG for 7 to 14 days. In addition, clients on tacrolimus may be given higher doses. Those on cyclosporine usually do not receive higher doses because of nephrotoxicity.

An additional consideration is that liver and biliary tract functions vary among clients. As a result, the pharmacokinetics of some immunosuppressant drugs are altered. Cyclosporine has been studied most in this setting. When liver function is impaired, for example, oral cyclosporine is poorly absorbed and higher oral doses or IV administration are required to maintain adequate blood levels. When liver function and bile flow are restored, absorption of oral cyclosporine is greatly improved and dosage must be substantially reduced to maintain stable blood concentrations. Absorption of other lipid-soluble drugs is also improved. In addition, serum albumin levels are usually decreased for months after transplantation, producing higher blood levels of drugs that normally bind to albumin.

Still another consideration is that neurologic adverse effects (eg, ataxia, psychosis, seizures) occur in almost half of liver transplant recipients. These effects have been associated with corticosteroids, cyclosporine, muromonab-CD3, and tacrolimus.

Bone marrow transplant recipients are usually given cyclosporine and a corticosteroid.

Laboratory Monitoring

With *azathioprine*, bone marrow depression (eg, severe leukopenia or thrombocytopenia) may occur. To monitor bone marrow function, CBC and platelet counts should be checked weekly during the first month, every 2 weeks during the second and third months, then monthly. If dosage is changed or a client's health status worsens at any time during therapy, more frequent blood tests are needed.

With oral *cyclosporine*, blood levels are monitored periodically for low or high values. Subtherapeutic levels may lead to organ transplant rejection. They are more likely to occur with the Sandimmune formulation than with Neoral because Sandimmune is poorly absorbed. High levels increase adverse effects. The blood levels are used to regulate dosage. In addition, renal (serum creatinine, blood urea nitrogen) and liver (bilirubin, aminotransferase enzymes) function tests should be performed regularly to monitor for nephrotoxicity and hepatotoxicity.

With *leflunomide*, renal and liver functions tests should be done periodically.

With *methotrexate*, CBC and platelet counts and renal and liver function tests should be done periodically.

With *muromonab-CD3*, WBC and differential counts should be performed periodically.

With *mycophenolate*, a CBC is recommended weekly during the first month, twice monthly during the second and third months, and monthly during the first year.

With *tacrolimus*, periodic measurements of serum creatinine, potassium, and glucose are recommended to monitor for the adverse effects of nephrotoxicity, hyperkalemia, and hyperglycemia.

Nursing Notes: Apply Your Knowledge

Jane Reily, a kidney transplant recipient taking corticosteroids and cyclosporine, comes to the clinic 6 months after transplantation. She complains of general malaise and not feeling well for the past week. Her temperature is 38°C (100.4°F). What additional information will you collect to differentiate between infection and organ rejection?

Use in Children

Most immunosuppressants are used in children for the same disorders and with similar effects as in adults. Corticosteroids impair growth in children. As a result, some transplantation centers avoid prednisone therapy until a first rejection episode occurs. When prednisone is used, administering it every other day may improve growth rates. *Cyclosporine* has been safely and effectively given to children as young as 6 months of age, but extensive studies have not been performed. *Muromonab-CD3* has been used successfully in children as young as 2 years of age; however, safety and efficacy for use in children have not been established. *Mycophenolate* has been used in a few children undergoing renal transplantation. In children with impaired renal function, recommended doses of mycophenolate cause a high incidence of adverse effects. Thus, dosage should be adjusted for the level of renal function. *Tacrolimus* has been used in children younger than 12 years of age who were undergoing liver transplantation. This usage indicates that children require higher doses to maintain therapeutic blood levels than adults because they metabolize the drug more rapidly.

Little information is available about the use of newer immunosuppressants in children. Safety and effectiveness have not been established for *basiliximab, daclizumab, infliximab,* or *leflunomide*. Leflunomide is not recommended for children under 18 years of age. *Etanercept* is approved for clients 4 to 17 years of age with juvenile rheumatoid arthritis. In clinical trials, effects in children were similar to those in adults. Most children in a 3-month study had an infection while receiving etanercept. The infections were usually mild and consistent with those commonly seen in outpatient pediatric settings. Children reported abdominal pain, nausea, vomiting, and headache more often than adults. Other medications (eg, a corticosteroid, methotrexate, a nonsteroidal anti-inflammatory drug, a salicylate, or an analgesic) may be continued during treatment.

Use in Older Adults

Immunosuppressants are used for the same purposes and produce similar therapeutic and adverse effects in older adults as in younger adults. Because older adults often have multiple disorders and organ impairments, it is especially important that drug choices, dosages, and monitoring tests are individualized. In addition, infections occur more commonly in older adults, and this tendency may be increased with immunosuppressant therapy.

Use in Renal Impairment

- *Azathioprine* metabolites are excreted in urine but they are inactive and the dose does not need to be reduced in clients with renal impairment.
- *Cyclosporine* is nephrotoxic but commonly used in clients with renal and other transplants. Nephrotoxicity has been noted in 25% of renal, 38% of cardiac, and 37% of liver transplant recipients, especially with high doses. It usually subsides with decreased dosage or stopping the drug.

  In renal transplant recipients, when serum creatinine and blood urea nitrogen levels remain elevated, a complete evaluation of the client must be done to differentiate cyclosporine-induced nephrotoxicity from a transplant rejection reaction (although up to 20% of clients may have simultaneous nephrotoxicity and rejection). If renal function is deteriorating from cyclosporine, dosage reduction may be needed. If dosage reduction does not improve renal function, another immunosuppressant is preferred.

  If renal function is deteriorating from a rejection reaction, decreasing cyclosporine dosage would increase the severity of the reaction. With severe rejection that does not respond to treatment with corticosteroids and monoclonal antibodies, it is preferable to allow the kidney transplant to be rejected and removed rather than increase cyclosporine dosage to high levels in an attempt to reverse the rejection.

  To decrease risks of nephrotoxicity, dosage is adjusted according to cyclosporine blood levels and renal function test results, and other nephrotoxic drugs should be avoided. An additional factor is the potential for significant drug interactions with microsomal enzyme inhibitors and inducers. Drugs that inhibit hepatic metabolism (eg, cimetidine) raise cyclosporine blood levels, whereas those that stimulate metabolism decrease levels.

- *Methotrexate* is mainly excreted in urine, so its half-life is prolonged in clients with renal impairment, with risks of accumulation to toxic levels and additional renal damage. However, the risks are less with the small doses used for treatment of rheumatoid arthritis than for the high doses used in cancer chemotherapy. To decrease these risks, adequate renal function should be documented before the drug is given and clients should be well hydrated.

- *Muromonab-CD3* has caused increased serum creatinine and decreased urine output in a few clients during the first 1 to 3 days of use. This was attributed to the release of cytokines with resultant renal function impairment or delayed renal allograft function. The renal function impairment was reversible. Overall, there is little information about the use of this drug in clients with renal impairment.

- *Mycophenolate* produces higher plasma levels in renal transplant recipients with severe, chronic renal impairment than in clients with less severe renal impairment and healthy volunteers. Doses higher than 1 g twice a day should be avoided in these clients. There is no information about mycophenolate use in cardiac transplant recipients with severe, chronic renal impairment.
- *Tacrolimus* is often associated with high rates of nephrotoxicity when given IV, so oral dosing is preferred. Renal impairment does not increase drug half-life.

No information is available about the use of basiliximab, etanercept, infliximab, or leflunomide in clients with renal impairment. However, leflunomide metabolites are partly excreted renally and the drug should be used cautiously. Daclizumab dosage does not need to be adjusted with renal impairment.

Use in Hepatic Impairment

- *Azathioprine* is normally metabolized to its active metabolite in the liver. As a result, pharmacologic action is decreased in clients with hepatic impairment. When azathioprine is used in liver transplantation, clients sometimes experience hepatotoxicity characterized by cholestasis, peliosis hepatis, nodular regenerative hyperplasia, and veno-occlusive disease. Liver function usually improves within a week if azathioprine is discontinued.
- *Cyclosporine* reportedly causes hepatotoxicity (eg, elevated serum aminotransferases and bilirubin) in approximately 4% of renal and liver transplant recipients and 7% of cardiac transplant recipients. This is most likely to occur during the first month of therapy, when high doses of cyclosporine are usually given, and usually subsides with reduced dosage.
- Methotrexate is metabolized in the liver and may cause hepatotoxicity, even in the low doses used in rheumatoid arthritis and psoriasis. Several studies indicate that these clients eventually sustain liver changes that may include fatty deposits, lobular necrosis, fibrosis, and cirrhosis. Progression to cirrhosis may be related to the deposition of methotrexate and its metabolites in the liver. Many clinicians recommend serial liver biopsies for clients on long-term, low-dose methotrexate (eg, after each cumulative dose of 1 to 1.5 g) because fibrosis and cirrhosis may not produce clinical manifestations.

In addition, in clients with or without initial liver impairment, liver function tests should be performed to monitor clients for hepatotoxicity and to guide drug dosage. In general, methotrexate dosage should be decreased by 25% if bilirubin (normal = 0.1 to 1.0 mg/dL) is between 3 and 5 mg/dL or aspartate aminotransferase (AST) (normal = 10 to 40 IU/L) is above 180 IU/L, and the drug should be omitted if bilirubin is above 5 mg/dL.

- *Muromonab-CD3* may cause a transient increase in liver aminotransferase enzymes (eg, AST, alanine aminotransferase [ALT]) with the first few doses. Overall, however, there is little information about drug effects or use in clients with liver impairment.
- *Mycophenolate* is metabolized in the liver to an active metabolite that is further metabolized to inactive metabolites. Liver impairment presumably could interfere with these processes and affect both action and elimination. However, there is no information about its use in clients with hepatic impairment.
- *Tacrolimus* is metabolized in the liver by the microsomal P450 enzyme system. Impaired liver function may decrease presystemic (first-pass) metabolism of oral tacrolimus and produce higher blood levels. Also, the elimination half-life is significantly longer for IV or oral drug. As a result, dosage must be decreased in clients with impaired liver function.

  An additional factor is the potential for significant drug interactions with microsomal enzyme inhibitors and inducers. Drugs that inhibit hepatic metabolism (eg, cimetidine) raise tacrolimus blood levels, whereas those that stimulate metabolism decrease levels.

There is no information about the use of *basiliximab, daclizumab, etanercept,* or *infliximab* in clients with liver impairment. *Leflunomide* may be hepatotoxic in clients with normal liver function and is not recommended for use in clients with liver impairment or positive serology tests for hepatitis B or C. Considerations and guidelines include the following:

1. Leflunomide is metabolized to an active metabolite. The site of metabolism is unknown, but thought to be the liver and the wall of the intestine. With liver impairment, less formation of the active metabolite may result in reduced therapeutic effect.
2. The active metabolite is further metabolized and excreted through the kidneys and biliary tract. Some of the drug excreted in bile is reabsorbed. Leflunomide's long half-life is attributed to this biliary recycling.
3. The role of the liver in drug metabolism and excretion in bile increases risks of hepatotoxicity. The drug increased liver enzymes (mainly AST and ALT) in clinical trials. Most elevations were mild and usually subsided with continued therapy. Higher elevations were infrequent and subsided if dosage was

reduced or the drug was discontinued. It is recommended that liver enzymes, especially ALT, be measured before starting leflunomide, every month during therapy until stable, then as needed.

4. When ALT elevation is more than twice the upper limits of normal (ULN), leflunomide dosage should be reduced to 10 mg/day (half the usual daily maintenance dose). If ALT levels are more than twice but not more than three times the ULN and persist despite dosage reduction, liver biopsy is recommended if continued drug use is desired. If elevations are more than three times the ULN and persist despite dosage reduction and cholestyramine (see later), leflunomide should be discontinued. ALT levels should be monitored and cholestyramine readministered as indicated.

5. When leflunomide is stopped because of liver impairment, a special procedure is recommended to eliminate the drug (otherwise it could take as long as 2 years). The procedure involves administration of cholestyramine (see Chap. 58) 8 g three times daily for 11 days (the 11 days do not need to be consecu-

tive unless blood levels need to be lowered rapidly). If plasma levels are still above the goal level of less than 0.02 µg/mL, additional cholestyramine may be needed.

Home Care

With clients who are taking immunosuppressant drugs, a major role of the home care nurse is to assess the environment for potential sources of infection, assist clients and other members of the household to understand the client's susceptibility to infection, and teach ways to decrease risks of infection. Although infections often develop from the client's own body flora, other potential sources include people with infections, caregivers, water or soil around live plants, and raw fruits and vegetables. Meticulous environmental cleansing, personal hygiene, and hand washing are required. In addition, the nurse may need to assist with clinic visits for monitoring and follow-up care.

(*text continues on page 695*)

NURSING ACTIONS	Immunosuppressants

NURSING ACTIONS	RATIONALE/EXPLANATION
1. Administer accurately	
a. For prepared intravenous (IV) solutions, check for appropriate dilution, discoloration, particulate matter, and expiration time. If okay, give by infusion pump, for the recommended time.	IV drugs should be reconstituted and diluted in a pharmacy and the manufacturers' instructions should be followed exactly. Once mixed, most of these drugs are stable only for a few hours. Also, some do not contain preservatives.
b. Give oral **azathioprine** in divided doses, after meals; give IV drug by infusion, usually over 30 to 60 min.	To decrease nausea and vomiting with oral drug
c. With **basiliximab**, infuse through a peripheral or central vein over 20–30 min. Use the reconstituted solution within 4 h at room temperature or 24 h if refrigerated.	The first dose is given within 2 h before transplantation surgery and the second dose 4 d after transplantation.
d. With **IV cyclosporine**, infuse over 2–6 h.	Intravenous drug is given to patients who are unable to take it orally; resume oral administration when feasible.
e. With **oral cyclosporine** solutions, measure doses with the provided syringe; add to room-temperature orange or apple juice (avoid grapefruit juice); stir well and have the patient drink at once (do not allow diluted solution to stand before drinking). Use a glass container, not plastic. Rinse the glass with more juice to ensure the total dose is taken. Do not rinse the dosing syringe with water or other cleaning agents. Give	These are the manufacturer's recommendations. Mixing with orange or apple juice improves taste; grapefruit juice should not be used because it affects metabolism of cyclosporine.
	The amount of fluid should be large enough to increase palatability, especially for children, but small enough to be consumed quickly. Rinsing ensures the entire dose is taken.
	(*continued*)

NURSING ACTIONS	RATIONALE/EXPLANATION
on a consistent schedule in relation to time of day and meals.	Oral cyclosporine may be given to clients who have had an anaphylactic reaction to the IV preparation, because the reaction is attributed to the oil diluent rather than the drug.
f. Infuse reconstituted and diluted **daclizumab** through a peripheral or central vein over 15 min. Once mixed, use within 4 h or refrigerate up to 24 h.	The first dose is given approximately 24 h before transplantation, followed by a dose every 2 wk for four doses (total of five doses).
g. With **etanercept**, slowly inject 1 mL of the supplied Sterile Bacteriostatic Water for Injection into the vial, without shaking (to avoid excessive foaming). Give subcutaneously, rotating sites so that a new dose is injected at least 1 inch from an old site and never into areas where the skin is tender, bruised, red, or hard.	This drug may be administered at home, by a client or a caregiver, with appropriate instructions and supervised practice in mixing and injecting the drug.
h. Infuse reconstituted and diluted **infliximab** over approximately 2 h, starting within 3 h of preparation (contains no antibacterial preservatives).	Infliximab should be prepared in a pharmacy because special equipment is required for administration.
i. Give **lymphocyte immune globulin, antithymocyte globulin** (diluted to a concentration of 1 mg/mL) into a large or central vein, using an in-line filter and infusion pump, over at least 4 h. Once diluted, use within 24 h.	Manufacturer's recommendations. Using a high-flow vein decreases phlebitis and thrombosis at the IV site. The filter is used to remove any insoluble particles.
j. Give **muromonab-CD3** in an IV bolus injection once daily. Do not give by IV infusion or mix with other drug solutions.	Manufacturer's recommendations
k. Infuse **IV mycophenolate** over approximately 2 h, within 4 h of solution preparation (contains no antibacterial preservatives).	The IV drug must be reconstituted and diluted with 5% dextrose to a concentration of 6 mg/mL (1 g in 140 mL or 1.5 g in 210 mL). Handle the drug cautiously to avoid contact with skin and mucous membranes. If such contact occurs, wash thoroughly with soap and water; rinse eyes with plain water.
l. Give **oral mycophenolate** on an empty stomach. Do not crush the tablets, do not open or crush the capsules, and ask clients to swallow the capsules whole, without biting or chewing.	Food decreases absorption. Avoid inhaling the powder from the capsules or getting on skin or mucous membranes. Such contacts produced teratogenic effects in animals.
m. Give **IV tacrolimus** as a continuous infusion by infusion pump.	
n. Give the first dose of **oral tacrolimus** 8–12 h after stopping the IV infusion.	Oral tacrolimus can usually be substituted for IV drug 2–3 d after transplantation.
2. **Observe for therapeutic effects**	
a. When a drug is given to suppress the immune response to organ transplants, therapeutic effect is the absence of signs and symptoms indicating rejection of the transplanted tissue.	
b. When azathioprine or methotrexate is given for rheumatoid arthritis, observe for decreased pain.	With azathioprine, therapeutic effects usually occur after 6–8 wk. If no response occurs within 12 wk, other treatment measures are indicated. With methotrexate, therapeutic effects usually occur within 3–6 wk.

(continued)

NURSING ACTIONS	RATIONALE/EXPLANATION
c. When etanercept is given for rheumatoid arthritis, observe for decreased symptoms and less joint destruction on x-ray reports.	
d. When infliximab is given for Crohn's disease, observe for decreased symptoms.	
3. **Observe for adverse effects**	
a. Observe for infection (fever, sore throat, wound drainage, productive cough, dysuria, and so forth).	Frequency and severity increase with higher drug dosages. Risks are high in immunosuppressed clients. Infections may be caused by almost any microorganism and may affect any part of the body, although respiratory and urinary tract infections may occur more often.
b. With azathioprine, observe for:	The incidence of adverse effects is high in renal transplant recipients. Dosage reduction or stopping azathioprine may be indicated.
(1) Bone marrow depression (anemia, leukopenia, thrombocytopenia, abnormal bleeding).	
(2) Nausea and vomiting	Can be reduced by dividing the daily dosage and giving after meals
c. With basiliximab and daclizumab, observe for gastrointestinal (GI) disorders (nausea, vomiting, diarrhea, heartburn, abdominal distention)	GI symptoms were often reported in clinical trials. Although adverse effects involving all body systems were reported, the number and type were similar for basiliximab, daclizumab, and placebo groups. All patients were also receiving cyclosporine and a corticosteroid.
d. With cyclosporine, observe for:	
(1) Nephrotoxicity (increased serum creatinine and blood urea nitrogen [BUN], decreased urine output, edema, hyperkalemia)	This is a major adverse effect, and it may produce signs and symptoms that are difficult to distinguish from those caused by renal graft rejection. Rejection usually occurs within the first month after surgery. If it occurs, dosage must be reduced and the patient observed for improved renal function.
	Also, note that graft rejection and drug-induced nephrotoxicity may be present simultaneously. The latter may be decreased by reducing dosage. Nephrotoxicity often occurs 2–3 mo after transplantation and results in a stable but decreased level of renal function (BUN of 35–45 mg/dL and serum creatinine of 2.0–2.5 mg/dL).
(2) Hepatotoxicity (increased serum enzymes and bilirubin)	The reported incidence is less than 8% after kidney, heart, or liver transplantation. It usually occurs during the first month, when high doses are used, and decreases with dosage reduction.
(3) Hypertension	This is especially likely to occur in clients with heart transplants and may require antihypertensive drug therapy. Do not give a potassium-sparing diuretic as part of the antihypertensive regimen because of increased risk of hyperkalemia.

(continued)

NURSING ACTIONS	RATIONALE/EXPLANATION
(4) Anaphylaxis (with IV cyclosporine) (urticaria, hypotension or shock, respiratory distress)	This is rare but may occur. The allergen is thought to be the polyoxyethylated castor oil because people who had allergic reactions with the IV drug have later taken oral doses without allergic reactions. During IV administration, observe the client continuously for the first 30 min and often thereafter. Stop the infusion if a reaction occurs, and give emergency care (eg, epinephrine 1:1000).
(5) Central nervous system (CNS) toxicity (confusion, depression, hallucinations, seizures, tremor)	These effects are relatively uncommon and may be caused by factors other than cyclosporine (eg, nephrotoxicity).
(6) Other (gingival hyperplasia, hirsutism)	Gingival hyperplasia can be minimized by thorough oral hygiene.
e. With infliximab, observe for:	
(1) Infusion reactions (fever, chills, pruritus, urticaria, chest pain)	
(2) GI upset (nausea, vomiting, abdominal pain)	
(3) Respiratory symptoms (bronchitis, chest pain, coughing, dyspnea)	
f. With leflunomide, observe for:	The drug was in general well tolerated in clinical trials, with the number and type of most adverse effects similar to those occurring with placebo.
(1) GI upset (nausea, diarrhea)	
(2) Hepatotoxicity (elevation of transaminases)	
(3) Skin (alopecia, rash)	
g. With lymphocyte immune globulin, antithymocyte globulin, observe for:	
(1) Anaphylaxis (chest pain, respiratory distress, hypotension or shock)	An uncommon but serious allergic reaction to the animal protein in the drug that may occur anytime during therapy. If it occurs, stop the drug infusion, inject 0.3 mL epinephrine 1:1000, and provide other supportive emergency care as indicated.
(2) Chills and fever	Fever occurs in approximately 50% of clients; it may be decreased by premedicating with acetaminophen, an antihistamine, or a corticosteroid.
h. With methotrexate, observe for:	
(1) GI disorders (nausea, vomiting, diarrhea, ulcerations, bleeding)	Monitor complete blood count (CBC) regularly. Bone marrow depression is less likely to occur with the small doses used for inflammatory disorders than with doses used in cancer chemotherapy.
(2) Bone marrow depression (anemia, neutropenia, thrombocytopenia)	Long-term, low-dose methotrexate may produce fatty changes, fibrosis, necrosis, and cirrhosis in the liver.
(3) Hepatotoxicity (yellow discoloration of skin or eyes, dark urine, elevated liver aminotransferases)	Progression to cirrhosis may involve deposition of the drug and its metabolites in the liver. Some clinicians recommend serial liver biopsies (with each cumulative dose of 1–1.5 g) because progression to cirrhosis may not cause symptoms.

(continued)

NURSING ACTIONS	RATIONALE/EXPLANATION

i. With muromonab-CD3, observe for:

(1) An acute reaction called the cytokine release syndrome (high fever, chills, chest pain, dyspnea, hypertension, nausea, vomiting, diarrhea)

This reaction is attributed to the release of cytokines by activated lymphocytes or monocytes. Symptoms may range from "flu-like" to a less frequent but severe, shock-like reaction that may include serious cardiovascular and CNS disorders.

(2) Hypersensitivity (edema, difficulty in swallowing or breathing, skin rash, urticaria, rapid heart beat)

Symptoms usually occur approximately 30–60 min after administration of a dose, especially the first dose, and may last several hours. The reaction usually subsides with later doses, but may recur with dosage increases or restarting after a period without the drug.

(3) Nausea, vomiting, diarrhea

Patients experiencing a hypersensitivity reaction should receive immediate treatment.

j. With mycophenolate, observe for:

(1) GI effects (nausea, vomiting, diarrhea)

GI effects are more likely when mycophenolate is started and may subside if dosage is reduced.

(2) Hematologic effects (anemia, neutropenia)

Monitor CBC reports regularly. Up to 2% of renal and 2.8% of cardiac transplant recipients taking mycophenolate have severe neutropenia (absolute neutrophil count <500/mm^3). The neutropenia may be related to mycophenolate, concomitant medications, viral infections, or a combination of these causes. If a client has neutropenia, interrupt drug administration or reduce the dose and initiate appropriate treatment as soon as possible.

(3) CNS effects (dizziness, headache, insomnia)

k. With tacrolimus, observe for;

(1) Nephrotoxicity

Nephrotoxicity (increased serum creatinine, decreased urine output) has occurred in one third or more of liver transplant recipients who received tacrolimus. The risk is greater with higher doses.

(2) Neurotoxicity—minor neurologic effects include insomnia, mild tremors, headaches, photophobia, nightmares; major effects include confusion, seizures, coma, expressive aphasia, psychosis, and encephalopathy.

Neurologic symptoms are common and occur in approximately 10%–20% of clients receiving tacrolimus.

(3) Infection—cytomegalovirus (CMV) infection and others

CMV infection commonly occurs.

(4) Hyperglycemia

Glucose intolerance may require insulin therapy.

4. Observe for drug interactions

Drug interactions have not been reported with the newer biologic immunosuppressants (basiliximab, daclizumab, etanercept, infliximab).

a. Drugs that *increase* effects of azathioprine:

(1) Allopurinol

Inhibits hepatic metabolism, thereby increasing pharmacologic effects. If the two drugs are given concomitantly, the dose of azathioprine should be reduced drastically to 25%–35% of the usual dose.

(*continued*)

NURSING ACTIONS	RATIONALE/EXPLANATION
(2) Corticosteroids	Increased immunosuppression and risk of infection
b. Drugs that *increase* effects of cyclosporine:	
(1) Aminoglycoside antibiotics (eg, gentamicin), antifungals (amphotericin B, ketoconazole)	Increased risk of nephrotoxicity. Avoid other nephrotoxic drugs when possible.
(2) Antifungals (fluconazole, itraconazole), calcium channel blockers (diltiazem, nicardipine, verapamil), cimetidine	Decreased hepatic metabolism, increased serum drug levels, and increased risk of toxicity.
(3) Erythromycin, metoclopramide	Increased GI absorption of cyclosporine
c. Drugs that *decrease* effects of cyclosporine:	
(1) Enzyme inducers, including anticonvulsants (carbamazepine, phenobarbital, phenytoin), rifampin, trimethoprim-sulfamethoxazole	Enzyme-inducing drugs stimulate hepatic metabolism of cyclosporine, thereby reducing blood levels. If concurrent administration is necessary, monitor cyclosporine blood levels to avoid subtherapeutic levels and decreased effectiveness.
d. Drugs that *increase* effects of leflunomide:	
(1) Rifampin	Rifampin induces liver enzymes and accelerates metabolism of leflunomide to its active metabolite.
(2) Hepatotoxic drugs (eg, methotrexate)	Additive hepatotoxicity
e. Drugs that *decrease* effects of leflunomide:	
(1) Charcoal	These drugs may be used to lower blood levels of leflunomide.
(2) Cholestyramine	
f. Drugs that *increase* effects of methotrexate:	Probenecid, salicylates, and sulfonamides may increase both therapeutic and toxic effects. The mechanism is unknown, but may involve slowing of methotrexate elimination through the kidneys or displacement of methotrexate from plasma protein binding sites.
(1) Probenecid	
(2) Salicylates	
(3) Sulfonamides	
(4) Nonsteroidal anti-inflammatory drugs (NSAIDs)	
(5) Procarbazine	NSAIDs are often used concomitantly with methotrexate by clients with rheumatoid arthritis. There may be an increased risk of GI ulceration and bleeding.
(6) Alcohol and other hepatotoxic drugs	Procarbazine may increase nephrotoxicity; hepatotoxic drugs increase hepatotoxicity.
g. Drug that *decreases* effects of methotrexate:	
(1) Folic acid	Methotrexate acts by blocking folic acid. Its effectiveness is decreased by folic acid supplementation, alone or in multivitamin preparations.
h. Drugs that *increase* effects of mycophenolate:	
(1) Acyclovir, ganciclovir	Increase blood levels of mycophenolate, probably by decreasing renal excretion
(2) Probenecid, salicylates	Increase blood levels
i. Drug that *decreases* effects of mycophenolate:	
(1) Cholestyramine	Decreases absorption

(continued)

NURSING ACTIONS	RATIONALE/EXPLANATION
j. Drugs that *increase* effects of tacrolimus:	
(1) Nephrotoxic drugs (eg, aminoglycoside antibiotics, amphotericin B, cisplatin, NSAIDs)	Increased risk of nephrotoxicity
(2) Antifungals (clotrimazole, fluconazole, itraconazole, ketoconazole); erythromycin and other macrolides; calcium channel blockers (diltiazem, verapamil), cimetidine, danazol, methylprednisolone, metoclopramide	These drugs may increase blood levels of tacrolimus, probably by inhibiting or competing for hepatic drug-metabolizing enzymes
(3) Angiotensin-converting enzyme inhibitors, potassium supplements	Increased risk of hyperkalemia. Serum potassium levels should be monitored closely.
k. Drugs that *decrease* effects of tacrolimus:	
(1) Antacids	With oral tacrolimus, antacids adsorb the drug or raise the pH of gastric fluids and increase its degradation. If ordered concomitantly, an antacid should be given at least 2 h before or after tacrolimus.
(2) Enzyme inducers—carbamazepine, phenobarbital, phenytoin, rifampin, rifabutin	Induction of drug-metabolizing enzymes in the liver may accelerate metabolism of tacrolimus and decrease its blood levels.

Nursing Notes: Apply Your Knowledge

Answer: Complete a total body assessment, looking for signs of infection. It is important to note that patients taking immunosuppressive drugs do not mount an effective immune response in the presence of infection. Her temperature, even though it is a low-grade fever, is very significant and supports that an infection might be present. Signs of organ rejection include fever, flank pain, and signs that indicate the kidney is no longer functioning well (increased creatinine and blood urea nitrogen [BUN], decreased urine output, weight gain). Provide Ms. Reily's transplant surgeon with the data you have collected. He or she will order laboratory tests, including white blood cell count and differential, creatinine, BUN, and a cyclosporine level.

▶ REVIEW AND APPLICATION EXERCISES

1. List clinical indications for use of immunosuppressant drug therapy.

2. How do the different types of drugs exert their immunosuppressant effects?

3. What are major adverse effects of immunosuppressant drugs?

4. When assessing a client receiving one or more immunosuppressant drugs, what specific signs and symptoms indicate adverse drug effects?

5. For a client taking one or more immunosuppressant drugs, prepare a teaching plan related to safe and effective drug therapy.

SELECTED REFERENCES

Burckart, G.J., Venkataramanan, R., & Ptachcinski, R.J. (1997). Overview of transplantation. In J.T. DiPiro, R.L. Talbert, G.C. Yee, G.R. Matzke, B.G. Wells, & L.M. Posey (Eds.), *Pharmacotherapy: A pathophysiologic approach*, 3rd ed., pp. 129–147. Stamford, CT: Appleton & Lange.

Butani, L., Plamer, J., Baluarte, H.J., & Polinsky, M.S. (1999). Adverse effects of mycophenolate mofetil in pediatric renal transplant recipients with presumed chronic rejection. *Transplantation, 68*, 83–86.

Chong, A.S., Huang, W., Liu, W., Luo, J., et al. (1999). In vivo activity of leflunomide: Pharmacokinetic analyses and mechanism of immunosuppression. *Transplantation, 68*, 100–109.

Diasio, R.B. & LoBuglio, A.F. (1996). Immunomodulators: Immunosuppressive agents and immunostimulants. In J.G. Hardman, L.E. Limbird, P.B. Molinoff, & R.W. Ruddon (Eds.), *Goodman & Gilman's The pharmacological basis of therapeutics*, 9th ed., pp. 1291–1308. New York: McGraw-Hill.

Drug facts and comparisons. (Updated monthly). St. Louis: Facts and Comparisons.

Guyton, A.C. & Hall, J.E. (Eds.). (1996). *Textbook of medical physiology*, 9th ed. Philadelphia: W.B. Saunders.

Kelley, W.N. (Ed.). (1997). *Textbook of internal medicine*, 3rd ed. Philadelphia: Lippincott-Raven.

Hirsch, F. & Kroemer, G. (1998). The immune system and immune modulation. In T.F. Kresina (Ed.), *Immune modulating agents*, pp. 1–19. New York: Marcel Dekker.

Lichtenstein, G.R. & MacDermott, R.P. (1999). The future has arrived: Biological therapy for Crohn's disease. Presented at the American Gastroenterological Association Clinical Symposium, Digestive Disease Week, Orlando, Florida, May, 1999. [Online: Available http://www.medscape.com. Accessed August 20, 1999.]

Munoz, S.J. (1996). Long-term management of the liver transplant recipient. *Medical Clinics of North America, 80*, 1103–1119.

Present, DH, Rutgeerts, P., & Targan, S. (1999). Infliximab for the treatment of fistulas in patients with Crohn's disease. *New England Journal of Medicine, 340*, 1398–1405.

Shah, S., Bousvaros, A., & Stevens, A.C. (1998). Immunomodulating agents in gastrointestinal disease. In T.F. Kresina (Ed.), *Immune modulating agents*, pp. 267–299. New York: Marcel Dekker.

Weinblatt, M.E., Kremer, J.M. Bankhurst, A.D., et al. (1999). A trial of etanercept, a recombinant tumor necrosis factor receptor:Fc fusion protein, in patients with rheumatoid arthritis receiving methotrexate. *New England Journal of Medicine, 340*, 253–259.

Drugs Affecting the Respiratory System

46

Physiology of the Respiratory System

Objectives

After studying this chapter, the student will be able to:

1. Review roles of the main respiratory tract structures in oxygenation of body tissues.

2. Describe the role of carbon dioxide in respiration.

3. List common signs and symptoms affecting respiratory function.

4. Identify general categories of drugs used to treat respiratory disorders.

THE RESPIRATORY SYSTEM

The respiratory system helps meet the basic human need for oxygen (O_2). Oxygen is necessary for the oxidation of foodstuffs, by which energy for cellular metabolism is produced. When the oxygen supply is inadequate, cell function is impaired; when oxygen is absent, cells die. Permanent brain damage occurs within 4 to 6 minutes of anoxia. In addition to providing oxygen to all body cells, the respiratory system also removes carbon dioxide (CO_2), a major waste product of cell metabolism. Excessive accumulation of CO_2 damages or kills body cells.

The efficiency of the respiratory system depends on the quality and quantity of air inhaled, the patency of air passageways, the ability of the lungs to expand and contract, and the ability of O_2 and CO_2 to cross the alveolar–capillary membrane. In addition to the respiratory system, the circulatory, nervous, and musculoskeletal systems have important functions in respiration. Additional characteristics of the respiratory system and the process of respiration are described in the following sections.

Respiration

Respiration is the process of gas exchange by which O_2 is obtained and CO_2 is eliminated. This gas exchange occurs between the lung and the blood across the alveolar–capillary membrane and between the blood and body cells. More specifically, the four parts of respiration are:

- *Ventilation*—the movement of air between the atmosphere and the alveoli of the lungs
- *Perfusion*—blood flow through the lungs
- *Diffusion*—the process by which O_2 and CO_2 are transferred between alveoli and blood and between blood and body cells
- *Regulation* of breathing by the respiratory muscles and nervous system

Respiratory Tract

The respiratory tract is a series of branching tubes with progressively smaller diameters. These tubes (nose, pharynx, larynx, trachea, bronchi, and bronchioles) function as air passageways and air "conditioners" that filter, warm, and humidify incoming air. Most of the conditioning is done by the ciliated mucous membrane that lines the entire respiratory tract except the pharynx and alveoli. *Cilia* are tiny, hair-like projections that sweep mucus toward the pharynx to be expectorated or swallowed. The mucous membrane secretes mucus, which forms a protective blanket and traps foreign particles, such as bacteria or dust.

When air is inhaled through the nose, it is conditioned by the nasal mucosa. When the nasal passages are blocked, the mouth serves as an alternate airway. The oral mucosa may warm and humidify air but cannot filter it.

Pharynx, Larynx, and Trachea

Air passes from the nasal cavities to the pharynx (throat). Pharyngeal walls are composed of skeletal muscle and their lining is composed of mucous membrane. The pharynx contains the palatine tonsils, which are large masses of lymphatic tissue. The pharynx is a passageway for food, fluids, and air. Food and fluids go from the pharynx to the esophagus, and air passes from the pharynx into the trachea.

The larynx is composed of nine cartilages joined by ligaments and controlled by skeletal muscles. It contains the vocal cords and forms the upper end of the trachea. It closes on swallowing to prevent aspiration of food and fluids into the lungs.

The trachea is the passageway between the larynx and the main stem bronchi. It is a cartilaginous tube lined with ciliated epithelium and mucus-secreting cells. Cilia and mucus help to protect and defend the lungs.

Lungs

The lungs begin where the trachea divides into the right and left mainstem *bronchi* and contain the remaining respiratory structures. They are divided into five lobes, each with a secondary bronchus. The lobes are further subdivided into bronchopulmonary segments supplied by smaller bronchi. The bronchopulmonary segments contain lobules, which are the functional units of the lung (the site where gas exchange takes place). Each lobule is supplied by a bronchiole, an arteriole, a venule, and a lymphatic vessel. Blood enters the lobules through a pulmonary artery and exits through a pulmonary vein. Lymphatic structures surround the lobule and aid in the removal of plasma proteins and other particles from interstitial spaces.

The mainstem bronchi branch into smaller bronchi, then into bronchioles. *Bronchioles* are approximately the size of a pencil lead and do not contain cartilage or mucus-secreting glands. The walls of the bronchioles contain smooth muscle, which is controlled by the autonomic nervous system. Parasympathetic nerves cause constriction; sympathetic nerves cause relaxation or dilation.

The epithelial lining of the bronchioles becomes thinner with progressive branchings until only one cell layer is apparent. The bronchioles give rise to the *alveoli*, which are grape-like clusters of air sacs surrounded by capillaries.

The alveoli are composed of two types of cells. Type I cells are flat, thin epithelial cells that fuse with capillaries to form the alveolar–capillary membrane across which gas exchange occurs. Oxygen enters the bloodstream to be transported to body cells; CO_2 enters the alveoli to be exhaled from the lungs. Type II cells produce surfactant, a lipoprotein substance that decreases the surface tension in the alveoli and aids lung inflation. The alveoli also contain macrophages that help to protect and defend the lungs.

The lungs are encased in a membrane called the *pleura*, which is composed of two layers. The inner layer, which adheres to the surface of the lung, is called the *visceral pleura*. The outer layer, which lines the thoracic cavity, is called the *parietal pleura*. The potential space between the layers is called the pleural cavity. It contains fluid that allows the layers to glide over each other and minimizes friction.

The lungs expand and relax in response to changes in pressure relationships (intrapulmonic and intrapleural pressures). Elastic tissue in the bronchioles and alveoli allows the lungs to stretch or expand to accommodate incoming air. This ability is called *compliance*. The lungs also recoil (like a stretched rubber band) to expel air. Some air remains in the lungs after expiration, which allows gas exchange to continue between respirations.

In addition to exchanging O_2 and CO_2, the lungs synthesize, store, release, remove, metabolize, or inactivate a variety of biologically active substances. These substances, which may be locally released or carried in blood or tissue fluids, participate in both physiologic and pathologic processes. Specific substances that may be released from the lungs include biogenic amines (eg, catecholamines, histamine, serotonin), arachidonic acid metabolites (eg, prostaglandins, leukotrienes), angiotensin converting enzyme, and heparin. The amines are important in regulating smooth muscle tone (ie, constriction or dilation) in the airways and blood vessels. Prostaglandins and leukotrienes are important in inflammatory processes. Angiotensin converting enzyme converts angiotensin I to angiotensin II, which is important in regulating blood pressure. Heparin helps to dissolve blood clots, especially in the capillaries, where small clots are trapped. The lungs also process peptides, lipids, hormones, and drugs and inactivate bradykinin.

Lung Circulation

The pulmonary circulatory system transports O_2 and CO_2. After oxygen enters the bloodstream across the alveolar–capillary membrane, it combines with hemoglobin in red blood cells for transport to body cells, where it is released. Carbon dioxide combines with hemoglobin in the cells for return to the lungs and elimination from the body.

The lungs receive the total cardiac output of blood and are supplied with blood from two sources, the pulmonary and bronchial circulations. The pulmonary circulation provides for gas exchange as the pulmonary arteries carry unoxygenated blood to the lungs and the pulmonary veins return oxygenated blood to the heart. The bronchial arteries arise from the thoracic aorta and supply the air passages and supporting structures. The bronchial circulation also warms and humidifies incoming air and can form new vessels and develop collateral circulation when normal vessels are blocked (eg, in pulmonary embolism). The latter ability helps to keep lung tissue alive until circulation can be restored.

Capillaries in the lungs are lined by a single layer of epithelial cells called endothelium. Once thought to be a passive conduit for blood, it is now known that the endothelium performs several important functions. First, it forms a barrier that prevents leakage of water and other substances into lung tissue. Second, it participates in the transport of respiratory gases, water, and solutes. Third, it secretes vasodilating substances such as nitric oxide and prostacyclin. Nitric oxide also regulates smooth muscle tone in the bronchi, and prostacyclin also inhibits platelet aggregation. When pulmonary endothelium is injured (eg, by endotoxins or drugs such as bleomycin, an anticancer drug), these functions are impaired.

Nervous System

The nervous system regulates the rate and depth of respiration by the respiratory center in the medulla oblongata, the pneumotaxic center in the pons, and the apneustic center in the reticular formation. The respiratory center is stimulated primarily by increased CO_2 in the fluids of the center. (However, excessive CO_2 depresses the respiratory center.) When the center is stimulated, the rate and depth of breathing are increased, and excessive CO_2 is exhaled. A lesser stimulus to the respiratory center is decreased oxygen in arterial blood.

The nervous system also operates several reflexes important to respiration. The cough reflex is especially important because it helps protect the lungs from foreign particles, air pollutants, bacteria, and other potentially harmful substances. A cough occurs when nerve endings in the respiratory tract mucosa are stimulated by dryness, pressure, cold, irritant fumes, and excessive secretions.

Musculoskeletal System

The musculoskeletal system participates in chest expansion and contraction. Normally, the diaphragm and external intercostal muscles expand the chest cavity and are called muscles of inspiration. The abdominal and internal intercostal muscles are the muscles of expiration.

Summary

Overall, normal respiration requires:

1. Atmospheric air containing at least 21% O_2
2. Adequate ventilation. Ventilation, in turn, requires patent airways, expansion and contraction of the chest, expansion and contraction of the lungs, and maintenance of a normal range of intrapulmonic and intrapleural pressures.
3. Adequate diffusion of O_2 and CO_2 through the alveolar–capillary membrane. Factors influencing diffusion include the thickness and surface area of

the membrane and pressure differences between gases on each side of the membrane.

4. Adequate perfusion or circulation of blood and sufficient hemoglobin to carry needed O_2

In addition, normal breathing occurs 16 to 20 times per minute and is quiet, rhythmic, and effortless. Approximately 500 mL of air is inspired and expired with a normal breath (tidal volume); deep breaths or "sighs" occur 6 to 10 times per hour to ventilate more alveoli. Fever, exercise, pain, and emotions such as anger increase respirations. Sleep or rest and various medications, such as tranquilizers, sedatives, and narcotic analgesics, slow respiration.

DISORDERS OF THE RESPIRATORY SYSTEM

The respiratory system is subject to many disorders that interfere with respiration and other lung functions. These disorders may be caused by agents that reach the system through inhaled air or through the bloodstream and include respiratory tract infections, allergic disorders, inflammatory disorders, and conditions that obstruct air flow (eg, excessive respiratory tract secretions, asthma, and other chronic obstructive pulmonary diseases). Injury to the lungs by various disorders (eg, anaphylaxis, asthma, mechanical stimulation such as hyperventilation, pulmonary thromboembolism, pulmonary edema, acute respiratory distress syndrome) is associated with the release of histamine and other biologically active chemical mediators from the lungs. These mediators often cause inflammation and constriction of the airways.

The ciliated epithelial cells of the larger airways, the type I epithelial cells of the alveoli, and the capillary endothelial cells of the alveolar area are especially susceptible to injury. Once injured, cellular functions are impaired (eg, decreased mucociliary clearance). Common signs and symptoms of respiratory disorders include cough, increased secretions, mucosal congestion, and bronchospasm. Severe disorders or inadequate treatment may lead to cell necrosis.

DRUG THERAPY

As a general rule, drug therapy is more effective in relieving respiratory symptoms than in curing the underlying disorders that cause the symptoms. Major drug groups used to treat respiratory symptoms are bronchodilating and other antiasthmatic agents (see Chap. 47), antihistamines (see Chap. 48), and nasal decongestants, antitussives, and cold remedies (see Chap. 49).

 REVIEW AND APPLICATION EXERCISES

1. What is the main function of the respiratory system?
2. Where does the exchange of oxygen and carbon dioxide occur?
3. List factors that stimulate rate and depth of respiration.
4. List factors that depress rate and depth of respiration.
5. What are common signs and symptoms of respiratory disorders for which drug therapy is often used?

SELECTED REFERENCES

Guyton, A.C. & Hall, J.E. (1996). *Textbook of medical physiology,* 9th ed. Philadelphia: W.B. Saunders.
Porth, C.M. (Ed.). (1998). *Pathophysiology: Concepts of altered health states,* 5th ed. Philadelphia: Lippincott Williams & Wilkins.
Smeltzer, S.C. & Bare, B.G. (1996). *Brunner and Suddarth's Textbook of medical-surgical nursing,* 8th ed. Philadelphia: Lippincott-Raven.

47

Bronchodilating and Other Antiasthmatic Drugs

Objectives

After studying this chapter, the student will be able to:

1. Differentiate the types of bronchodilating and anti-inflammatory drugs used in the treatment of asthma and related disorders.

2. Differentiate between short-acting and long-acting inhaled beta$_2$-adrenergic agonists in terms of uses and nursing process implications.

3. Describe theophylline preparations in terms of indications for use, routes of administration, adverse effects, and nursing process implications.

4. Compare adrenergic and xanthine bronchodilators in terms of therapeutic and adverse effects and nursing process implications.

5. Discuss the uses of corticosteroids, leukotriene inhibitors, and mast cell stabilizers in the treatment of asthma and other bronchoconstrictive respiratory disorders.

6. Discuss principles of therapy and nursing process for a client with an acute asthma attack.

7. Discuss principles of therapy and nursing process for a client with chronic bronchoconstrictive disorders.

8. Discuss the use of bronchodilators and other antiasthmatic drugs in special populations.

Gwen, a 12-year-old middle schooler, was recently diagnosed with asthma. She uses two inhalers four times a day, in addition to using a rescue inhaler during periods of dyspnea. She also is taking peak flow measurements. As the school nurse, you are responsible for overseeing Gwen's care while she is in school.

Reflect on:

▶ The developmental level of 12-year-olds. How might this affect Gwen's feelings about having asthma and complying with treatment?

▶ What asthma triggers might be present in the school environment?

▶ School regulations usually require that all medication be kept in the nurse's office. What impact might this have if Gwen experiences an asthma attack?

▶ Develop an educational program on asthma for middle schoolers. How might Gwen and other students with asthma participate?

RESPIRATORY DISORDERS

Bronchodilating and antiasthmatic agents are used in the treatment of respiratory disorders characterized by bronchoconstriction or bronchospasm, inflammation, mucosal edema, and excessive mucus production (asthma, bronchitis, and emphysema). Bronchoconstriction involves narrowing of the airways, which is aggravated by the inflammation, mucosal edema, and excessive mucus. Resultant symptoms include dyspnea, wheezing, coughing, and other signs of respiratory distress.

Bronchoconstriction may be precipitated by respiratory infections, odors, smoke, chemical fumes or other air pollutants, cold air, exercise, tartrazine (a yellow dye found in many foods and drugs), and some drugs (eg, beta-adrenergic blocking agents, aspirin, and nonsteroidal anti-inflammatory agents). When lung tissues are exposed to these stimuli, mast cells release histamine and other substances that cause bronchoconstriction and inflammation. Mast cells are found throughout the body in connective tissues and are abundant in tissues surrounding capillaries in the lungs.

Bronchoconstrictive and proinflammatory substances include acetylcholine, cyclic guanosine monophosphate (GMP), histamine, leukotrienes, prostaglandins, serotonin, and others. These substances are antagonized by cyclic adenosine monophosphate (cyclic AMP). Cyclic AMP is an intracellular substance that initiates various intracellular activities, depending on the type of cell. In lung cells, cyclic AMP inhibits release of bronchoconstrictive substances and thus indirectly promotes bronchodilation.

Asthma

Asthma is a group of airway disorders characterized by inflammation, bronchoconstriction, and hyperreactivity to various stimuli. Inflammation and damaged airway mucosa are chronically present, even when clients appear symptom free. Bronchoconstriction is usually recurrent and reversible, either spontaneously or with drug therapy. Hyperreactivity may initiate both inflammation and bronchoconstriction. These characteristics all contribute to airway obstruction and other symptoms of asthma attacks (labored, wheezing respirations, chest tightness, and cough). Acute episodes of asthma are often triggered by exposure to airway irritants (eg, allergens, chemicals, smoke) or viral infections of the respiratory tract and they may last minutes to hours. Asthma may occur at any age but is especially common in childhood and early adulthood. Children who are exposed to allergens and airway irritants such as tobacco smoke during infancy are at high risk for development of asthma.

When sensitized mast cells in the lungs or eosinophils in the blood are exposed to allergens or irritants, multiple cytokines and other chemical mediators (eg, histamine, interleukins, leukotrienes) are synthesized and released. These chemicals act directly on target tissues of the airways, causing smooth muscle constriction, increased capillary permeability and fluid leakage, and changes in the mucus-secreting properties of the airway epithelium. Although multiple chemical mediators are involved in any asthmatic reaction, different mediators may predominate in individual clients.

Chronic Bronchitis and Emphysema

In *chronic bronchitis* and *emphysema*, commonly called chronic obstructive pulmonary disease (COPD), bronchoconstriction and inflammation are more constant and less reversible than with asthma. Anatomic and physiologic changes occur over several years and lead to increasing dyspnea and activity intolerance. These conditions usually affect middle-aged or older adults.

DRUG THERAPY

Bronchodilators are used to prevent and treat bronchoconstriction associated with asthma, acute and chronic bronchitis, and emphysema. Anti-inflammatory drugs are used to prevent and treat inflammation of the airways. Reducing inflammation also reduces bronchoconstriction by decreasing mucosal edema and mucus secretions that narrow airways and by decreasing airway hyperreactivity to various stimuli. The drugs are described in the following sections; dosage ranges of individual drugs are listed in Tables 47-1 and 47-2.

Bronchodilators

Adrenergics

Adrenergic drugs (see Chap. 18) stimulate beta$_2$-adrenergic receptors in the smooth muscle of bronchi and bronchioles. The receptors, in turn, stimulate the enzyme adenyl cyclase to increase production of cyclic AMP. The increased cyclic AMP produces bronchodilation. Some beta-adrenergic drugs (eg, epinephrine) also stimulate beta$_1$-adrenergic receptors in the heart to increase the rate and force of contraction. Cardiac stimulation is an adverse effect when the drugs are given for bronchodilation. These drugs are contraindicated in clients with cardiac tachyarrhythmias and severe coronary artery disease; they should be used cautiously in clients with hypertension, hyperthyroidism, diabetes mellitus, and seizure disorders.

Epinephrine may be injected subcutaneously in an acute attack of bronchoconstriction, with therapeutic effects in approximately 5 minutes and lasting for approximately 4 hours. The drug is also available without pre-

TABLE 47-1   **Bronchodilating Drugs**

Generic/Trade Names	Routes and Dosage Ranges	
	Adults	**Children**
Bronchodilators		
ADRENERGICS		
Epinephrine (Adrenalin, Bronkaid)	Aqueous solution (epinephrine 1 : 1000), SC 0.2–0.5 mL; dose may be repeated after 20 min if necessary Aqueous suspension (Sus-Phrine 1 : 200), SC 0.1–0.3 mL; dose may be repeated after 4 h if necessary Inhalation by inhaler, one or two inhalations four to six times per day Inhalation by nebulizer, 0.25–0.5 mL of 2.25% racemic epinephrine in 2.5 mL normal saline	Aqueous solution (epinephrine 1 : 1000), SC 0.01 mL/kg q4h as needed. A single dose should not exceed 0.5 mL. Aqueous suspension (Sus-Phrine 1 : 200), SC 0.005 mL/kg q8–12h if necessary Inhalation, same as adults for both inhaler and nebulizer
Albuterol (Proventil, others)	PO 2–4 mg three or four times per day Inhalation,* one or two inhalations (90 µg/puff) q4–6h	Safety and effectiveness in children <12 y have not been established.
Bitolterol (Tornalate)	Treatment, two inhalations (0.37 mg/puff) at least 1–3 min apart, followed by a third if necessary Prophylaxis, two inhalations q8h; maximum recommended dose, three inhalations q6h or two inhalations q4h	Children >12 y: Same as adults
Isoproterenol (Isuprel)	Inhalation by nebulizer, 0.25– 0.5 mL of 1 : 200 Isuprel solution in 2.5 mL saline Inhalation by inhaler,* one or two inhalations (0.075–0.125 mg/puff) four times per day; maximum dose, three inhalations per attack of bronchospasm	Same as adults
Levalbuterol (Xopenex)	Nebulizer, 0.63–1.25 mg three times daily, q6–8h	≥12 y: Same as adults
Metaproterenol (Alupent)	Inhalation,* 1–3 puffs (0.65 mg/dose), four times per day; maximum dose, 12 inhalations/d PO 10–20 mg q6–8h	Inhalation, not recommended for use in children <12 y ≤9 y or weight under 27 kg, PO 10 mg q6–8h >9 y or weight over 27 kg, PO 20 mg q6–8h
Pirbuterol (Maxair)	Inhalation,* two puffs (0.4 mg/dose), four to six times per day; maximum dose, 12 inhalations/d	>12 y: Same as adults; not recommended for use in children <12 y
Salmeterol (Serevent)	Oral inhalation, two inhalations (42 µg), q12h	Dosage not established
Terbutaline (Brethine)	PO 2.5–5 mg q6–8h; maximum dose, 15 mg/d SC 0.25 mg, repeated in 15–30 min if necessary, q4–6h Inhalation,* two inhalations (400 µg/dose) q4–6h	PO 2.5 mg three times per day for children ≥12 y; maximum dose, 7.5 mg/d SC dosage not established Inhalation, same as adults for children ≥12 y
ANTICHOLINERGIC		
Ipratropium bromide (Atrovent)	Two inhalations (36 µg) from the metered-dose inhaler four times per day	Dosage not established
Ipratropium/Albuterol combination (Combivent)	Two inhalations four times daily	Dosage not established
Xanthines		
Short-acting Theophylline (Aminophylline)	PO, 500 mg initially, then 200–300 mg q6–8h; IV infusion, 6 mg/kg over 30 min, then 0.1–1.2 mg/kg/h	PO, 7.5 mg/kg initially, then 5–6 mg/kg q6–8h; IV infusion, 6 mg/kg over 30 min, then 0.6–0.9 mg/kg/h
Long-acting Theophylline (Theo-Dur, others)	PO, 150–300 mg q8–12h; maximal dose 13 mg/kg or 900 mg daily, whichever is less	PO, 100–200 mg q8–12h; maximal dose, 24 mg/kg/d

IV, intravenous; PO, oral; SC, subcutaneous.
* Adrenergic bronchodilators are used mainly by inhalation, as needed, rather than on a regular schedule.

TABLE 47-2 **Anti-inflammatory Antiasthmatic Drugs**

Generic/Trade Names	Routes and Dosage Ranges	
	Adults	Children
Corticosteroids		
Beclomethasone (Beclovent, Vanceril)	Oral inhalation, two inhalations (0.84 mg/dose) three or four times daily; maximum, 20 inhalations/24 h Nasal inhalation (Vanceril nasal inhaler), one inhalation (0.42 mg) in each nostril two to four times per day	6–12 y: Oral inhalation, one or two inhalations three or four times per day; maximum dose, 10 inhalations/24 h >12 y: Nasal inhalation, same as adults
Budesonide (Pulmocort Turbuhaler)	Oral inhalation, 200–400 µg twice daily	≥6 y: Oral inhalation 200 µg twice daily
Flunisolide (AeroBid)	Oral inhalation, two inhalations (0.50 mg/dose) twice daily, morning and evening; maximum dose, four inhalations twice daily (2 mg) Nasal inhalation (Nasalide), two sprays in each nostril twice daily; maximum dose, eight sprays in each nostril per day	6–15 y: Oral inhalation, two inhalations twice daily Nasal inhalation, one spray in each nostril three times per day, or two sprays twice daily; maximum dose, four sprays in each nostril per day
Fluticasone aerosol (Flovent)	Aerosol, 220–440 µg twice daily	Dosage not established
Fluticasone powder (Flovent Rotadisk)	Powder, 100–500 µg twice daily	4–11 y: Powder, 50–100 µg twice daily
Hydrocortisone sodium phosphate and sodium succinate	IV 100–200 mg q4–6h initially, then decreased or switched to an oral dosage form	IV 1–5 mg/kg q4–6h
Methylprednisolone sodium succinate	IV 10–40 mg q4–6h for 48–72 h	IV 0.5 mg/kg q4–6h
Prednisone	PO 20–60 mg/d	PO 2 mg/kg/d initially
Triamcinolone (Azmacort)	Oral inhalation, two inhalations three or four times per day; maximum dose, 16 inhalations/24 h	6–12 y: one or two inhalations three or four times per day; maximum dose, 12 inhalations/24 h
Leukotriene Inhibitors		
Montelukast (Singulair)	PO 10 mg once daily in the evening	≥15 y: Same as adults 6–14 y: PO 5 mg once daily in the evening 2–5 y: 4 mg once daily
Zafirlukast (Accolate)	PO 20 mg twice daily, 1 h before or 2 h after a meal	≥12 y: Same as adults <12 y: Dosage not established
Zileuton (Zyflo)	PO 600 mg four times daily	≥12 y: Same as adults <12 y: Dosage not established
Mast Cell Stabilizers		
Cromolyn (Intal)	Nebulizer solution, oral inhalation, 20 mg four times daily Aerosol spray, oral inhalation, two sprays four times daily	≥2 y: Same as adults ≥5 y: Same as adults
(Nasalcrom)	One spray in each nostril three to six times per day at regular intervals	≥6 y: Same as adults
Nedocromil (Tilade)	Inhalation, 4 mg q6–12h	>12 y: Same as adults

IV, intravenous; PO, oral.

scription in a pressurized aerosol form (eg, Primatene). Almost all over-the-counter aerosol products promoted for use in asthma contain epinephrine. These products are often abused and may delay the client from seeking medical attention. Clients should be cautioned that excessive use may produce hazardous cardiac stimulation and other adverse effects.

Albuterol, bitolterol, levalbuterol, and **pirbuterol** are short-acting beta$_2$-adrenergic agonists used for prevention and treatment of bronchoconstriction. These drugs act more selectively on beta$_2$ receptors and cause fewer cardiac effects than epinephrine. They are usually self-administered by metered-dose inhalation devices. Although most drug references still list a regular dosing schedule (eg, every 4 to 6 hours), asthma experts recommend that the drugs be used when needed (eg, to prevent dyspnea during exercise or to treat acute dyspnea that occurs during treatment with salmeterol). If these drugs are overused, they lose their bronchodilating effects because the beta$_2$-adrenergic receptors become unresponsive to stimulation. This tolerance does not occur with salmeterol.

Salmeterol is a long-acting beta$_2$-adrenergic agonist used only for *prophylaxis* of acute bronchoconstriction. It is not effective in acute attacks because it has a slow onset of action (approximately 20 minutes). Effects last 12 hours and the drug should not be taken more frequently. If additional bronchodilating medication is needed, a short-acting agent (eg, albuterol) should be used.

Isoproterenol is a short-acting bronchodilator and cardiac stimulant. When used for treatment of bronchospasm, isoproterenol is given by inhalation, alone or in combination with other agents.

Metaproterenol is a relatively selective, intermediate-acting beta$_2$-adrenergic agonist that may be given orally or by metered-dose inhaler. It is used to treat acute bronchospasm and to prevent exercise-induced asthma. In high doses, metaproterenol loses some of its selectivity and may cause cardiac and central nervous system (CNS) stimulation.

Terbutaline is a relatively selective beta$_2$-adrenergic agonist that is a long-acting bronchodilator. When given subcutaneously, terbutaline loses its selectivity and has little advantage over epinephrine. Muscle tremor is the most frequent side effect with this agent.

Xanthines

Xanthines (eg, theophylline) increase cyclic AMP by inhibiting the enzyme phosphodiesterase, which metabolizes cyclic AMP. Several other mechanisms of action (eg, increasing endogenous catecholamines, inhibiting calcium ion movement into smooth muscle, inhibiting prostaglandin synthesis and release, or inhibiting the release of bronchoconstrictive substances from mast cells and leukocytes) have also been proposed. In addition to bronchodilation, other effects that may be beneficial in asthma include inhibiting pulmonary edema by decreasing vascular permeability, increasing the ability of cilia to clear mucus from the airways, and strengthening contractions of the diaphragm. Xanthines also increase cardiac output, cause peripheral vasodilation, exert a mild diuretic effect, and stimulate the CNS. The cardiovascular and CNS effects are adverse effects. Serum drug levels should be monitored to help regulate dosage and avoid adverse effects. These drugs are contraindicated in clients with acute gastritis and peptic ulcer disease; they should be used cautiously in those with cardiovascular disorders that could be aggravated by drug-induced cardiac stimulation.

Theophylline may be used in the prevention and treatment of bronchoconstriction associated with asthma, bronchitis, and emphysema. Numerous dosage forms are available. Theophylline ethylenediamine (aminophylline) contains approximately 85% theophylline and is the only formulation that can be given intravenously (IV). It may be used for acute bronchoconstriction. Oral theophylline preparations are used for long-term treatment of chronic disorders. Most formulations contain anhydrous theophyl-

line (100% theophylline) as the active ingredient, and sustained-action tablets (eg, Theo-Dur, Theobid) are more commonly used than other formulations. Theophylline is metabolized in the liver; metabolites and some unchanged drug are excreted through the kidneys.

Anticholinergic

Anticholinergics (see Chap. 21) block the action of acetylcholine in bronchial smooth muscle when given by inhalation. This action reduces intracellular GMP, a bronchoconstrictive substance.

Ipratropium was formulated to be taken by inhalation for maintenance therapy of bronchoconstriction associated with chronic bronchitis and emphysema. Improved pulmonary function usually occurs within 15 minutes, peaks in 1 to 2 hours, and lasts approximately 4 hours. Ipratropium acts synergistically with adrenergic bronchodilators and may be used concomitantly. However, it is ineffective in acute bronchospasm when a rapid response is required. It should be used with caution in clients with narrow-angle glaucoma and prostatic hypertrophy. The most common adverse effects are cough, nervousness, nausea, gastrointestinal upset, headache, and dizziness.

Anti-inflammatory Agents
Corticosteroids

Corticosteroids are used in the treatment of acute and chronic asthma and other bronchoconstrictive disorders, in which they have two major actions. First, they suppress inflammation in the airways by inhibiting the following processes: movement of fluid and protein into tissues; migration and function of neutrophils and eosinophils; synthesis of histamine in mast cells; and production of proinflammatory substances (eg, prostaglandins, leukotrienes, several interleukins, and others). Beneficial effects of suppressing airway inflammation include decreased mucus secretion, decreased edema of airway mucosa, and repair of damaged epithelium, with subsequent reduction of airway reactivity. A second action is to increase the number and sensitivity of beta$_2$-adrenergic receptors, which restores or increases the effectiveness of beta$_2$-adrenergic bronchodilators. The number of beta$_2$ receptors increases within approximately 4 hours, and improved responsiveness to beta$_2$ agonists occurs within approximately 2 hours.

These drugs should be used with caution in clients with peptic ulcer disease, inflammatory bowel disease, hypertension, congestive heart failure, and thromboembolic disorders.

Beclomethasone, **budesonide**, **flunisolide**, **fluticasone**, and **triamcinolone** are topical corticosteroids for inhalation. Topical administration minimizes systemic absorption and adverse effects. These preparations may substitute for or allow reduced dosage of systemic corticosteroids. In people with asthma who are taking an oral corticosteroid, the oral dosage is reduced slowly (over weeks to months) when an inhaled corticosteroid is added. The goal is to give the lowest oral dose necessary to control symptoms. Beclomethasone, flunisolide, and fluticasone also are available in nasal solutions for treatment of allergic rhinitis, which may play a role in bronchoconstriction. Because systemic absorption occurs in clients using inhaled corticosteroids, fluticasone and high doses of the other drugs should be reserved for those otherwise requiring oral corticosteroids.

Hydrocortisone, prednisone, and **methylprednisolone** are given to clients who require systemic corticosteroids. Corticosteroids may be given IV in acute, severe attacks of asthma or bronchospasm; they may be given orally in chronic asthma or bronchospasm.

Leukotriene Inhibitors

Leukotrienes are strong chemical mediators of bronchoconstriction and inflammation (see Chap. 1), the major pathologic features of asthma. They also increase mucus secretion and mucosal edema in the respiratory tract. Leukotriene-inhibitor drugs were developed to counteract these effects and are indicated for the prophylaxis and chronic treatment of asthma in adults and children 12 years of age and older. Although the drugs are not effective in relieving acute asthma attacks, they may be continued concurrently with other drugs during acute episodes.

The leukotriene-inhibitor drugs include three agents with two different mechanisms of action. **Zileuton** inhibits lipoxygenase and thereby reduces formation of leukotrienes; **montelukast** and **zafirlukast** inhibit leukotriene receptors and are classified as leukotriene receptor antagonists. The drugs are used for *prevention* of asthma attacks; they are not effective in relieving bronchospasm in acute asthma attacks. The drugs can be used alone or combined with low doses of corticosteroids. They are contraindicated in clients with hypersensitivity to the drugs, and zileuton is contraindicated in clients with active liver disease or substantially elevated liver enzymes (three times the upper limit of normal values).

Montelukast and zafirlukast are well absorbed with oral administration. They are metabolized in the liver by the cytochrome P450 enzyme system and may interact with other drugs metabolized by this system. Most metabolites are excreted in the feces. Zafirlukast is excreted in breast milk and should not be taken during lactation. The most common adverse effects reported in clinical trials were headache, nausea, diarrhea, and infection.

Zileuton is well absorbed, highly bound to serum albumin (93%), and metabolized by the cytochrome P450 liver enzymes; metabolites are excreted mainly in urine. Hepatic aminotransferase enzymes should be monitored during zileuton therapy and the drug should be discontinued if enzyme levels reach five times the normal values or if symptoms of liver dysfunction develop. Elevation of liver enzymes was the most serious adverse effect during clinical trials; other adverse effects include headache, pain, and nausea. Zileuton increases serum concentrations of propranolol, theophylline, and warfarin.

Mast Cell Stabilizers

Cromolyn and **nedocromil** stabilize mast cells and prevent the release of bronchoconstrictive and inflammatory substances when mast cells are confronted with allergens and other stimuli. The drugs are indicated only for prophylaxis of acute asthma attacks in clients with chronic asthma; they are not effective in acute bronchospasm or status asthmaticus and should not be used in these conditions. Use of one of these drugs may allow reduced dosage of bronchodilators and corticosteroids.

The drugs are taken by inhalation. Cromolyn is available in a metered-dose aerosol and a solution for use with a power-operated nebulizer. A nasal solution is also available for prevention and treatment of allergic rhinitis. Nedocromil is available in a metered-dose aerosol.

Mast cell stabilizers are contraindicated in clients who are hypersensitive to the drugs. They should be used with caution in clients with impaired renal or hepatic function. Also, the propellants in the aerosols may aggravate coronary artery disease or arrhythmias.

NURSING PROCESS

Assessment

Assess the client's pulmonary function:

- General assessment factors include rate and character of respiration, skin color, arterial blood gas analysis, and pulmonary function tests. Abnormal breathing patterns (eg, rate below 12 or above 24 per minute, dyspnea, cough, orthopnea, wheezing, "noisy" respirations) may indicate respiratory distress. Severe respiratory distress is characterized by tachypnea, dyspnea, use of accessory muscles of respiration, and hypoxia. Early signs of hypoxia include mental confusion, restlessness, anxiety, and increased blood pressure and pulse rate. Late signs include cyanosis and decreased blood pressure and pulse. Hypoxemia is confirmed if arterial blood gas analysis shows decreased partial pressure of oxygen (Po_2).
- In acute bronchospasm, a medical emergency, the client is in obvious and severe respiratory distress. A characteristic feature of bronchospasm is forceful expiration or wheezing.
- If the client has chronic asthma, try to determine the frequency and severity of acute attacks, factors that precipitate or relieve acute attacks,

antiasthmatic medications taken occasionally or regularly, allergies, and condition between acute attacks, such as restrictions in activities of daily living due to asthma.

- If the client has chronic bronchitis or emphysema, assess for signs of respiratory distress, hypoxia, cough, amount and character of sputum, exercise tolerance (eg, dyspnea on exertion, dyspnea at rest), medications, and nondrug treatment measures (eg, breathing exercises, chest physiotherapy).

Nursing Diagnoses

- Impaired Gas Exchange related to bronchoconstriction and excessive mucus production
- Ineffective Breathing Pattern related to bronchoconstriction
- Activity Intolerance related to fatigue
- Self Care Deficit related to impaired gas exchange
- Altered Nutrition: Less Than Body Requirements related to fatigue
- Risk for Injury: Respiratory infection
- Anxiety related to chronic illness
- Altered Tissue Perfusion related to bronchodilator-induced cardiac stimulation and arrhythmias
- Noncompliance: Overuse of adrenergic bronchodilators
- Sleep Pattern Disturbance: Insomnia with adrenergic and xanthine bronchodilators
- Altered Thought Processes: Confusion and nervousness related to CNS stimulation with adrenergic and xanthine bronchodilators
- Knowledge Deficit: Factors precipitating bronchoconstriction
- Knowledge Deficit: Measures to avoid precipitating factors and respiratory infection
- Knowledge Deficit: Accurate self-administration of drugs, including use of inhalers

Planning/Goals

The client will:

- Self-administer bronchodilating and other drugs accurately
- Experience relief of symptoms
- Avoid preventable adverse drug effects
- Avoid overusing bronchodilating drugs
- Avoid exposure to stimuli that cause bronchospasm when possible
- Avoid respiratory infections when possible

Interventions

Use measures to prevent or relieve bronchoconstriction when possible. General measures include those to prevent respiratory disease or promote an adequate airway. Some specific measures include the following:

- Use mechanical measures for removing respiratory tract secretions and preventing their retention. Effective measures include coughing, deep breathing, percussion, and postural drainage.
- Help the client identify and avoid exposure to conditions that precipitate bronchoconstriction. For example, allergens may be removed from the home, school, or work environment. When bronchospasm is precipitated by exercise, prophylaxis by prior inhalation of bronchodilating agents is better than avoiding exercise, especially in children.
- Assist clients with asthma to identify early signs of difficulty, including increased need for beta-adrenergic agonists, activity limitations, and waking at night with asthma symptoms.
- Monitor peak expiratory flow rate (PEFR) when indicated. Portable meters are available for use in clinics, physicians' offices, and clients' homes. This is an objective measure of airflow/airway obstruction and helps to evaluate the client's treatment regimen.
- Assist clients with moderate to severe asthma in obtaining meters and learning to measure PEFR. Clients with a decreased PEFR may need treatment to prevent acute, severe respiratory distress.
- Assist clients and at least one family member in managing acute attacks of bronchoconstriction, including when to seek emergency care.
- Try to prevent or reduce anxiety, which may aggravate bronchospasm. Stay with the client during an acute asthma attack if feasible. Clients experiencing severe and prolonged bronchospasm (status asthmaticus) should be admitted or transferred to a hospital intensive care unit.

Evaluation

- Observe for relief of symptoms and improved arterial blood gas values.
- Interview and observe for correct drug administration, including use of inhalers.
- Interview and observe for tachyarrhythmias, nervousness, insomnia, and other adverse drug effects.
- Interview about and observe behaviors to avoid stimuli that cause bronchoconstriction and respiratory infections.

CLIENT TEACHING GUIDELINES
Antiasthmatic Drugs

General Considerations

✔ Asthma and other chronic lung diseases are characterized by constant inflammation of the airways and periodic or persistent labored breathing from constriction or narrowing of the airways. Antiasthmatic drugs are often given in combination to combat these problems. Thus, it is extremely important to know the type and purpose of each drug.

✔ Except for the short-acting, inhaled bronchodilators (eg, albuterol), antiasthmatic medications are used long term to control symptoms and prevent acute asthma attacks. This means they must be taken on a regular schedule and continued when symptom free.

✔ When an asthma attack (ie, acute bronchospasm with shortness of breath, wheezing respirations, cough) occurs, the only fast-acting, commonly used medication to relieve these symptoms is an inhaled bronchodilator (eg, albuterol). Other inhaled and oral drugs are not effective and should not be used.

✔ Try to prevent symptoms. For example, respiratory infections can precipitate difficulty in breathing. Avoiding infections (eg, by good hand washing, avoiding people with infections, annual influenza vaccinations, and other measures) can prevent acute asthma attacks. If you are allergic to tobacco smoke, perfume, or flowers, try to avoid or minimize exposure.

✔ A common cause of acute asthma attacks is not taking medications correctly. Some studies indicate that one third to two thirds of clients with asthma do not comply with instructions for using their medications. Factors that contribute to noncompliance with drug therapy include long-term use, expense, and adverse effects. If you have difficulty taking medications as prescribed, discuss the situation with a health care provider. Cheaper medications or lower doses may be effective alternatives. Just stopping the medications may precipitate acute breathing problems.

✔ If unable to prevent symptoms, early recognition and treatment may help prevent severe distress and hospitalizations. Signs of impending difficulty include increased needs for bronchodilator inhalers, activity limitations, waking at night because of asthma symptoms, and variability in the peak expiratory flow rate (PEFR), if you use a PEFR meter at home. The first treatment is to use a short-acting, inhaled bronchodilator. If this does not improve breathing, seek emergency care.

✔ Keep adequate supplies of medications on hand. Missing a few doses of "preventive" medications may precipitate an acute asthma attack; not using an inhaled bronchodilator for early breathing difficulty may lead to more severe problems and the need for emergency treatment or hospitalization.

✔ Be sure you can use your metered-dose inhalers correctly. Many patients do not.

✔ Drinking 2 to 3 quarts of fluids daily helps thin secretions in the throat and lungs and makes them easier to remove.

✔ Avoid tobacco smoke and other substances that irritate breathing passages (eg, aerosol hair spray, antiperspirants, and cleaning products) when possible.

✔ Avoid excessive intake of coffee, tea, and cola drinks. These caffeine-containing beverages may increase bronchodilation but also may increase nervousness and insomnia with bronchodilating drugs.

✔ Take influenza vaccine annually and pneumococcal vaccine once if you have chronic lung disease.

✔ Inform all health care providers about the medications you are taking and do not take over-the-counter drugs without consulting a health care provider. Some drugs can decrease beneficial effects or increase adverse effects of antiasthmatic medications. For example, over-the-counter nasal decongestants, asthma remedies, cold remedies, and antisleep medications can increase the rapid heartbeat, palpitations, and nervousness often associated with bronchodilators.

Self-administration

✔ Follow instructions carefully. Better breathing with minimal adverse effects depends on accurate use of prescribed medications. If help is needed with metered-dose inhalers, consult a health care provider.

✔ Use short-acting bronchodilator inhalers as needed, not on a regular schedule. If desired effects are not achieved or if symptoms worsen, inform the prescribing physician. Do not increase dosage or frequency of taking medication.

✔ If taking salmeterol, a long-acting bronchodilator inhaler, do not use more often than every 12 hours. If constricted breathing occurs, use a short-acting bronchodilator inhaler. Salmeterol does not relieve acute shortness of breath because it takes approximately 20 minutes to start acting and 1 to 4 hours to achieve maximal bronchodilating effects.

✔ If taking an oral or inhaled corticosteroid, take on a regular schedule, approximately the same time each day. The purpose of these drugs is to relieve inflammation in the airways and *prevent* acute respiratory distress. They are not effective unless taken regularly.

✔ If taking oral theophylline, take fast-acting preparations before meals with a full glass of water, at regular intervals around the clock. If gastrointestinal upset occurs, take with food. Take long-acting preparations every 8 to 12 hours; do not chew or crush.

✔ Take zafirlukast 1 hour before or 2 hours after a meal; montelukast and zileuton may be taken with or without food.

(continued)

CLIENT TEACHING GUIDELINES
Antiasthmatic Drugs (continued)

✔ Use inhalers correctly:
1. Shake well immediately before each use.
2. Remove the cap from the mouthpiece.
3. Exhale to the end of a normal breath.
4. With the inhaler in the upright position, place the mouthpiece just inside the mouth, and use the lips to form a tight seal or hold the mouthpiece approximately two finger-widths from the open mouth.
5. While pressing down on the inhaler, take a slow, deep

breath for 3 to 5 seconds, hold the breath for approximately 10 seconds, and exhale slowly.
6. Wait 3 to 5 min before taking a second inhalation of the drug.
7. Rinse the mouth with water after each use.
8. Rinse the mouthpiece and store the inhaler away from heat.
9. If you have difficulty using an inhaler, ask your physician about a spacer device (a tube attached to the inhaler that makes it easier to use).

PRINCIPLES OF THERAPY

Drug Selection and Administration

Choice of drug and route of administration are determined largely by the severity of the disease process and the client's response to therapy. Some guidelines include the following:

1. A selective, short-acting, inhaled beta$_2$-adrenergic agonist (eg, albuterol) is the initial drug of choice for acute bronchospasm. The long-acting drug salmeterol should *not* be used because its slow onset of action makes it ineffective in acute bronchospasm.
2. Because aerosol products act directly on the lungs, drugs given by inhalation can usually be given in smaller doses and produce fewer adverse effects than oral or parenteral drugs.
3. Theophylline is usually given orally in an extended-release formulation for chronic disorders, such as COPD. Although IV aminophylline has been used to treat acute asthma attacks, some studies indicate no benefit from its addition to inhaled beta$_2$ agonists and systemic corticosteroids.
4. Ipratropium, the anticholinergic bronchodilator, is most useful in the long-term management of COPD. It is ineffective in relieving acute bronchospasm.

How Can You Avoid This Medication Error?

Keith Wilson, 66 years of age, has worsening chronic obstructive pulmonary disease. At his last office visit, his physician added ipratropium bromide (Atrovent) and beclomethasone (Vanceril) to his beta-adrenergic (Alupent) inhaler. He visits the office complaining of severe dyspnea. You quickly grab his Atrovent inhaler to administer a PRN dose and try to get him to relax. What drug error has occurred, and how could this error be avoided?

5. Cromolyn and nedocromil are used prophylactically; they are ineffective in acute bronchospasm.
6. Because inflammation has been established as a major component of asthma and other bronchoconstrictive respiratory disorders, inhaled corticosteroids are being used early in the disease process, often with bronchodilators or mast cell stabilizers. In acute bronchoconstriction, a corticosteroid is often given orally or IV for several days.

   In chronic disorders, inhaled corticosteroids should be taken on a regular schedule. These drugs may be effective when used alone or with relatively small doses of an oral corticosteroid. Optimal schedules of administration are not clearly established, but more frequent dosing (eg, every 6 hours) may be more effective than less frequent dosing (eg, every 12 hours), even if the total amount is the same. As with systemic glucocorticoid therapy, the recommended dose is the lowest amount required to control symptoms. High doses (>1500 μg daily in adults and 800 μg daily in children) suppress adrenocortical function, but much less than systemic drugs. Small doses (eg, 600 μg of beclomethasone daily) may impair bone metabolism and predispose adults to osteoporosis by decreasing calcium deposition and increasing calcium resorption from bone. In children, chronic administration of corticosteroids may retard growth. Local adverse effects (oropharyngeal candidiasis, hoarseness) can be decreased by reducing the dose, administering less often, rinsing the mouth after use, or using a spacer device. These measures decrease the amount of drug deposited in the oral cavity. The inhaled drugs seem to be well tolerated with chronic use.
7. Using a combination of drugs may be more effective than using a single agent. One advantage of a multidrug regimen is that smaller doses of each agent usually can be given. This may decrease adverse effects and allow dosages to be increased when exacerbation of symptoms occurs.

8. A common regimen for treatment of asthma is an inhaled corticosteroid on a regular schedule, two to four times daily, and an inhaled beta$_2$-adrenergic agonist as needed for prevention or treatment of bronchoconstriction. When leukotriene inhibitors are added to a regimen, they reduce the need for corticosteroids and as-needed inhaled bronchodilators.

Dosage Factors

Dosage of bronchodilators, corticosteroids, and mast cell stabilizers must be individualized so the smallest effective amounts are given. With theophylline preparations, guidelines include the following:

1. Dosage should be individualized. One way is to start with a low dose and gradually increase the amount according to symptom relief and serum theophylline levels. Serum levels should be monitored because of individual differences in hepatic metabolism; therapeutic range is 5 to 15 μg/mL. Serum levels of 20 μg/mL or above are associated with a high incidence of toxicity. Blood for serum levels should be drawn 1 to 2 hours after immediate-release dosage forms and 4 hours after sustained-release forms.
2. Children and cigarette smokers usually need higher doses to maintain therapeutic blood levels because they metabolize theophylline rapidly.
3. Clients who have liver disease, congestive heart failure, chronic pulmonary disease, or acute viral infections usually need smaller doses because these conditions impair theophylline metabolism.
4. For obese clients, theophylline dosage should be calculated on the basis of lean or ideal body weight because theophylline is not highly distributed in fatty tissue.

Use in Children

Antiasthmatic medications are used in children and adolescents for the same indications as for adults. With adrenergic bronchodilators, recommendations for use vary according to route of administration and age of the child.

Nursing Notes: Apply Your Knowledge

Gwen, 12 years of age, has just been diagnosed with asthma. She states, "I will use the inhalers at home, but I don't want to take them to school." How will you develop a plan to teach Gwen to use her inhalers and evaluate her ability to do so effectively?

Inhalation of albuterol, bitolterol, metaproterenol, and terbutaline is not recommended in children younger than 12 years of age. In addition, extended-release tablets of albuterol are not recommended for children younger than 12 years, and the syrup formulation is not recommended for children younger than 2 years of age. Metaproterenol oral tablets are not recommended for children younger than 6 years, and terbutaline oral tablets are not recommended for children younger than 12 years of age.

With theophylline, use in children should be closely monitored because dosage needs and rates of metabolism vary widely. In children younger than 6 months, especially premature infants and neonates, drug elimination may be prolonged because of immature liver function. Except for preterm infants with apnea, theophylline preparations are not recommended for use in this age group. Children 6 months to 16 years of age, approximately, metabolize theophylline more rapidly than younger or older clients. Thus, they may need higher doses than adults in proportion to size and weight. If the child is obese, the dosage should be calculated on the basis of lean or ideal body weight because the drug is not highly distributed in fatty tissue. Long-acting dosage forms are not recommended for children younger than 6 years of age. Children may become hyperactive and disruptive from the CNS-stimulating effects of theophylline. Tolerance to these effects usually develops with continued use of the drug.

Corticosteroids are being used earlier in children as in adults. The effectiveness and safety of inhaled corticosteroids in children older than 3 years of age is well established; few data are available on the use of inhaled drugs in those younger than 3 years. A major concern in children is impairment of bone growth, even with inhaled drugs. Bone growth should be monitored closely, especially in children between 4 and 10 years of age.

Leukotriene inhibitors have not been extensively studied in children and adolescents. With montelukast, the 10-mg film-coated tablet is recommended for adolescents 15 years of age and older and a 4-mg chewable tablet is recommended for children 2 to 5 years of age. Safety and effectiveness of zafirlukast in children younger than 12 years have not been established.

Cromolyn aerosol solution may be used in children 5 years of age and older, and nebulizer solution is used with children 2 years and older. Nedocromil is not established as safe and effective in children younger than 12 years of age.

Use in Older Adults

Older adults often have pulmonary disorders for which bronchodilators and antiasthmatic medications are used. As with other populations, administering the medications by inhalation and giving the lowest effective dose decrease adverse effects. The main risks with adrenergic broncho-dilators are excessive cardiac and CNS stimulation.

Theophylline use must be carefully monitored because drug effects are unpredictable. On the one hand, cigarette smoking and drugs that stimulate drug-metabolizing enzymes in the liver (eg, phenobarbital, phenytoin) increase the rate of metabolism and therefore dosage requirements. On the other hand, impaired liver function, decreased blood flow to the liver, and some drugs (eg, cimetidine, erythromycin) impair metabolism and therefore decrease dosage requirements. Adverse effects include cardiac and CNS stimulation. Safety can be increased by measuring serum drug levels and adjusting dosage to maintain therapeutic levels of 5 to 15 μg/mL. If the client is obese, dosage should be based on lean or ideal body weight because theophylline is not highly distributed in fatty tissue.

Corticosteroids increase the risks of osteoporosis and cataracts in older adults. Leukotriene inhibitors usually are well tolerated by older adults, with pharmacokinetics and effects similar to those in younger adults. With zafirlukast, however, blood levels are higher and elimination is slower than in younger adults. Zileuton is contraindicated in older adults with underlying hepatic dysfunction.

Use in Renal Impairment

Bronchodilating and anti-inflammatory drugs can usually be used without dosage adjustments in clients with impaired renal function. Beta agonists may be given by inhalation or parenteral routes. Theophylline can be given in usual doses, but serum drug levels should be monitored periodically. Most corticosteroids are eliminated by hepatic metabolism, and dosage reductions are not needed in clients with renal impairment. No data are available about the use of montelukast, and no dosage adjustments are recommended for zafirlukast or zileuton.

Cromolyn is eliminated by renal and biliary excretion; the drug should be given in reduced doses, if at all, in clients with renal impairment.

Use in Hepatic Impairment

Montelukast and zafirlukast produce higher blood levels and are eliminated more slowly in clients with hepatic impairment. However, no dosage adjustment is recommended for clients with mild to moderate hepatic impairment. Zileuton is associated with hepatotoxicity and contraindicated in clients with active liver disease or aminotransferase elevations of three times the upper limit of normal or higher. Recommendations to avoid hepatotoxicity include measuring hepatic aminotransferases (eg, alanine aminotransferase) before starting zileuton, once a month for the first 3 months of therapy, every 2 to

3 months for the remainder of the first year, and periodically thereafter. The drug should be discontinued if symptoms of liver dysfunction develop (eg, right upper quadrant pain, nausea, fatigue, pruritus, jaundice, or flu-like symptoms) or aminotransferase levels increase to more than five times the upper limit of normal.

Cromolyn is eliminated by renal and biliary excretion; the drug should be given in reduced doses, if at all, in clients with hepatic impairment.

Use in Critical Illness

Acute, severe asthma (status asthmaticus) is characterized by severe respiratory distress and requires emergency treatment. Beta$_2$ agonists should be given in high doses and as often as every 20 minutes for 1 to 2 hours (by metered-dose inhalers with spacer devices or by compressed-air nebulization). Then, dosage can usually be reduced and dosing intervals extended. High doses of corticosteroids are also given for several days, usually IV initially, then orally.

When respiratory function improves, efforts to prevent future episodes are needed. These efforts may include identifying and avoiding suspected triggers, evaluation and possible adjustment of the client's treatment regimen, and assessment of the client's adherence to the prescribed regimen.

 Home Care

All of the drugs discussed in this chapter are used in the home setting. A major role of the home care nurse is to assist clients in using the drugs safely and effectively. Several studies have indicated that many people do not use metered-dose inhalers and other devices correctly. The home care nurse needs to observe a client using an inhalation device when possible. If errors in technique are assessed, teaching or reteaching may be needed. With inhaled medications, a spacer device may be useful, especially for children and older adults, because less muscle coordination is required to administer a dose. Adverse effects may be minimized as well.

For clients with asthma, especially children, assess the environment for potential triggers of acute bronchospasm, such as cigarette smoking. In addition, assist clients to recognize and treat (or get help for) exacerbations before respiratory distress becomes severe.

With theophylline, the home care nurse needs to assess the client and the environment for substances that may affect metabolism of theophylline and decrease therapeutic effects or increase adverse effects. In addition, the nurse needs to reinforce the importance of not exceeding the prescribed dose, not crushing long-acting formulations, reporting adverse effects, and keeping appointments for follow-up care.

NURSING ACTIONS	RATIONALE/EXPLANATION

1. Administer accurately

a. Be sure clients have adequate supplies of inhaled bronchodilators and corticosteroids available for self-administration. Observe technique of self-administration for accuracy and assist if needed.

b. Give immediate-release oral theophylline before meals with a full glass of water, at regular intervals around the clock. If gastrointestinal upset occurs, give with food.

To promote dissolution and absorption. Taking with food may decrease nausea and vomiting.

c. Give sustained-release theophylline q8–12h, with instructions not to chew or crush.

Sustained-release drug formulations should never be chewed or crushed because doing so causes immediate release of potentially toxic doses.

d. Give intravenous (IV) aminophylline no faster than 25 mg/min.

IV aminophylline is usually given as a loading dose for faster effects, followed by a maintenance infusion. Rapid administration may cause toxic effects.

e. Give zafirlukast 1 h before or 2 h after a meal; montelukast and zileuton may be given with or without food.

The bioavailability of zafirlukast is reduced approximately 40% if taken with food. Food does not significantly affect the bioavailability of montelukast and zileuton.

2. Observe for therapeutic effects

a. Decreased dyspnea, wheezing, and respiratory secretions

b. Reduced rate and improved quality of respirations

c. Reduced anxiety and restlessness

d. Therapeutic serum levels of theophylline (5–15 µg/mL)

e. Improved arterial blood gas levels (normal values: PO_2 80 to 100 mm Hg; PCO_2 35 to 45 mm Hg; pH, 7.35 to 7.45)

f. Improved exercise tolerance

g. Decreased incidence and severity of acute attacks of bronchospasm with chronic administration of drugs

Relief of bronchospasm and wheezing should be evident within a few minutes after giving subcutaneous epinephrine, IV aminophylline, or aerosolized adrenergic bronchodilators.

3. Observe for adverse effects

a. With adrenergic bronchodilators, observe for tachycardia, arrhythmias, palpitations, restlessness, agitation, insomnia.

These signs and symptoms result from cardiac and central nervous system (CNS) stimulation.

b. With ipratropium, observe for cough or exacerbation of symptoms.

Ipratropium produces few adverse effects because it is not absorbed systemically.

c. With xanthine bronchodilators, observe for tachycardia, arrhythmias, palpitations, restlessness, agitation, insomnia, nausea, vomiting, convulsions.

Theophylline causes cardiac and CNS stimulation. Convulsions occur at toxic serum concentrations (>20 µg/mL). They may occur without preceding

(continued)

NURSING ACTIONS	RATIONALE/EXPLANATION
	symptoms of toxicity and may result in death. IV diazepam (Valium) may be used to control seizures. Theophylline also stimulates the chemoreceptor trigger zone in the medulla oblongata to cause nausea and vomiting.
d. With inhaled corticosteroids, observe for hoarseness, cough, throat irritation, and fungal infection of mouth and throat.	Inhaled corticosteroids are unlikely to produce the serious adverse effects of long-term systemic therapy (see Chap. 24).
e. With leukotriene inhibitors, observe for headache, infection, nausea, pain, elevated liver enzymes (eg, alanine aminotransferase [ALT]), and liver dysfunction.	These drugs are usually well tolerated. A highly elevated ALT and liver dysfunction are more likely to occur with zileuton.
f. With cromolyn, observe for arrhythmias, hypotension, chest pain, restlessness, dizziness, convulsions, CNS depression, anorexia, nausea and vomiting. Sedation and coma may occur with overdosage.	Some of the cardiovascular effects are thought to be caused by the propellants used in the aerosol preparation.
4. Observe for drug interactions	
a. Drugs that *increase* effects of bronchodilators:	
(1) Monoamine oxidase inhibitors	These drugs inhibit the metabolism of catecholamines. The subsequent administration of bronchodilators may increase blood pressure.
(2) Erythromycin, clindamycin, cimetidine	These drugs may decrease theophylline clearance and thereby increase plasma levels.
b. Drugs that *decrease* effects of bronchodilators:	
(1) Lithium	Lithium may increase excretion of theophylline and therefore decrease therapeutic effectiveness.
(2) Phenobarbital	This drug may increase the metabolism of theophylline by way of enzyme induction.
(3) Propranolol, other nonselective beta blockers	These drugs may cause bronchoconstriction and oppose effects of bronchodilators.
c. Drugs that alter effects of zafirlukast:	
(1) Aspirin	Increases blood levels
(2) Erythromycin, theophylline	Decrease blood levels

How Can You Avoid This Medication Error?

Answer: Only short-acting beta-adrenergic bronchodilators should be used for acute dyspnea. Alupent, not Atrovent, is indicated. When patients have more than one inhaler, they should be taught which inhaler to use in emergency situations. The canister should be a different color (many manufacturers consider this) or clearly marked with tape, so that quick identification can occur in an emergency. Additional teaching may be indicated for the nurse and the patient regarding the action of each inhaler.

Nursing Notes: Apply Your Knowledge

Answer: First, it is very important to listen to Gwen's concerns about using her inhalers in school. Do not minimize her feelings, and try to understand why she feels the way she does. Adolescents do not like to feel different, and peer acceptance is very important. Ultimately, the decision will be Gwen's. It is important that she understand the consequences should she

(*continued*)

decide not to use her inhalers at school (exacerbation of her asthma; acute, embarrassing attack at school), but do not threaten or beg. It is important that Gwen feel responsible for managing this chronic condition. Assure her that there will be a room where she can use her inhalers privately, after calling the school nurse to make sure that this is true.

Proper technique in using an inhaler is important to ensure that medication reaches the lung parenchyma. Shake the canister and remove the cap from the mouthpiece. Stress the importance of good posture (sitting or standing) so lungs can expand fully, and have Gwen exhale completely. Holding the inhaler in an upright position 1 to 2 inches from her mouth, Gwen should coordinate pressing the canister down as she inhales. Encourage Gwen to hold her breath for 10 seconds (if possible) to optimize medication delivery. She should wait 3 to 5 minutes before administering the second dose or using a different inhaler. Make sure you clearly mark which inhaler should be used in an emergency. To evaluate Gwen's technique, watch her use the inhaler. You will observe to see if she is able to coordinate her breathing with medication delivery. If this coordination is a problem, a spacer can be ordered. This allows the medication to sit in a cylinder so that it can be inhaled fully when inhaling over time.

REVIEW AND APPLICATION EXERCISES

1. What are some causes of bronchoconstriction, and how can they be prevented or minimized?

2. How do beta-adrenergic agonists and theophylline act as bronchodilators?

3. What adverse effects are associated with bronchodilators, and how can they be prevented or minimized?

4. What is the therapeutic range of serum theophylline levels, and why should they be monitored?

5. For what effects are corticosteroids used in the treatment of bronchoconstrictive respiratory disorders?

6. For what effects are leukotriene inhibitors used in the treatment of asthma?

7. How do cromolyn and nedocromil act to prevent acute asthma attacks?

8. What are the main elements of treating respiratory distress from acute bronchospasm?

SELECTED REFERENCES

Busse, W.W. (1996). Long- and short-acting beta₂-adrenergic agonists. *Archives of Internal Medicine, 156*, 1514–1520.

Cockcroft, D.W. (1999). Pharmacologic therapy for asthma: Overview and historical perspective. *Journal of Clinical Pharmacology, 39*, 216–222.

Cockcroft, D.W. & Kalra, S. (1996). Outpatient asthma management. *Medical Clinics of North America, 80*, 701–718.

Drug facts and comparisons. (Updated monthly). St. Louis: Facts and Comparisons.

Guyton, A.C. & Hall, J.E. (1996). *Textbook of medical physiology*, 9th ed. Philadelphia: W.B. Saunders.

Kelly, H.W. & Kamada, A.K. (1997). Asthma. In J.T. DiPiro, R.L. Talbert, G.C. Yee, G.R. Matzke, B.G. Wells, & L.M. Posey (Eds.), *Pharmacotherapy: A pathophysiologic approach*, 3rd ed., pp. 553–590. Stamford, CT: Appleton & Lange.

Larsen, G.L. (1999). Pediatric asthma: Towards the millennium. An update from the 1999 American Lung Association/American Thoracic Society international conference. [Online: Available *http://www.medscape.com/Medscape/RespiratoryCare/TreatmentUpdate/1999/tu01/public/toc-tu01.html.* Accessed September 11, 1999.]

Middleton, A.D. (1997). Managing asthma: It takes teamwork. *American Journal of Nursing, 97*(1), 39–43.

Noyes, M.A. & Stratton, M.A. (1997). Chronic obstructive lung disease. In J.T. DiPiro, R.L. Talbert, G.C. Yee, G.R. Matzke, B.G. Wells, & L.M. Posey (Eds.), *Pharmacotherapy: A pathophysiologic approach*, 3rd ed., pp. 591–613. Stamford, CT: Appleton & Lange.

Owen, C.L. (1999). New directions in asthma management. *American Journal of Nursing, 99*(3), 26–33

Pittman, A. & Tillinghast, J. (1998). Allergy and immunology. In C.F. Carey, H.H. Lee, & K.F. Woeltje (Eds.), *The Washington manual of medical therapeutics*, 29th ed., pp. 213–226. Philadelphia: Lippincott Williams & Wilkins.

Porth, C.M. (Ed.). (1998). *Pathophysiology: Concepts of altered health states*, 5th ed. Philadelphia: Lippincott Williams & Wilkins.

Taylor, D.R., Sears, M.R., & Cockcroft, D.W. (1997). The beta-agonist controversy. *Medical Clinics of North America, 80*, 719–748.

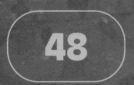

48

Antihistamines

Objectives

After studying this chapter, the student will be able to:

1. Delineate effects of histamine on selected body tissues.

2. Differentiate histamine receptors.

3. Describe the types of hypersensitivity or allergic reactions.

4. Discuss allergic rhinitis, allergic contact dermatitis, and drug allergies as conditions for which antihistamines are commonly used.

5. Identify the effects of histamine that are blocked by histamine-1 receptor antagonist drugs.

6. Differentiate first- and second-generation antihistamines.

7. Describe antihistamines in terms of indications for use, adverse effects, and nursing process implications.

8. Discuss the use of antihistamines in special populations.

You are working at the college health center. John, a freshman, comes to the clinic complaining of seasonal pollen allergies that have worsened significantly since his relocation at college. He has been self-treating with over-the-counter (OTC) medications a friend in the dorms gave him.

Reflect on:

▶ Assessment of John's allergy history and factors that may have increased John's allergic response.

▶ Appropriate teaching about the allergic response and how antihistamines work.

▶ Informed use of OTC allergy medications to manage symptoms, including side effects and interactions.

▶ Nonpharmacologic methods to prevent or limit allergic reactions.

Antihistamines are drugs that antagonize the action of histamine. Thus, to understand the use of these drugs, it is necessary to understand histamine and its effects on body tissues, characteristics of allergic reactions, and selected conditions for which antihistamines are used.

HISTAMINE AND ITS RECEPTORS

Histamine, the first chemical mediator to be released, is very important in immune and inflammatory responses. It is synthesized and stored in most body tissues, with high concentrations in tissues exposed to environmental substances (eg, the skin and mucosal surfaces of the eye, nose, lungs, and gastrointestinal [GI] tract). It is also found in the central nervous system (CNS). In these tissues, histamine is located mainly in secretory granules of mast cells (tissue cells surrounding capillaries) and basophils (circulating blood cells).

Histamine is discharged from mast cells and basophils in response to certain stimuli (eg, allergic reactions, cellular injury, extreme cold). Once released, it diffuses rapidly into other tissues, where it interacts with three types of histamine receptors on target organs, called H_1, H_2, and H_3. H_1 receptors are located mainly on smooth muscle cells in blood vessels and the respiratory and GI tracts. When histamine binds with these receptors and stimulates them, effects include:

- Contraction of smooth muscle in the bronchi and bronchioles (producing bronchoconstriction and respiratory distress)
- Stimulation of vagus nerve endings to produce reflex bronchoconstriction and cough
- Increased permeability of veins and capillaries, which allows fluid to flow into subcutaneous tissues and form edema.
- Increased secretion of mucous glands. Mucosal edema and increased nasal mucus produce the nasal congestion characteristic of allergic rhinitis and the common cold.
- Stimulation of sensory peripheral nerve endings to cause pain and pruritus. Pruritus is especially prominent with allergic skin disorders.
- Dilation of capillaries in the skin, to cause flushing

When H_2 receptors are stimulated, the main effects are increased secretion of gastric acid and pepsin, increased rate and force of myocardial contraction, and decreased immunologic and proinflammatory reactions (eg, decreased release of histamine from basophils, decreased movement of neutrophils and basophils into areas of injury, inhibited T- and B-lymphocyte function). Stimulation of both H_1 and H_2 receptors causes peripheral vasodilation (with hypotension, headache, and skin flushing) and increases bronchial, intestinal, and salivary secretion of mucus.

The H_3 receptor functions as a negative-feedback mechanism to inhibit histamine synthesis and release in many body tissues. Stimulation of H_3 receptors opposes the effects produced by stimulation of H_1 receptors. In addition, stimulation of H_3 receptors on nerve terminals of the sympathetic nervous system inhibits vasoconstriction and slows heart rate.

HYPERSENSITIVITY (ALLERGIC) REACTIONS

Hypersensitivity or allergic reactions are immune responses (see Chap. 42) in which a person's body overreacts to an environmental or ingested substance that does not cause a reaction in most people. That is, the person is hypersensitive or allergic to the substance (called an antigen, allergen, or immunogen). Allergic reactions may result from specific antibodies, sensitized T lymphocytes, or both, formed during exposure to an antigen.

Types of Allergic Reactions

- *Type I* (also called immediate hypersensitivity because it occurs within minutes of exposure to the antigen) is an immunoglobulin E (IgE)-induced response that causes release of histamine and other mediators. For example, *anaphylaxis* is a type I response that may be mild (characterized mainly by urticaria, other dermatologic manifestations, or rhinitis) or severe and life threatening (characterized by respiratory distress and cardiovascular collapse). It is uncommon and does not occur on first exposure to an antigen; it occurs with a second or later exposure, after antibodies were induced by an earlier exposure. Severe anaphylaxis (sometimes called anaphylactic shock; see Chap. 54) is characterized by cardiovascular collapse from profound vasodilation and pooling of blood in the splanchnic system so that the patient has severe hypotension and functional hypovolemia. Respiratory distress often occurs from laryngeal edema and bronchoconstriction. Urticaria often occurs because the skin has many mast cells to release histamine. Anaphylaxis is a systemic reaction that usually involves the respiratory, cardiovascular, and dermatologic systems. Severe anaphylaxis may be fatal if not treated promptly and effectively.
- *Type II* responses are mediated by IgG or IgM. They produce direct damage to the cell surface. These cytotoxic reactions include blood transfusion reactions, hemolytic disease of newborns, autoimmune hemolytic anemia, and some drug reactions.
- *Type III* is an IgG- or IgM-mediated reaction characterized by formation of antigen–antibody complexes that induce an acute inflammatory reaction in the tissues. *Serum sickness*, the prototype of these reactions,

occurs when excess antigen combines with antibodies to form immune complexes. The complexes then diffuse into affected tissues, where they cause tissue damage by activating the complement system and initiating the inflammatory response. If small amounts of immune complexes are deposited locally, the antigenic material can be phagocytized and digested by white blood cells and macrophages without tissue destruction. If large amounts are deposited locally or reach the bloodstream and become deposited in blood vessel walls, the lysosomal enzymes released during phagocytosis may cause permanent tissue destruction.

- *Type IV* hypersensitivity (also called delayed hypersensitivity because it usually occurs several hours or days after exposure to the antigen) is a cell-mediated response in which sensitized T lymphocytes react with an antigen to cause inflammation mediated by release of lymphokines, direct cytotoxicity, or both.

Allergic Rhinitis

Allergic rhinitis is inflammation of nasal mucosa caused by a type I hypersensitivity reaction to inhaled allergens. It is a very common disorder characterized by nasal congestion, itching, sneezing, and watery drainage. Itching of the throat, eyes, and ears often occurs as well.

There are two types of allergic rhinitis. Seasonal disease (often called hay fever) produces acute symptoms in response to the protein components of airborne pollens from trees, grasses and weeds, mainly in spring or fall. Perennial disease produces chronic symptoms in response to nonseasonal allergens such as dust mites, animal dander, and molds. Actually, mold spores can cause both seasonal and perennial allergies because they are present year round, with seasonal increases. Some people have both types, with chronic symptoms plus acute seasonal symptoms.

People with a personal or family history of other allergic disorders are likely to have allergic rhinitis. Once the nasal mucosa is inflamed, symptoms can be worsened by nonallergenic irritants such as tobacco smoke, strong odors, air pollution, and climatic changes.

Allergic rhinitis is an immune response in which normal nasal breathing and filtering of air brings inhaled antigens into contact with mast cells and basophils in nasal mucosa, blood vessels, and submucosal tissues. With initial exposure, the inhaled antigens are processed by lymphocytes that produce IgE, an antigen-specific antibody that binds to mast cells. With later exposures, the IgE interacts with inhaled antigens and triggers the breakdown of the mast cell. This breakdown causes the release of histamine and other inflammatory mediators such as prostaglandins and leukotrienes (Fig. 48-1). These mediators, of

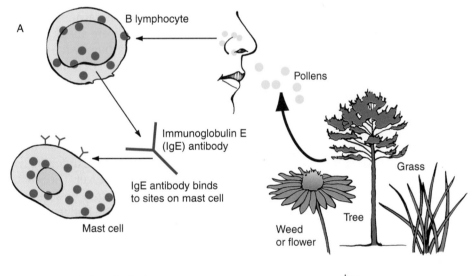

FIGURE 48–1 Type I hypersensitivity reaction: allergic rhinitis. (**A**) The first exposure of mast cells in nasal mucosa to inhaled antigens (eg, pollens from weeds, grasses, trees) leads to the formation of immunoglobulin E (IgE) antibody molecules. These molecules then bind to the surface membranes of mast cells. This process sensitizes mast cells to the effects of inhaled antigens (allergens). (**B**) When sensitized mast cells are re-exposed to inhaled pollens or other antigens, they release histamine and other chemical mediators which then act on nasal mucosa to produce characteristic symptoms of allergic rhinitis.

which histamine may be the most important, dilate and engorge blood vessels to produce nasal congestion, stimulate secretion of mucus, and attract inflammatory cells (eg, eosinophils, lymphocytes, monocytes, macrophages). In people with allergies, mast cells and basophils are increased in both number and reactivity. Thus, they may be capable of releasing large amounts of histamine and other mediators.

Allergic rhinitis that is not effectively treated may lead to chronic fatigue, impaired ability to perform usual activities of daily living, difficulty sleeping, sinus infections, postnasal drip, cough, and headache. In addition, this condition is a strong risk factor for asthma.

Allergic Contact Dermatitis

Allergic contact dermatitis is a type IV hypersensitivity reaction resulting from direct contact with antigens to which a person has previously become sensitized (eg, poison ivy or poison oak, cosmetics, hair dyes, metals, drugs applied topically to the skin). This reaction, which may be acute or chronic, usually occurs more than 24 hours after re-exposure to an antigen and may last from days to weeks.

Affected areas of the skin are usually inflamed, warm, edematous, intensely pruritic, and tender to touch. Skin lesions are usually erythematous macules, papules, and vesicles (blisters) that may drain, develop crusts, and become infected. Lesion location may indicate the causative antigen.

Allergic Drug Reactions

Virtually any drug may induce an immunologic response in susceptible people, and any body tissues may be affected. Allergic drug reactions are complex and diverse and may include any of the types of hypersensitivity described previously. A single drug may induce one or more of these states and multiple symptoms. There are no specific characteristics that identify drug-related reactions, although some reactions commonly attributed to drugs (eg, skin rashes, drug fever, hematologic reactions, hepatic reactions) rarely occur with plant pollens and other naturally occurring antigens. Usually, however, the body responds to a drug as it does to other foreign materials (antigens). In addition, some reactions may be caused by coloring agents, preservatives, and other additives rather than the drug itself.

Allergic drug reactions should be considered when new signs and symptoms develop or when they differ from the usual manifestations of the illness being treated, especially if a reaction:

- Follows ingestion of a drug, especially one known to produce allergic reactions
- Is unpredictable and occurs in only a few clients when many clients receive the suspected drug

- Occurs approximately 7 to 10 days after initial exposure to the suspected drug (to allow antibody production)
- Follows a previous exposure to the same or similar drug (sensitizing exposure)
- Occurs minutes or hours after a second or subsequent exposure
- Occurs after small doses (reduces the likelihood that the reaction is due to dose-related drug toxicity)
- Occurs with other drugs that are chemically or immunologically similar to the suspected drug
- Produces signs and symptoms that differ from the usual pharmacologic actions of the suspected drug
- Produces signs and symptoms usually considered allergic in nature (eg, anaphylaxis, urticaria, serum sickness)
- Produces similar signs and symptoms to previous allergic reactions to the same or a similar drug
- Increases eosinophils in blood or tissue
- Resolves within a few days of discontinuing the suspected drug

Virtually all drugs have been implicated in **anaphylactic reactions**. Penicillins and other antimicrobials, radiocontrast media, aspirin and other nonsteroidal antiinflammatory drugs, and antineoplastics such as asparaginase and cisplatin are more common offenders. Less common causes include anesthetics (local and general), opioid analgesics, skeletal muscle relaxants used with general anesthetics, and vaccines. Approximately 10% of severe anaphylactic reactions are fatal. In many cases, it is unknown whether clinical manifestations are immunologic or nonimmunologic in origin.

Serum sickness is a delayed hypersensitivity reaction most often caused by drugs, such as antimicrobials. In addition, many drugs that produce anaphylaxis also produce serum sickness. With initial exposure to the antigen, symptoms usually develop within 7 to 10 days and include urticaria, lymphadenopathy, myalgia, arthralgia, and fever. The reaction usually resolves within a few days but may be severe or even fatal. With repeated exposure to the antigen, after prior sensitization of the host, accelerated serum sickness may develop within 2 to 4 days, with similar but often more severe signs and symptoms.

Systemic lupus erythematosus (SLE) is an autoimmune disorder that may be induced by hydralazine, procainamide, isoniazid, and other drugs. Clinical manifestations vary greatly, depending on the location and severity of the inflammatory and immune processes, and may include skin lesions, fever, pneumonia, anemia, arthralgia, arthritis, nephritis and others. Drug-induced lupus produces less renal and CNS involvement than idiopathic SLE.

Fever often occurs with allergic drug reactions. It may occur alone, with a skin rash and eosinophilia, or with other drug-induced allergic reactions such as serum sickness, SLE, vasculitis and hepatitis.

Dermatologic conditions (eg, skin rash, urticaria, inflammation) commonly occur with allergic drug reactions and may be the first and most visible manifestation.

Pseudoallergic Drug Reactions

Pseudoallergic drug reactions resemble immune responses (because histamine and other chemical mediators are released) but they do not produce antibodies or sensitized T lymphocytes. **Anaphylactoid reactions** are like anaphylaxis in terms of immediate occurrence, symptoms, and life-threatening severity. The main difference is that they are not antigen–antibody reactions and therefore may occur on first exposure to the causative agent. The drugs bind directly to mast cells, activate the cells, and cause the release of histamine and other vasoactive chemical mediators. Contrast media for radiologic diagnostic tests are often implicated.

ANTIHISTAMINES

The term *antihistamines* generally indicates classic or traditional drugs. With increased knowledge about histamine receptors, these drugs are often called H_1 receptor antagonists. These drugs prevent or reduce most of the physiologic effects that histamine normally induces at H_1 receptor sites. Thus, they

- Inhibit smooth muscle constriction in blood vessels and the respiratory and GI tracts
- Decrease capillary permeability
- Decrease salivation and tear formation

The drugs are similar in effectiveness as histamine antagonists but differ in adverse effects. These are the antihistamines discussed in this chapter. Cimetidine (Tagamet), ranitidine (Zantac), famotidine (Pepcid), and nizatidine (Axid) are H_2 receptor antagonists or blocking agents used to prevent or treat peptic ulcer disease. These are discussed in Chapter 60. H_3 receptor agonists and antagonists are being investigated, but none is available for clinical use. Selected H_1 antagonists are described in the following sections and in Table 48-1.

First-Generation H_1 Receptor Antagonists

These chemically diverse antihistamines bind to both central and peripheral H_1 receptors and can cause CNS depression or stimulation. They usually cause CNS depression (drowsiness, sedation) with usual therapeutic doses and

TABLE 48-1 Commonly Used Antihistamines

Generic/Trade Name	Indications for Use	Routes and Dosage Ranges Adults	Children
First Generation			
Azatadine (Optimine)	Allergic rhinitis Chronic urticaria	PO 1–2 mg q12h	≥12 y: Same as adults
Azelastine (Astelin)	Allergic rhinitis	Nasal inhalation, two sprays per nostril q12h	≥12 y: Same as adults
Brompheniramine (Dimetane)	Hypersensitivity reactions (eg, allergic reactions to blood or plasma, allergic rhinitis)	Immediate allergic reactions, IV, IM, SC, 10 mg q12h; maximal dose 40 mg in 24 h Allergic rhinitis PO 4 mg q4–6h	<12 y, IV, IM, SC, 0.5 mg/kg/d or 15 mg/m²/d, divided into three or four doses ≥12 y: PO same as adults
Chlorpheniramine (Chlor-Trimeton)	Allergic rhinitis	PO 4 mg q4–6h; maximal dose, 24 mg in 24 h Timed-release forms, PO 8 mg q8–12h or 12 mg q12h; maximal dose, 24 mg in 24 h	≥12 y: Same as adults 6–12 y: PO 2 mg q4–6h; maximal dose, 12 mg in 24h 2–6 y: PO 1 mg q4–6h Timed-release forms, ≥12 y: PO 8 mg q8–12h or 12 mg q12h; maximal dose, 24 mg in 24h
Clemastine (Tavist)	Allergic rhinitis Urticaria/angioedema	Allergic rhinitis, PO 1.34 mg twice daily, increased up to a maximum of 8.04 mg daily, if necessary Urticaria/angioedema, PO 2.68 mg one to three times daily	Allergic rhinitis, 6–12 y (syrup only): PO 0.67 mg twice daily, increased up to a maximum of 4.02 mg daily, if necessary Urticaria/angioedema, 6–12 y (syrup only): PO 1.34 mg twice daily
Cyproheptadine (Periactin)	Hypersensitivity reactions (allergic rhinitis, conjunctivitis, dermatitis)	PO 4 mg q8h initially, increase if necessary. Maximal dose 0.5 mg/kg/d	(Calculate total daily dosage as 0.25 mg/kg or 8 mg/m²) 7–14 y: PO 4 mg q8–12h; maximal dose, 16 mg/d 2–6 y: 2 mg q8–12h; maximal dose, 12 mg/d *(continued)*

TABLE 48-1) **Commonly Used Antihistamines** (*continued*)

Generic/Trade Name	Indications for Use	Routes and Dosage Ranges	
		Adults	Children
Dexchlorpheniramine (Polaramine)	Hypersensitivity reactions (allergic rhinitis, conjunctivitis, dermatitis)	Regular tablets and syrup, PO 2 mg q4–6h Timed-release tablets, PO 4–6 mg at bedtime or q8–12h	≥12 y: Same as adults 6–11 y: PO 1 mg q4–6h 2–5 y: PO 0.5 mg q4–6h Timed-release tablets, ≥12 y: Same as adults 6–12 y: 4 mg once daily, at bedtime
Diphenhydramine (Benadryl)	Hypersensitivity reactions (allergic rhinitis, conjunctivitis, dermatitis) Motion sickness Parkinsonism Insomnia Antitussive (syrup only)	Hypersensitivity reaction, motion sickness, parkinsonism, PO 25–50 mg q4–8h; IV or deep IM 10–50 mg, increased if necessary to a maximal daily dose of 400 mg Insomnia, PO 50 mg at bedtime Syrup for cough, PO 25 mg (10 mL) q4h, not to exceed 100 mg (40 mL) in 24 h	Weight >10 kg (22 lbs): PO 12.5–25 mg q6–8h, 5 mg/kg/d, or 150 mg/m^2/d; IV 5 mg/kg/d, or 150 mg/m^2/d. Maximum oral or parenteral dosage, 300 mg daily Insomnia, ≥12 y: Same as adults Syrup for cough, 6–12 y: PO 12.5 mg (5 mL) q4h, not to exceed 50 mg (20 mL) in 24 h 2–6 y: PO 6.25 mg (2.5 mL) q4h, not to exceed 25 mg (10 mL) in 24 h
Hydroxyzine (Vistaril, Atarax)	Pruritus Sedation Antiemetic	PO 25 mg q6–8h; IM 25–100 mg as needed	>6 y: PO 50–100 mg daily in divided doses <6 y: PO 50 mg daily in divided doses
Phenindamine (Nolahist)	Allergic rhinitis	PO 25 mg q4–6h; maximal dose 150 mg in 24 h	≥12 y: Same as adults 6–11 y: PO 12.5 mg q4–6h; maximal dose 75 mg in 24 h
Promethazine (Phenergan)	Hypersensitivity reactions (allergic rhinitis, conjunctivitis, dermatitis) Sedation Antiemetic Motion sickness	PO, IM, rectally, 25 mg q4–6h as needed	≥2 y: 12.5 mg q4–6h as needed
Tripelennamine (PBZ)	Hypersensitivity reactions (allergic rhinitis, conjunctivitis, dermatitis)	PO 25–50 mg q4–6h Extended-release tablets, PO 100 mg q12h	PO 5 mg/kg/d or 150 mg/m^2/d in four to six divided doses Do not use extended-release tablets.
Second Generation			
Cetirizine (Zyrtec)	Allergic rhinitis Chronic idiopathic urticaria	PO 5–10 mg once daily Renal or hepatic impairment: PO 5 mg once daily	≥6 y: Same as adults
Fexofenadine (Allegra)	Allergic rhinitis	PO 60 mg twice daily Renal impairment: PO 60 mg once daily	≥12 y: Same as adults 6–11 y: PO 30 mg twice daily
Loratadine (Claritin)	Allergic rhinitis Chronic idiopathic urticaria	PO 10 mg once daily Renal or hepatic impairment: PO 10 mg every other day	≥6 y: Same as adults

IM, intramuscular; IV, intravenous; PO, oral; SC, subcutaneous.

may cause CNS stimulation (anxiety, agitation) with excessive doses, especially in children. They also have substantial anticholinergic effects (eg, cause dry mouth, urinary retention, constipation, blurred vision). **Azelastine**, **brompheniramine**, **chlorpheniramine**, and **dexchlorpheniramine** cause minimal drowsiness. **Diphenhydramine** (Benadryl), the prototype of first-generation antihistamines, causes a high incidence of

drowsiness and anticholinergic effects. **Hydroxyzine** and **promethazine** are strong CNS depressants and cause extensive drowsiness.

First-generation antihistamines are usually well absorbed after oral administration. Immediate-release oral forms act within 15 to 60 minutes and last approximately 4 to 6 hours. Enteric-coated or sustained-release preparations last 8 to 12 hours. Most drugs are given orally; a few may be given parenterally. These drugs are primarily metabolized by the liver, with metabolites and small amounts of unchanged drug excreted in urine within 24 hours. **Azelastine**, which is applied topically to nasal mucosa, produces peak levels in 2 to 3 hours. It is metabolized in the liver to an active metabolite and is excreted mainly in feces. Several of these drugs are available without prescription, including **brompheniramine**, **chlorpheniramine**, and **diphenhydramine**, alone, in combination with adrenergic nasal decongestants, and in combination with other ingredients (eg, analgesics and allergy, cold, and sinus remedies).

Second-Generation H₁ Receptor Antagonists

Second-generation H₁ antagonists were developed mainly to produce less sedation than the first-generation drugs. They cause less CNS depression because they are selective for peripheral H₁ receptors and do not cross the blood–brain barrier.

These drugs are well absorbed with oral administration and have a rapid onset of action. **Cetirizine** is an active metabolite of hydroxyzine that causes less drowsiness than hydroxyzine. It reaches maximal serum concentration in 1 hour, is approximately 93% protein bound, and approxi-

mately half is metabolized in the liver and approximately half is excreted unchanged in the urine. **Fexofenadine** reaches peak serum concentrations in approximately 2.5 hours, is 60% to 70% protein bound, and 95% is excreted unchanged in bile and urine. **Loratadine** effects occur within 1 to 3 hours, reach a maximum in 8 to 12 hours, and last 24 hours or longer. It is metabolized in the liver and its long duration of action is due, in part, to an active metabolite. These drugs are available only by prescription.

Mechanism of Action

Antihistamines are structurally related to histamine and occupy the same receptor sites as histamine, which prevents histamine from acting on target tissues (Fig. 48-2). Thus, the drugs are effective in inhibiting vascular permeability, edema formation, bronchoconstriction, and pruritus associated with histamine release. They do not prevent histamine release or reduce the amount released.

Indications for Use

Antihistamines are used for a variety of allergic and non-allergic disorders to prevent or reverse target organ inflam-

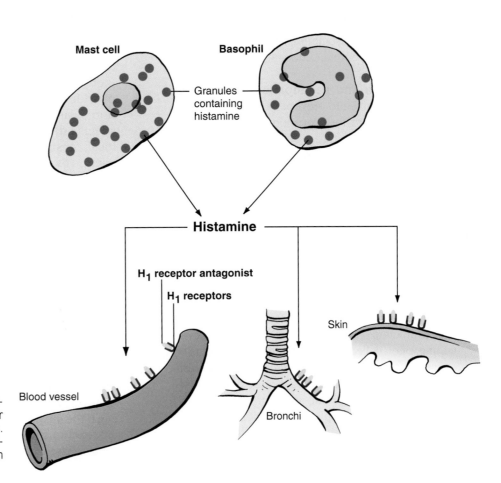

FIGURE 48–2 Action of antihistamine drugs. Histamine₁ (H₁) receptor antagonists bind to H₁ receptors. This prevents histamine from binding to its receptors and acting on target tissues.

Jane Morgan is admitted to the oncology unit for chemotherapy. Before administering a chemotherapeutic agent that is known to cause allergic symptoms in some patients, diphenhydramine (Benadryl) is ordered. Discuss the rationale for this order. If anaphylaxis developed in this client, would administering additional Benadryl help?

mation and its effects on organ function. The drugs can relieve symptoms but do not relieve the hypersensitivity.

- **Allergic rhinitis.** Of people with seasonal allergic rhinitis, 75% to 95% experience some relief of sneezing, rhinorrhea, nasal airway obstruction, and conjunctivitis with the use of antihistamines. People with perennial allergic rhinitis usually experience decreased nasal congestion and drying of nasal mucosa.
- **Anaphylaxis.** Antihistamines are helpful in treating urticaria and pruritus but are less effective in treating bronchoconstriction and hypotension. Epinephrine, rather than an antihistamine, is the drug of choice for treating severe anaphylaxis.
- **Allergic conjunctivitis.** This condition, which is characterized by redness, itching, and tearing of the eyes, is often associated with allergic rhinitis. Antihistamine eye medications may be given (see Chap. 65).
- **Drug allergies and pseudoallergies.** Antihistamines may be given to prevent or treat reactions to drugs. When used for prevention, they should be given before exposure (eg, before a diagnostic test that uses an iodine preparation as contrast media; before an IV infusion of amphotericin B). When used for treatment, giving an antihistamine and stopping the causative drug usually relieve signs and symptoms within a few days.
- **Transfusions of blood and blood products.** Premedication with an antihistamine is often used to prevent allergic reactions.
- **Dermatologic conditions.** Antihistamines are the drugs of choice for treatment of allergic contact dermatitis and acute urticaria (a vascular reaction of the skin characterized by papules or wheals and severe itching, often called *hives*). Urticaria often occurs because the skin has many mast cells to release histamine. Other indications for use include drug-induced skin reactions, pruritus ani, and pruritus vulvae. Systemic drugs are used; topical preparations are not recommended because they often induce skin rashes themselves. With pruritus, oral cyproheptadine and hydroxyzine are especially effective.

- **Miscellaneous.** Some antihistamines are commonly used for nonallergic disorders, such as motion sickness, nausea and vomiting (eg, promethazine, hydroxyzine; see Chap. 63), and sleep (eg, diphenhydramine). The active ingredient in over-the-counter (OTC) sleep aids (eg, Compoz, Sominex) is a sedating antihistamine. Antihistamines are also common ingredients in OTC cold remedies (see Chap. 49).

Contraindications to Use

Antihistamines are contraindicated or must be used with caution in clients with hypersensitivity to the drugs, narrow-angle glaucoma, prostatic hypertrophy, stenosing peptic ulcer, and bladder neck obstruction, and during pregnancy.

NURSING PROCESS

Assessment

- Assess the client's condition in relation to disorders for which antihistamines are used. For the client with known allergies, try to determine the factors that precipitate or relieve allergic reactions and specific signs and symptoms experienced during a reaction.
- Assess every client for a potential hypersensitivity reaction. For example, it is standard practice on first contact to ask a client if he or she has any food, drug, or other allergies. The health care provider is likely to get more complete information by asking clients about allergic reactions to specific drugs (eg, antibiotics such as penicillin, local anesthetics) rather than asking if they are allergic to or cannot take any drugs.

  If a drug allergy is identified, ask about specific signs and symptoms as well as any drugs currently taken. With previous exposure and sensitization to the same or a similar drug, immediate allergic reactions may occur. With a new drug, antibody formation and allergic reactions usually require a week or longer. Most reactions appear within a month of starting a drug.

  When a suspected allergic reaction occurs (eg, skin rash, fever, edema, dyspnea), interview the client or consult medical records about the drug, dose, route, and time of administration. In addition, evaluate all the drugs a client is taking as a potential cause of the reaction. This assessment may involve searching drug literature to see if the suspected drug is associated with allergic reactions and discussion with physicians and pharmacists.

Nursing Diagnoses

- Ineffective Airway Clearance related to thick respiratory secretions
- Risk for Injury related to drowsiness and dizziness
- Knowledge Deficit: Safe and accurate drug use
- Knowledge Deficit: Ways of preventing conditions for which antihistamines are used

Planning/Goals

The client will:

- Experience relief of symptoms
- Take antihistamines accurately
- Avoid hazardous activities if sedated from antihistamines
- Avoid preventable adverse drug effects
- Avoid taking sedative-type antihistamines with alcohol or other sedative drugs

Interventions

- For clients with known allergies, assist in identifying and avoiding precipitating factors when possible. If it is a drug allergy, encourage the client to carry a medical alert device that identifies the drug.

- Monitor the client closely for excessive drowsiness during the first few days of therapy with antihistamines known to cause sedation.
- Encourage a fluid intake of 2000 to 3000 mL daily, if not contraindicated.
- Because antihistamines are most effective before exposure to the stimulus that causes histamine release, assist clients in learning when to take the drugs (eg, during seasons of high pollen and mold counts).
- When indicated, obtain an order and administer an antihistamine before situations known to elicit allergic reactions (eg, blood transfusions, diagnostic tests that involve contrast media).
- For clients who have experienced an allergic or pseudoallergic drug reaction, assist them in learning about the drug thought responsible (including the generic and commonly used trade names), suitable alternatives for future drug therapy, and potential sources of the drug.

Evaluation

- Observe for relief of symptoms.
- Interview and observe for correct drug usage.
- Interview and observe for excessive drowsiness.

CLIENT TEACHING GUIDELINES
Antihistamines

General Considerations

✔ Some antihistamines should not be taken by people with glaucoma, peptic ulcer, urinary retention, or pregnancy. Inform your physician if you have any of these conditions or, for over-the-counter (OTC) antihistamines, read the label to see if you should avoid a particular drug.

✔ Antihistamines may dry and thicken respiratory tract secretions and make them more difficult to remove. Thus, do not take diphenhydramine (Benadryl), which is available OTC, if you have active asthma, bronchitis, or pneumonia.

✔ Some antihistamines cause drowsiness or dizziness and impair mental alertness, judgment, and physical coordination, especially during the first few days. Do not smoke, drive a car, operate machinery, or perform other tasks requiring alertness and physical dexterity until drowsiness has worn off, to avoid injury.

✔ Avoid using sedating antihistamines with other sedative-type drugs (eg, alcohol, medications to relieve nervousness or produce sleep), to avoid adverse effects and dangerous drug interactions. Alcohol and other drugs that depress brain function may cause excessive sedation, respiratory depression, and death.

✔ Do not take more than one antihistamine at a time (eg, two prescription drugs, two OTC drugs, or a combination of prescription and OTC drugs) because adverse effects are likely. If you do not know whether a particular medication is an antihistamine, consult a health care provider. For example, many OTC cold remedies and "nighttime" or "PM" allergy or sinus preparations contain an antihistamine. In addition, the active ingredient in OTC sleep aids is a sedating antihistamine, usually diphenhydramine (Benadryl).

✔ Avoid prolonged exposure to sunlight and use sunscreens and protective clothing; some antihistamines may increase sensitivity to sunlight and risks of skin damage from sunburn.

✔ Report adverse effects, such as excessive drowsiness. The physician may be able to change drugs or dosages to decrease adverse effects.

✔ Store antihistamines out of reach of children to avoid accidental ingestion.

✔ If you experience an allergic reaction to a medication, obtain information about the drug thought responsible (including its various names), acceptable alternatives for

CLIENT TEACHING GUIDELINES
Antihistamines (continued)

future drug therapy, and potential sources of the drug. For example, Ecotrin is a coated form of aspirin (to reduce stomach upset) that is often used to treat heart attack and stroke. In addition, read the list of ingredients on labels of OTC drug preparations, inform all health care providers about the drug reaction before taking any newly prescribed drug, and wear a medical alert device that lists drugs to be avoided. Note that people may be allergic to additives (eg, dyes, binders, others) rather than the active drug.

Self-administration

✔ Take antihistamines only as prescribed or as instructed on packages of OTC preparations to increase beneficial

effects and decrease adverse effects. If you miss a dose, do not take a double dose.

✔ Take most antihistamines with meals to decrease stomach upset. Take loratadine (Claritin) on an empty stomach for better absorption; cetirizine (Zyrtec) may be taken with or without food.

✔ When taking an antihistamine to prevent motion sickness, take it 30 to 60 minutes before travel.

✔ Do not chew or crush sustained-release tablets and do not open sustained-release capsules. Such actions can cause rapid drug absorption, high blood levels, and serious adverse effects, rather than the slow absorption and prolonged action intended with these products.

PRINCIPLES OF THERAPY

Prevention of Histamine-Releasing Reactions

When possible, avoiding exposure to known allergens can prevent allergic reactions. If antihistamine therapy is required, it is more effective if started before exposure to allergens because the drugs can then occupy receptor sites before histamine is released.

Drug Selection and Usage

- Choosing an antihistamine is based on the desired effect, duration of action, adverse effects, and other characteristics of available drugs. For most people, a second-generation drug is the first drug of choice. However, they are quite expensive. If costs are prohibitive for a client, a first-generation drug may be used with minimal daytime sedation if taken at bedtime or in low initial doses, with gradual increases over a week or two. Azelastine nasal spray also causes little sedation, but it leaves an unpleasant taste. Overall, safety should be the determining factor. Some studies have shown performance impairment with the first-generation drugs even when the person does not feel drowsy or impaired.
- For treatment of acute allergic reactions, a rapid-acting agent of short duration is preferred.
- For chronic allergic symptoms (eg, allergic rhinitis), long-acting preparations provide more consistent relief. A client may respond better to one antihistamine than to another. Thus, if one does not relieve symptoms or produces excessive sedation, another may be effective.

- For treatment of the common cold, studies have demonstrated that antihistamines do not relieve symptoms and are not recommended. However, an antihistamine is often included in prescription and OTC combination products for the common cold.

Use in Children

First-generation antihistamines (eg, diphenhydramine) may cause drowsiness and decreased mental alertness in children as in adults. Young children may experience paradoxical excitement. These reactions may occur with therapeutic dosages. In overdosage, hallucinations, convulsions, and death may occur. Close supervision and appropriate dosages are required for safe drug usage in children.

Diphenhydramine is not recommended for use in premature or full-term newborn infants or children with chickenpox or a flu-like infection. When used in young children, doses should be small because of drug effects on the brain and nervous system. **Promethazine** should not be used in children with hepatic disease, Reye's syndrome, a history of sleep apnea, or a family history of sudden infant death syndrome.

The second-generation drugs, **cetirizine, loratadine, and fexofenadine** may be used in children 6 years of age and older.

How Can You Avoid This Medication Error?

You are the phone resource nurse for an urgent care center. Mrs. Doe calls you, very upset, explaining that her 2-year-old son has just swallowed what was remaining in a bottle of an over-the-counter (OTC) cold remedy. What advice should you give Mrs. Doe? How can this error be prevented in the future?

Use in Older Adults

First-generation antihistamines (eg, **diphenhydramine**) may cause confusion (with impaired thinking, judgment, and memory), dizziness, hypotension, sedation, syncope, unsteady gait, and paradoxical CNS stimulation in older adults. These effects, especially sedation, may be misinterpreted as senility or mental depression. Older men with prostatic hypertrophy may have difficulty voiding while taking these drugs. Some of these adverse reactions derive from anticholinergic effects of the drugs and are likely to be more severe if the client is also taking other drugs with anticholinergic effects (eg, tricyclic antidepressants, antipsychotic drugs, some antiparkinson drugs). Despite the increased risk of adverse effects, however, diphenhydramine is sometimes prescribed as a sleep aid for occasional use in older adults. As with many other drugs, smaller-than-usual dosages are indicated.

Use in Renal Impairment

Little information is available about using antihistamines in clients with impaired renal function. With **diphenhydramine**, the dosing interval should be extended to 12 to 18 hours in clients with severe kidney failure. With **cetirizine** (5 mg once daily), **fexofenadine** (60 mg once daily), and **loratadine** (10 mg every other day), recommended doses for initial use are approximately one-half of those used for young and middle-aged adults.

Use in Hepatic Impairment

Little information is available about using antihistamines in clients with impaired hepatic function. With **diphenhydramine,** single doses are probably safe but the effects of multiple doses have not been studied in this population. With **promethazine**, cholestatic jaundice has been reported and the drug should be used with caution. With **cetirizine** (5 mg once daily) and **loratadine** (10 mg every other day), smaller-than-usual doses are recommended.

Use in Critical Illness

Antihistamines are not often used in the treatment of clients with critical illness. Most are given orally, and many critically ill clients are unable to take oral drugs. **Diphenhydramine** may be given by injection, usually as a single dose, to a client who is having a blood transfusion or a diagnostic test, to prevent allergic reactions. **Hydroxyzine** or **promethazine** may be given by injection for nausea and vomiting or to provide sedation, but are not usually the first drugs of choice for these indications.

 Home Care

Antihistamines are often taken in the home setting, especially for allergic rhinitis and other allergic disorders. Most people are familiar with the use and side effects of first-generation drugs; they may be less familiar with the second-generation drugs. The home care nurse is unlikely to be involved in antihistamine drug therapy unless visiting a client for other care and purposes. If a first-generation drug is being used, the home care nurse needs to assess for drowsiness and safety hazards in the environment (eg, operating a car or other potentially hazardous machinery). In most people, tolerance develops to the sedative effects within a few days if they are not taking other sedative-type drugs or alcoholic beverages.

NURSING ACTIONS — Antihistamines	
NURSING ACTIONS	**RATIONALE/EXPLANATION**
1. Administer accurately	
a. Give most oral antihistamines with food; give loratadine on an empty stomach; give cetirizine with or without food.	To decrease gastrointestinal (GI) effects of the drugs
b. Give intramuscular antihistamines deeply into a large muscle mass.	To decrease tissue irritation
c. Inject intravenous (IV) antihistamines slowly, over a few minutes.	Severe hypotension may result from rapid IV injection.
d. When a drug is used to prevent motion sickness, give it 30–60 min before travel.	*(continued)*

NURSING ACTIONS	RATIONALE/EXPLANATION
2. Observe for therapeutic effects	Therapeutic effects depend on the reason for use.
a. A verbal statement of therapeutic effect (relief of symptoms)	
b. Decreased nausea and vomiting when given for antiemetic effects	
c. Decreased dizziness and nausea when taken for motion sickness	
d. Drowsiness or sleep when given for sedation	
3. Observe for adverse effects	
a. First-generation drugs	
(1) Sedation	Drowsiness due to central nervous system (CNS) depression is the most common adverse effect.
(2) Paradoxical excitation—restlessness, insomnia, tremors, nervousness, palpitations	This reaction is more likely to occur in children. It may result from the anticholinergic effects of antihistamines.
(3) Convulsive seizures	Antihistamines, particularly the phenothiazines, may lower the seizure threshold.
(4) Dryness of mouth, nose, and throat, blurred vision, urinary retention, constipation	Due to anticholinergic effects
(5) GI distress—anorexia, nausea, vomiting	
b. Second-generation drugs	Adverse effects are few and mild.
(1) Drowsiness	Drowsiness and dry mouth are more likely to occur with cetirizine; headache is more likely to occur with loratadine; fexofenadine produces minimal adverse effects.
(2) Dry mouth	
(3) Fatigue	
(4) Headache	
(5) GI upset	
4. Observe for drug interactions	
a. Drugs that *increase* effects of first-generation antihistamines:	
(1) Ethyl alcohol, CNS depressants (eg, antianxiety and antipsychotic agents, opioid analgesics, sedative-hypnotics)	Additive CNS depression. Concomitant use may lead to drowsiness, lethargy, stupor, respiratory depression, coma, and death.
(2) Monoamine oxidase inhibitors	Inhibit metabolism of antihistamines, leading to an increased duration of action; increased incidence and severity of anticholinergic adverse effects.
(3) Tricyclic antidepressants	Additive anticholinergic side effects
b. Drugs that *increase* plasma levels of loratadine:	These drugs increase loratadine levels by decreasing its metabolism.
(1) Macrolide antibacterials (azithromycin, clarithromycin, erythromycin)	
(2) Azole antifungals (fluconazole, itraconazole, ketoconazole, miconazole)	
(3) Cimetidine	

Nursing Notes: Apply Your Knowledge

Answer: Benadryl, an antihistamine, blocks histamine-1 receptors, thus decreasing histamine-induced symptoms such as rash, pruritus, cough, and swelling. If an allergic, histamine-related response occurs, the symptoms will be less severe if Benadryl has been previously administered. If a severe allergic reaction involving bronchospasm and hypotension occurs, epinephrine should be administered to reverse these potentially life-threatening symptoms.

How Can You Avoid This Medication Error?

Answer: Mrs. Doe needs to induce her son to vomit to prevent additional absorption of the cold remedy. Syrup of ipecac can be used to promote vomiting, which usually occurs 20 to 30 minutes after ingestion. If vomiting cannot be induced, instruct Mrs. Doe to bring her son to the urgent care center where gastric lavage can be used to empty the stomach.

Question Mrs. Doe regarding the time that has elapsed since ingestion, the amount of the medication ingested, medications contained in the cold remedy, and any symptoms her son is exhibiting.

Teaching is essential to prevent future accidental poisonings. All medication, even OTC and herbal remedies, must be kept out of reach of all children and have childproof tops. Toddlers are especially prone to accidental poisoning because they are inquisitive and like to put things in their mouths, and cannot understand the danger such a situation poses. Children need constant supervision and should not be left alone. Make sure that Mrs. Doe has syrup of ipecac on hand and the phone number of the poison control center posted.

REVIEW AND APPLICATION EXERCISES

1. Describe several factors that cause histamine release from cells.

2. What signs and symptoms are produced by the release of histamine?

3. How do antihistamines act to block the effects of histamine?

4. Differentiate between H_1 and H_2 receptor antagonists in terms of pharmacologic effects and clinical indications for use.

5. In general, when should an antihistamine be taken to prevent or treat allergic disorders?

6. Compare and contrast the first- and second-generation antihistamines.

SELECTED REFERENCES

Drug facts and comparisons. (Updated monthly). St. Louis: Facts and Comparisons.

Guyton, A.C. & Hall, J.E. (1996). *Textbook of medical physiology*, 9th ed. Philadelphia: W.B. Saunders.

Lieberman, P. (1996). Antihistamines. In R.R. Rich, T.A. Fleisher, B.D. Schwartz, W.T. Sehearer, & W. Strober (Eds.), *Clinical immunology: Principles and practice*. St. Louis: C.V. Mosby.

May, J.R., Feger, T.A., & Guill, M.F. (1997). Allergic rhinitis. In J.T. DiPiro, R.L. Talbert, G.C. Yee, G.R. Matzke, B.G. Wells, & L.M. Posey (Eds.), *Pharmacotherapy: A pathophysiologic approach*, 3rd ed., pp. 1801–1813. Stamford, CT: Appleton & Lange.

Porth, C.M. (Ed.). (1998). *Pathophysiology: Concepts of altered health states*, 5th ed. Philadelphia: Lippincott Williams & Wilkins.

49

Nasal Decongestants, Antitussives, Mucolytics, and Cold Remedies

Objectives

After studying this chapter, the student will be able to:

1. Describe characteristics of selected upper respiratory disorders and symptoms.

2. Review decongestant effects of adrenergic drugs.

3. Describe general characteristics and effects of antitussive agents.

4. Discuss the advantages and disadvantages of using combination products in treatment of the common cold.

5. Evaluate over-the-counter cough, cold, and sinus remedies for personal or clients' use.

New parents bring their 5-month-old into the clinic with symptoms of a cold. The mother states her daughter has a slight fever, a runny nose, and a cough. The baby has had difficulty sleeping and has been keeping the mother awake with her fussing. The baby's appetite has also decreased.

Reflect on:

▶ Worries and concerns new parents are likely to have about their sick infant.

▶ The effectiveness of an infant's immune system in resisting infection.

▶ How nasal stuffiness may affect smaller anatomic structures of the infant.

▶ Nonpharmacologic interventions to decrease cold symptoms.

DESCRIPTION

The drugs discussed in this chapter are used to treat upper respiratory disorders and symptoms such as the common cold, sinusitis, nasal congestion, cough, and secretions. Some of these diverse drugs are discussed more extensively in other chapters; they are discussed here in relation to their use in upper respiratory conditions.

THE COMMON COLD

The common cold, a viral infection of the upper respiratory tract, is the most common respiratory tract infection. Adults usually have 2 to 4 colds per year; schoolchildren may have as many as 10 per year. A cold often begins with dry, stuffy feelings in the nose and throat, an increased amount of clear nasal secretions, and tearing of the eyes. As the mucous membranes of the nose and throat become more inflamed, other common symptoms include sore throat, hoarseness, headache, and general malaise. Colds can be caused by several types of virus, most often the rhinovirus. Shedding of these viruses, mainly from nasal mucosa, can result in rapid spread to other people. The major mode of transmission is contamination of skin or environmental surfaces. The uninfected person touches contaminated surfaces with the fingers and then transfers the viruses by touching nasal or eye mucosal membranes. Cold viruses can survive for several hours on the skin and hard surfaces, such as wood and plastic. Once the viruses gain entry, the incubation period is approximately 5 days, the most contagious period is approximately 3 days after symptoms begin, and the cold usually lasts approximately 7 days. Because of the way cold viruses are spread, frequent and thorough hand washing (by both infected and uninfected people) is the most important protective and preventive measure.

SINUSITIS

Sinusitis is inflammation of the paranasal sinuses, air cells that connect with the nasal cavity and are lined by similar mucosa. As in other parts of the respiratory tract, ciliated mucous membranes help move fluid and microorganisms out of the sinuses and into the nasal cavity. This movement becomes impaired when sinus openings are blocked by nasal swelling, and the impairment is considered a major cause of sinus infections. Another contributing factor is a lower oxygen content in the sinuses, which aids the growth of microorganisms and impairs local defense mechanisms. Rhinitis (inflammation and congestion of nasal mucosa) and upper respiratory tract infections are the most common causes of sinusitis. Symptoms may include moderate to severe headache, tenderness or pain in the affected sinus area, and fever.

COMMON SIGNS AND SYMPTOMS OF RESPIRATORY DISORDERS

- **Nasal congestion** is manifested by obstructed nasal passages ("stuffy nose") and nasal drainage ("runny nose"). It is a prominent symptom of the common cold and rhinitis (including allergic rhinitis; see Chap. 48). Nasal congestion results from dilation of the blood vessels in the nasal mucosa and engorgement of the mucous membranes with blood. At the same time, nasal membranes are stimulated to increase mucus secretion. Related symptomatic terms are *rhinorrhea* (the discharge of mucus from the nose), *rhinitis* (inflammation of the mucous membrane of the nose), and *coryza* (profuse discharge from the mucous membrane of the nose).
- **Cough** is a forceful expulsion of air from the lungs. It is normally a protective reflex for removing foreign bodies, environmental irritants, or accumulated secretions from the respiratory tract. The cough reflex involves central and peripheral mechanisms. Centrally, the cough center in the medulla oblongata receives stimuli and initiates the reflex response (deep inspiration, closed glottis, buildup of pressure within the lungs, and forceful exhalation). Peripherally, cough receptors in the pharynx, larynx, trachea, or lungs may be stimulated by air, dryness of mucous membranes, or excessive secretions. A cough is productive when secretions are expectorated; it is nonproductive when it is dry and no sputum is expectorated.

  Cough is a prominent symptom of respiratory tract infections (eg, influenza, bronchitis, pharyngitis) and chronic obstructive pulmonary diseases (eg, emphysema, chronic bronchitis).
- **Increased secretions** may result from excessive production or decreased ability to cough or otherwise remove secretions from the respiratory tract. Secretions may seriously impair respiration by obstructing airways and preventing air flow to and from alveoli, where gas exchange occurs. Secretions also may cause atelectasis and cause or aggravate infections by supporting bacterial growth.

  Respiratory disorders characterized by retention of secretions include influenza, pneumonia, upper respiratory infections, acute and chronic bronchitis, emphysema, and acute attacks of asthma. Nonrespiratory conditions that predispose to secretion retention include immobility, debilitation, cigarette smoking, and postoperative status. Surgical procedures involving the chest or abdomen are most likely to be associated with retention of secretions because pain may decrease the client's ability to cough, breathe deeply, and ambulate.

DRUGS FOR RESPIRATORY DISORDERS

Numerous drugs are available and widely used to treat these symptoms. Many are nonprescription drugs and can be obtained alone or in combination products. Available products include nasal decongestants, antitussives, and expectorants.

Nasal Decongestants

Nasal decongestants are used to relieve nasal obstruction and discharge. Adrenergic (sympathomimetic) drugs are most often used for this purpose (see Chap. 18). These agents relieve nasal congestion and swelling by constricting arterioles and reducing blood flow to nasal mucosa. Some nasal decongestants are applied topically to the nasal mucosa as sprays or drops (eg, phenylephrine); most are taken orally (eg, phenylpropanolamine, pseudoephedrine). Rebound nasal swelling can occur with excessive use of nasal drops and sprays.

Nasal decongestants are most often used to relieve rhinitis associated with respiratory infections or allergies. They also may be used to reduce local blood flow before nasal surgery and to aid visualization of the nasal mucosa during diagnostic examinations.

These drugs are contraindicated in clients with severe hypertension or coronary artery disease because of their cardiac stimulating and vasoconstricting effects. They also are contraindicated for clients with narrow-angle glaucoma and those taking tricyclic or monoamine oxidase inhibitor antidepressants. They must be used with caution in the presence of cardiac arrhythmias, hyperthyroidism, diabetes mellitus, glaucoma, and prostatic hypertrophy.

Antitussives

Antitussive agents suppress cough by depressing the cough center in the medulla oblongata or the cough

receptors in the throat, trachea, or lungs. Centrally acting antitussives include narcotics (eg, codeine) and non-narcotics (eg, dextromethorphan). Peripherally acting agents (eg, glycerin, ammonium chloride) usually contain demulcents or local anesthetics to decrease irritation of pharyngeal mucosa. These agents are used as gargles, lozenges, and syrups. Flavored syrups are often used as vehicles for other drugs. Lozenges and hard candy increase the flow of saliva, which also soothes pharyngeal mucosa and may suppress cough.

The major clinical indication for use of antitussives is a dry, hacking, nonproductive cough that interferes with rest and sleep. It is not desirable to suppress a productive cough.

Expectorants

Expectorants are agents given orally to liquefy respiratory secretions and allow for their easier removal. Guaifenesin is an ingredient in many combination cough and cold remedies, although many authorities question its effectiveness.

Mucolytics

Mucolytics are administered by inhalation to liquefy mucus in the respiratory tract. Solutions of mucolytic drugs may be nebulized into a face mask or mouthpiece or instilled directly into the respiratory tract through a tracheostomy. Sodium chloride solution and acetylcysteine (Mucomyst) are the only agents recommended for use as mucolytics. Acetylcysteine is effective within 1 minute after inhalation, and maximal effects occur within 5 to 10 minutes. It is effective immediately after direct instillation. Oral acetylcysteine is widely used in the treatment of acetaminophen overdosage (see Chap. 7).

Cold Remedies

Many combination products are available for treating symptoms of the common cold. Most of the products contain an antihistamine, a nasal decongestant, and an analgesic. Some contain antitussives, expectorants, and other agents as well. Many cold remedies are over-the-counter (OTC) formulations. Commonly used ingredients include chlorpheniramine (antihistamine), pseudoephedrine or phenylpropanolamine (adrenergic nasal decongestants), acetaminophen or ibuprofen (analgesics), dextromethorphan (antitussive), and guaifenesin (expectorant). Although antihistamines are popular OTC drugs because they dry nasal secretions, they are not recommended because they can also dry lower respiratory secretions and worsen secretion retention and cough.

> ### How Can You Avoid This Medication Error?
>
> Mr. Fell, an elderly man with a history of hypertension and diabetes, has a cold. A resident, who does not know Mr. Fell well, prescribes pseudoephedrine (Sudafed) to relieve nasal congestion. You administer this medication as ordered. Discuss the error and the impact it will have on Mr. Fell.

Some products come in several formulations, with different ingredients, and are advertised for different purposes. For example, "nondrowsy" or "daytime" formulas contain a nasal decongestant, but do not contain an antihistamine. PM or "night" formulas contain a sedating antihistamine to promote sleep. "Maximum strength" preparations often contain 1000 mg of acetaminophen per dose. Pseudoephedrine is the nasal decongestant in oral Afrin; oxymetazoline is the decongestant in Afrin solutions for nasal spray and drops. In addition, labels on OTC combination products list ingredients by generic name, without identifying the type of drug. As a result of these bewildering products, consumers, including nurses and other health care providers, may not know what medications they are taking or whether some drugs increase or block the effects of other drugs.

INDIVIDUAL DRUGS

Individual decongestants, antitussives, expectorants, and mucolytics are listed in Table 49-1; selected combination products are listed in Table 49-2.

Nursing Notes: Apply Your Knowledge

Joan, a college student, comes to the health clinic with cold symptoms (productive cough, low-grade fever, continuous nasal discharge, and general malaise and discomfort). She states she went to the drugstore to buy some cold medicine, but there were so many different preparations that she was confused. Discuss your recommendations for Joan, with their underlying rationale.

NURSING PROCESS

Assessment

Assess the client's condition in relation to disorders for which the drugs are used.

- With nasal congestion, observe for decreased ability to breathe through the nose. If nasal discharge is present, note the amount, color, and thickness. Question the client about the duration and extent of nasal congestion and factors that precipitate or relieve the symptom.
- With coughing, a major assessment factor is whether the cough is productive of sputum or dry and hacking. If the cough is productive, note the color, odor, viscosity, and amount of sputum. In addition, assess factors that stimulate or relieve cough and the client's ability and willingness to cough effectively.

Nursing Diagnoses

- Risk for Injury related to cardiac arrhythmias, hypertension, and other adverse effects of nasal decongestants
- Noncompliance: Overuse of nasal decongestant and antitussive drugs
- Ineffective Airway Clearance related to suppression of a productive cough
- Knowledge Deficit: Appropriate use of single- and combination-drug formulations

Planning/Goals

The client will:

- Experience relief of symptoms
- Take drugs accurately and safely
- Avoid overuse of decongestants and antitussives
- Avoid preventable adverse drug effects
- Act to avoid recurrence of symptoms

Interventions

Encourage clients to use measures to prevent or minimize the incidence and severity of symptoms:

- Avoid smoking cigarettes. Cigarette smoke irritates respiratory tract mucosa, and this irritation causes cough, increased secretions, and decreased effectiveness of cilia in cleaning the respiratory tract.
- Avoid exposure to crowds, especially during winter when the incidence of influenza is high.
- Avoid contact with people who have colds or other respiratory infections. This is especially important for clients with chronic lung disease because upper respiratory infections may precipitate acute attacks of asthma or bronchitis.
- Maintain a fluid intake of 2000 to 3000 mL daily unless contraindicated by cardiovascular or renal disease.
- Maintain nutrition, rest, activity, and other general health measures.
- Practice good hand washing techniques.
- Annual vaccination for influenza is recommended for clients who are elderly or have chronic respiratory, cardiovascular, or renal disorders.

Evaluation

- Interview and observe for relief of symptoms.
- Interview and observe for tachycardia, hypertension, drowsiness, and other adverse drug effects.
- Interview and observe for compliance with instructions about drug use.

TABLE 49-1 **Nasal Decongestants, Antitussives, and Expectorants**

Generic/Trade Name	Routes and Dosage Ranges	
	Adults	Children
Nasal Decongestants		
Ephedrine	PO 25–50 mg q3–4h Topically, 1–2 drops of 1%–3% solution as needed	
Naphazoline (Privine)	Topically, 1–2 drops or 2 spray inhalations no more often than q4–6h	>6 y, topically, same as adults <6 y, not recommended
Oxymetazoline (Afrin)	Topically, 2–4 drops or 2–3 spray inhalations in each nostril, morning and bedtime	>6 y, topically, same as adults <6 y, 2–3 drops of 0.025% solution twice daily
Phenylephrine (Neo-Synephrine)	PO 10 mg three times daily Topically, 2–3 drops of 0.25%–1% solution in each nostril as needed	>6 y, PO 5 mg three times daily: topically, same as adults Infants, topically, 1–2 drops of 0.125% solution as needed
Phenylpropanolamine (Propagest)	PO 25 mg q4h or 75 mg (sustained release) q12h; maximal dose 150/d	6–12 y, PO 12.5 mg q4h; maximal dose 75 mg/d 2–6 y, PO 6.25 mg q4h
Propylhexedrine (Benzedrex)	Topically, 2 inhalations (0.6–0.8 mg) in each nostril as needed	
Pseudoephedrine (Sudafed)	PO 60 mg three or four times daily Sustained-release preparations, PO 120 mg twice daily	>6 y, PO 60 mg three or four times daily 4 mo–6 y, PO 30 mg three or four times daily
Tetrahydrozoline (Tyzine)	Topically, 2–3 drops or 1–2 sprays of 0.1% solution instilled in each nostril, no more often than q3h	≥6 y, topically, 1–3 drops of 0.05% solution in each nostril q4–6h <6 y, not recommended
Xylometazoline (Otrivin)	Topically, 2–4 drops or inhalations of 0.1% solution in each nostril two or three times daily	6 mo–12 y, topically, 2–3 drops of 0.05% solution in each nostril two or three times daily <6 mo, topically, 1 drop of 0.05% solution in each nostril two to three times daily
Narcotic Antitussive		
Codeine	PO 10–20 mg q4–6h as needed; maximal dose 120 mg/24 h	Age 6–12 y, PO 1–1.5 mg/kg/d in six divided doses as needed
Nonnarcotic Antitussive		
Dextromethorphan (Benylin DM, others)	PO 10–30 mg three or four times daily. Maximum dose 120 mg/24 h	2–6 y, PO 2.5–7.5 mg q4–8h. Maximum dose, 30 mg/24h 6–12 y, PO 5–10 mg q4h or 15 mg q6–8h Maximum dose, 60 mg/24h
Expectorant		
Guaifenesin (glyceryl guaiacolate) (Robitussin)	PO 200 mg (2 tsp) q4h	≥12 y, PO 200 mg (2 tsp) q4h 6–12 y, PO 100 mg (1 tsp) q4h 2–6 y, PO 50 mg (½ tsp) q4h
Mucolytic		
Acetylcysteine (Mucomyst)	Nebulization, 1–10 mL of a 20% solution or 2–20 mL of a 10% solution q2–6h Instillation, 1–2 mL of a 10% or 20% solution q1–4h Acetaminophen overdosage, PO 140 mg/kg initially, then 70 mg/kg q4h for 17 doses; dilute a 10% or 20% solution to a 5% solution with cola, fruit juice, or water	

PO, oral.

PRINCIPLES OF THERAPY

Drug Selection and Administration

Choice of drugs and routes of administration are influenced by several client- and drug-related variables. Some guidelines include the following:

1. Single-drug formulations allow flexibility and individualization of dosage, whereas combination products may contain unneeded ingredients and are more expensive. However, many people find combination products more convenient to use.

2. With nasal decongestants, topical preparations (ie, nasal solutions or sprays) are often preferred for

TABLE 49-2 Nonprescription Cold, Cough, and Sinus Remedies

	Ingredients				
Trade Name	Antihistamine	Nasal Decongestant	Analgesic	Antitussive	Expectorant
Actifed	Triprolidine 2.5 mg/tab or cap	Pseudoephedrine 60 mg/tab or cap			
Advil Cold and Sinus Caplets		Pseudoephedrine 30 mg	Ibuprofen 200 mg		
Allerest	Chlorpheniramine 2 mg/tab	Phenylpropanol- amine 18.7 mg/ tab			
Allerest (children's preparation)	Chlorpheniramine 1 mg/tab	Phenylpropanol- amine 9.4 mg/tab			
Cheracol D Cough Liquid				Dextromethorphan 10 mg/5 mL	Guaifenesin 100 mg/ 5 mL
Comtrex	Chlorpheniramine 2 mg/cap	Phenylpropanol- amine 12.5 mg/ cap	Acetaminophen 325 mg/cap	Dextromethorphan 10 mg/cap	
Contac	Chlorpheniramine 8 mg/cap	Phenylpropanol- amine 75 mg/cap			
Coricidin	Chlorpheniramine 2 mg/tab		Acetaminophen 325 mg/tab		
Coricidin D	Chlorpheniramine 2 mg/tab	Phenylpropanol- amine 12.5 mg/ tab	Acetaminophen 325 mg/tab		
CoTylenol cold formula	Chlorpheniramine 2 mg/tab or cap	Pseudoephedrine 30 mg/tab or cap	Acetaminophen 325 mg/tab or cap	Dextromethorphan 15 mg/tab or cap	
CoTylenol liquid (children's preparation)	Chlorpheniramine 1 mg/5 mL	Phenylpropanol- amine 6.25 mg/ 5 mL	Acetaminophen 160 mg/5 mL		
Dimetapp Elixir	Brompheniramine 2 mg/5 mL	Phenylpropanol- amine 12.5 mg/ 5 mL			
Dimetapp Tablets	Brompheniramine 4 mg/tab	Phenylpropanol- amine 25 mg/tab			
Dimetapp Extentabs	Brompheniramine 12 mg/tab	Phenylpropanol- amine 75 mg/tab			
Dimetapp Sinus Caplets		Pseudoephedrine 30 mg	Ibuprofen 200 mg		
Dristan	Chlorpheniramine 2 mg/cap or tab	Phenylephrine 5 mg/ cap or tab	Acetaminophen 325 mg/cap or tab		
Dristan Sinus Caplets		Pseudoephedrine 30 mg			
Drixoral	Dexbrompheni- ramine 6 mg/tab	Pseudoephedrine 120 mg/tab			
Motrin IB Sinus Caplets		Pseudoephedrine 30 mg	Ibuprofen 200 mg		
Robitussin-CF		Phenylpropanol- amine 12.5 mg/ 5 mL		Dextromethorphan 10 mg/5 mL	Guaifenesin 100 mg/ 5 mL
Robitussin-DM				Dextromethorphan 15 mg/5 mL	Guaifenesin 100 mg/ 5 mL
Sinutab	Chlorpheniramine 2 mg/tab	Pseudoephedrine 30 mg/tab	Acetaminophen 325 mg/tab		
TheraFlu flu, cold, and cough powder	Chlorpheniramine 4 mg/pack	Pseudoephedrine 60 mg/pack	Acetaminophen 650 mg/pack	Dextromethorphan 20 mg/pack	
Vicks NyQuil	Doxylamine 7.5 mg/oz	Pseudoephedrine 60 mg/oz	Acetaminophen 1000 mg/oz	Dextromethorphan 30 mg/oz	

CLIENT TEACHING GUIDELINES
Nasal Decongestants, Anticough Medications, and Multi-ingredient Cold Remedies

General Considerations

✔ These drugs may relieve symptoms but do not cure the disorder causing the symptoms.

✔ An adequate fluid intake, humidification of the environment, and sucking on hard candy or throat lozenges can help to relieve mouth dryness and cough.

✔ Over-the-counter (OTC) cold remedies should not be used longer than 1 week. Do not use nose drops more often than recommended or for longer than 7 consecutive days. Excessive or prolonged use may damage nasal mucosa and produce chronic nasal congestion.

✔ Do not increase dosage if symptoms are not relieved by recommended amounts.

✔ See a health care provider if symptoms persist longer than 1 week.

✔ Read the labels of OTC allergy, cold, and sinus remedies for information about ingredients, dosages, conditions, or other medications with which the drugs should not be taken, and adverse effects.

✔ Do not combine two drug preparations containing the same or similar active ingredients. For example, phenylpropanolamine is the nasal decongestant component of numerous OTC multi-ingredient cold remedies (Allerest, Comtrex, Contac, Dimetapp, others). These preparations should not be combined with each other, with other preparations containing pseudoephedrine (a drug with similar effects), or with OTC appetite suppressants such as Acutrim or Dexatrim (the active ingredient is phenylpropanolamine).

✔ Note that many combination products contain acetaminophen or ibuprofen as pain relievers. If you are taking another form of one of these drugs (eg, Tylenol or Advil), there is a risk of overdosage and adverse effects. Acetaminophen can cause liver damage; ibuprofen is a relative of aspirin that can cause gastrointestinal upset and bleeding. Thus, you need to be sure your total daily dosage is not excessive (with Tylenol, above four to six doses of 1000 mg each; with ibuprofen, above 2400 mg).

Self-administration

✔ Take medications as prescribed or as directed on the labels of OTC preparations. Taking excessive amounts or taking recommended amounts too often can lead to serious adverse effects.

✔ Do not chew or crush long-acting tablets or capsules (eg, those taken once or twice daily). Such actions can cause rapid drug absorption, high blood levels, and serious adverse effects, rather than the slow absorption and prolonged action intended with these products.

✔ For OTC drugs available in different dosage strengths, start with lower recommended doses rather than "maximum strength" formulations or the highest recommended doses. It is safer to see how the drugs affect you, then increase doses if necessary and not contraindicated.

✔ With topical nasal decongestants:
1. Use only preparations labeled for intranasal use. For example, phenylephrine (Neo-Synephrine) is available in both nasal and eye formulations. The two types of solutions *cannot* be used interchangeably. In addition, phenylephrine preparations may contain 0.125%, 0.25%, 0.5%, or 1% of drug. Be sure the concentration is appropriate for the person to receive it (eg, an infant, young child, or older adult).
2. Blow the nose gently before instilling nasal solutions or sprays. This clears nasal passages and increases effectiveness of medications.
3. To instill nose drops, lie down or sit with the neck hyperextended and instill medication without touching the dropper to the nostrils (to avoid contamination of the dropper and medication). Rinse the medication dropper after each use.
4. For nasal sprays, sit or stand, squeeze the container once to instill medication, avoid touching the spray tip to the nostrils, and rinse the spray tip after each use. Most nasal sprays are designed to deliver one dose when used correctly. If necessary, secretions may be cleared and a second spray used.
5. Give decongestant nose drops to infants 20 to 30 minutes before feeding. Nasal congestion interferes with an infant's ability to suck.

✔ Take or give cough syrups undiluted and avoid eating and drinking for approximately 30 minutes. Part of the beneficial effect of cough syrups stems from soothing effects on pharyngeal mucosa. Food or fluid removes the medication from the pharynx.

✔ Report palpitations, dizziness, drowsiness, or rapid pulse. These effects may occur with nasal decongestants and cold remedies and may indicate excessive dosage.

---

short-term use. They are rapidly effective because they come into direct contact with nasal mucosa. If used longer than 7 days or in excessive amounts, however, these products may produce rebound nasal congestion. Oral drugs are preferred for long-term use (>7 days). For clients with cardiovascular disease, topical nasal decongestants are preferred.

Oral agents are usually contraindicated because of cardiovascular effects (eg, increased force of myocardial contraction, increased heart rate, increased blood pressure).

3. Most antitussives are given orally as tablets or cough syrups. Syrups serve as vehicles for antitussive drugs and may exert antitussive effects of their own by

soothing irritated pharyngeal mucosa. Dextromethorphan is the antitussive drug of choice in most circumstances (often designated by DM on the product label). It is as effective as codeine without the disadvantages of a narcotic preparation. Dextromethorphan has no analgesic effect, does not produce tolerance or dependence, and does not depress respiration.

4. For treatment of excessive respiratory tract secretions, mechanical measures (eg, coughing, deep breathing, ambulation, chest physiotherapy, forcing fluids) are more likely to be effective than expectorant drug therapy.

Use in Children

Upper respiratory infections with nasal congestion, cough, and increased secretions are common in children. The drugs described in this chapter are often used, and general principles apply.

Nasal congestion may interfere with an infant's ability to nurse. Phenylephrine nasal solution, applied just before feeding time, is usually effective.

Excessive amounts or too frequent administration of topical agents may result in rebound nasal congestion and systemic effects of cardiac and central nervous system stimulation. Despite these potential difficulties, topical drugs are less likely to cause systemic effects than oral agents.

Use in Older Adults

Older adults are at high risk of adverse effects (eg, hypertension, arrhythmias, nervousness, insomnia) from oral nasal decongestants. Adverse effects from topical agents are less likely, but rebound nasal congestion and systemic effects may occur with overuse. Older adults with significant cardiovascular disease should usually avoid the drugs.

 Home Care

Clients and others in home settings may ask the home care nurse for advice about OTC cold remedies. Before recommending a particular product, the nurse needs to assess the intended recipient for conditions or other medications that contraindicate the product's use. For example, the nasal decongestant component may cause or aggravate cardiovascular disorders (eg, hypertension). In addition, other medications the client is taking need to be evaluated in terms of potential drug interactions with the cold remedy.

The home care nurse also must emphasize the need to read the label of any OTC medication for administration instructions, precautions, contraindications, and so forth.

(*text continues on page 739*)

NURSING ACTIONS	Nasal Decongestants, Antitussives, and Cold Remedies

NURSING ACTIONS	**RATIONALE/EXPLANATION**
1. Administer accurately	
a. With topical nasal decongestants:	
(1) Use only preparations labeled for intranasal use.	Intranasal preparations are usually dilute, aqueous solutions prepared specifically for intranasal use. Some agents (eg, phenylephrine) are available in ophthalmic solutions as well. The two types of solutions *cannot* be used interchangeably.
(2) Use the drug concentration ordered.	Some drug preparations are available in several concentrations. For example, phenylephrine preparations may contain 0.125%, 0.25%, 0.5%, or 1% of drug.
(3) For instillation of nose drops, have the client lie down or sit with the neck hyperextended. Instill medication without touching the dropper to the nares. Rinse the medication dropper after each use.	To avoid contamination of the dropper and medication
(4) For nasal sprays, have the client sit, squeeze the container once to instill medication, avoid touching the spray tip to the nares, and rinse the spray tip after each use.	Most nasal sprays are designed to deliver one dose when used correctly. If necessary, secretions may be cleared and a second spray used. Correct usage and cleansing prevents contamination and infection.

(*continued*)

NURSING ACTIONS	RATIONALE/EXPLANATION
(5) Give nasal decongestants to infants 20–30 min before feeding.	Nasal congestion interferes with an infant's ability to suck.
b. Administer cough syrups undiluted and instruct the client to avoid eating and drinking for approximately 30 min.	Part of the therapeutic benefit of cough syrups stems from soothing effects on pharyngeal mucosa. Food or fluid removes the medication from the pharynx.
2. Observe for therapeutic effects	Therapeutic effects depend on the reason for use.
a. When nasal decongestants are given, observe for decreased nasal obstruction and drainage.	
b. With antitussives, observe for decreased coughing.	The goal of antitussive therapy is to suppress non-purposeful coughing, not productive coughing.
c. With cold and allergy remedies, observe for decreased nasal congestion, rhinitis, muscle aches, and other symptoms.	
3. Observe for adverse effects	
a. With nasal decongestants, observe for:	
(1) Tachycardia, cardiac arrhythmias, hypertension	These effects may occur with any of the adrenergic drugs (see Chap. 18). When adrenergic drugs are used as nasal decongestants, cardiovascular effects are more likely to occur with oral agents. However, topically applied drugs also may be systemically absorbed through the nasal mucosa or by being swallowed and absorbed through the gastrointestinal tract.
(2) Rebound nasal congestion, chronic rhinitis, and possible ulceration of nasal mucosa	Adverse effects on nasal mucosa are more likely to occur with excessive or long-term (>10 d) use.
b. With antitussives, observe for:	
(1) Excessive suppression of the cough reflex (inability to cough effectively when secretions are present)	This is a potentially serious adverse effect because retained secretions may lead to atelectasis, pneumonia, hypoxia, hypercarbia, and respiratory failure.
(2) Nausea, vomiting, constipation, dizziness, drowsiness, pruritus, and drug dependence	These are adverse effects associated with narcotic agents (see Chap. 6). When narcotics are given for antitussive effects, however, they are given in relatively small doses and are unlikely to cause adverse reactions.
(3) Nausea, drowsiness, and dizziness with non-narcotic antitussives	Adverse effects are infrequent and mild with these agents.
c. With combination products (eg, cold remedies), observe for adverse effects of individual ingredients (ie, antihistamines, adrenergics, analgesics, and others)	Adverse effects are rarely significant when the products are used as prescribed. There may be subtherapeutic doses of one or more component drugs, especially in over-the-counter formulations. Also, the drowsiness associated with antihistamines may be offset by stimulating effects of adrenergics. Ephedrine, for example, has central nervous system (CNS)–stimulating effects.
4. Observe for drug interactions	
a. Drugs that *increase* effects of nasal decongestants:	These interactions are more likely to occur with oral decongestants than topically applied drugs.

(continued)

NURSING ACTIONS	RATIONALE/EXPLANATION
(1) Cocaine, digoxin, general anesthetics, monoamine oxidase (MAO) inhibitors, other adrenergic drugs, thyroid preparations, and xanthines	Increased risks of cardiac arrhythmias
(2) Antihistamines, epinephrine, ergot alkaloids, MAO inhibitors, methylphenidate	Increased risks of hypertension due to vasoconstriction
b. Drugs that *increase* antitussive effects of codeine:	
(1) CNS depressants (alcohol, antianxiety agents, barbiturates, and other sedative-hypnotics)	Additive CNS depression. Codeine is given in small doses for antitussive effects, and risks of significant interactions are minimal.
c. Drugs that alter effects of dextromethorphan:	
(1) MAO inhibitors	This combination is contraindicated. Apnea, muscular rigidity, hyperpyrexia, laryngospasm, and death may occur.
d. Drugs that may alter effects of combination products for coughs, colds, and allergies:	Interactions depend on the individual drug components of each formulation. Risks of clinically significant drug interactions are increased with use of combination products.
(1) Adrenergic (sympathomimetic) agents (see Chap. 18)	
(2) Antihistamines (see Chap. 48)	
(3) CNS depressants (see Chaps. 6, 8, and 13)	
(4) CNS stimulants (see Chap. 16)	

How Can You Avoid This Medication Error?

Answer: Sudafed is an adrenergic agent whose use is contraindicated in hypertensive clients because it significantly increases blood pressure. It is the nurse's responsibility to know contraindications to any medication she or he administers. When requesting an order from a physician who does not know the patient well, it is helpful to briefly outline significant medical problems or medications that may interact. Because Mr. Fell's blood pressure and pulse rate are likely to go up, monitor vital signs more frequently and request a PRN order for an antihypertensive agent if necessary.

 REVIEW AND APPLICATION EXERCISES

1. How do adrenergic drugs relieve nasal congestion?
2. Who should usually avoid OTC nasal decongestants and cold remedies?
3. What are advantages and disadvantages of multi-ingredient cold remedies?
4. What is usually the antitussive of choice?
5. When is an antitussive contraindicated or undesirable?
6. Given a client with a productive cough, what are non-drug interventions to promote removal of secretions?

Nursing Notes: Apply Your Knowledge

Answer: Joan has the symptoms of a cold. Tell her to avoid combination products that may include medications she does not need and are generally more expensive. Because her cough is productive, an antitussive agent (cough suppressant) is contraindicated because expectorating retained secretions promotes recovery and prevents pneumonia and other respiratory complications. An expectorant, such as guaifenesin, would help liquefy respiratory secretions and aid their removal. A nasal decongestant could be used to decrease nasal stuffiness and discharge. Acetaminophen can be taken to reduce generalized discomfort. In addition to discussing medications, stress the importance of getting adequate rest and drinking lots of fluids.

SELECTED REFERENCES

Drug facts and comparisons. (Updated monthly). St. Louis: Facts and Comparisons.
Guyton, A.C. & Hall, J.E. (1996). *Textbook of medical physiology*, 9th ed. Philadelphia: W.B. Saunders.
Porth, C.M. (Ed.). (1998). *Pathophysiology: Concepts of altered health states*, 5th ed. Philadelphia: Lippincott Williams & Wilkins.

Drugs Affecting the Cardiovascular System

50

Physiology of the Cardiovascular System

Objectives

After studying this chapter, the student will be able to:

1. Review roles of the heart, blood vessels, and blood in supplying oxygen and nutrients to body tissues.

2. Describe the role of vascular endothelium in maintaining homeostasis.

3. Discuss atherosclerosis as the basic disorder causing many cardiovascular disorders for which drug therapy is required.

4. List cardiovascular disorders for which drug therapy is a major treatment modality.

5. Identify general categories of drugs used to treat cardiovascular disorders.

The cardiovascular or circulatory system is composed of the heart, blood vessels, and blood. The general functions of the system are to carry oxygen, nutrients, hormones, antibodies, and other substances to all body cells and to remove waste products of cell metabolism (carbon dioxide and others). The efficiency of the system depends on the heart's ability to pump blood, the patency and functions of blood vessels, and the quality and quantity of blood.

HEART

The heart is a hollow, muscular organ that functions as an electrical double pump to circulate 5 to 6 liters of blood through the body every minute. Major components and characteristics are described in the following sections.

Chambers

The heart has four chambers: two atria and two ventricles. The *atria* are receiving chambers. The right atrium receives deoxygenated blood from the upper part of the body by way of the superior vena cava, from the lower part of the body by way of the inferior vena cava, and from veins and sinuses within the heart itself. The left atrium receives oxygenated blood from the lungs through the pulmonary veins. The *ventricles* are distributing chambers. The right ventricle sends deoxygenated blood through the pulmonary circulation. It is small and thin walled because it contracts against minimal pressure. The left ventricle pumps oxygenated blood through the systemic circuit. It is much more muscular and thick walled because it contracts against relatively high pressure. The right atrium and right ventricle form one pump, and the left atrium and left ventricle form another. The right and left sides of the heart are separated by a strip of muscle called the *septum*.

Layers

The layers of the heart are the endocardium, myocardium, and epicardium. The *endocardium* is the membrane lining the heart chambers. It is continuous with the endothelial lining of blood vessels entering and leaving the heart and covers the heart valves. The *myocardium* is the strong muscular layer of the heart that provides the pumping power of the circulation. The *epicardium* is the outer, serous layer of the heart. The heart is enclosed in a fibroserous sac called the *pericardium*.

Valves

Heart valves function to guide the one-way flow of blood and prevent backflow. The *mitral* valve separates the left atrium and left ventricle. The *tricuspid* valve separates the right atrium and right ventricle. The *pulmonic* valve separates the right ventricle and pulmonary artery. The *aortic* valve separates the left ventricle and aorta.

Conduction System

The heart contains special cells that can carry electrical impulses much more rapidly than ordinary muscle fibers. This special conduction system consists of the sinoatrial (SA) node, the atrioventricular node, bundle of His, right and left bundle branches, and Purkinje fibers. The SA node, the normal pacemaker of the heart, can be compared with a battery. It originates a burst of electrical energy approximately 70 to 80 times each minute under normal circumstances. The electrical current flows over the heart in an orderly way to produce contraction of both atria, then both ventricles.

A unique characteristic of the heart is that each part can generate its own electrical impulse to contract. For example, the ventricles can beat independently, but at a rate of only 30 to 40 beats per minute. In addition, the heart does not require nervous stimulation to contract. However, the autonomic nervous system does influence heart rate. Sympathetic nerves increase heart rate; parasympathetic nerves (by way of the vagus nerve) decrease heart rate.

Blood Supply

The heart receives its blood supply from the coronary arteries. Coronary arteries branch off the aorta and fill during *diastole*, the resting or filling phase of the cardiac cycle. Coronary arteries branch into "end arteries," which supply certain parts of the myocardium without an overlapping supply from other branches. However, there are many artery-to-artery anastomoses between adjacent vessels. The anastomotic arteries do not supply sufficient blood to the heart if a major artery is suddenly occluded, but they may dilate into arteries of considerable size when disease (usually coronary atherosclerosis) develops slowly. The resultant *collateral circulation* may provide sufficient blood for myocardial function, at least during rest.

BLOOD VESSELS

There are three types of blood vessels, the arteries, veins, and capillaries. Arteries and veins are similar in that they have three layers. The *intima*, the inner lining, has an elastic layer that joins the media and a layer of endothelial cells that lies next to the blood. The endothelial layer provides a smooth inner surface for the vessel. The *media* is the middle layer of muscle and elastic tissue. The *adventitia* is the outer layer of connective tissue.

Blood vessel walls are composed of two types of cells, *smooth muscle cells* and *endothelial cells*. Vascular smooth muscle functions to maintain blood pressure and blood flow. It contracts and relaxes in response to numerous stimuli, including local and circulating mediators. Contractile properties also vary among locations, with some blood vessels being more responsive to some stimuli than others. Overall, regulation of tone in vascular smooth muscle depends on the intracellular concentration of calcium ions. Increased intracellular calcium leads to increased vascular tone. There are several mechanisms by which calcium ions can enter the cell.

Endothelial cells, once thought to be passive conduits for blood flow, are now known to perform two extremely important functions in maintaining homeostatic processes. One function is structural, in which the cells act as a permeability barrier and regulate passage of molecules and cells across the blood vessel wall. The second function is metabolic, in which the cells secrete opposing mediators that maintain a balance between bleeding and clotting of blood (including activation and inhibition of platelet functions and fibrinolysis), constriction and dilation of blood vessels, and promotion and inhibition of vascular cell growth and inflammation. Selected mediators are listed in Table 50-1; some are discussed in more detail in later chapters.

Arteries

Arteries and arterioles contain a well-developed layer of smooth muscle (the media) and are sometimes called *resistance* vessels. Their efficiency depends on their patency and ability to constrict or dilate in response to various stimuli. The degree of constriction or dilation (vasomotor tone) determines peripheral vascular resistance, which is a major determinant of blood pressure.

Veins

Veins and venules have a thin media and valves that assist blood flow against gravity. They are sometimes called *capacitance* vessels, because blood may accumulate in various parts of the venous system. Their efficiency depends on patency, competency of valves, and the pumping action of muscles around veins.

Capillaries

Capillaries, the smallest blood vessels, connect the arterial and venous portions of the circulation. They consist of a single layer of connected endothelial cells and a few smooth muscle cells. Gases, nutrients, cells, and waste products are exchanged between blood and extracellular fluid across capillary walls. The endothelial lining acts as a semipermeable membrane to regulate the exchange of plasma solutes with extracellular fluid. Lipid-soluble materials diffuse directly through the capillary cell membrane; water and water-soluble materials enter and leave the capillary through the junctions or gaps between endothelial cells.

TABLE 50-1 Endothelial Mediators that Regulate Cardiovascular Function

Promoting Factors	Inhibiting Factors
Vasomotor Tone	
Vasodilators	**Vasoconstrictors**
Endothelial-derived hyperpolarizing factor (EDHF)	Angiotensin II
Nitric oxide (also called endothelial-derived relaxing factor, or EDRF)	Endothelin
	Endothelium-derived constricting factor
Prostacyclin (prostaglandin I$_2$)	Platelet-derived growth factor
	Thromboxane A$_2$
Blood Coagulation	
Procoagulants	**Anticoagulants**
Tissue factor	Heparin sulfate
Von Willebrand factor	Thrombomodulin
Platelet activators	**Platelet inhibitors**
Platelet-activating factor	Nitric oxide
Von Willebrand factor	Prostacyclin
Profibrinolytic factors	**Antifibrinolytic factor**
Tissue plasminogen activator (t-PA)	Plasminogen activator inhibitor-1
Urokinase-type plasminogen activator	
Cell Growth	
Angiotensin II	Heparan
Endothelin	Nitric oxide
Platelet-derived growth factor	Prostacyclin
Inflammation	
Proinflammatory factors	**Anti-inflammatory factors**
Cellular and intercellular adhesion molecules	Nitric oxide
Monocyte chemotactic protein-1	
Interleukin-8	

Lymphatics

Lymphatic vessels, which are composed mainly of endothelium, parallel the veins and empty into the venous system. They drain tissue fluid that has filtered through the endothelium of capillaries and venules from the plasma. They then carry lymphocytes, large molecules of protein and fat, microorganisms, and other materials to regional lymph nodes.

BLOOD

Blood functions to nourish and oxygenate body cells, protect the body from invading microorganisms, and initiate hemostasis when a blood vessel is injured. Specific functions and components are listed in the following sections.

Functions

- Transports oxygen to cells and carbon dioxide from cells to lungs for removal from the body
- Carries absorbed food products from the gastrointestinal tract to tissues; at the same time, it carries metabolic wastes from tissues to the kidneys, skin, and lungs for excretion
- Carries hormones from endocrine glands to other parts of the body
- Carries leukocytes and antibodies to sites of injury, infection, and inflammation
- Helps regulate body temperature by transferring heat produced by cell metabolism to the skin, where it can be released
- Carries platelets to injured areas for hemostasis

Components

- *Plasma* comprises approximately 55% of the total blood volume, and it is more than 90% water. Other ingredients are
  - Serum albumin, which helps maintain blood volume by exerting colloid osmotic pressure
  - Fibrinogen, which is necessary for hemostasis
  - Gamma globulin, which is necessary for defense against microorganisms
  - Less than 1% antibodies, nutrients, metabolic wastes, respiratory gases, enzymes, and inorganic salts
- *Solid particles* or cells comprise approximately 45% of total blood volume. Cells include erythrocytes (red blood cells or RBCs); leukocytes (white blood cells or WBCs); and thrombocytes (platelets). The bone marrow produces all RBCs, 60% to 70% of WBCs, and all platelets. Lymphatic tissues (spleen and lymph nodes) produce 20% to 30% of the WBCs, and reticuloendothelial tissues (spleen, liver, lymph nodes) produce 4% to 8% of WBCs. Cell characteristics include the following:
  - Erythrocytes function mainly to transport oxygen. Almost all oxygen (95% to 97%) is transported in combination with hemoglobin; very little is dissolved in blood. The lifespan of a normal RBC is approximately 120 days.
  - Leukocytes function mainly as a defense mechanism against microorganisms. They leave the bloodstream to enter injured tissues and phagocytize the injurious agent. They also produce antibodies. The lifespan of a normal WBC is a few hours.
  - Platelets are fragments of large cells, called megakaryocytes, found in the bone marrow. Platelets are essential to blood coagulation. For example, when a blood vessel is injured, platelets adhere to each other and the edges of the injury to form a cluster of activated platelets (ie, a platelet throm-

bus or "plug") that sticks to the vessel wall and prevents leakage of blood. In addition, the clustered platelets release substances (eg, adenosine diphosphate, thromboxane A_2, von Willebrand factor) that promote recruitment and aggregation of new platelets.

Platelets have no nucleus and cannot replicate. If not used, they circulate for approximately a week before being removed by phagocytic cells of the spleen.

CARDIOVASCULAR DISORDERS

Cardiovascular disorders, which are common causes of morbidity and mortality, often stem from blood vessel abnormalities. In turn, most vascular diseases result from the malfunction of endothelial cells or smooth muscle cells. In fact, dysfunctional endothelium is considered a major factor in atherosclerosis, angina pectoris, myocardial infarction, hypertension, and thromboembolic disorders. The main cause of endothelial dysfunction is injury to the blood vessel wall from trauma or disease processes. The injury unbalances the normal regulatory forces and leads to vasospasm, thrombosis, growth of the intimal layer of the blood vessel, rupture of atherosclerotic plaque, tissue ischemia and infarction, and arrhythmias. Pathologic changes in the structure of the capillary and venular endothelium also result in the accumulation of excess fluid in interstitial space (edema), a common symptom of cardiovascular and other disorders.

Overall, cardiovascular disorders may involve any structure or function of the cardiovascular system. Because the circulatory system is a closed system, a disorder in one part of the system eventually disturbs the function of all other parts.

DRUG THERAPY IN CARDIOVASCULAR DISORDERS

Cardiovascular disorders usually treated with drug therapy include atherosclerosis, heart failure, cardiac arrhythmias, angina pectoris, myocardial infarction, hypertension, hypotension, and shock. Peripheral vascular disease and valvular disease are usually treated surgically. Blood disorders that respond to drug therapy include certain types of anemia and coagulation disorders.

The goal of drug therapy in cardiovascular disorders is often to restore homeostasis or physiologic balance between opposing factors (eg, coagulant vs. anticoagulant, vasoconstriction vs. vasodilation). Thus, cardiovascular drugs may be given to increase or decrease cardiac output, blood pressure, and heart rate; to alter heart rhythm; increase or decrease blood clotting; alter the quality of blood; and decrease chest pain of cardiac origin. In addition, these drugs are often given for palliation of symptoms. For example, in angina pectoris, hypertension, and heart failure, the drugs relieve symptoms but do not alter the underlying disease process.

 REVIEW AND APPLICATION EXERCISES

1. How does the heart muscle differ from skeletal muscle?

2. What is the normal pacemaker of the heart?

3. In what circumstances do other parts of the heart take over as pacemaker?

4. What is the effect of parasympathetic (vagal) stimulation on the heart?

5. What is the effect of sympathetic stimulation on the heart and blood vessels?

6. How does low or high blood volume influence blood pressure?

7. List five chemical mediators produced by endothelial cells and their roles in maintaining cardiovascular function.

8. How does endothelial cell dysfunction contribute to cardiovascular disorders?

SELECTED REFERENCES

Gokce, N., Keaney, J.F., Jr., & Vita, J.A. (1998). Endotheliopathies: Clinical manifestations of endothelial dysfunction. In J. Loscalzo & A.I. Schafer (Eds.), *Thrombosis and hemorrhage,* 2nd ed., pp. 901–924. Baltimore: Williams & Wilkins.

Guyton, A.C. & Hall, J.E. (1996). *Textbook of medical physiology,* 9th ed. Philadelphia: W.B. Saunders.

Hathaway, D.R. & Marach, K.L. (1997). Vascular biology. In W.N. Kelley (Ed.), *Textbook of internal medicine,* 3rd ed., pp. 66–72. Philadelphia: Lippincott-Raven.

Porth, C.M. (Ed.). (1998). *Pathophysiology: Concepts of altered health states,* 5th ed. Philadelphia: Lippincott Williams & Wilkins.

Selwyn, A.P. (1998). Coronary physiology and pathophysiology. In D.L. Brown (Ed.), *Cardiac intensive care,* pp. 63–65. Philadelphia: W.B. Saunders.

Smeltzer, S.C. & Bare, B.G. (1996). *Brunner and Suddarth's Textbook of medical-surgical nursing,* 8th ed. Philadelphia: Lippincott-Raven.

51

Drug Therapy of Heart Failure

Objectives

After studying this chapter, the student will be able to:

1. Describe major manifestations of heart failure (HF).

2. Discuss the role of endothelial dysfunction in HF.

3. Differentiate the types of drugs used to treat HF.

4. List characteristics of digoxin in terms of effects on myocardial contractility and cardiac conduction, indications for use, principles of therapy, and nursing process implications.

5. Differentiate therapeutic effects of digoxin in HF and atrial fibrillation.

6. Differentiate digitalizing and maintenance doses of digoxin.

7. Identify therapeutic and excessive serum digoxin levels.

8. Identify clients at risk for development of digoxin toxicity.

9. Discuss interventions to prevent or minimize digoxin toxicity.

10. Explain the roles of potassium chloride, lidocaine, atropine, and digoxin immune fab in the treatment of digoxin toxicity.

11. Teach clients ways to increase safety and effectiveness of digoxin.

12. Discuss important elements of using digoxin in special populations.

George Sweeney, a 72-year-old retired carpenter, was recently hospitalized with heart failure and started on captopril, an angiotensin-converting enzyme (ACE) inhibitor. You are a staff nurse assigned to his care. He has many questions about his new diagnosis and the captopril.

Reflect on:

▶ Physiologically, what happens when the heart fails to pump adequately, and what symptoms are seen in the client?

▶ How ACE inhibitors decrease the workload of the heart.

▶ What criteria (objective and subjective) will you use to evaluate whether the ACE inhibitor is effectively managing Mr. Sweeney's heart failure?

HEART FAILURE

Heart failure (HF), also called congestive heart failure (CHF), is a common condition that occurs when the heart cannot pump enough blood to meet tissue needs for oxygen and nutrients. It may result from impaired myocardial contraction during systole (systolic dysfunction), impaired filling of ventricles during diastole (diastolic dysfunction), or a combination of systolic and diastolic dysfunction.

Causes

At the cellular level, HF stems from dysfunction of contractile myocardial cells and the endothelial cells that line the heart and blood vessels (see Chap. 50). Endothelial dysfunction allows processes that narrow the blood vessel lumen (eg, buildup of atherosclerotic plaque, growth of cells, inflammation, activation of platelets) and lead to blood clot formation and vasoconstriction that further narrow the blood vessel lumen. These are major factors in coronary artery disease and hypertension, the most common conditions leading to HF.

Other causative factors include hyperthyroidism, excessive intravenous (IV) fluids or blood transfusions, and drugs that decrease the force of myocardial contraction (eg, antiarrhythmic drugs) or cause retention of sodium and water (eg, corticosteroids, estrogens, nonsteroidal anti-inflammatory agents). These factors impair the pumping ability or increase the workload of the heart so an adequate cardiac output cannot be maintained.

Compensatory Mechanisms

When HF develops, the low cardiac output and inadequately filled arteries activate compensatory mechanisms that help the body maintain blood flow to tissues. One mechanism is increased sympathetic activity and circulating catecholamines, which increases the force of myocardial contraction, increases heart rate, and causes vasoconstriction. Another mechanism is activation of the renin-angiotensin-aldosterone system. Renin is an enzyme produced in the kidney in response to impaired blood flow and tissue perfusion. When released into the blood-

stream, it stimulates the production of angiotensin II, a powerful vasoconstrictor.

Arterial vasoconstriction impairs heart function by increasing the impedance (afterload) against which the ventricle ejects blood. This raises filling pressures inside the heart, increases stretch and stress on the myocardial wall, and predisposes to subendocardial ischemia. In addition, clients with severe HF have constricted arterioles in cerebral, myocardial, renal, hepatic, and mesenteric vascular beds. This results in increased organ hypoperfusion and dysfunction. Venous vasoconstriction limits venous capacitance, resulting in venous congestion and increased diastolic ventricular filling pressures (preload).

The adrenal cortex is also stimulated to increase production of aldosterone, and aldosterone increases reabsorption of sodium and water in renal tubules. Secretion of vasopressin (antidiuretic hormone) also increases. These mechanisms combine to increase blood volume and pressure in the heart chambers, stretch muscle fibers, and produce dilation, hypertrophy, and changes in the shape of the heart (a process called cardiac or ventricular remodeling) that make it contract less efficiently. Overall, the compensatory mechanisms increase preload (amount of venous blood returning to the heart), workload of the heart, afterload (amount of resistance in the aorta and peripheral blood vessels that the heart must overcome to pump effectively), and blood pressure.

Signs and Symptoms

Clients with compensated HF usually have no symptoms at rest and no edema; dyspnea and fatigue occur only with activities involving moderate or higher levels of exertion. Symptoms that occur with minimal exertion or at rest and are accompanied by ankle edema and distention of the jugular vein (from congestion of veins and leakage of fluid into tissues) reflect decompensation. Acute, severe cardiac decompensation is manifested by pulmonary edema, a medical emergency that requires immediate treatment. Clients with chronic HF are often classified according to the New York Heart Association grouping that separates clients into four groups according to symptoms and activity tolerance (Box 51-1). These categories are often used in research studies, to help evaluate results of therapy, and

BOX 51-1   NEW YORK HEART ASSOCIATION CLASSIFICATION OF PATIENTS WITH HEART DISEASE

Class I. No limitations of physical activity; ordinary physical activity does not cause dyspnea, fatigue, or palpitations.

Class II. Slight limitations of physical activity. Patients are comfortable at rest but have dyspnea, fatigue, palpitations, or chest pain (angina) with ordinary physical activity.

Class III. Marked limitations of physical activity. Patients are comfortable at rest but develop symptoms with less than ordinary physical activity.

Class IV. Patients are unable to perform any physical activity without discomfort. Symptoms of heart failure or angina are present even at rest. If any physical activity is undertaken, discomfort increases.

in literature about heart disease, to indicate a client's functional status.

DRUG THERAPY

For many years, a digitalis glycoside (eg, digoxin) and a diuretic (eg, hydrochlorothiazide or furosemide) were the main drugs used in the treatment of both acute and chronic HF. Now, various drugs are used to treat acute HF, and a combination of an angiotensin-converting enzyme (ACE) inhibitor and a diuretic is first-line therapy for chronic failure. Increasingly, digoxin, a beta-adrenergic blocking agent, or spironolactone is being added to the ACE inhibitor and diuretic regimen.

Drug therapy of HF continues to evolve as the pathophysiologic mechanisms are better understood and research studies indicate more effective regimens. Combinations of drugs are commonly used in efforts to improve circulation, alter the compensatory mechanisms, and reverse heart damage in affected clients. Most of the drugs used to treat HF are also used in other disorders and are discussed mainly in other chapters; their effects in HF are described in Box 51-2. The primary focus of this chapter is digoxin; amrinone and milrinone are also discussed.

BOX 51-2   DRUGS USED TO TREAT HEART FAILURE

Adrenergics

Dopamine or dobutamine (see Chaps. 18 and 54) may be used in acute, severe heart failure (HF) when circulatory support is required, usually in an intensive care unit. Given by intravenous (IV) infusion, these drugs strengthen myocardial contraction (inotropic or cardiotonic effects) and increase cardiac output. Dosage or flow rate is titrated to hemodynamic effects; minimal effective doses are recommended because of vasoconstrictive effects. They may also cause tachycardia and hypertension and increase cardiac workload and oxygen consumption.

Angiotensin-converting Enzyme (ACE) Inhibitors

Captopril and other ACE inhibitors (see Chap. 55) are drugs of first choice in treating patients with all four New York Heart Association (NYHA) classifications of chronic HF. For patients with moderate or severe symptomatic HF (NYHA class III or IV), the standard of care includes an ACE inhibitor and a loop diuretic with or without digoxin.

These drugs improve cardiac function and decrease mortality. They also relieve symptoms, increase exercise tolerance, and delay further impairment of myocardial function and progression of HF (ie, ventricular remodeling). They act mainly to decrease activation of the renin-angiotensin-aldosterone system, a major pathophysiologic mechanism in HF. More specifically, the drugs prevent inactive angiotensin I from being converted to angiotensin II. Angiotensin II produces vasoconstriction and retention of sodium and water; inhibition of angiotensin II decreases vasoconstriction and retention of sodium and water. Thus, major effects of the drugs are dilation of both veins and arteries, decreased preload and afterload, decreased workload of the heart, and increased perfusion of body organs and tissues.

An ACE inhibitor is usually given in combination with a diuretic. Apparently all of the drugs have similar effects, but captopril, enalapril, lisinopril, and quinapril are approved by the Food and Drug Administration (FDA) for treatment of HF. Some clinicians use captopril initially because it has a short half-life and is rapidly eliminated when stopped, then switch to a long-acting drug if captopril is tolerated by the client. Digoxin, a beta-adrenergic blocking agent, or spironolactone may be added to the ACE inhibitor/diuretic regimen.

During ACE inhibitor therapy, clients usually need to see a health care provider frequently for dosage titration and monitoring of serum creatinine and potassium levels for increases. Elevated creatinine levels may indicate impaired renal function, in which case dosage needs to be reduced; elevated potassium levels indicate hyperkalemia, an adverse effect of the drugs.

Angiotensin Receptor Antagonists

Losartan and other angiotensin receptor antagonists (see Chap. 55) are similar to the ACE inhibitors in their effects on cardiac function, although they are not FDA approved for treatment of HF. Some clinicians prescribe one of these drugs for clients who are unable to tolerate an ACE inhibitor (eg, development of a cough, a common adverse effect of ACE inhibitors).

Beta-adrenergic Blocking Agents

Although beta blockers (see Chaps. 19, 52, and 55) were formerly considered contraindicated, numerous research studies indicate they decrease morbidity (ie, symptoms and hospitalizations) and mortality in clients with chronic HF. The change evolved from a better understanding of chronic HF (ie, that it involves more than a weak pumping mechanism).

Beta blockers suppress activation of the sympathetic nervous system and the resulting catecholamine excess that eventually damages myocardial cells, reduces

(continued)

BOX 51–2 **DRUGS USED TO TREAT HEART FAILURE** (continued)

myocardial beta receptors, and reduces cardiac output. As a result, over time, ventricular dilatation and enlargement (ventricular remodeling) regress, the heart returns toward a more normal shape and function, and cardiac output increases. Most studies were done with clients in NYHA class II or III; effects in class IV clients are being studied.

Beta blockers are not recommended for clients in acute HF because of the potential for an initial decrease in myocardial contractility. A beta blocker may be started once normal blood volume is restored and edema and other symptoms are relieved. The goal of beta blocker therapy is to shrink the ventricle back to its normal size (reverse remodeling). The beta blocker is added to the ACE inhibitor/diuretic regimen, usually near the end of a hospital stay or as outpatient therapy. Most studies have been done with bisoprolol, carvedilol, or metoprolol; it is not yet known whether some beta blockers are more effective than others. When one of the drugs is used in clients with chronic HF, recommendations include starting with a low dose (because symptoms may initially worsen in some clients), titrating the dose upward at approximately 2-week intervals, and monitoring closely. Significant hemodynamic improvement usually requires 2 to 3 months of therapy, but effects are long lasting. Beneficial effects can be measured by increases in the left ventricular ejection fraction (ie, cardiac output).

Diuretics

Diuretics (see Chap. 56) are used in treating both acute and chronic HF. Thiazides (eg, hydrochlorothiazide) can be used for mild diuresis in clients with normal renal function; loop diuretics (eg, furosemide) should be used in clients who need strong diuresis or who have impaired renal function.

In acute failure, which is characterized by fluid accumulation, a diuretic is the initial treatment. It acts to decrease plasma volume (extracellular fluid volume) and increase excretion of sodium and water, thereby decreasing preload. With early or mild HF, starting or increasing the dose of an oral thiazide may be effective. With moderate to severe HF (pulmonary edema), an intravenous loop diuretic is indicated. IV furosemide also has a vasodilatory effect that helps relieve vasoconstriction (afterload). Although diuretic therapy relieves symptoms, it does not improve left ventricular function and decrease mortality rates. Thus, an ACE inhibitor is usually added. Some clients may also need drugs to increase myocardial contractility and vasodilators to decrease preload, afterload, or both.

In chronic HF, an oral diuretic is a common component of treatment regimens. Depending on the sever-

ity of symptoms or degree of HF, the regimen may also include an ACE inhibitor, a beta blocker, and digoxin. Increasingly, spironolactone is also being added for clients with moderate to severe HF. Increased aldosterone is a major factor in the pathophysiology of HF; spironolactone is an aldosterone antagonist that reduces the aldosterone-induced retention of sodium and water and impaired vascular function. Although ACE inhibitors also decrease aldosterone initially, this effect is transient. Spironolactone is usually given in a daily dose of 12.5 to 25 mg, along with standard doses of an ACE inhibitor, a loop diuretic, and usually digoxin. In clients with adequate renal function (ie, serum creatinine ≤2.5 mg/dL), the addition of spironolactone usually allows smaller doses of loop diuretics and potassium supplements. Overall, studies indicate that the addition of spironolactone improves cardiac function and reduces symptoms, hospitalizations, and mortality.

Potassium-sparing diuretics (eg, amiloride, triamterene) are often given concurrently with potassium-losing diuretics (eg, thiazides or loop diuretics) to help maintain normal serum potassium levels. Concomitant use of ACE inhibitors and nonsteroidal anti-inflammatory drugs and the presence of diabetes mellitus increase risks of hyperkalemia.

With all diuretic therapy, serum potassium levels must be measured periodically to monitor for hypokalemia and hyperkalemia. Both hypokalemia and hyperkalemia are cardiotoxic or impair heart function.

Vasodilators

Vasodilators are essential components of treatment regimens for HF, and the beneficial effects of ACE inhibitors and angiotensin receptor antagonists stem significantly from their vasodilating effects (ie, preventing or decreasing angiotensin-induced vasoconstriction). Other vasodilators may also be used. Venous dilators (eg, nitrates) decrease preload; arterial dilators (eg, hydralazine) decrease afterload. Isosorbide dinitrate and hydralazine may be combined to decrease both preload and afterload. The combination has similar effects to those of an ACE inhibitor or an angiotensin receptor antagonist, but may not be as well tolerated by clients. Nitrates are discussed in Chapter 53; hydralazine and other vasodilators are discussed in Chapter 55.

Oral vasodilators usually are used in clients with chronic HF and parenteral agents are reserved for those who have severe HF or are unable to take oral medications. They should be started at low doses, titrated to desired hemodynamic effects, and discontinued slowly to avoid rebound vasoconstriction.

Digoxin

Digoxin (Lanoxin) is the only commonly used digitalis glycoside. In the following discussion, the terms *digitalization* and *digitalis toxicity* refer to digoxin.

General Characteristics

When digoxin is given orally, absorption varies among available preparations. Lanoxicaps, which are liquid-filled capsules, and the elixir used for children are better absorbed than tablets. With tablets, the most frequently used formulation, differences in bioavailability are important because a person who is stabilized on one formulation may be underdosed or overdosed if another formulation is taken. Differences are attributed to the rate and extent of tablet dissolution rather than amounts of digoxin. In addition to drug dosage forms, other factors that may decrease digoxin absorption include the presence of food in the gastrointestinal tract, delayed gastric emptying, malabsorption syndromes, and concurrent administration of some drugs (eg, antacids, cholestyramine).

Digoxin is distributed to most body tissues and high concentrations are found in the myocardium, brain, liver, and skeletal muscle. It also crosses the placenta, and serum levels in newly delivered neonates are similar to those in the mother. It circulates mainly in a free state, with only 20% to 30% bound to serum proteins. Therapeutic serum levels of digoxin are 0.5 to 2 ng/mL; toxic serum levels are above 2 ng/mL. However, toxicity may occur at virtually any serum level.

Most (60% to 70%) of the digoxin is excreted unchanged by the kidneys. Dosage must be reduced in the presence of renal failure to prevent drug accumulation and toxicity. The remainder is metabolized or excreted by nonrenal routes.

Mechanisms of Action

In HF, digoxin exerts a cardiotonic or positive inotropic effect that improves the pumping ability of the heart. Increased myocardial contractility allows the ventricles to empty more completely with each heartbeat. With improved cardiac output, heart size, heart rate, end-systolic and end-diastolic pressures, vasoconstriction, sympathetic nerve stimulation, and venous congestion decrease. The mechanism by which digoxin increases the force of myocardial contraction is thought to be inhibition of Na, K-adenosine triphosphatase (Na,K-ATPase), an enzyme in cardiac cell membranes that decreases the movement of sodium out of myocardial cells after contraction. As a result, calcium enters the cell in exchange for sodium, causing additional calcium to be released from intracellular binding sites. With the increased intracellular concentration of free calcium ions, more calcium is available to activate the contractile proteins actin and myosin, and increase myocardial contractility. Overall, digoxin helps to relieve symptoms and decrease hospitalizations, but

does not prolong survival. It is given concomitantly with a diuretic and an ACE inhibitor.

In atrial arrhythmias, digoxin slows the rate of ventricular contraction (negative chronotropic effect). Negative chronotropic effects are probably caused by several factors. First, digoxin has a direct depressant effect on cardiac conduction tissues, especially the atrioventricular node. This action decreases the number of electrical impulses allowed to reach the ventricles from supraventricular sources. Second, digoxin indirectly stimulates the vagus nerve. Third, increased efficiency of myocardial contraction and vagal stimulation decrease compensatory tachycardia resulting from the sympathetic nervous system response to inadequate circulation.

Indications for Use

The clinical uses of digoxin are treatment of HF, atrial fibrillation, and atrial flutter. Digoxin may be used in acute or chronic conditions, for digitalization, or for maintenance therapy.

Contraindications to Use

Digoxin is contraindicated in severe myocarditis, ventricular tachycardia, or ventricular fibrillation and must be used cautiously in clients with acute myocardial infarction, heart block, Adams-Stokes syndrome, Wolff-Parkinson-White syndrome (risk of fatal arrhythmias), electrolyte imbalances (hypokalemia, hypomagnesemia, hypercalcemia), and renal impairment.

Administration and Digitalization

Digoxin is given orally or IV. Although it can be given intramuscularly, this route is not recommended because pain and muscle necrosis may occur at injection sites. When given orally, onset of action occurs in 30 minutes to 2 hours, and peak effects occur in approximately 6 hours. When given IV, the onset of action occurs within 10 to 30 minutes, and maximal effects occur in 1 to 5 hours.

In the heart, maximum drug effect occurs when a steady-state tissue concentration has been achieved. This occurs in approximately 1 week (five half-lives) unless loading doses are given for more rapid effects. Traditionally, a loading dose is called a *digitalizing dose*. Digitalization (administration of an amount sufficient to produce therapeutic effects) may be accomplished rapidly by giving approximately 0.75 to 1 mg of digoxin in divided doses 6 to 8 hours apart over a 24-hour period. Because rapid digitalization engenders higher risks of toxicity, it is usually done for atrial tachyarrhythmias rather than for HF. Slow digitalization may be accomplished by initiating therapy with a maintenance dose of digoxin. When digoxin is discontinued, the drug is eliminated from the body in approximately 1 week.

ROUTES AND DOSAGE RANGES

Adults and children >10 y: Digitalizing dose, oral (PO) 0.75–1 mg in three or four divided doses over 24 h; IV 0.5–0.75 mg in divided doses over 24 h

Maintenance dose, PO, IV 0.125–0.5 mg/d (average, 0.25)

Children 2–10 y: Digitalizing dose, PO 0.02–0.04 mg/kg in four divided doses q6h; IV 0.015–0.035 mg/kg in four divided doses q6h

Maintenance dose, PO, IV approximately 20%–35% of the digitalizing dose or a maximum dosage of 100–150 µg/d

Children 1 mo–2 y: Digitalizing dose, PO 0.035–0.06 mg/kg in four divided doses q6h; IV 0.035–0.05 mg/kg in four divided doses q6h

Maintenance dose, PO, IV approximately 20%–35% of the digitalizing dose

Newborns: Digitalizing dose, PO 0.025–0.035 mg/kg in four divided doses q6h; IV 0.02–0.03 mg/kg in four divided doses q6h

Maintenance dose, PO, IV approximately 20%–35% of the digitalizing dose

Digoxin Toxicity

Digoxin has a low therapeutic index (ie, a dose adequate for therapeutic effects may be accompanied by signs of toxicity). Digoxin toxicity may result from many contributing factors:

1. Accumulation of larger-than-necessary maintenance doses
2. Rapid loading or digitalization, whether by one or more large doses or frequent administration of small doses
3. Impaired renal function, which delays excretion of digoxin
4. Age extremes (young or old)
5. Electrolyte imbalance (eg, hypokalemia, hypomagnesemia, hypercalcemia)
6. Hypoxia due to heart or lung disease, which increases myocardial sensitivity to digoxin
7. Hypothyroidism, which slows digoxin metabolism and may cause accumulation
8. Concurrent treatment with other drugs affecting the heart, such as quinidine, verapamil, or nifedipine

Nursing Notes: Apply Your Knowledge

Your assessment of Pamela Kindra reveals the following: 118/92, 110, 32 and labored. Respiratory assessment reveals coarse rhonchi and wheezing bilaterally. Urine output has been less than 30 cc per hour and she has gained 12 pounds over the last 2 days. You place Ms. Kindra in a high-Fowler's position and call her physician. After examining her, he orders digoxin 0.5 mg IV STAT: repeat in 4 hours; then give 0.25 mg qd. Do you feel this is a safe dosage of digoxin to give? Discuss the rationale for your answer.

Phosphodiesterase Inhibitors

Amrinone (Inocor) and **milrinone IV** (Primacor) are cardiotonic-inotropic agents used in short-term management of acute, severe HF that is not controlled by digoxin, diuretics, and vasodilators. The drugs increase levels of cyclic adenosine monophosphate (cAMP) in myocardial cells by inhibiting phosphodiesterase, the enzyme that normally metabolizes cAMP. They also relax vascular smooth muscle to produce vasodilation and decrease preload and afterload. In HF, inotropic and vasodilator effects increase cardiac output. The effects of these drugs are additive to those of digoxin and may be synergistic with those of adrenergic drugs (eg, dobutamine). There is a time delay before the drugs reach therapeutic serum levels and interindividual variability in therapeutic doses.

Compared with amrinone, milrinone is more potent as an inotropic agent and causes fewer adverse effects. Both drugs are given IV by bolus injection followed by continuous infusion. Flow rate is titrated to maintain adequate circulation. Milrinone can be used alone or with other drugs such as dobutamine and nitroprusside. Its dosage should be reduced in the presence of renal impairment. Dose-limiting adverse effects of the drugs include tachycardia, atrial or ventricular arrhythmias, and hypotension. Hypotension is more likely to occur in clients who are hypovolemic. Milrinone has a long half-life of approximately 80 hours and may accumulate with prolonged infusions.

Amrinone

ROUTE AND DOSAGE RANGES

Adults: IV injection (loading dose), 0.75 mg/kg slowly, over 2–3 min

IV infusion (maintenance dose), 5–10 µg/kg/min, diluted in 0.9% or 0.45% NaCl solution to a concentration of 1–3 mg/mL; maximum dosage, 10 mg/kg/d

Milrinone

ROUTE AND DOSAGE RANGES

Adults: IV bolus infusion (loading dose), 50 µg/kg over 10 min

IV continuous infusion (maintenance dose), 0.375–0.75 µg/kg/min, diluted in 0.9% or 0.45% NaCl solution or 5% dextrose injection

NURSING PROCESS

Assessment

Assess clients for current or potential HF:

- Identify risk factors for HF:
  - **Cardiovascular disorders:** atherosclerosis, hypertension, coronary artery disease, myo-

cardial infarction, cardiac arrhythmias, cardiac valvular disease.

- ○ **Noncardiovascular disorders:** severe infections, hyperthyroidism, pulmonary disease (eg, cor pulmonale–right-sided HF resulting from lung disease)
- ○ **Other factors:** excessive amounts of IV fluids, rapid infusion of IV fluids or blood transfusions, advanced age
- ○ A **combination** of any of the preceding factors
- Interview and observe for signs and symptoms of chronic HF. Within the clinical syndrome of HF, clinical manifestations vary from few and mild to many and severe, including the following:
  - ○ **Mild HF.** Common signs and symptoms of mild HF are ankle edema, dyspnea on exertion, and easy fatigue with exercise. Edema results from increased venous pressure, which allows fluids to leak into tissues; dyspnea and fatigue result from tissue hypoxia.
  - ○ **Moderate or severe HF.** More extensive edema, dyspnea, and fatigue at rest are likely to occur. Additional signs and symptoms include orthopnea, postnocturnal dyspnea, and cough (from congestion of the respiratory tract with venous blood); mental confusion (from cerebral hypoxia); oliguria and decreased renal function (from decreased blood flow to the kidneys); and anxiety.
- Observe for signs and symptoms of acute HF. Acute pulmonary edema indicates acute HF and is a medical emergency. Causes include acute myocardial infarction, cardiac arrhythmias, severe hypertension, acute fluid or salt overload, and certain drugs (eg, quinidine and other cardiac depressants, propranolol and other antiadrenergics, and phenylephrine, norepinephrine, and other alpha-adrenergic stimulants). Pulmonary edema occurs when left ventricular failure causes blood to accumulate in pulmonary veins and tissues. As a result, the person experiences severe dyspnea, hypoxia, hypertension, tachycardia, hemoptysis, frothy respiratory tract secretions, and anxiety.

Assess clients for signs and symptoms of atrial tachyarrhythmias:

- Record the rate and rhythm of apical and radial pulses. Atrial fibrillation, the most common atrial arrhythmia, is characterized by tachycardia, pulse deficit (faster apical rate than radial rate) and a very irregular rhythm. Fatigue, dizziness, and fainting may occur.
- Check the electrocardiogram (ECG) for abnormal P waves, rapid rate of ventricular contraction, and QRS complexes of normal configuration but irregular intervals.

Assess baseline vital signs; weight; edema; laboratory results for potassium, magnesium, and cal-

cium levels; and other tests of cardiovascular function when available.

Assess a baseline ECG before digoxin therapy when possible. If a client is in normal sinus rhythm, later ECGs may aid recognition of digitalis toxicity (ie, drug-induced arrhythmias). If a client has an atrial tachyarrhythmia and is receiving digoxin to slow the ventricular rate, later ECGs may aid recognition of therapeutic and adverse effects. For clients who are already receiving digoxin at the initial contact, a baseline ECG can still be valuable because changes in later ECGs may promote earlier recognition and treatment of drug-induced arrhythmias.

Nursing Diagnoses

- Altered Tissue Perfusion related to decreased cardiac output
- Activity Intolerance related to decreased cardiac output
- Self Care Deficit related to dyspnea and fatigue
- Anxiety related to chronic illness and lifestyle changes
- Impaired Gas Exchange related to venous congestion and fluid accumulation in lungs
- Decreased Cardiac Output related to drug-induced arrhythmias
- Sensory/Perceptual Alterations related to drug-induced changes in vision
- Altered Nutrition: Less Than Body Requirements related to digoxin-induced anorexia, nausea, and vomiting
- Noncompliance related to the need for long-term drug therapy and regular medical supervision
- Knowledge Deficit: Managing drug therapy regimen safely and effectively

Planning/Goals

The client will:

- Take digoxin and other medications safely and accurately
- Experience improved breathing and less fatigue and edema
- Maintain serum digoxin levels within therapeutic ranges
- Be closely monitored for therapeutic and adverse effects, especially during digitalization, when dosage is being changed, and when other drugs are added to or removed from the treatment regimen
- Keep appointments for follow-up monitoring of vital signs, serum potassium levels, serum digoxin levels, and renal function

Interventions

Use measures to prevent or minimize HF and atrial arrhythmias. In the broadest sense, preventive measures include sensible eating habits (a balanced diet, avoiding excess saturated fat and salt, weight control), avoiding cigarette smoking, and regular exercise. In the client at risk for development of HF and arrhythmias, preventive measures include the following:

- Treatment of hypertension
- Avoidance of hypoxia
- Weight control
- Avoidance of excess sodium in the diet
- Avoidance of fluid overload, especially in elderly clients
- Maintenance of treatment programs for HF, atrial arrhythmias, and other cardiovascular or noncardiovascular disorders

Monitor vital signs, weight, urine output, and serum potassium regularly, and compare with baseline values.

Monitor ECG when available, and compare with baseline or previous tracings.

Evaluation

- Interview and observe for relief of symptoms (weight loss, increased urine output, less extremity edema, easier breathing, improved activity tolerance and self-care ability, slower heart rate).
- Observe serum drug levels for normal or abnormal values, when available.
- Interview regarding compliance with instructions for taking the drug.
- Interview and observe for adverse drug effects, especially cardiac arrhythmias.

CLIENT TEACHING GUIDELINES
Digoxin

General Considerations

✔ This drug is prescribed for two types of heart disease. One type is heart failure, in which digoxin strengthens your heartbeat and helps to relieve such symptoms as ankle swelling, shortness of breath, and fatigue. The other type is a fast heartbeat called atrial fibrillation, in which digoxin slows the heartbeat and decreases symptoms such as fatigue. Because these are chronic conditions, digoxin therapy is usually long term. Ask your health care provider why you are being given digoxin and what effects you can expect, both beneficial and adverse.

✔ It is extremely important to take digoxin (and other cardiovascular medications) as prescribed, usually once daily. The drug must be taken regularly to maintain therapeutic blood levels, but overuse can cause serious adverse effects.

✔ Precautions to increase the drug's safety and effectiveness include the following:

✔ As a general rule, *do not* miss a dose. It is helpful to develop a routine of taking the medication approximately the same time each day and maintain a written record, such as a dated check list. If you forget a dose at the usual time and remember it within a few hours (approximately 6), go ahead and take the daily dose.

✔ *Do not* take an extra dose. For example, do not take a double dose to make up for a missed dose.

✔ *Do not* take other prescription or nonprescription (eg, antacids, cold remedies, diet pills) drugs without consulting the physician who prescribed digoxin. Several drugs interact with digoxin to increase or decrease its effects.

✔ You will need periodic physical examinations, electrocardiograms, and blood tests to check digoxin and electrolyte (sodium, potassium, magnesium) levels to monitor your response to digoxin and see whether changes in dosage are needed.

✔ Digoxin is often one drug in a treatment regimen of several drugs for heart disease. The drugs are all needed to help the heart and blood vessels work better. Together, the drugs help to maintain a balance in the cardiovascular system. As a result, changing any aspect of one of the drugs can upset the balance and lead to symptoms. For example, stopping one drug because of real or perceived adverse effects can lead to problems. If you think a drug needs to be stopped or its dosage reduced, talk with a health care provider. *Do not* make changes on your own; serious illness or even death could result.

✔ Small doses (eg, 0.125 milligrams [125 micrograms] daily or every other day) are usually given to older adults, who often have impaired kidney function, and other people with impaired kidney function. Digoxin is eliminated through the kidneys; it can accumulate and cause adverse effects if dosage is not reduced with kidney impairment.

✔ You may need to limit your salt (sodium chloride) intake and get an adequate supply of potassium. Follow your health care provider's recommendations about any diet changes. People taking digoxin are often taking a diuretic, a drug that takes sodium and potassium out of the body. If potassium levels get too low, adverse effects of digoxin are more likely to occur. However, too much potassium can also be harmful. Do not use salt substitutes (potassium chloride) without consulting a health care provider.

✔ Report adverse drug effects (eg, undesirable changes in heart rate or rhythm, nausea and vomiting, or visual problems) to a health care provider. These symptoms may indicate that digoxin dosage needs to be reduced.

✔ Use the same brand and type of digoxin all the time. For example, whether using generic digoxin or trade-name Lanoxin tablets, get the same one each time a prescription is refilled. In addition, there is a capsule form and a liquid form. These forms and concentrations are different and cannot be used interchangeably. Underdoses

(continued)

CLIENT TEACHING GUIDELINES
Digoxin (*continued*)

and overdoses may occur. Lanoxin tablets are the most commonly used formulation.

Self- or Caregiver Administration

✔ If instructed to do so by your health care provider, count your pulse before each dose. In some circumstances, you may be advised to skip that scheduled dose. *Do not* skip doses unless specifically instructed to do so.

✔ Take or give digoxin tablets approximately the same time each day to maintain more even blood levels and help

in remembering to take the drug. The tablets may be crushed and can be taken with or after food, if desired, although milk and dairy products may delay absorption.

✔ Digoxin capsules should be swallowed whole.

✔ If taking or giving a liquid form of digoxin, it is extremely important to measure it accurately. A few drops more could produce overdosage, with serious adverse effects; a few drops less could produce underdosage, with a loss or decrease of therapeutic effects.

PRINCIPLES OF THERAPY

Goals of Treatment

The goals for clients with asymptomatic (compensated) HF are to maintain function as nearly normal as possible and to prevent symptomatic (acute, congestive, or decompensated) HF, hospitalizations, and death. When symptoms or decompensation occurs, the goals are to relieve symptoms, restore function, and prevent progressive cardiac deterioration.

Nonpharmacologic Treatment Measures

1. Prevent or treat conditions that precipitate cardiac decompensation and failure (eg, fluid and sodium retention, factors that impair myocardial contractility or increase cardiac workload).
2. Reduce physical activity in clients with symptomatic HF. This decreases the workload and oxygen consumption of the myocardium. If bed rest is instituted, heparin should be given to prevent deep vein thrombosis.
3. Restrict dietary sodium intake to reduce edema and other symptoms and allow a decrease in diuretic dosage. For most clients, sodium restriction need not be severe. A common order, "no added salt," may be accomplished by avoiding obviously salty food (eg, ham, potato chips, snack foods) and by not adding salt during cooking or eating. For clients with more severe HF, dietary intake may be more restricted (eg, ≤2 g daily). A major source of sodium intake is table salt: a level teaspoonful contains 2300 mg of sodium.
4. If hyponatremia (serum sodium <130 mEq/L) develops from sodium restrictions and diuretic therapy,

fluids may need to be restricted (eg, ≤1.5 L/day) until the serum sodium level increases. Severe hyponatremia (<125 mEq/L) may lead to arrhythmias.
5. For clients who are obese, weight loss is desirable to decrease systemic vascular resistance and myocardial oxygen demand.
6. Administer oxygen, if needed, to relieve dyspnea, improve oxygen delivery, reduce the work of breathing, and decrease constriction of pulmonary blood vessels (which occurs in clients with hypoxemia).

Pharmacologic Treatment

A combination of drugs is the standard of care for both acute and chronic HF. Specific drug components of the combinations depend on the client's symptoms and hemodynamic status.

1. For **acute HF**, the first drugs of choice may include an IV loop diuretic, a cardiotonic-inotropic agent (eg, digoxin, dobutamine, or milrinone), and vasodilators (eg, nitroglycerin and hydralazine or nitroprusside). This combination reduces preload and afterload and increases myocardial contractility.
2. For **chronic HF**, an ACE inhibitor and a diuretic are the basic standard of care. Digoxin, a beta-adrenergic blocking agent, and spironolactone may also be added. Although the use of digoxin in clients with normal sinus rhythm has been questioned, studies indicate improved ejection fraction and exercise tolerance in clients who receive digoxin. In addition, in clients stabilized on digoxin, a diuretic, and an ACE inhibitor, symptoms worsen if digoxin is discontinued.

   Overall, these drugs improve clients' quality of life by decreasing their symptoms and increasing their ability to function in activities of daily living. They also decrease hospitalizations and deaths from HF.

3. Electrolyte balance must be monitored and maintained during digoxin therapy, particularly normal serum levels of potassium (3.5 to 5 mEq/L), magnesium (1.5 to 2.5 mg/100 mL), and calcium (8.5 to 10 mg/100 mL). Hypokalemia and hypomagnesemia increase cardiac excitability and ectopic pacemaker activity, leading to arrhythmias; hypercalcemia enhances the effects of digoxin. These electrolyte abnormalities increase the risk of digoxin toxicity. Hypocalcemia increases excitability of nerve and muscle cell membranes and causes myocardial contraction to be weak (leading to a decrease in digoxin effect).

In acute HF, there is a high risk of hypokalemia because large doses of potassium-losing diuretics are often given. Serum potassium levels should be monitored regularly and supplemental potassium may be needed. In chronic HF, hypokalemia may be less likely to occur than formerly because lower doses of potassium-losing diuretics are usually being given. In addition, there may be more extensive use of potassium-sparing diuretics (eg, amiloride or triamterene) and spironolactone. Note, however, that hyperkalemia must also be prevented because it is cardiotoxic.

Guidelines for Individualizing Digoxin Dosage

1. Digoxin dosages are usually stated as the average amounts needed for digitalization and maintenance therapy. These dosages must be interpreted with consideration of specific client characteristics. Digitalizing or loading doses are safe *only* for a short period, usually 24 hours. In addition, loading doses should be used cautiously in clients who have taken digoxin within the previous 2 or 3 weeks. Maintenance doses, which are much smaller than digitalizing doses, may be safely used to initiate digoxin therapy and are always used for long-term therapy.

2. In general, larger doses are needed to slow the heart rate in atrial tachyarrhythmias than to increase myocardial contractility in HF. Larger doses may also be needed to reach therapeutic serum levels of digoxin in a small group of clients (approximately 10%) who have digoxin-metabolizing bacteria in their colons. Members of this group are at risk for development of digoxin toxicity if they are given antibacterial drugs that destroy colonic bacteria.

3. Smaller doses (loading and maintenance) should be given to clients who are elderly or have hypothyroidism. Because metabolism and excretion of digoxin are delayed in such people, the drug may accumulate and cause toxicity if dosage is not reduced. Dosage also should be reduced in clients with hypokalemia, extensive myocardial damage,

or cardiac conduction disorders. These conditions increase risks of digoxin-induced arrhythmias.

4. Dosage can be titrated according to client response. In HF, severity of symptoms, ECG, and serum drug concentrations are useful. In atrial fibrillation, dosage can be altered to produce the desired decrease in the ventricular rate of contraction. Optimal dosage is the lowest amount that relieves signs and symptoms of HF or alters heart rate and rhythm toward normal without producing toxicity.

5. IV dosage of digoxin should be 20% to 30% less than oral dosage.

6. Dosage of digoxin must be reduced by approximately half in clients with renal failure to avoid drug accumulation and toxicity. Dosage should be based on signs and symptoms of toxicity, creatinine clearance, and serum drug levels.

7. Dosage of digoxin must be reduced by approximately half when certain drugs are given concurrently, to avoid drug accumulation and toxicity. For example, amiodarone, quinidine, nifedipine, and verapamil slow digoxin excretion and increase serum digoxin levels.

8. When a hospitalized client is unable to take a daily maintenance dose of digoxin at the scheduled time because of diagnostic tests, treatment measures, or other reasons, the dose should usually be given later rather than omitted. If the client is having surgery, the nurse often must ask the physician whether the drug should be given on the day of surgery (ie, orally with a small amount of water or parenterally) and whether the drug should be reordered after surgery. Many clients require continued digoxin therapy. However, if a dose is missed, probably no ill effects will occur because the pharmacologic actions of digoxin persist longer than 24 hours.

Recognition and Treatment of Digoxin Toxicity

Recognition of digoxin toxicity may be difficult because of nonspecific early manifestations (eg, anorexia, nausea, confusion) and the similarity between the signs and symptoms of heart disease for which digoxin is given and the signs and symptoms of digoxin intoxication. Continued atrial fibrillation with a rapid ventricular response may indicate inadequate dosage. However, other arrhythmias may indicate toxicity. Premature ventricular contractions commonly occur. Serum drug levels and ECG may be helpful in verifying suspected toxicity. Serum digoxin levels should be drawn just before a dose. Drug distribution to tissues requires approximately 6 hours after a dose is given; if the blood is drawn before 6 hours, the level may be high.

When signs and symptoms of digoxin toxicity occur, treatment may include any or all of the following interventions, depending on the client's condition:

1. Digoxin should be discontinued, not just reduced in dosage. Most clients with mild or early toxicity recover completely within a few days after the drug is stopped.

2. If serious cardiac arrhythmias are present, several drugs may be used, including:

   a. **Potassium chloride**, a myocardial depressant that acts to decrease myocardial excitability. The dose depends on the severity of toxicity, serum potassium level, and client response. Potassium is contraindicated in renal failure and should be used with caution in the presence of cardiac conduction defects.

   b. **Lidocaine**, an antiarrhythmic local anesthetic agent used to decrease myocardial irritability.

   c. **Atropine** or **isoproterenol**, used in the treatment of bradycardia or conduction defects

   d. **Other antiarrhythmic drugs** may be used, but are in general less effective in digoxin-induced arrhythmias than in arrhythmias due to other causes.

   e. **Digoxin immune fab** (Digibind, Digidote) is a digoxin-binding antidote derived from anti-digoxin antibodies produced in sheep. It is recommended only for serious toxicity. It combines with digoxin and pulls digoxin out of tissues and into the bloodstream. This causes serum digoxin levels to be high, but the drug is bound to the antibody and therefore inactive. Digoxin immune fab is given IV, as a bolus injection, if the client is in danger of immediate cardiac arrest, but preferably over 15 to 30 minutes. Dosage varies and is calculated according to the amount of digoxin ingested (see manufacturers' instructions). Each 40-mg vial neutralizes approximately 0.6 mg of digoxin.

Use in Children

Digoxin is commonly used in children for the same indications as for adults and should be prescribed by or supervised by a pediatric cardiologist when possible. The response to a given dose varies with age, size, and renal and hepatic function. There may be little difference between a therapeutic dose and a toxic dose. Very small amounts are often given to children. These factors increase the risks of dosage errors in children, and, in hospitalized children, each dose should be verified with another nurse before it is administered. ECG monitoring is desirable when digoxin therapy is started.

As in adults, dosage of digoxin should be individualized and carefully titrated. Digoxin is primarily excreted by the kidneys, and dosage must be reduced with impaired renal function. In general, divided daily doses should be given to infants and children younger than 10 years, and

adult dosages adjusted to their weight should be given to children older than 10 years of age. Larger doses are usually needed to slow a too-rapid ventricular rate in children with atrial fibrillation or flutter. Differences in bioavailability of different preparations (parenterals, capsules, elixirs, and tablets) must be considered when switching from one preparation to another.

Neonates vary in tolerance of digoxin depending on their degree of maturity. Premature infants are especially sensitive to drug effects. Dosage must be reduced, and digitalization should be even more individualized and cautiously approached than in more mature infants and children. Early signs of toxicity in newborns are undue slowing of sinus rate, sinoatrial arrest, and prolongation of the PR interval.

Use in Older Adults

Digoxin is widely used and a frequent cause of adverse effects in older adults. The most commonly recommended dose is 0.125 mg daily. Reduced dosages are usually required because of decreased liver or kidney function, decreased lean body weight, and advanced cardiovascular disease. All of these characteristics are common in older adults. Impaired renal function leads to slower drug excretion and increased risk of accumulation, so smaller doses are needed. Dosage must be reduced by approximately 50% with renal failure or concurrent administration of amiodarone, quinidine, nifedipine, or verapamil. These drugs increase serum digoxin levels and increase risks of toxicity if dosage is not reduced. Antacids decrease absorption of oral digoxin and should not be given at the same time.

Use in Renal Impairment

Digoxin should be used cautiously, in reduced dosages, because renal impairment delays its excretion. Both loading and maintenance doses should be reduced. Clients with advanced renal impairment can achieve therapeutic serum concentrations with a dosage of 0.125 mg three to five times per week.

In addition, in clients with reduced blood flow to the kidneys (eg, fluid volume depletion or acute HF), digoxin may be reabsorbed in renal tubules. As a result, less digoxin is excreted through the kidneys and maintenance doses may need even greater decreases than those calculated according to creatinine clearance. Thus, digoxin toxicity develops more often and lasts longer in renal impairment. Clients with renal impairment who are receiving digoxin, even in small doses, should be monitored closely for adverse effects, and serum digoxin levels should be monitored periodically.

There is no information available about the use of amrinone in renal impairment. However, pharmacokinetic data indicate higher plasma levels with HF-induced reductions in renal perfusion. Also, the drug and its metabolites are excreted primarily by the kidneys.

With milrinone, which is also excreted primarily by the kidneys, renal impairment significantly increases elimination half-life, drug accumulation, and adverse effects. Dosage should be reduced according to creatinine clearance (see manufacturer's instructions).

Use in Hepatic Impairment

Hepatic impairment has little effect on digoxin clearance, and no dosage adjustments are needed. Amrinone is extensively metabolized in the liver and may be hepatotoxic. If significant increases in liver enzymes and clinical symptoms occur, amrinone should be discontinued. If smaller increases in liver enzymes occur without clinical symptoms, amrinone may be continued with reduced dosage or discontinued, depending on the client's need for the drug.

Use in Critical Illness

Critically ill clients often have multiple cardiovascular and other disorders that require drug therapy. Acute HF may be the primary critical illness. It may also be precipitated by other illnesses or treatments that alter fluid balance, impair myocardial contractility, or increase the workload of the heart beyond its capacity to accommodate. Treatment is often symptomatic, with choice of drug and dosage requir-

ing careful titration and frequent monitoring of the client's response. Cardiotonic, diuretic, and vasodilator drugs are often required. All of the drugs should be used with caution in critically ill clients.

 ## Home Care

Most digoxin is taken at home, and the home care nurse shares responsibility for teaching clients how to use the drug effectively and circumstances to be reported to a health care provider. Accurate dosing is vitally important because underuse may cause recurrence of symptoms and overuse may cause toxicity. Either condition may be life threatening and require emergency care. The home care nurse also needs to monitor clients' responses to the drug and changes in conditions or drug therapy that increase risks of toxicity.

When clients are receiving a combination of drugs for treatment of HF, the nurse needs to assist them in understanding that the different types of drugs perform different jobs, so to speak. As a result, they work together to be more effective and maintain a more balanced state of cardiovascular function. Changing drugs or dosages can upset the balance and lead to acute and severe symptoms that require hospitalization and may even cause death from HF. Thus, it is extremely important that they take all the medications as prescribed. If unable to take the medications for any reason, the client or a caregiver should notify the prescribing physician. Tell them not to wait until symptoms become severe before seeking care.

(text continues on page 763)

NURSING ACTIONS	Cardiotonic-Inotropic Drugs

NURSING ACTIONS	RATIONALE/EXPLANATION
1. Administer accurately	
a. With digoxin:	
(1) Read the drug label and the physician's order carefully when preparing a dose.	For accurate administration
(2) Give only the ordered dosage form (eg, tablet, Lanoxicap, or elixir).	Digoxin formulations vary in concentration and bioavailability and *cannot* be used interchangeably.
(3) Check the apical pulse before each dose. If the rate is below 60 in adults or 100 in children, omit the dose, and notify the physician.	Bradycardia is an adverse effect.
(4) Have the same nurse give digoxin to the same clients when possible because it is important to detect *changes* in rate and rhythm (see *Observe for therapeutic effects* and *Observe for adverse effects*, later).	

(continued)

NURSING ACTIONS	RATIONALE/EXPLANATION
(5) Give oral digoxin with food or after meals.	This may minimize gastric irritation and symptoms of anorexia, nausea, and vomiting. However, these symptoms probably arise from drug stimulation of chemoreceptors in the medulla rather than a direct irritant effect of the drug on the gastrointestinal (GI) tract.
(6) Inject intravenous (IV) digoxin slowly (over at least 5 min).	Digoxin should be given slowly because the diluent, propylene glycol, has toxic effects on the cardiac conduction system if given too rapidly. Digoxin may be given undiluted or diluted with a fourfold or greater volume of sterile water for injection, 0.9% sodium chloride injection, or 5% dextrose injection. If diluted, use the solution immediately.
b. With amrinone:	
(1) Give undiluted or diluted to a concentration of 1 to 3 mg/mL.	
(2) Dilute with 0.9% or 0.45% sodium chloride solution, and use the diluted solution within 24 h. Do not dilute with solutions containing dextrose.	Amrinone may be injected into IV tubing containing a dextrose solution because contact is brief. However, a chemical interaction occurs with prolonged contact.
(3) Give bolus injections into the tubing of an IV infusion, over 2 to 3 min.	
(4) Administer maintenance infusions at a rate of 5 to 10 μg/kg/min.	
c. With milrinone:	
(1) Dilute with 0.9% or 0.45% sodium chloride or 5% dextrose solution.	Manufacturer's recommendations
(2) Give the loading dose by bolus infusion over 10 min.	
(3) Give maintenance infusions at a standard rate of 0.5 μg/kg/min; this rate may be increased or decreased according to response.	
2. Observe for therapeutic effects	
a. When the drugs are given in heart failure (HF), observe for:	
(1) Fewer signs and symptoms of pulmonary congestion (dyspnea, orthopnea, cyanosis, cough, hemoptysis, rales, anxiety, restlessness)	The pulmonary symptoms that develop with HF are a direct result of events initiated by inadequate cardiac output. The left side of the heart is unable to accommodate incoming blood flow from the lungs. The resulting back pressure in pulmonary veins and capillaries causes leakage of fluid from blood vessels into tissue spaces and alveoli. Fluid accumulation may result in severe respiratory difficulty and pulmonary edema, a life-threatening development. The improved strength of myocardial contraction resulting from cardiotonic-inotropic drugs reverses this potentially fatal chain of events.

(*continued*)

NURSING ACTIONS	RATIONALE/EXPLANATION
(2) Decreased edema—absence of pitting, decreased size of ankles or abdominal girth, decreased weight	Diuresis and decreased edema result from improved circulation and increased renal blood flow.
(3) Increased tolerance of activity	Indicates a more adequate supply of blood to tissues
b. When digoxin is given in atrial arrhythmias, observe for:	
(1) Gradual slowing of the heart rate to 70 to 80 beats/min	
(2) Elimination of the pulse deficit	In clients with atrial fibrillation, slowing of the pulse rate and elimination of the pulse deficit are rough guides that digitalization has been achieved.
(3) Change in rhythm from irregular to regular	
3. Observe for adverse effects	
a. With digoxin observe for:	There is a high incidence of adverse effects with digoxin therapy. Therefore, every client receiving digoxin requires close observation. Severity of adverse effects can be minimized with early detection and treatment.
(1) Cardiac arrhythmias:	Digoxin toxicity may cause any type of cardiac arrhythmia. These are the most serious adverse effects associated with digoxin therapy. They are detected as abnormalities in electrocardiograms and in pulse rate or rhythm.
(a) Premature ventricular contractions (PVCs)	PVCs are among the most common digoxin-induced arrhythmias. They are not specific for digoxin toxicity because there are many possible causes. They are usually perceived as "skipped" heartbeats.
(b) Bradycardia	Excessive slowing of the pulse rate is an extension of the drug's therapeutic action of slowing conduction through the atrioventricular (AV) node and probably depressing the sinoatrial node as well.
(c) Paroxysmal atrial tachycardia with heart block	
(d) AV nodal tachycardia	
(e) AV block (second- or third-degree heart block)	
(2) Anorexia, nausea, vomiting	These GI effects commonly occur with digoxin therapy. Because they are caused at least in part by stimulation of the vomiting center in the brain, they occur with parenteral and oral administration. The presence of these symptoms raises suspicion of digitalis toxicity, but they are not specific because many other conditions may cause anorexia, nausea, and vomiting. Also, clients receiving digoxin are often taking other medications that cause these side effects, such as diuretics and potassium supplements.

(continued)

NURSING ACTIONS	RATIONALE/EXPLANATION
(3) Headache, drowsiness, confusion	These central nervous system effects are most common in older adults.
(4) Visual disturbances (eg, blurred vision, photophobia, altered perception of colors, flickering dots)	These are due mainly to drug effects on the retina and may indicate acute toxicity.
b. With amrinone, observe for:	
(1) Thrombocytopenia	Thrombocytopenia is more likely to occur with prolonged therapy and is usually reversible if dosage is reduced or the drug is discontinued.
(2) Anorexia, nausea, vomiting, abdominal pain	GI symptoms can be decreased by reducing drug dosage.
(3) Hypotension	Hypotension probably results from vasodilatory effects of amrinone.
(4) Hepatotoxicity	If marked changes in liver enzymes occur in conjunction with clinical symptoms, the drug should be discontinued.
c. With milrinone, observe for ventricular arrhythmias, hypotension, and headache	Ventricular arrhythmias reportedly occur in 12% of clients, hypotension and headache in approximately 3% of clients.
4. Observe for drug interactions	Most significant drug interactions increase risks of toxicity. Some alter absorption or metabolism to produce under-digitalization and decreased therapeutic effect.
a. Drugs that *increase* effects of digoxin:	
(1) Adrenergic drugs (eg, ephedrine, epinephrine, isoproterenol), succinylcholine	Increase risks of cardiac arrhythmias
(2) Antiarrhythmics (eg, amiodarone, propafenone, quinidine)	Decrease clearance of digoxin, thereby increasing serum digoxin levels and risks of toxicity. Dosage of digoxin should be reduced if one of these drugs is given concurrently (approximately 25% with propafenone and approximately 50% with amiodarone and quinidine).
(3) Anticholinergics	Increase absorption of oral digoxin by slowing transit time through the GI tract
(4) Calcium preparations	Increase risks of cardiac arrhythmias. IV calcium salts are contraindicated in digitalized clients.
(5) Calcium channel blockers (eg, diltiazem, felodipine, nifedipine, verapamil)	Decrease clearance of digoxin, thereby increasing serum digoxin levels and risks of toxicity. Dosage of digoxin should be reduced approximately 25% if verapamil is given concurrently.
b. Drugs that *decrease* effects of digoxin:	
(1) Antacids, cholestyramine, colestipol, laxatives, oral aminoglycosides (eg, neomycin)	Decrease absorption of oral digoxin

Nursing Notes: Apply Your Knowledge

Answer: Ms. Kindra's symptoms are consistent with acute heart failure and may indicate she is experiencing pulmonary edema. Administering digoxin is appropriate in the situation. The dose is a loading dose, rather than a maintenance dose. The digoxin is given IV and a loading dosage is used to achieve a therapeutic level more quickly so that adequate cardiac output can be restored. A loading dose should not exceed 1 mg/24 hours. Maintenance doses for digoxin are 0.125 to 0.50 mg/day, with the most common daily maintenance dose being 0.25 mg.

REVIEW AND APPLICATION EXERCISES

1. What signs and symptoms usually occur with HF? How would you assess for these?

2. What are the physiologic effects of digoxin on the heart?

3. How does digoxin produce or assist diuresis?

4. What is digitalization?

5. Differentiate between a digitalizing dose of digoxin and a daily maintenance dose.

6. Why do nurses need to check heart rate and rhythm before giving digoxin?

7. When is it appropriate to withhold a dose of digoxin?

8. What are adverse effects associated with digoxin, and how may they be prevented or minimized?

9. For clients with renal failure who need digoxin, what are the options for safe, effective therapy?

10. Why is it important to maintain a therapeutic serum potassium level during digoxin therapy?

11. What is the specific antidote for severe digoxin toxicity?

SELECTED REFERENCES

Brater, D.C. (1997). Clinical pharmacology of cardiovascular drugs. In W.N. Kelley (Ed.), *Textbook of internal medicine*, 3rd ed., pp. 552–569. Philadelphia: Lippincott-Raven.

Cody, R.J. (1998). Intensive diuretic therapy for acute cardiac decompensation. In D.L. Brown (Ed.), *Cardiac intensive care*, pp. 555–562. Philadelphia: W.B. Saunders.

Cohn, J.N. (1997). Approach to the patient with heart failure. In W.N. Kelley (Ed.), *Textbook of internal medicine*, 3rd ed., pp. 322–328. Philadelphia: Lippincott-Raven.

Drug facts and comparisons. (Updated monthly). St. Louis: Facts and Comparisons.

Ewald, G.A. & Rogers, J.G. (1998). Heart failure, cardiomyopathy, and valvular heart disease. In C.F. Carey, H.H. Lee, & K.F. Woeltje (Eds.), *The Washington manual of medical therapeutics*, 29th ed. pp. 109–129. Philadelphia: Lippincott Williams & Wilkins.

Givertz, M.M. & Colucci, W.S. (1998). Inotropic and vasoactive agents in the cardiac intensive care unit. In D.L. Brown (Ed.), *Cardiac intensive care*, pp. 545–553. Philadelphia: W.B. Saunders.

Guyton, A.C. & Hall, J.E. (1996). *Textbook of medical physiology*, 9th ed. Philadelphia: W.B. Saunders.

Johnson, J.A. & Lalonde, R.L. (1997). Congestive heart failure. In J.T. DiPiro, R.L. Talbert, G.C. Yee, G.R. Matzke, B.G. Wells, & L.M. Posey (Eds.), *Pharmacotherapy: A pathophysiologic approach*, 3rd ed., pp. 219–256. Stamford, CT: Appleton & Lange.

O'Laughlin, M.P. (1999). Congestive heart failure in children. *Pediatric Clinics of North America, 46,* 263–273.

Pitt, B., Zannad, F., Remme, W.J., Cody, T., et al. (1999). The effect of spironolactone on morbidity and mortality in patients with severe heart failure. *New England Journal of Medicine, 341,* 709–717.

Porth, C.M. (Ed.). (1998). *Pathophysiology: Concepts of altered health states,* 5th ed. Philadelphia: Lippincott Williams & Wilkins.

Schrier, R.W. & Abraham, W.T. (1999). Hormones and hemodynamics in heart failure. *New England Journal of Medicine, 341,* 577–585.

Smeltzer, S.C. & Bare, B.G. (1996). *Brunner and Suddarth's Textbook of medical-surgical nursing,* 8th ed. Philadelphia: Lippincott-Raven.

Weber, K.T. (1999). Aldosterone and spironolactone in heart failure [Editorial]. *New England Journal of Medicine, 341,* 753–755.

52

Antiarrhythmic Drugs

Objectives

After studying this chapter, the student will be able to:

1. Differentiate between supraventricular and ventricular dysrhythmias in terms of etiology and hemodynamic effects.

2. Describe nonpharmacologic measures to prevent or minimize tachyarrhythmias.

3. Discuss the roles of beta-adrenergic blocking agents, calcium channel blockers, digoxin, and quinidine in the treatment of supraventricular tachyarrhythmias.

4. Discuss the effects of lidocaine in the treatment of ventricular tachycardia.

5. Describe adverse effects and nursing process implications related to the use of selected antiarrhythmic drugs.

Seventy-nine-year-old Elmer Fitzgerald was recently diagnosed with atrial fibrillation. His heart rate is irregularly irregular, ranging between 120 and 160 beats per minute. At times, Mr. Fitzgerald is very symptomatic, experiencing weakness, dizziness, and syncope. His physician prescribes verapamil, a calcium channel blocker.

Reflect on:

▶ The emotional impact of the diagnosis of a serious cardiac problem, such as an arrhythmia.

▶ How atrial fibrillation affects cardiac function and the ability to oxygenate effectively.

▶ How the resulting symptoms of weakness, dizziness, and syncope may affect Mr. Fitzgerald's daily functioning.

▶ How verapamil would work to improve cardiac function.

Antiarrhythmic agents are diverse drugs used for prevention and treatment of cardiac arrhythmias. Arrhythmias, also called dysrhythmias, are abnormalities in heart rate or rhythm. They become significant when they interfere with cardiac function and ability to perfuse body tissues. To aid in understanding of arrhythmias and antiarrhythmic drug therapy, the physiology of cardiac conduction and contractility is reviewed.

CARDIAC ELECTROPHYSIOLOGY

The heart is an electrical pump. The "electrical" activity resides primarily in the specialized tissues that can generate and conduct an electrical impulse. Although impulses are conducted through muscle cells, the rate is much slower. The mechanical or "pump" activity resides in contractile tissue. Normally, these activities result in effective cardiac contraction and distribution of blood throughout the body. Each heartbeat or cardiac cycle occurs at regular intervals and consists of four events. These are *stimulation* from an electrical impulse, *transmission* of the electrical impulse to adjacent conductive or contractile tissue, *contraction* of atria and ventricles, and *relaxation* of atria and ventricles, during which they refill with blood in preparation for the next contraction.

Automaticity

Automaticity is the heart's ability to generate an electrical impulse. Any part of the conduction system can spontaneously start an impulse, but the sinoatrial (SA) node normally has the highest degree of automaticity and therefore the highest rate of spontaneous impulse formation. With its faster rate of electrical discharge or depolarization, the SA node serves as pacemaker and controls heart rate and rhythm.

Initiation of an electrical impulse depends on the movement of sodium and calcium ions into a myocardial cell and movement of potassium ions out of the cell. Normally, the cell membrane becomes more permeable to sodium and opens pores or channels to allow its rapid movement into the cell. Calcium ions follow sodium ions into the cell at a slower rate. As sodium and calcium ions move into cells, potassium moves out of cells. The movement of the ions changes the membrane from its resting state of electrical neutrality to an activated state of electrical energy buildup. When the electrical energy is discharged (depolarization), muscle contraction occurs.

Some cells in the cardiac conduction system depolarize in response to the entry of calcium ions rather than entry of sodium ions. In these calcium-respondent cells, which are found mainly in the SA and atrioventricular (AV) nodes, the electrical impulse is conducted more slowly and recovery of excitability takes longer than in sodium-respondent cells. Overall, activation of the SA and AV nodes depends on a slow depolarizing current through calcium channels and activation of the atria and ventricles depends on a rapid depolarizing current through sodium channels. These two types of conduction tissues are often called slow and fast channels, respectively, and they differ markedly in their responses to drugs that affect conduction of electrical impulses.

The ability of a cardiac muscle cell to respond to an electrical stimulus is called *excitability* or *irritability*. The stimulus must reach a certain intensity or threshold to cause contraction. After contraction, there is a period of decreased excitability (called the *refractory period*) during which the cell cannot respond to a new stimulus. During the refractory period, sodium and calcium ions return to the extracellular space, potassium ions return to the intracellular space, muscle relaxation occurs, and the cell prepares for the next electrical stimulus and contraction.

Conductivity

Conductivity is the ability of cardiac tissue to transmit electrical impulses. Although the electrophysiology of a single myocardial cell can assist understanding of the process, the orderly, rhythmic transmission of impulses to all cells results in effective myocardial contraction.

Normally, electrical impulses originate in the SA node and are transmitted to atrial muscle, where they cause atrial contraction, and then to the AV node, bundle of His, bundle branches, Purkinje fibers, and ventricular muscle, where they cause ventricular contraction. The cardiac conduction system is shown in Figure 52-1.

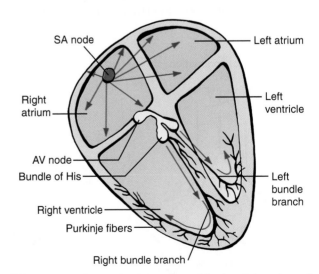

FIGURE 52–1 The conducting system of the heart. Impulses originating in the SA node are transmitted through the atria, into the AV node to the bundle of His, and by way of Purkinje fibers through the ventricles.

CARDIAC ARRHYTHMIAS

Cardiac arrhythmias can originate in any part of the conduction system or from atrial or ventricular muscle. They result from disturbances in electrical impulse formation (automaticity), conduction (conductivity), or both. The characteristic of automaticity allows myocardial cells other than the SA node to depolarize and initiate the electrical impulse that culminates in atrial and ventricular contraction. This may occur when the SA node fails to initiate an impulse or does so too slowly. When the electrical impulse arises anywhere other than the SA node, it is an abnormal or ectopic focus. If the ectopic focus depolarizes at a rate faster than the SA node, the ectopic focus becomes the dominant pacemaker. Ectopic pacemakers may arise in the atria, AV node, Purkinje fibers, or ventricular muscle. They may be activated by hypoxia, ischemia, or hypokalemia. Ectopic foci indicate myocardial irritability (increased responsiveness to stimuli) and potentially serious impairment of cardiac function.

A common mechanism by which abnormal conduction causes arrhythmias is called *reentry excitation*. With normal conduction, the electrical impulse moves freely down the conduction system until it reaches recently excited tissue that is refractory to stimulation. This causes the impulse to be extinguished. The SA node then recovers, fires spontaneously, and the conduction process starts over again. Reentry excitation means that an impulse continues to reenter an area of the heart rather than becoming extinguished. For this to occur, the impulse must encounter an obstacle in the normal conducting pathway. The obstacle is usually an area of damage, such as myocardial infarction. The damaged area allows conduction in only one direction and causes a circular movement of the impulse (Fig. 52-2).

Arrhythmias may be mild or severe, acute or chronic, episodic or relatively continuous. They are clinically significant if they interfere with cardiac function (ie, the heart's ability to pump sufficient blood to body tissues). The normal heart can maintain an adequate cardiac output with ventricular rates ranging from 40 to 180 beats per minute. The diseased heart, however, may not be able to maintain an adequate cardiac output with heart rates below 60 or above 120. Arrhythmias are usually categorized by rate, location, or patterns of conduction. Common types of arrhythmias are described in Box 52-1.

ANTIARRHYTHMIC DRUGS

Antiarrhythmic drugs alter the heart's electrical conduction system. Atropine for bradyarrhythmias is discussed in Chapter 21; digoxin and its use in treating atrial fibrillation are discussed in Chapter 51. The focus of this chapter is the drugs used for tachyarrhythmias. These drugs are described in the following sections and listed in Table 52-1.

Clinical use of antiarrhythmic drugs for tachyarrhythmias has undergone significant changes. One change is that the goal of drug therapy is to prevent or relieve symptoms or prolong survival, not just suppress arrhythmias. This change resulted from studies in which clients treated for some arrhythmias had a higher mortality rate than clients who did not receive antiarrhythmic drug therapy. The higher mortality rate was attributed to proarrhythmic effects (ie, worsening existing arrhythmias or causing new arrhythmias). Overall, there is decreasing use of class I drugs (eg, quinidine) and increasing use of class II (beta blockers) and class III drugs (eg, amiodarone).

Another change is the greater use of nonpharmacologic treatment of arrhythmias. These methods include destroying arrhythmogenic foci in the heart with radio waves (radiofrequency catheter ablation) or surgical procedures and implanting devices for sensing, cardioverting, defibrillating, or pacing (eg, the implantable cardioverter-defibrillator or ICD).

(*text continues on page 770*)

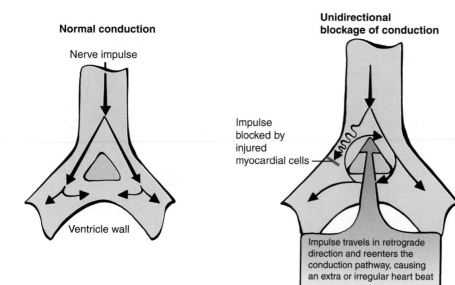

Normal conduction

Nerve impulse

Ventricle wall

Unidirectional blockage of conduction

Impulse blocked by injured myocardial cells

Impulse travels in retrograde direction and reenters the conduction pathway, causing an extra or irregular heart beat

FIGURE 52–2 Reentry excitation of arrhythmias.

BOX 52–1 **TYPES OF ARRHYTHMIAS**

Sinus arrhythmias are usually significant only if they are severe or prolonged. Tachycardia increases the workload of the heart and may lead to heart failure or angina pectoris. Sinus tachycardia may cause anginal pain (myocardial ischemia) by two related mechanisms. One mechanism involves increased myocardial oxygen consumption. The other mechanism involves a shortened diastole so that coronary arteries may not have adequate filling time between heartbeats. Thus, additional blood flow to the myocardium is required at the same time that a decreased blood supply is delivered.

Sinus tachycardia may be caused by numerous conditions such as fever, hypotension, heart failure, thyrotoxicosis, stimulation of the sympathetic nervous system (eg, stress or drugs, including asthma remedies and nasal decongestants), and lifestyle drugs such as alcohol, caffeine, and nicotine. Thus, the initial assessment of a client with sinus tachycardia should include a search for underlying causes. The rate usually may be slowed by treating the underlying cause or by stimulating the vagus nerve (eg, by carotid sinus massage or Valsalva's maneuver).

Sinus bradycardia may occur with excessive vagal stimulation, deficient sympathetic tone, and sinus node dysfunction. It often occurs in healthy young adults, especially in athletes and during sleep. Other conditions associated with sinus bradycardia include hypothyroidism, hypothermia, vasovagal reactions, and drugs such as beta-adrenergic blocking agents, amiodarone, diltiazem, lithium, and verapamil. Thus, as with sinus tachycardia, efforts to identify the underlying cause are needed. Asymptomatic sinus bradycardia does not require treatment. Acute, symptomatic sinus bradycardia can be treated with atropine or a temporary transvenous pacemaker. Chronic symptomatic sinus bradycardia requires insertion of a permanent pacemaker.

Atrial arrhythmias are most significant in the presence of underlying heart disease. Atrial fibrillation and atrial flutter commonly occur, especially in older adults. Numerous conditions may lead to these arrhythmias, including myocardial ischemia or infarction, hypertension, cardiomyopathy, valvular disorders, pulmonary embolus, pulmonary hypertension, thyrotoxicosis, alcohol withdrawal, sepsis, or excessive physical exertion. One characteristic of *atrial fibrillation* is disorganized, tremor-like movement of the atria. This lack of effective atrial contraction impairs ventricular filling, decreases cardiac output, and may lead to the formation of atrial thrombi, with a high potential for embolization. Another characteristic is a very rapid atrial rate (400 to 600 beats/minute). Some of the atrial impulses penetrate the atrioventricular (AV) conduction system to reach the ventricles, and some do not. This results in irregular activation of the ventricles and a slower ventricular rate (120 to 180 beats/minute) than atrial rate.

Atrial flutter occurs less often than atrial fibrillation but causes similar symptoms. Atrial flutter is characterized by a rapid (270 to 330 atrial beats/minute) but regular atrial activation and a regular ventricular pulse rate.

For some patients, the main goal of treatment for atrial fibrillation or flutter is restoration of sinus rhythm by pharmacologic or electrical cardioversion. Then, long-term drug therapy is usually given to prevent recurrence. For patients who are not considered candidates for conversion to normal sinus rhythm, the goals are to slow the ventricular response rate (with antiarrhythmic medication) and to prevent stroke or other thromboembolic complications (eg, with aspirin, warfarin, or both).

Nodal arrhythmias may involve tachycardia and increased workload of the heart or bradycardia from heart block. Either tachycardia or bradycardia may decrease cardiac output. Heart block involves impaired conduction of the electrical impulse through the AV node. With first-degree heart block, conduction is slowed, but not significantly. With second-degree heart block, every second, third, or fourth atrial impulse is blocked and does not reach the ventricles (2:1, 3:1, or 4:1 block). Thus, atrial and ventricular rates differ. Second-degree heart block may interfere with cardiac output or progress to third-degree block. Third-degree is the most serious type of heart block because no impulses reach the ventricles. As a result, ventricles beat independently at a rate of 30 to 40 per minute. This slow ventricular rate severely reduces cardiac output.

Ventricular arrhythmias include premature ventricular contractions (PVCs), ventricular tachycardia, and ventricular fibrillation. PVCs occur in healthy people as well as those with heart disease and may cause no symptoms or only mild palpitations. Serious PVCs often occur with ischemic heart disease, especially after acute myocardial infarction. PVCs are considered serious if they produce significant symptoms (eg, anginal pain, dyspnea, or syncope), occur more than five times per minute, are coupled or grouped, are multifocal, or occur during the resting phase of the cardiac cycle. Serious PVCs indicate a high degree of myocardial irritability and may lead to life-threatening ventricular tachycardia, ventricular fibrillation, or asystole. The goal of treatment is to decrease myocardial irritability, relieve symptoms, and prevent progression to more serious arrhythmias.

(*continued*)

BOX 52–1   TYPES OF ARRHYTHMIAS (continued)

Ventricular tachycardia (VT) is characterized by a ventricular rate of 160 to 250 beats/minute. It is diagnosed when three or more PVCs occur in a row at a rate greater than 100 beats/minute. VT may be sustained (lasts longer than 30 seconds or requires termination because of hemodynamic collapse) or nonsustained (stops spontaneously in less than 30 seconds). Occasional brief episodes of VT may be asymptomatic; frequent or relatively long episodes may result in hemodynamic collapse, a life-threatening situation. An acute episode most often occurs during an acute myocardial infarction. Other precipitating factors include severe electrolyte imbalances (eg, hypokalemia), hypoxemia, or digoxin toxicity. Correction of these precipitating factors usually prevents recurrences of VT. Clients with organic heart disease may have a chronic recurrent form of VT. Torsades de pointes is an especially serious type of VT that may deteriorate into ventricular fibrillation. Predisposing factors include severe bradycardia, electrolyte deficiencies (eg, hypokalemia, hypomagnesemia), and several drug groups (eg, class IA antiarrhythmics, phenothiazine antipsychotics, and tricyclic antidepressants). VT can be treated with lidocaine (a loading dose and continuous infusion), direct-current countershock, or insertion of a transvenous pacing wire for overdrive pacing.

Ventricular fibrillation (VF) produces ineffective myocardial contraction so that there is no cardiac output. Death results unless effective cardiopulmonary resuscitation or defibrillation is instituted within approximately 4 to 6 minutes. It most often occurs in clients with ischemic heart disease, especially acute myocardial infarction. Direct-current countershock and antiarrhythmic drugs are used to restore a functional heart rhythm. After successful resuscitation, antiarrhythmic drug therapy should be continued until the client's rhythm and clinical status stabilize. Then, the client should be monitored closely for recurrence of VT or VF. Myocardial revascularization surgery or ablation of the arrhythmogenic focus may be effective in controlling VT/VF. However, transvenous implantable cardioverter-defibrillators (ICDs) are being used more frequently for antitachycardia pacing, cardioversion, defibrillation, and ventricular pacing (if asystole occurs). It is not yet known whether the ICDs are more effective than beta blockers, sotalol, or amiodarone in reducing total mortality. Reducing mortality is the goal of antiarrhythmic therapy for life-threatening ventricular arrhythmias.

TABLE 52–1   Antiarrhythmic Drugs

	Routes and Dosage Ranges	
Drugs for Tachyarrhythmias	**Adults**	**Children**

Class 1 Sodium Channel Blockers

CLASS 1A: TREATMENT OF SYMPTOMATIC PREMATURE VENTRICULAR CONTRACTIONS, SUPRAVENTRICULAR TACHYCARDIA, AND VENTRICULAR TACHYCARDIA; PREVENTION OF VENTRICULAR FIBRILLATION

Quinidine (Cardioquin, Quinaglute)	PO 200–600 mg q6h; maximum dose, 3–4 g/d Maintenance dose, PO 200–600 mg q6h, or 1 or 2 extended-action tablets, two or three times per day IM (quinidine gluconate) 600 mg initially, then 400 mg q4–6h	PO 6 mg/kg q4–6h
Procainamide (Pronestyl, Procanbid)	PO 1 g loading dose initially, then 250–500 mg q3–4h (q6h for sustained-release tablets) IM loading dose, 500–1000 mg followed by oral maintenance doses IV 25–50 mg/min; maximum dose, 1000 mg	PO 50 mg/kg/d in four to six divided doses
Disopyramide (Norpace)	PO loading dose, 300 mg, followed by 150 mg q6h; usual dose, PO 400–800 mg/d in four divided doses	

CLASS 1B: TREATMENT OF SYMPTOMATIC PREMATURE VENTRICULAR CONTRACTIONS AND VENTRICULAR TACHYCARDIA; PREVENTION OF VENTRICULAR FIBRILLATION

Lidocaine (Xylocaine)	IV 1–2 mg/kg, not to exceed 50–100 mg, as a single bolus Injection over 2 min, followed by a continuous infusion (1 g of lidocaine in 500 mL of 5% dextrose in water) at a rate to deliver 1–4 mg/min; maximum dose, 300 mg/h. IM 4–5 mg/kg as a single dose; may repeat in 60–90 min	IV injection 1 mg/kg, followed by IV infusion of 20–50 µg/kg/min

TABLE 52-1 **Antiarrhythmic Drugs** (*continued*)

Drugs for Tachyarrhythmias	Routes and Dosage Ranges	
	Adults	Children
Mexiletine (Mexitil)	PO 200 mg q8h initially, increased by 50–100 mg every 2–3 d if necessary to a maximum of 1200 mg/d	
Tocainide (Tonocard)	PO 400 mg q8h initially, increased up to 1800 mg/d in three divided doses if necessary	
Phenytoin (Dilantin)	PO, loading dose 13 mg/kg (approximately 1000 mg) first day, 7.5 mg/kg second and third days; maintenance dose 4–6 mg/kg/d (average 400 mg) in one or two doses starting on the fourth day IV 100 mg every 5 min until the arrhythmia is reversed or toxic effects occur; maximum dose, 1 g/24 h	

CLASS 1C: TREATMENT OF LIFE-THREATENING VENTRICULAR TACHYCARDIA OR FIBRILLATION AND SUPRAVENTRICULAR TACHYCARDIA UNRESPONSIVE TO OTHER DRUGS

Flecainide (Tambocor)	PO 100 mg q12h initially, increased by 50 mg q12h every 4 d until effective; maximum dose, 400 mg/d	
Propafenone (Rythmol)	PO 150 mg q8h initially, increased to a maximum dose of 1200 mg/d if necessary; usual maintenance dose 150–300 mg q8h	

CLASS 1 MISCELLANEOUS: TREATMENT OF LIFE-THREATENING VENTRICULAR ARRHYTHMIAS

Moricizine (Ethmozine)	PO 200–300 mg q8h	

Class II Beta Blockers: Treatment of Supraventricular Tachycardia

Acebutolol (Sectral)	PO 200 mg twice daily, increased gradually until optimal response is obtained (usually 600–1200 mg/d)	
Esmolol (Brevibloc)	IV infusion 500 µg/kg/min initially as a loading dose, followed by a maintenance dose of 50 µg/kg/min over 4 min. Repeat the same loading dose, and increase maintenance doses in 50 µg/kg increments every 5–10 min until therapeutic effects are obtained. Average maintenance dose, 100 µg/kg/min.	
Propranolol (Inderal)	IV injection 1–3 mg at a rate of 1 mg/min PO 10–20 mg three or four times per day	

Class III Potassium Channel Blockers: Treatment of Ventricular Tachycardia and Fibrillation; Conversion of Atrial Fibrillation or Flutter to Sinus Rhythm; Maintenance of Sinus Rhythm (Amiodarone)

Amiodarone (Cordarone)	Loading dose, IV, 150 mg over 10 min (15 mg/min), then 360 mg over the next 6 h (1 mg/min), then 540 mg over the next 18 h (0.5 mg/min) Maintenance dose, IV, 720 mg/24 h (0.5 mg/min) Loading dose, PO, 800–1600 mg/d for 1–3 wk, with a gradual decrease to 600–800 mg/d for 1 mo Maintenance dose, PO 400 mg/d	
Bretylium (Bretylol)	IM 5 mg/kg, repeated in 1–2 h then q6–8h IV 5–10 mg/kg (diluted in at least 50 mL of IV fluid and infused over 10–20 min). During cardiopulmonary resuscitation, IV 5 mg/kg given by direct injection (undiluted); may be repeated every 15–30 min to a maximum total dose of 30 mg/kg.	
Ibutilide (Corvert)	Weight ≥60 kg: IV infusion over 10 min, 1 mg Weight <60 kg: IV infusion over 10 min, 0.01 mg/kg The dose can be repeated once, after 10 min, if necessary.	

(continued)

TABLE 52-1   **Antiarrhythmic Drugs (*continued*)**

| Drugs for Tachyarrhythmias | Routes and Dosage Ranges | |
	Adults	Children
Sotalol (Betapace)	PO 80 mg q12h initially, titrated to response; average dose; 160–320 mg daily. See manufacturer's recommendations for dosing in renal failure.	
Class IV Calcium Channel Blockers: Treatment of Supraventricular Tachycardia		
Diltiazem (Cardizem)	IV injection 0.25 mg/kg (average dose 20 mg) over 2 min. A second dose of 0.35 mg/kg (average, 25 mg) may be given in 15 min, and an IV infusion of 5–15 mg/h may be given up to 24 h, if necessary.	
Verapamil (Calan, Isoptin)	PO 40–120 mg q6–8h IV 5–10 mg initially, then 10 mg 30 min later, if necessary	<1 y: IV injection 0.1–0.2 mg/kg (usual range, 0.75–2.0 mg for a single dose) over 2 min with continuous ECG monitoring 1–15 y: IV injection 0.1–0.3 mg/kg (usual range 2–5 mg for a single dose) over 2 min with continuous ECG monitoring; repeat in 30 min if necessary
Unclassified: Adenosine is Used to Treat Supraventricular Tachycardia; Magnesium Sulfate is Used to Treat Torsades de Pointes		
Adenosine (Adenocard)	IV 6 mg given rapidly over 1–2 sec. If first dose does not slow the supraventricular tachycardia within 1–2 min, give 12 mg rapidly, and repeat one time, if necessary.	
Magnesium sulfate	IV 1–2 g (2–4 mL of 50% solution), diluted in 10 mL of 5% dextrose solution	

ECG, electrocardiogram; IM, intramuscular; IV, intravenous; PO, oral.

Indications for Use

Antiarrhythmic drug therapy usually is indicated in the following conditions:

1. To convert atrial fibrillation (AF) or flutter to normal sinus rhythm (NSR)
2. To maintain NSR after conversion from AF or flutter
3. When the ventricular rate is so fast or irregular that cardiac output is impaired. Decreased cardiac output leads to symptoms of decreased systemic, cerebral, and coronary circulation.
4. When dangerous arrhythmias occur and may be fatal if not quickly terminated. For example, ventricular tachycardia may cause cardiac arrest.

Mechanisms of Action

Drugs used for rapid arrhythmias mainly *reduce automaticity* (spontaneous depolarization of myocardial cells, including ectopic pacemakers), *slow conduction* of electrical impulses through the heart, and *prolong the refractory period* of myocardial cells (so they are less likely to be prematurely activated by adjacent cells). Several different groups of drugs perform one or more of these actions. They are classified according to their mechanisms of action and

effects on the conduction system, even though they differ in other respects. In addition, some drugs have characteristics of more than one classification.

CLASSIFICATIONS AND INDIVIDUAL DRUGS

Class I Sodium Channel Blockers

Class I drugs block the movement of sodium into cells of the cardiac conducting system. This results in a membrane-stabilizing effect and decreased formation and conduction of electrical impulses. This group of drugs is declining in clinical use, mainly because of proarrhythmic effects and resultant increased mortality rates. The higher mortality rates occur most often in clients with significant structural heart disease.

Class IA

Class IA drugs have a broad spectrum of antiarrhythmic effects and are used for both supraventricular and ventricular arrhythmias. **Quinidine**, the prototype, reduces automaticity, slows conduction, and prolongs the refractory period. It has long been used to maintain NSR in clients with AF or flutter who have been converted to NSR with digoxin or electrical cardioversion. However, such use is declining because clients may have recurrent AF and have higher mortality rates with long-term quinidine therapy.

Quinidine is well absorbed after oral administration. Therapeutic serum levels (2 to 6 µg/mL) are attained within 1 hour and persist for 6 to 8 hours. Quinidine is highly bound to serum albumin and has a half-life of approximately 6 hours. It is metabolized by the liver (approximately 80%) and excreted in the urine (approximately 20%). In alkaline urine (ie, pH >7), renal excretion of quinidine decreases, and serum levels may rise. Serum levels greater than 8 µg/mL are toxic.

Quinidine's low therapeutic ratio and high incidence of adverse effects limit its clinical usefulness. The drug is usually contraindicated in clients with severe, uncompensated congestive heart failure or with heart block because it depresses myocardial contractility and conduction through the AV node.

Quinidine salts used clinically include quinidine gluconate (Quinaglute), quinidine sulfate (Quinora), and quinidine polygalacturonate (Cardioquin). These salts differ in the amount of active drug (quinidine base) they contain and the rate of absorption with oral administration. The sulfate salt contains 83% quinidine base, and peak effects occur in 0.5 to 1.5 hours (4 hours for sustained-release forms). The gluconate salt contains 62% active drug, and peak effects occur in 3 to 4 hours. The polygalacturonate salt contains 60% active drug, and peak effects occur in approximately 6 hours. Quinidine preparations are usually given orally. The gluconate and polygalacturonate salts reportedly cause less gastrointestinal (GI) irritation than quinidine sulfate; this is probably related to their lower quinidine content. Oral extended-action preparations of quinidine (Quinidex Extentabs, Quinaglute Dura-Tabs) also are available.

Disopyramide is similar to quinidine in pharmacologic actions and may be given orally to adults with ventricular tachyarrhythmias. It is well absorbed after oral administration and reaches peak serum levels (2 to 8 µg/mL) within 30 to 60 minutes. Drug half-life is 5 to 8 hours. Disopyramide is excreted by the kidneys and the liver in almost equal proportions. Dosage must be reduced in renal insufficiency.

Procainamide is related to the local anesthetic procaine and is similar to quinidine in actions and uses. Quinidine may be preferred for long-term use because procainamide produces a high incidence of adverse effects, including a syndrome resembling lupus erythematosus. Procainamide has a short duration of action (3 to 4 hours); sustained-release tablets (Procanbid) prolong action to approximately 6 hours. Therapeutic serum levels are 4 to 8 µg/mL.

Class IB

Lidocaine, a local anesthetic (see Chap. 14), is the prototype of class IB. It is the drug of choice for treating serious ventricular arrhythmias associated with acute myocardial infarction, cardiac surgery, cardiac catheterization, and electrical cardioversion. Lidocaine decreases myocardial irritability (automaticity) in the ventricles. It has little effect on atrial tissue and is not useful in treating atrial arrhythmias. It differs from quinidine in that:

1. It must be given by injection.
2. It does not decrease AV conduction or myocardial contractility with usual therapeutic doses.
3. It has a rapid onset and short duration of action. After intravenous (IV) administration of a bolus dose, therapeutic effects occur within 1 to 2 minutes and last approximately 20 minutes. This characteristic is advantageous in emergency treatment but limits lidocaine use to intensive care settings.
4. It is metabolized in the liver. Dosage must be reduced in clients with hepatic insufficiency or congestive heart failure to avoid drug accumulation and toxicity.
5. It is less likely to cause heart block, cardiac asystole, ventricular arrhythmias, and congestive heart failure.

Therapeutic serum levels of lidocaine are 2 to 5 µg/mL. Lidocaine may be given intramuscularly (IM) in emergencies when IV administration is impossible. When given IM, therapeutic effects occur in approximately 15 minutes and last approximately 90 minutes. Lidocaine is contraindicated in clients allergic to related local anesthetics (eg, procaine). Anaphylactic reactions may occur in sensitized people.

Mexiletine and **tocainide** are oral analogs of lidocaine with similar pharmacologic actions. They are used to suppress ventricular fibrillation or ventricular tachycardia. They are well absorbed from the GI tract, and peak serum levels are obtained within 3 hours. Taking the drug with food delays but does not decrease absorption.

Phenytoin, an anticonvulsant (see Chap. 11), may be used to treat arrhythmias produced by digoxin intoxication. Phenytoin decreases automaticity and improves conduction through the AV node. Decreased automaticity helps control arrhythmias, whereas enhanced conduction may improve cardiac function. Further, because heart block may result from digoxin, quinidine, or procainamide, phenytoin may relieve arrhythmias without intensifying heart block. Phenytoin is not a cardiac depressant. Its only quinidine-like action is to suppress automaticity; otherwise, it counteracts the effects of quinidine and procainamide largely by increasing the rate of conduction. Phenytoin also has a longer half-life (22 to 36 hours) than other antiarrhythmic drugs. Given IV, a therapeutic plasma level (10 to 20 µg/mL) can be obtained rapidly. Given orally, however, the drug may not reach a steady-state concentration for approximately 1 week unless loading doses are given initially.

Class IC

Flecainide and **propafenone** are oral agents that greatly decrease conduction in the ventricles. They may initiate new arrhythmias or aggravate pre-existing arrhythmias, sometimes causing sustained ventricular tachycardia or ventricular fibrillation. These effects are more likely to occur with high doses and rapid dose increases. The drugs are recommended for use only in life-threatening ventricular arrhythmias.

Miscellaneous Class I Drug

Moricizine is a class I agent with properties of the other subclasses (ie, IA, IB, and IC). It is indicated for treatment of life-threatening ventricular arrhythmias, such as sustained ventricular tachycardia, and contraindicated in clients with heart block, cardiogenic shock, and hypersensitivity reactions to the drug. After oral administration, onset of action occurs within 2 hours, and duration of action is 10 to 24 hours. The drug is 95% protein bound, extensively metabolized in the liver, and excreted in the urine. Because moricizine may cause new arrhythmias or aggravate pre-existing arrhythmias, therapy should be initiated in hospitalized clients with continuous electrocardiographic (ECG) monitoring.

Class II Beta-Adrenergic Blockers

These agents (see Chap. 19) exert antiarrhythmic effects by blocking sympathetic nervous system stimulation of beta receptors in the heart and decreasing risks of ventricular fibrillation. Blockage of receptors in the SA node and ectopic pacemakers decreases automaticity, and blockage of receptors in the AV node increases the refractory period. The drugs are effective for treatment of supraventricular arrhythmias and those resulting from excessive sympathetic activity. Thus, they are most often used to slow the ventricular rate of contraction in supraventricular tachyarrhythmias (eg, AF, atrial flutter, paroxysmal supraventricular tachycardia [PSVT]).

As a class, beta blockers are being used more extensively because of their effectiveness and their ability to reduce mortality in a variety of clinical settings, including post-myocardial infarction and heart failure. Reduced mortality may result from the drugs' ability to prevent ventricular fibrillation. Only four of the beta blockers marketed in the United States are approved by the Food and Drug Administration (FDA) for treatment of arrhythmias. **Acebutolol** may be given orally for chronic therapy to prevent ventricular arrhythmias, especially those precipitated by exercise. **Esmolol** has a rapid onset and short duration of action. It is given IV for supraventricular tachyarrhythmias, especially during anesthesia, surgery, or other emergency situations when the ventricular rate must be reduced rapidly. It is not used for chronic therapy. **Propranolol** may be given orally for chronic therapy to prevent ventricular arrhythmias, especially those precipitated by exercise. It may be given IV for life-threatening arrhythmias or those occurring during anesthesia. **Sotalol** is a noncardioselective beta blocker (class II) that also

has properties of class III antiarrhythmic drugs. Because its class III characteristics are considered more important in its antiarrhythmic effects, it is a class III drug (see next section).

Class III Potassium Channel Blockers

These drugs act to prolong duration of the action potential, slow repolarization, and prolong the refractory period in both atria and ventricles. Although the drugs share a common mechanism of action, they are very different drugs. As with beta blockers, clinical use of class III agents is increasing because they are associated with less ventricular fibrillation and decreased mortality compared with class I drugs.

Although classified as a potassium channel blocker, **amiodarone** also has electrophysiologic characteristics of sodium channel blockers, beta blockers, and calcium channel blockers. Thus, it has vasodilating effects and decreases systemic vascular resistance; it prolongs conduction in all cardiac tissues and decreases heart rate; and it decreases contractility of the left ventricle.

Intravenous and oral amiodarone differ in their electrophysiologic effects. When given IV, the major effect is slowing conduction through the AV node and prolonging the effective refractory period. Thus, it is given IV mainly for acute suppression of refractory, hemodynamically destabilizing ventricular tachycardia and ventricular fibrillation. It is given orally to treat recurrent ventricular tachycardia or ventricular fibrillation and to maintain a NSR after conversion of AF and flutter. Low doses (100 to 200 mg/day) may prevent recurrence of AF with less toxicity than higher doses of amiodarone or usual doses of other agents, including quinidine.

Amiodarone is extensively metabolized in the liver and produces active metabolites. The drug and its metabolites accumulate in the liver, lung, fat, skin, and other tissues. With IV administration, the onset of action usually occurs within several hours. With oral administration, the action may be delayed from a few days up to a week or longer. Because of its long serum half-life, loading doses are usually given and higher loading doses reduce the time required for therapeutic effects. Also, effects may persist for several weeks after the drug is discontinued.

Adverse effects include hypothyroidism, hyperthyroidism, pulmonary fibrosis, myocardial depression, hypotension, bradycardia, hepatic dysfunction, central nervous system (CNS) disturbances (depression, insomnia, nightmares, hallucinations), peripheral neuropathy and muscle weakness, bluish discoloration of skin and corneal deposits that may cause photosensitivity, appearance of colored halos around lights, and reduced visual acuity. Most adverse effects are considered dose dependent and reversible.

When oral amiodarone is used long-term, it also increases the effects of numerous drugs, including anticoagulants, beta blockers, calcium channel blockers, class I antiarrhythmics (quinidine, flecainide, lidocaine, procainamide), cyclosporine, digoxin, methotrexate, phenytoin, and theophylline.

Bretylium initially increases release of catecholamines and therefore increases heart rate, blood pressure, and myocardial contractility. This is followed in a few minutes by a decrease in vascular resistance, blood pressure, and heart rate. It is used primarily for acute control of recurrent ventricular fibrillation, especially in clients with recent myocardial infarction, in intensive care settings. It is given by IV infusion, with a loading dose followed by a maintenance dose, or in repeated IV injections. Because it is excreted almost entirely by the kidney, drug half-life is prolonged with renal impairment and dosage must be reduced. Adverse effects include hypotension and arrhythmias.

Ibutilide is indicated for treatment of recent onset of AF or atrial flutter, in which the goal is conversion to NSR. Ibutilide is widely distributed and has an elimination half-life of approximately 6 hours. Most of a dose is metabolized, and the metabolites are excreted in urine and feces. Adverse effects include supraventricular and ventricular arrhythmias and hypotension. Ibutilide should be administered in a setting with personnel and equipment available for emergency use.

Sotalol has both beta-adrenergic blocking and potassium channel blocking activity. Beta-blocking effects predominate at lower doses and class III effects predominate at higher doses. The drug is well absorbed after oral administration, and peak serum level is reached in 2 to 4 hours. It has an elimination half-life of approximately 12 hours, and 80% to 90% is excreted unchanged by the kidneys. Sotalol is approved for prevention or treatment of ventricular tachycardia and fibrillation. It has also been used, usually in smaller doses, to prevent or treat AF. It is contraindicated in clients with asthma, sinus bradycardia, heart block, cardiogenic shock, heart failure, and previous hypersensitivity to sotalol. Dosage should be individualized, reduced with renal impairment, and increased slowly (eg, every 2 to 3 days with normal renal function, at longer intervals with impaired renal function). Arrhythmogenic effects are most likely to occur when therapy is started or when dosage is increased. Heart failure may occur in clients with markedly depressed left ventricular systolic function. Most adverse effects are attributed to beta-blocking activity.

Like amiodarone, sotalol may be preferred over a class I agent because it is more effective in reducing recurrent ventricular tachycardia, ventricular fibrillation, and death.

Class IV Calcium Channel Blockers

Calcium channel blockers (see Chap. 53) block the movement of calcium into conductile and contractile myocardial cells. As antiarrhythmic agents, they act primarily against tachycardias at SA and AV nodes because the cardiac cells and slow channels that depend on calcium influx are found mainly at these sites. Thus, they reduce automaticity of the SA and AV nodes, slow conduction,

and prolong the refractory period in the AV node. They are effective only in supraventricular tachycardias.

Diltiazem and **verapamil** are the only calcium channel blockers approved for treatment of arrhythmias. Both drugs may be given IV to terminate acute PSVT, usually within 2 minutes, and in AF and flutter. They are also effective in exercise-related tachycardias. When given IV, the drugs act within 15 minutes and last up to 6 hours. Oral verapamil may be used in the chronic treatment of the aforementioned arrhythmias. Diltiazem and verapamil are metabolized by the liver, and metabolites are primarily excreted by the kidneys. The drugs are contraindicated in digoxin toxicity because they may worsen heart block. If used with propranolol or digoxin, caution must be exercised to avoid further impairment of myocardial contractility. *Do not* use IV verapamil with IV propranolol; potentially fatal bradycardia and hypotension may occur.

Unclassified

Adenosine, a naturally occurring component of all body cells, differs chemically from other antiarrhythmic drugs but acts like the calcium channel blockers. It depresses conduction at the AV node and is used to restore NSR in clients with PSVT; it is ineffective in other arrhythmias. The drug has a very short duration of action (serum half-life is less than 10 seconds) and a high degree of effectiveness. It must be given by a rapid bolus injection, preferably through a central venous line. If given slowly, it is eliminated before it can reach cardiac tissues and exert its action.

Magnesium sulfate is given IV in the treatment of several arrhythmias, including prevention of recurrent episodes of torsades de pointes and treatment of digitalis-induced arrhythmias. Its antiarrhythmic effects may derive from imbalances of magnesium, potassium, and calcium.

Hypomagnesemia increases myocardial irritability and is a risk factor for both atrial and ventricular arrhythmias. Thus, serum magnesium levels should be monitored in clients at risk and replacement therapy instituted when indicated. However, in some instances, the drug seems to have antiarrhythmic effects even when serum magnesium levels are normal.

NURSING PROCESS

Assessment

Assess the client's condition in relation to cardiac arrhythmias:

- Identify conditions or risk factors that may precipitate arrhythmias. These include the following:
  - Hypoxia
  - Electrolyte imbalances (eg, hypokalemia, hypomagnesemia)

- Acid–base imbalances
- Ischemic heart disease (angina pectoris, myocardial infarction)
- Cardiac valvular disease
- Febrile illness
- Respiratory disorders (eg, chronic lung disease)
- Exercise
- Emotional upset
- Excessive ingestion of caffeine-containing beverages (eg, coffee, tea, colas)
- Cigarette smoking
- Drug therapy with digoxin, antiarrhythmic drugs, CNS stimulants, anorexiants, and tricyclic antidepressants
- Hyperthyroidism
- Observe for clinical signs and symptoms of arrhythmias. Mild or infrequent arrhythmias may be perceived by the client as palpitations or skipped heartbeats. More severe arrhythmias may produce manifestations that reflect decreased cardiac output and other hemodynamic changes, as follows:
  - Hypotension, bradycardia or tachycardia, and irregular pulse
  - Shortness of breath, dyspnea, and cough from impaired respiration
  - Syncope or mental confusion from reduced cerebral blood flow
  - Chest pain from decreased coronary artery blood flow. Angina pectoris or myocardial infarction may occur.
  - Oliguria from decreased renal blood flow
- When ECGs are available (eg, 12-lead ECG or continuous ECG monitoring), assess for indications of arrhythmias.

Nursing Diagnoses

- Decreased Cardiac Output related to ineffective pumping action of the heart
- Altered Tissue Perfusion related to decreased cardiac output
- Altered Tissue Perfusion related to drug-induced hypotension
- Activity Intolerance related to weakness and fatigue
- Self Care Deficit related to decreased tissue perfusion and fatigue
- Impaired Gas Exchange related to decreased tissue perfusion
- Anxiety related to potentially serious illness
- Knowledge Deficit: Pharmacologic and nonpharmacologic management of arrhythmias
- Fluid Volume Excess: Peripheral edema and pulmonary congestion related to decreased cardiac output
- Noncompliance: Underuse of drugs related to adverse drug effects

Planning/Goals

The client will:

- Receive or take antiarrhythmic drugs accurately
- Avoid conditions that precipitate arrhythmias, when feasible
- Experience improved heart rate, circulation, and activity tolerance
- Be closely monitored for therapeutic and adverse drug effects
- Avoid preventable adverse drug effects
- Have adverse drug effects promptly recognized and treated if they occur
- Keep follow-up appointments for monitoring responses to treatment measures

---

CLIENT TEACHING GUIDELINES
Antiarrhythmic Drugs

General Considerations

✔ A fast heartbeat normally occurs in response to exercise, fever, and other conditions so that more blood can be pumped and carried to body tissues. An irregular heartbeat occurs occasionally in most people. However, when you are prescribed a long-term medication to slow or regularize your heartbeat, this means that you have a potentially serious condition. In addition, the medications can cause potentially serious adverse effects. Thus, it is extremely important that you take

the medications exactly as prescribed. Taking extra doses is dangerous; skipping doses or waiting longer between doses may lead to loss of control of the heart problem.

✔ You may be given a drug classified as an antiarrhythmic or a drug from another group that has antiarrhythmic effects (eg, a beta blocker such as propranolol, a calcium channel blocker such as verapamil or diltiazem, or digoxin). Instructions should be provided for the specific drug ordered.

(continued)

CLIENT TEACHING GUIDELINES
Antiarrhythmic Drugs (continued)

✔ Be sure you know the names (generic and brand) of the medication, why you are receiving it, and what effects you can expect (therapeutic and adverse).

✔ You will need continued medical supervision, along with periodic measurements of heart rate and blood pressure, blood tests, and electrocardiograms.

✔ Try to learn the triggers for your irregular heartbeats and avoid them when possible (eg, excessive caffeinated beverages, strenuous or excessive exercise).

✔ Avoid over-the-counter cold and asthma remedies, appetite suppressants, and antisleep preparations. These drugs are stimulants that can cause or aggravate irregular heartbeats.

Self- or Caregiver Administration

✔ Take or give medications at evenly spaced intervals to maintain adequate blood levels.

✔ Take or give amiodarone, mexiletine, quinidine, and tocainide with food to decrease gastrointestinal symptoms.

✔ Do not crush or chew sustained-release tablets or capsules.

✔ Report dizziness or fainting spells. This may mean the medication is decreasing your blood pressure, which is more likely to occur when starting or increasing the dose of an antiarrhythmic drug. Drug dosage may need to be adjusted.

Interventions

Use measures to prevent or minimize arrhythmias:

- Treat underlying disease processes that contribute to arrhythmia development. These include cardiovascular (eg, acute myocardial infarction) and noncardiovascular (eg, chronic lung disease) disorders.

- Prevent or treat other conditions that predispose to arrhythmias (eg, hypoxia, electrolyte imbalance).

Nursing Notes: Ethical/Legal Dilemma

You are working on a surgical unit, caring for Betty Kelman 1 day after her major abdominal surgery. During your assessment, you note her pulse rate is very rapid (over 150 beats/minute) with a very irregular rhythm. The resident orders an electrocardiogram that identifies a serious arrhythmia. He gives you a verbal order for lidocaine, first IV push then followed by a continuous IV infusion. You have never given this drug before and feel uncomfortable administering it to Ms. Kelman.

Reflect on:

- Identify factors in this situation that contributed to the nurse's reluctance to administer the drug.

- Does a nurse have a right to refuse to administer a medication?

- Explore the consequences of refusing to give this medication for the nurse, the patient, and the physician.

- What supports might be available in an acute care facility for the nurse in this situation?

- Help the client avoid cigarette smoking, overeating, excessive coffee drinking, and other habits that may cause or aggravate arrhythmias. Long-term supervision and counseling may be needed.

- For the client receiving antiarrhythmic drugs, implement the preceding measures to minimize the incidence and severity of acute arrhythmias, and help the client comply with drug therapy.

- Monitor heart rate and rhythm and blood pressure every 4 to 6 hours.

- Check laboratory reports of serum electrolytes and serum drug levels when available. Report abnormal values.

Evaluation

- Check vital signs for improved heart rate and rhythm.

- Interview and observe for relief of symptoms and improved functioning in activities of daily living.

- Interview and observe for hypotension and other adverse drug effects.

- Interview and observe for compliance with instructions for taking antiarrhythmic drugs and other aspects of care.

PRINCIPLES OF THERAPY

Nonpharmacologic Treatment of Arrhythmias

Nonpharmacologic treatment is preferred, at least initially, for several arrhythmias. For example, sinus tachycardia usually results from such disorders as infection, dehydration, or hypotension, and treatment should be aimed toward relieving the underlying cause. For PSVT with mild or moderate symptoms, Valsalva's maneuver, carotid sinus massage, or other measures to increase vagal tone are preferred. For ventricular fibrillation, immediate defibrillation by electrical countershock is the initial treatment of choice.

In addition to these strategies, others are being increasingly used. The impetus for nonpharmacologic treatments developed mainly from studies demonstrating that antiarrhythmic drugs could worsen existing arrhythmias, cause new arrhythmias, and cause higher mortality rates in clients receiving the drugs than clients not receiving the drugs. Current technology allows clinicians to insert pacemakers and defibrillators (eg, ICD) to control bradyarrhythmias or tachyarrhythmias and to use radio waves (radiofrequency catheter ablation) or surgery to deactivate ectopic foci.

Pharmacologic Treatment of Arrhythmias

Rational drug therapy for cardiac arrhythmias requires accurate identification of the arrhythmia, understanding of the basic mechanisms causing the arrhythmia, observation of the hemodynamic and ECG effects of the arrhythmia, knowledge of the pharmacologic actions of specific antiarrhythmic drugs, and the expectation that therapeutic effects will outweigh potential adverse effects. Even when these criteria are met, antiarrhythmic drug therapy is somewhat empiric. Although some arrhythmias usually respond to particular drugs, different drugs or combinations of drugs are often required. General trends and guidelines for drug therapy of supraventricular and ventricular arrhythmias are described in the following sections.

General Trends

1. There is a relative consensus of opinion among clinicians about appropriate treatment for acute, symptomatic arrhythmias, in which the goals are to abolish the abnormal rhythm, restore NSR, and prevent recurrence of the arrhythmia. There is less agreement about long-term use of the drugs, which is probably indicated only for clients who experience recurrent symptomatic episodes.
2. Class I agents do not prolong survival in any group of clients and their use is declining. For example, quinidine is no longer recommended to slow heart rate or prevent recurrence of AF. Some clinicians recommend restricting their use to clients without structural heart disease, who are less likely to experience increased mortality than others.
3. Class II and class III drugs are being used increasingly, because of demonstrated benefits in relieving symptoms and decreasing mortality rates in clients with heart disease.

Supraventricular Tachyarrhythmias

1. **Propranolol** and other beta blockers are being increasingly used for tachyarrhythmias, especially in clients with myocardial infarction, heart failure, or exercise-induced arrhythmias. In addition to controlling arrhythmias, the drugs decrease the mortality rate in these clients. Also, a beta blocker is the treatment of choice if a rapid heart rate is causing angina or other symptoms in a client with known coronary artery disease.
2. **Atrial fibrillation** is the most common arrhythmia. Treatment may involve conversion to NSR by electrical or pharmacologic means or long-term drug therapy to slow the rate of ventricular response. Advantages of conversion to NSR include improvement of symptoms and decreased risks of heart failure or thromboembolic problems. If pharmacologic conversion is chosen, IV **adenosine, dofetilide, ibutilide, verapamil**, or **diltiazem** may be used. Once converted to NSR, clients usually require long-term drug therapy. Low-dose **amiodarone** seems to be emerging as the drug of choice for preventing recurrent AF after electrical or pharmacologic conversion. The low doses cause fewer adverse effects than the higher ones used for life-threatening ventricular arrhythmias.

   When clients are not converted to NSR, drugs are given to slow the heart rate. This strategy is used for clients who:
   a. Have chronic AF but are asymptomatic
   b. Have had AF for longer than 1 year
   c. Are elderly
   d. Have not responded to multiple drugs

   In addition to amiodarone, other drugs used to slow the heart rate include a **beta blocker, digoxin, verapamil**, or **diltiazem.** In most clients, a beta blocker, verapamil, or diltiazem may be preferred. In clients with heart failure, digoxin may be preferred. In addition, the class IC agents **flecainide** or **propafenone** may be used to suppress paroxysmal atrial flutter and fibrillation in clients with minimal or no heart disease.
3. IV **adenosine, ibutilide, verapamil**, or **diltiazem** may be used to convert PSVT to a NSR. These drugs block conduction across the AV node.

Nursing Notes: *Apply Your Knowledge*

You are working on a telemetry unit. The monitor indicates that your patient, Mr. Sweeny, is experiencing paroxysmal supraventricular tachycardia. You have a standing order to treat this arrhythmia with a calcium channel blocker, diltiazem, 20 mg, IV push. How will you proceed to administer this medication safely?

Ventricular Arrhythmias

1. Treatment of asymptomatic PVCs and nonsustained ventricular tachycardia (formerly standard practice with lidocaine in clients post-myocardial infarction) is not recommended.
2. A **beta blocker** may be preferred as a first-line drug for symptomatic ventricular arrhythmias. **Amiodarone**, **bretylium**, **flecainide**, **propafenone**, and **sotalol** are also used in the treatment of life-threatening ventricular arrhythmias, such as sustained ventricular tachycardia. Class I agents (eg, **lidocaine**, **mexiletine**, **tocainide**) may be used in clients with structurally normal hearts. Lidocaine may also be used for treating digoxin-induced ventricular arrhythmias.
3. **Amiodarone**, **sotalol**, or **a beta blocker** may be used to prevent recurrence of ventricular tachycardia or fibrillation in clients resuscitated from cardiac arrest.
4. **Moricizine** is infrequently used in the United States but may be used to treat life-threatening ventricular arrhythmias such as sustained ventricular tachycardia.

Use in Children

Antiarrhythmic drugs are less often needed in children than in adults, and their use has decreased with increased use of catheter ablative techniques. Catheter ablation uses radio waves to destroy arrhythmia-producing foci in cardiac tissue and reportedly causes fewer adverse effects and complications than long-term antiarrhythmic drug therapy.

Antiarrhythmic drug therapy is also less clear-cut in children. The only antiarrhythmic drug that is FDA approved for use in children is digoxin. However, pediatric cardiologists have used various drugs and developed guidelines for their use, especially dosages. As with adults, the drugs should be used only when clearly indicated, and children should be monitored closely because all of the drugs can cause adverse effects, including hypotension and new or worsened arrhythmias.

Supraventricular tachyarrhythmias are the most common sustained arrhythmias in children. IV **adenosine**, **digoxin**, **procainamide**, or **propranolol** can be used acutely to terminate supraventricular tachyarrhythmias. IV verapamil, which is often used in adults to terminate supraventricular tachyarrhythmias, is contraindicated in infants and small children. Although it can be used cautiously in older children, some clinicians recommend that IV verapamil be avoided in the pediatric population. **Digoxin** or a **beta blocker** may be used for long-term treatment of supraventricular tachyarrhythmias.

Propranolol is the beta blocker most commonly used in children. It is one of the few antiarrhythmic drugs available in a liquid solution. Propranolol has a shorter half-life (3 to 4 hours) in infants than in children older than 1 to 2 years of age and adults (6 hours). When given IV, antiarrhythmic effects are rapid, and clients require careful monitoring for bradycardia and hypotension. **Esmolol** is being used more frequently to treat tachyarrhythmias in children, especially those occurring after surgery.

Lidocaine may be used to treat ventricular arrhythmias precipitated by cardiac surgery or digitalis toxicity. Class I or III drugs are usually started in a hospital setting, at lower dosage ranges, because of proarrhythmic effects. Proarrhythmia is more common in children with structural heart disease or significant arrhythmias. As a general rule, serum levels should be monitored with class IA and IC drugs and IV lidocaine. Flecainide is the class IC drug most commonly used in children. Class III drugs are used in pediatrics mainly to treat life-threatening refractory tachyarrhythmias.

As in adults, most antiarrhythmic drugs and their metabolites are excreted through the kidneys and may accumulate in clients with impaired renal function.

Use in Older Adults

Cardiac arrhythmias are common in older adults, but in general only those causing symptoms of circulatory impairment should be treated with antiarrhythmic drugs. Compared with younger adults, older adults are more likely to experience serious adverse drug effects, including aggravation of existing arrhythmias, production of new arrhythmias, hypotension, and heart failure. Cautious use is required, and dosage usually needs to be reduced to compensate for heart disease or impaired drug elimination processes.

Use in Renal Impairment

Antiarrhythmic drug therapy in clients with renal impairment should be very cautious, with close monitoring of drug effects (eg, plasma drug levels, ECG changes, symptoms that may indicate drug toxicity). Most antiarrhythmic drugs and their metabolites are excreted renally. As a result, decreased renal perfusion or other renal impairment can reduce drug elimination and lead to accumulation and adverse effects if dosage is not reduced. As a general rule, dosage of bretylium, digoxin, disopyramide, flecainide, lidocaine, moricizine, procainamide, propafenone, quinidine, sotalol, and tocainide should be reduced in clients with significant impairment of renal function. Dosage of adenosine, amiodarone, ibutilide, and mexiletine does not require reduction.

Use in Hepatic Impairment

As with renal impairment, antiarrhythmic drug therapy in clients with hepatic impairment should be very cautious, with close monitoring of drug effects (eg, plasma drug levels, ECG changes, symptoms that may indicate drug toxicity).

Amiodarone may be hepatotoxic and cause serious, sometimes fatal, liver disease. Hepatic enzyme levels are often elevated without accompanying symptoms of liver impairment. However, liver enzymes should be monitored regularly, especially in clients receiving relatively high maintenance doses. If enzyme levels are above three times the normal range or double in a client whose baseline levels were elevated, dosage reduction or drug discontinuation should be considered.

Hepatic impairment increases plasma half-life of several antiarrhythmic drugs, and dosage usually should be reduced. These include disopyramide, flecainide, lidocaine, mexiletine, moricizine, procainamide, propafenone, quinidine, and tocainide.

Dosages of adenosine and ibutilide are unlikely to need reductions in clients with hepatic impairment.

Use in Critical Illness

Critically ill clients often have multiple cardiovascular and other disorders that increase their risks for development of acute, serious, and potentially life-threatening arrhythmias. They may also have refractory arrhythmias that require strong, potentially toxic antiarrhythmic drugs. Thus, antiarrhythmic drugs are often given IV in critical care settings for rapid reversal of a fast rhythm. This may be followed by IV or oral drugs to prevent recurrence of the arrhythmia.

Because serious problems may stem from either arrhythmias or their treatment, health care providers should be adept in preventing, recognizing, and treating conditions that predispose to the development of serious arrhythmias (eg, electrolyte imbalances, hypoxia). If arrhythmias cannot be prevented, early recognition and treatment are needed.

Overall, any antiarrhythmic drug therapy in critically ill clients is preferably performed or at least initiated in critical care units or other facilities with appropriate equipment and personnel. For example, nurses who work in emergency departments or critical care units must be certified in cardiopulmonary resuscitation and advanced cardiac life support (ACLS). With ACLS, algorithms have been developed by the American Heart Association and others to guide drug therapy of arrhythmias.

 Home Care

Clients receiving chronic antiarrhythmic drug therapy are likely to have significant cardiovascular disease. With each visit, the home care nurse needs to assess the client's physical, mental, and functional status and evaluate pulse and blood pressure. In addition, clients and caregivers should be taught to report symptoms (eg, dizziness or fainting, chest pain) and avoid over-the-counter drugs unless discussed with a health care provider.

(*text continues on page 781*)

NURSING ACTIONS	Antiarrhythmic Drugs

NURSING ACTIONS	**RATIONALE/EXPLANATION**
1. **Administer accurately**	
a. Check apical and radial pulses before each dose. Withhold the dose and report to the physician if marked changes are noted in rate, rhythm, or quality of pulses.	Bradycardia may indicate impending heart block or cardiovascular collapse.
b. Check blood pressure at least once daily in hospitalized clients.	To detect hypotension. Hypotension is most likely to occur when antiarrhythmic drug therapy is being initiated or altered.
c. During intravenous (IV) administration of antiarrhythmic drugs, maintain continuous cardiac monitoring and check blood pressure about every 5 min.	For early detection of hypotension and impending cardiac collapse. These drug side effects are more likely to occur with IV use.
d. Give oral drugs at evenly spaced intervals.	To maintain adequate blood levels
e. With oral amiodarone, give once daily or in two divided doses if gastrointestinal (GI) upset occurs.	
f. With IV amiodarone, mix and give loading and maintenance infusions according to the manufacturer's instructions.	Specific instructions are required for accurate mixing and administration, partly because concentra-
	(*continued*)

NURSING ACTIONS	**RATIONALE/EXPLANATION**

tions and infusion rates vary. The drug should be given in an intensive care setting, by experienced personnel, preferably through a central venous catheter.

g. Give mexiletine, quinidine, and tocainide with food.

To decrease GI symptoms

h. Give lidocaine parenterally only, as a bolus injection or a continuous drip. Use only solutions labeled "For cardiac arrhythmias," and do *not* use solutions containing epinephrine. Give an IV bolus over 2 min.

Lidocaine solutions that contain epinephrine are used for local anesthesia only. They should *never* be given intravenously in cardiac arrhythmias because the epinephrine can cause or aggravate arrhythmias. Rapid injection (within approximately 30 sec) produces transient blood levels several times greater than therapeutic range limits. Therefore, there is increased risk of toxicity without a concomitant increase in therapeutic effectiveness.

2. Observe for therapeutic effects

a. Conversion to normal sinus rhythm

b. Improvement in rate, rhythm, and quality of apical and radial pulses and the electrocardiogram (ECG)

c. Signs of increased cardiac output—blood pressure near normal range, urine output more adequate, no complaints of dizziness.

After a single oral dose, peak plasma levels are reached in approximately 1–4 h with quinidine, procainamide, and propranolol and in 6–12 h with phenytoin. A state of equilibrium between plasma and tissue levels is reached in 1 or 2 d with quinidine, procainamide, and propranolol; in approximately 1 wk with phenytoin; in 1–3 wk with amiodarone; and in just a few minutes with IV lidocaine. Although this information may be helpful in determining when therapeutic effects are most likely to appear, remember that many other factors influence therapeutic effects, such as dose, frequency of administration, presence of conditions that alter drug metabolism, arterial blood gases, serum electrolyte levels, and myocardial status.

d. Serum drug levels within therapeutic ranges.

Serum drug levels must be interpreted in light of the client's clinical status.

Class IA
Quinidine	2–6	μg/mL
Disopyramide	2–8	μg/mL
Procainamide	4–8	μg/mL

Class IB
Lidocaine	1.5–6	μg/mL
Mexiletine	0.5–2	μg/mL
Phenytoin	10–20	μg/mL
Tocainide	4–10	μg/mL

Class IC
Flecainide	0.2–1	μg/mL
Propafenone	0.06–1	μg/mL

Class II
Propranolol	0.05–0.1	μg/mL

Class III
Amiodarone	0.5–2.5	μg/mL
Bretylium	0.5–1.5	μg/mL

Class IV
Verapamil	0.08–0.3	μg/mL

(continued)

NURSING ACTIONS	RATIONALE/EXPLANATION
3. Observe for adverse effects	
a. Heart block—may be indicated on the ECG by a prolonged PR interval, prolonged QRS complex, or absence of P waves	Owing to depressant effects on the cardiac conduction system
b. Arrhythmias—aggravation of existing arrhythmia, tachycardia, bradycardia, premature ventricular contractions, ventricular tachycardia or fibrillation	Because they affect the cardiac conduction system, antiarrhythmic drugs may worsen existing arrhythmias or cause new arrhythmias.
c. Hypotension	Owing to decreased cardiac output
d. Additional adverse effects with specific drugs:	
(1) Disopyramide—mouth dryness, blurred vision, urinary retention, other anticholinergic effects	These effects commonly occur.
(2) Lidocaine—drowsiness, paresthesias, muscle twitching, convulsions, changes in mental status (eg, confusion), hypersensitivity reactions (eg, urticaria, edema, anaphylaxis)	Most adverse reactions result from drug effects on the central nervous system (CNS). Convulsions are most likely to occur with high doses. Hypersensitivity reactions may occur in people who are allergic to related local anesthetic agents.
(3) Phenytoin—nystagmus, ataxia, slurring of speech, tremors, drowsiness, confusion, gingival hyperplasia	CNS changes are caused by depressant effects.
(4) Propranolol—weakness or dizziness, especially with activity or exercise	The beta-adrenergic blocking action of propranolol blocks the normal sympathetic nervous system response to activity and exercise. Clients may have symptoms caused by deficient blood supply to body tissues.
(5) Quinidine—hypersensitivity and cinchonism (tinnitus, vomiting, severe diarrhea, vertigo, headache)	
(6) Tocainide—lightheadedness, dizziness, nausea, paresthesia, tremor	These are the most frequent adverse effects. They may be reversed by decreasing dosage, administering with food, or discontinuing the drug.
4. Observe for drug interactions	
a. Drugs that *increase* effects of antiarrhythmics:	These drugs may potentiate therapeutic effects or increase risk of toxicity.
(1) Antiarrhythmic agents	When antiarrhythmic drugs are combined, there are additive cardiac depressant effects.
(2) Antihypertensives, diuretics, phenothiazine antipsychotic agents	Additive hypotension
(3) Cimetidine	Increases effects by inhibiting hepatic metabolism of quinidine, procainamide, lidocaine, tocainide, flecainide, and phenytoin
b. Drugs that *decrease* effects of antiarrhythmic agents:	
(1) Atropine sulfate	Atropine is used to reverse propranolol-induced bradycardia.
(2) Phenytoin, rifampin	Decrease effects by inducing drug-metabolizing enzymes in the liver and accelerating the metabolism of quinidine, disopyramide, and mexiletine

Nursing Notes: Apply Your Knowledge

Answer: Research the correct administration time and time it carefully with the second hand of your watch. It is usually given over 2 minutes. Too rapid injection can result in serious side effects. Make sure the patient is monitored during administration so that you can quickly detect severe bradycardia or heart block. Because severe hypotension can occur, monitor blood pressure before administration and at 5-minute intervals. Observe the patient for improved heart rate and rhythm.

REVIEW AND APPLICATION EXERCISES

1. Which tissues in the heart are able to generate an electrical impulse and therefore serve as a pacemaker?

2. What risk factors predispose a client to development of arrhythmias?

3. Name interventions that clients or health care providers can perform to decrease risks of arrhythmias.

4. Differentiate the hemodynamic effects of common arrhythmias.

5. What are the classes of antiarrhythmic drugs?

6. How do beta-adrenergic blocking agents act on the conduction system to slow heart rate?

7. Why are class I drugs being used less often and class II and class III drugs being used more often?

8. What are common and potentially serious adverse effects of antiarrhythmic drugs?

SELECTED REFERENCES

Advani, S.V. & Singh, B.N. (1998). Antiarrhythmic therapies. In D.L. Brown (Ed.), *Cardiac intensive care*, pp. 563–589. Philadelphia: W.B. Saunders.

Bauman, J.L. & Schoen, M.D. (1997). The arrhythmias. In J.T. DiPiro, R.L. Talbert, G.C. Yee, G.R. Matzke, B.G. Wells, & L.M. Posey (Eds.), *Pharmacotherapy: A pathophysiologic approach*, 3rd ed., pp. 323–359. Stamford, CT: Appleton & Lange.

Botteron, G.W. & Smith, J.M. (1998). Cardiac arrhythmias. In C.F. Carey, H.H. Lee, & K.F. Woeltje (Eds.), *The Washington manual of medical therapeutics*, 29th ed., pp. 130–156. Philadelphia: Lippincott Williams & Wilkins.

Brater, D.C. (1997). Clinical pharmacology of cardiovascular drugs. In W.N. Kelley (Ed.), *Textbook of internal medicine*, 3rd ed., pp. 552–569. Philadelphia: Lippincott-Raven.

Case, C.L. (1999). Diagnosis and treatment of pediatric arrhythmias. *Pediatric Clinics of North America, 46*, 347–354.

Conti, C.R. (1996). Re-examining the clinical safety and roles of calcium antagonists in cardiovascular medicine. *American Journal of Cardiology, 79*(suppl 9A), 13–18.

Davenport, J. & Morton, P.G. (1997). Identifying nonischemic causes of life-threatening arrhythmias. *American Journal of Nursing, 97*(11), 50–55.

Drug facts and comparisons. (Updated monthly). St. Louis: Facts and Comparisons.

Grant, A.O. (1999). Very new antiarrhythmic drugs. Presented at the 20th Annual Scientific Sessions of the North American Society of Pacing and Electrophysiology, May 12, 1999, Toronto, Canada. [Online: Available http://www.medscape.com/Medscape/CNO/1999/NASPE/Story.cfm?story_id=573. Accessed October 20, 1999.]

Guyton, A.C. & Hall, J.E. (1996). *Textbook of medical physiology*, 9th ed. Philadelphia: W.B. Saunders.

Hilleman, D.E. & Seyedroudbari, A. (1999). Arrhythmias: Clinical perspectives for pharmacists. *Drug Topics, 143*(4), 69–76.

Perry, J.C. (1998). Pharmacologic therapy of arrhythmias. In B.J. Deal, G.S. Wolff, & H. Gelband (Eds.), *Current concepts in diagnosis and management in infants and children*, pp. 267–305. Armonk, NY: Futura.

Porth, C.M. (Ed.). (1998). *Pathophysiology: Concepts of altered health states*, 5th ed. Philadelphia: Lippincott Williams & Wilkins.

Roden, D.M. (1996). Antiarrhythmic drugs. In J.G. Hardman, L.E. Limbird, P.B. Molinoff, & R.W. Ruddon (Eds.), *Goodman & Gilman's The pharmacological basis of therapeutics*, 9th ed., pp. 839–874. New York: McGraw-Hill.

Strimike, C.L. & Wojcik, J.M. (1998). Stopping atrial fibrillation with ibutilide. *American Journal of Nursing, 98*(1), 32–34.

53

Antianginal Drugs

Objectives

After studying this chapter, the student will be able to:

1. Describe the types, causes, and effects of angina pectoris.

2. Describe general characteristics and types of antianginal drugs.

3. Discuss nitrate antianginals in terms of indications for use, routes of administration, adverse effects, nursing process implications, and drug tolerance.

4. Differentiate between short-acting and long-acting dosage forms of nitrate antianginal drugs.

5. Discuss calcium channel blockers in terms of their effects on body tissues, clinical indications for use, common adverse effects, and nursing process implications.

6. Teach clients ways to prevent, minimize, or treat acute anginal attacks.

Mrs. Sinatro, a 56-year-old housewife, experiences chest pressure after exercise. She is the mother of six and works 30 hours a week word-processing documents for a law firm. When she is told that her chest discomfort is probably secondary to coronary artery disease, she cannot believe it. She states, "I'm just too young to have heart problems!" Mrs. Sinatro is referred to her primary care physician and given sublingual nitroglycerin tablets to use PRN for chest pain.

Reflect on:

▶ What assessment questions will you ask to determine Mrs. Sinatro's risk factors for heart disease?

▶ Evaluate Mrs. Sinatro's reaction to her new diagnosis and implications this may have for patient teaching.

▶ What lifestyle modifications would help minimize progression of coronary artery blockage?

ANGINA PECTORIS

Angina pectoris is a clinical syndrome characterized mainly by episodes of chest pain. It occurs when there is a deficit in myocardial oxygen supply (myocardial ischemia) in relation to myocardial oxygen demand. It is most often caused by atherosclerotic plaque formation in the coronary arteries. Atherosclerotic plaque narrows the lumen, decreases elasticity, and impairs dilation of coronary arteries. The result is impaired blood flow to the myocardium, especially with exercise or other factors that increase the cardiac workload and need for oxygen.

Anginal pain is usually described as constricting, squeezing, or suffocating. It is usually located in the substernal area of the chest and may radiate to the left jaw, shoulder, arm, or other areas of the chest. It is sometimes mistaken for arthritis or indigestion. It is usually brief, with a duration of 5 minutes or less. There are three main types of angina: classic angina, variant angina, and unstable angina (Box 53-1). The Canadian Cardiovascular Society classifies clients with angina according to the amount of physical activity they can tolerate before anginal pain occurs (Box 53-2). These categories can assist in clinical assessment and evaluation of therapy.

BOX 53-1 TYPES OF ANGINA PECTORIS

Classic

Classic angina (also called stable, typical, or exertional angina) occurs when atherosclerotic plaque obstructs coronary arteries and the heart requires more oxygenated blood than the blocked arteries can deliver. Chest pain is usually precipitated by situations that increase the workload of the heart, such as physical exertion, exposure to cold, and emotional upset. Recurrent episodes of classic angina usually have the same pattern of onset, duration, and intensity of symptoms. Pain is usually relieved by rest or a fast-acting preparation of nitroglycerin.

Variant

Variant angina (also called atypical, Prinzmetal's, or vasospastic angina) is caused by spasms of the coronary artery that are strong enough to decrease blood flow to the myocardium. The spasms occur most often in coronary arteries that are already partly blocked by atherosclerotic plaque. Variant angina usually occurs during rest or with minimal exercise and often occurs at night. It often occurs at the same time each day. Pain is usually relieved by nitroglycerin. Long-term management includes avoidance of conditions that precipitate vasospasm, when possible (eg, exposure to cold, smoking, and emotional stress), as well as antianginal drugs.

Unstable

Unstable angina (also called rest, preinfarction, and crescendo angina) is a type of myocardial ischemia that falls between classic angina and myocardial infarction. It usually occurs in clients with advanced coronary atherosclerosis and produces increased frequency, intensity, and duration of symptoms. It often leads to myocardial infarction.

Unstable angina usually develops when a minor injury ruptures atherosclerotic plaque. The resulting injury to the endothelium causes platelets to aggregate at the site of injury, form a thrombus, and release chemical mediators that cause vasoconstriction (eg, thromboxane, serotonin, platelet-derived growth factor). The disrupted plaque, thrombus, and vasoconstriction combine to obstruct blood flow further in the affected coronary artery. When the plaque injury is mild, blockage of the coronary artery may be intermittent and cause silent myocardial ischemia or episodes of anginal pain at rest. Thrombus formation and vasoconstriction may progress until the coronary artery is completely occluded, producing myocardial infarction. Endothelial injury, with subsequent thrombus formation and vasoconstriction, may also result from therapeutic procedures (eg, balloon angioplasty, atherectomy).

The Agency for Healthcare Research and Quality (formerly the Agency for Health Care Policy and Research), in its clinical practice guidelines for the management of angina, defines unstable angina as meeting one or more of the following criteria:

- Anginal pain at rest that usually lasts longer than 20 minutes
- Recent onset (<2 months) of exertional angina of at least Canadian Cardiovascular Society Classification (CCSC) class III severity
- Recent (<2 months) increase in severity as indicated by progression to at least CCSC class III.

However, myocardial ischemia may also be painless or silent in a substantial number of patients. Overall, the diagnosis is usually based on chest pain history, electrocardiographic evidence of ischemia, and other signs of impaired cardiac function (eg, heart failure).

Because unstable angina often occurs hours or days before acute myocardial infarction, early recognition and effective treatment are extremely important in preventing progression to infarction, heart failure, or sudden cardiac death.

BOX 53–2   **CANADIAN CARDIOVASCULAR SOCIETY CLASSIFICATION OF PATIENTS WITH ANGINA PECTORIS**

Class I: Ordinary physical activity (eg, walking, climbing stairs) does not cause angina. Angina occurs with strenuous, rapid, or prolonged exertion at work or recreation.

Class II: Slight limitation of ordinary activity. Angina occurs on walking or climbing stairs rapidly, walking uphill, walking or stair climbing after meals, or in cold, in wind, or under emotional stress. Walking more than two blocks on the level and climbing more than one flight of ordinary stairs at a normal pace and in normal conditions can elicit angina.

Class III: Marked limitations of ordinary physical activity. Angina occurs on walking one or two blocks on the level and climbing one flight of stairs in normal conditions and at a normal pace.

Class IV: Inability to carry on any physical activity without discomfort—anginal symptoms may be present at rest.

Numerous overlapping factors (eg, myocardial ischemia, coronary atherosclerosis, other cardiovascular impairments) contribute to the development and progression of angina. To aid understanding of drug therapy for angina, these factors are described in the following sections.

Myocardial Ischemia

Myocardial ischemia occurs when the coronary arteries are unable to provide sufficient blood and oxygen for normal cardiac functions. It is also called ischemic heart disease, coronary artery disease (CAD), and coronary heart disease. There are three main consequences of myocardial ischemia. One is angina pectoris, with the occurrence of pain (symptomatic myocardial ischemia). A second is silent or asymptomatic ischemia (without chest pain), which is demonstrated by ischemic changes on electrocardiograms (ECGs) or cardiac monitoring. A third is myocardial infarction, which occurs when the ischemia is persistent or severe. Both symptomatic and silent myocardial ischemia are important indicators of active CAD and increased risk of myocardial infarction or sudden cardiovascular death.

Myocardial ischemia is most often caused by atherosclerotic plaque in the coronary arteries, which narrows the lumen, decreases elasticity, and impairs dilation. The result is impaired blood flow to the myocardium, especially with exercise, mental stress, exposure to cold, or other factors that increase the cardiac workload. Most people (≥90%) with myocardial ischemia have advanced coronary atherosclerosis. Hypertension is also a major risk factor for myocardial ischemia.

Coronary Atherosclerosis

Atherosclerosis (see Chap. 58) begins with accumulation of lipid-filled macrophages (ie, foam cells) on the inner lining of coronary arteries. Foam cells, which promote growth of atherosclerotic plaque, develop in response to elevated blood cholesterol levels. Initially, white blood cells (monocytes) become attached to the endothelium and move through the endothelial layer into subendothelial spaces, where they ingest lipid and become foam cells. These early lesions progress to fibrous plaques containing foam cells covered by smooth muscle cells and connective tissue. Advanced lesions also contain hemorrhages, ulcerations, and scar tissue.

Factors contributing to plaque development and growth include endothelial injury, lipid infiltration (ie, cholesterol), recruitment of inflammatory cells (mainly monocytes and T lymphocytes), and smooth muscle cell proliferation. Endothelial injury may be the initiating factor in plaque formation because it allows monocytes, platelets, cholesterol, and other blood components to come in contact with and stimulate abnormal growth of smooth muscle cells and connective tissue in the arterial wall.

Atherosclerosis commonly develops in the coronary arteries. As the plaque lesions develop over time, they become larger and extend farther into the lumen of the artery. The lesions may develop for decades before they produce symptoms of reduced blood flow. Eventually, such events as plaque rupture, mural hemorrhage, formation of a thrombus that partly or completely occludes an artery, and vasoconstriction precipitate myocardial ischemia. Thus, serious impairment of blood flow may occur with a large atherosclerotic plaque or a relatively small plaque with superimposed vasospasm and thrombosis. If stenosis blocks approximately 80% of the artery, blood flow cannot increase in response to increased need; if stenosis blocks approximately 90% or more of the artery, blood flow is impaired when the client is at rest.

When coronary atherosclerosis develops slowly, collateral circulation develops to increase blood supply to the heart. Collateral circulation develops from anastomotic channels that connect the coronary arteries and allow perfusion of an area by more than one artery. When one artery becomes blocked, the anastomotic channels become larger and allow blood from an unblocked artery to perfuse the area normally supplied by the occluded artery. Endothelium-derived relaxing factors such as nitric oxide (NO) can dilate collateral vessels and facilitate regional myocardial blood flow. Although collateral circulation may prevent myocardial ischemia in the client at rest, it has limited ability to increase myocardial perfusion with increased cardiac workload.

Cardiovascular Impairments

1. With normal cardiac function, coronary blood flow can increase to meet needs for an increased oxygen supply with exercise or other conditions that increase cardiac workload. When coronary arteries are partly blocked by atherosclerotic plaque, vasospasm, or thrombi, blood flow may not be able to increase sufficiently.
2. The endothelium of normal coronary arteries synthesizes numerous substances (see Chap. 50) that protect against vasoconstriction and vasospasm, bleeding and clotting, inflammation, and excessive cell growth. Impaired endothelium (eg, by rupture of atherosclerotic plaque or the shear force of hypertension) leads to vasoconstriction, vasospasm, clot formation, formation of atherosclerotic plaque, and growth of smooth muscle cells in blood vessel walls.

   One important substance produced by the endothelium of coronary arteries is nitric oxide (also called endothelium-derived relaxing factor). Nitric oxide, which is synthesized from the amino acid arginine, is released by shear stress on the endothelium, sympathetic stimulation of exercise, and interactions with acetylcholine, histamine, prostacyclin, serotonin, thrombin, and other chemical mediators. Nitric oxide relaxes vascular smooth muscle and inhibits adhesion and aggregation of platelets. When the endothelium is damaged, these vasodilating and antithrombotic effects are lost. At the same time, production of strong vasoconstrictors (eg, angiotensin II, endothelin-1, thromboxane A_2) is increased. In addition, inflammatory cells enter the injured area and growth factors stimulate growth of smooth muscle cells. All of these factors participate in blocking coronary arteries.
3. Sympathetic nervous system stimulation normally produces dilation of coronary arteries, tachycardia, and increased myocardial contractility to handle an increased need for oxygenated blood. Atherosclerosis of coronary arteries, especially if severe, may cause vasoconstriction as well as decrease blood flow by obstruction.

Nonpharmacologic Management of Angina

For clients with CAD at any stage of development and with or without symptoms of myocardial ischemia, optimal

management involves lifestyle changes and medications, if necessary, to control or reverse risk factors for disease progression. Risk factors that can be altered include smoking, hypertension, hyperlipidemia, obesity, sedentary lifestyle, stress, and the use of drugs that increase cardiac workload (eg, adrenergics, corticosteroids). Thus, efforts are needed to assist clients in reducing blood pressure, weight, and serum cholesterol levels, when indicated, and developing an exercise program.

In addition, clients should avoid circumstances known to precipitate acute attacks, and those who smoke should stop. Smoking is harmful to clients because:

- Nicotine increases heart rate and blood pressure.
- Carbon monoxide inhaled in smoke, which forms carboxyhemoglobin, decreases delivery of blood and oxygen to the heart, decreases myocardial contractility, and increases the risks of life-threatening cardiac arrhythmias (eg, ventricular fibrillation) during ischemic episodes.
- Both nicotine and carbon monoxide increase platelet adhesiveness and aggregation, thereby promoting thrombosis.
- Smoking increases the risks for myocardial infarction, sudden cardiac death, cerebrovascular disease (eg, stroke), peripheral vascular disease (eg, arterial insufficiency), and hypertension. It also reduces high-density lipoprotein, the "good" cholesterol.

Additional nonpharmacologic treatment includes surgical revascularization (eg, coronary artery bypass graft). However, most clients must still take antianginal and other cardiovascular medications.

ANTIANGINAL DRUGS

Drugs used in angina pectoris are the organic nitrates, the beta-adrenergic blocking agents, and the calcium channel blocking agents. These drugs relieve anginal pain by decreasing myocardial demand for oxygen or increasing blood supply to the myocardium. Nitrates and beta blockers are described in the following sections and dosage ranges are listed in Table 53-1. Calcium channel blockers are described in a following section; indications for use and dosage ranges are listed in Table 53-2.

Organic Nitrates

Organic nitrates relax smooth muscle in blood vessel walls. This action produces vasodilation, which relieves anginal pain by several mechanisms. First, dilation of veins reduces venous pressure and venous return to the heart. This decreases blood volume and pressure within the heart (preload), which in turn decreases cardiac workload and oxygen demand. Second, nitrates dilate coronary arteries and can increase blood flow to ischemic areas of the

TABLE 53-1	Nitrate and Beta-Blocker Antianginal Drugs	
Generic/Trade Name	**Indications for Use**	**Routes and Dosage Ranges**
Nitrates		
Nitroglycerin (Nitro-Bid, others)	Relieve acute angina Prevent exercise-induced angina Long-term prophylaxis to decrease the frequency and severity of acute anginal episodes	PO Immediate-release tablets, 2.5–9 mg two or three times per day PO Sustained-release tablets or capsules, 2.5 mg three or four times per day SL 0.15–0.6 mg PRN for chest pain Translingual spray, one or two metered doses (0.4 mg/dose) sprayed onto oral mucosa at onset of anginal pain, to a maximum of three doses in 15 min Transmucosal tablet, 1 mg q3–5h while awake, placed between upper lip and gum or cheek and gum Topical ointment, ½–2 inches q4–8h; do not rub in Topical transdermal disc, applied once daily IV 5–10 μg/min initially, increased in 10- to 20-μg/min increments up to 100 μg/min or more if necessary to relieve pain
Isosorbide dinitrate (Isordil, Sorbitrate)	Treatment and prevention of angina	SL 2.5–10 mg PRN or q2–4h PO Regular tablets, 10–60 mg q4–6h PO Chewable tablets, 5–10 mg q2–3h PO Sustained-release capsules, 40 mg q6–12h
Isosorbide mononitrate (Ismo, Imdur)	Treatment and prevention of angina	PO 20 mg twice daily, with first dose on arising and the second dose 7 h later PO Extended-release tablets (Imdur), 30–60 mg once daily in the morning, increased after several days to 120 mg once daily if necessary
Beta Blockers		
Propranolol (Inderal)	Long-term management of angina, to reduce frequency and severity of anginal episodes	PO 10–80 mg two to four times per day IV 0.5–3 mg q4h until desired response is obtained
Atenolol (Tenormin)	Same as propranolol	PO 50 mg once daily, initially, increased to 100 mg/d after 1 wk if necessary
Metoprolol (Lopressor)	Same as propranolol	PO 50 mg twice daily initially, increased up to 400 mg daily if necessary
Nadolol (Corgard)	Same as propranolol	PO 40–240 mg/d in a single dose

IV, intravenous; PO, oral; PRN, as needed; SL, sublingual.

myocardium. Third, nitrates dilate arterioles, which lowers peripheral vascular resistance (afterload). This results in lower systolic blood pressure and, consequently, reduced cardiac workload. The prototype and most widely used nitrate is nitroglycerin.

Nitrates are converted to NO in vascular smooth muscle. Nitric oxide activates guanylate cyclase, an enzyme that catalyzes formation of cyclic guanine monophosphate, which decreases calcium levels in vascular smooth muscle cells. Because intracellular calcium is required for contraction of vascular smooth muscle, the result of decreased calcium is vasodilation. The NO derived from nitrate medications can be considered a replacement or substitute for the NO that a damaged endothelium can no longer produce.

Clinical indications for nitroglycerin and other nitrates are treatment and prevention of acute chest pain caused by myocardial ischemia. For acute angina and prophylaxis before a situation deemed likely to precipitate acute angina, fast-acting preparations (sublingual or chewable tablets, transmucosal spray or tablet) are used. For management of recurrent angina, long-acting preparations (oral and sustained-release tablets or transdermal ointment and discs) are used. Intravenous (IV) nitroglycerin is used to treat angina that is unresponsive to organic nitrates or beta-adrenergic blocking agents. It also may be used to control blood pressure in perioperative or emergency situations and to reduce preload and afterload in severe congestive heart failure.

Contraindications include hypersensitivity reactions, severe anemia, hypotension, and hypovolemia. The drugs should be used cautiously in the presence of head injury or cerebral hemorrhage because they may increase intracranial pressure.

Individual Nitrates

Nitroglycerin (Nitro-Bid, others), the prototype drug, is used to relieve acute angina pectoris, prevent exercise-induced angina, and decrease the frequency and severity

TABLE 53-2	Calcium Channel Blockers	
Generic/Trade Name	**Indications**	**Routes and Dosage Ranges**
Amlodipine (Norvasc)	Angina Hypertension	PO 5–10 mg once daily
Bepridil (Vascor)	Angina	PO 200 mg/d initially, increased to 300 mg daily after 10 d if necessary; maximum dose, 400 mg daily
Diltiazem (Cardizem)	Angina Hypertension Atrial fibrillation and flutter PSVT	Angina or hypertension, immediate-release, PO 60–90 mg four times daily before meals and at bedtime Hypertension, sustained-release only, PO 120–180 mg twice daily Arrhythmias (Cardizem IV only) IV injection 0.25 mg/kg (average dose 20 mg) over 2 min with a second dose of 0.35 mg/kg (average dose 25 mg) in 15 min if necessary, followed by IV infusion of 5–15 mg/h up to 24 h
Felodipine (Plendil)	Hypertension	PO 5–10 mg once daily
Isradipine (DynaCirc)	Hypertension	PO 2.5–5 mg twice daily
Nicardipine (Cardene)	Angina Hypertension	Angina, immediate-release only, PO 20–40 mg three times daily Hypertension, immediate-release, same as for angina, above; sustained-release, PO 30–60 mg twice daily
Nifedipine (Adalat, Procardia)	Angina Hypertension	Angina, immediate-release, PO 10–30 mg three times daily; sustained-release, PO 30–60 mg once daily Hypertension, sustained-release only, 30–60 mg once daily
Nimodipine (Nimotop)	Subarachnoid hemorrhage	PO 60 mg q4h for 21 consecutive d. If patient unable to swallow, aspirate contents of capsule into a syringe with an 18-gauge needle, administer by nasogastric tube, and follow with 30 mL normal saline.
Nisoldipine (Sular)	Hypertension	PO, initially 20 mg once daily, increased by 10 mg/wk or longer intervals to a maximum of 60 mg daily. Average maintenance dose, 20–40 mg daily. Adults with liver impairment or >65 y, PO, initially 10 mg once daily
Verapamil (Calan, Isoptin)	Angina Atrial fibrillation or flutter PSVT Hypertension	Angina, PO 80–120 mg three times daily Arrhythmias, PO 80–120 mg three to four times daily; IV injection, 5–10 mg over 2 min or longer, with continuous monitoring of electrocardiogram and blood pressure Hypertension, PO 80 mg three times daily or 240 mg (sustained release) once daily

IV, intravenous; PO, oral; PSVT, paroxysmal supraventricular tachycardia.

of acute anginal episodes. Oral dosage forms are rapidly metabolized in the liver, and relatively small proportions of doses reach the systemic circulation. In addition, oral doses act slowly and do not help relieve acute chest pain.

For these reasons, several alternative dosage forms have been developed, including transmucosal tablets and sprays administered sublingually or buccally, transdermal ointments and adhesive discs applied to the skin, and an IV preparation. When given sublingually, nitroglycerin is absorbed directly into the systemic circulation. It acts within 1 to 3 minutes and lasts approximately 30 to 60 minutes. When applied topically to the skin, nitroglycerin is also absorbed directly into the systemic circulation. However, absorption occurs at a slower rate, and topical nitroglycerin has a longer duration of action than other forms. It is available in an ointment, which is effective for 4 to 8 hours, and a transdermal disc, which is effective for approximately 12 hours. An IV form of nitroglycerin is used to relieve acute anginal pain that does not respond to other agents.

Isosorbide dinitrate (Isordil, Sorbitrate) is used to reduce the frequency and severity of acute anginal episodes. When given sublingually or in chewable tablets, it acts in approximately 2 minutes, and its effects last approximately 2 to 3 hours. When higher doses are given orally, more drug escapes metabolism in the liver and produces systemic effects in approximately 30 minutes. Therapeutic effects last approximately 4 hours after oral administration. The effective oral dose is usually determined by increasing the dose until headache occurs, indicating the maximum tolerable dose. Sustained-release capsules also are available.

Isosorbide mononitrate (Ismo, Imdur) is the metabolite and active component of isosorbide dinitrate. It is well absorbed after oral administration and almost 100% bioavailable. Unlike other oral nitrates, this drug is not subject to first-pass hepatic metabolism. Onset of action occurs within 1 hour, peak effects occur between 1 and 4 hours, and the elimination half-life is approximately 5 hours. It is used only for prophylaxis of angina; it does not act rapidly enough to relieve acute attacks.

Beta-Adrenergic Blocking Agents

Beta-adrenergic blocking agents, of which propranolol is the prototype, are often prescribed in a variety of clinical conditions. Their actions, uses, and adverse effects are discussed in Chapter 19. In this chapter, the drugs are discussed only in relation to their use in angina pectoris.

Sympathetic stimulation of beta receptors in the heart increases heart rate and force of myocardial contraction, both of which increase myocardial oxygen demand and may precipitate acute anginal attacks. Beta-blocking drugs prevent or inhibit sympathetic stimulation. Thus, the drugs reduce heart rate and myocardial contractility, particularly when sympathetic output is increased during exercise. A slower heart rate may improve coronary blood flow to the ischemic area. Beta blockers also reduce blood pressure, which in turn decreases myocardial workload and oxygen demand. In angina pectoris, beta-adrenergic blocking agents are used in long-term management to decrease the frequency and severity of anginal attacks, decrease the need for sublingual nitroglycerin, and increase exercise tolerance. When a beta blocker is being discontinued after prolonged use, it should be tapered in dosage and gradually discontinued. If this is not done, rebound angina can occur.

These drugs should not be given to clients with known or suspected coronary artery spasms because they may intensify the frequency and severity of vasospasm. This probably results from unopposed stimulation of alpha-adrenergic receptors, which causes vasoconstriction, when beta-adrenergic receptors are blocked by the drugs.

Propranolol, the prototype beta blocker, is used to reduce the frequency and severity of acute attacks of angina. It is usually added to the antianginal drug regimen when nitrates do not prevent anginal episodes. It is especially useful in preventing exercise-induced tachycardia, which can precipitate anginal attacks.

Propranolol is well absorbed after oral administration. It is then metabolized extensively in the liver; a relatively small proportion of an oral dose (approximately 30%) reaches the systemic circulation. For this reason, oral doses of propranolol are much higher than IV doses. Onset of action is 30 minutes after oral administration and 1 to 2 minutes after IV injection. Because of variations in the degree of hepatic metabolism, clients vary widely in the dosages required to maintain a therapeutic response.

Atenolol, **metoprolol**, and **nadolol** have the same actions, uses, and adverse effects as propranolol, but they have long half-lives and can be given once daily. They are excreted by the kidneys, and dosage must be reduced in clients with renal impairment.

Calcium Channel Blocking Agents

Calcium channel blockers act on contractile and conductive tissues of the heart and on vascular smooth muscle. For these cells to function normally, the concentration of intracellular calcium must be increased. This is usually accomplished by movement of extracellular calcium ions into the cell (through calcium channels in the cell membrane) and release of bound calcium from the sarcoplasmic reticulum in the cell. Thus, calcium plays an important role in maintaining vasomotor tone, myocardial contractility, and conduction. Calcium channel blocking agents prevent the movement of extracellular calcium into the cell. As a result, coronary and peripheral arteries are dilated, myocardial contractility is decreased, and the conduction system is depressed in relation to impulse formation (automaticity) and conduction velocity (Fig. 53-1).

In angina pectoris, the drugs improve the blood supply to the myocardium by dilating coronary arteries and decrease the workload of the heart by dilating peripheral arteries. In atrial fibrillation or flutter and other supraventricular tachyarrhythmias, diltiazem and verapamil slow the rate of ventricular response. In hypertension, the

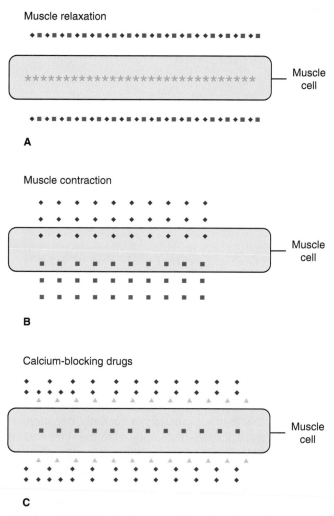

FIGURE 53–1 Calcium channel blockers: mechanism of action. (**A**) During muscle relaxation, potassium ions are inside the muscle cell and calcium and sodium ions are outside the muscle cell. (**B**) For muscle contraction to occur, potassium ions leave the cell and sodium and calcium ions enter the cell through open channels in the cell membrane. (**C**) When calcium channels are blocked by drug molecules, muscle contraction is decreased because calcium ions cannot move through the cell membrane into the muscle cell. (Calcium ions = ◆; sodium ions = ■; potassium ions = *; calcium channel blocking drugs = ▲.)

drugs lower blood pressure primarily by dilating peripheral arteries.

Calcium channel blockers are well absorbed after oral administration but undergo extensive first-pass metabolism in the liver. Most of the drugs are more than 90% protein bound and reach peak plasma levels within 1 to 2 hours (≥6 hours for sustained-release forms). Most also have short elimination half-lives (<5 hours), so doses must be given three or four times daily unless sustained-release formulations are used. Amlodipine (30 to 50 hours), bepridil (24 hours), and felodipine (11 to 16 hours) have long elimination half-lives and therefore can be given once daily. The drugs are metabolized in the liver, and dosage should be reduced in clients with severe liver disease. Dosage reductions are not required with renal disease.

The calcium channel blockers approved for use in the United States vary in their chemical structures and effects on body tissues. Seven of these are chemically dihydropyridines, of which nifedipine is the prototype. Bepridil, diltiazem, and verapamil differ chemically from the dihydropyridines and each other. Nifedipine and related drugs act mainly on vascular smooth muscle to produce vasodilation, whereas verapamil and diltiazem have greater effects on the cardiac conduction system.

The drugs also vary in clinical indications for use; most are used for angina or hypertension, and only diltiazem and verapamil are used to treat supraventricular tachyarrhythmias. In addition, nimodipine is approved for use only in subarachnoid hemorrhage to decrease spasm in cerebral blood vessels and thereby limit the extent of brain damage. In animal studies, nimodipine exerted greater effects on cerebral arteries than on other arteries, probably because it is highly lipid soluble and penetrates the blood–brain barrier.

Contraindications include second- or third-degree heart block, cardiogenic shock, and severe bradycardia, congestive heart failure, or hypotension. The drugs should be used cautiously with milder bradycardia, congestive heart failure, or hypotension and with renal or hepatic impairment.

Adjunctive Antianginal Drugs

In addition to antianginal drugs, several other drugs may be used to control risk factors and prevent progression of myocardial ischemia to myocardial infarction and sudden cardiac death. These may include:

- **Aspirin.** This drug has become the standard of care because of its antiplatelet (ie, antithrombotic) effects. Recommended doses vary from 81 mg daily to 325 mg daily or every other day; apparently all are beneficial.
- **Antilipemics.** These drugs (see Chap. 58) may be needed by clients who are unable to lower serum cholesterol levels sufficiently with a low-fat diet. Lovastatin or a related "statin" is often used. The goal is usually to reduce serum cholesterol to below 200 mg/dL and low-density lipoprotein cholesterol to below 130 mg/dL.
- **Antihypertensives.** These drugs (see Chap. 55) may be needed for clients with hypertension. Because beta blockers and calcium channel blockers are used to treat hypertension as well as angina, one of these drugs may be effective for both disorders.

NURSING PROCESS

Assessment

Assess the client's condition in relation to angina pectoris. Specific assessment data vary with each client but usually should include the following:

- During the initial nursing history interview, try to answer the following questions:
  - How long has the client been taking antianginal drugs? For what purpose are they being taken (prophylaxis, treatment of acute attacks, or both)?
  - What is the frequency and duration of acute anginal attacks? Has either increased recently? (An increase could indicate worsening coronary atherosclerosis and increased risk of myocardial infarction.)
  - Do symptoms other than chest pain occur during acute attacks (eg, sweating, nausea)?
  - Are there particular activities or circumstances that provoke acute attacks? Do attacks ever occur when the client is at rest? Where does the client fit in the Canadian classification system?
  - What relieves symptoms of acute angina?
  - If the client takes nitroglycerin, ask how often it is required, how many tablets are needed for relief of pain, how often the supply is replaced, and where the client stores or carries the drug.
- Assess blood pressure and pulse, ECG reports, serum cholesterol, and cardiac enzyme reports. Elevated cholesterol is a significant risk factor for coronary atherosclerosis and angina and the risk is directly related to the degree of elevation. Cardiac enzyme levels, such as creatine phosphokinase (CPK), lactate dehydrogenase (LDH), and aspartate aminotransferase (AST), should all be normal in clients with angina.
- During an acute attack, assess the following:
  - Location and quality of the pain. Chest pain is nonspecific. It may be a symptom of numerous disorders, such as pulmonary embolism, esophageal spasm or inflammation (heartburn), costochondritis, or anxiety. Chest pain of cardiac origin is caused by myocardial ischemia and may indicate angina pectoris or myocardial infarction.
  - Precipitating factors. For example, what was the client doing, thinking, or feeling just before the onset of chest pain?

○ Has the client had invasive procedures to diagnose or treat his CAD (eg, cardiac catheterization, angioplasty, revascularization surgery)?

Nursing Diagnoses

- Decreased Cardiac Output related to disease process or drug therapy
- Altered Tissue Perfusion: Cerebral and peripheral, related to drug-induced hypotension
- Pain in chest related to inadequate perfusion of the myocardium
- Pain (headache) related to vasodilating effects of nitrate antianginal drugs
- Activity Intolerance related to chest pain
- Risk for Injury related to hypotension and syncope from antianginal drugs
- Noncompliance related to drug therapy and lifestyle changes
- Impaired Tissue Integrity related to skin irritation from topical nitroglycerin preparations
- Constipation related to drug therapy with calcium channel blockers
- Knowledge Deficit related to management of disease process and drug therapy
- Ineffective Individual Coping related to chronic disease process
- Social Isolation related to activity intolerance
- Body Image Disturbance related to inability to perform usual activities of daily living
- Sexual Dysfunction related to fear of precipitating chest pain

Planning/Goals

The client will:

- Receive or take antianginal drugs accurately
- Experience relief of acute chest pain
- Have fewer episodes of acute chest pain
- Have increased activity tolerance
- Identify and avoid or learn to manage situations that precipitate anginal attacks
- Be closely monitored for therapeutic and adverse effects, especially when drug therapy is started
- Avoid preventable adverse effects
- Verbalize essential information about the disease process, needed dietary and lifestyle changes to improve health status, and drug therapy
- Keep appointments for follow-up care and monitoring

Interventions

Use the following measures to prevent acute anginal attacks:

- Assist in preventing, recognizing, and treating contributory disorders, such as atherosclerosis, hypertension, hyperthyroidism, hypoxia, and anemia. For example, hypertension is a common risk factor for CAD and morbidity and mortality increase progressively with the degree of either systolic or diastolic elevation. Treatment of hypertension reduces morbidity and mortality rates. However, most studies indicate that the reductions stem more from fewer strokes, less renal failure, and less heart failure, than from less CAD.
- Help the client recognize and avoid precipitating factors (eg, heavy meals, strenuous exercise) when possible. If anxiety is a factor, relaxation techniques or psychological counseling may be helpful.
- Help the client to develop a more healthful lifestyle in terms of diet and weight control, adequate rest and sleep, regular exercise, and not smoking. Ideally, these self-help interventions are practiced before illness occurs and they can help prevent or delay illness. However, most people are unmotivated until illness develops, and perhaps after it develops as well. These interventions are beneficial at any stage of CAD. For example, for a client who already has angina, a supervised exercise program helps to develop collateral circulation. Smoking has numerous ill effects on the client with angina and decreases effectiveness of antianginal drugs.

During an acute anginal attack in a client known to have angina or CAD:

- Assume that any chest pain may be of cardiac origin.
- Have the client lie down or sit down to reduce cardiac workload and provide rest.
- Check vital signs and compare them with baseline values.
- Record characteristics of chest pain and the presence of other signs and symptoms.
- Have the client take a fast-acting nitroglycerin preparation (previously prescribed), up to three sublingual tablets or three oral sprays within 15 minutes, if necessary.
- If chest pain is not relieved with rest and nitroglycerin, assume that a myocardial infarction has occurred until proven otherwise. Keep the client at rest and notify the physician immediately.
- Leave sublingual nitroglycerin at the bedside of hospitalized clients. The tablets or spray should be within reach so they can be used immediately. Record the number of tablets used daily, and ensure an adequate supply is available.

Evaluation

- Observe and interview for relief of acute chest pain.
- Observe and interview regarding the number of episodes of acute chest pain.
- Interview regarding diet, weight, and lifestyle factors that relate to angina.
- Interview regarding compliance with drug therapy.

CLIENT TEACHING GUIDELINES
Antianginal Drugs

General Considerations

✔ Angina is chest pain that occurs because your heart is not getting enough blood and oxygen. The most common causes are hypertension and atherosclerosis of the coronary arteries. The chest pain usually lasts less than 5 minutes and episodes can be managed for years without causing permanent heart damage. If it is severe or prolonged, however, it may result in a heart attack and heart damage. You need to seek information about your heart condition to prevent or decrease episodes of angina and prevent a heart attack.

✔ Several types of drugs are used in angina, and you may need a combination of drugs for the best effects. Most clients take one or more long-acting drugs to prevent anginal attacks and a fast, short-acting drug (usually nitroglycerin tablets that you dissolve under your tongue, or a nitroglycerin solution that you spray into your mouth) to relieve acute attacks. You should seek medical or emergency care immediately if your chest pain is not relieved by rest and three sublingual tablets or oral sprays 5 minutes apart. The long-acting medications are not effective in relieving sudden anginal pain.

✔ As with any medications for serious or potentially serious conditions, it is extremely important to take antianginal medications as prescribed. Do not increase dosage or discontinue the drugs without specific instructions from the physician.

✔ With sublingual nitroglycerin tablets, keep them in the original container, carry them so that they are always within reach but not where they are exposed to body heat, and replace them approximately every 6 months because they become ineffective.

✔ It may be helpful to record the number and severity of anginal episodes, the number of nitroglycerin tablets required to relieve the attack, and the total number of tablets taken daily. Such a record can help your physician know when to change your medications or your dosages.

✔ Headache and dizziness may occur with nitrate antianginal drugs, especially sublingual nitroglycerin. These effects are usually temporary and dissipate with continued therapy. If dizziness occurs, avoid strenuous activity and stand up slowly for approximately an hour after taking the drugs. If headache is severe, you may take aspirin or acetaminophen with the nitrate drug. Do not reduce drug dosage or take the drug less often to avoid headache. Loss of effectiveness may occur.

✔ Keep family members or support people informed about the location and use of antianginal medications in case help is needed.

✔ Avoid over-the-counter decongestants, cold remedies, and diet pills, which stimulate the heart and constrict blood vessels and thus may cause angina.

✔ With nitrate antianginal drugs, avoid alcohol. Both the drugs and alcohol dilate blood vessels and an excessive reduction in blood pressure (with dizziness and fainting) may occur with the combination.

✔ Several calcium channel blockers are available in both immediate-acting and long-acting (sustained-release) forms. The brand names often differ very little (eg, Procardia is a brand name of immediate-release nifedipine; Procardia XL is a long-acting formulation). It is extremely important that the correct formulation is used consistently.

Self- or Caregiver Administration

✔ Take or give as instructed; specific instructions differ with the type of antianginal drug being taken.

✔ Take or give antianginal drugs on a regular schedule, at evenly spaced intervals. This increases drug effectiveness in preventing acute attacks of angina.

✔ With nitroglycerin and other nitrate preparations:
  ✔ Use according to instructions for the particular dosage form. The dosage forms were developed for specific routes of administration and are not interchangeable.
  ✔ For sublingual nitroglycerin tablets, place them under the tongue until they dissolve. Take at the first sign of an anginal attack, before severe pain develops. If chest pain is not relieved in 5 minutes, dissolve a second tablet under the tongue. If pain is not relieved within another 5 minutes, dissolve a third tablet. If pain continues or becomes more severe, notify your physician immediately or report to the nearest hospital emergency room. Sit down when you take the medications. This may help to relieve your pain and prevent dizziness from the drug.
  ✔ For the translingual solution of nitroglycerin, spray onto or under the tongue; do not inhale the spray.
  ✔ For transmucosal tablets of nitroglycerin, place them under the upper lip or between the cheek and gum and allow them to dissolve slowly over 3 to 5 hours. Do not chew or swallow the tablets.
  ✔ Take oral nitrates on an empty stomach with a glass of water. Oral isosorbide dinitrate is available in regular and chewable tablets; be sure each type is taken appropriately. Do not crush or chew sustained-release nitroglycerin tablets.
  ✔ For sublingual isosorbide dinitrate tablets, place them under the tongue until they dissolve.
  ✔ If an oral nitrate and topical nitroglycerin are being used concurrently, stagger the times of administration. This minimizes dizziness from low blood pressure and headache, which are common adverse effects of nitrate drugs.
  ✔ For nitroglycerin ointment, use the special paper to measure the dose. Place the ointment on a nonhairy

(continued)

CLIENT TEACHING GUIDELINES
Antianginal Drugs (continued)

part of the body and apply with the applicator paper. Cover the area with plastic wrap or tape. Rotate application sites. The measured paper must be used for accurate dosage. The paper is used to apply the ointment because the drug is readily absorbed through the skin. Skin contact should be avoided except on the designated area of the body. Plastic wrap or tape aids absorption and prevents removal of the drug. It also prevents soiling of clothes and linens. Application sites should be rotated because the ointment can irritate the skin.

✔ For nitroglycerin patches, apply at the same time each day to clean, dry, hairless areas on the upper body or arms. Rotate sites. Avoid applying below the knee or elbow or in areas of skin irritation or scar tissue. Correct application is necessary to promote effective and consistent drug absorption. The drug is not as well absorbed from distal portions of the extremities because of decreased blood flow. Rotation of sites decreases skin irritation. Also, used patches must be disposed of properly because there is enough residual nitroglycerin to be harmful, especially to children and pets.

✔ With sustained-release forms of calcium channel blockers, which are usually taken once daily, do not take more often than prescribed and do not crush or chew.

PRINCIPLES OF THERAPY

Goals of Therapy

The goals of drug therapy are to relieve acute anginal pain; reduce the number and severity of acute anginal attacks; improve exercise tolerance and quality of life; delay progression of CAD; prevent myocardial infarction; and prevent sudden cardiac death.

Choice of Drug and Dosage Form

For relief of acute angina and prophylaxis before events that cause acute angina, nitroglycerin (sublingual tablets or translingual spray) is usually the drug of first choice. Sublingual or chewable tablets of isosorbide dinitrate also may be used. For long-term prevention or management of recurrent angina, oral or topical nitrates, beta-adrenergic blocking agents, or calcium channel blocking agents are used. Combination drug therapy with a nitrate and one of the other drugs is common and effective. Clients taking one or more long-acting antianginal drugs should carry a short-acting drug as well, to be used for acute attacks.

Titration of Dosage

Dosage of all antianginal drugs should be individualized to achieve optimal benefit and minimal adverse effects. This is usually accomplished by starting with relatively small doses and increasing them at appropriate intervals if necessary. Doses may vary widely among individuals.

Tolerance to Long-Acting Nitrates

Clients who take long-acting dosage forms of nitrates on a regular schedule develop tolerance to the vasodilating (antianginal) effects of the drug. Although this decreases the adverse effects of hypotension, dizziness,

---

Nursing Notes: Apply Your Knowledge

Mrs. Sinatro, a patient with newly diagnosed coronary artery disease (CAD), has been started on a nitroglycerin patch that she is to apply in the morning and remove before going to bed at night. Sublingual nitroglycerin, PRN, is ordered for episodes of chest pain. Discuss appropriate teaching for Mrs. Sinatro.

How Can You Avoid This Medication Error?

Mr. Ely has Nitropaste (nitroglycerin ointment), 1 inch, ordered every 6 hours to decrease blood pressure and control angina. The nurse carefully measures out 1 inch of ointment on the measuring paper and spreads the ointment with her finger. Before she is able to administer the medication, she feels dizzy and unwell. She hands the medication to another nurse and asks her to give it. Identify the error and how it could be prevented.

and headache, therapeutic effects also may be decreased. As a result, episodes of chest pain may occur more often or be more severe than expected. In addition, short-acting nitrates may be less effective in relieving acute pain.

Opinions seem divided about the best way to prevent or manage nitrate tolerance. Some authorities recommend using short-acting nitrates when needed and avoiding the long-acting forms. Others recommend using the long-acting forms for approximately 12 to 16 hours daily during active periods and omitting them during inactive periods or sleep. Thus, a dose of an oral nitrate or topical ointment would be given every 6 hours for three doses daily, allowing a rest period of 6 hours without a dose. Transdermal discs should be removed at bedtime.

Use in Children

The safety and effectiveness of antianginal drugs have not been established for children. Nitroglycerin has been given IV for congestive heart failure and intraoperative control of blood pressure, with the initial dose adjusted for weight and later doses titrated to response.

Use in Older Adults

Antianginal drugs are often used because cardiovascular disease and myocardial ischemia are common problems in older adults. Adverse drug effects, such as hypotension and syncope, are likely to occur, and they may be more severe than in younger adults. Blood pressure and ability to ambulate safely should be closely monitored, especially when drug therapy is started or dosages are increased. Ambulatory clients also should be monitored for their ability to take the drugs correctly.

With calcium channel blockers, older adults may have higher plasma concentrations of verapamil, diltiazem, nifedipine, and amlodipine. This is attributed to decreased hepatic metabolism of the drugs, probably because of decreased hepatic blood flow. In addition, older adults may experience more hypotension with verapamil, nifedipine, and felodipine than younger clients. Blood pressure should be monitored with these drugs.

Use in Renal Impairment

Little information is available about the use of antianginal drugs in clients with impaired renal function. A few studies indicate that advanced renal failure may alter the pharmacokinetics of calcium channel blockers. Although the pharmacokinetics of diltiazem and verapamil are quite similar in clients with normal and impaired renal function, caution is still advised. With verapamil, approximately 70% of a dose is excreted as metabolites in urine.

Dosage reductions are considered unnecessary with verapamil and diltiazem but may be needed with nifedipine and several other dihydropyridine derivatives. With nifedipine, protein binding is decreased and the elimination half-life is prolonged with renal impairment. In a few clients, reversible elevations in blood urea nitrogen and serum creatinine have occurred. With nicardipine, plasma concentrations are higher in clients with renal impairment, and dosage should be reduced. Bepridil should be used with caution because its metabolites are excreted mainly in urine.

Use in Hepatic Impairment

Nitrates, beta blockers (see Chap. 19), and calcium channel blockers are metabolized in the liver, and all should be used with caution in clients with significant impairment of hepatic function from reduced blood flow or disease processes.

With oral nitrates, it is difficult to predict effects. On the one hand, first-pass metabolism is reduced, which increases bioavailability (amount of active drug) of a given dose. On the other hand, the nitrate reductase enzymes that normally deactivate the drug may increase if large doses are given. In this case, more enzymes are available and the drug is metabolized more rapidly, possibly reducing therapeutic effects of a given dose. Relatively large doses of oral nitrates are sometimes given to counteract the drug tolerance (reduced hemodynamic effects) associated with chronic use. In addition, metabolism of nitroglycerin and isosorbide dinitrate normally produces active metabolites. Thus, if metabolism is reduced by liver impairment, drug effects may be decreased and shorter in duration.

With calcium channel blockers, impairment of liver function has profound effects on the pharmacokinetics and pharmacodynamics of most of these drugs. Thus, the drugs should be used with caution, dosages should be substantially reduced, and clients should be closely monitored for drug effects (including periodic measurements of liver enzymes). These recommendations stem from the following effects:

- An impaired liver produces fewer drug-binding plasma proteins such as albumin. This means that a greater proportion of a given dose is unbound and therefore active.
- In clients with cirrhosis, bioavailability of oral drugs is greatly increased and metabolism (of both oral and parenteral drugs) is greatly decreased. Both of these effects increase plasma levels of drug from a given dose (essentially an overdose). The effects result from shunting of blood around the liver so that drug molecules circulating in the bloodstream do not come in contact with drug-metabolizing enzymes and therefore are not metabolized. For example, the bioavailability of verapamil, nifedipine, felodipine,

and nisoldipine is approximately double and their clearance is approximately one third that of clients without cirrhosis.

- Although hepatotoxicity is uncommon, clinical symptoms of hepatitis, cholestasis, or jaundice and elevated liver enzymes (eg, alkaline phosphatase, CPK, LDH, AST, alanine aminotransferase) have occurred, mainly with diltiazem, nifedipine, and verapamil. These changes resolve if the causative drug is stopped.

Use in Critical Illness

Antianginal drugs have multiple cardiovascular effects and may be used alone or in combination with other cardiovascular drugs in clients with critical illness. They are probably used most often to treat severe angina, severe hypertension, or serious cardiac arrhythmias. For example, IV nitroglycerin may be used for angina and hypertension; an IV beta blocker or calcium channel blocker may be used for angina, hypertension, or supraventricular tachyarrhythmias that impair cardiovascular function. With any of these drugs, dosage must be carefully titrated

and clients must be closely monitored for hypotension and other drug effects.

In addition, absorption of oral drugs or topical forms of nitroglycerin may be impaired in clients with extensive edema, heart failure, hypotension, or other conditions that impair blood flow to the gastrointestinal tract or skin.

 Home Care

The role of the home care nurse may vary, depending largely on the severity of the client's illness. Initially, the nurse should assess the frequency and severity of anginal attacks and how the attacks are managed. In addition, the nurse can assess the home setting for lifestyle and environmental factors that may precipitate myocardial ischemia. When causative factors are identified, plans can be developed to avoid or minimize them. Other aspects of home care may include monitoring the client's response to antianginal medications; teaching clients and caregivers how to use, store, and replace medications to ensure a constant supply; and discussing circumstances for which the client should seek emergency care.

(*text continues on page 797*)

NURSING ACTIONS   ## Antianginal Drugs

NURSING ACTIONS	RATIONALE/EXPLANATION
1. Administer accurately	
a. Check blood pressure and heart rate before each dose of an antianginal drug. Withhold the drug if systolic blood pressure is below 90 mm Hg. If the dose is omitted, record and report to the physician.	Hypotension is an adverse effect of antianginal drugs. Bradycardia is an adverse effect of propranolol and nadolol. Dosage adjustments may be necessary if these effects occur.
b. Give antianginal drugs on a regular schedule, at evenly spaced intervals.	To increase effectiveness in preventing acute attacks of angina
c. If oral nitrates and topical nitroglycerin are being used concurrently, stagger times of administration.	To minimize risks of additive hypotension and headache
d. For sublingual nitroglycerin and isosorbide dinitrate, instruct the client to place the tablets under the tongue until they dissolve.	
e. For oral isosorbide dinitrate, regular and chewable tablets are available. Be sure each type of tablet is taken appropriately.	
f. For sublingual nitroglycerin, check the expiration date on the container.	Sublingual tablets of nitroglycerin are volatile. Once the bottle has been opened, they become ineffective after approximately 6 mo and should be replaced.

(*continued*)

NURSING ACTIONS	RATIONALE/EXPLANATION
g. To apply nitroglycerin ointment, use the special paper to measure the dose. Place the ointment on a nonhairy part of the body, and apply with the applicator paper. Cover the area with plastic wrap or tape. Rotate application sites.	The measured paper must be used for accurate dosage. The paper is used to apply the ointment because the drug is readily absorbed through the skin. Skin contact should be avoided except on the designated area of the body. Plastic wrap or tape aids absorption and prevents removal of the drug. It also prevents soiling of clothes and linens. Application sites should be rotated because the ointment can irritate the skin.
h. For nitroglycerin patches, apply at the same time each day to clean, dry, hairless areas on the upper body or arms. Rotate sites. Avoid applying below the knee or elbow or in areas of skin irritation or scar tissue.	To promote effective and consistent drug absorption. The drug is not as well absorbed from distal portions of the extremities because of decreased blood flow. Rotation of sites decreases skin irritation.
i. For intravenous (IV) nitroglycerin, dilute the drug and give by continuous infusion, with frequent monitoring of blood pressure and heart rate. Use only with the special administration set supplied by the manufacturer to avoid drug adsorption onto tubing.	The drug should not be given by direct IV injection. The drug is potent and may cause hypotension. Dosage (flow rate) is adjusted according to response (pain relief or drop in systolic blood pressure of 20 mm Hg).
j. With IV verapamil, inject slowly, over 2–3 min.	To decrease hypotension and other adverse effects
2. Observe for therapeutic effects	
a. Relief of chest pain with acute attacks	Sublingual nitroglycerin usually relieves pain within 5 min. If pain is not relieved, two additional tablets may be given, 5 min apart. If pain is not relieved after three tablets, report to the physician.
b. Reduced incidence and severity of acute attacks with prophylactic antianginal drugs	
c. Increased exercise tolerance	
3. Observe for adverse effects	
a. With nitrates, observe for hypotension, dizziness, lightheadedness, tachycardia, palpitations, and headache	Adverse effects are extensions of pharmacologic action. Vasodilation causes hypotension, which in turn causes dizziness from cerebral hypoxia and tachycardia from compensatory sympathetic nervous system stimulation. Hypotension can decrease blood flow to coronary arteries and precipitate angina pectoris or myocardial infarction. Hypotension is most likely to occur within an hour after drug administration. Vasodilation also causes headache, the most common adverse effect of nitrates.
b. With beta-adrenergic blocking agents, observe for hypotension, bradycardia, bronchospasm, and congestive heart failure.	Beta blockers lower blood pressure by decreasing myocardial contractility and cardiac output. Excessive bradycardia may contribute to hypotension and cardiac arrhythmias. Bronchospasm is more likely to occur in clients with asthma or other chronic respiratory problems.
c. With calcium channel blockers, observe for hypotension, dizziness, lightheadedness, weakness, peripheral edema, headache, congestive	Adverse effects result primarily from reduced smooth muscle contractility. These effects, except constipation, are much more likely to occur with

(continued)

NURSING ACTIONS	RATIONALE/EXPLANATION
heart failure, pulmonary edema, nausea, and constipation. Bradycardia may occur with verapamil and diltiazem; tachycardia may occur with nifedipine and nicardipine.	nifedipine and other dihydropyridines. Nifedipine may cause profound hypotension, which activates the compensatory mechanisms of the sympathetic nervous system and the renin-angiotensin-aldosterone system. Peripheral edema may require the administration of a diuretic. Constipation is more likely to occur with verapamil. Diltiazem reportedly causes few adverse effects.
4. Observe for drug interactions	
a. Drugs that *increase* effects of antianginal drugs:	
(1) Antiarrhythmics, antihypertensive drugs, diuretics, phenothiazine antipsychotic agents	Additive hypotension
(2) Cimetidine	May increase beta-blocking effects of propranolol by slowing its hepatic clearance and elimination. Increases effects of all calcium channel blockers by inhibiting hepatic metabolism and increasing serum drug levels.
(3) Digoxin	Additive bradycardia when given with beta-blocking agents
b. Drugs that *decrease* effects of antianginal drugs:	
(1) Adrenergic drugs (eg, epinephrine, isoproterenol)	Adrenergic drugs, which stimulate beta receptors, can reverse bradycardia induced by beta blockers.
(2) Anticholinergic drugs	Drugs with anticholinergic effects can increase heart rate, offsetting slower heart rates produced by beta blockers.
(3) Calcium salts	May decrease therapeutic effectiveness of calcium channel blockers
(4) Carbamazepine, phenobarbital, phenytoin, rifampin	May decrease effects of calcium channel blockers by inducing hepatic enzymes and thereby increasing their rate of metabolism

Nursing Notes: Apply Your Knowledge

Answer: Assess Mrs. Sinatro's knowledge about CAD and her readiness to learn about her new medications and other methods to manage this problem. Give Mrs. Sinatro written handouts about CAD and written information about her antianginal medications. Demonstrate how to apply the patch, stressing to rotate sites and not use hairy or scarred areas because they may decrease drug absorption. The patch is removed at night because the oxygen demand of the heart is usually less at rest, and continuous application can increase the development of drug tolerance. Discuss side effects, including headache and hypotension, that can cause dizziness and falls.

Teaching must include how to manage an episode of chest pain. First stress the importance of *never* ignoring chest pain. Some patients may deny they are experiencing chest pain and delay treatment. Tell her to rest if chest pain occurs. If pain does not subside, place a nitroglycerin tablet under the tongue to dissolve. Do not swallow. Repeat every 5 minutes. If the pain has not subsided with rest and three nitroglycerin tablets, call 911. Do not drive yourself to the hospital or clinic because you may be having a heart attack (myocardial infarction). Also stress the importance of keeping nitroglycerin with her at all times and making sure the prescription is refilled before it reaches the expiration date. The tablets should be kept in the amber bottle to protect them from sunlight and stored away from moisture and excessive heat.

How Can You Avoid This Medication Error?

Answer: Actually, there are two errors in this situation. A nurse can only safely administer medication that she has prepared. In this situation, after the medication has been spread on the paper, the dosage will be unclear. Also, a nurse should never touch Nitropaste without wearing gloves. This potent vasodilator absorbs through the nurse's skin, causing systemic effects such as dizziness and headache.

REVIEW AND APPLICATION EXERCISES

1. What is angina pectoris?
2. What is the role of endothelial dysfunction in the development of coronary artery atherosclerosis and myocardial ischemia?
3. How do nitrates relieve angina?
4. Develop a teaching plan for a client who is beginning nitrate therapy.
5. How do beta blockers relieve angina?
6. Why should beta blockers be tapered and discontinued slowly in clients with angina?
7. How do calcium channel blockers relieve angina?
8. Develop a teaching plan for a client taking a calcium channel blocker.

SELECTED REFERENCES

Brater, D.C. (1997). Clinical pharmacology of cardiovascular drugs. In W.N. Kelley (Ed.), *Textbook of internal medicine*, 3rd ed., pp. 552–569. Philadelphia: Lippincott-Raven.

Drug facts and comparisons. (Updated monthly). St. Louis: Facts and Comparisons.

Elliott, H.L., Meredith, P.A., & Reid, J.L. (1998). Calcium antagonists. In M. Epstein (Ed.), *Calcium antagonists in clinical medicine*, 2nd ed., pp. 35–56. Philadelphia: Hanley and Belfus.

Jugdutt, B.I. (1998). Adjunctive pharmacologic therapies in acute myocardial infarction. In D.L. Brown, *Cardiac intensive care*, pp. 181–186. Philadelphia: W.B. Saunders.

Porth, C.M. (Ed.). (1998). *Pathophysiology: Concepts of altered health states*, 5th ed., pp. 485–526. Philadelphia: Lippincott Williams & Wilkins.

Robertson, R.M. & Robertson, D. (1996). Drugs used for the treatment of myocardial ischemia. In J.G. Hardman, L.E. Limbird, P.B. Molinoff, & R.W. Ruddon (Eds.), *Goodman & Gilman's The pharmacological basis of therapeutics*, 9th ed., pp. 759–779. New York: McGraw-Hill.

Rockett, J.L. (1999). Endothelial dysfunction and the promise of ACE inhibitors. *American Journal of Nursing, 99*(10), 44–49.

Talbert, R.L. (1997). Ischemic heart disease. In J.T. DiPiro, R.L. Talbert, G.C. Yee, G.R. Matzke, B.G. Wells, & L.M. Posey (Eds.), *Pharmacotherapy: A pathophysiologic approach*, 3rd ed., pp. 257–294. Stamford, CT: Appleton & Lange.

Willerson, J.T. (1998). Recognition and treatment of unstable angina. In D.L. Brown (Ed.), *Cardiac intensive care*, pp. 337–346. Philadelphia: W.B. Saunders.

Winters, K.J. & Eisenberg, P.R. (1998). Ischemic heart disease. In C.F. Carey, H.H. Lee, & K.F. Woeltje (Eds.), *The Washington manual of medical therapeutics*, 29th ed., pp. 81–108. Philadelphia: Lippincott Williams & Wilkins.

54

Drugs Used in Hypotension and Shock

Objectives

After studying this chapter, the student will be able to:

1. Identify clients at risk for development of hypovolemia and shock.

2. Identify common causes of hypotension and shock.

3. Discuss assessment of a client in shock.

4. Describe therapeutic and adverse effects of vasopressor drugs used in the treatment of hypotension and shock.

Betty Smith is in the cardiac care unit being treated for cardiogenic shock. She is currently on the following IV infusion: dobutamine (Dobutrex) 5 μg/kg/min and dopamine hydrochloride (Intropin) 5 μg/kg/min.

Reflect on:

▶ Define shock. How does cardiogenic shock differ from hypovolemic shock, and how will this affect treatment?

▶ What symptoms would likely occur when a client is experiencing cardiogenic shock?

▶ Review the autonomic nervous system (ANS). Describe the ANS effects of Mrs. Smith's medications and how they will be used to manage shock.

▶ Dopamine's effects differ depending on dosage. What effects will you most likely see in Mrs. Smith?

HYPOTENSION AND SHOCK

Shock is a clinical syndrome characterized by decreased blood supply to body tissues. Clinical symptoms depend on the degree of impaired perfusion of vital organs (eg, brain, heart, and kidneys). Common signs and symptoms include oliguria, heart failure, mental confusion, cool extremities, and coma. Most, but not all, people in shock are hypotensive. In a previously hypertensive person, shock may be present if a drop in blood pressure of greater than 50 mm Hg has occurred, even if current blood pressure readings are "normal."

An additional consequence of inadequate blood flow to tissues is that cells change from aerobic (oxygen-based) to anaerobic metabolism. Lactic acid produced by anaerobic metabolism leads to generalized metabolic acidosis and eventually to organ failure and death if blood flow is not promptly restored.

Types of Shock

There are three general categories of shock that are based on the circulatory mechanisms involved. These mechanisms are intravascular volume, the ability of the heart to pump, and vascular tone.

Hypovolemic shock involves a loss of intravascular fluid volume that may be due to actual blood loss or relative loss from fluid shifts within the body.

Cardiogenic shock, also called *pump failure*, occurs when the myocardium has lost its ability to contract efficiently and maintain an adequate cardiac output.

Distributive or *vasogenic shock* is characterized by severe, generalized vasodilation, which results in severe hypotension and impairment of blood flow. Distributive shock is further divided into anaphylactic, neurogenic, and septic shock.

- *Anaphylactic shock* results from a hypersensitivity (allergic) reaction to drugs or other substances (see Chap. 18).
- *Neurogenic shock* results from inadequate sympathetic nervous system (SNS) stimulation. The SNS normally maintains sufficient vascular tone (ie, a small amount of vasoconstriction) to support adequate blood circulation. Neurogenic shock may occur with depression of the vasomotor center in the brain or decreased sympathetic outflow to blood vessels.
- *Septic shock* results from bacterial infections that gain access to the bloodstream.

It is important to know the etiology of shock because treatment varies among the types. The types of shock, with their causes and symptoms, are summarized in Table 54-1.

TABLE 54-1 Types of Shock

Types of Shock	Possible Causes	Clinical Manifestations
Hypovolemic	Trauma Gastrointestinal bleed Ruptured aneurysms Third spacing Dehydration	Hypotension Tachycardia Cool, clammy skin Diaphoresis Pallor Oliguria
Cardiogenic	Acute myocardial infarction Cardiac surgery Arrhythmias Cardiomyopathy	Signs and symptoms of heart failure Signs and symptoms of decreased cardiac output
Distributive Neurogenic	Spinal cord damage Spinal anesthesia Severe pain Drugs	Hypotension Bradycardia Warm, dry skin
Septic	Infection (eg, urinary tract, upper respiratory infections) Invasive procedures	Hypotension Cool or warm dry skin Hypothermia or hyperthermia
Anaphylactic	Contrast dyes Drugs Insect bites Foods	Hypotension Hives Bronchospasms

ANTISHOCK DRUGS

Drugs used in the treatment of shock are primarily the adrenergic drugs, which are discussed more extensively in Chapter 18. In this chapter, the drugs are discussed only in relation to their use in hypotension and shock. In these conditions, drugs with alpha-adrenergic activity (eg, norepinephrine, phenylephrine) are used to increase peripheral vascular resistance and raise blood pressure. Drugs with beta-adrenergic activity (eg, dobutamine, isoproterenol) are used to increase myocardial contractility and heart rate, which in turn raises blood pressure. Some drugs have both alpha- and beta-adrenergic activity (eg, dopamine, epinephrine). In many cases, a combination of drugs is used, depending on the type of shock and the client's response to treatment.

Adrenergic drugs with beta activity may be relatively contraindicated in shock states precipitated or complicated by cardiac arrhythmias. Beta-stimulating drugs also should be used cautiously in cardiogenic shock after myocardial infarction because increased contractility and heart rate can increase myocardial oxygen consumption and extend the area of infarction.

Individual drugs are described in the following section; indications for use and dosage ranges are listed in Table 54-2.

TABLE 54-2   **Drugs Used for Hypotension and Shock**

| Generic/Trade Names | Indications for Use | Routes and Dosage Ranges | |
		Adults	Children
Dopamine (Intropin)	Increase cardiac output Treat hypotension Increase urine output	IV 2 to 5 µg/kg/min initially, gradually increasing to 20–50 µg/kg/min if necessary. Prepare by adding 200 mg of dopamine to 250 mL of IV fluid for a final concentration of 800 µg/mL or to 500 mL IV fluid for a final concentration of 400 µg/mL.	Same as adults
Dobutamine (Dobutrex)	Increase cardiac output	IV 2.5–15 µg/kg/min, increased to 40 µg/kg/min if necessary. Reconstitute the 250-mg vial with 10 mL of sterile water or 5% dextrose injection. The resulting solution should be diluted to at least 50 mL with IV solution before administering (5000 µg/mL). Add 250 mg of drug to 500 mL of diluent for a concentration of 500 µg/mL.	
Epinephrine (Adrenalin)	Treat anaphylactic shock Reverse bronchoconstriction Increase cardiac output Treat cardiac arrest	IV 1–4 µg/min. Prepare the solution by adding 2 mg (2 mL) of epinephrine injection 1:1000 to 250 or 500 mL of IV fluid. The final concentration is 8 or 4 µg/mL, respectively. IV direct injection, 100–1000 µg of 1:10,000 injection, every 5–15 min, injected slowly. Prepare the solution by adding 1 mL epinephrine 1:1000 to 9 mL sodium chloride injection. The final concentration is 100 µg/mL. Cardiac arrest, IV injection, 0.5–1.0 mg of 1:10,000 solution, repeated every 5 min as needed	IV infusion, 0.025 to 0.3 µg/kg/min IV direct injection, 5 to 10 µg/kg, slowly SC, 0.01 mg/kg of 1:1000 solution
Isoproterenol (Isuprel)	Treat atropine-refractory brady-cardias	IV infusion, 0.5–10 µg/min. Prepare solution by adding 2 mg to 250 mL of IV fluid. Final concentration is 8 µg/mL.	IV infusion, 0.05–0.3 µg/kg/min
Metaraminol (Aramine)	Treat hypotension due to spinal anesthesia	IM 2–10 mg IV injection, 0.5–5 mg IV infusion, add 15–500 mg of metaraminol to 250 or 500 mL of IV fluid. Adjust flow rate (dosage) to maintain the desired blood pressure.	IM 0.1 mg/kg IV injection, 0.01 mg/kg IV infusion, 1 mg/25 mL of dilu-ent. Adjust flow rate to main-tain the desired blood pressure.
Milrinone (Primacor)	Increase cardiac output in cardio-genic shock	IV injection (loading dose), 50 µg/kg over 10 min IV infusion (maintenance, dose), 0.375–0.75 µg/kg/min diluted in 0.9% or 0.45% sodium chloride or 5% dex-trose solution. Maximum dose, 1.13 mg/kg/d.	
Norepinephrine (Levophed)	Treat hypotension Increase cardiac output	IV infusion, 2–4 µg/min, to a maximum of 20 µg/min. Pre-pare solution by adding 2 mg	IV infusion, 0.03–0.1 µg/kg/min

TABLE 54-2 **Drugs Used for Hypotension and Shock** (*continued*)

Generic/Trade Names	Indications for Use	Routes and Dosage Ranges	
		Adults	Children
Phenylephrine (Neo-Synephrine)	Treat hypotension	to 500 mL of IV fluid. Final concentration is 4 µg/mL. IV infusion, 100–180 µg/min initially, then 40–60 µg/min. Prepare solution by adding 10 mg of phenylephrine to 250 or 500 mL of IV fluid. Final concentration is 20 or 40 µg/mL, respectively. IV injection, 0.1–0.5 mg every 10–15 min	SC, IM 0.5–1 mg/25 lbs

IM, intramuscular; IV, intravenous; SC, subcutaneous.

INDIVIDUAL DRUGS

Dopamine is a naturally occurring catecholamine that functions as a neurotransmitter. Dopamine exerts its actions by stimulating alpha, beta, or dopaminergic receptors, depending on the dose being used. In addition, dopamine acts indirectly by releasing norepinephrine from sympathetic nerve endings and the adrenal glands. Peripheral dopamine receptors are located in splanchnic and renal vascular beds. At low doses (2.5 to 10 µg/kg/minute), dopamine stimulates dopaminergic receptors. At moderate doses (10 to 20 µg/kg/minute), dopamine also stimulates beta receptors and increases heart rate, myocardial contractility, and blood pressure. At high doses (20 to 50 µg/kg/minute), beta activity remains, but increasing alpha stimulation (vasoconstriction) may overcome the dopaminergic actions.

It has long been accepted that stimulation of dopamine receptors by low doses of exogenous dopamine produces vasodilation in the renal circulation and increases urine output. More recent studies indicate that low-dose dopamine enhances renal function only when cardiac function is improved.

Dopamine is useful in hypovolemic and cardiogenic shock. Adequate fluid therapy is necessary for the maximal pressor effect of dopamine. Acidosis decreases the effectiveness of dopamine.

Dobutamine is a synthetic catecholamine developed to provide less vascular activity than dopamine. It acts mainly on beta$_1$ receptors in the heart to increase the force of myocardial contraction with a minimal increase in heart rate. Dobutamine also may increase blood pressure with large doses. It is less likely to cause tachycardia, arrhythmias, and increased myocardial oxygen demand than dopamine and isoproterenol. It is most useful in cases of shock that require increased cardiac output without the need for blood pressure support. It is recommended for short-term use only. It may be used with dopamine to augment the beta$_1$ activity that is sometimes overridden

by alpha effects when dopamine is used alone at doses greater than 10 µg/kg/minute.

Dobutamine has a short plasma half-life and therefore must be administered by continuous intravenous (IV) infusion. A loading dose is not required because the drug has a rapid onset of action and reaches steady state within approximately 10 minutes after the infusion is begun. It is rapidly metabolized to inactive metabolites.

Epinephrine is a naturally occurring catecholamine produced by the adrenal glands. At low doses, epinephrine stimulates beta receptors, which increases cardiac output by increasing the rate and force of myocardial contractility. It also causes bronchodilation. Larger doses act on alpha receptors to increase blood pressure.

Epinephrine is the drug of choice for treatment of anaphylactic shock because of its rapid onset of action and antiallergic effects. It prevents the release of histamine and other mediators that cause symptoms of anaphylaxis, thereby reversing vasodilation and bronchoconstriction. In early treatment of anaphylaxis, it may be given subcutaneously to produce therapeutic effects within 5 to 10 minutes, with peak activity in approximately 20 minutes. It is usually given by continuous IV infusion to treat shock. However, bolus doses may be given in emergencies, such as cardiac arrest.

The use of epinephrine in other types of shock is limited because it may produce excessive cardiac stimulation, ventricular arrhythmias, and reduced renal blood flow. In addition, more potent vasoconstrictors are available (eg, norepinephrine).

Epinephrine has an elimination half-life of approximately 2 minutes and is rapidly inactivated to metabolites, which are then excreted by the kidneys.

Isoproterenol is a synthetic catecholamine that acts exclusively on beta receptors to increase heart rate, myocardial contractility, and systolic blood pressure. However, it also stimulates vascular beta$_2$ receptors, which causes vasodilation, and may decrease diastolic blood pressure. For this reason, isoproterenol has limited usefulness as a pressor agent. It also may increase myocardial oxygen consumption and decrease coronary artery blood flow, which in turn causes myocardial ischemia. Cardiac arrhythmias may result from excessive beta stimulation. Because of these limitations, use of isoproterenol is limited to shock associated with slow heart rates and myocardial depression.

Metaraminol is used mainly for hypotension associated with spinal anesthesia. It acts indirectly by releasing norepinephrine from sympathetic nerve endings. Thus, its vasoconstrictive actions are similar to those of norepinephrine, except that metaraminol is less potent and has a longer duration of action.

Milrinone is discussed in Chapter 51 as a treatment for congestive heart failure. It is also used to treat cardiogenic shock in combination with other inotropes or vasopressors. It increases cardiac output and decreases systemic vascular resistance without significantly increasing heart rate or myocardial oxygen consumption. The increased cardiac output improves renal blood flow, which then leads to increased urine output, decreased circulating blood volume, and decreased cardiac workload.

Norepinephrine is a pharmaceutical preparation of the naturally occurring catecholamine norepinephrine. It stimulates alpha-adrenergic receptors and thus increases blood pressure primarily by vasoconstriction. It also stimulates beta$_1$ receptors and therefore increases heart rate and force of myocardial contraction. It is useful in cardiogenic and septic shock, but reduced renal blood flow limits its prolonged use. Norepinephrine is used mainly with clients who are unresponsive to dopamine or dobutamine. Blood pressure should be monitored frequently during infusion.

Phenylephrine (Neo-Synephrine) is an adrenergic drug that stimulates alpha-adrenergic receptors. As a result, it constricts arterioles and raises systolic and diastolic blood pressures. Phenylephrine resembles epinephrine but has fewer cardiac effects and a longer duration of action. Reduction of renal and mesenteric blood flow limits prolonged use.

Nursing Notes: Apply Your Knowledge

Your client in the intensive care unit (ICU) is receiving two medications to treat hypovolemic shock. What evaluation criteria will you use to determine the effectiveness of this drug therapy?

NURSING PROCESS

Assessment

Assess the client's condition in relation to hypotension and shock.

- Check blood pressure; heart rate; urine output; skin temperature and color of extremities; level of consciousness; orientation to person, place, and time; and adequacy of respiration. Abnormal values are not specific indicators of hypotension and shock, but they may indicate a need for further evaluation. In general, report blood pressure below 90/60, heart rate above 100, and urine output below 50 mL/hour.
- Check electrocardiograms, cardiac monitors, and hemodynamic monitors for indications of impaired cardiac function, when available.
- Monitor available laboratory reports for abnormal values (eg, decreased oxygen saturation levels indicate decreased oxygenation of tissues; abnormal arterial blood gases may indicate metabolic acidosis; an increased hematocrit may indicate hypovolemia; an increased eosinophil count may indicate anaphylaxis; the presence of bacteria in blood cultures may indicate sepsis; an increased serum creatinine and blood urea nitrogen may indicate impending renal failure).

Nursing Diagnoses

- Decreased Cardiac Output related to hypotension and vasoconstriction
- Altered Tissue Perfusion: Decreased related to decreased cardiac output
- Fluid Volume Deficit related to fluid loss or vasodilation
- Anxiety related to potentially life-threatening illness
- Risk for Injury: Myocardial infarction, stroke, or renal damage related to decreased blood flow to vital organs

Planning/Goals

The client will:
- Have improved tissue perfusion and relief of symptoms
- Have improved vital signs
- Be guarded against recurrence of hypotension and shock if possible
- Be monitored for therapeutic and adverse effects of adrenergic drugs
- Avoid preventable adverse effects of adrenergic drugs

Interventions

Use measures to prevent or minimize hypotension and shock.

- General measures include those to maintain airway, maintain fluid balance, control hemorrhage, treat infections, prevent hypoxia, and control other causative factors.

- Learn to recognize impending shock so treatment can be initiated early. Do not wait until symptoms are severe. The earlier the treatment, the greater the likelihood of reversing shock.
- Assist in recognizing and treating the underlying cause of shock in a particular client (eg, replacing fluids; preventing further loss of blood or other body fluids).

Monitor clients during shock and vasopressor drug therapy.

- Titrate adrenergic drug infusions to maintain blood pressure and tissue perfusion without causing hypertension.
- Check blood pressure and pulse constantly or at least every 5 to 15 minutes during acute shock and vasopressor drug therapy.
- Monitor distal pulses, urine output, and skin temperature and color closely to assess tissue perfusion.
- Check venipuncture sites frequently for infiltration or extravasation. Have phentolamine (Regitine), an alpha-adrenergic blocking agent that reverses vasoconstriction, readily available in any setting where IV adrenergic drugs are used.
- Keep family members informed about treatment measures, including drug therapy, monitoring equipment, and the need for close observation of vital signs, IV infusion site, urine output, and so forth.

Evaluation

Observe for improved vital signs, color and temperature of skin, urine output, and responsiveness.

PRINCIPLES OF THERAPY

Goal of Therapy

The goal of adrenergic drug therapy in hypotension and shock is to restore and maintain adequate tissue perfusion, especially to vital organs.

How Can You Avoid This Medication Error?

Your postoperative patient is hypotensive and has low urine output. When a fluid bolus does not produce a significant increase in urine output, the physician orders low-dose IV dopamine. After the dopamine has infused for 2 hours, the patient complains of burning at the infusion site. When you assess the site, you do not detect swelling or warmth. You decide to continue to monitor the IV site rather than change it because you know starting another IV will be very difficult.

Choice of Drug

The choice of drug depends primarily on the pathophysiology involved. For cardiogenic shock and decreased cardiac output, dopamine or dobutamine is given. With severe congestive heart failure characterized by decreased cardiac output and high peripheral vascular resistance, vasodilator drugs (eg, nitroprusside, nitroglycerin) may be given along with the cardiotonic drug. The combination increases cardiac output and decreases cardiac workload by decreasing preload and afterload. However, vasodilators should not be used alone because of the risk of severe hypotension and further compromising tissue perfusion. Milrinone may be given when other drugs fail.

For distributive shock characterized by severe vasodilation and decreased peripheral vascular resistance, a vasoconstrictor or vasopressor drug, such as norepinephrine, is the drug of first choice. Drug dosage must be carefully titrated to avoid excessive vasoconstriction and hypertension, which causes impairment rather than improvement in tissue perfusion.

Guidelines for Treatment of Hypotension and Shock

- Vasopressor drugs are less effective in the presence of inadequate blood volume, electrolyte abnormalities, and acidosis. These conditions also must be treated if present. In addition, normalizing the blood pH and body temperature facilitates the release of oxygen from hemoglobin to the cells.
- Minimal effective doses of adrenergic drugs are recommended because of their extreme vasoconstrictive effects. Dosage can be easily controlled by varying the flow rate of IV infusions because catecholamine drugs have short half-lives. Dosage and flow rate usually are titrated to maintain a low-normal blood pressure. Such titration depends on frequent and accurate blood pressure measurements.
- Septic shock requires appropriate antibiotic therapy in addition to other treatment measures. If an abscess is the source of infection, it must be surgically drained.
- Hypovolemic shock is most effectively treated by IV fluids that replace the type of fluid lost; that is, blood loss should be replaced with whole blood, and gastrointestinal losses should be replaced with solutions containing electrolytes (eg, Ringer's lactate or sodium chloride solutions with added potassium chloride).
- Cardiogenic shock may be complicated by pulmonary congestion, for which diuretic drugs are indicated and IV fluids are contraindicated (except to maintain a patent IV line).

- Anaphylactic shock is often treated by nonadrenergic drugs as well as epinephrine. For example, the histamine-induced cardiovascular symptoms (eg, vasodilation and increased capillary permeability) are thought to be mediated through both types of histamine receptors. Thus, treatment may include a histamine-1 receptor blocker (eg, diphenhydramine 1 mg/kg IV) and a histamine-2 receptor blocker (eg, cimetidine 4 mg/kg IV), given over at least 5 minutes. In addition, IV corticosteroids are frequently given, such as methylprednisolone (20 to 100 mg) or hydrocortisone (100 to 500 mg). Doses may need to be repeated every 2 to 4 hours. Corticosteroids increase tissue responsiveness to adrenergic drugs in approximately 2 hours but do not produce anti-inflammatory effects for several hours.

Use in Children

Little information is available about adrenergic drugs for the treatment of hypotension and shock in children. In general, treatment is the same as for adults, with drug dosages adjusted for weight.

Use in Older Adults

The use of adrenergic drugs to manage hypotension and shock in the older adult is essentially the same as for younger adults. Older adults often have disorders such as atherosclerosis, peripheral vascular disease, and diabetes mellitus. When adrenergic drugs are given, their vasoconstricting effects may decrease blood flow and increase risks of tissue ischemia and thrombosis. Careful monitoring of pulses and skin color and temperature, especially in the extremities, is required.

Use in Renal Impairment

Although adrenergic drugs may be life saving, they can reduce renal blood flow and cause renal failure because of their vasoconstrictive effects. Renal impairment may occur in clients with previously normal renal function and may be worsened in clients whose renal function is already impaired. Dopamine is often used to increase renal perfusion, but the effectiveness of this practice is being questioned.

In men with benign prostatic hypertrophy, oliguric renal failure may need to be differentiated from urinary retention because some adrenergic drugs (eg, epinephrine, norepinephrine, phenylephrine) can cause urinary retention.

Most adrenergic drugs are metabolized in the liver and the metabolites are excreted in the urine. However, little accumulation of the drugs or metabolites is likely because the drugs have short half-lives.

Use in Hepatic Impairment

Catecholamine drugs are metabolized by monoamine oxidase (MAO) and catechol-O-methyl transferase (COMT). MAO is widely distributed in most body tissues, whereas COMT is located mainly in the liver. Thus, the drugs are eliminated mainly by liver metabolism and must be used cautiously in clients with impaired liver function. Clients should be monitored closely and drug dosage should be adjusted as symptoms warrant. However, the half-life of most adrenergic drugs is very brief, and this decreases the chances of drug accumulation in hepatically impaired clients.

Use in Critical Illness

The adrenergic catecholamines (eg, dopamine, dobutamine, epinephrine, norepinephrine) are widely used in clients with a low cardiac output that persists despite adequate fluid replacement and correction of electrolyte imbalance. By improving circulation, the drugs also help to prevent tissue injury from ischemia (eg, renal failure).

Although the drugs may be used initially in almost any setting, most clients with hypotension and shock are treated in critical care units. Dobutamine and dopamine are usually the cardiotonic agents of choice in critically ill clients. Dopamine varies in clearance rate in both adult and pediatric clients in critical care units. However, this variance may result from the use of non–steady-state plasma concentrations in calculating the clearance rate. When a dopamine IV infusion is started, it may take 1 to 2 hours to achieve a steady-state plasma level. Relatively large doses of dopamine are given for cardiotonic and vasoconstrictive effects.

Epinephrine and norepinephrine are also widely used in critically ill clients. However, their pharmacokinetics have not been studied in this population. Recommended infusion rates in critically ill clients vary from 0.01 to 0.15 µg/kg/minute for epinephrine and from 0.06 to 0.15 µg/kg/minute for norepinephrine. All clients receiving drugs for treatment of hypotension and shock should be closely monitored regarding drug dosage, vital signs, relevant laboratory test results, and other indicators of clinical status. This is especially true of critically ill clients, who often have multiple organ impairments and are clinically unstable.

(*text continues on page 807*)

NURSING ACTIONS	Drugs Used in Hypotension and Shock

NURSING ACTIONS	RATIONALE/EXPLANATION
1. Administer accurately	
a. Use a large vein for the venipuncture site.	To decrease risks of extravasation
b. Dilute drugs for continuous infusion in 250 or 500 mL of intravenous (IV) fluid. A 5% dextrose injection is compatible with all of the drugs and is most often used. For use of other IV fluids, consult drug manufacturers' literature. Dilute drugs for bolus injections to at least 10 mL with sodium chloride or water for injection.	To avoid adverse effects, which are more likely to occur with concentrated drug solutions
c. Use a separate IV line or a "piggyback" IV setup.	This allows the adrenergic drug solution to be regulated or discontinued without disruption of other IV lines.
d. Use an infusion pump	To administer the drug at a consistent rate. This helps to prevent wide fluctuations in blood pressure and other cardiovascular functions.
e. Discard any solution with a brownish color or precipitate.	Most of the solutions are stable for 24–48 h. Epinephrine and isoproterenol decompose on exposure to light, producing a brownish discoloration.
f. Start the adrenergic drug slowly, and increase as necessary to obtain desired responses in blood pressure and other parameters of cardiovascular function.	Flow rate (dosage) is titrated according to client response.
g. Stop the drug gradually.	Abrupt discontinuance of pressor drugs may cause rebound hypotension.
h. Treat the client, not the monitor.	Abnormal monitor readings (ie, blood pressure monitors) should be confirmed with a manual reading before making a medication dosage adjustment.
2. Observe for therapeutic effects	
a. Systolic blood pressure of 80–100 mm Hg	These levels are adequate for tissue perfusion. Higher levels may increase cardiac workload, resulting in reflex bradycardia and decreased cardiac output. However, higher levels may be necessary to maintain cerebral blood flow in older adults.
b. Heart rate of 60–100, improved quality of peripheral pulses	These indicate improved tissue perfusion and cardiovascular function.
c. Improved urine output	Increased urine output indicates improved blood flow to the kidneys.
d. Improved skin color and temperature	These indicate improved peripheral tissue perfusion.
e. Pulmonary capillary wedge pressure between 15 and 20 mm Hg in cardiogenic shock	Normal pulmonary capillary wedge pressure is 6–12 mm Hg. Higher levels are required to maintain cardiac output in cardiogenic shock.
3. Observe for adverse effects	
a. Bradycardia	Reflex bradycardia may occur with norepinephrine, metaraminol, and phenylephrine.

(continued)

NURSING ACTIONS	RATIONALE/EXPLANATION
b. Tachycardia	This is most likely to occur with isoproterenol, but may occur with dopamine and epinephrine.
c. Arrhythmias	Serious arrhythmias may occur with any of the agents used in hypotension and shock. Causes may include high doses that result in excessive adrenergic stimulation of the heart, low doses that result in inadequate perfusion of the myocardium, or the production of lactic acid by ischemic tissue.
d. Hypertension	This is most likely to occur with high doses of norepinephrine, metaraminol, and phenylephrine.
e. Hypotension	This is most likely to occur with low doses of dopamine and isoproterenol, owing to vasodilation.
f. Angina pectoris—chest pain, dyspnea, palpitations	All pressor agents may increase myocardial oxygen consumption and induce myocardial ischemia.
g. Tissue necrosis if extravasation occurs	This may occur with extravasation of solutions containing dopamine, norepinephrine, metaraminol, and phenylephrine, owing to local vasoconstriction and impaired blood supply. Tissue necrosis may be prevented by injecting 5–10 mg of phentolamine (Regitine), subcutaneously, around the area of extravasation. Regitine is most effective if injected within 12 h after extravasation.
4. Observe for drug interactions	
a. Drugs that *increase* effects of pressor agents:	
(1) General anesthetics (eg, halothane)	Halothane and other halogenated anesthetics increase cardiac sensitivity to sympathomimetic drugs and increase the risks of cardiac arrhythmias.
(2) Anticholinergic drugs (eg, atropine)	Atropine and other drugs with anticholinergic activity may potentiate the tachycardia that often occurs with pressor agents, especially isoproterenol.
(3) Monoamine oxidase (MAO) inhibitors (eg, tranylcypromine)	All effects of exogenously administered adrenergic drugs are magnified in clients taking MAO inhibitors because MAO is the circulating enzyme responsible for metabolism of adrenergic agents.
(4) Oxytocics (eg, oxytocin)	The risk of severe hypertension is increased.
b. Drugs that *decrease* effects of pressor agents:	
(1) Beta-blocking agents (eg, propranolol)	Beta-blocking agents antagonize the cardiac stimulation produced by some pressor agents (eg, dobutamine, isoproterenol). Decreased heart rate, myocardial contractility, and blood pressure may result.

Nursing Notes: Apply Your Knowledge

Answer: Vital signs should be continuously monitored for clients in the ICU. Systolic blood pressure should be kept between 80 and 100 mm Hg. This provides adequate pressure to perfuse vital organs with blood. Using drugs to raise the blood pressure to significantly higher levels may increase the workload of the heart. For the ICU client experiencing shock, pulmonary capillary wedge pressures are often monitored. Normal values are 6 to 12 mm Hg, but they may need to be higher for the client in cardiogenic shock. Pulse rates should normalize between 60 and 100, with a regular rhythm. Urine output should be monitored at least hourly. An output of 30 mL/hour indicates adequate perfusion to the kidneys. Improved skin color and temperature, lack of diaphoresis, and alert mental status all indicate adequate organ and tissue perfusion.

How Can You Avoid This Medication Error?

Answer: Considering that extravasation of this medication can cause very significant tissue damage, this was a very poor decision. IV medications sometimes infuse at very slow rates, so that swelling is not present when the IV solution has infiltrated. It is the responsibility of the nurse to be knowledgeable concerning which drugs are vesicants and take special precautions. Vasopressor agents significantly constrict the vessels of the surrounding tissue, thus impeding blood flow and causing necrosis. Whenever possible, infuse these medications into central lines. When extravasation occurs, phentolamine (Regitine), an alpha adrenergic blocker, can be injected into the tissue to reverse vasoconstriction and restore blood flow.

 REVIEW AND APPLICATION EXERCISES

1. How do adrenergic drugs improve circulation in hypotension and shock?

2. Which adrenergic drug should be readily available for treatment of anaphylactic shock?

3. What are major adverse effects of adrenergic drugs?

4. How would you assess the client for therapeutic or adverse effects of an adrenergic drug being given by continuous IV infusion?

5. Why is it important to prevent extravasation of adrenergic drug infusions into tissues surrounding the vein?

6. In hypovolemic shock, should fluid volume be replaced before or after an adrenergic drug is given? Why?

SELECTED REFERENCES

Bailey, J.M., Miller, B.E., Lu, W., Kanter, K.R., & Tam, V.K. (1999). The pharmacokinetics of milrinone in pediatric patients after cardiac surgery. *Anesthesiology, 90*, 1012–1018.

Benowitz, N.L. (1999). Therapeutic drugs and antidotes: Epinephrine. In K.R. Olson (Ed.), *Poisoning and drug overdose*, 3rd ed., pp. 365–366. Stamford, CT: Appleton & Lange.

Dax, J.M. & Hermey, C.L. (2000). Shock and multiple organ dysfunction syndrome. In S.M. Lewis, M.M. Heitkemper, & S.R. Dirksen (Eds.), *Medical-surgical nursing: Assessment and management of clinical problems*, 5th ed., pp 1865–1894. St. Louis: Mosby.

Hatzizacharias, A., Makris, T., Krespi, P., Triposkiadis, F., Voyatzi, P., Dalianis, N., & Kyriakidis, M. (1999). Intermittent milrinone effect on long-term hemodynamic profile in patients with severe congestive heart failure. *American Heart Journal, 138*, 241–246.

Hoffman, B.B. & Lefkowitz, R.J. (1996). Catecholamines, sympathomimetic drugs, and adrenergic receptor antagonists. In J.G. Hardman, L.E. Limbird, P.B. Molinoff, & R.W. Ruddon (Eds.), *Goodman & Gilman's The pharmacological basis of therapeutics*, 9th ed., pp. 199–248. New York: McGraw-Hill.

Karch, A.M. (2000). *Lippincott's 2000 nursing drug guide*. Philadelphia: Lippincott Williams & Wilkins.

Perdue, P.W., Blaser, J.R., Lipsett, P.A., & Breslow, M.J. (1998). "Renal dose" dopamine in surgical patients: Dogma or science? *Annals of Surgery, 227*, 470–473.

Sypniewski, E., Jr. (1997). Hypovolemic and cardiogenic shock. In J.T. DiPiro, R.L. Talbert, G.C. Yee, G.R. Matzke, B.G. Wells, & L.M. Posey (Eds.), *Pharmacotherapy: A pathophysiologic approach*, 3rd ed., pp. 509–541. Stamford, CT: Appleton & Lange.

Urban, N. (1998). Heart failure and circulatory shock. In C.M. Porth (Ed.), *Pathophysiology: Concepts of altered health states*, 5th ed., pp. 427–456. Philadelphia: Lippincott Williams & Wilkins.

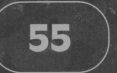

55

Antihypertensive Drugs

Objectives

After studying this chapter, the student will be able to:

1. Describe factors that control blood pressure.

2. Define/describe hypertension.

3. Identify clients at risk for development of hypertension and its sequelae.

4. Discuss nonpharmacologic measures to control hypertension.

5. Review the effects of alpha-adrenergic blockers, beta-adrenergic blockers, and calcium channel blockers in hypertension.

6. Discuss angiotensin-converting enzyme inhibitors and angiotensin II receptor antagonists in terms of mechanisms of action, indications for use, adverse effects, and nursing process implications.

7. Describe the rationale for using combination drugs in the treatment of hypertension.

8. Discuss interventions to increase therapeutic effects and minimize adverse effects of antihypertensive drugs.

9. Discuss the use of antihypertensive drugs in special populations.

Wally Ramos, a 36-year-old man, returns to the clinic for his third blood pressure check. Because his blood pressure is still elevated (178/96), the physician decides to start him on an angiotensin-converting enzyme inhibitor, captopril. He states, "I just can't believe I have high blood pressure. I feel just fine. I have heard stories that these medications have lots of undesirable side effects."

Reflect on:

▶ An appropriate teaching plan discussing hypertension and its effects.

▶ An appropriate teaching plan discussing non-pharmacologic strategies to decrease blood pressure.

▶ How you will address Mr. Ramos' concerns about potential side effects.

▶ Factors that could affect compliance with anti-hypertensive therapy.

Antihypertensive drugs are used to treat hypertension, a common, chronic disorder affecting an estimated 50 to 60 million adults and an unknown number of children and adolescents in the United States. Hypertension increases risks of myocardial infarction, heart failure, cerebral infarction and hemorrhage, and renal disease. To understand hypertension and antihypertensive drug therapy, it is necessary first to understand the physiologic mechanisms that normally control blood pressure, characteristics of hypertension, and characteristics of antihypertensive drugs.

REGULATION OF ARTERIAL BLOOD PRESSURE

Arterial blood pressure reflects the force exerted on arterial walls by blood flow. Blood pressure normally stays relatively constant because of homeostatic mechanisms that adjust blood flow to meet tissue needs. The two major determinants of arterial blood pressure are cardiac output (systolic pressure) and peripheral vascular resistance (diastolic pressure).

Cardiac output equals the product of the heart rate and stroke volume (CO = HR × SV). Stroke volume is the amount of blood ejected with each heartbeat (approximately 60 to 90 mL). Thus, cardiac output depends on the force of myocardial contraction, blood volume, and other factors. Peripheral vascular resistance is determined by local blood flow and the degree of constriction or dilation in arterioles and arteries (vascular tone).

Autoregulation of Blood Flow

Autoregulation is the ability of body tissues to regulate their own blood flow. Local blood flow is regulated mainly by nutritional needs of the tissue, such as lack of oxygen or accumulation of products of cellular metabolism (eg, carbon dioxide, lactic acid). Local tissues can form vasodilating and vasoconstricting substances to reg-

ulate local blood flow. Important tissue factors include histamine, bradykinin, serotonin, and prostaglandins.

Histamine is found mainly in mast cells surrounding blood vessels and released when these tissues are injured. In some tissues, such as skeletal muscle, mast cell activity is mediated by the sympathetic nervous system (SNS) and histamine is released when SNS stimulation is blocked or withdrawn. In this case, vasodilation results from increased histamine release and the withdrawal of SNS vasoconstrictor activity. *Bradykinin* is released from a protein in body fluids. It dilates arterioles, increases capillary permeability, and constricts venules. *Serotonin* is released from aggregating platelets during blood coagulation. It causes vasoconstriction and plays a major role in control of bleeding. *Prostaglandins* are formed in response to tissue injury and include vasodilators (eg, prostacyclin) and vasoconstrictors (eg, thromboxane A$_2$).

An important component of regulating local blood flow is the production of several vasoactive substances by the endothelial cells that line blood vessels. Vasoconstricting substances, which increase vascular tone and blood pressure, include angiotensin II, endothelin-1, and thromboxane A$_2$. Vasodilating substances, which decrease vascular tone and blood pressure, include nitric oxide and prostacyclin. Excessive vasoconstrictors or deficient vasodilators may contribute to the development of atherosclerosis, hypertension, and other diseases. Injury to the endothelial lining of blood vessels (eg, by the shear force of blood flow with hypertension or by rupture of atherosclerotic plaque) leads to vasoconstriction, vasospasm, thrombus formation, and thickening of the blood vessel wall. All of these factors make the blood flow through a narrow lumen and increase peripheral vascular resistance.

Overall, regulation of blood pressure involves a complex, interacting, overlapping network of hormonal, neural, and vascular mechanisms, and any condition that affects heart rate, stroke volume, or peripheral vascular resistance affects arterial blood pressure. Many of these mechanisms are compensatory effects that try to restore balance when hypotension or hypertension occurs. The mechanisms are further described in Box 55-1 and referred to in the following discussion of antihypertensive drugs and their actions in lowering high blood pressure.

BOX 55-1   MECHANISMS THAT REGULATE BLOOD PRESSURE

Neural
Neural regulation of blood pressure mainly involves the sympathetic nervous system (SNS). In the heart, SNS neurons control heart rate and force of contraction. In blood vessels, SNS neurons control muscle tone by maintaining a state of partial contraction, with additional constriction or dilation accomplished by altering this basal state. When hypotension and inadequate tis-

sue perfusion occur, the SNS is activated and produces secretion of epinephrine and norepinephrine by the adrenal medulla, constriction of blood vessels in the skin, gastrointestinal tract, and kidneys, and stimulation of beta-adrenergic receptors in the heart, which increases heart rate and force of myocardial contraction. All of these mechanisms act to increase blood pressure and tissue perfusion, especially of the brain and heart.

(continued)

BOX 55–1   **MECHANISMS THAT REGULATE BLOOD PRESSURE** (*continued*)

The SNS is activated by the vasomotor center in the brain, which constantly receives messages from baroreceptors and chemoreceptors located in the circulatory system. Adequate function of these receptors is essential for rapid and short-term regulation of blood pressure. The vasomotor center interprets the messages from these receptors and modifies cardiovascular functions to maintain adequate blood flow.

More specifically, baroreceptors detect changes in pressure or stretch. For example, when a person moves from a lying to a standing position, blood pressure falls and decreases stretch in the aorta and arteries. This elicits increased heart rate and vasoconstriction to restore adequate circulation. The increased heart rate occurs rapidly and blood pressure is adjusted within a minute or two. This quick response prevents orthostatic hypotension with dizziness and possible syncope. (Antihypertensive medications may blunt this response and cause orthostatic hypotension.)

Chemoreceptors, which are located in the aorta and carotid arteries, are in close contact with arterial blood and respond to changes in the oxygen, carbon dioxide, and hydrogen ion content of blood. Although their main function is to regulate ventilation, they also communicate with the vasomotor center and can induce vasoconstriction. Chemoreceptors are stimulated when blood pressure drops to a certain point because oxygen is decreased and carbon dioxide and hydrogen ions are increased in arterial blood.

The central nervous system (CNS) also regulates vasomotor tone and blood pressure. Inadequate blood flow to the brain can cause ischemia of the vasomotor center. When this happens, neurons in the vasomotor center stimulate widespread vasoconstriction in an attempt to raise blood pressure and restore blood flow. This reaction is called the CNS ischemic response, an emergency measure to preserve blood flow to vital brain centers. If blood flow is not restored within approximately 3 to 10 minutes, the neurons of the vasomotor center are unable to function, the impulses that maintain vascular muscle tone stop, and blood pressure drops to a fatal level.

Hormonal

The renin-angiotensin-aldosterone (RAA) system and vasopressin are important hormonal mechanisms in blood pressure regulation.

The *RAA system* is activated in response to hypotension and acts as a compensatory mechanism to restore adequate blood flow to body tissues. Renin is an enzyme that is synthesized, stored, and released from the kidneys in response to decreased blood pressure,

SNS stimulation, or decreased sodium concentration in extracellular fluid. When released into the bloodstream, where its action lasts approximately 30 to 60 minutes, renin converts a plasma protein (angiotensinogen) to angiotensin I. Then, angiotensin-converting enzyme (ACE) in the endothelium of pulmonary blood vessels acts on angiotensin I to produce angiotensin II. Angiotensin II strongly constricts arterioles (and weakly constricts veins), increases peripheral resistance, and increases blood pressure by direct vasoconstriction, stimulation of the SNS, and stimulation of catecholamine release from the adrenal medulla. It also stimulates secretion of aldosterone from the adrenal cortex, which then causes the kidneys to retain sodium and water. Retention of sodium and water increases blood volume, cardiac output, and blood pressure. *Vasopressin*, also called antidiuretic hormone or ADH, is a hormone from the posterior pituitary gland that regulates reabsorption of water by the kidneys. It is released in response to decreased blood volume and decreased blood pressure. It causes retention of body fluids and vasoconstriction, both of which act to raise blood pressure.

Vascular

The endothelial cells that line blood vessels synthesize and secrete several substances that play important roles in regulating cardiovascular functions, including blood pressure. These substances normally maintain a balance between vasoconstriction and vasodilation. When the endothelium is damaged (eg, by trauma, hypertension, hypercholesterolemia, or atherosclerosis), the resulting imbalance promotes production of vasoconstricting substances and also causes blood vessels to lose their ability to relax in response to dilator substances. In addition, changes in structure of endothelial and vascular smooth muscle cells (vascular remodeling, see later) further impair vascular functions.

Vasoconstrictors increase vascular tone (ie, constrict or narrow blood vessels so that higher blood pressure is required to pump blood to body tissues). Vasoconstricting substances produced by the endothelium include angiotensin II, endothelin-1, platelet-derived growth factor (PDGF), and thromboxane A_2. Endothelin-1 is the strongest endogenous vasoconstrictor known. Angiotensin II and thromboxane A_2 can also be produced by other types of cells, but endothelial cells can produce both. Thromboxane A_2, a product of arachidonic acid metabolism, also promotes platelet aggregation and thrombosis.

Vasodilators decrease vascular tone and blood pressure. Major vasodilating substances produced by the

(*continued*)

BOX 55–1 MECHANISMS THAT REGULATE BLOOD PRESSURE (*continued*)

endothelium include nitric oxide (NO) and prostacyclin (prostaglandin I_2)

NO is a gas that can diffuse through cell membranes, trigger biochemical reactions, and then dissipate rapidly. It is formed by the action of the enzyme nitric oxide synthase on the amino acid L-arginine and continually released by normal endothelium. Its production is tightly regulated and depends on the amount of ionized calcium in the fluid portion of endothelial cells. Several substances (eg, acetylcholine, bradykinin, catecholamines, substance P, and products of aggregating platelets such as adenosine diphosphate and serotonin) act on receptors in endothelial cell membranes to increase the cytosolic concentration of ionized calcium, activate nitric oxide synthase, and increase NO production. In addition, increased blood flow or blood pressure increases shear stress at the endothelial surface and stimulates production of NO.

Once produced, endothelium-derived NO produces vasodilation primarily by activating guanylyl cyclase in vascular smooth muscle cells and increasing intracellular cyclic 3,5′-guanosine monophosphate as a second messenger. NO also inhibits platelet aggregation and production of platelet-derived vasoconstricting substances. Because NO is released into the vessel wall (to relax smooth muscle) and into the vessel lumen (to inactivate platelets), it is thought to have protective effects against vasoconstriction and thrombosis.

NO is also produced in leukocytes, fibroblasts, and vascular smooth muscle cells and may have pathologic effects when large amounts are produced. In these tissues, nitric oxide seems to have other functions, such as modifying nerve activity in the nervous system.

Prostacyclin is synthesized and released from endothelium in response to stimulation by several factors (eg, bradykinin, interleukin-1, serotonin, thrombin, PDGF). It produces vasodilation by activating adenylyl cyclase and increasing levels of cyclic adenosine monophosphate in smooth muscle cells. In addition, like NO, prostacyclin also inhibits platelet aggregation and production of platelet-derived vasoconstricting substances. The vasodilating effects of prostacyclin may occur independently or in conjunction with NO.

Overall, excessive vasoconstrictors or deficient vasodilators may contribute to the development of atherosclerosis, hypertension, and other diseases. Injury to the endothelial lining of blood vessels (eg, by the shear force of blood flow with hypertension or by rupture of atherosclerotic plaque) decreases vasodilators and leads to vasoconstriction, vasospasm, thrombus formation, and thickening of the blood vessel wall. All of these factors require the blood to flow through a narrowed lumen and increase blood pressure.

Vascular Remodeling

Vascular remodeling is similar to the left ventricular remodeling that occurs in heart failure (see Chap. 51). It results from endothelial dysfunction and produces a thickening of the blood vessel wall and a narrowing of the blood vessel lumen. Thickening of the wall makes blood vessels less flexible and less able to respond to vasodilating substances. There are also changes in endothelial cell structure (ie, the connections between endothelial cells become looser) that lead to increased permeability. The mechanisms of these vascular changes, which promote and aggravate hypertension, are described below.

As discussed in previous chapters, normal endothelium helps maintain a balance between vasoconstriction and vasodilation, procoagulation and anticoagulation, proinflammation and anti-inflammation, and progrowth and antigrowth. In the inflammatory process, normal endothelium acts as a physical barrier against the movement of leukocytes into the subendothelial space. Endothelial products such as NO may also inhibit leukocyte activity. However, inflammatory cytokines such as tumor necrosis factor-alpha and interleukin-1 activate endothelial cells to produce adhesion molecules (which allow leukocytes to adhere to the endothelium), interleukin-8 (which attracts leukocytes to the endothelium and allows them to accumulate in subendothelial cells), and foam cells (lipid-filled monocyte/macrophages that form fatty streaks, the beginning lesions of atherosclerotic plaque). Although activation of endothelial cells may be a helpful component of the normal immune response, the resulting inflammation may contribute to disease development.

In terms of cell growth, normal endothelium limits the growth of vascular smooth muscle that underlies the endothelium and forms the vessel wall. Growth-inhibiting products of the endothelium include NO, which also inhibits platelet activation and production of growth-promoting substances. When the endothelium is damaged, endothelial cells become activated and also produce growth-promoting products. Other endothelial products (eg, angiotensin II and endothelin-1) may also stimulate growth of vascular smooth muscle cells. Thus, damage or loss of endothelial cells stimulates growth of smooth muscle cells in the intimal layer of the blood vessel wall.

Response to Hypotension

When hypotension (and decreased tissue perfusion) occurs, the SNS is stimulated, the hormones epinephrine and norepinephrine are secreted by the adrenal medulla, angiotensin II and aldosterone are formed, and the kidneys retain fluid. These compensatory mechanisms raise the blood pressure. Specific effects include the following:

1. Constriction of arterioles, which increases peripheral vascular resistance
2. Constriction of veins and increased venous tone
3. Stimulation of cardiac beta-adrenergic receptors, which increases heart rate and force of myocardial contraction
4. Activation of the renin-angiotensin-aldosterone mechanism

Response to Hypertension

When arterial blood pressure is elevated, the following sequence of events occurs:

1. Kidneys excrete more fluid (increase urine output).
2. Fluid loss reduces both extracellular fluid volume and blood volume.
3. Decreased blood volume reduces venous blood flow to the heart and therefore decreases cardiac output.
4. Decreased cardiac output reduces arterial blood pressure.
5. The vascular endothelium produces vasodilating substances (eg, nitric oxide, prostacyclin), which reduce blood pressure.

HYPERTENSION

Hypertension is persistently high blood pressure that results from abnormalities in regulatory mechanisms. It is usually defined as a systolic pressure above 140 mm Hg or a diastolic pressure above 90 mm Hg on multiple blood pressure measurements.

Primary or essential hypertension (that for which no cause can be found) makes up 90% to 95% of known cases. Secondary hypertension may result from renal, endocrine, or central nervous system disorders and from drugs that stimulate the SNS or cause retention of sodium and water. Primary hypertension can be controlled with appropriate therapy; secondary hypertension can sometimes be cured by surgical therapy.

The Sixth Report of the Joint National Committee on Detection, Evaluation, and Treatment of High Blood Pressure, published in 1997, classified blood pressures in adults (in mm of Hg), as follows:

- Normal = systolic 130 or below; diastolic 85 or below
- High normal = systolic 130 to 139; diastolic 85 to 89

- Stage 1 hypertension (mild) = systolic 140 to 159; diastolic 90 to 99
- Stage 2 hypertension (moderate) = systolic 160 to 179; diastolic 100 to 109
- Stage 3 hypertension (severe) = systolic 180 to 209; diastolic 110 to 119
- Stage 4 hypertension (very severe) = systolic 210 or above; diastolic 120 or above

A systolic pressure of 140 or above with a diastolic pressure below 90 is usually called isolated systolic hypertension.

Hypertension profoundly alters cardiovascular function by increasing the workload of the heart and causing thickening and sclerosis of arterial walls. As a result of increased cardiac workload, the myocardium hypertrophies as a compensatory mechanism. However, heart failure eventually occurs. As a result of endothelial dysfunction and arterial changes (vascular remodeling), the arterial lumen is narrowed, blood supply to tissues is decreased, and risks of thrombosis are increased. In addition, necrotic areas may develop in arteries, and these may rupture with sustained high blood pressure. The areas of most serious damage are the heart, brain, kidneys, and eyes. These are often called *target organs*.

Initially and perhaps for years, primary hypertension may produce no symptoms. If symptoms occur, they are usually vague and nonspecific. Hypertension may go undetected, or it may be incidentally discovered when blood pressure measurements are taken as part of a routine physical examination, screening test, or assessment of other disorders. Eventually, symptoms reflect target organ damage. Not infrequently, hypertension is discovered after a person experiences angina pectoris, myocardial infarction, heart failure, stroke, or renal disease.

Hypertensive emergencies are episodes of severely elevated blood pressure that may be an extension of malignant (rapidly progressive) hypertension or caused by cerebral hemorrhage, dissecting aortic aneurysm, renal disease, pheochromocytoma, or eclampsia. These require immediate treatment, usually intravenous (IV) antihypertensive drugs, to lower blood pressure. Symptoms include severe headache, nausea, vomiting, visual disturbances, neurologic disturbances, disorientation, and decreased level of consciousness (drowsiness, stupor, coma). Hypertensive urgencies are episodes of less severe hypertension often managed with oral drugs. The goal of treatment is to lower blood pressure within 24 hours. In most instances, it is better to lower blood pressure gradually (rather than precipitously) and to avoid wide fluctuations in blood pressure.

ANTIHYPERTENSIVE DRUGS

Drugs used in the treatment of primary hypertension belong to several different groups, including angiotensin-converting enzyme (ACE) inhibitors, angiotensin II receptor antagonists (AIIRAs), antiadrenergics, calcium channel blockers, diuretics, and direct vasodilators. In general, these drugs act to decrease blood pressure by decreasing cardiac output or peripheral vascular resistance.

Angiotensin-Converting Enzyme Inhibitors

Angiotensin-converting enzyme (also called kininase) is mainly located in the endothelial lining of blood vessels, and this is where most angiotensin II is produced. This same enzyme also metabolizes bradykinin, an endogenous substance with strong vasodilating properties.

ACE inhibitors block the enzyme that normally converts angiotensin I to the potent vasoconstrictor angiotensin II. By blocking production of angiotensin II, the drugs decrease vasoconstriction (thereby having a vasodilating effect) and decrease aldosterone production (thereby reducing retention of sodium and water). In addition to inhibiting formation of angiotensin II, the drugs also inhibit the breakdown of bradykinin, thereby prolonging its vasodilating effects. These effects and possibly others help to prevent or reverse the remodeling of heart muscle and blood vessel walls that impairs cardiovascular function and exacerbates cardiovascular disease processes. Because of their effectiveness in hypertension and beneficial effects on the heart, blood vessels, and kidneys, these drugs are increasing in importance, number, and use. Widely used to treat heart failure and hypertension, the drugs may also decrease morbidity and mortality in other cardiovascular disorders. For example, they improve survival in clients post-myocardial infarction when added to standard therapy of aspirin, a beta blocker, and a thrombolytic.

ACE inhibitors may be used alone or in combination with other antihypertensive agents, such as thiazide diuretics. Although the drugs can cause or aggravate proteinuria and renal damage in nondiabetic people, they decrease proteinuria and slow the development of nephropathy in diabetic clients.

Most ACE inhibitors (captopril, enalapril, fosinopril, lisinopril, ramipril, and quinapril) also are used in the treatment of heart failure because they decrease peripheral vascular resistance, cardiac workload, and ventricular remodeling. Captopril is also indicated for the treatment of diabetic nephropathy, in which it slows progression of renal impairment. Captopril's "renal protective" effects are thought to be greater than its antihypertensive effects because other antihypertensive agents do not slow nephropathy. Although other ACE inhibitors are not approved by the Food and Drug Administration for this indication, presumably they would have similar effects.

ACE inhibitors are well absorbed with oral administration, produce effects within 1 hour that last approximately 24 hours, have prolonged serum half-lives with impaired renal function, and most are metabolized to active metabolites that are excreted in urine and feces. These drugs are

well tolerated, with a low incidence of serious adverse effects (eg, neutropenia, agranulocytosis, proteinuria, glomerulonephritis, and angioedema). However, a persistent cough develops in approximately 10% to 20% of clients and may lead to stopping the drug. Also, acute hypotension may occur when an ACE inhibitor is started, especially in clients with fluid volume deficit. This reaction may be prevented by starting with a low dose, taken at bedtime, or by stopping diuretics and reducing dosage of other antihypertensive drugs temporarily. Hyperkalemia may develop in clients who have diabetes mellitus or renal impairment or who are taking nonsteroidal anti-inflammatory drugs, potassium supplements, or potassium-sparing diuretics.

These drugs are contraindicated during pregnancy because serious illnesses, including renal failure, have been identified in neonates whose mothers took an ACE inhibitor during the second and third trimesters.

Angiotensin II Receptor Antagonists

Angiotensin II receptor antagonists were developed to block the strong blood pressure–raising effects of angiotensin II. Instead of decreasing production of angiotensin II, as the ACE inhibitors do, these drugs compete with angiotensin II for tissue binding sites and prevent angiotensin II from combining with its receptors in body tissues. Although multiple types of receptors have been identified, the AT1 receptors located in brain, renal, myocardial, vascular, and adrenal tissue determine most of the effects of angiotensin II on cardiovascular and renal functions. AIIRAs block the angiotensin II AT1 receptors and decrease arterial blood pressure by decreasing systemic vascular resistance (Fig. 55-1).

These drugs are similar to ACE inhibitors in their effects on blood pressure and hemodynamics and are as effective as ACE inhibitors in the treatment of hypertension and probably heart failure. They do not cause a cough and are less likely to cause hyperkalemia than ACE inhibitors. Overall, the drugs are well tolerated, and the incidence of most adverse effects is similar to that of placebo.

Losartan, the first AIIRA, is readily absorbed and rapidly metabolized by the cytochrome P450 liver enzymes to an active metabolite. Both losartan and the metabolite are highly bound to plasma albumin, and losartan has a shorter duration of action than its metabolite. When losartan therapy is started, maximal effects on blood pressure usually occur within 3 to 6 weeks. If losartan alone does not control blood pressure, a low dose of a diuretic may be added. A combination product with 50 mg of losartan and 12.5 mg of hydrochlorothiazide is available.

Antiadrenergics

Antiadrenergic (sympatholytic) drugs inhibit activity of the SNS. When the SNS is stimulated (see Chap. 17), the

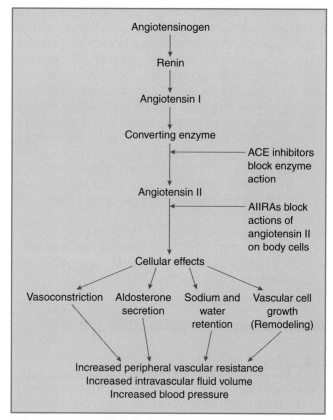

FIGURE 55–1 Angiotensin-converting enzyme inhibitors inhibit angiotensin-converting enzyme and thereby prevent formation of angiotensin II; angiotensin II receptor antagonists (AIIRAs) prevent angiotensin II from connecting with its receptors and thereby prevent it from acting on body tissues containing those receptors (eg, blood vessels, adrenal cortex).

nerve impulse travels from the brain and spinal cord to the ganglia. From the ganglia, the impulse travels along postganglionic fibers to effector organs (eg, heart, blood vessels). Although SNS stimulation produces widespread effects in the body, the effects relevant to this discussion are the increases in heart rate, force of myocardial contraction, cardiac output, and blood pressure that occur. When the nerve impulse is inhibited or blocked at any location along its pathway, the result is decreased blood pressure (see Chap. 19).

Alpha$_1$-adrenergic receptor blocking agents (eg, prazosin) dilate blood vessels and decrease peripheral vascular resistance. These drugs can be used alone or in multidrug regimens. One adverse effect, called the *first-dose phenomenon*, involves orthostatic hypotension with palpitations, dizziness, and perhaps syncope 1 to 3 hours after the first dose or an increased dose. To prevent this effect, first doses and first increased doses are taken at bedtime. Another effect, associated with long-term use or higher doses, leads to sodium and fluid retention and a need for concurrent diuretic therapy. Alpha$_2$ receptor agonists (eg, clonidine) stimulate presynaptic alpha$_2$ receptors in the brain. As a result, less norepinephrine is released and sympathetic outflow from the vasomotor center is re-

duced. Stimulation of presynaptic alpha$_2$ receptors peripherally may also contribute to the decreased sympathetic activity. Reduced sympathetic activity leads to decreased cardiac output, heart rate, peripheral vascular resistance, and blood pressure. Chronic use of clonidine and related drugs may result in sodium and fluid retention, especially with higher doses.

Beta-adrenergic blocking agents (eg, propranolol) decrease heart rate, force of myocardial contraction, cardiac output, and renin release from the kidneys. Other antiadrenergic drugs include guanethidine and related drugs, which act at postganglionic nerve endings; and two other alpha blockers (phentolamine and phenoxybenzamine), which occasionally are used in hypertension resulting from catecholamine excess. The latter two drugs are discussed in Chapter 19.

Calcium Channel Blocking Agents

Calcium channel blockers (eg, verapamil) are used for several cardiovascular disorders. Their mechanism of action and use in the treatment of tachyarrhythmias and angina pectoris are discussed in Chapters 52 and 53, respectively. In hypertension, they mainly dilate peripheral arteries and decrease peripheral vascular resistance.

Most of the available drugs are approved for use in hypertension. Nifedipine has been used to treat hypertensive emergencies or urgencies, often by puncturing the capsule and squeezing the contents under the tongue or having the client bite and swallow the capsule. Such use is declining, mainly because of reports of increased morbidity with precipitous lowering of blood pressure with this drug. In addition, nifedipine is not absorbed through oral mucosa and its effects result from the swallowed drug.

Diuretics

Antihypertensive effects of diuretics are usually attributed to sodium and water depletion. In fact, diuretics usually produce the same effects as severe dietary sodium restriction. In many cases of hypertension, diuretic therapy alone may lower blood pressure. When diuretic therapy is begun, blood volume and cardiac output decrease. With long-term administration of a diuretic, cardiac output returns to normal, but there is a persistent decrease in peripheral vascular resistance. This has been attributed to a persistent small reduction in extracellular water and plasma volume, decreased receptor sensitivity to vasopressor substances such as angiotensin, direct arteriolar vasodilation, and arteriolar vasodilation secondary to electrolyte depletion in the vessel wall.

In moderate or severe hypertension that does not respond to a diuretic alone, the diuretic may be continued and another antihypertensive drug added, or monotherapy with a different type of antihypertensive drug may be tried.

The most commonly used diuretics are the thiazides (eg, hydrochlorothiazide). Others are useful in particular circumstances; see Chapter 56 for more information regarding diuretic drugs.

Vasodilators (Direct Acting)

Vasodilator antihypertensive drugs directly relax smooth muscle in blood vessels to cause dilation and decreased peripheral vascular resistance. They also reduce afterload and may be used in treatment of heart failure. Hydralazine and minoxidil act mainly on arterioles; nitroprusside acts on arterioles and venules. These drugs have a limited effect on hypertension when used alone because the vasodilating action that lowers blood pressure also stimulates the SNS and arouses reflexive compensatory mechanisms (vasoconstriction, tachycardia, and increased cardiac output), which raise blood pressure. This effect can be prevented during long-term therapy by also giving a drug that prevents excessive sympathetic stimulation (eg, propranolol). These drugs also cause sodium and water retention, which may be minimized by giving a diuretic concomitantly.

INDIVIDUAL DRUGS

Diuretics are discussed in Chapter 56 and listed in Table 56-1. Antihypertensive agents are shown in Table 55-1; antihypertensive–diuretic combination products are listed in Table 55-2.

NURSING PROCESS

Assessment

Assess the client's condition in relation to hypertension.

- Identify conditions and risk factors that may lead to hypertension. These include:
  - Obesity
  - Elevated serum cholesterol (total and low-density lipoprotein) and triglycerides
  - Cigarette smoking
  - Sedentary lifestyle
  - Family history of hypertension or other cardiovascular disease
  - African-American race
  - Renal disease (eg, renal artery stenosis)
  - Adrenal disease (eg, hypersecretion of aldosterone, pheochromocytoma)
  - Other cardiovascular disorders (eg, atherosclerosis, left ventricular hypertrophy)
  - Diabetes mellitus
  - Oral contraceptives, corticosteroids, appetite suppressants, nasal decongestants, nonsteroidal anti-inflammatory agents
  - Neurologic disorders (eg, brain damage)
- Observe for signs and symptoms of hypertension.
  - Check blood pressure accurately and repeatedly. As a rule, multiple measurements in which systolic pressure is above 140 mm Hg, diastolic pressure is above 90 mm Hg, or both are necessary to establish a diagnosis of hypertension.

    The importance of accurate blood pressure measurements cannot be overemphasized because there are many possibilities for errors. Some ways to improve accuracy and validity include using correct equipment (eg, proper cuff size), having the client rested and in the same position each time blood pressure is measured (eg, sitting or supine with arm at heart level), and using the same arm for repeated measurements.
  - In most cases of early hypertension, elevated blood pressure is the only clinical manifestation. If symptoms do occur, they are usually nonspecific (eg, headache, weakness, fatigue, tachycardia, dizziness, palpitations, epistaxis).
  - Eventually, signs and symptoms occur as target organs are damaged. Heart damage is often reflected as angina pectoris, myocardial infarction, or heart failure. Chest pain, tachycardia, dyspnea, fatigue, and edema may occur. Brain damage may be indicated by transient ischemic attacks or strokes of varying severity with symptoms ranging from syncope to hemiparesis. Renal damage may be reflected by proteinuria, increased blood urea nitrogen (BUN), and increased serum creatinine. Ophthalmoscopic examination may reveal hemorrhages, sclerosis of arterioles, and inflammation of the optic nerve (papilledema). Because arterioles can be visualized in the retina of the eye, damage to retinal vessels may indicate damage to arterioles in the heart, brain, and kidneys.

Nursing Diagnoses

- Decreased Cardiac Output related to disease process or drug therapy
- Anxiety related to fear of myocardial infarction or stroke
- Ineffective Individual Coping related to long-term lifestyle changes and drug therapy
- Noncompliance related to lack of knowledge about hypertension and its management, costs and adverse effects of drug therapy, and psychosocial factors

(*text continues on page 820*)

TABLE 55-1	Antihypertensive Drugs	
	Routes and Dosage Ranges	
Generic/Trade Name	**Adults**	**Children***

Angiotensin-Converting Enzyme (ACE) Inhibitors

Generic/Trade Name	Adults	Children*
Benazepril (Lotensin)	PO 10 mg once daily initially, increased to 40 mg daily if necessary, in one or two doses	
Captopril (Capoten)	PO 25 mg two to three times daily initially, increased after 1–2 wk if necessary to 50 mg two to three times daily, then to 100 mg two to three times daily, then to 150 mg two to three times daily. Maximal dose, 450 mg/d.	Children PO initially 1.5 mg/kg/d in divided doses, q8h; maximum dose 6 mg/kg/d Neonates PO 0.03–0.15 mg/kg/d, q8–24h. Maximum dose, 2 mg/kg/d
Enalapril (Vasotec)	PO 5 mg once daily, increased to 10–40 mg daily, in one or two doses, if necessary	PO 0.15 mg q12–24h
Fosinopril (Monopril)	Same as benazepril, above	
Lisinopril (Prinivil, Zestril)	PO 10 mg once daily, increased to 40 mg if necessary	
Moexipril (Univasc)	PO, initial dose 7.5 mg (3.75 mg for those who have renal impairment or are taking a diuretic). Maintenance dose 7.5–30 mg daily, in one or two divided doses, adjusted according to blood pressure control.	
Quinapril (Accupril)	PO 10 mg once daily initially, increased to 20, 40, or 80 mg daily if necessary, in one or two doses. Wait at least 2 wk between dose increments	
Perindopril (Aceon)	PO 4–16 mg daily, in one or two doses	
Ramipril (Altace)	PO 2.5 mg once daily, increased to 20 mg daily if necessary, in one or two doses	
Trandolapril (Mavik)	PO, initial dose 1 mg once daily (0.5 mg for those who have hepatic or renal impairment or are taking a diuretic; 2 mg for African Americans). Usual maintenance dose 2–4 mg daily, in a single dose, adjusted according to blood pressure control	

Angiotensin II Receptor Antagonists

Generic/Trade Name	Adults	Children*
Candesartan (Atacand)	PO, initial dose 16 mg once daily, increased to a maximum daily dosage of 32 mg in one or two doses	
Irbesartan (Avapro)	PO, initial dose 150 mg once daily, increased up to 300 mg once daily, if necessary	
Losartan (Cozaar)	PO, initial dose 50 mg daily (25 mg for those who have hepatic impairment or are taking a diuretic) Maintenance dose 35–100 mg daily, in a single dose or two divided doses, adjusted according to blood pressure control	
Telmisartan (Micardis)	PO, initial dose 40 mg daily, increased to a maximum of 80 mg daily if necessary	
Valsartan (Diovan)	PO, initially 80 mg daily, when used as monotherapy in clients who are not volume depleted. Maintenance dose increased up to a maximum dose of 320 once daily, if necessary. However, adding a diuretic has better antihypertensive effect than increasing dose beyond 80 mg.	

Antiadrenergic Agents

ALPHA₁-BLOCKING AGENTS

Generic/Trade Name	Adults	Children*
Doxazosin (Cardura)	PO 1 mg once daily initially, increased to 2 mg, then to 4, 8, and 16 mg if necessary	
Prazosin (Minipress)	PO 1 mg two to three times daily initially, increased if necessary to a total daily dose of 20 mg in divided doses. Average maintenance dose, 6–15 mg/d.	
Terazosin (Hytrin)	PO 1 mg at bedtime initially, increased gradually to maintenance dose, usually 1–5 mg once daily	

(continued)

TABLE 55-1 **Antihypertensive Drugs** (*continued*)

	Routes and Dosage Ranges	
Generic/Trade Name	Adults	Children*
ALPHA₂ AGONISTS		
Clonidine (Catapres)	PO 0.1 mg two times daily initially, gradually increased if necessary up to 2.4 mg/d. Average maintenance dose, 0.2–0.8 mg/d.	PO 5–25 µg/kg/d, in divided doses, q6h; increase at 5- to 7-d intervals, if needed
Guanabenz (Wytensin)	PO 4 mg twice daily, increased by 4–8 mg daily every 1–2 wk if necessary to a maximal dose of 32 mg twice daily	
Guanfacine (Tenex)	PO 1 mg daily at bedtime, increased to 2 mg after 3–4 wk, then to 3 mg if necessary	
Methyldopa (Aldomet)	PO 250 mg two or three times daily initially, increased gradually at intervals of not less than 2 d until blood pressure is controlled or a daily dose of 3 g is reached	PO 10 mg/kg/d in two to four divided doses initially, increased or decreased according to response. Maximal dose, 65 mg/kg/d or 3 g daily, whichever is less.
POSTGANGLIONIC-ACTIVE DRUGS		
Guanadrel (Hylorel)	PO 10 mg daily initially. Usual dosage range, 20–75 mg daily in divided doses.	
Guanethidine sulfate (Ismelin)	PO 10 mg daily initially, increased every 5–7 d to a maximal daily dose of 300 mg if necessary. Usual daily dose, 25–50 mg. For hospitalized clients, therapy may be initiated with 25–50 mg daily and increased every 1–2 d.	PO 0.2 mg/kg/d initially, increased by the same amount every 7–10 d if necessary to a maximum dose of 3 mg/kg/d
Reserpine (Serpasil)	PO 0.25-0.5 mg daily initially for 1–2 wk, reduced slowly to 0.1–0.25 mg daily for maintenance	
BETA-ADRENERGIC BLOCKING AGENTS		
Acebutolol (Sectral)	PO 400 mg once daily initially, increased to 800 mg daily if necessary	
Atenolol (Tenormin)	PO 50 mg once daily initially, increased in 1–2 wk to 100 mg once daily, if necessary	
Betaxolol (Kerlone)	PO 10–20 mg daily	
Bisoprolol (Zebeta)	PO 5 mg once daily, increased to a maximum dose of 20 mg daily if necessary	
Carteolol (Cartrol)	PO 2.5 mg once daily initially, gradually increased to a maximum daily dose of 10 mg if necessary. Usual maintenance dose, 2.5–5 mg once daily. Extend dosage interval to 48 h for a creatinine clearance of 20–60 mL/min and to 72 h for a creatinine clearance below 20 mL/min.	
Metoprolol (Lopressor)	PO 50 mg twice daily, gradually increased in weekly or longer intervals if necessary, to maximal daily dose of 450 mg	
Nadolol (Corgard)	PO 40 mg daily initially, gradually increased if necessary, by 40–80 mg daily. Average daily dose, 80–320 mg.	
Penbutolol (Levatol)	PO 20 mg once daily	
Pindolol (Visken)	PO 5 mg two or three times daily initially, increased by 10 mg/d at 3- to 4-wk intervals to a maximal daily dose of 60 mg	
Propranolol (Inderal)	PO 40 mg twice daily initially, gradually increased to 160–640 mg daily	PO 1 mg/kg/d initially, gradually increased to a maximum dose of 10 mg/kg/d
Timolol (Blocadren)	PO 10 mg twice daily initially, increased gradually if necessary. Average daily dose, 20–40 mg; maximal daily dose, 60 mg.	
ALPHA-BETA-ADRENERGIC-BLOCKING AGENTS		
Carvedilol (Coreg)	PO 6.25 mg twice daily for 7–14 d, then increase to 12.5 mg twice daily for 7–14 d, then increase to a maximal dose of 25 mg twice daily if tolerated and needed	
Labetalol (Trandate, Normodyne)	PO 100 mg twice daily, increased by 100 mg twice daily every 2–3 d if necessary. Usual maintenance dose, 200–400 mg twice daily. Severe hypertension may require 1200–2400 mg daily.	

(continued)

TABLE 55-1) **Antihypertensive Drugs** (*continued*)

Generic/Trade Name	Routes and Dosage Ranges	
	Adults	**Children***
	IV injection, 20 mg slowly over 2 min, followed by 40–80 mg every 10 min until the desired blood pressure is achieved or 300 mg has been given. IV infusion, add 200 mg to 250 mL of 5% dextrose or 0.9% sodium chloride solution (concentration 2 mg/3 mL) and infuse at a rate of 3 mL/min. Adjust flow rate according to blood pressure, and substitute oral labetalol when blood pressure is controlled.	
Calcium Channel Blocking Agents		
Amlodipine (Norvasc)	PO 5–10 mg once daily	
Diltiazem (sustained release) (Cardizem SR)	PO 60–120 mg twice daily	
Felodipine (Plendil)	PO 5–10 mg once daily. Extended-release tablets; swallow whole, do not crush or chew.	
Isradipine (DynaCirc)	PO 2.5–5 mg twice daily	
Nicardipine (Cardene, Cardene SR, Cardene IV)	PO 20–40 mg three times daily; sustained-release, PO 30–60 mg twice daily; IV infusion 5–15 mg/h	
Nifedipine (Adalat, Procardia, Procardia XL)	Immediate-release, PO 10 mg for hypertensive crisis (have client bite and swallow capsule); sustained-release, PO 30–60 mg once daily, increased over 1–2 wk if necessary	
Nisoldipine (Sular)	PO, initially 20 mg once daily, increased by 10 mg/wk or longer intervals to a maximum of 60 mg daily. Average maintenance dose, 20–40 mg daily. Adults with liver impairment or >65 y, PO, initially 10 mg once daily	
Verapamil (Calan, Isoptin, Calan SR, Isoptin SR)	Immediate-release, PO 80 mg three times daily; sustained-release, PO 240 mg once daily	
Other Vasodilators		
Fenoldopam (Corlopam)	IV infusion, initial dose based on body weight, then flow rate titrated to achieve desired response. Mix with 0.9% sodium chloride or 5% dextrose to a concentration of 40 μg/mL (eg, 40 mg of drug [4 mL of concentrate] in 1000 mL of IV fluid.	
Hydralazine (Apresoline)	Chronic hypertension, PO 10 mg four times daily for 2–4 d, increased to 25 mg four times daily for 2–4 d if necessary, then increased to 50 mg four times daily if necessary, to a maximal dose of 300 mg/d Hypertensive crisis, IM, IV 10–20 mg, increased to 40 mg if necessary. Repeat dose as needed.	Chronic hypertension, 0.75 mg/kg/d initially in four divided doses. Gradually increased over 3–4 wk to a maximal dose of 7.5 mg/kg/d if necessary Hypertensive crisis, IM, IV 0.1–0.2 mg/kg per dose every 4–6 h as needed
Minoxidil (Loniten)	PO 5 mg once daily initially, increased gradually until blood pressure is controlled. Average daily dose, 10–40 mg; maximal daily dose, 100 mg in single or divided doses	<12 y, PO 0.2 mg/kg/d initially as a single dose, increased gradually until blood pressure is controlled. Average daily dose, 0.25–1.0 mg/kg; maximal dose, 50 mg/d
Sodium nitroprusside (Nipride)	IV infusion at a flow rate to deliver 0.5–10 μg/kg/min. Average dose is 3 μg/kg/min. Prepare solution by adding 50 mg of sodium nitroprusside to 250–1000 mL of 5% dextrose in water, and wrap promptly in aluminum foil to protect from light.	Same as for adults.

IM, intramuscular; IV, intravenous; PO, oral.

*Children's dosages from *Drug Facts and Comparisons* (1996) and the National High Blood Pressure Education Program Working Group on Hypertension Control in Children and Adolescents (1996).

TABLE 55-2 Oral Antihypertensive Combination Products*

	Components						
Trade Name	Angiotensin II Receptor Antagonist	Angiotensin-Converting Enzyme Inhibitor	Beta Blocker	Calcium Channel Blocker	Diuretic	Non–Beta-Blocker Antiadrenergic	Dosage Ranges
Aldoril					HCTZ 15, 25, 30, or 50 mg	Methyldopa 250 or 500 mg	1 tablet two to three times daily for 48 h, then adjusted according to response
Capozide		Captopril 25 or 50 mg			HCTZ 15 or 25 mg		1 tablet two to three times daily
Combipres					Chlorthalidone 15 mg	Clonidine 0.1, 0.2, or 0.3 mg	1 tablet twice daily
Corzide			Nadolol 40 or 80 mg		Bendroflumethiazide 5 mg		1 tablet daily
Diovan HCT	Valsartan 80 or 160 mg				HCTZ 12.5 mg		1 tablet daily
Hyzaar	Losartan 50 mg				HCTZ 12.5 mg		1 tablet once daily
Inderide			Propranolol 40 or 80 mg		HCTZ 25 mg		1–2 tablets twice daily
Inderide LA			Propranolol 80, 120, or 160 mg		HCTZ 50 mg		1 capsule once daily
Lopressor HCT			Metoprolol 50 or 100 mg		HCTZ 25 or 50 mg		1–2 tablets daily
Lotensin HCT		Benazepril 5, 10, or 20 mg			HCTZ 12.5 or 25 mg		1 tablet daily
Lotrel		Benazepril 10 or 20 mg		Amlodipine 2.5 or 5 mg			1 capsule daily
Minizide					Polythiazide 0.5 mg	Prazosin 1, 2, or 5 mg	1 capsule two to three times daily
Prinzide		Lisinopril 20 mg			HCTZ 12.5 or 25 mg		1 tablet daily
Tarka		Trandolapril 1, 2, or 4 mg		Verapamil 180 or 240 mg			1 tablet daily
Tenoretic			Atenolol 50 or 100 mg		Chlorthalidone 25 mg		1 tablet daily
Timolide			Timolol 10 mg		HCTZ 25 mg		1–2 tablets one or two times daily
Vaseretic		Enalapril			HCTZ 25 mg		1–2 tablets daily
Zestoretic		Lisinopril 10 or 20 mg			HCTZ 12.5 or 25 mg		1 tablet daily
Ziac		Bisoprolol 2.5, 5, or 10 mg			HCTZ 6.25 mg		1 tablet daily

HCTZ, hydrochlorothiazide.
*Note that one trade name product may be available in multiple formulations, with variable amounts of antihypertensive, diuretic or both components.

- Body Image Disturbance related to the need for long-term treatment and medical supervision
- Fatigue related to antihypertensive drug therapy
- Knowledge Deficit related to hypertension, antihypertensive drug therapy, and nondrug lifestyle changes
- Sexual Dysfunction related to adverse drug effects
- Risk for Injury related to drug-induced hypotension and dizziness

Planning/Goals

The client will:

- Receive or take antihypertensive drugs correctly
- Be monitored closely for therapeutic and adverse drug effects, especially when drug therapy is started, when changes are made in drugs, and when dosages are increased or decreased
- Use nondrug measures to assist in blood pressure control
- Avoid, manage, or report adverse drug reactions
- Verbalize or demonstrate knowledge of prescribed drugs and recommended lifestyle changes
- Keep follow-up appointments

Interventions

Implement measures to prevent or minimize hypertension. Preventive measures are mainly lifestyle changes to reduce risk factors. These measures should be started in childhood and continued throughout life. Once hypertension is diagnosed, lifetime adherence to a therapeutic regimen may be necessary to control the disease and prevent complications. The nurse's role is important in the prevention, early detection, and treatment of hypertension. Some guidelines for intervention at community, family, and personal levels include the following:

- Participate in programs to promote healthful lifestyles (eg, improving eating habits, increasing exercise, managing stress more effectively, and avoiding cigarette smoking).
- Participate in community screening programs, and make appropriate referrals when abnormal blood pressures are detected. If hypertension develops in women taking oral contraceptives, the drug is usually discontinued for 3 to 6 months to see whether blood pressure decreases without antihypertensive drugs.
- Help the hypertensive client comply with prescribed therapy. Noncompliance is high among clients with hypertension. Reasons often given for noncompliance include lack of symptoms, lack of motivation and self-discipline to make

needed lifestyle changes (eg, lose weight, stop smoking, restrict salt intake), perhaps experiencing more symptoms from medications than from hypertension, the cost of therapy, and the client's failure to realize the importance of treatment, especially as related to prevention of major cardiovascular diseases (myocardial infarction, stroke, and death). In addition, several studies have shown that compliance decreases as the number of drugs and number of doses increase.

The nurse can help increase compliance by teaching the client about hypertension, helping the client make necessary lifestyle changes, and maintaining supportive interpersonal relationships. Losing weight, stopping smoking, and other changes are most likely to be effective if attempted one at a time.

- Use recommended techniques for measuring blood pressure. Poor techniques are too often used (eg, the client's arm up or down rather than at heart level; cuff applied over clothing, too loosely, deflated too rapidly, or reinflated before completely deflated; a regular-sized cuff used on large arms that need a large cuff). It is worrisome to think that antihypertensive drugs may be prescribed and dosages changed on the basis of inaccurate blood pressures.

Evaluation

- Observe for blood pressure measurements within goal or more nearly normal ranges.
- Observe and interview regarding compliance with instructions about drug therapy and lifestyle changes.
- Observe and interview regarding adverse drug effects.

PRINCIPLES OF THERAPY

Therapeutic Regimens

Once the diagnosis of hypertension is established, a therapeutic regimen must be designed and implemented.

The goal of treatment for most clients is to achieve and maintain normal blood pressure range (below 140/90 mm Hg). If this goal cannot be achieved, lowering blood pressure to any extent is still considered beneficial in decreasing the incidence of coronary artery disease and stroke.

The Joint National Committee on Detection, Evaluation, and Treatment of High Blood Pressure recommends a treatment algorithm in which initial interventions are lifestyle modifications (ie, reduction of weight and sodium

CLIENT TEACHING GUIDELINES
Antihypertensive Medications

General Considerations

✔ Hypertension is a major risk factor for heart attack, stroke (sometimes called brain attack), and kidney failure. Although it rarely causes symptoms unless complications occur, it can be controlled by appropriate treatment. Consequently, you need to learn all you can about the disease process, the factors that cause or aggravate it, and its treatment. In few other conditions is your knowledge and understanding about your condition as important as with hypertension.

✔ For many people, lifestyle changes (ie, a diet to avoid excessive salt and control weight and fat intake, regular exercise, and avoiding smoking) may be sufficient to control blood pressure. If drug therapy is prescribed, these measures should be continued.

✔ When drug therapy is needed, your physician will try to choose a drug and develop a regimen that works for you. There are numerous antihypertensive drugs and many can be taken once a day, which makes their use more convenient and less disruptive of your usual activities of daily living. You may need several office visits to find the right drug or combination of drugs and the right dosage. Changes in drugs or dosages may also be needed later, especially if you develop other conditions or take other drugs that alter your response to the antihypertensive drugs.

✔ Antihypertensive drug therapy is usually long term, may require more than one drug, and may produce side effects. You need to know the brand and generic names of any prescribed drugs and how to take each drug for optimal benefit and minimal adverse effects.

✔ Antihypertensive drugs must be taken as prescribed for optimal benefits, even if you do not feel well when a medication is started or when dosage is increased. *No antihypertensive drug should be stopped abruptly.* If problems develop, they should be discussed with the clinician who is treating the hypertension. If treatment is stopped, blood pressure usually increases gradually as the medication(s) are eliminated from the body. Sometimes, however, blood pressure rapidly increases to pretreatment levels or even higher. With any of these situations, you are at risk of a heart attack or stroke. In addition, stopping one drug of a multidrug regimen may lead to increased adverse effects as well as decreased antihypertensive effectiveness. To avoid these problems, antihypertensive drugs should be tapered in dosage and discontinued gradually.

✔ Blood pressure measurements are the only way you can tell if your medication is working. Thus, you may want to monitor your blood pressure at home, especially when starting drug therapy, changing medications, or changing dosages. If so, a blood pressure machine may be purchased at a medical supply store. Follow instructions regarding use, take your blood pressure approximately the same time(s) each day (eg, before morning and evening meals), and keep a record to show to your physician.

✔ People sometimes feel dizzy or faint while taking antihypertensive medications. This usually means your blood pressure drops momentarily and is most likely to occur when you start a medication, increase dosage, or stand up suddenly from a sitting or lying position. This can be prevented or decreased by moving to a standing position slowly, sleeping with the head of the bed elevated, wearing elastic stockings, exercising legs, avoiding prolonged standing, and avoiding hot baths. If episodes still occur, you should sit or lie down to avoid a fall and possible injury.

✔ It is very important to keep appointments for follow-up care.

Self- or Caregiver Administration

✔ Take or give antihypertensive drugs at prescribed time intervals, about the same time each day. For example, take once-daily drugs as close to every 24 hours as you can manage; twice-a-day drugs should be taken every 12 hours. If ordered four times daily, take approximately every 6 hours. Taking doses too close together can increase dizziness, weakness, and other adverse effects. Taking doses too far apart may not control blood pressure adequately and may increase risks of heart attack or stroke.

✔ Take oral captopril on an empty stomach. Food decreases drug absorption.

✔ Take most oral antihypertensive agents with or after food intake to decrease gastric irritation. Candesartan, irbesartan, losartan, telmisartan, and valsartan may be taken with or without food.

✔ With prazosin, doxazosin, or terazosin, take the first dose and the first increased dose at bedtime to prevent dizziness and possible fainting.

✔ With the clonidine skin patch, apply to a hairless area on the upper arm or torso once every 7 days. Rotate sites.

intake, regular physical activity, moderate alcohol intake, and no smoking). If these modifications do not produce goal blood pressure or substantial progress toward goal blood pressure within 3 to 6 months, they should be continued along with an antihypertensive drug. Although the Committee recommends monotherapy (use of one antihypertensive drug) with a diuretic or a beta blocker because research studies demonstrate reduced morbidity and mortality with these agents, a drug from another classification (eg, ACE inhibitors, AIIRAs, calcium channel blockers, alpha₁-adrenergic blockers) may also be used effectively. Studies also indicate decreased cardiovascular morbidity and mortality with ACE inhibitors.

If the initial drug (and dose) does not produce the desired blood pressure, options for further treatment include increasing the drug dose, substituting another drug, or adding a second drug from a different group. If the response is still inadequate, a second or third drug may be added, including a diuretic if not previously prescribed. When current treatment is ineffective, reassess the client's compliance with lifestyle modifications and drug therapy. In addition, review other factors that may be sabotaging the therapeutic regimen, such as over-the-counter appetite suppressants or nasal decongestants, which raise blood pressure.

The World Health Organization and the International Society of Hypertension guidelines for treatment of hypertension include considering age, ethnicity, and concomitant cardiovascular disorders when choosing an antihypertensive drug; starting with a single drug, in the lowest available dose; changing to a drug from a different group, rather than increasing dosage of the first drug or adding a second drug, if the initial drug is ineffective or not well tolerated; and using long-acting drugs (ie, a single dose effective for 24 hours). However, the guidelines also note that many clients require two or more drugs to achieve adequate blood pressure control. When this is the case, fixed-dose combinations may be preferred.

Drug Selection

Because many effective antihypertensive drugs are available, choices depend primarily on client characteristics and responses. Some general guidelines include the following:

1. **Angiotensin-converting enzyme inhibitors** may be effective alone in white hypertensive clients or in combination with a diuretic in African-American hypertensive clients. They are also recommended for hypertensive adults with diabetes mellitus and kidney damage. Based on research studies that indicate reduced morbidity and mortality from cardiovascular diseases, these drugs are increasingly being prescribed as a component of a multidrug regimen.

2. **Angiotensin II receptor antagonists** have therapeutic effects similar to those of ACE inhibitors, with fewer adverse effects. They may be used in most clients with hypertension.

3. **Antiadrenergics** may be effective in any hypertensive population. **Alpha agonists** and **antagonists** are most often used in multidrug regimens for stages 2, 3, or 4 because they may cause postural hypotension and syncope. Clonidine is available in a skin patch that is applied once a week and reportedly reduces adverse effects and increases compliance. An additional advantage of transdermal clonidine is that it can be used by clients who cannot take oral medications. A disadvantage of this system is a delayed onset of effect (2 to 3 days), so other antihypertensive medications must also be given during the first 2 to 3 days of clonidine transdermal therapy. Other disadvantages include cost, a 20% incidence of local skin rash or irritation, and a 2- to 3-day delay in "offset" of action when transdermal therapy is discontinued. **Beta blockers** are the drugs of first choice for clients younger than 50 years of age with high-renin hypertension, tachycardia, angina pectoris, myocardial infarction, or left ventricular hypertrophy. Most beta blockers are approved for use in hypertension and are probably equally effective. However, the cardioselective drugs (see Chap. 19) are preferred for hypertensive clients who also have asthma, peripheral vascular disease, or diabetes mellitus.

4. **Calcium channel blockers** may be used for monotherapy or in combination with other drugs. They may be especially useful for hypertensive clients who also have angina pectoris or other cardiovascular disorders. Note that sustained-release forms of nifedipine, diltiazem, and verapamil and other long-acting drugs (eg, amlodipine, felodipine) are recommended.

5. **Diuretics** are usually preferred for initial therapy in older clients and African-American hypertensive clients. They are usually included in any multidrug regimen for these and other populations. Thiazide and related diuretics are equally effective. Hydrochlorothiazide is commonly used.

6. **Vasodilators** are usually used in combination with a beta blocker and a diuretic to prevent hypotension-induced compensatory mechanisms (stimulation

of the SNS and fluid retention) that raise blood pressure.

7. **Combination products** usually combine two drugs with different mechanisms of action (eg, a thiazide or related diuretic plus a beta blocker or other anti-adrenergic, an ACE inhibitor, an AIIRA, or a calcium channel blocker). Most are available in various formulations (see Table 55-2). Potential advantages of fixed-dose combination products include comparable or improved effectiveness, smaller doses of individual components, fewer adverse effects, improved compliance, and possibly decreased costs.

Dosage Factors

1. Dosage of antihypertensive drugs must be titrated according to individual response. Dosage usually is started at minimal levels and increased if necessary. Lower doses decrease the incidence and severity of adverse effects.

2. For many clients, it may be more beneficial to change drugs or add another drug rather than increase dosage. Two or three drugs in small doses may be effective and cause fewer adverse effects than a single drug in large doses. When two or more drugs are given, the dose of each drug may need to be reduced.

Duration of Therapy

Clients who maintain control of their blood pressure for 1 year or so may be candidates for reduced dosages or reduced numbers of drugs. Any such adjustments must be gradual and carefully supervised by a health care provider. Expected benefits include fewer adverse effects and greater compliance.

Sodium Restriction

Any therapeutic regimen for hypertension includes sodium restriction. Severe restrictions usually are not acceptable to clients; however, moderate restrictions (avoiding heavily salted foods, such as cured meats, sandwich meats, pretzels, and potato chips, and not adding salt to food at the table) are beneficial and more easily implemented. These statements are based on research studies that indicate the following:

1. Sodium restriction alone reduces blood pressure.
2. Sodium restriction potentiates the antihypertensive actions of diuretics and other antihypertensive drugs. Conversely, excessive sodium intake decreases the antihypertensive actions of all antihypertensive drugs. Clients with unrestricted salt intake who are taking thiazides may lose excessive potassium and become hypokalemic.
3. Sodium restriction may decrease dosage requirements of antihypertensive drugs, thereby decreasing the incidence and severity of adverse effects.

Genetic/Ethnic Considerations

For most antihypertensive drugs, there have been few research studies comparing their effects in different genetic or ethnic groups. However, several studies indicate that beta blockers have greater effects in people of Asian heritage compared with their effects in white people. For hypertension, Asians in general need much smaller doses because they metabolize and excrete beta blockers slowly. In African Americans, diuretics are effective and recommended as initial drug therapy; calcium channel blockers, alpha$_1$ receptor blockers, and the alpha–beta blocker labetalol are reportedly equally effective in African-American and white people. ACE inhibitors, some AIIRAs (eg, losartan, telmisartan), and beta blockers are less effective as monotherapy in African Americans. When beta blockers are used, they are usually one component of a multidrug regimen, and higher doses may be required. Overall, African Americans are more likely to have severe hypertension and require multiple drugs.

Use in Surgical Clients

The Joint National Committee on Detection, Evaluation, and Treatment of High Blood Pressure recommends that drug therapy be continued until surgery and restarted as soon as possible after surgery. If clients cannot take drugs orally, parenteral diuretics, antiadrenergic agents, ACE inhibitors, calcium blockers, or vasodilators may be given to avoid the rebound hypertension associated with abrupt discontinuance of some antiadrenergic antihypertensive agents. Transdermal clonidine also may be used. The anesthesiologist and surgeon must be informed about the client's medication status.

Use in Children

Most principles of managing adult hypertension apply to managing childhood and adolescent hypertension; some additional elements include the following:

1. Children may have primary or secondary hypertension, but the incidence is unknown and treatment is not well defined. In recent years, increased blood pressure measurements during routine pediatric examinations have led to the discovery of significant asymptomatic hypertension and the realization that mild elevations in blood pressure are more common

during childhood, especially in adolescents, than previously thought. Hypertension in children and adolescents may indicate underlying disease processes (eg, cardiac, endocrine, renovascular, or renal parenchymal disorders) or the early onset of primary hypertension. Routine blood pressure measurement is especially important for children who are overweight or who have a hypertensive parent. Increased blood pressure in children often correlates with hypertension in young adults.

2. National norms have been established for blood pressure in children and adolescents of comparable age, body size (height and weight), and sex. Normal blood pressure is defined as systolic and diastolic values less than the 90th percentile; hypertension is defined as an average of systolic or diastolic pressures that equals or exceeds the 95th percentile on three or more occasions. Blood pressure values obtained with a child or adolescent should be compared with the norms and recorded in permanent health care records. Multiple accurate measurements are especially important in diagnosing hypertension because blood pressure may be more labile in children and adolescents.

3. Children have a greater incidence of secondary hypertension than adults. In general, the higher the blood pressure and the younger the child, the greater the likelihood of secondary hypertension. Diagnostic tests may be needed to rule out renovascular disease or coarctation of the aorta in those younger than 18 years of age with blood pressure above 140/90 mm Hg and young children with blood pressures above the 95th percentile for their age group. Oral contraceptives may cause secondary hypertension in adolescents.

4. The goals of treatment are to reduce blood pressure to below the 95th percentile and prevent the long-term effects of persistent hypertension. As in adults, prevention of obesity, avoiding excessive sodium intake, and exercise are important nonpharmacologic measures. Obese adolescents who lose weight also lower their blood pressure, especially when they also increase physical activity.

   Most children with secondary hypertension require drug therapy, which should be directed at the cause of hypertension if known. Drug therapy should be cautious and conservative because few studies have been done in children and long-term effects are unknown. The fewest drugs and the lowest doses should be used. Thus, if an initial drug is ineffective, it may be better to give a different single drug than to add a second drug to the regimen.

5. Some guidelines for choosing drugs are as follows:
   a. Beta blockers are used in children of all ages; they should probably be avoided in children with resting pulse rates under 60.
   b. Thiazide diuretics may be used, and they do not commonly produce hyperglycemia, hyper-

uricemia, or hypercalcemia in children as they do in adults.
   c. Angiotensin II receptor antagonists have not been established as safe and effective for use in children younger than 18 years of age.
   d. Although ACE inhibitors have been used to treat hypertension in children, their safety and efficacy have not been established. Most clinical experience has been with captopril, with which hemodynamic effects are stronger and last longer in newborns and young infants than in older children. Also, excessive and prolonged hypotension, with oliguria and seizures, has occurred. In general, captopril should be used in children only when other measures for controlling blood pressure are ineffective. Also, because of teratogenic effects, these drugs should be used very cautiously, if at all, in adolescent girls who may be sexually active.
   e. Calcium channel blockers are used in treating acute and chronic childhood hypertension. With chronic hypertension, immediate-release forms have a short duration of action and require frequent administration, and long-acting forms contain dosages that are not suitable for young children.
   f. Hydralazine seems to be less effective in childhood and adolescent hypertension than in adult disease.

6. Although all clients with primary hypertension need regular supervision and assessment of blood pressure, this is especially important with young children and adolescents because of growth and developmental changes.

Use in Older Adults

Most principles of managing hypertension in other populations apply to older adults (>65 years). In addition, the following factors require consideration:

1. There are basically two types of hypertension in older adults. One is systolic hypertension, in which systolic blood pressure is above 160 mm Hg, but diastolic pressure is below 95 mm Hg or normal. The other type, systolic-diastolic hypertension, involves elevations of both systolic and diastolic pressures.

   Both types increase cardiovascular morbidity and mortality, especially heart failure and stroke, and should be treated.

2. Nonpharmacologic treatments should be tried alone or with drug therapy. For example, weight reduction and moderate sodium restriction may be the initial treatment of choice if the client is hypertensive and overweight.

3. If antihypertensive drug therapy is required, drugs used for younger adults may be used alone or in

combination. A diuretic is usually the drug of first choice in older adults and may be effective alone. ACE inhibitors and calcium channel blocking agents may also be effective as monotherapy; beta blockers are usually less effective as monotherapy. Some ACE inhibitors (eg, lisinopril, ramipril, quinapril, moexipril) or their active metabolites produce higher plasma concentrations in older adults than in younger ones. This is attributed to decreased renal function rather than age itself. Additional guidelines include the following:

a. The goal of drug therapy for systolic-diastolic hypertension is usually a systolic pressure below 140 mm Hg and a diastolic below 90 mm Hg in clients with no other complications. For those with diabetes or renal failure, the goal is a systolic pressure below 130 mm Hg and a diastolic below 85 mm Hg. However, the latter goal may be difficult for most clients to meet because it requires rather stringent lifestyle restrictions and may require two or more antihypertensive drugs.

b. Older adults may be especially susceptible to the adverse effects of antihypertensive drugs because their homeostatic mechanisms are less efficient. For example, if hypotension occurs, the mechanisms that raise blood pressure are less efficient and syncope may occur. In addition, renal and liver function may be reduced, making accumulation of drugs more likely.

c. Initial drug doses should be approximately half of the recommended doses for younger adults, and increases should be smaller and spaced at longer intervals. Lower drug doses (eg, hydrochlorothiazide 12.5 mg daily) are often effective and reduce risks of adverse effects.

d. Blood pressure should be reduced slowly to facilitate adequate blood flow through arteriosclerotic vessels. Rapid lowering of blood pressure may produce cerebral insufficiency (syncope, transient ischemic attacks, stroke).

e. If blood pressure control is achieved and maintained for approximately 6 to 12 months, drug dosage should be gradually reduced, if possible.

Use in Renal Impairment

Antihypertensive drugs are frequently required by clients with renal impairment ranging from mild insufficiency to end-stage failure. A temporary decrease in renal function may occur in these clients when the blood pressure is initially lowered. Guidelines include the following:

1. In hypertensive clients with primary renal disease or diabetic nephropathy, drug therapy may slow progression of renal impairment.

2. Diuretics are usually required because sodium retention is an important element of hypertension in these clients. Thiazides are usually contraindicated because they are ineffective if serum creatinine is above 2 mg/dL. However, metolazone, a thiazide-related drug, may be used and relatively large doses may be required. Loop diuretics, such as furosemide, are more often used, and relatively large doses may be required.

3. Angiotensin-converting enzyme inhibitors are usually effective in clients with renal impairment, but responses may vary and the following factors should be considered.

a. When a client with renal impairment is started on an ACE inhibitor, careful monitoring is required, especially during the first few weeks of therapy, to prevent irreversible renal failure. For some clients, it may not be possible to normalize blood pressure and maintain adequate renal perfusion.

b. In clients with severe atherosclerosis, especially those with unilateral or bilateral stenosis of renal arteries, ACE inhibitors can impair renal blood flow and worsen renal impairment (ie, increase BUN and serum creatinine). This may require stopping the drug. In addition, some clients without renal artery stenosis have developed increased BUN and serum creatinine levels. Although these are usually minor and transient, the drug may need to be discontinued or reduced in dosage.

c. Approximately 25% of clients taking an ACE inhibitor for heart failure experience increases in BUN and serum creatinine levels. These clients usually do not require drug discontinuation unless they have severe, preexisting renal impairment. In clients with severe heart failure, whose renal function may depend on the activity of the renin-angiotensin-aldosterone system, treatment with an ACE inhibitor may worsen renal impairment. However, acute renal failure rarely occurs.

d. The mechanisms are unclear, but ACE inhibitors also have renal protective effects in hypertensive clients with some renal impairment and clients with diabetic nephropathy. A possible mechanism is less damage to the endothelium and less vascular remodeling (ie, less narrowing of the lumen and less thickening of the wall).

e. The elimination half-life of most ACE inhibitors and their active metabolites is prolonged in clients with renal impairment. Dosage may need to be reduced with benazepril, lisinopril, quinapril, and ramipril.

4. Angiotensin II receptor antagonists also inhibit the renin-angiotensin-aldosterone system and may produce effects similar to those of the ACE inhibitors. As with ACE inhibitors, some clients with severe heart failure have had oliguria or worsened renal impairment. These drugs are also likely to increase BUN and serum creatinine in clients with stenosis of one or both renal arteries.

Dosage reductions usually are not required for clients with renal impairment. However, fluid volume deficits (eg, from diuretic therapy) should be corrected before starting the drug, and blood pressure should be monitored closely during drug therapy. Clients on hemodialysis may have orthostatic hypotension with telmisartan and possibly other drugs of this group.

5. Most beta blockers are eliminated primarily by the kidneys and serum half-life is prolonged in clients with renal impairment. Thus, most of the drugs should be used with caution and in reduced dosages. Dosage of metoprolol does not need to be reduced. An additional consideration is that cardiac output and blood pressure should not be lowered enough to impair renal blood flow and aggravate renal impairment.

6. Calcium channel blockers are often used in clients with renal impairment because, in general, they are effective and well tolerated; they maintain renal blood flow even during blood pressure reduction in most clients; and they are mainly eliminated by hepatic metabolism. However, cautious use is still recommended because several agents produce active metabolites that are excreted by the kidneys (see section on Use in Renal Impairment, Chap. 53).

Use in Hepatic Impairment

Little information is available about the use of antihypertensive drugs in clients with impaired hepatic function. However, many of the drugs are metabolized in the liver and hepatic impairment can increase and prolong plasma concentrations.

1. Angiotensin-converting enzyme inhibitors have occasionally been associated with a syndrome that started with cholestatic jaundice and progressed to hepatic necrosis and sometimes death. The mechanism of liver impairment is unknown. Clients who have jaundice or marked elevations of hepatic enzymes while taking an ACE inhibitor should have the drug discontinued. In addition, therapeutic effects can be decreased with several of the drugs (eg, fosinopril, quinapril, ramipril) because less of a given dose is converted to an active metabolite. Clearance of fosinopril, quinapril, and probably other ACE inhibitors that are metabolized is reduced in clients with alcoholic or biliary cirrhosis.

2. Angiotensin II receptor antagonists should be used cautiously in clients with biliary tract obstruction or hepatic impairment. For some of these drugs (eg, candesartan, irbesartan, valsartan), dosage reduction is unnecessary. However, a lower starting dose is recommended for losartan because plasma concentrations of the drug and its active metabolite are increased and clearance is decreased approxi-

mately 50%. With telmisartan, plasma concentrations are increased and bioavailability approaches 100%. In addition, the drug is eliminated mainly by biliary excretion and clients with biliary tract obstruction or hepatic impairment have reduced clearance. The drug should be used with caution, but dosage forms that allow dosage reduction below 40 mg are not available. Thus, an alternative drug should probably be considered for clients with hepatic impairment.

3. Beta blockers that normally undergo extensive first-pass hepatic metabolism (eg, acebutolol, metoprolol, propranolol, timolol) may produce excessive blood levels in clients with cirrhosis because the blood containing the drug is shunted around the liver into the systemic circulation. Dosage should be started at a low dose and titrated carefully in these clients. Dosage of bisoprolol and pindolol should also be reduced in clients with cirrhosis or other hepatic impairment.

4. Calcium channel blockers should be used with caution, dosages should be substantially reduced, liver enzymes should be monitored periodically, and clients should be closely monitored for drug effects (see section on Use in Hepatic Impairment, Chap. 53).

Use in Critical Illness

Antihypertensive drugs are frequently prescribed for clients with critical illness and must be used cautiously, usually with reduced dosages and careful monitoring of responses. In many cases, the drugs are continued during critical illnesses caused by both cardiovascular and noncardiovascular disorders. If the client cannot take oral drugs, drug choices are narrowed because many commonly used drugs are not available in a dosage form that can be given parenterally, by gastrointestinal tube, or topically (eg, like a clonidine skin patch). Thus, clients' drug therapy must usually be retitrated. In one way, this may be more difficult, because critically ill clients are often unstable in their conditions and responses to drug therapy. In another way, it may be easier in a critical care unit, where hemodynamic monitoring is commonly used. The goal of treatment is usually to maintain adequate tissue perfusion while avoiding both hypotension and hypertension.

Antihypertensive drugs are also used to treat hypertensive urgencies and emergencies, which involve dangerously high blood pressures and actual or potential damage to target organs. Although there are risks with severe hypertension, there are also risks associated with lowering blood pressure excessively or too rapidly, including stroke, myocardial infarction, and acute renal failure. Thus, the goal of treatment is usually to lower blood pressure over several minutes to several hours, with careful titration of drug dosage to avoid precipitous drops.

Urgencies can be treated with oral antihypertensive agents such as **captopril** 25 to 50 mg every 1 to 2 hours; **clonidine** 0.2 mg initially, then 0.1 mg hourly until diastolic blood pressure falls below 110 mm Hg or 0.7 mg has been given; and **nifedipine** 10 mg (often given sublingually, but nifedipine is not absorbed across the mucosa and must be swallowed; rapid effects are obtained by perforating the capsule or having the client bite the capsule).

A hypertensive emergency, defined as a diastolic pressure of 120 mm Hg or higher and target organ damage, requires an IV drug. The goal of treatment is usually to lower diastolic pressure to 100 to 110 mm Hg and maintain it there for several days to allow adjustment of the physiologic mechanisms that normally regulate blood pressure. Then, the blood pressure can be lowered to normotensive levels.

Several drugs can be given to treat a hypertensive emergency. **Fenoldopam** is a fast-acting drug indicated only for short-term use (≤48 hours) in hospitalized clients. Dosage is calculated according to body weight and desired effects on blood pressure. It is given by an infusion pump, with frequent monitoring of blood pressure. **Nitroglycerin** is especially beneficial in clients with both severe hypertension and myocardial ischemia. The dose is titrated according to blood pressure response and may range from 5 to 100 µg/minute. Tolerance develops to IV nitroglycerin over 24 to 48 hours. **Nitroprusside**, which has a rapid onset and short duration of action, is given as a continuous infusion at a rate of 0.5 to 8.0 µg/kg/minute. Intra-arterial blood pressure should be monitored during the infusion. Nitroprusside is metabolized to thiocyanate, and serum thiocyanate levels should be measured if the drug is given longer than 72 hours. The infusion should be stopped after 72 hours if the serum thiocyanate level is more than 12 mg/dL; it should be stopped at 48 hours in clients with renal impairment. Symptoms of thiocyanate toxicity, including nausea, vomiting, myoclonus, and seizures, can be reversed with hemodialysis. Other drugs that may be used include IV **hydralazine**, **labetalol**, and **nicardipine**; see Table 55-1 for dosages.

 Home Care

Antihypertensive drugs are commonly self-administered in the home setting. The home care nurse is most likely to be involved when making home visits for other reasons. Whether the client or another member of the household is taking antihypertensive medications, the home care nurse may be helpful in teaching about the drugs, monitoring for drug effects, and promoting compliance with the prescribed regimen (pharmacologic and lifestyle modifications).

Noncompliance with prescribed antihypertensive drug therapy is a major problem, and consequences may be catastrophic. The home care nurse is well situated to assess for actual or potential barriers to compliance. For example, several antihypertensive medications are quite expensive and clients may not take the drugs at all or they may take fewer than the prescribed number of doses. If the nurse's assessment reveals this sort of situation, he or she may contact the prescribing physician and discuss the possibility of using less expensive drugs. If the physician is unwilling to try alternative drugs, the nurse may be able to identify resources for obtaining the needed medications.

NURSING ACTIONS	Antihypertensive Drugs

NURSING ACTIONS	RATIONALE/EXPLANATION
1. Administer accurately	
a. Give oral captopril and moexipril on an empty stomach, 1 h before meals.	Food decreases drug absorption.
b. Give most other oral antihypertensives with or after food intake.	To decrease gastric irritation
c. Give angiotensin II receptor antagonists with or without food.	Food does not impair drug absorption.
d. For intravenous injection of propranolol or labetalol, the client should be attached to a cardiac monitor. In addition, parenteral atropine and isoproterenol (Isuprel) must be readily available.	For early detection and treatment of excessive myocardial depression and arrhythmias. Atropine may be used to treat excessive bradycardia. Isoproterenol may be used to stimulate myocardial contractility and increase cardiac output.
e. Give the first dose and the first increased dose of prazosin, doxazosin, and terazosin at bedtime.	To prevent orthostatic hypotension and syncope

(continued)

NURSING ACTIONS	RATIONALE/EXPLANATION
f. For administration of fenoldopam and nitro-prusside, use the manufacturers' instructions to develop a unit protocol for preparation of infusion solutions, dosages, flow rates, durations of use, and monitoring of blood pressure during infusion.	These drugs are used to lower blood pressure rapidly in hypertensive emergencies, usually in an emergency department or critical care unit. They also have specific requirements for preparation and administration. A protocol established beforehand can save valuable time in an emergency situation.
2. Observe for therapeutic effects	The choice of drugs and drug dosages often requires adjustment to maximize beneficial effects and minimize adverse effects. Thus, optimal therapeutic effects may not occur immediately after drug therapy is begun.
a. Decreased blood pressure. The usual goal is a normal blood pressure (ie, below 140/90).	
3. Observe for adverse effects	Adverse effects are most likely to occur in clients who are elderly, have impaired renal function, and are receiving multiple antihypertensive drugs or large doses of antihypertensive drugs.
a. Postural hypotension, dizziness, weakness	This is an extension of the expected pharmacologic action. Postural hypotension results from drug blockage of compensatory reflexes (vasoconstriction, decreased venous pooling in extremities and increased venous return to the heart) that normally maintain blood pressure in the upright position. This adverse reaction may be aggravated by other conditions that cause vasodilation (eg, exercise, heat or hot weather, and alcohol consumption). Postural hypotension is more likely to occur with guanethidine, methyldopa, and reserpine.
b. Sodium and water retention, increased plasma volume, perhaps edema and weight gain	These effects result from decreased renal perfusion. This reaction can be prevented or minimized by concurrent administration of a diuretic.
c. Prolonged atrioventricular conduction, bradycardia	Owing to increased vagal tone and stimulation
d. Gastrointestinal disturbances, including nausea, vomiting, and diarrhea	These effects are more likely to occur with hydralazine, methyldopa, propranolol, and captopril.
e. Mental depression (with reserpine)	Apparently caused by decreased levels of catecholamines and serotonin in the brain
f. Bronchospasm (with nonselective beta blockers)	The drugs may cause bronchoconstriction and are contraindicated in patients with asthma and other bronchoconstrictive lung disorders.
g. Hypertensive crisis (with abrupt withdrawal of clonidine or guanabenz).	This may be prevented by tapering the prescribed dosage over a period of at least 2–4 days before discontinuing the drug.
h. Cough and hyperkalemia with angiotensin-converting enzyme (ACE) inhibitors	A chronic, nonproductive cough is a relatively common adverse effect. Hyperkalemia has been reported with 1%–4% of clients.
4. Observe for drug interactions	
a. Drugs that *increase* effects of antihypertensives:	
(1) Other antihypertensive agents	Combinations of two or three drugs with different mechanisms of action are often given for their addi-

(continued)

NURSING ACTIONS	RATIONALE/EXPLANATION
	tive effects and efficacy in controlling blood pressure when a single drug is ineffective.
(2) Alcohol, other central nervous system depressants (eg, narcotic analgesics, phenothiazine antipsychotics)	These drugs have hypotensive effects when used alone and increased hypotension occurs when they are combined with antihypertensive drugs.
(3) Digoxin	Additive bradycardia with beta blockers
b. Drugs that *decrease* effects of antihypertensives:	
(1) Adrenergics	These drugs stimulate the sympathetic nervous system and raise blood pressure. They include over-the-counter nasal decongestants, cold remedies, bronchodilators, and appetite suppressants.
(2) Antacids	May decrease bioavailability of ACE inhibitors, especially captopril. Give antacids 2 h before or after ACE inhibitors.
(3) Nonsteroidal anti-inflammatory drugs, oral contraceptives	These drugs tend to increase blood pressure by causing retention of sodium and water.

How Can You Avoid This Medication Error?

Answer: If Mr. Simosa is having trouble swallowing, oral medications may not be safely taken at this time. Crushing the medications is also not indicated because Cardizem SR and Slow-K are sustained-release products. If Cardizem SR is crushed, the sustained-release properties will be lost. Immediately after administration, you will see a significant hypotensive effect because all the medication will be absorbed. Because none of the medication's absorption will be delayed, you may see a rebound hypertension at a later time. Slow-K will also lose the ability to absorb slowly, which might cause it to be excreted by the diuretic effects of the Lasix, which is not affected by crushing.

REVIEW AND APPLICATION EXERCISES

1. Describe the physiologic mechanisms that control blood pressure.

2. What are common factors that raise blood pressure?

3. What signs and symptoms occur with hypertension, and how would you assess for them?

4. Why is it important to measure blood pressure accurately and repeatedly?

5. Does all hypertension require nonpharmacologic or pharmacologic treatment? Justify your answer.

6. What are the potential consequences of untreated or inadequately treated hypertension?

7. How do ACE inhibitors, AIIRAs, alpha- and beta-adrenergic blockers, calcium channel blockers, and direct vasodilators lower blood pressure?

8. What are adverse effects of each group of antihypertensive drugs, and how may they be prevented or minimized?

9. For a client newly diagnosed with hypertension, outline a teaching plan for lifestyle and pharmacologic interventions.

10. List interventions by health care providers that may help hypertensive clients adhere to their treatment regimens and maintain quality of life.

11. List at least two major considerations in using antihypertensive drugs in children, older adults, and clients who have renal or hepatic impairment.

12. Mentally rehearse your assessment and interventions for a client with a hypertensive urgency or emergency.

13. How would you assess a client being treated for hypertension for compliance with the prescribed lifestyle and drug therapy regimen?

SELECTED REFERENCES

Applegate, W.B. (1997). Approach to the elderly patient with hypertension. In W.N. Kelley (Ed.), *Textbook of internal medicine*, 3rd ed., pp. 2482–2488. Philadelphia: Lippincott-Raven.

Brater, D.C. (1997). Clinical pharmacology of cardiovascular drugs. In W.N. Kelley (Ed.), *Textbook of internal medicine*, 3rd ed., pp. 552–569. Philadelphia: Lippincott-Raven.

Bartosh, S.M. & Aronson, A.J. (1999). Childhood hypertension: An update on etiology, diagnosis, and treatment. *Pediatric Clinics of North America, 46*, 235–252.

Drug facts and comparisons. (Updated monthly). St. Louis: Facts and Comparisons.

Hall, W.D. (1999). A rational approach to the treatment of hypertension in special populations. *American Family Physician, 60,* 156–162.

Hawkins, D.W., Bussey, H.I., & Prisant, L.M. (1997). Hypertension. In J.T. DiPiro, R.L. Talbert, G.C. Yee, G.R. Matzke, B.G. Wells, & L.M. Posey (Eds.), *Pharmacotherapy: A pathophysiologic approach,* 3rd ed., pp. 195–218. Stamford, CT: Appleton & Lange.

Jackson, E.K. & Garrison, J.C. (1996). Renin and angiotensin. In J.G. Hardman, L.E. Limbird, P.B. Molinoff, & R.W. Ruddon (Eds.), *Goodman & Gilman's The pharmacological basis of therapeutics,* 9th ed., pp. 733–758. New York: McGraw-Hill.

Joint National Committee on Detection, Evaluation, and Treatment of High Blood Pressure. (1997). *The sixth report of the Joint National Committee on Detection, Evaluation, and Treatment of High Blood Pressure* (NIH Publication No. 98-4080). Bethesda, MD: National Institutes of Health, National Heart, Lung and Blood Institute.

Kaplan, N.M. (1999). Angiotensin II receptor antagonists in the treatment of hypertension. *American Family Physician, 60,* 1185–1190.

Kirk, J.K. (1999). Angiotensin-II receptor antagonists: Their place in therapy. *American Family Physician, 59,* 3140–3148.

McHugh, J. & Cheek, D.J. (1998). Nitric oxide and regulation of vascular tone: Pharmacological and physiological considerations. *American Journal of Critical Care, 7,* 131–140.

Naftilan, A.J. (1998). Angiotensin II receptor inhibitors. *Clinical Reviews, Winter,* 28–30. [Online: Available http://www.medscape.com/SMA/ ClinicalReviews/1998/winter98/crW98.08.naft/crW98.08.naft-01.html. Accessed October 10, 1999.]

National High Blood Pressure Education Program Working Group. (1996). Update on the 1987 task force report on high blood pressure in children and adolescents. *Pediatrics, 98,* 649–658.

Oates, J.A. (1996). Antihypertensive agents and the drug therapy of hypertension. In J.G. Hardman, L.E. Limbird, P.B. Molinoff, & R.W. Ruddon (Eds.), *Goodman & Gilman's The pharmacological basis of therapeutics,* 9th ed., pp. 780–808. New York: McGraw-Hill.

Porth, C.M. (1998). Alterations in blood pressure: Hypertension and orthostatic hypotension. In C.M. Porth (Ed.), *Pathophysiology: Concepts of altered health states,* 5th ed., pp. 363–384. Philadelphia: Lippincott Williams & Wilkins.

Rockett, J.L. (1999). Endothelial dysfunction and the promise of ACE inhibitors. *American Journal of Nursing, 99*(10), 44–49.

Weinberger, M.H. (1997). Systemic hypertension. In W.N. Kelley (Ed.), *Textbook of internal medicine,* 3rd ed., pp. 175–183. Philadelphia: Lippincott-Raven.

Woods, A.D. (1999). Managing hypertension. *Nursing99, 29*(3), 41–46.

The World Health Organization and the International Society of Hypertension (1999). Clinical update: 1999 Guidelines for hypertension management. *Clinician Reviews 9*(6), 123–126. [Online: Available http://www.medscape.com/CPG/Clin/Reviews/1999/v09.n06/C0906.02/c0906.02-01.html. Accessed November 4, 1999.]

56

Diuretics

Objectives

After studying this chapter, the student will be able to:

1. List characteristics of diuretics in terms of mechanism of action, indications for use, principles of therapy, and nursing process implications.

2. Discuss major adverse effects of thiazide, loop, and potassium-sparing diuretics.

3. Identify clients at risk for development of adverse reactions to diuretic administration.

4. Recognize commonly used potassium-losing and potassium-sparing diuretics.

5. Discuss the rationale for using combination products containing a potassium-losing and a potassium-sparing diuretic.

6. Discuss the rationale for concomitant use of a loop diuretic and a thiazide or related diuretic.

7. Teach clients to manage diuretic therapy effectively.

8. Discuss important elements of diuretic therapy in special populations.

Jennie Masury, an 82-year-old widow, is started on a thiazide diuretic to control her hypertension. She also has a history of osteoarthritis. She lives alone with her two cats and manages independently with only a little help from her neighbors. Her children live out-of-state, but she talks with them on the phone weekly.

Reflect on:

▶ How diuretics work to decrease blood pressure.

▶ How a diuretic and its effects may affect activities and normal daily functions.

▶ Factors, including diuretic therapy, that may pose safety risks for this widow. How might you minimize these risks?

▶ An appropriate teaching plan for this patient regarding her diuretic therapy.

DESCRIPTION

Diuretics are drugs that increase renal excretion of water, sodium, and other electrolytes, thereby increasing urine formation and output. They are important therapeutic agents widely used in the treatment of edematous (eg, heart failure, renal and hepatic disease) and nonedematous (eg, hypertension, ophthalmic surgery) conditions. To aid understanding of diuretic drug therapy, renal physiology related to drug action and characteristics of edema are reviewed. Types of diuretics are then described, and individual drugs are listed in Table 56-1.

RENAL PHYSIOLOGY

The primary function of the kidneys is to regulate the volume, composition, and pH of body fluids. The kidneys receive approximately 25% of the cardiac output. From this large amount of blood flow, the normally functioning kidney is efficient in retaining substances needed by the body and eliminating those not needed.

The Nephron

The nephron is the functional unit of the kidney; each kidney contains approximately 1 million nephrons. Each nephron is composed of a glomerulus and a tubule (Fig. 56-1). The glomerulus is a network of capillaries that receives blood from the renal artery. Bowman's capsule is a thin-walled structure that surrounds the glomerulus, then narrows and continues as the tubule. The tubule is a thin-walled structure of epithelial cells surrounded by peritubular capillaries. The tubule is divided into three main segments, the proximal tubule, loop of Henle, and distal tubule, which differ in structure and function. The tubules are often called *convoluted tubules* because of their many twists and turns. The convolutions provide a large surface area that brings the blood flowing through the peritubular capillaries and the glomerular filtrate flowing through the tubular lumen into close proximity. Consequently, substances can be readily exchanged through the walls of the tubules.

The nephron functions by three processes: glomerular filtration, tubular reabsorption, and tubular secretion. These processes normally maintain the fluid volume, electrolyte concentration, and pH of body fluids within a relatively narrow range. They also remove waste products of cellular metabolism. A minimum daily urine output of approximately 400 mL is required to remove normal amounts of metabolic end products.

Glomerular Filtration

Arterial blood enters the glomerulus by the afferent arteriole at the relatively high pressure of approximately 70 mm Hg. This pressure pushes water, electrolytes, and other solutes out of the capillaries into Bowman's capsule and then to the proximal tubule. This fluid, called *glomerular filtrate*, contains the same components as blood except for blood cells, fats, and proteins.

The glomerular filtration rate (GFR) is approximately 180 L/day, or 125 mL/minute. Most of this fluid is reabsorbed as the glomerular filtrate travels through the tubules. The end product is approximately 2 L of urine daily. Urine flows into collecting tubules, which carry it to the renal pelvis. From the renal pelvis, urine flows through the ureters, bladder, and urethra for elimination from the body.

Blood that does not become part of the glomerular filtrate travels out of the glomerulus through the efferent arteriole. The efferent arteriole branches into the peritubular capillaries, which eventually empty into veins and return the blood to the systemic circulation.

Tubular Reabsorption

The term *reabsorption*, in relation to renal function, indicates movement of substances from the tubule (glomerular filtrate) to the blood in the peritubular capillaries. Most reabsorption occurs in the proximal tubule. Almost all glucose and amino acids are reabsorbed; approximately 80% of water, sodium, potassium, chloride, and most other substances is reabsorbed. As a result, approximately 20% of the glomerular filtrate enters the loop of Henle. In the descending limb of the loop of Henle, water is reabsorbed; in the ascending limb, sodium is reabsorbed. A large fraction of the total amount of sodium (up to 30%) filtered by the glomeruli is reabsorbed in the loop of Henle. Additional sodium is reabsorbed in the distal tubule, primarily by the exchange of sodium ions for potassium ions secreted by epithelial cells of tubular walls. Final reabsorption of water occurs in the distal tubule and small collecting tubules. The remaining water and solutes are now correctly called *urine*.

Antidiuretic hormone from the posterior pituitary gland promotes reabsorption of water from the distal tubules and the collecting ducts of the kidneys. This conserves water needed by the body and produces a more concentrated urine. Aldosterone, a hormone from the adrenal cortex, promotes sodium–potassium exchange mainly in the distal tubule and collecting ducts. Thus, aldosterone promotes sodium reabsorption and potassium loss.

Tubular Secretion

The term *secretion*, in relation to renal function, indicates movement of substances from blood in the peritubular capillaries to glomerular filtrate flowing through the renal tubules. Secretion occurs in the proximal and distal tubules, across the epithelial cells that line the tubules. In the proximal tubule, uric acid, creatinine, hydrogen ions, and ammonia are secreted; in the distal tubule, potassium ions, hydrogen ions, and ammonia are secreted. Secretion of

TABLE 56-1 **Diuretic Agents**

Generic/Trade Name	Routes and Dosage Ranges	
	Adults	Children

Thiazide and Related Diuretics

Generic/Trade Name	Adults	Children
Bendroflumethiazide (Naturetin)	PO 5 mg daily initially. For maintenance, 2.5–20 mg daily or intermittently	PO up to 0.4 mg/kg/d initially, in two divided doses. For maintenance, 0.05–0.1 mg/kg/d in a single dose.
Benzthiazide (Exna)	PO 50–200 mg daily for several days initially, depending on response. For maintenance, dosage is gradually reduced to the minimal effective amount.	PO 1–4 mg/kg/d initially, in three divided doses. For maintenance, dosage is reduced to the minimal effective amount.
Chlorothiazide (Diuril)	PO 500–1000 mg one or two times daily IV 500 mg twice daily	PO 22 mg/kg/d in two divided doses Infants <6 mo, up to 33 mg/kg/d in two divided doses IV not recommended
Chlorthalidone (Hygroton)	PO 25–100 mg daily	PO 3 mg/kg three times weekly, adjusted according to response
Hydrochlorothiazide (HydroDIURIL, Esidrix, Oretic)	PO 25–100 mg one or two times daily Elderly, 12.5–25 mg daily	PO 2 mg/kg/d in two divided doses Infants <6 mo, up to 3.3 mg/kg/d in two divided doses
Hydroflumethiazide (Saluron)	PO 25–200 mg daily	PO 1 mg/kg/d
Indapamide (Lozol)	PO 2.5–5 mg daily	Dosage not established
Methyclothiazide (Enduron)	PO 2.5–10 mg daily	PO 0.05–0.2 mg/kg/d
Metolazone (Zaroxolyn, Mykrox)	PO 5–20 mg daily, depending on severity of condition and response	
Polythiazide (Renese)	PO 1–4 mg daily, depending on severity of condition and response	PO 0.02–0.08 mg/kg/d
Quinethazone (Hydromox)	PO 50–200 mg daily	Dosage not established
Trichlormethiazide (Metahydrin, Naqua)	PO 2–4 mg one or two times daily initially. For maintenance, 1–4 mg once daily	PO 0.07 mg/kg/d in single or divided doses

Loop Diuretics

Generic/Trade Name	Adults	Children
Bumetanide (Bumex)	PO 0.5–2 mg daily as a single dose. May be repeated q4–6h to a maximal dose of 10 mg, if necessary. Giving on alternate days or for 3–4 d with rest periods of 1–2 d is recommended for long-term control of edema. IV, IM 0.5–1 mg, repeated in 2–3 h if necessary, to a maximal daily dose of 10 mg. Give IV injections over 1–2 min.	Not recommended for children <18 y
Ethacrynic acid (Edecrin)	Edema, PO 50–100 mg daily, increased or decreased according to severity of condition and response, maximal daily dose, 400 mg Rapid mobilization of edema, IV 50 mg or 0.5–1 mg/kg injected slowly to a maximum of 100 mg/dose	PO 25 mg daily No recommended parenteral dose in children
Furosemide (Lasix)	Edema, PO 20–80 mg as a single dose initially. If an adequate diuretic response is not obtained, dosage may be gradually increased by 20- to 40-mg increments at intervals of 6–8 h. For maintenance, dosage range and frequency of administration vary widely and must be individualized. Maximal daily dose, 600 mg. Hypertension, PO 40 mg twice daily, gradually increased if necessary Rapid mobilization of edema, IV 20–40 mg initially, injected slowly. This dose may be repeated in 2 h. With acute pulmonary edema, initial dose is usually 40 mg, which may be repeated in 60–90 min. Acute renal failure, IV 40 mg initially, increased if necessary. Maximum dose, 1–2 g/24 h Hypertensive crisis, IV 40–80 mg injected over 1–2 min. With renal failure, much larger doses may be needed.	PO 2 mg/kg one or two times daily initially, gradually increased by increments of 1–2 mg/kg per dose if necessary at intervals of 6–8 h. Maximal daily dose, 6 mg/kg IV 1 mg/kg initially. If diuretic response is not adequate, increase dosage by 1 mg/kg no sooner than 2 h after previous dose. Maximal dose, 6 mg/kg
Torsemide (Demadex)	PO, IV 5–20 mg once daily	

(continued)

TABLE 56-1	**Diuretic Agents** (*continued*)	
	Routes and Dosage Ranges	
Generic/Trade Name	**Adults**	**Children**
Potassium-Sparing Diuretics		
Amiloride (Midamor)	PO 5–20 mg daily	Dosage not established
Spironolactone (Aldactone)	PO 25–200 mg daily	PO 3.3 mg/kg/d in divided doses
Triamterene (Dyrenium)	PO 100–300 mg daily in divided doses	PO 2–4 mg/kg/d in divided doses
Osmotic Agents		
Glycerin (Osmoglyn)	PO 1–1.5 g/kg of body weight, usually given as a 50% or 75% solution, 1–2 h before ocular surgery	Same as adults
Isosorbide (Ismotic)	PO 1.5–3 g/kg, up to four times daily if necessary for glaucoma or ocular surgery	
Mannitol (Osmitrol)	Diuresis, IV infusion 50–200 g over 24 h, flow rate adjusted to maintain a urine output of 30–50 mL/h Oliguria and prevention of renal failure, IV 50–100g Reduction of intracranial or intraocular pressure, IV 1.5–2 g/kg, given as a 20% solution, over 30–60 min	Same as adults

IM, intramuscular; IV, intravenous; PO, oral.

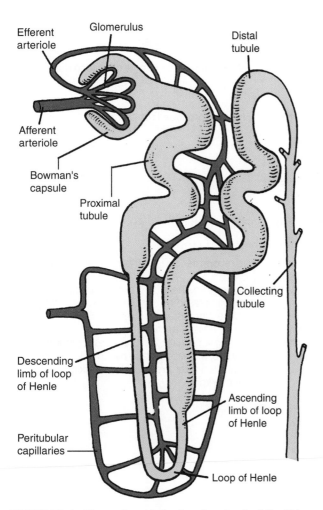

FIGURE 56–1 The nephron is the functional unit of the kidney.

hydrogen ions is important in maintaining acid–base balance in body fluids.

ALTERATIONS IN RENAL FUNCTION

Many clinical conditions alter renal function. In some conditions, excessive amounts of substances (eg, sodium and water) are retained; in others, needed substances (eg, potassium, proteins) are eliminated. These conditions include cardiovascular, renal, hepatic, and other disorders that may be treated with diuretic drugs.

Edema

Edema is the excessive accumulation of fluid in body tissues. It is a symptom of many disease processes and may occur in any part of the body. Additional characteristics include the following:

1. Edema formation results from one or more of the following mechanisms that allow fluid to leave the bloodstream (intravascular compartment) and enter interstitial spaces.
   a. Increased capillary permeability occurs as part of the response to tissue injury. Thus, edema may occur with burns and trauma or allergic and inflammatory reactions.
   b. Increased capillary hydrostatic pressure results from a sequence of events in which increased blood volume (from fluid overload or sodium

and water retention) or obstruction of venous blood flow causes a high venous pressure and a high capillary pressure. This is the primary mechanism for edema formation in congestive heart failure, pulmonary edema, and renal failure.

  c. Decreased plasma oncotic pressure may occur with decreased synthesis of plasma proteins (caused by liver disease or malnutrition) or increased loss of plasma proteins (caused by burn injuries or the nephrotic syndrome). Plasma proteins are important in keeping fluids within the bloodstream. When plasma proteins are lacking, fluid seeps through the capillaries and accumulates in tissues.

2. Edema interferes with blood flow to tissues. Thus, it interferes with delivery of oxygen and nutrients and removal of metabolic waste products. If severe, edema may distort body features, impair movement, and interfere with activities of daily living.

3. Specific manifestations of edema are determined by its location and extent. A common type of localized edema occurs in the feet and ankles (dependent edema), especially with prolonged sitting or standing. A less common but more severe type of localized edema is pulmonary edema, a life-threatening condition that occurs with circulatory overload (eg, of intravenous [IV] fluids or blood transfusions) or acute heart failure. Generalized massive edema (anasarca) interferes with the functions of many body organs and tissues.

DIURETIC DRUGS

Diuretic drugs act on the kidneys to decrease reabsorption of sodium, chloride, water, and other substances. Major subclasses are the thiazides and related diuretics, loop diuretics, and potassium-sparing diuretics, which act at different sites in the nephron (Fig. 56-2).

Major clinical indications for diuretics are edema, heart failure, and hypertension. In edematous states, diuretics mobilize tissue fluids by decreasing plasma volume. In hypertension, the exact mechanism by which diuretics lower blood pressure is unknown, but antihypertensive action is usually attributed to sodium depletion. Initially, diuretics decrease blood volume and cardiac output. With chronic use, cardiac output returns to normal, but there is a persistent decrease in plasma volume and peripheral vascular resistance. Sodium depletion may have a vasodilating effect on arterioles.

Use of diuretic agents in the treatment of heart failure and hypertension is discussed further in Chapters 51 and 55, respectively.

Thiazide and Related Diuretics

Thiazide diuretics are synthetic drugs that are chemically related to the sulfonamides and differ mainly in their duration of action. Hydrochlorothiazide is the most commonly used; chlorothiazide is the only one that can be given IV. Related diuretics are nonthiazides whose pharmacologic actions are essentially the same as those of the thiazides; they include chlorthalidone, metolazone, and quinethazone.

Thiazides and related diuretics are frequently prescribed in the long-term management of heart failure and hypertension. They act to decrease reabsorption of sodium, water, chloride, and bicarbonate in the distal convoluted tubule. Most sodium is reabsorbed before it reaches the distal convoluted tubule and only a small amount is reabsorbed at this site. Thus, these drugs are not strong diuretics. In addition, they are ineffective when immediate diuresis is required and are relatively ineffective with decreased renal function.

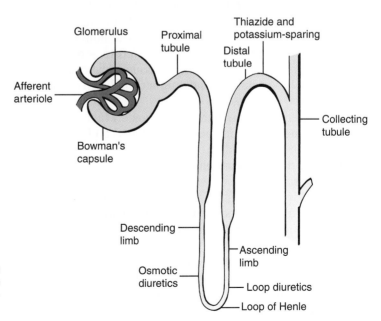

FIGURE 56–2 Diuretic sites of action in the nephron. Diuretics act at different sites in the nephron to decrease reabsorption of sodium and water and increase urine output.

These drugs are well absorbed, widely distributed in body fluids, and highly bound to plasma proteins. They accumulate only in the kidneys. Diuretic effects usually occur within 2 hours, peak at 4 to 6 hours, and last 6 to 24 hours. Antihypertensive effects usually last long enough to allow use of a single daily dose. Most of the drugs are excreted unchanged by the kidneys within 3 to 6 hours; some (eg, polythiazide, chlorthalidone) have longer durations of action (approximately 48 to 72 hours), attributed to slower excretion.

Thiazides and related drugs are contraindicated in clients allergic to sulfonamide drugs. They must be used cautiously during pregnancy because they cross the placenta and may have adverse effects on the fetus.

Loop Diuretics

Loop diuretics inhibit sodium and chloride reabsorption in the ascending limb of the loop of Henle, where reabsorption of most filtered sodium occurs. Thus, these potent drugs produce significant diuresis, with their saluretic (sodium-losing) effect up to 10 times greater than that of thiazide diuretics. They also are called high-ceiling diuretics because their dosage can be increased to produce greater diuretic effects (in contrast, increasing the dosage of thiazides beyond a certain point does not increase diuretic effects). Loop diuretics are the most effective and versatile diuretics available for clinical use.

Loop diuretics may be given orally or IV. After oral administration, diuretic effects occur within 30 to 60 minutes, peak in 1 to 2 hours, and last 6 to 8 hours. After IV administration, diuretic effects occur within 5 minutes, peak within 30 minutes, and last approximately 2 hours. Thus, the drugs produce extensive diuresis for short periods, after which the kidney tubules regain their ability to reabsorb sodium. Actually, the kidneys reabsorb more sodium than usual during this postdiuretic phase, so a high dietary intake of sodium can cause sodium retention and reduce or cancel the diuretic-induced sodium loss. Thus, dietary sodium restriction is required to achieve optimum therapeutic benefits. The drugs are metabolized and excreted by the kidneys, and drug accumulation does not occur even with repeated doses.

Loop diuretics are the diuretics of choice when rapid effects are required (eg, in pulmonary edema) and when renal function is impaired (creatinine clearance <30 mL/minute). The drugs are contraindicated during pregnancy unless necessary.

Furosemide is the most commonly used loop diuretic. Bumetanide may be used to produce diuresis in some clients who are allergic to or no longer respond to furosemide. It is more potent than furosemide on a weight basis, and large doses can be given in small volumes. These drugs differ mainly in potency and produce similar effects at equivalent doses (eg, furosemide 40 mg = bumetanide 1 mg).

Potassium-Sparing Diuretics

Sodium is normally reabsorbed in the distal tubule in exchange for potassium and hydrogen ions. Potassium-sparing diuretics act at the distal tubule to decrease sodium reabsorption and potassium excretion. This group includes three drugs. One is spironolactone, an aldosterone antagonist. Aldosterone is a hormone secreted by the adrenal cortex. It promotes retention of sodium and water and excretion of potassium by stimulating the sodium–potassium exchange mechanism in the distal tubule. Spironolactone blocks the sodium-retaining effects of aldosterone, and aldosterone must be present for spironolactone to be effective. The other two drugs, amiloride and triamterene, act directly on the distal tubule to decrease the exchange of sodium for potassium, and have similar diuretic activity.

Potassium-sparing diuretics are weak diuretics when used alone. Thus, they are usually given in combination with potassium-losing diuretics to increase diuretic activity and decrease potassium loss. They are contraindicated in the presence of renal insufficiency because their use may cause hyperkalemia. Hyperkalemia is the major adverse effect of these drugs; clients receiving potassium-sparing diuretics should *not* be given potassium supplements, encouraged to eat foods high in potassium, or allowed to use salt substitutes. Salt substitutes contain potassium chloride rather than sodium chloride.

Osmotic Diuretics

Osmotic agents produce rapid diuresis by increasing the solute load (osmotic pressure) of the glomerular filtrate. The increased osmotic pressure causes water to be pulled from extravascular sites into the bloodstream, thereby increasing blood volume and decreasing reabsorption of water and electrolytes in the renal tubules. Mannitol is useful in treating oliguria or anuria, and it may prevent acute renal failure during prolonged surgery, trauma, or infusion of cisplatin, an antineoplastic agent. Mannitol is effective even when renal circulation and GFR are reduced (eg, in hypovolemic shock, trauma, or dehydration). Other important clinical uses of hyperosmolar agents include reduction of intracranial pressure before or after neurosurgery, reduction of intraocular pressure before certain types of ophthalmic surgery, and urinary excretion of toxic substances. Other osmotic agents are listed in Table 56-1.

Combination Products

Thiazide and related diuretics are available in numerous fixed-dose combinations with nondiuretic antihypertensive agents (see Chap. 55) and with potassium-sparing diuretics (Table 56-2). A major purpose of the antihypertensive combinations is to increase client convenience and compliance with drug therapy regimens. A major purpose of the diuretic combinations is to prevent potassium imbalances.

TABLE 56-2 | **Combination Diuretic Products**

Trade Name	Thiazide (Potassium-Losing) Diuretic	Potassium-Sparing Diuretic	Adult Dosage
Aldactazide 25/25	HCTZ 25 mg	Spironolactone 25 mg	PO 1–8 tablets daily
Aldactazide 50/50	HCTZ 50 mg	Spironolactone 50 mg	PO 1–4 tablets daily
Dyazide, Maxzide 25 mg	HCTZ 25 mg	Triamterene 37.5 mg	Hypertension, PO 1 capsule bid initially, then adjusted according to response Edema, PO 1–2 capsules bid
Maxzide	HCTZ 50 mg	Triamterene 75 mg	PO 1 tablet daily
Moduretic	HCTZ 50 mg	Amiloride 5 mg	PO 1–2 tablets daily with meals

HCTZ, hydrochlorothiazide; PO, oral.

NURSING PROCESS

Assessment

Assess the client's status in relation to baseline data and conditions in which diuretic drugs are used.

- Useful baseline data include serum electrolytes, creatinine, glucose, blood urea nitrogen (BUN), and uric acid, because diuretics may alter these values. Other data are blood pressure readings, weight, amount and appearance of urine output, and measurement of edematous areas, such as ankles or abdomen.
- Observe for edema. Visible edema often occurs in the feet and legs of ambulatory clients. Rapid weight gain may indicate fluid retention.
  - With congestive heart failure, numerous signs and symptoms result from edema of various organs and tissues. For example, congestion in the gastrointestinal tract may cause nausea and vomiting, liver congestion may cause abdominal pain and tenderness, and congestion in the lungs (pulmonary edema) causes rapid, labored breathing, hypoxemia, frothy sputum, and other manifestations of severe respiratory distress.
  - Cerebral edema may be manifested by confusion, headache, dizziness, convulsions, unconsciousness, bradycardia, or failure of the pupils to react to light.
  - Ascites, which occurs with hepatic cirrhosis, is an accumulation of fluid in the abdominal cavity. The abdomen appears much enlarged.
- With congestive heart failure, fatigue and dyspnea, in addition to edema, are common symptoms.
- Hypertension (blood pressure above 140/90 mm Hg on several measurements) may be the only clinical manifestation present.

Nursing Diagnoses

- Fluid Volume Excess in edematous clients, related to retention of sodium and water

- Fluid Volume Deficit related to increased urine output during diuretic drug therapy
- Altered Urinary Elimination: Increased frequency
- Altered Nutrition: Less Than Body Requirements related to excessive loss of potassium with thiazide and loop diuretics
- Risk for Injury: Hypotension and dizziness as adverse drug effects
- Knowledge Deficit related to the need for and correct usage of diuretics
- Sexual Dysfunction related to adverse drug effects

Planning/Goals

The client will:

- Take or receive diuretic drugs as prescribed
- Experience reduced edema and improved control of blood pressure
- Reduce dietary intake of sodium and increase dietary intake of potassium
- Avoid preventable adverse drug effects
- Keep appointments for follow-up monitoring of blood pressure, edema, and serum electrolytes

Interventions

Promote measures to prevent or minimize conditions for which diuretic drugs are used.

- With edema, helpful measures include the following:
  - Decreasing dietary sodium intake
  - Losing weight, if obese
  - Elevating legs when sitting
  - Avoiding prolonged standing or sitting
  - Wearing support hose or elastic stockings
  - Treating the condition causing edema
- With congestive heart failure and in older adults, administer IV fluids or blood transfusions carefully to avoid fluid overload and pulmonary edema. Fluid overload may occur with rapid administration or excessive amounts of IV fluids.
- With hypertension, helpful measures include decreasing dietary sodium intake, exercising regularly, and losing weight, if obese.

- With edematous clients, interventions to monitor fluid losses include weighing under standardized conditions, measuring urine output, and measuring edematous sites such as the ankles or the abdomen. Once the client reaches "dry weight," these measurements stabilize and can be done less often.
- With clients who are taking digoxin, a potassium-losing diuretic, and a potassium supplement, assist them to understand that the drugs act together to increase therapeutic effectiveness and avoid adverse effects (eg, hypokalemia and digoxin toxicity). Thus, stopping or changing

dosage of one of these drugs can lead to serious illness.

Evaluation

- Observe for reduced edema and body weight.
- Observe for reduced blood pressure.
- Observe for increased urine output.
- Monitor serum electrolytes for normal values.
- Interview regarding compliance with instructions for diet and drug therapy.
- Monitor compliance with follow-up appointments in outpatients.

CLIENT TEACHING GUIDELINES
Diuretics

General Considerations

✔ Diuretics increase urine output and are commonly used to treat hypertension, heart failure, and edema (swelling) from heart, kidney, liver, and other disorders.

✔ While taking a diuretic drug, you need to maintain regular medical supervision so drug effects can be monitored and dosages adjusted when indicated.

✔ Reducing sodium intake in your diet helps diuretic drugs be more effective and allows smaller doses to be taken. Smaller doses are less likely to cause adverse effects. Thus, you need to avoid excessive table salt and obviously salty foods (eg, ham, packaged sandwich meats, potato chips, dill pickles, most canned soups). These foods may aggravate edema or hypertension by causing sodium and water retention.

✔ Diuretics may cause blood potassium imbalances, and either too little or too much damages heart function. Periodic measurements of blood potassium and other substances is one of the major reasons for regular visits to a health care provider.

Too little potassium (hypokalemia) is probably more common and may result from the use of such potassium-losing diuretics as hydrochlorothiazide, Lasix, and several others. To prevent or treat hypokalemia, your doctor may prescribe a potassium chloride supplement or a combination of a potassium-losing and a potassium-saving diuretic (either separately or as a combined product such as Dyazide, Maxzide, or Aldactazide). He or she may also recommend increased dietary intake of potassium-containing foods (eg, bananas, orange juice).

Too much potassium (hyperkalemia) can result from the use of potassium-saving diuretics, the overuse of potassium supplements, or from the use of salt substitutes. Potassium-saving diuretics are not a major cause of hyperkalemia because they are usually given along with a potassium-losing diuretic. If potassium supplements are prescribed, they should be taken as directed.

You should **not** use salt substitutes without consulting your primary health care provider because they contain potassium chloride instead of sodium chloride. Hyperkalemia is most likely to occur in people with decreased kidney function, which often occurs in older adults and people with diabetes.

✔ With diuretic therapy, you will have increased urination, which usually lasts only a few days or weeks if you do not have edema. If you do have edema (eg, in your ankles), you can expect weight loss and decreased swelling as well as increased urination. It is a good idea to check and record your weight two or three times per week. Rapid changes in weight often indicate gain or loss of fluid.

✔ Some commonly used diuretics may increase blood sugar levels and cause or aggravate diabetes. If you have diabetes, you may need larger doses of your antidiabetic medications.

✔ Diuretics may cause sensitivity to sunlight. Thus, you need to avoid prolonged exposure to sunlight, use sunscreens, and wear protective clothing.

✔ Do not drink alcoholic beverages or take other medications without the approval of your health care provider.

✔ If you are taking a diuretic to lower your blood pressure, especially with other antihypertensive drugs, you may feel dizzy or faint when you stand up suddenly. This can be prevented or decreased by changing positions slowly. If dizziness is severe, notify your health care provider.

Self- or Caregiver Administration

✔ Take or give a diuretic early in the day, if ordered daily, to decrease nighttime trips to the bathroom. Fewer bathroom trips means less interference with sleep and less risk of falls. Ask someone to help you to the bathroom if you are elderly, weak, dizzy, or unsteady in walking (or use a bedside commode).

(continued)

✔ Take or give most diuretics with or after food to decrease stomach upset. Torsemide (Demadex) may be taken without regard to meals.

✔ If you are taking digoxin, a potassium-losing diuretic, and a potassium supplement, it is very important that you take these drugs as prescribed. This is a com-

mon combination of drugs for clients with congestive heart failure and the drugs work together to increase beneficial effects and avoid adverse effects. Stopping or changing the dose of one of these medications while continuing the others can lead to serious illness.

Nursing Notes: Apply Your Knowledge

You are caring for a patient with severe heart disease who is being treated for hypertension and congestive heart failure. Medications include enalapril (Vasotec) 10 mg qd and Lasix 40 mg bid. What assessment data are important to collect before administering these medications?

PRINCIPLES OF THERAPY

Drug Selection

The choice of diuretic drug depends primarily on the client's condition.

1. **Thiazides and related diuretics** are the drugs of choice for most clients who require diuretic therapy, especially for long-term treatment of heart failure and hypertension. All the drugs in this group have similar effects. For most clients, short-acting (eg, bendroflumethiazide) or intermediate-acting (eg, hydrochlorothiazide) agents are preferred. Although long-acting drugs (eg, several other thiazides and metolazone) may increase client compliance by requiring less frequent administration, they also may cause more hypokalemia. Some of the drugs are also more expensive than others.

2. A **loop diuretic** (eg, furosemide) is preferred when rapid diuretic effects are required or when renal impairment is present.

3. A **potassium-sparing diuretic** may be given concurrently with a potassium-losing diuretic to prevent or treat hypokalemia and to augment the diuretic effect. The two drugs can be given separately or in a fixed-dose combination product (see Table 56-2).

4. Two **potassium-losing diuretics** are sometimes given concurrently when an inadequate diuretic response occurs with one of the drugs. The combination of a loop and a thiazide diuretic has syn-

ergistic effects because the drugs act in different segments of the renal tubule. The synergistic effects probably result from the increased delivery of sodium to the distal tubule (where thiazides act) as sodium reabsorption in the loop of Henle is blocked by a loop diuretic. A commonly used combination is furosemide and hydrochlorothiazide (chlorothiazide can be given IV in clients who are unable to take an oral drug). Furosemide and metolazone have also been used. Because a thiazide–loop diuretic combination can induce profound diuresis, with severe sodium, potassium, and volume depletion, its use should be reserved for hospitalized clients who can be closely monitored. If used for ambulatory clients, the thiazide diuretic should be given in very low doses or only occasionally, to avoid serious adverse events.

Dosage Factors

Dosage of diuretics depends largely on the client's condition and response and should be individualized to administer the minimal effective amount.

1. With hydrochlorothiazide, smaller doses (eg, 12.5 to 25 mg daily) are effective for most people and produce fewer adverse effects (eg, hypokalemia) than larger doses. Some of the fixed-dose combinations of hydrochlorothiazide and a potassium-sparing diuretic contain 50 mg of hydrochlorothiazide. As a result, despite the convenience of a combination product, it may be better to give the drugs separately so that dosage can be titrated to the client's needs.

2. Clients who do not achieve an adequate diuretic response with usual doses of an oral drug may need larger doses or an IV drug.

3. With torsemide, which is highly bioavailable after both oral and IV administration, oral and IV doses are equivalent and clients may be switched from one route to the other without changing dosage.

4. In liver disease, small doses of all diuretics are usually indicated because diuretic-induced electrolyte imbalances may precipitate or aggravate hepatic coma.

5. In renal disease, furosemide is often given in large doses to achieve a diuretic response. Bumetanide may be a useful alternative, because it can be given in smaller dose volumes.

6. When metolazone is given concurrently with furosemide, the initial dose is usually metolazone 2.5 to 10 mg. The dose is then doubled every 24 hours until the desired response is achieved. If an adequate diuretic effect occurs with the first dose of metolazone, the dose of furosemide can be decreased. Hydrochlorothiazide 50 mg may also be used with furosemide and may be safer than metolazone because of its shorter duration of action.

Use in Edema

When diuretics are used to treat clients with edema, the underlying cause of the edema should be addressed, not just the edema itself. When treating such clients, it is preferable to aim for a weight loss of approximately 2 lb (approximately 1 kg) per day. Rapid and excessive diuresis may cause dehydration and decreased blood volume with circulatory collapse. In some clients, giving a diuretic every other day or 3 to 5 days per week may be effective and is less likely to cause electrolyte imbalances.

Use With Digoxin

When digoxin and diuretics are given concomitantly, as is common when treating clients with heart failure, the risk of digoxin toxicity is increased. Digoxin toxicity is related to diuretic-induced hypokalemia. Potassium is a myocardial depressant and antiarrhythmic; it has essentially opposite cardiac effects to those of digoxin. In other words, extracellular potassium decreases the excitability of myocardial tissue, but digoxin increases excitability. The higher the serum potassium, the less effective a given dose of digoxin will be. Conversely, decreased serum potassium increases the likelihood of digoxin-induced cardiac arrhythmias, even with small doses and therapeutic serum levels of digoxin.

How Can You Avoid This Medication Error?

You are working on a cardiac unit, caring for clients after bypass surgery. Mr. Vellara has Lasix 80 mg ordered bid to pull off extra fluid that is retained from the surgery. After administering the medication, you look through the chart as you document the medication you gave. You note that the nursing assistant has charted the following:

Vital signs: 142/88 (lying) 108/60 (sitting), AP 96 and regular, R 18.
Daily weight—164 lb (a 9-lb drop from yesterday)
Yesterday's intake 1565 mL, output 3590 mL
Serum K+, 2.8 mEq/L

Were you wrong to administer the Lasix, and if so, why?

Supplemental potassium chloride, a potassium-sparing diuretic, and other measures to prevent hypokalemia are often used to maintain normal serum potassium levels (3.5 to 5.0 mEq/L).

Prevention and Treatment of Potassium Imbalances

Potassium imbalances (see Chap. 32) may occur with diuretic therapy. Hypokalemia and hyperkalemia are cardiotoxic and should be prevented when possible.

1. **Hypokalemia** (serum potassium level <3.5 mEq/L) may occur with potassium-losing diuretics (eg, hydrochlorothiazide, furosemide). Measures to prevent or treat hypokalemia include the following:
   a. Giving low doses of the diuretic (eg, 12.5 to 25 mg daily of hydrochlorothiazide; 25 mg daily of chlorthalidone)
   b. Giving supplemental potassium, usually potassium chloride, in an average dosage range of 20 to 60 mEq daily. Sustained-release tablets are usually better tolerated than liquid preparations.
   c. Giving a potassium-sparing diuretic along with the potassium-losing drug
   d. Increasing food intake of potassium. Many texts advocate this approach as preferable to supplemental potassium or combination diuretic therapy, but its effectiveness is not clearly established. Although the minimal daily requirement of potassium is unknown, usual recommendations are 40 to 50 mEq daily for the healthy adult. Potassium loss with diuretics may be several times this amount.

   Some foods (eg, bananas) have undeserved reputations for having high potassium content; actually, large amounts must be ingested. To provide 50 mEq of potassium daily, estimated amounts of certain foods include 1000 mL of orange juice, 1600 mL of apple or grape juice, 1200 mL of pineapple juice, four to six bananas, or 30 to 40 prunes. Some of these foods are high in calories and may be contraindicated, at least in large amounts, for obese clients.
   e. Restricting dietary sodium intake. This reduces potassium loss by decreasing the amount of sodium available for exchange with potassium in renal tubules.

2. **Hyperkalemia** (serum potassium level >5 mEq/L) may occur with potassium-sparing diuretics. The following measures help prevent hyperkalemia:
   a. Avoiding use of potassium-sparing diuretics and potassium supplements in clients with renal impairment
   b. Avoiding excessive amounts of potassium chloride supplements
   c. Avoiding salt substitutes
   d. Maintaining urine output, the major route for eliminating potassium from the body

Use in Children

Although they have not been extensively studied in children, diuretics are commonly used to treat heart failure, which often results from congenital heart disease; hypertension, which is usually related to cardiac or renal dysfunction; bronchopulmonary dysplasia and respiratory distress syndrome, which are often associated with pulmonary edema; and edema, which may occur with cardiac or renal disorders such as the nephrotic syndrome.

With most thiazides, safety and effectiveness have not been established for use in children. **Hydrochlorothiazide** is used in doses of approximately 2.2 mg/kg/day. IV chlorothiazide usually is not recommended. Thiazides do not commonly cause hyperglycemia, hyperuricemia, or hypercalcemia in children, as they do in adults.

Although **metolazone**, a thiazide-related drug, is not usually recommended, it is sometimes used. Metolazone has some advantages over a thiazide because it is a stronger diuretic, causes less hypokalemia, and can produce diuresis in renal failure. In children, it is most often used with furosemide, in which case it is most effective when given 30 to 60 minutes before the furosemide.

Furosemide is the loop diuretic used most often in children. Oral therapy is preferred when feasible, and doses above 6 mg/kg/day are not recommended. In preterm infants, furosemide stimulates production of prostaglandin E_2 in the kidneys and may increase the incidence of patent ductus arteriosus and neonatal respiratory distress syndrome. In neonates, furosemide may be given with indomethacin to prevent nonsteroidal anti-inflammatory drug–induced nephrotoxicity during therapeutic closure of a patent ductus arteriosus. In both preterm and full-term infants, furosemide half-life is prolonged but becomes shorter as renal and hepatic functions develop.

Adverse effects of furosemide include fluid and electrolyte imbalances (eg, hyponatremia, hypokalemia, fluid volume deficit) and ototoxicity. Serum electrolytes should be closely monitored in children because of frequent changes in kidney function and fluid distribution associated with growth and development. Ototoxicity, which is associated with high plasma drug levels (>50 µg/mL), can usually be avoided by dividing oral doses, and by slow injection or continuous infusion of IV doses.

Safety and effectiveness of bumetanide, ethacrynic acid, and torsemide have not been established. However, **bumetanide** may cause less ototoxicity and thus may be preferred for children who are taking other ototoxic drugs (eg, premature and ill neonates are often given gentamicin, an aminoglycoside antibiotic). Bumetanide may also cause less hypokalemia. The half-life of bumetanide is approximately 2 hours in critically ill infants and approximately 1 hour in children.

Spironolactone is the most widely used potassium-sparing diuretic in children. It is used with other diuretics to decrease potassium loss and hypokalemia. Spironolactone accumulates in renal failure, and dosage should be reduced. It usually should not be used in severe renal failure.

Use in Older Adults

Thiazide diuretics are often prescribed for the treatment of hypertension and heart failure, which are common in older adults. Older adults are especially sensitive to adverse drug effects, such as hypotension and electrolyte imbalance. Thiazides may aggravate renal or hepatic impairment. With rapid or excessive diuresis, myocardial infarction, renal impairment, or cerebral thrombosis may occur from fluid volume depletion and hypotension. The smallest effective dose is recommended, usually a daily dose of 12.5 to 25 mg of hydrochlorothiazide or equivalent doses of other thiazides and related drugs. Risks of adverse effects may exceed benefits at doses greater than 25 mg.

With loop diuretics, older adults are at greater risk of excessive diuresis, hypotension, fluid volume deficit, and possibly thrombosis or embolism. Rapid diuresis may cause urinary incontinence. With potassium-sparing diuretics, hyperkalemia is more likely to occur in older adults because of the renal impairment that occurs with aging.

Use in Renal Impairment

Most clients with renal impairment require diuretics as part of their drug therapy regimens. In these clients, the diuretic response may be reduced and edema of the gastrointestinal tract may limit absorption of oral medications.

Thiazides may be useful in treating edema due to renal disorders such as nephrotic syndrome and acute glomerulonephritis. However, their effectiveness decreases as the GFR decreases, and the drugs become ineffective when the GFR is less than 30 mL/minute. The drugs may accumulate and increase adverse effects in clients with impaired renal function. Thus, renal function tests should be performed periodically. If progressive renal impairment becomes evident (eg, a rising serum creatinine or BUN), a thiazide usually should be discontinued and metolazone, indapamide, or a loop diuretic may be given. Metolazone and indapamide are thiazide-related diuretics that may be effective in clients with significantly impaired renal function.

Loop diuretics are effective in clients with renal impairment. However, in chronic renal failure, they have lower peak concentrations at their site of action, which decreases diuresis. Renal elimination of the drugs is also prolonged. If renal dysfunction becomes more severe during treatment (eg, oliguria, increases in BUN or creatinine) the diuretic may need to be discontinued. If high doses of furosemide are used, a volume-controlled IV infusion at a rate of 4 mg/minute or less may be used. If IV bumetanide is given to clients with chronic renal impairment, a continuous infusion (eg, 12 mg over 12 hours) produces more diuresis than equivalent-dose intermittent injections. Continuous infusion also produces lower serum drug levels and therefore may decrease adverse effects.

Potassium-sparing diuretics are contraindicated in clients with renal impairment because of the high risk of hyperkalemia. If they are used at all, frequent monitoring of serum electrolytes, creatinine, and BUN is needed.

Use in Hepatic Impairment

Diuretics are often used to treat edema and ascites in clients with hepatic impairment. They must be used with caution because diuretic-induced fluid and electrolyte imbalances may precipitate or worsen hepatic encephalopathy and coma. In clients with cirrhosis, diuretic therapy should be initiated in a hospital setting, with small doses and careful monitoring. To prevent hypokalemia and metabolic alkalosis, supplemental potassium or spironolactone may be needed.

Use in Critical Illness

Fast-acting, potent diuretics such as furosemide and bumetanide are the most likely diuretics to be used in critically ill clients (eg, those with extensive edema, including pul-

monary edema). In clients with severe renal impairment, high doses are required to produce diuresis. Large doses may produce fluid volume depletion and worsen renal function. Although IV bolus doses of the drugs are often given, continuous IV infusions may be more effective and less likely to produce adverse effects in critically ill clients.

Home Care

Diuretics are often taken in the home setting. The home care nurse may need to assist clients and caregivers in using the drugs safely and effectively, monitor client responses (eg, assess nutritional status, blood pressure, weight, and use of over-the-counter medications that may aggravate edema or hypertension with each home visit), and provide information as indicated. In some cases, the home care nurse may need to assist the client in obtaining medications or blood tests (eg, serum potassium levels).

(*text continues on page 846*)

NURSING ACTIONS   Diuretics

NURSING ACTIONS	RATIONALE/EXPLANATION
1. Administer accurately	
a. Give in the early morning if ordered daily.	So that peak action will occur during waking hours and not interfere with sleep
b. Take safety precautions. Keep a bedpan or urinal within reach. Keep the call light within reach, and be sure the client knows how to use it. Assist to the bathroom anyone who is elderly, weak, dizzy, or unsteady in walking.	Mainly to avoid falls
c. Give amiloride and triamterene with or after food	To decrease gastrointestinal (GI) upset
d. Give intravenous (IV) injections of furosemide and bumetanide over 1–2 min; give torsemide over 2 min.	To decrease or avoid high peak serum levels, which increase risks of adverse effects, including ototoxicity
e. Give high-dose furosemide continuous IV infusions at a rate of 4 mg/min or less	
2. Observe for therapeutic effects	
a. Decrease or absence of edema, increased urine output, decreased blood pressure	Most oral diuretics act within approximately 2 h; IV diuretics act within minutes. Antihypertensive effects may not be evident for several days, with optimal effects in approximately 2–4 wk.
(1) Weigh the client daily while edema is present and two or three times weekly thereafter. Weigh under standard conditions: early morning before eating or drinking, after	Body weight is a very good indicator of fluid gain or loss. A weight change of 2.2 lb (1 kg) may indicate a gain or loss of 1000 mL of fluid. Also, weighing assists in dosage regulation to maintain thera-

(continued)

NURSING ACTIONS	RATIONALE/EXPLANATION
urination, with the same amount of clothing, and using the same scales.	peutic benefit without excessive or too rapid fluid loss.
(2) Record fluid intake and output every shift.	Normally, oral fluid intake approximates urinary output (1500 mL/24 h). With diuretic therapy, urinary output may exceed intake, depending on the amount of edema or fluid retention, renal function, and diuretic dosage. All sources of fluid gain, including IV fluids, must be included; all sources of fluid loss (perspiration, fever, wound drainage, GI tract drainage) are important. Clients with abnormal fluid losses have less urine output with diuretic therapy. Oliguria (decreased excretion of urine) may require stopping the drug. Output greater than 100 mL/h may indicate that side effects are more likely to occur.
(3) Observe and record characteristics of urine.	Excessively dilute urine may indicate excessive fluid intake or greater likelihood of fluid and electrolyte imbalance due to rapid diuresis. Concentrated urine may mean oliguria or decreased fluid intake.
(4) Check daily for edema: ankles for the ambulatory client, sacral area and posterior thighs for clients at bed rest. Also, it is often helpful to measure abdominal girth, ankles, and calves to monitor gain or loss of fluid.	Expect a decrease in visible edema and size of measured areas. If edema reappears or worsens, a thorough reassessment of the client is in order. Questions to be answered include the following:\n\n(1) Is the prescribed diuretic being taken correctly?\n\n(2) What type of diuretic and what dosage is ordered?\n\n(3) Is there worsening of the underlying condition(s) that contributed to edema formation in the first place?\n\n(4) Has other disease developed?
(5) In clients with congestive heart failure or acute pulmonary edema, observe for decreased dyspnea, rales, cyanosis, and cough.	Decreased fluid in the lungs leads to dramatic improvement in respirations as more carbon dioxide and oxygen gas exchange takes place and greater tissue oxygenation occurs.
(6) Record blood pressure two to four times daily when diuretic therapy is initiated.	Although thiazide diuretics apparently do not lower normal blood pressure, other diuretics may, especially with excessive or rapid diuresis.
3. Observe for adverse effects	Major adverse effects are fluid and electrolyte imbalances.
a. With potassium-losing diuretics (thiazides, bumetanide, furosemide, ethacrynic acid), observe for:	
(1) Hypokalemia	Potassium is required for normal muscle function. Thus, potassium depletion causes weakness of cardiovascular, respiratory, digestive, and skeletal muscles. Clients most likely to have hypokalemia are those who are taking large doses of diuretics, potent diuretics (eg, furosemide), or adrenal cortico-
(a) Serum potassium levels below 3.5 mEq/L	
(b) Electrocardiographic (ECG) changes (eg, low voltage, flattened T wave, depressed ST segment)	

(continued)

NURSING ACTIONS	RATIONALE/EXPLANATION
(c) Cardiac arrhythmias; weak, irregular pulse	steroids; those who have decreased food and fluid intake; or those who have increased potassium losses through vomiting, diarrhea, chronic laxative or enema use, or GI suction. Clinically significant symptoms are most likely to occur with a serum potassium level below 3 mEq/L.
(d) Hypotension	
(e) Weak, shallow respirations	
(f) Anorexia, nausea, vomiting	
(g) Decreased peristalsis or paralytic ileus	
(h) Skeletal muscle weakness	
(i) Confusion, disorientation	
(2) Hyponatremia, hypomagnesemia, hypochloremic alkalosis, changes in serum and urinary calcium levels	In addition to potassium, sodium chloride, magnesium, and bicarbonate also are lost with diuresis. Thiazides and related diuretics cause hypercalcemia and hypocalciuria. They have been used to prevent calcium nephrolithiasis (kidney stones). Furosemide and other loop diuretics tend to cause hypocalcemia and hypercalciuria.
(3) Dehydration	Fluid volume depletion occurs with excessive or rapid diuresis. If it is prolonged or severe, hypovolemic shock may occur.
(a) Poor skin turgor, dry mucous membranes	
(b) Oliguria, urine of high specific gravity	
(c) Thirst	
(d) Tachycardia; hypotension	
(e) Decreased level of consciousness	
(f) Elevated hematocrit (above 45%)	
(4) Hyperglycemia—blood glucose above 120 mg/100 mL, polyuria, polydipsia, polyphagia, glycosuria	Hyperglycemia is more likely to occur in clients with known or latent diabetes mellitus. Larger doses of hypoglycemic agents may be required. The hyperglycemic effect may be reversible when diuretic therapy is discontinued. Long-term use of a thiazide or loop diuretic may alter glucose metabolism. One mechanism is thought to involve diuretic-induced hypokalemia and hypomagnesemia, which then leads to decreased postprandial insulin release. Another mechanism may be development or worsening of insulin resistance. Because glucose intolerance is an important risk factor for coronary artery disease, diuretics should be used with caution in prediabetic or diabetic hypertensive clients.
(5) Hyperuricemia—serum uric acid above 7.0 mg/100 mL	Hyperuricemia is usually asymptomatic except for clients with gout, a predisposition toward gout, or chronic renal failure. Apparently, decreased renal excretion of uric acid allows its accumulation in the blood.

(continued)

NURSING ACTIONS	**RATIONALE/EXPLANATION**
(6) Pulmonary edema (with osmotic diuretics)	Pulmonary edema is most likely to occur in clients with congestive heart failure who cannot tolerate the increased blood volume produced by the drugs.
(7) Ototoxicity (with furosemide and ethacrynic acid)	Reversible or transient hearing impairment, tinnitus, and dizziness are more common, although irreversible deafness may occur. Ototoxicity is more likely to occur with high serum drug levels (eg, high doses or use in clients with severe renal impairment) or when other ototoxic drugs (eg, aminoglycoside antibiotics) are being taken concurrently.
b. With potassium-sparing diuretics (spironolactone, triamterene, amiloride), observe for:	
(1) Hyperkalemia	Hyperkalemia is most likely to occur in clients with impaired renal function or those who are ingesting additional potassium (eg, salt substitutes)
(a) Serum potassium levels above 5 mEq/L	
(b) ECG changes (ie, prolonged P-R interval; wide QRS complex; tall, peaked T wave; depressed ST segment)	
(c) Cardiac arrhythmias, which may progress to ventricular fibrillation and asystole	
4. Observe for drug interactions	
a. Drugs that *increase* effects of diuretics:	
(1) Aminoglycoside antibiotics	Additive ototoxicity with ethacrynic acid
(2) Antihypertensive agents	Additive hypotensive effects. In addition, angiotensin-converting enzyme inhibitor therapy significantly increases risks of hyperkalemia with spironolactone.
(3) Corticosteroids	Additive hypokalemia
b. Drugs that *decrease* effects of diuretics:	
(1) Nonsteroidal anti-inflammatory drugs (eg, aspirin, ibuprofen, others)	These drugs cause retention of sodium and water.
(2) Oral contraceptives	Retention of sodium and water
(3) Vasopressors (eg, epinephrine, norepinephrine)	These drugs may antagonize hypotensive effects of diuretics by decreasing responsiveness of arterioles.

Nursing Notes: Apply Your Knowledge

Answer: Assess blood pressure and compare this value with baseline blood pressure readings over the last few days. If blood pressure is significantly different from baseline (very high—greater than 180/90, or very low—less than 100/60), notify the physician because adjustment of medications may be indicated. Postural blood pressure should be monitored because orthostatic hypotension is likely for patients on these medications. When orthostatic hypotension is present, make sure to have the patient rise slowly, sitting until dizziness has passed. Daily weight and intake and output records should also be assessed to evaluate whether drug treatment is effective. Check for signs of hypokalemia and serum potassium levels. This is especially important because the client is on a high dose (80 mg/day) of a potassium-wasting diuretic without potassium supplementation. Hypokalemia can increase the risk of cardiac arrhythmias.

How Can You Avoid This Medication Error?

Answer: The purpose of the diuretic therapy is to pull off excessive fluid, but the assessment data gathered from Mr. Vallera (significant weight loss—almost 10 lb in 1 day; orthostatic B/P with elevated pulse, which indicates volume depletion; and hypokalemia) indicate that diuresis is occurring too rapidly. It is always important to evaluate assessment data before giving a medication, so that a medication can be held if the client's condition warrants it.

REVIEW AND APPLICATION EXERCISES

1. What are clinical indications for the use of diuretics?

2. What is the general mechanism by which diuretics act?

3. How can you assess a client for therapeutic effects of a diuretic?

4. Compare and contrast the main groups of diuretics in terms of adverse effects.

5. Why should serum potassium levels be monitored during diuretic therapy?

6. Which prescription and over-the-counter drugs may decrease the effects of a diuretic?

7. For a client who is starting diuretic therapy, what are important points to teach the client about safe and effective drug usage?

8. For a client who is taking a potassium-losing diuretic and a potassium chloride supplement, explain the possible consequences of discontinuing one drug while continuing the other.

SELECTED REFERENCES

Applegate, W.B. (1997). Approach to the elderly patient with hypertension. In W.N. Kelley (Ed.), *Textbook of internal medicine*, 3rd ed., pp. 2482–2488. Philadelphia: Lippincott-Raven.

Brater, D.C. (1997). Clinical pharmacology of cardiovascular drugs. In W.N. Kelley (Ed.), *Textbook of internal medicine*, 3rd ed., pp. 552–569. Philadelphia: Lippincott-Raven.

Cody, R.J. (1998). Intensive diuretic therapy for acute cardiac decompensation. In D.L. Brown (Ed.), *Cardiac intensive care*, pp. 555–562. Philadelphia: W.B. Saunders.

Drug facts and comparisons. (Updated monthly). St. Louis: Facts and Comparisons.

Guyton, A.C. & Hall, J.E. (1996). *Textbook of medical physiology*, 9th ed. Philadelphia: W.B. Saunders.

Hawkins, D.W., Bussey, H.I., & Prisant, L.M. (1997). Hypertension. In J.T. DiPiro, R.L. Talbert, G.C. Yee, G.R. Matzke, B.G. Wells, & L.M. Posey (Eds.), *Pharmacotherapy: A pathophysiologic approach*, 3rd ed., pp. 195–218. Stamford, CT: Appleton & Lange.

Jackson, E.K. (1996). Diuretics. In J.G. Hardman, L.E. Limbird, P.B. Molinoff, & R.W. Ruddon (Eds.), *Goodman & Gilman's The pharmacological basis of therapeutics*, 9th ed., pp. 685–713. New York: McGraw-Hill.

Johnson, J.A. & LaLonde, R.L. (1997). Congestive heart failure. In J.T. DiPiro, R.L. Talbert, G.C. Yee, G.R. Matzke, B.G. Wells, & L.M. Posey (Eds.), *Pharmacotherapy: A pathophysiologic approach*, 3rd ed., pp. 219–256. Stamford, CT: Appleton & Lange.

Porth, C.M. (Ed.). (1998). *Pathophysiology: Concepts of altered health states*, 5th ed. Philadelphia: Lippincott Williams & Wilkins.

Yunis, C. & Buckalew, V.M. (1998). Diuretic therapy. *Clinical Reviews*, Winter, 20–22. [Online: Available http://www.medscape.com/SMA/ClinicalReviews/1998/winter98/crW98.06.yuni/crW98.06.yuni-01.html. Accessed November 14, 1999.]

57

Drugs That Affect Blood Coagulation

Objectives

After studying this chapter, the student will be able to:

1. Describe important elements in the physiology of hemostasis and thrombosis.

2. Discuss potential consequences of blood clotting disorders.

3. Discuss characteristics and uses of anticoagulant, antiplatelet, and thrombolytic agents.

4. Compare and contrast heparin and warfarin in terms of indications for use, onset and duration of action, route of administration, blood tests used to monitor effects, and nursing process implications.

5. Teach clients on long-term warfarin therapy protective measures to prevent abnormal bleeding.

6. Discuss antiplatelet agents in terms of indications for use and effects on blood coagulation.

7. With aspirin, contrast the dose and frequency of administration for antiplatelet effects with those for analgesic, antipyretic, and anti-inflammatory effects.

8. Describe thrombolytic agents in terms of indications and contraindications for use, routes of administration, and major adverse effects.

9. Discuss the use of anticoagulant, antiplatelet, and thrombolytic drugs in special populations.

10. Describe systemic hemostatic agents for treating overdoses of anticoagulant and thrombolytic drugs.

Juan Sanchez, a 56-year-old migrant farmer without health insurance, is admitted to the hospital after an episode of syncope. He is diagnosed with atrial fibrillation and is started on a calcium channel blocker and Coumadin. Before his discharge, you are responsible for patient teaching.

Reflect on:

- Assessment data that would be helpful to individualize your teaching plan.

- Discuss the rationale for use of Coumadin for clients with atrial fibrillation.

- Identify side effects of Coumadin therapy.

- Consider strategies that might help Mr. Sanchez comply with therapy and experience limited side effects.

DESCRIPTION

Anticoagulant, antiplatelet, and thrombolytic drugs are used in the prevention and treatment of thrombotic and thromboembolic disorders. Thrombosis involves the formation (thrombogenesis) or presence of a blood clot (thrombus) in the vascular system. Blood clotting is a normal body defense mechanism to prevent blood loss. Thus, thrombogenesis may be life saving when it occurs as a response to hemorrhage; however, it may be life threatening when it occurs at other times, because the thrombus can obstruct a blood vessel and block blood flow to tissues beyond the clot. When part of a thrombus breaks off and travels to another part of the body, it is called an *embolus*.

Atherosclerosis is the basic disease process that often leads to pathologic thrombosis. It begins with accumulation of lipid-filled macrophages (ie, foam cells) on the inner lining of arteries. Foam cells develop in response to elevated blood lipid levels and eventually become fibrous plaques (ie, foam cells covered by smooth muscle cells and connective tissue). Advanced atherosclerotic lesions also contain hemorrhages, ulcerations, and scar tissue.

Atherosclerosis can affect any organ or tissue, but often involves the arteries supplying the heart, brain, and legs. Over time, plaque lesions become larger and extend farther into the lumen of the artery. Eventually, a thrombus may develop at plaque sites and partly or completely occlude an artery. In coronary arteries, a thrombus may precipitate myocardial ischemia (angina or infarction) (see Chap. 53); in carotid or brain arteries, a thrombus may precipitate a stroke; in peripheral arteries, a thrombus may cause intermittent claudication (pain in the legs with exercise) or acute occlusion. Thus, serious impairment of blood flow may occur with a large atherosclerotic plaque or a relatively small plaque with superimposed vasospasm and thrombosis. Consequences and clinical manifestations of thrombi and emboli depend primarily on their location and size.

Normally, thrombi are constantly being formed and dissolved (thrombolysis), but the blood stays fluid and blood flow is not significantly obstructed. If the balance between thrombogenesis and thrombolysis is upset, thrombotic or bleeding disorders result. Thrombotic disorders occur much more often than bleeding disorders and are emphasized here; bleeding disorders may result from excessive amounts of drugs that inhibit clotting. To aid understanding of drug therapy for thrombotic disorders, normal hemostasis, endothelial functions in relation to blood clotting, platelet functions, blood coagulation, and characteristics of arterial and venous thrombosis are described.

HEMOSTASIS

Hemostasis means prevention or stoppage of blood loss from an injured blood vessel. It involves activation of several mechanisms, including vasoconstriction, formation of a platelet plug (a cluster of aggregated platelets), sequential activation of clotting factors in the blood (Table 57-1), and growth of fibrous tissue (fibrin) into the blood clot to make it more stable and to repair the hole in the blood vessel. Overall, normal hemostasis is a complex process involving numerous interacting activators and inhibitors, including endothelial factors, platelets, and blood coagulation factors (Box 57-1).

CLOT LYSIS

When a blood clot is being formed, plasminogen (an inactive protein found in many body tissues and fluids) is bound to fibrin and becomes a component of the clot. After the outward blood flow is stopped and the rent in the blood vessel repaired, plasminogen is activated by plasminogen activator (produced by endothelial cells or the coagulation cascade) to produce plasmin. Plasmin is

TABLE 57-1	**Blood Coagulation Factors**	
Number	**Name**	**Functions**
I	Fibrinogen	Forms fibrin, the insoluble protein strands that compose the supporting framework of a blood clot. Thrombin and calcium are required for the conversion.
II	Prothrombin	Forms thrombin, which catalyzes the conversion of fibrinogen to fibrin
III	Thromboplastin	Converts prothrombin to thrombin
IV	Calcium	Catalyzes the conversion of prothrombin to thrombin
V	Labile factor	Required for formation of active thromboplastin
VII	Proconvertin or stable factor	Accelerates action of tissue thromboplastin
VIII	Antihemophilic factor	Promotes breakdown of platelets and formation of active platelet thromboplastin
IX	Christmas factor	Similar to factor VIII
X	Stuart factor	Promotes action of thromboplastin
XI	Plasma thromboplastin antecedent	Promotes platelet aggregation and breakdown, with subsequent release of platelet thromboplastin
XII	Hageman factor	Similar to factor XI
XIII	Fibrin-stabilizing factor	Converts fibrin meshwork to the dense, tight mass of the completely formed clot

BOX 57–1   HEMOSTASIS AND THROMBOSIS

The blood vessels and blood normally maintain a balance between procoagulant and anticoagulant factors that favors anticoagulation and keeps the blood fluid. Injury to blood vessels and tissues causes complex reactions and interactions among vascular endothelial cells, platelets, and blood coagulation factors that shift the balance toward procoagulation and thrombosis.

Endothelial cells

Endothelial cells play a role in all aspects of hemostasis and thrombosis. Normal endothelium helps to prevent thrombosis by producing anticoagulant factors, inhibiting platelet reactivity, and inhibiting activation of the coagulation cascade. However, endothelium promotes thrombosis when its continuity is lost (eg, the blood vessel wall is torn by rupture of atherosclerotic plaque, hypertension, trauma), its function is altered, or when blood flow is altered or becomes static. After a blood clot is formed, the endothelium also induces its dissolution and restoration of blood flow.

Antithrombotic Functions

- Synthesizes and releases prostacyclin (prostaglandin I_2), which inhibits platelet aggregation
- Releases endothelium-derived relaxing factor (nitric oxide), which inhibits platelet adhesion and aggregation
- Blocks platelet exposure to subendothelial collagen and other stimuli for platelet aggregation
- May inhibit platelet reactivity by inactivating adenosine diphosphate (ADP), a platelet product that promotes platelet aggregation.
- Produces plasminogen activators (eg, tissue-type or tPA) in response to shear stress and such agonists as histamine and thrombin. These activators convert inactive plasminogen to plasmin, which then breaks down fibrin and dissolves blood clots (fibrinolytic effects).
- Produces thrombomodulin, a protein that helps prevent formation of intravascular thrombi by inhibiting thrombin-mediated platelet aggregation. Thrombomodulin also reacts with thrombin to activate proteins C and S, which inhibit the plasma cascade of clotting factors.

Prothrombotic Functions

- Produces antifibrinolytic factors. Normally, the balance between profibrinolysis and antifibrinolysis favors fibrinolysis (clot dissolution). In pathologic conditions, including atherosclerosis, fibrinolysis may be limited and thrombosis enhanced.
- In pathologic conditions, may induce synthesis of prothrombotic factors such as von Willebrand factor. Von

Willebrand factor serves as a site for subendothelial platelet adhesion and as a carrier for blood coagulation factor VIII in plasma. Several disease states are associated with increased or altered production of von Willebrand factor, including atherosclerosis.

- Produces tissue factor, which activates the extrinsic coagulation pathway after exposure to oxidized low-density lipoprotein cholesterol, homocysteine, and cytokines (eg, interleukin-1, tumor necrosis factor-alpha)

Platelets

Platelets (also called *thrombocytes*) are fragments of large cells called *megakaryocytes*. They are produced in the bone marrow and released into the bloodstream, where they circulate for approximately 7 to 10 days before they are removed by the spleen. They contain no nuclei and therefore cannot repair or replicate themselves.

The cell membrane of a platelet contains a coat of glycoproteins that prevents the platelet from adhering to normal endothelium but allows it to adhere to damaged areas of endothelium and subendothelial collagen in the blood vessel wall. It also contains receptors for ADP, collagen, blood coagulation factors such as fibrinogen, and other substances. Breakdown of the cell membrane releases arachidonic acid (which can be metabolized to produce thromboxane A_2) and allows leakage of platelet contents (eg, thromboplastin and other clotting factors), which serve various functions to stop bleeding

The cytoplasm of a platelet contains storage granules with ADP, fibrinogen, histamine, platelet-derived growth factor, serotonin, von Willebrand factor, enzymes that produce thromboxane A_2, and other substances. The cytoplasm also contains contractile proteins that contract storage granules so they empty their contents and help a platelet plug to retract and plug a hole in a torn blood vessel.

The only known function of platelets is hemostasis. When platelets come in contact with a damaged vascular surface, they become activated and undergo changes in structure and function. They enlarge, express receptors on their surfaces, release mediators from their storage granules, become sticky so that they stick to endothelial and collagen cells, and form a platelet thrombus (ie, a cluster or aggregate of activated platelets) within seconds. The thrombus blocks the blood vessel and prevents further leakage of blood. Platelets usually disappear from a blood clot within 24 hours and are replaced by fibrin.

(continued)

BOX 57–1   HEMOSTASIS AND THROMBOSIS *(continued)*

Formation of a platelet thrombus proceeds through the phases of activation, adhesion, aggregation, and procoagulation.

Activation

Platelet activation occurs when agonists such as thrombin, collagen, ADP, or epinephrine bind to their specific receptors on the platelet cell membrane surface. Activated platelets release von Willebrand factor, which aids platelet adhesion to blood vessel walls. They also secrete ADP and thromboxane A_2 into the blood. The ADP and thromboxane A_2 activate and recruit nearby platelets.

Adhesion

Platelet adhesion involves changes in platelets that allow them to adhere to endothelial cells and subendothelial collagen exposed by damaged endothelium. Adhesion is mediated by interactions between platelets and substances in the subendothelial tissues. Platelets contain binding sites for several subendothelial tissue proteins, including collagen and von Willebrand factor. In capillaries, where blood shear rates are high, platelets also can bind indirectly to collagen through von Willebrand factor. Von Willebrand factor is synthesized by endothelial cells and megakaryocytes. Although it contains binding sites for platelets and collagen, it does not normally bind with platelets until they are activated.

Aggregation

Aggregation involves the accumulation of platelets at a site of injury to a blood vessel wall and is stimulated by ADP, collagen, thromboxane A_2, thrombin, and other factors. It requires the binding of extracellular fibrinogen to platelet fibrinogen receptors. The fibrinogen receptor is located on a complex of two glycoproteins (GPIIb and IIIa) in the platelet cell membrane. Although many GP IIb/IIIa complexes are on the surface of each platelet, they do not function as fibrinogen receptors until the platelet is activated by an agonist. Each activated GP IIb/IIIa complex is capable of binding a single fibrinogen molecule. However, a fibrinogen molecule may bind to receptors on adjacent activated platelets, thus acting as a bridge to connect the platelets. Activated GP IIb/IIIa complexes can also bind von Willebrand factor and promote platelet aggregation when fibrinogen is lacking.

Aggregated platelets produce and release thromboxane A_2, which acts with ADP from platelet storage granules to promote additional GP IIb/IIIa activation, platelet secretion, and aggregate formation. The exposure of functional GP IIb/IIIa complexes is also stimulated by thrombin, which can directly stimulate thromboxane A_2

synthesis and granule secretion without initial aggregation. Collagen stimulates additional aggregation by increasing the production of thromboxane A_2 and storage granule secretion.

Overall, aggregated platelets release substances that recruit new platelets and stimulate additional aggregation. This activity helps the platelet plug become large enough to block blood flow out of a damaged blood vessel. If the opening is small, the platelet plug can stop blood loss. If the opening is large, a platelet plug and a blood clot are both required to stop the bleeding.

Procoagulant Activity

In addition to forming a platelet thrombus, platelets also activate and interact with circulating blood coagulation factors to form a larger, more stable blood clot. Activation of the previously inactive blood coagulation factors leads to formation of fibrin threads that attach to the platelets and form a tight meshwork of a fully developed blood clot.

More specifically, the platelet plug provides a surface on which coagulation enzymes, substrates, and cofactors interact at high local concentrations. These interactions lead to activation of coagulation factor X and the conversion of prothrombin to thrombin.

Blood Coagulation

The blood coagulation process causes hemostasis within 1 to 2 minutes. It involves sequential activation of clotting factors that are normally present in blood and tissues as inactive precursors and formation of a meshwork of fibrin strands that cements blood components together to form a stable, dense clot. Major phases include release of thromboplastin by disintegrating platelets and damaged tissue; conversion of prothrombin to thrombin, which requires thromboplastin and calcium ions; and conversion of fibrinogen to fibrin by thrombin.

Blood coagulation results from activation of the intrinsic or extrinsic coagulation pathway. Both pathways, which are activated when blood passes out of a blood vessel, are needed for normal hemostasis. The intrinsic pathway occurs in the vascular system; the extrinsic pathway occurs in the tissues. Although the pathways are initially separate, the terminal steps (ie, activation of factor X and thrombin-induced formation of fibrin) are the same.

The intrinsic pathway is activated when blood comes in contact with collagen in the injured vessel wall and coagulation factor XII interacts with biologic surfaces. The normal endothelium prevents factor XII from interacting with such surfaces. The activated form of factor XII is a protease that starts the interactions among fac-

(continued)

BOX 57–1   HEMOSTASIS AND THROMBOSIS (*continued*)

tors involved in the intrinsic pathway (eg, prekallikrein, factor IX, factor VIII).

The extrinsic pathway is activated when blood is exposed to tissue extracts and tissue factor interacts with circulating coagulation factor VII. Activated factors VII and IX both act on factor X to produce activated factor X, which then interacts with factor V, calcium, and platelet factor 3. Platelet factor 3, a component of the platelet cell membrane, becomes available on the platelet surface only during platelet activation. The interactions among these substances lead to formation of thrombin, which then activates fibrinogen to form fibrin, and the clot is complete.

---

an enzyme that breaks down the fibrin meshwork that stabilizes the clot; this fibrinolytic or thrombolytic action dissolves the clot.

THROMBOTIC AND THROMBOEMBOLIC DISORDERS

Thrombosis may occur in both arteries and veins. Arterial thrombosis is usually associated with atherosclerotic plaque, hypertension, and turbulent blood flow. These conditions damage arterial endothelium and activate platelets to initiate the coagulation process. Arterial thrombi cause disease by obstructing blood flow. If the obstruction is incomplete or temporary, local tissue ischemia (deficient blood supply) occurs. If the obstruction is complete or prolonged, local tissue death or infarction occurs.

Venous thrombosis is usually associated with venous stasis. When blood flows slowly, thrombin and other procoagulant substances present in the blood become concentrated in local areas and initiate the clotting process. With a normal rate of blood flow, these substances are rapidly removed from the blood, primarily by Kupffer cells in the liver. A venous thrombus is less cohesive than an arterial thrombus, and an embolus can easily become detached and travel to other parts of the body.

Venous thrombi cause disease by two mechanisms. First, thrombosis causes local congestion, edema, and perhaps inflammation by impairing normal outflow of venous blood (eg, thrombophlebitis, deep vein thrombosis [DVT]). Second, embolization obstructs the blood supply when the embolus becomes lodged. The pulmonary arteries are common sites of embolization.

DRUGS USED IN THROMBOTIC AND THROMBOEMBOLIC DISORDERS

Drugs given to prevent or treat thrombosis alter some aspect of the blood coagulation process. Anticoagulants are widely used in thrombotic disorders. They are more effective in preventing venous thrombosis than arterial thrombosis. Antiplatelet drugs are used to prevent arterial thrombosis. Thrombolytic agents are used to dissolve thrombi and limit tissue damage in selected thromboembolic disorders. These drugs are described in the following sections and in Table 57-2.

Anticoagulants

Anticoagulant drugs are given to prevent formation of new clots and extension of clots already present. They do not dissolve formed clots, improve blood flow in tissues around the clot, or prevent ischemic damage to tissues beyond the clot. Heparins and warfarin are commonly used anticoagulants; danaparoid and lepirudin are newer agents. Clinical indications include prevention or treatment of thromboembolic disorders, such as thrombophlebitis, DVT, and pulmonary embolism. The main adverse effect is bleeding.

Heparin

Heparin is a pharmaceutical preparation of the natural anticoagulant produced primarily by mast cells in pericapillary connective tissue. Endogenous heparin is found in various body tissues, most abundantly in the liver and lungs. Exogenous heparin is obtained from bovine lung or porcine intestinal mucosa and standardized in units of biologic activity.

Heparin combines with antithrombin III (a natural anticoagulant in the blood) to inactivate clotting factors IX, X, XI, and XII, inhibit the conversion of prothrombin to thrombin, and prevent thrombus formation. After thrombosis has developed, heparin can inhibit additional coagulation by inactivating thrombin, preventing the conversion of fibrinogen to fibrin, and inhibiting factor XIII (the fibrin-stabilizing factor). Other effects include inhibiting factors V and VIII and platelet aggregation.

Heparin acts immediately after intravenous (IV) and within 20 to 30 minutes after subcutaneous injection. It is metabolized in the liver and excreted in the urine, primarily as inactive metabolites. Heparin does not cross the placental barrier and is not secreted in breast milk. Disadvantages of heparin are its short duration of action and the subsequent need for frequent administration, the necessity for parenteral injection (because it is not absorbed

TABLE 57-2 Anticoagulant, Antiplatelet, and Thrombolytic Agents

Generic/Trade Name	Indications for Use	Dosage
Anticoagulants		
Heparin	Prevention and treatment of thromboembolic disorders (eg, deep vein thrombosis, pulmonary embolism, atrial fibrillation with embolization)	*Adults*, IV injection, 5000 units initially, followed by 5000–10,000 units q4–6h, to a maximum dose of 25,000 units/d DIC, IV injection, 50–100 units/kg q4h; IV infusion, 20,000–40,000 units/d at initial rate of 0.25 units/kg/min, then adjusted according to APTT SC 10,000–12,000 units q8h, or 14,000–20,000 units q12h Low-dose prophylaxis, SC 5000 units 2 h before surgery, then q12h until discharged from hospital or fully ambulatory *Children*, DIC, IV injection, 25–50 units/kg q4h IV infusion, 50 units/kg initially, followed by 100 units/kg q4h or 20,000 units/m² over 24 h
Ardeparin (Normiflo)	Prophylaxis of DVT in clients having knee replacement surgery	SC 50 U/kg q12h, starting evening of surgery or next morning and continuing for 14 d or less, until the client is fully ambulatory
Dalteparin (Fragmin)	Prophylaxis of DVT in clients having hip replacement surgery; also clients at high risk of thromboembolic disorders who are having abdominal surgery	Abdominal surgery, SC 2500 IU 1–2 h before surgery and then once daily for 5–10 d after surgery Hip replacement surgery, SC 2500 IU 1–2 h before surgery and the evening of surgery (at least 6 h after first dose) and then 5000 IU once daily for 5 d
Danaparoid (Orgaran)	Prophylaxis of DVT in clients having hip replacement surgery	SC 750 IU twice daily, with first dose 1–24 h before surgery, then daily for 7–14 d after surgery
Enoxaparin (Lovenox)	Prevention and treatment of DVT and pulmonary embolism Treatment of unstable angina, to prevent myocardial infarction	DVT prophylaxis in clients having hip or knee replacement surgery, SC 30 mg twice daily, with first dose within 12–24 h after surgery and continued for approximately 7–10 d Abdominal surgery, SC 40 mg once daily with first dose given 2 h before surgery, for 7–10 d DVT/pulmonary embolism treatment, outpatients, SC 1 mg/kg q12h; inpatients, 1 mg/kg q12h or 1.5 mg/kg q24h Unstable angina 1 mg/kg q12h in conjunction with oral aspirin (100–325 mg once daily)
Lepirudin (Refludan)	Heparin alternative for anticoagulation of clients with heparin-induced thrombocytopenia and associated thromboembolic disorders	IV injection, 0.4 mg/kg over 15–20 sec, followed by continuous IV infusion of 0.15 mg/kg for 2–10 d or longer if needed
Warfarin (Coumadin)	Long-term prevention or treatment of venous thromboembolic disorders, including deep vein thrombosis, pulmonary embolism, and embolization associated with atrial fibrillation and prosthetic heart valves. May also be used after myocardial infarction to decrease reinfarction, stroke, venous thromboembolism, and death	PO 5–10 mg/d for 2–3 d, then adjusted according to the international normalized ratio (INR); average maintenance dose, 2–5 mg/d
Antiplatelet Agents		
Aspirin	Prevention of myocardial infarction Prevention of thromboembolic disorders in clients with prosthetic heart valves or transient ischemic attacks	PO 81–325 mg/d
Abciximab (ReoPro)	Used with PTCA to prevent rethrombosis of treated arteries Intended for use with aspirin and heparin	IV bolus injection, 0.25 mg/kg 10–60 min before starting PCTA, then a continuous IV infusion of 10 μg/min for 12 h
Anagrelide (Agrylin)	Essential thrombocythemia, to reduce the elevated platelet count, the risk of thrombosis, and associated symptoms	PO 0.5 mg four times daily or 1 mg twice daily initially, then titrate to lowest dose effective in maintaining platelet count <600,000/mm³

TABLE 57-2	Anticoagulant, Antiplatelet, and Thrombolytic Agents (continued)	
Generic/Trade Name	**Indications for Use**	**Dosage**
Cilostazol (Pletal)	Intermittent claudication, to increase walking distance (before leg pain occurs)	PO 100 mg twice daily approximately 30 min before or 2 h after breakfast and dinner; reduce to 50 mg twice daily with concurrent use of ketoconazole, itraconazole, erythromycin, or diltiazem
Clopidogrel (Plavix)	Reduction of atherosclerotic events (myocardial infarction, stroke, vascular death) in clients with atherosclerosis documented by recent stroke, recent myocardial infarction, or established peripheral artery disease	PO 75 mg once daily with or without food
Dipyridamole (Persantine)	Prevention of thromboembolism after cardiac valve replacement, given with warfarin	PO 25–75 mg three times per day, 1 h before meals
Eptifibatide (Integrilin)	Acute coronary syndromes, including clients who are to be managed medically and those undergoing PTCA	IV bolus injection, 180 µg/kg, followed by continuous infusion of 2 µg/kg/min. See manufacturer's instructions for preparation and administration.
Ticlopidine (Ticlid)	Prevention of thrombosis in clients with coronary artery or cerebral vascular disease (eg, clients who have had stroke precursors or a completed thrombotic stroke)	PO 250 mg twice daily with food
Tirofiban (Aggrastat)	Acute coronary syndromes, with heparin, for clients who are to be managed medically or those undergoing PTCA	IV infusion, 0.4 µg/kg/min for 30 min, then 0.1 µg/kg/min. Patients with severe renal impairment (creatinine clearance <30 mL/min) should receive half the usual rate of infusion. See manufacturer's instructions for preparation and administration.
Thrombolytic Agents		
Alteplase (Activase)	Acute myocardial infarction Pulmonary embolism Acute ischemic stroke	IV infusion, 100 mg over 3 h (first hour, 60 mg with a bolus of 6–10 mg over 1–2 min initially; second hour, 20 mg; third hour, 20 mg)
Anistreplase, recombinant (Eminase)	Acute myocardial infarction	IV injection, 30 units over 2–5 min
Reteplase, recombinant (Retavase)	Acute myocardial infarction	IV injection, 10 units over 2 min, repeated in 30 min. Inject into a flowing IV infusion line that contains no other medications.
Streptokinase (Streptase)	Treatment of acute pulmonary emboli or iliofemoral thrombophlebitis when these conditions are severe and life threatening Used to dissolve clots in arterial or venous cannulas or catheters May be injected into a coronary artery to dissolve a thrombus if done within 6 h of onset of symptoms	IV 250,000 units over 30 min, then 100,000 units/h for 24–72 h
Urokinase (Abbokinase)	Coronary artery thrombi Pulmonary emboli Clearance of clogged IV catheters	IV 4400 units/kg over 10 min, followed by continuous infusion of 4400 units/kg/h for 12 h For clearing IV catheters, see manufacturer's instructions

APTT, activated partial thromboplastin time; DIC, disseminated intravascular coagulation; DVT, deep vein thrombosis; IV, intravenous; PTCA, percutaneous transluminal coronary angioplasty or atherectomy; SC, subcutaneous.

Nursing Notes: Apply Your Knowledge

You are caring for a patient who is in traction. He is receiving 5000 units of subcutaneous heparin bid. Discuss the reason why this patient is receiving heparin and how you will safely administer the medication.

from the gastrointestinal [GI] tract), and local tissue reactions at injection sites.

Prophylactically, low doses of heparin are given to prevent DVT and pulmonary embolism in clients at risk for development of these disorders, such as the following:

1. Those with major illnesses (eg, acute myocardial infarction, heart failure, serious pulmonary infections, stroke)

2. Those having major abdominal or thoracic surgery
3. Those with a history of thrombophlebitis or pulmonary embolism, including pregnant women
4. Those having gynecologic surgery, especially if they have been taking estrogens or oral contraceptives or have other risk factors for DVT
5. Those expected to be on bed rest or to have limited activity for longer than 5 days

Low-dose heparin prophylaxis is either ineffective or contraindicated in major orthopedic surgery, abdominal prostatectomy, and brain surgery.

Therapeutically, heparin is used for treatment of acute thromboembolic disorders (eg, DVT, thrombophlebitis, pulmonary embolism). In these conditions, the aim of therapy is to prevent further thrombus formation and embolization. Heparin is also used in disseminated intravascular coagulation (DIC), a life-threatening condition characterized by widespread clotting, which depletes the blood of coagulation factors. The depletion of coagulation factors then produces widespread bleeding. The goal of heparin therapy in DIC is to prevent blood coagulation long enough for clotting factors to be replenished and thus be able to control hemorrhage.

Heparin is also used to prevent clotting during cardiac and vascular surgery, extracorporeal circulation, hemodialysis, blood transfusions, and in blood samples to be used in laboratory tests.

Contraindications include GI ulcerations (eg, peptic ulcer disease, ulcerative colitis), blood dyscrasias, severe kidney or liver disease, severe hypertension, polycythemia vera, and recent surgery of the eye, spinal cord, or brain. It should be used with caution in clients with hypertension, renal or hepatic disease, alcoholism, history of GI ulcerations, drainage tubes (eg, nasogastric tubes, indwelling urinary catheters), and any occupation with high risks of traumatic injury.

Low–Molecular-Weight Heparins

Standard heparin is a mixture of high– and low–molecular-weight fractions, but most anticoagulant activity is attributed to the low–molecular-weight portion. **Low–molecular-weight heparins** (LMWH) (eg, enoxaparin) contain the low–molecular-weight fraction and are as effective as IV heparin in treating thrombotic disorders. Indications for use include prevention or treatment of thromboembolic complications associated with surgery or ischemic complications of unstable angina and myocardial infarction. LMWH differ from standard heparin and each other; they cannot be used interchangeably (ie, unit for unit).

In addition, LMWH are given subcutaneously and do not require close monitoring of blood coagulation tests. These characteristics allow outpatient anticoagulant therapy, an increasing trend. LMWH are also associated with less thrombocytopenia than standard heparin. However, platelet counts should be monitored during therapy.

Warfarin

Warfarin is the most commonly used oral anticoagulant. It acts in the liver to prevent synthesis of vitamin K–dependent clotting factors (ie, factors II, VII, IX, and X). Warfarin is similar to vitamin K in structure and therefore acts as a competitive antagonist to hepatic use of vitamin K. Anticoagulant effects do not occur for approximately 3 to 5 days after warfarin is started because clotting factors already in the blood follow their normal pathway of elimination. Warfarin has no effect on circulating clotting factors or on platelet function.

Warfarin is well absorbed after oral administration. It is highly bound to plasma proteins (approximately 98%), mainly albumin. It is metabolized in the liver and primarily excreted as inactive metabolites by the kidneys.

Warfarin is most useful in long-term prevention or treatment of venous thromboembolic disorders, including DVT, pulmonary embolism, and embolization associated with atrial fibrillation and prosthetic heart valves. In addition, warfarin therapy after myocardial infarction may decrease reinfarction, stroke, venous thromboembolism, and death. Smaller doses are being used now than formerly, with similar antithrombotic effects and decreased risks of bleeding.

Like heparin, warfarin is contraindicated in clients with GI ulcerations, blood disorders associated with bleeding, severe kidney or liver disease, severe hypertension, and recent surgery of the eye, spinal cord, or brain. It should be used cautiously with mild hypertension, renal or hepatic disease, alcoholism, history of GI ulcerations, drainage tubes (eg, nasogastric tubes, indwelling urinary catheters), and occupations with high risks of traumatic injury. In addition, warfarin is contraindicated during pregnancy.

Other Anticoagulant Drugs

Danaparoid is a low–molecular-weight, heparin-like drug derived from porcine mucosa. It has antithrombotic effects and is given subcutaneously to prevent postoperative thromboembolism in clients having hip replacement surgery. It cannot be used interchangeably with standard heparin or LMWH.

Lepirudin is a recombinant form of hirudin, an anticoagulant secreted by leeches. It prevents blood coagulation by inactivating thrombin. It is used as a heparin substitute for clients who need anticoagulation but have thrombocytopenia with heparin.

Antiplatelet Drugs

Antiplatelet drugs prevent one or more steps in the prothrombotic activity of platelets. As described previously, platelet activity is very important in both physiologic hemostasis and pathologic thrombosis. Arterial thrombi, which are composed primarily of platelets, may form on top of atherosclerotic plaque and block blood flow in the artery. They may also form on heart walls and valves and embolize to other parts of the body.

Drugs used clinically for antiplatelet effects act by a variety of mechanisms to inhibit platelet activation, adhesion, aggregation, or procoagulant activity. These include drugs that block platelet receptors for thromboxane A$_2$, adenosine diphosphate (ADP), glycoprotein (GP) IIb/IIIa, and phosphodiesterase.

Thromboxane A$_2$ Inhibitors

Aspirin is a commonly used analgesic–antipyretic–anti-inflammatory drug (see Chap. 7) with potent antiplatelet effects. Aspirin exerts pharmacologic actions by inhibiting synthesis of prostaglandins. In this instance, aspirin acetylates cyclooxygenase, the enzyme in platelets that normally synthesizes thromboxane A$_2$, a prostaglandin product that causes platelet aggregation. Thus, aspirin prevents formation of thromboxane A$_2$ and thromboxane A$_2$-induced platelet aggregation and thrombus formation. A single dose of 300 to 600 mg or multiple doses of 30 mg (eg, daily for several days) inhibit the cyclooxygenase in circulating platelets almost completely. These antithrombotic effects persist for the life of the platelet (7 to 10 days). Aspirin may be used long term for prevention of myocardial infarction or stroke, and in clients with prosthetic heart valves. It is also increasingly being used for initial treatment of acute myocardial infarction (eg, when thrombolytic drugs are contraindicated or when thrombolytics or angioplasty cannot be started early enough to decrease infarction or reperfusion injury) and transient ischemic attacks (TIAs) or evolving thrombotic strokes. Adverse effects are uncommon with the small doses used for antiplatelet effects. However, there is an increased risk of bleeding, including hemorrhagic stroke. Because approximately 85% of strokes are thrombotic, the benefits of aspirin or other antiplatelet agents are thought to outweigh the risks of hemorrhagic strokes (approximately 15%).

Nonsteroidal anti-inflammatory drugs (NSAIDs), including ibuprofen and many other aspirin-related drugs, inhibit cyclooxygenase reversibly. Their antiplatelet effects subside when the drugs are eliminated from the circulation and the drugs usually are not used for antiplatelet effects. However, clients who take an NSAID daily (eg, for arthritis pain) may not need to take additional aspirin for antiplatelet effects. Acetaminophen does not affect platelets in usual doses.

Adenosine Diphosphate Receptor Antagonists

Ticlopidine inhibits platelet aggregation by preventing ADP-induced binding between platelets and fibrinogen. This reaction inhibits platelet aggregation irreversibly, and effects persist for the lifespan of the platelet. The drug is indicated for prevention of thrombotic stroke in people who have had stroke precursor events (eg, TIAs) or a completed thrombotic stroke. Ticlopidine is considered a second-line drug for clients who cannot take aspirin, mainly because of adverse effects (eg, neutropenia, diarrhea, skin rashes) and greater cost. Contraindications include active bleeding disorders (eg, GI bleeding from peptic ulcer or intracranial bleeding), neutropenia, thrombocytopenia, severe liver disease, and hypersensitivity to the drug.

Ticlopidine is rapidly absorbed after oral administration and reaches peak plasma levels approximately 2 hours after a dose. It is highly protein bound (98%), extensively metabolized in the liver, and excreted in urine and feces. As with other antiplatelet drugs, there is increased risk of bleeding with ticlopidine.

Clopidogrel is a newer drug that is chemically related to ticlopidine and causes similar effects. It is indicated for reduction of myocardial infarction, stroke, and vascular death in clients with atherosclerosis and reportedly causes fewer or less severe adverse effects than ticlopidine.

Glycoprotein IIb/IIIa Receptor Antagonists

Abciximab is a monoclonal antibody that prevents the binding of fibrinogen, von Willebrand factor, and other molecules to GP IIb/IIIa receptors on activated platelets. This action inhibits platelet aggregation.

Abciximab is used with percutaneous transluminal coronary angioplasty or removal of atherosclerotic plaque to prevent rethrombosis of treated arteries. It is used with aspirin and heparin and is contraindicated in clients who have recently received an oral anticoagulant or IV Dextran. Other contraindications include active bleeding, thrombocytopenia, history of a serious stroke, surgery or major trauma within the previous 6 weeks, uncontrolled hypertension, or hypersensitivity to drug components.

Eptifibatide and **tirofiban** inhibit platelet aggregation by preventing activation of GP IIb/IIIa receptors on the platelet surface and the subsequent binding of fibrinogen and von Willebrand factor to platelets. Antiplatelet effects occur during drug infusion and stop when the drug is stopped. The drugs are indicated for acute coronary syndrome (eg, unstable angina, myocardial infarction) in clients who are to be managed medically or by angioplasty or atherectomy.

Drug half-life is approximately 2.5 hours for eptifibatide and 2 hours for tirofiban; the drugs are cleared mainly by renal excretion. With tirofiban, plasma clearance is approximately 25% lower in older adults and approximately 50% lower in clients with severe renal impairment (creatinine clearance <30 mL/minute).

The drugs are contraindicated in clients with hypersensitivity to any component of the products; current or previous bleeding (within the previous 30 days); a history of thrombocytopenia after previous exposure to tirofiban; a history of stroke within 30 days or any history of hemorrhagic stroke; major surgery or severe physical trauma within the previous month; severe hypertension (systolic blood pressure >180 mm Hg with tirofiban or >200 mm Hg with eptifibatide, or diastolic blood pressure >110 mm Hg with either drug); a history of intracranial hemorrhage, neoplasm, arteriovenous malformation, or aneurysm; a platelet count less than 100,000 mm^3; serum creatinine 2 mg/dL or above (for the 180 μg/kg bolus and the 2 μg/kg/minute infusion) or 4 mg/dL or above (for the 135 μg/kg bolus and the 0.5 μg/kg/minute infusion); or dependency on dialysis (eptifibatide).

Bleeding is the most common adverse effect, with most major bleeding occurring at the arterial access site for cardiac catheterization. If bleeding occurs and cannot be controlled with pressure, the drug infusion and heparin should be discontinued.

These drugs should be used cautiously if given with other drugs that affect hemostasis (eg, warfarin, thrombolytics, other antiplatelet drugs).

Phosphodiesterase Inhibitor

Cilostazol inhibits phosphodiesterase, an enzyme that metabolizes cyclic adenosine monophosphate (cAMP). The inhibition increases intracellular cAMP, which then inhibits platelet aggregation and produces vasodilation. The drug reversibly inhibits platelet aggregation induced by various stimuli (eg, thrombin, ADP, collagen, arachidonic acid, epinephrine, and shear stress). It is indicated for treatment of intermittent claudication. Symptoms usually improve within 2 to 4 weeks, but may take as long as 12 weeks. The drug is contraindicated in clients with heart failure.

Cilostazol is highly protein bound (95% to 98%), mainly to albumin, extensively metabolized by hepatic cytochrome P450 enzymes, and excreted in urine (74%) and feces. The drug and two active metabolites accumulate with chronic administration and reach steady state within a few days. The most common adverse effects are diarrhea and headache.

Miscellaneous Agents

Anagrelide inhibits platelet aggregation induced by cAMP phosphodiesterase, ADP, and collagen. However, it is indicated only to reduce platelet counts for clients with essential thrombocythemia (a disorder characterized by excessive numbers of platelets). Doses to reduce platelet production are smaller than those required to inhibit platelet aggregation.

Dipyridamole inhibits platelet adhesion, but its mechanism of action is unclear. It is used for prevention of thromboembolism after cardiac valve replacement. It is given with warfarin.

Thrombolytic Agents

Thrombolytic agents are given to dissolve thrombi. They stimulate conversion of plasminogen to plasmin (also called fibrinolysin), a proteolytic enzyme that breaks down fibrin, the framework of a thrombus. The main use of thrombolytic agents is for treatment of acute, severe thromboembolic disease, such as myocardial infarction, pulmonary embolism, and iliofemoral thrombosis.

The goal of thrombolytic therapy is to reestablish blood flow and prevent or limit tissue damage. Heparin and warfarin are given after therapy is finished. The drugs also are used to dissolve clots in intravascular catheters.

Alteplase, which is produced by recombinant deoxyribonucleic acid technology, is a tissue plasminogen activator and is often called tPA. It is used in acute myocardial infarction to dissolve clots obstructing coronary arteries and reestablish perfusion of tissues beyond the thrombotic area. The drug binds to fibrin in a clot and acts locally to dissolve the clot. It has fewer systemic effects than streptokinase.

The most common adverse effect is bleeding, which may be internal (eg, intracranial, GI, genitourinary) or external (eg, venous or arterial puncture sites, surgical incisions). The drug is contraindicated in the presence of bleeding, a history of stroke, central nervous system surgery or trauma within the previous 2 months, and severe hypertension.

Anistreplase is a combination of human plasminogen and streptokinase. Like alteplase, it breaks down fibrin and is used to lyse coronary artery clots in acute myocardial infarction. Adverse effects and contraindications are the same as for other thrombolytic agents. An advantage is that anistreplase can be given in a single IV injection.

Streptokinase, a protein derived from streptococci, promotes dissolution of blood clots by interacting with a plasminogen proactivator. The resulting substance catalyzes the conversion of plasminogen to plasmin. Plasmin breaks down fibrin. Streptokinase may be used for treatment of acute pulmonary emboli or iliofemoral thrombophlebitis when these conditions are severe and life threatening. Bleeding, fever, and allergic reactions may occur. Streptokinase also may be injected directly into a coronary artery to dissolve a thrombus if done within 6 hours of onset of symptoms. An additional use is to dissolve clots in arterial or venous cannulas or catheters.

Urokinase is a proteolytic enzyme that catalyzes the conversion of plasminogen to plasmin. Plasmin breaks down fibrin and thereby promotes dissolution of blood clots. Urokinase is recommended for use in clients allergic to streptokinase. It is contraindicated in children, pregnant women, and clients with wounds, malignancies, and recent strokes. In addition, all other contraindications to heparin and warfarin therapy apply to urokinase. Urokinase causes a high incidence of bleeding and is more expensive than other thrombolytics.

Drugs Used to Control Bleeding

Anticoagulant, antiplatelet, and thrombolytic drugs profoundly affect hemostasis, and their major adverse effect is bleeding. As a result, systemic hemostatic agents (antidotes) may be needed to prevent or treat bleeding episodes. Antidotes should be used cautiously because overuse can increase risks of recurrent thrombotic disorders. The drugs are described in this section and in Table 57-3.

Aminocaproic acid and **tranexamic acid** are used to stop bleeding caused by overdoses of thrombolytic agents. Aminocaproic acid also may be used in other bleeding disorders caused by hyperfibrinolysis (eg, cardiac surgery, blood disorders, hepatic cirrhosis, prostatectomy, neoplastic disorders). Tranexamic acid also is used for short periods (2 to 8 days) in clients with hemophilia to prevent or decrease bleeding from tooth extraction. Dosage of tranexamic acid should be reduced in the presence of moderate or severe renal impairment.

Aprotinin is a natural protease inhibitor obtained from bovine lung that has a variety of effects on blood coagulation. It inhibits plasmin and kallikrein, thus inhibiting fibrinolysis, and inhibits breakdown of blood clotting factors. It is used to decrease bleeding in selected clients undergoing coronary artery bypass surgery.

Protamine sulfate is an antidote for standard heparin and LMWH. Because heparin is an acid and protamine sulfate is a base, protamine neutralizes heparin activity. Protamine dosage depends on the amount of heparin administered during the previous 4 hours. Each milligram of protamine neutralizes approximately 100 units of heparin (or 100 units of ardeparin and dalteparin) and 1 mg of enoxaparin. A single dose should not exceed 50 mg.

The drug is given by slow IV infusion over at least 10 minutes (to prevent or minimize adverse effects of hypotension, bradycardia, and dyspnea). Protamine effects occur immediately and last for approximately 2 hours. A second dose may be required because heparin activity lasts approximately 4 hours.

Protamine sulfate can cause severe hypotensive and anaphylactoid reactions. Thus, it should be given in settings with equipment and personnel for resuscitation and treatment of anaphylactic shock.

Vitamin K is the antidote for warfarin overdosage. An oral dose of 10 to 20 mg usually stops minor bleeding and returns the international normalized ratio (INR) (see section on Regulation of Heparin and Warfarin Dosage, later) to a normal range within 24 hours.

NURSING PROCESS

Assessment

Assess the client's status in relation to thrombotic and thromboembolic disorders.

- Risk factors for thromboembolism include:
  - Immobility (eg, limited activity or bed rest for more than 5 days)
  - Obesity
  - Cigarette smoking
  - History of thrombophlebitis, DVT, or pulmonary emboli
  - Congestive heart failure
  - Pedal edema
  - Lower limb trauma
  - Myocardial infarction
  - Atrial fibrillation
  - Mitral or aortic stenosis
  - Prosthetic heart valves
  - Abdominal, thoracic, pelvic, or major orthopedic surgery
  - Atherosclerotic heart disease or peripheral vascular disease
  - Use of oral contraceptives
- Signs and symptoms of thrombotic and thromboembolic disorders depend on the location and size of the thrombus.

TABLE 57-3	Systemic Hemostatic Drugs	
Generic/Trade Name	**Indications for Use**	**Dosage**
Aminocaproic acid (Amicar)	Control bleeding caused by overdoses of thrombolytic agents or bleeding disorders caused by hyperfibrinolysis (eg, cardiac surgery, blood disorders, hepatic cirrhosis, prostatectomy, neoplastic disorders)	PO, IV infusion, 5 g initially, followed by 1.0 to 1.25 g/h for 8 h or until bleeding is controlled; maximum dose, 30 g/24 h
Aprotinin (Trasylol)	Used in selected clients undergoing coronary artery bypass graft surgery to decrease blood loss and blood transfusions	See manufacturer's literature
Protamine sulfate	Treatment of heparin overdosage	Depends on the amount of heparin given within the previous 4 h
Tranexamic acid (Cyklokapron)	Control bleeding caused by overdoses of thrombolytic agents Prevent or decrease bleeding from tooth extraction in clients with hemophilia	PO 25 mg/kg three to four times daily, starting 1 d before surgery, or IV 10 mg/kg immediately before surgery, followed by 25 mg/kg PO three to four times daily for 2–8 d
Vitamin K (Mephyton)	Antidote for warfarin overdosage	PO 10–20 mg in a single dose

IV, intravenous; PO, oral.

○ DVT and thrombophlebitis usually occur in the legs. The conditions may be manifested by edema (the affected leg is often measurably larger than the other) and pain, especially in the calf when the foot is dorsiflexed (Homans' sign). If thrombophlebitis is superficial, it may be visible as a red, warm, tender area following the path of a vein.

○ Pulmonary embolism, if severe enough to produce symptoms, is manifested by chest pain, cough, hemoptysis, tachypnea, and tachycardia. Massive emboli cause hypotension, shock, cyanosis, and death.

○ DIC is usually manifested by bleeding, which may range from petechiae or oozing from a venipuncture site to massive internal bleeding or bleeding from all body orifices.

Nursing Diagnoses

- Altered Tissue Perfusion related to thrombus or embolus
- Pain related to tissue ischemia
- Impaired Physical Mobility related to bed rest and pain
- Altered Tissue Perfusion related to drug-induced bleeding
- Decreased Cardiac Output related to hemorrhage and volume depletion
- Anxiety related to fear of myocardial infarction or stroke
- Ineffective Individual Coping related to the need for long-term prophylaxis of thromboembolic disorders or fear of excessive bleeding
- Noncompliance related to anxiety, the need for periodic blood tests, and lack of knowledge about therapy
- Knowledge Deficit related to anticoagulant or antiplatelet drug therapy
- Risk for Injury related to drug-induced impairment of blood coagulation

Planning/Goals

The client will:

- Receive or take anticoagulant and antiplatelet drugs correctly
- Be monitored closely for therapeutic and adverse drug effects, especially when drug therapy is started and when changes are made in drugs or dosages
- Use nondrug measures to decrease venous stasis and prevent thromboembolic disorders
- Act to prevent trauma from falls and other injuries
- Inform any health care provider when taking an anticoagulant or antiplatelet drug
- Avoid or report adverse drug reactions
- Verbalize or demonstrate knowledge of safe management of anticoagulant drug therapy

- Keep follow-up appointments for tests of blood coagulation and drug dosage regulation
- Avoid preventable bleeding episodes

Interventions

Use measures to prevent thrombotic and thromboembolic disorders.

- Have the client ambulate and exercise legs regularly, especially after surgery.
- For clients who cannot ambulate or do leg exercises, do passive range-of-motion and other leg exercises several times daily when changing the client's position or performing other care.
- Have the client wear elastic stockings. Elastic stockings should be removed every 8 hours and replaced after inspecting the skin. Improperly applied elastic stockings can impair circulation rather than aid it. For clients on bed rest, intermittent pneumatic compression devices can also be used.
- Avoid trauma to lower extremities.
- Maintain adequate fluid intake (1500 to 3000 mL/day) to avoid dehydration and hemoconcentration.
- Assist clients to promote good blood circulation (eg, exercise) and avoid situations that impair circulation (eg, wearing tight clothing, crossing the legs at the knees, prolonged sitting or standing, bed rest, and placing pillows under the knees when in bed).

For the client receiving anticoagulant therapy, implement safety measures to prevent trauma and bleeding.

- For clients who cannot ambulate safely because of weakness, sedation, or other conditions, keep the call light within reach, keep bedrails elevated, and assist in ambulation.
- Provide an electric razor for shaving.
- Avoid intramuscular injections, venipunctures, and arterial punctures when possible.
- Avoid intubations when possible (eg, nasogastric tubes, indwelling urinary catheters).

For the client receiving tirofiban or eptifibatide:

- Monitor the femoral artery access site closely. This is the most common site of bleeding.
- Avoid invasive procedures as much as possible (eg, arterial and venous punctures, intramuscular injections, urinary catheters, nasotracheal suction, nasogastric tubes). If venipuncture must be done, avoid sites where pressure cannot be applied (eg, subclavian or jugular veins).
- While the vascular sheath is in place, keep clients on complete bed rest with the head of the bed elevated 30 degrees and the affected limb restrained in a straight position.
- Discontinue heparin for 3 to 4 hours and be sure the activated clotting time is less than 180 sec-

onds or the activated partial thromboplastin time (APTT) is below 45 seconds before removing the vascular sheath.

- After the vascular sheath is removed, apply pressure to the site and observe closely. For outpatients, be sure there is no bleeding for at least 4 hours before hospital discharge.

For the client receiving a thrombolytic drug or a revascularization procedure for acute myocardial infarction:

- Monitor closely for bleeding.
- Assist the client and family to understand the importance of diligent efforts to reverse risk factors contributing to coronary artery disease (eg, diet and perhaps medication to lower serum cholesterol to below 200 mg/dL and low-density lipoprotein cholesterol to below 130 mg/dL, weight reduction if overweight, control

of blood pressure if hypertensive, avoidance of smoking, stress reduction techniques, exercise program designed and supervised by a health care provider).

- Assist the client and family to understand the importance of complying with medication orders to prevent reinfarction and other complications, and continued medical supervision.

Evaluation

- Observe for signs and symptoms of thromboembolic disorders or bleeding.
- Check blood coagulation tests for therapeutic ranges.
- Observe and interview regarding compliance with instructions about drug therapy.
- Observe and interview regarding adverse drug effects.

CLIENT TEACHING GUIDELINES
Drugs to Prevent or Treat Blood Clots

General Considerations

✔ Antiplatelet and anticoagulant drugs are given to people who have had, or who are at risk of having, a heart attack, stroke, or other problems from blood clots. For prevention of a heart attack or stroke, you are most likely to be given an antiplatelet drug (eg, aspirin, clopidogrel) or warfarin (Coumadin). For home treatment of deep vein thrombosis, which usually occurs in the legs, you are likely to be given warfarin for long-term therapy and heparin injections for a few days. These medications help to prevent the blood clot from getting larger, traveling to your lungs, or recurring later.

✔ All of these drugs can increase your risk of bleeding, so you need to take safety precautions to prevent injury.

✔ To help prevent blood clots from forming and decreasing blood flow through your arteries, you need to reduce risk factors that contribute to cardiovascular disease. This can be done by a low-fat, low-cholesterol diet (and medication if needed) to lower total cholesterol to below 200 mg/dL and low-density lipoprotein cholesterol to below 130 mg/dL; weight reduction if overweight; control of blood pressure if hypertensive; avoidance of smoking; stress reduction techniques; and regular exercise.

✔ To help prevent blood clots from forming in your leg veins, avoid or minimize situations that slow blood circulation, such as wearing tight clothing; crossing the legs at the knees; prolonged sitting or standing; and bed rest. For example, on automobile trips, stop and walk around every 1 to 2 hours; on long plane trips, exercise your feet and legs at your seat and walk around when you can.

✔ Following instructions regarding these medications is extremely important. Too little medication increases

your risk of problems from blood clot formation; too much medication can cause bleeding.

✔ While taking any of these medications, you need regular medical supervision and periodic blood tests. The blood tests can help your physician regulate drug dosage and maintain your safety.

✔ You need to take the drugs as directed; avoid taking other drugs without the physician's knowledge and consent; inform any physician, surgeon, or dentist that you are taking an antiplatelet or anticoagulant drug before any treatments are begun; and keep all appointments for continuing care.

✔ With warfarin therapy, you need to avoid walking barefoot; avoid contact sports; use an electric razor; avoid injections when possible; and carry an identification card, necklace, or bracelet (eg, MedicAlert) stating the name of the drug and the physician's name and telephone number. Also, avoid large amounts of green, leafy vegetables (eg, spinach), tomatoes, bananas, or fish; these foods contain vitamin K and may decrease anticoagulant effects.

✔ For home treatment of deep vein thrombosis, both warfarin and enoxaparin (Lovenox) are given for approximately 5 days. With Lovenox, you need an injection, usually every 12 hours. You or someone close to you may be instructed in injecting the medication, or a visiting nurse may do the injections, if necessary.

Even if a nurse is not needed to give the injections, one will usually visit your home each day to perform a fingerstick blood test. The results of this test determine your daily dose of warfarin. Once the blood test and the warfarin dose stabilize, the blood tests are done less often (eg, every 2 weeks).

(continued)

CLIENT TEACHING GUIDELINES
Drugs to Prevent or Treat Blood Clots (continued)

✔ Report any sign of bleeding (eg, excessive bruising of the skin, blood in urine or stool). If superficial bleeding occurs, apply direct pressure to the site for 3 to 5 minutes or longer if necessary.

Self-administration

✔ Take aspirin with food or after meals, with 8 oz of water, to decrease gastrointestinal (GI) upset. However, GI upset is uncommon with the small doses used for antiplatelet effects. Do not crush or chew coated tablets (long-acting preparations).

✔ Take cilostazol (Pletal) approximately 30 minutes before or 2 hours after morning and evening meals for better absorption and effectiveness.

✔ Take ticlopidine (Ticlid) with food or after meals to decrease GI upset. Clopidogrel (Plavix) may be taken with or without food.

✔ With Lovenox, wash hands and cleanse skin to prevent infection; inject deep under the skin, around the navel, upper thigh, or buttocks; and change the injection site daily. If excessive bruising occurs at the injection site, rubbing an ice cube over an area before the injection may be helpful.

PRINCIPLES OF THERAPY

Drug Selection

Choices of anticoagulant and antiplatelet drugs depend on the reason for use and other drug and client characteristics.

1. Heparin is the anticoagulant of choice in acute venous thromboembolic disorders because the anticoagulant effect begins immediately with IV administration.
2. Warfarin is the anticoagulant of choice for long-term maintenance therapy (ie, several weeks or months) because it can be given orally.
3. Aspirin has long been the most widely used antiplatelet drug for prevention of myocardial reinfarction and arterial thrombosis in clients with TIAs and prosthetic heart valves. However, some of the newer drugs (eg, clopidogrel) are being used and may be more effective than aspirin.
4. When anticoagulation is required during pregnancy, heparin is used because it does not cross the placenta. Warfarin is contraindicated during pregnancy.
5. Various combinations of antithrombotic drugs are used concomitantly or sequentially (eg, abciximab is used with aspirin and heparin; thrombolytic drugs are usually followed with heparin and warfarin).

Regulation of Heparin and Warfarin Dosage

Heparin dosage is regulated by the APTT, which is sensitive to changes in blood clotting factors, except factor VII. Thus, normal or control values indicate normal blood coagulation; therapeutic values indicate low levels of clotting factors and delayed blood coagulation. During heparin therapy, the APTT should be maintained at

How Can You Avoid This Medication Error?

Helen Innes is admitted to your medical unit for treatment of bacterial pneumonia. She has been on oral antibiotics for 7 days but her respiratory condition has not improved. In addition to her intravenous antibiotics, you administer her usual dose of Coumadin that she takes for a history of pulmonary emboli. When you document the medications given, you notice that her international normalized ratio (INR) is 6.

approximately 1.5 to 2 times the control or baseline value. The normal control value is 25 to 35 seconds; therefore, therapeutic values are 45 to 70 seconds, approximately. With continuous IV infusion, blood for the APTT may be drawn at any time; with intermittent administration, blood for the APTT should be drawn approximately 1 hour before a dose of heparin is scheduled. APTT is not necessary with low-dose standard heparin given subcutaneously for prophylaxis of thromboembolism or with the LMWH (eg, enoxaparin).

Warfarin dosage is regulated according to the INR, for which therapeutic values are 2.0 to 3.0 in most conditions. An average maintenance dose of 4 to 5 mg daily maintains a therapeutic INR; stopping warfarin returns an elevated INR to normal in approximately 4 days in most clients.

The INR is based on prothrombin time (PT). PT is sensitive to changes in three of the four vitamin K–dependent coagulation factors. Thus, normal or control values indicate normal levels of these factors; therapeutic values indicate low levels of the factors and delayed blood coagulation. A normal baseline or control PT is approximately 12 seconds; a therapeutic value is approximately 1.5 times the control, or 18 seconds.

When warfarin is started, PT and INR should be assessed daily until a stable daily dose is reached (the dose that maintains PT and INR within therapeutic ranges and does not cause bleeding). Thereafter, PT and INR are determined every 2 to 4 weeks for the duration of oral anticoagulant drug therapy. If the warfarin dose is changed, PT and INR are needed more often until a stable daily dose is again reached.

For many years, the PT was used to regulate warfarin dosage. PT is determined by adding a mixture of thromboplastin and calcium to citrated plasma and measuring the time (in seconds) it takes for the blood to clot. However, values vary among laboratories according to the type of thromboplastin and the instrument used to measure PT. The INR system standardizes the PT by comparing a particular thromboplastin with a standard thromboplastin designated by the World Health Organization. Advantages of the INR include consistent values among laboratories, more consistent warfarin dosage with less risk of bleeding or thrombosis, and more consistent reports of clinical trials and other research studies. Some laboratories report both PT and INR.

Warfarin dosage may need to be reduced in clients with biliary tract disorders (eg, obstructive jaundice), liver disease (eg, hepatitis, cirrhosis), malabsorption syndromes (eg, steatorrhea), and hyperthyroidism or fever. These conditions increase anticoagulant drug effects by reducing absorption of vitamin K, decreasing hepatic synthesis of blood clotting factors, or increasing the breakdown of clotting factors. Despite these influencing factors, however, the primary determinant of dosage is the PT and INR.

Warfarin interacts with many other drugs to cause increased, decreased, or unpredictable anticoagulant effects. Thus, warfarin dosage may need to be increased or decreased when other drugs are given concomitantly. Most drugs can be given if warfarin dosage is carefully titrated according to the PT or INR and altered appropriately when an interacting drug is added or stopped. INR or PT measurements and vigilant observation are needed whenever a drug is added to or removed from a drug therapy regimen containing warfarin.

Thrombolytic Therapy

1. Thrombolytic therapy should be performed only by experienced personnel in an intensive care setting with cardiac and other monitoring devices in place.

2. All of the available agents are effective with recommended uses. Thus, the choice of a thrombolytic agent depends mainly on risks of adverse effects and costs. All of the drugs may cause bleeding. Alteplase and anistreplase may act more specifically on the fibrin in a clot and cause less systemic depletion of fibrinogen, but these agents are very expensive. Streptokinase, the least expensive agent, may cause allergic reactions because it is a foreign protein. Combination therapy (eg, with alteplase and streptokinase) may also be used.

3. Before a thrombolytic agent is begun, INR, APTT, platelet count, and fibrinogen should be checked to establish baseline values and to determine if a blood coagulation disorder is present. Two or 3 hours after thrombolytic therapy is started, the fibrinogen level can be measured to determine that fibrinolysis is occurring. Alternatively, INR or APTT can be checked for increased values because the breakdown products of fibrin exert anticoagulant effects.

4. Major factors in decreasing risks of bleeding are selecting recipients carefully, avoiding invasive procedures when possible, and omitting anticoagulant or antiplatelet drugs while thrombolytics are being given. If bleeding does occur, it is most likely from a venipuncture or invasive procedure site, and local pressure may control it. If bleeding cannot be controlled or involves a vital organ, the thrombolytic drug should be stopped and fibrinogen replaced with whole blood plasma or cryoprecipitate. Aminocaproic acid or tranexamic acid may also be given.

5. When the drugs are used in acute myocardial infarction, cardiac arrhythmias may occur when blood flow is reestablished. Therefore, antiarrhythmic drugs should be readily available.

Use in Children

Little information is available about the use of anticoagulants in children. Heparin solutions containing benzyl alcohol as a preservative should not be given to premature infants because fatal reactions have been reported. When given for systemic anticoagulation, heparin dosage should be based on the child's weight (approximately 50 units/kg). Safety and effectiveness of LMWH (eg, enoxaparin) have not been established in children.

Warfarin is given to children after cardiac surgery to prevent thromboembolism, but doses and guidelines for safe, effective use have not been developed. Accurate drug administration, close monitoring of blood coagulation tests, safety measures to prevent trauma and bleeding, avoiding interacting drugs, and informing others in the child's environment (eg, teachers, babysitters, health care providers) are necessary.

Antiplatelet and thrombolytic drugs have no established indications for use in children.

Use in Older Adults

Older adults often have atherosclerosis and thrombotic disorders, including myocardial infarction, thrombotic stroke, and peripheral arterial insufficiency, for which they receive an anticoagulant or an antiplatelet drug. They are more likely than younger adults to experience bleeding and other complications of anticoagulant and antiplatelet drugs. For example, aspirin or clopidogrel is commonly used to prevent thrombotic stroke, but both drugs increase risks of hemorrhagic stroke.

With standard heparin, general principles for safe and effective use apply. With LMWH, elimination may be delayed in older adults with renal impairment and the drugs should be used cautiously. They should also be used with caution in clients taking a platelet inhibitor (eg, aspirin, clopidogrel) to prevent myocardial infarction or thrombotic stroke or an NSAID for arthritis pain. NSAIDs, which are commonly used by older adults, also have antiplatelet effects. Clients who take an NSAID daily may not need low-dose aspirin for antithrombotic effects.

With warfarin, dosage should be reduced because impaired liver function and decreased plasma proteins increase the risks of bleeding. Also, many drugs interact with warfarin to increase or decrease its effect, and older adults often take multiple drugs. Starting or stopping any drug may require that warfarin dosage be adjusted.

Use in Renal Impairment

Most anticoagulant, antiplatelet, and thrombolytic drugs may be used in clients with impaired renal function. For example, heparin and warfarin can be used in usual dosages, and thrombolytic agents (eg, streptokinase and urokinase) may be used to dissolve clots in IV catheters or vascular access sites for hemodialysis. Dosage of LMWH should be reduced in clients with severe renal impairment (creatinine clearance <30 mL/minute) because they are excreted by the kidneys and elimination is slowed. In addition, home treatment of DVT with LMWH and warfarin is contraindicated in clients with severe renal impairment. Guidelines for the use of other drugs include the following:

- *Anagrelide* may be given to clients with renal impairment (eg, serum creatinine ≥2 mg/dL) if potential benefits outweigh risks. Clients receiving this medication should be monitored closely for signs of renal toxicity.
- *Cilostazol* is probably safe to use in clients with mild or moderate renal impairment. However, severe renal impairment alters drug protein binding and increases blood levels of metabolites.
- *Clopidogrel* does not need dosage reduction in clients with renal impairment.
- *Danaparoid* is excreted mainly by the kidneys and dosage may need to be reduced in clients with severe renal impairment. Monitor serum creatinine during therapy.
- *Eptifibatide* does not need dosage reduction in clients with mild to moderate renal impairment. No data are available for clients with severe impairment or those on hemodialysis.
- *Lepirudin* is excreted by the kidneys and may accumulate in clients with impaired renal function. Dosage should be reduced.
- *Ticlopidine* may be more likely to cause bleeding in clients with renal impairment because the plasma drug concentration is increased and elimination is slower.
- *Tirofiban* clearance from plasma is decreased approximately 50% in clients with severe renal impairment (eg, creatinine clearance <30 mL/minute), including those receiving hemodialysis. Dosage must be reduced by approximately 50%.

Use in Hepatic Impairment

Little information is available about the use of most anticoagulant, antiplatelet, and thrombolytic drugs in clients with impaired liver function. However, such drugs should be used very cautiously because these clients may already be predisposed to bleeding because of decreased hepatic synthesis of clotting factors. Additional considerations include the following:

- *Warfarin* is more likely to cause bleeding in clients with liver disease, because of decreased synthesis of vitamin K. In addition, warfarin is eliminated only by hepatic metabolism and may accumulate with liver impairment.
- *Low–molecular-weight heparins* are contraindicated for home treatment of DVT in clients with severe liver disease because of high risks of excessive bleeding.
- *Anagrelide* is metabolized in the liver and may accumulate with hepatic impairment. Clients with evidence of impairment (eg, bilirubin or aspartate aminotransferase more than 1.5 times the upper limit of normal) should receive anagrelide only if potential benefits outweigh potential risks. When anagrelide is given, clients should be closely monitored for signs of hepatotoxicity.
- *Clopidogrel* is metabolized in the liver and may accumulate with hepatic impairment. It should be used cautiously.
- *Dipyridamole* is metabolized in the liver and excreted in bile.
- *Ticlopidine* plasma concentrations may be increased.

 Home Care

Antiplatelet agents and warfarin are used for long-term prevention or treatment of thromboembolism and are often taken at home. For prevention, antiplatelet agents and warfarin are usually self-administered at home, with periodic office or clinic visits for blood tests and other follow-up care.

For home treatment of DVT, warfarin may be self-administered, but a nurse usually visits, performs a finger-stick INR, and notifies the physician, who then prescribes the daily dose of warfarin. Precautions are needed to decrease risks of bleeding. The risk of bleeding has lessened in recent years because of lower doses of warfarin. In addition, bleeding during warfarin therapy may be caused by medical conditions other than anticoagulation.

Heparin may also be taken at home. Standard heparin may be taken subcutaneously, but LMWH for home treatment of venous thrombosis is becoming standard practice. Enoxaparin is approved by the Food and Drug Administration for outpatient treatment. Daily visits by a home care nurse may be needed if the client or a family member is unable or unwilling to inject the medication. Platelet counts should be done before and every 2 to 3 days during heparin therapy. Heparin should be discontinued if the platelet count falls below 100,000 or to less than half the baseline value.

Most home treatment regimens involve a structured protocol. Clients and family members should be educated about the disorder (usually DVT), including the potential consequences of either overcoagulation or undercoagulation, and the need for blood tests.

The home care nurse needs to assess clients in relation to knowledge about prescribed drugs and ability and willingness to comply with instructions for taking the drugs, obtaining blood tests when indicated, and taking safety precautions. In addition, assess the environment for risk factors for injury. Interventions vary with clients, environments, and assessment data, but may include reinforcing instructions for safe use of the drugs, assisting clients to obtain laboratory tests, and teaching how to observe for signs and symptoms of bleeding.

(text continues on page 867)

NURSING ACTIONS — Drugs That Affect Blood Coagulation

NURSING ACTIONS	RATIONALE/EXPLANATION
1. Administer accurately	
a. With standard heparin:	
(1) When handwriting a heparin dose, write out "units" rather than using the abbreviation "U."	This is a safety precaution to avoid erroneous dosage. For example, 1000 U (1000 units) may be misread as 10,000 units.
(2) Check dosage and vial label carefully.	Underdosage may cause thromboembolism, and overdosage may cause bleeding. In addition, heparin is available in several concentrations (1000, 2500, 5000, 10,000, 15,000, 20,000, and 40,000 units/mL).
(3) For subcutaneous (SC) heparin:	
(a) Use a 26-gauge, ½-inch needle.	To minimize trauma and risk of bleeding
(b) Grasp a skinfold and inject the heparin into it, at a 90-degree angle, without aspirating.	To give the drug in a deep subcutaneous or fat layer, with minimal trauma
(4) For intermittent intravenous (IV) administration:	
(a) Give by direct injection into a heparin lock or tubing injection site.	These methods prevent repeated venipunctures.
(b) Dilute the dose in 50 to 100 mL of any IV fluid (usually 5% dextrose in water).	
(5) For continuous IV administration:	This is usually the preferred method because it maintains consistent serum drug levels and decreases risks of bleeding.
(a) Use a volume-control device and an infusion-control device.	To regulate dosage and flow rate accurately
(b) Add only enough heparin for a few hours. One effective method is to fill the volume-control set (eg, Volutrol) with 100 mL of 5% dextrose in water and add 5000 units of heparin to yield a concentration of 50 units/mL. Dosage is regulated by varying the flow rate. For example, administration of 1000 units/h requires a flow rate of 20 mL/h. Another method is to add 25,000 units of heparin to 500 mL of IV solution.	To avoid inadvertent administration of large amounts. Whatever method is used, it is desirable to standardize concentration of heparin solutions within an institution. Standardization is safer, because it reduces risks of errors in dosage.

(continued)

NURSING ACTIONS	RATIONALE/EXPLANATION
b. With low–molecular-weight heparins:	
(1) Give by deep SC injection, into an abdominal skin fold, with the patient lying down. Do not rub the injection site.	To decrease bruising
(2) Rotate sites.	
c. After the initial dose of warfarin, check the international normalized ratio (INR) before giving a subsequent dose. Do not give the dose if the INR is above 3.0. Notify the physician.	The INR is measured daily until a maintenance dose is established, then periodically throughout warfarin therapy. An elevated INR indicates a high risk of bleeding.
d. Give ticlopidine with food or after meals; give cilostazol 30 min before or 2 h after morning and evening meals; give clopidogrel with or without food.	
e. With eptifibatide, tirofiban, and thrombolytic agents, follow manufacturers' instructions for reconstitution and administration.	These drugs require special preparation and administration techniques.
2. Observe for therapeutic effects	
a. With prophylactic heparins and warfarin, observe for the absence of signs and symptoms of thrombotic disorders.	
b. With therapeutic heparins and warfarin, observe for decrease or improvement in signs and symptoms (eg, less edema and pain with deep vein thrombosis, less chest pain and respiratory difficulty with pulmonary embolism).	
c. With prophylactic or therapeutic warfarin, observe for an INR between 2.0 and 3.0.	Frequency of INR determinations varies, but the test should be done periodically in all clients taking warfarin.
d. With therapeutic heparin, observe for an activated partial thromboplastin time of 1.5 to 2 times the control value.	
e. With anagrelide, observe for a decrease in platelet count.	Platelet counts should be done every 2 d during the first week of treatment and weekly until a maintenance dose is reached. Counts usually begin to decrease within the first 2 wk of therapy.
f. With aspirin, clopidogrel, and other antiplatelet drugs, observe for the absence of thrombotic disorders (eg, myocardial infarction, stroke)	
g. With cilostazol, observe for ability to walk farther without leg pain (intermittent claudication).	Improvement may occur within 2 to 4 wk or take as long as 12 wk.
3. Observe for adverse effects	
a. Bleeding:	Bleeding is the major adverse effect of anticoagulant drugs. It may occur anywhere in the body, spontaneously or in response to minor trauma.
	With eptifibatide and tirofiban, most major bleeding occurs at the arterial access site for cardiac catheterization.
(1) Record vital signs regularly.	Hypotension and tachycardia may indicate internal bleeding.

(continued)

NURSING ACTIONS	RATIONALE/EXPLANATION
(2) Check stools for blood (melena).	Gastrointestinal (GI) bleeding is fairly common; risks are increased with intubation. Blood in stools may be bright red, tarry (blood that has been digested by GI secretions), or occult (hidden to the naked eye but present with a guaiac test). Hematemesis also may occur.
(3) Check urine for blood (hematuria).	Genitourinary bleeding also is fairly common; risks are increased with catheterization or instrumentation. Urine may be red (indicating fresh bleeding) or brownish or smokey gray (indicating old blood). Or bleeding may be microscopic (red blood cells are visible only on microscopic examination during urinalysis).
(4) Inspect the skin and mucous membranes daily.	Bleeding may occur in the skin as petechiae, purpura, or ecchymoses. Surgical wounds, skin lesions, parenteral injection sites, the nose, and gums may be bleeding sites.
(5) Assess for excessive menstrual flow.	
b. Other adverse effects:	
(1) With heparin, tissue irritation at injection sites, transient alopecia, reversible thrombocytopenia, paresthesias, and hypersensitivity	These effects are uncommon. They are more likely to occur with large doses or prolonged administration.
(2) With warfarin, dermatitis, diarrhea, and alopecia	These effects occur only occasionally. Warfarin has been given for prolonged periods without toxicity.
(3) With anagrelide, adverse cardiovascular effects (eg, tachycardia, vasodilation, heart failure)	These effects are most likely to occur in clients with known heart disease.
(4) With clopidogrel and ticlopidine, GI upset, skin rash, neutropenia, and thrombocytopenia	Neutropenia and thrombocytopenia are more likely to occur with ticlopidine than clopidogrel.
c. With thrombolytic drugs, observe for bleeding with all uses and reperfusion arrhythmias when used for acute myocardial infarction.	Bleeding is most likely to occur at sites of venipuncture or other invasive procedures. Reperfusion arrhythmias may occur when blood supply is restored to previously ischemic myocardium.
4. Observe for drug interactions	
a. Drugs that *increase* risks of bleeding with anticoagulant, antiplatelet, and thrombolytic agents:	These drugs are often used concurrently or sequentially to decrease risks of myocardial infarction or stroke.
(1) Any one of these drugs in combination with any other drug that affects hemostasis	
(2) A combination of these drugs	
b. Drugs that *increase* effects of heparins:	
(1) Antiplatelet drugs (eg, aspirin, clopidogrel, others)	
(2) Warfarin	Additive anticoagulant effects and increased risks of bleeding
(3) Parenteral penicillins and cephalosporins	Some may affect blood coagulation and increase risks of bleeding

(*continued*)

NURSING ACTIONS	RATIONALE/EXPLANATION
c. Drugs that *decrease* effects of heparins:	
(1) Antihistamines, digoxin, tetracyclines	These drugs antagonize the anticoagulant effects of heparin. Mechanisms are not clear.
(2) Protamine sulfate	The antidote for heparin overdose
d. Drugs that *increase* effects of warfarin:	Mechanisms by which drugs may increase effects of warfarin include inhibiting warfarin metabolism, displacing warfarin from binding sites on serum albumin, causing antiplatelet effects, inhibiting bacterial synthesis of vitamin K in the intestinal tract, and others.
(1) Analgesics (eg, acetaminophen, aspirin and other nonsteroidal anti-inflammatory drugs)	
(2) Androgens and anabolic steroids	
(3) Antibacterial drugs (eg, aminoglycosides, erythromycin, fluoroquinolones, isoniazid, metronidazole, penicillins, cephalosporins, trimethoprim-sulfamethoxazole, tetracyclines)	
(4) Antifungal drugs (eg, fluconazole, ketoconazole, miconazole)	
(5) Antiseizure drugs (eg, phenytoin)	
(6) Cardiovascular drugs (eg, amiodarone, beta blockers, loop diuretics, gemfibrozil, lovastatin, propafenone, quinidine)	
(7) Gastrointestinal drugs (eg, cimetidine, omeprazole)	
(8) Thyroid preparations (eg, levothyroxine)	
e. Drugs that *decrease* effects of warfarin:	
(1) Antacids and griseofulvin	May decrease GI absorption
(2) Barbiturates and other sedative-hypnotics, carbamazepine, disulfiram, rifampin	These drugs activate liver metabolizing enzymes, which accelerate the rate of metabolism of warfarin.
(3) Cholestyramine	Decreases absorption
(4) Diuretics	Increase synthesis and concentration of blood clotting factors
(5) Estrogens, including oral contraceptives	Increase synthesis of clotting factors and have thromboembolic effect
(6) Vitamin K	Restores prothrombin and other vitamin K-dependent clotting factors in the blood. Antidote for overdose of warfarin.
f. Drug that may *increase* or *decrease* effects of warfarin:	
(1) Alcohol	Alcohol may induce liver enzymes, which *decrease* effects by accelerating the rate of metabolism of the anticoagulant drug. However, with alcohol-induced liver disease (ie, cirrhosis), effects may be *increased* owing to impaired metabolism of warfarin.
g. Drugs that *increase* effects of cilostazol:	
(1) Diltiazem	These drugs inhibit the main cytochrome P450 enzyme (CYP3A4) that metabolizes cilostazol. Grapefruit juice also inhibits drug metabolism and should be avoided.
(2) Erythomycin	
(3) Itraconazole, ketoconazole	

Nursing Notes: Apply Your Knowledge

Answer: Low-dose subcutaneous heparin is administered prophylactically to prevent deep vein thrombosis, which is associated with prolonged immobility. Partial thromboplastin time (PTT) levels may be assessed before beginning therapy, but routine PTT assessment and dosage adjustments are not required for low-dose heparin therapy. When giving the injection, care is taken to prevent trauma and subsequent bruising. A small, 26-gauge ½-inch needle is used. The area is cleansed and grasped firmly and the needle is inserted at a 90-degree angle. Do not aspirate or rub the area because this fosters bruising. Avoid injection within 2 inches of incisions or the umbilicus and any areas that are scarred or abnormal. Although research indicates that various sites (abdomen, arms, and legs) can be used, the preferred site is the abdomen. Observe and report any signs of bleeding.

How Can You Avoid This Medication Error?

Answer: Ms. Innes' INR is too high, which could significantly increase her risk for bleeding. Therapeutic INR levels are usually between 2 and 3. Before giving anticoagulants, it is important to check lab work (activated partial thromboplastin time for heparin, prothrombin time or INR for Coumadin) to determine whether the dose should be administered. For Ms. Innes, antibiotic therapy may have interfered with the synthesis of vitamin K in the intestine, thus increasing the risk of bleeding. Notify Ms. Innes' physician. Because no signs of bleeding have been noted, he or she may decrease the Coumadin dosage.

 REVIEW AND APPLICATION EXERCISES

1. What are the major functions of the endothelium, platelets, and coagulation factors in hemostasis and thrombosis?

2. What are the indications for use of heparin and warfarin?

3. How do heparin and warfarin differ in mechanism of action, onset and duration of action, and method of administration?

4. List interventions to protect clients from anticoagulant-induced bleeding.

5. When is it appropriate to use protamine sulfate as an antidote for heparin?

6. When is it appropriate to use vitamin K as an antidote for warfarin?

7. How do antiplatelet drugs differ from heparin and warfarin?

8. For what conditions are antiplatelet drugs indicated?

9. How do thrombolytic drugs act to dissolve blood clots?

10. When is it appropriate to use a thrombolytic drug?

11. How do aminocaproic acid and tranexamic acid stop bleeding induced by thrombolytics?

12. Compare and contrast nursing care needs of clients receiving anticoagulant therapy in hospital and home settings.

SELECTED REFERENCES

Brater, D.C. (1997). Clinical pharmacology of cardiovascular drugs. In W.N. Kelley (Ed.), *Textbook of internal medicine*, 3rd ed., pp. 552–569. Philadelphia: Lippincott-Raven.

Cohen, M. (1999). Treatment of unstable angina: The role of platelet inhibitors and anticoagulants. *Journal of Invasive Cardiology, 11*(3), 147–159. [Online: Available http://www.medscape.com/HMP/JIC/1999/v11.n03/jic1103.06.chohe/jic1103.06.cohe-01.html. Accessed November, 1999.]

Drug facts and comparisons. (Updated monthly). St. Louis: Facts and Comparisons.

Dunn, A.S. & Coller, B. (1999). Outpatient treatment of deep vein thrombosis: Translating clinical trials into practice. *American Journal of Medicine, 106*, 660–669.

Erdman, S.M., Rodvold, K.A., & Friedenberg, W.R. (1997). Thromboembolic disorders. In J.T. DiPiro, R.L. Talbert, G.C. Yee, G.R. Matzke, B.G. Wells, & L.M. Posey (Eds.), *Pharmacotherapy: A pathophysiologic approach*, 3rd ed., pp. 399–433. Stamford, CT: Appleton & Lange.

Ezekowitz, M.D. & Hirsh, J. (1997). Use of anticoagulant drugs. In W.N. Kelley (Ed.), *Textbook of internal medicine*, 3rd ed., pp. 569–578. Philadelphia: Lippincott-Raven.

Guyton, A.C. & Hall, J.E. (1996). *Textbook of medical physiology*, 9th ed. Philadelphia: W.B. Saunders.

Hochman, J.S., Wali, A.U., Gavrila, D., Sim, M.J., Malhotra, S., Palazzo, A.M., & De La Fuente, B. (1999). A new regimen for heparin use in acute coronary syndromes. *American Heart Journal, 138*, 313–318. [Online: Available http://www.medscape.com/mosby/AmHeartJ/1999/v138.n02/ahj1382.12.hock/ahj/1382.12.hock-01.html. Accessed November, 1999.]

Kearon, C. & Hirsh, J. (1998). Anticoagulation: Heparin and warfarin. In D.L. Brown (Ed.), *Cardiac intensive care*, pp. 533–544. Philadelphia: W.B. Saunders.

Majerus, P.W., Broze, G.J., Jr., Miletich, J.P., & Tollefsen, D.M. (1996). Anticoagulant, thrombolytic, and antiplatelet drugs. In J.G. Hardman, L.E. Limbird, P.B. Molinoff, & R.W. Ruddon (Eds.), *Goodman & Gilman's The pharmacological basis of therapeutics*, 9th ed., pp. 1341–1359. New York: McGraw-Hill.

Porsche, R. & Brenner, Z.R. (1999). Allergy to protamine sulfate. *Heart and Lung, 28*, 418–428.

Porth, C.M. (Ed.). (1998). *Pathophysiology: Concepts of altered health states*, 5th ed. Philadelphia: Lippincott Williams & Wilkins.

Sachdev, G.P., Ohlrogge, K.D., & Johnson, C.L. (1999). Review of the Fifth American College of Chest Physicians Consensus Conference on Antithrombotic Therapy: Outpatient management for adults. *American Journal of Health-System Pharmacy, 56*, 1505–1514.

White, R.H., Beyth, R.J., Zhou, H., & Romano, P.S. (1999). Major bleeding after hospitalization for deep-venous thrombosis. *American Journal of Medicine, 107*, 414–424.

58

Drugs for Hyperlipidemia

Objectives

After studying this chapter, the student will be able to:

1. Discuss the role of hyperlipidemia in the etiology of atherosclerosis.

2. Identify sources and functions of cholesterol and triglycerides.

3. Describe antilipemic drugs in terms of mechanism of action, indications for use, major adverse effects, and nursing process implications.

4. Teach clients pharmacologic and nonpharmacologic measures to prevent or reduce hyperlipidemia.

During a routine physical examination, 26-year-old William Halls is diagnosed with hyperlipidemia. His father died at 46 years of age of a massive myocardial infarction (MI). William jogs 3 miles three to four times a week. He eats out, mostly at fast-food places. He is very serious when he listens to the doctor explain his diagnosis. He responds by asking, "Does this mean I am going to die young like my dad?"

Reflect on:

▶ The emotional impact of this diagnosis for a young man, in light of his family history.

▶ The underlying pathophysiology of athero-sclerosis. What are possible consequences of atherosclerosis other than MI?

▶ Ways to explain the significance of laboratory values (cholesterol, low-density lipoproteins, high-density lipoproteins, triglycerides).

▶ A plan for teaching and follow-up regarding lifestyle modification.

ANTILIPEMIC DRUGS

Antilipemic drugs are used in the treatment of clients with elevated blood lipids, a major risk factor for atherosclerosis and vascular disorders such as coronary artery disease, strokes, and peripheral arterial insufficiency. These drugs have proven efficacy and are being used increasingly to reduce morbidity and mortality from coronary heart disease and other atherosclerosis-related cardiovascular disorders. To understand clinical use of these drugs, it is necessary to understand atherosclerosis, characteristics of blood lipids, and types of blood lipid disorders.

ATHEROSCLEROSIS

Atherosclerosis is a major cause of ischemic heart disease (eg, angina pectoris, myocardial infarction), heart failure, stroke, peripheral vascular disease, and death (see Chaps. 53 and 57). It is a systemic disease characterized by lesions in the endothelial lining of arteries throughout the body. These lesions (called fatty plaques or atheromas) start with injury to the endothelium and involve progressive accumulation of lipids (eg, cholesterol), vascular smooth muscle cells, macrophages, lymphocytes, and connective tissue proteins. Over time, the lesions interfere with nutrition of the blood vessel lining, the normally smooth endothelium becomes roughened, and thrombi, necrosis, scarring, and calcification occur. As the lesions develop and enlarge, they protrude into the lumen of the artery, reduce the size of the lumen, reduce blood flow, and may eventually occlude the artery. Severely impaired blood flow leads to damage or death of tissue supplied by the artery. Clinical manifestations vary according to the arteries involved and the extent of vessel obstruction.

BLOOD LIPIDS

Blood lipids, which include cholesterol, phospholipids, and triglycerides, are derived from the diet or synthesized by the liver and intestine. Most cholesterol is found in body cells, where it is a component of cell membranes and performs other essential functions. In cells of the adrenal glands, ovaries, and testes, cholesterol is required for the synthesis of steroid hormones (eg, cortisol, estrogen, progesterone, and testosterone). In liver cells, cholesterol is used to form cholic acid. The cholic acid is then conjugated with other substances to form bile salts, which promote absorption and digestion of fats. In addition, a small amount is found in blood serum. Serum cholesterol is the portion of total body cholesterol involved in formation of atherosclerotic plaques. Unless a person has a genetic disorder of lipid metabolism, the amount of cho-

lesterol in the blood is strongly related to dietary intake of saturated fat. Phospholipids are essential components of cell membranes, and triglycerides provide energy for cellular metabolism.

Blood lipids are transported in plasma by specific proteins called *lipoproteins*. Each lipoprotein contains cholesterol, phospholipid, and triglyceride bound to protein. The lipoproteins vary in density and amounts of lipid and protein. Density is determined mainly by the amount of protein, which is more dense than fat. Thus, density increases as the proportion of protein increases. The lipoproteins are differentiated according to these properties, which can be measured in the laboratory. For example, high-density lipoprotein (HDL) cholesterol contains larger amounts of protein and smaller amounts of lipid; low-density lipoprotein (LDL) cholesterol contains less protein and larger amounts of lipid. Other plasma lipoproteins are chylomicrons and very–low-density lipoproteins (VLDL). Additional characteristics of lipoproteins are described in Box 58-1.

The National Cholesterol Education Program Expert Panel on Detection, Evaluation and Treatment of High Blood Cholesterol in Adults classifies blood lipid levels as follows:

> **Total serum cholesterol** (mg/dL)
> Normal or desirable = less than 200
> Borderline high = 200 to 239
> High = 240 or above
> **LDL cholesterol** (mg/dL)
> Normal or desirable = less than 130
> Borderline high = 130 to 159
> High = 160
> **HDL cholesterol** (mg/dL)
> High = more than 60
> Low = less than 35
> **Triglycerides** (mg/dL)
> Normal or desirable = less than 200
> Borderline high = 200 to 400
> High = 400 to 1000
> Very high = more than 1000

Overall, the most effective blood lipid profile for prevention or treatment of atherosclerosis and its sequelae is a high HDL cholesterol, a low LDL cholesterol, and a low total cholesterol. A low triglyceride level is also desirable. For accurate interpretation of a client's lipid profile, blood samples for laboratory testing of triglycerides should be drawn after the client has fasted approximately 12 hours. Fasting is not required for cholesterol testing.

HYPERLIPIDEMIA

Hyperlipidemia (also called dyslipidemia) is associated with atherosclerosis and its many pathophysiologic effects (eg, myocardial ischemia and infarction, stroke, peripheral arterial occlusive disease). Ischemic heart disease has

BOX 58–1 TYPES OF LIPOPROTEINS

Chylomicrons, the largest lipoprotein molecules, are synthesized in the wall of the small intestine. They carry recently ingested dietary cholesterol and triglycerides that have been absorbed from the gastrointestinal tract. Hyperchylomicronemia normally occurs after a fatty meal reaches peak levels in 3 to 4 hours, and subsides within 12 to 14 hours. Chylomicrons carry triglycerides to fat and muscle cells, where the enzyme lipoprotein lipase breaks down the molecule and releases fatty acids to be used for energy or stored as fat. This process leaves a remnant containing cholesterol, which is then transported to the liver. Thus, chylomicrons transport triglycerides to peripheral tissues and cholesterol to the liver.

Low-density lipoprotein (LDL) cholesterol, sometimes called "bad cholesterol," transports approximately 75% of serum cholesterol and carries it to peripheral tissues and the liver. LDL cholesterol is removed from the circulation by receptor and nonreceptor mechanisms. The receptor mechanism involves the binding of LDL cholesterol to receptors on cell surface membranes. The bound LDL molecule is then engulfed into the cell, where it is broken down by enzymes and releases free cholesterol into the cytoplasm.

Most LDL cholesterol receptors are located in the liver. However, nonhepatic tissues (eg, adrenal glands, smooth muscle cells, endothelial cells, and lymphoid cells) also have receptors by which they obtain the cholesterol needed for building cell membranes and synthesizing hormones. These cells can regulate their cholesterol intake by adding or removing LDL receptors.

Approximately two thirds of the LDL cholesterol is removed from the bloodstream by the receptor-dependent mechanism. The number of LDL receptors on cell membranes determines the amount of LDL degradation (ie, the more receptors on cells, the more LDL is broken down). Conditions that decrease the number or function of receptors (eg, high dietary intake of cholesterol, saturated fat, or calories), increase blood levels of LDL.

The remaining one third is removed by mechanisms that do not involve receptors. Nonreceptor uptake occurs in various cells, especially when levels of circulating LDL cholesterol are high. For example, macrophage cells in arterial walls can attach LDL, thereby promoting accumulation of cholesterol and the development of atherosclerosis. The amount of LDL cholesterol removed by nonreceptor mechanisms is increased with inadequate numbers of receptors or excessive amounts of LDL cholesterol.

A high serum level of LDL cholesterol is atherogenic and a strong risk factor for coronary heart disease. The body normally attempts to compensate for high serum levels by inhibiting hepatic synthesis of cholesterol and cellular synthesis of new LDL receptors.

Very–low-density lipoprotein (VLDL) contains approximately 75% triglycerides and 25% cholesterol. It transports endogenous triglycerides (those synthesized in the liver and intestine, not those derived exogenously, from food) to fat and muscle cells. There, as with chylomicrons, lipoprotein lipase breaks down the molecule and releases fatty acids to be used for energy or stored as fat. The removal of triglycerides from VLDL leaves a cholesterol-rich remnant, which returns to the liver. Then the cholesterol is secreted into the intestine, mostly as bile acids, or it is used to form more VLDL and recirculated.

High-density lipoprotein (HDL) cholesterol, often referred to as "good cholesterol," is a small but very important lipoprotein. It is synthesized in the liver and intestine and some is derived from the enzymatic breakdown of chylomicrons and VLDL. It contains moderate amounts of cholesterol. However, this cholesterol is transported from blood vessel walls to the liver for catabolism and excretion. This reverse transport of cholesterol has protective effects against coronary heart disease.

The mechanisms by which HDL cholesterol exerts protective effects are unknown. Possible mechanisms include clearing cholesterol from atheromatous plaque; increasing excretion of cholesterol so less is available for reuse in the formation of LDL cholesterol; and inhibiting cellular uptake of LDL cholesterol. Regular exercise and moderate alcohol consumption are associated with increased levels of HDL cholesterol; obesity, diabetes mellitus, genetic factors, smoking, and some medications (eg, steroids and beta blockers) are associated with decreased levels. HDL cholesterol levels are not directly affected by diet.

a high rate of morbidity and mortality. Elevated total cholesterol and LDL cholesterol and reduced HDL cholesterol are the abnormalities that are major risk factors for coronary artery disease. Elevated triglycerides also play a role in cardiovascular disease. For example, high blood levels reflect excessive caloric intake (excessive dietary fats are stored in adipose tissue; excessive proteins and carbohydrates are converted to triglycerides and also stored in adipose tissue) and obesity. High caloric intake also increases the conversion of VLDL to LDL cholesterol, and high dietary intake of triglycerides and saturated fat decreases the activity of LDL receptors and increases synthesis of cholesterol. Very high triglyceride levels are associated with acute pancreatitis.

Hyperlipidemia may be primary (ie, genetic or familial) or secondary to dietary habits, other diseases (eg, diabetes mellitus, alcoholism, hypothyroidism, obesity, obstructive liver disease), and medications (eg, beta blockers, cyclosporine, oral estrogens, glucocorticoids, sertraline, thiazide diuretics, anti–human immunodeficiency virus protease inhibitors). Types of hyperlipidemias (also called hyperlipoproteinemias because increased blood levels of lipoproteins accompany increased blood lipid levels) are described in Box 58-2. Although hypercholesterolemia is usually emphasized, hypertriglyceridemia is also associated with most types of hyperlipoproteinemia.

INITIAL MANAGEMENT OF HYPERLIPIDEMIA

The National Cholesterol Education Program recommends treatment of clients according to their blood levels of total and LDL cholesterol and their risk factors for cardiovascular disease (Table 58-1). Note that both dietary and drug therapy are recommended at lower serum cholesterol levels in clients who already have cardiovascular disease or diabetes mellitus. Also, the target LDL serum level is lower in these clients. Guidelines include the following:

- Assess for, and treat, if present, conditions known to increase blood lipids (eg, diabetes mellitus, hypothyroidism).
- Stop medications known to increase blood lipids, if possible.
- Start a low-fat diet. A Step I diet contains no more than 30% of calories from fat, less than 10% of calories from saturated fats (eg, meat, dairy products), and less than 300 mg of cholesterol per day. A Step II diet contains no more than 30% of calories from

fat, less than 7% of calories from saturated fat, and less than 200 mg of cholesterol per day. The Step II diet is more stringent and may be used initially in clients with more severe hyperlipidemia, cardiovascular disease, or diabetes mellitus. It can decrease LDL cholesterol levels by 8% to 15%. Diets with more stringent fat restrictions than the Step II diet are not recommended because they produce little additional reduction in LDL cholesterol, they raise serum triglyceride levels, and they lower HDL cholesterol concentrations.

- Use the "Mediterranean diet," which includes moderate amounts of monounsaturated fats (eg, chicken, olive oil) and polyunsaturated fats (eg, safflower, corn, cottonseed, sesame, soybean, sunflower oils), to also decrease risks of cardiovascular disease.
- Increase dietary intake of soluble fiber (eg, psyllium preparations, oat bran, pectin, fruits and vegetables). This diet lowers serum LDL cholesterol by 5% to 10%.
- Start a weight reduction diet if the client is overweight or obese. Weight loss can increase HDL and decrease LDL.
- Emphasize regular aerobic exercise (usually 30 minutes at least three times weekly). This increases blood levels of HDL.
- If the client smokes, assist to develop a cessation plan. In addition to numerous other benefits, HDL levels are higher in nonsmokers.
- If the client is postmenopausal, hormone replacement therapy can raise HDL and lower LDL.
- If the client has elevated serum triglycerides, initial treatment includes efforts to achieve desirable body weight, ingest low amounts of saturated fat and cholesterol, exercise regularly, stop smoking, and reduce

---

BOX 58–2 **TYPES OF HYPERLIPIDEMIAS**

Type I is characterized by elevated or normal serum cholesterol, elevated triglycerides, and chylomicronemia. This rare condition may occur in infancy and childhood.

Type IIa (familial hypercholesterolemia) is characterized by a high level of low-density lipoprotein (LDL) cholesterol, a normal level of very–low-density lipoprotein (VLDL), and a normal or slightly increased level of triglycerides. It occurs in children and is a definite risk factor for development of atherosclerosis and coronary artery disease.

Type IIb (combined familial hyperlipoproteinemia) is characterized by increased levels of LDL, VLDL, cholesterol, and triglycerides and lipid deposits (xanthomas) in the feet, knees, and elbows. It occurs in adults.

Type III is characterized by elevations of cholesterol and triglycerides plus abnormal levels of LDL and

VLDL. This type usually occurs in middle-aged adults (40 to 60 years) and is associated with accelerated coronary and peripheral vascular disease.

Type IV is characterized by normal or elevated cholesterol levels, elevated triglycerides, and increased levels of VLDL. This type usually occurs in adults and may be the most common form of hyperlipoproteinemia. Type IV is often secondary to obesity, excessive intake of alcohol, or other diseases. Ischemic heart disease may occur at 40 to 50 years of age.

Type V is characterized by elevated cholesterol and triglyceride levels with an increased level of VLDL and chylomicronemia. This uncommon type usually occurs in adults. Type V is not associated with ischemic heart disease. Instead, it is associated with fat and carbohydrate intolerance, abdominal pain, and pancreatitis, which are relieved by lowering triglyceride levels.

TABLE 58-1 **National Cholesterol Education Program Recommendations for Treatment of Hyperlipidemia**

Patient's Cardiovascular Disease Status	Diet Therapy		Drug Therapy		Goal of Therapy (mg/dL)
	Total Cholesterol (mg/dL)	LDL Cholesterol (mg/dL)	Total Cholesterol (mg/dL)	LDL Cholesterol (mg/dL)	
No or one risk factor	240	160	275	190	LDL <160
More than two risk factors	200	130	240	160	LDL <130
Has cardiovascular disease	160	100	200	130	LDL <100

LDL, low-density lipoprotein.

alcohol intake, if indicated. The goal is to reduce serum triglyceride levels to 200 mg/dL or less.

DRUG THERAPY OF HYPERLIPIDEMIA

Antilipemic drugs are used to decrease blood lipids, to prevent or delay the development of atherosclerotic plaque, promote the regression of existing atherosclerotic plaque, and reduce morbidity and mortality from cardiovascular disease. The drugs act by altering the production, metabolism, or removal of lipids and lipoproteins. Drug therapy is recommended when approximately 6 months of dietary and other lifestyle changes fail to decrease hyperlipidemia to an acceptable level. It is also recommended for clients with signs and symptoms of coronary heart disease, a strong family history of coronary heart disease or hyperlipidemia, or other risk factors for atherosclerotic vascular disease (eg, hypertension, diabetes mellitus, cigarette smoking). Although several antilipemic drugs are available, none is effective in all types of hyperlipidemia. Types of drugs are described in the rest of this section; individual drugs are listed in Table 58-2.

The **HMG-CoA reductase inhibitors** or statins (eg, lovastatin) inhibit an enzyme (hydroxymethylglutaryl-coenzyme A reductase) required for hepatic synthesis of cholesterol. By decreasing production of cholesterol, these drugs decrease total serum cholesterol, LDL cholesterol, VLDL cholesterol, and triglycerides. They reduce LDL cholesterol within 2 weeks and reach maximal effects in approximately 4 to 6 weeks. HDL cholesterol levels remain unchanged or increase.

Overall, these drugs are useful in treating most of the major types of hyperlipidemia and are the most widely used antilipemics. Studies indicate that these drugs can reduce the incidence of coronary artery disease by 25% to 60% and the risk of death from any cause by approximately 30%. They also reduce the risk of angina pectoris, stroke, and peripheral arterial disease as well as the need for angioplasty and coronary artery grafting to increase or restore blood flow to the myocardium.

Statins are usually well tolerated; the most common adverse effects (nausea, constipation, diarrhea, abdominal cramps or pain, headache, skin rash) are usually mild

and transient. More serious reactions include rare occurrences of hepatotoxicity and myopathy.

Bile acid sequestrants (eg, cholestyramine) bind bile acids in the intestinal lumen. This causes the bile acids to be excreted in feces and prevents their being recirculated to the liver. Loss of bile acids stimulates hepatic synthesis of more bile acids from cholesterol. As more hepatic cholesterol is used to produce bile acids, more serum cholesterol moves into the liver to replenish the supply, thereby lowering serum cholesterol (especially LDL). LDL cholesterol levels decrease within a week of starting one of these drugs and reach maximal reductions within a month. When the drugs are stopped, pretreatment LDL cholesterol levels return within a month.

These drugs are used mainly to reduce LDL cholesterol further in clients who are already receiving a statin drug. The inhibition of cholesterol synthesis by a statin makes bile acid–binding drugs more effective. In addition, the combination increases HDL cholesterol and can further reduce the risk of cardiovascular disorders.

These drugs are not absorbed systemically and their main adverse effects are abdominal fullness, flatulence, and constipation. They may decrease absorption of many oral medications (eg, digoxin, folic acid, glipizide, propranolol, tetracyclines, thiazide diuretics, thyroid hormones, fat-soluble vitamins, and warfarin). Other drugs should be taken at least 1 hour before or 4 hours after cholestyramine or colestipol. In addition, dosage of the interactive drug may need to be changed when a bile acid sequestrant is added or withdrawn.

Fibrates are derivatives of fibric acid (eg, gemfibrozil, fenofibrate) and are similar to endogenous fatty acids. The drugs increase the oxidation of fatty acids in liver and muscle tissue and thereby decrease hepatic production of triglycerides, decrease VLDL cholesterol, and increase HDL cholesterol. These are the most effective drugs for reducing serum triglyceride levels, and their main indication for use is high serum triglyceride levels (>1000 mg/dL). They are also useful for clients with low HDL cholesterol levels. In clients with coronary artery disease, treatment with gemfibrozil is associated with regression of atherosclerotic lesions on angiography.

The main adverse effects are gastrointestinal discomfort and diarrhea, which may occur less often with feno-

TABLE 58-2 **Antilipemic Agents**

Generic/Trade Name	Clinical Indications (Type of Hyperlipidemia)	Routes and Dosage Ranges	
		Adults	Children
HMG-CoA Reductase Inhibitors (Statins)			
Atorvastatin (Lipitor)	Types IIa and IIb	PO 10 mg daily initially, increased up to 80 mg daily if necessary	
Cerivastatin (Baycol)	Types IIa and IIb	PO 0.3 mg daily	
Fluvastatin (Lescol)	Types IIa and IIb	PO 20–40 mg once daily at bedtime	
Lovastatin (Mevacor)	Types IIa and IIb	PO 20 mg daily with a meal, initially, increased up to 80 mg daily if necessary. Dosage increments should be at least 4 wk apart.	
Pravastatin (Pravachol)	Types IIa and IIb	PO 10–40 mg once daily at bedtime Elderly, PO 10 mg once daily at bedtime	
Simvastatin (Zocor)	Types IIa and IIb	PO 5–40 mg once daily in the evening Elderly, PO 5–20 mg once daily in the evening	
Fibrates			
Fenofibrate (Tricor)	Types IV and V (hyper-triglyceridemia)	PO 67 mg daily, increased if necessary to a maximum dose of 201 mg daily	
Gemfibrozil (Lopid)	Types IV, V (hypertri-glyceridemia)	PO 900–1500 mg daily, usually 1200 mg in two divided doses, 30 min before morning and evening meals	
Bile Acid Sequestrants			
Cholestyramine (Questran)	Type IIa	PO tablets 4 g once or twice daily initially, gradually increased at monthly intervals to 8–16 g daily in two divided doses. Maximum daily dose, 24 g. PO powder 4 g one to six times daily	
Colestipol	Type IIa	PO tablets 2 g once or twice daily initially, gradually increased at 1- to 2-mo intervals, up to 16 g daily PO granules 5 g daily initially, gradually increased at 1- to 2-mo intervals, up to 30 g daily in single or divided doses	
Miscellaneous			
Nicotinic acid (niacin)	Types II, III, IV, V	PO 2–6 g daily, in three or four divided doses, with or just after meals	PO 55–87 mg/kg/d, in three or four divided doses, with or just after meals

PO, oral.

fibrate than with gemfibrozil. The drugs may also increase cholesterol concentration in the biliary tract and cause gallstones. For clients receiving warfarin, warfarin dosage should be substantially decreased because fibrates displace warfarin from binding sites on serum albumin.

Niacin (nicotinic acid) decreases both cholesterol and triglycerides. It inhibits mobilization of free fatty acids from peripheral tissues, thereby reducing hepatic synthesis of triglycerides and secretion of VLDL, which leads to decreased production of LDL cholesterol. It also increases HDL cholesterol by reducing its catabolism. Disadvantages of niacin are the high doses required for antilipemic effects and the subsequent adverse effects. Niacin commonly causes skin flushing, pruritus, and gastric irritation and may cause hyperglycemia, hyperuricemia, elevated hepatic aminotransferase enzymes, and hepatitis. Flushing can be reduced by starting with small doses, gradually increasing doses, taking doses with meals, and taking aspirin 325 mg approximately 30 minutes before niacin doses.

Niacin is most effective in preventing heart disease when used in combination with another antilipemic drug such as a bile acid sequestrant or a fibrate. Its use with a statin lowers serum LDL cholesterol more than either drug alone, but the combination has not been studied in relation to preventing cardiovascular disease.

NURSING PROCESS

Assessment

Assess the client's status in relation to atherosclerotic vascular disease.

- Identify risk factors:
  - Hypertension
  - Diabetes mellitus
  - High intake of dietary fat and refined sugars
  - Obesity
  - Inadequate exercise
  - Cigarette smoking
  - Family history of atherosclerotic disorders
  - Hyperlipidemia
- Signs and symptoms depend on the specific problem:
  - **Hyperlipidemia** is manifested by elevated serum cholesterol (>240 mg/100 mL) or triglycerides (>200 mg/100 mL), or both.
  - **Coronary artery atherosclerosis** is manifested by myocardial ischemia (angina pectoris, myocardial infarction).
  - **Cerebrovascular insufficiency** may be manifested by syncope, memory loss, transient ischemic attacks (TIAs), or cerebrovascular accidents. Impairment of blood flow to the brain is caused primarily by atherosclerosis in the carotid, vertebral, or cerebral arteries.
  - **Peripheral arterial insufficiency** is manifested by impaired blood flow in the legs (weak or absent pulses; cool, pale extremities; intermittent claudication; leg pain at rest; and development of gangrene, usually in the toes because they are most distal to blood supply). This condition results from atherosclerosis in the distal abdominal aorta, the iliac arteries, and the femoral and smaller arteries in the legs.

Nursing Diagnoses

- Altered Tissue Perfusion related to atherosclerotic plaque in coronary, cerebral, or peripheral arteries
- Altered Nutrition: More Than Body Requirements of fats and calories
- Anxiety related to risks of atherosclerotic cardiovascular disease
- Body Image Disturbance related to the need for lifestyle changes
- Noncompliance related to dietary restrictions and adverse drug reactions
- Knowledge Deficit related to drug and diet therapy of hyperlipidemia

Planning/Goals

The client will:

- Take lipid-lowering drugs as prescribed
- Decrease dietary intake of saturated fats and cholesterol
- Lose weight if obese and maintain the lower weight
- Have periodic measurements of blood lipids
- Avoid preventable adverse drug effects
- Receive positive reinforcement for efforts to lower blood lipid levels
- Feel less anxious and more in control as risks of atherosclerotic cardiovascular disease are decreased

Interventions

Use measures to prevent, delay, or minimize atherosclerosis.

- Help clients to control risk factors. Ideally, primary prevention begins in childhood with healthful eating habits (ie, avoiding excessive fats, meat, and dairy products; obtaining adequate amounts of all nutrients, including dietary fiber; avoiding obesity), exercise, and avoiding cigarette smoking. However, changing habits to a more healthful lifestyle is helpful at any time, before or after disease manifestations appear. Weight loss often reduces blood lipids and lipoproteins to a normal range. Changing habits is difficult for most people, even those with severe symptoms.
- Use measures to increase blood flow to tissues:
  - Exercise is helpful in developing collateral circulation in the heart and legs. Collateral circulation involves use of secondary vessels in response to tissue ischemia related to obstruction of the principal vessels. Clients with angina pectoris or previous myocardial infarction require a carefully planned and supervised program of progressive exercise. Those with peripheral arterial insufficiency usually can increase exercise tolerance by walking regularly. Distances should be determined by occurrence of pain and must be individualized.
  - Posture and position may be altered to increase blood flow to the legs in peripheral arterial insufficiency. Elevating the head of the bed and having the legs horizontal or dependent may help. Elevating the feet is usually con-

traindicated unless edema is present or likely to develop.

- Although drug therapy is being increasingly used to prevent or treat atherosclerotic disorders, a major treatment of occlusive vascular disease is surgical removal of atherosclerotic plaque or revascularization procedures. Thus, severe angina pectoris may be relieved by a coronary artery bypass procedure that detours blood flow around occluded vessels. This procedure also may be done after a myocardial infarction. The goal is to prevent infarction or reinfarction. TIAs may be relieved by carotid endarterectomy; the goal is to prevent a stroke. Peripheral arterial insufficiency may be relieved by aortofemoral, femoropopliteal, or other bypass grafts that detour around occluded vessels. Although these procedures increase blood flow to ischemic tissues, they do not halt progression of atherosclerosis.

    The nursing role in relation to these procedures is to provide excellent preoperative and postoperative nursing care to promote healing, prevent infection, maintain patency of grafts, and help the client to achieve optimum function.

- Any antilipemic drug therapy must be accompanied by an appropriate diet; refer clients to a nutritionist. Overeating or gaining weight may decrease or cancel the lipid-lowering effects of the drugs.

- Encourage adult clients to have their serum cholesterol measured at least once every 5 years. Adults and children with a personal or family history of hyperlipidemia or other risk factors should be tested more often.

- The most effective measures for preventing hyperlipidemia and atherosclerosis are those related to a healthful lifestyle (diet low in cholesterol and saturated fats, weight control, exercise).

- Assist clients and family members to understand the desirability of lowering high blood lipid levels before serious cardiovascular diseases develop.

Evaluation

- Observe for decreased blood levels of total and LDL cholesterol and triglycerides; observe for increased levels of HDL cholesterol.
- Observe and interview regarding compliance with instructions for drug, diet, and other therapeutic measures.
- Observe and interview regarding adverse drug effects.
- Validate the client's ability to identify foods high and low in cholesterol and saturated fats.

CLIENT TEACHING GUIDELINES
Antilipemic Drugs

General Considerations

✔ Heart and blood vessel disease causes a great deal of illness and many deaths. The basic problem is usually atherosclerosis, in which the arteries are partly blocked by cholesterol deposits. Cholesterol, a waxy substance made in the liver, is necessary for normal body functioning. However, excessive amounts in the blood increase the likelihood of having a heart attack, stroke, or leg pain from inadequate blood flow. One type of cholesterol (low-density lipoprotein [LDL] or "bad") attaches to artery walls, where it can enlarge over time and block blood flow. The other type (high-density lipoprotein [HDL] or "good") carries cholesterol away from the artery and back to the liver, where it can be broken down. Thus, the healthiest blood cholesterol levels are low total cholesterol (<200 mg/dL), low LDL (<130 mg/dL) and high HDL (>35 mg/dL). High levels of blood triglycerides, another type of fat, are also unhealthy.

✔ Antilipemic drugs are given to lower high concentrations of fats (total cholesterol, LDL cholesterol, and triglycerides) in your blood. The goal of treatment is to prevent heart attack, stroke, and peripheral arterial disease. If you already have heart and blood vessel disease, the drugs can improve your symptoms, activity level, and quality of life.

✔ A low-fat diet is needed. This is often the first step in treating high cholesterol or triglyceride levels, and may be prescribed for 6 months or longer before drug therapy is begun. When drug therapy is prescribed, the diet should be continued. An important part is reducing the amount of saturated fat (from meats, dairy products). In addition, eating a bowl of oat cereal daily can help lower cholesterol by 5% to 10%. Diet counseling by a dietitian or nutritionist can be helpful in developing guidelines that fit your needs and lifestyle. Overeating or gaining weight may decrease or cancel the lipid-lowering effects of the drugs.

✔ Other lifestyle changes that can help improve cholesterol levels include regular aerobic exercise (raises HDL); losing weight (raises HDL, lowers LDL); and not smoking (HDL levels are higher in nonsmokers).

✔ Adults should have measurements of total cholesterol and HDL cholesterol at least once every 5 years. People with a personal or family history of hyperlipidemia or other risk factors for cardiovascular disease should be tested more often.

✔ Atorvastatin and other statin-type antilipemic drugs may increase sensitivity to sunlight. Avoid prolonged exposure to the sun, use sunscreens, and wear protective clothing.

(continued)

CLIENT TEACHING GUIDELINES
Antilipemic Drugs (continued)

✔ Gemfibrozil may cause dizziness or blurred vision and should be used cautiously while driving or performing other tasks that require alertness, coordination, or physical dexterity. It also may cause abdominal pain, diarrhea, nausea or vomiting. Notify a health care provider if these symptoms become severe.

✔ Skin flushing may occur with niacin. If it is distressing, taking one regular aspirin tablet (325 mg) approximately 30 to 60 minutes before the niacin dose may decrease this reaction. Flushing usually decreases in a few days, but may recur when niacin dosage is increased. Ask your physician if there is any reason you should not take aspirin.

✔ Cholestyramine and colestipol can cause constipation. Increasing intake of dietary fiber can help prevent this adverse effect.

Self-administration

✔ Take lovastatin with food; take atorvastatin, cerivastatin, fluvastatin, pravastatin, or simvastatin in the evening, with or without food. Food decreases stomach upset associated with lovastatin. All of these drugs are more effective

if taken in the evening or at bedtime, probably because more cholesterol is produced at nighttime and the drugs block cholesterol production.

✔ Take fenofibrate with food; food increases drug absorption.

✔ Take gemfibrozil on an empty stomach, approximately 30 minutes before morning and evening meals.

✔ Take immediate-release niacin with meals to decrease stomach upset; take timed-release niacin without regard to meals.

✔ Mix cholestyramine powder and colestipol granules with water or other fluids, soups, cereals, or fruits such as applesauce or crushed pineapple and follow with more fluid. These drug forms should not be taken dry.

✔ Do not take cholestyramine or colestipol with other drugs because they may prevent absorption of the other drugs. If taking other drugs, take them 1 hour before or 4 to 6 hours after cholestyramine or colestipol.

✔ Swallow colestipol tablets whole; do not cut, crush, or chew.

How Can You Avoid This Medication Error?

Mrs. Gribble, a 79-year-old nursing home resident, likes to take all of her medications together. You mix up her cholestyramine (Questran) in a large glass of orange juice and give it to her with her digoxin, Lasix, captopril, and Slow-K. You monitor her pulse and blood pressure before administration and they are within normal limits. What, if any, additional precautions should be used when Questran is administered?

Nursing Notes: Apply Your Knowledge

John Dwyer, 55 years of age, visits his primary health care provider. His cholesterol level (306 mg/dL) has been elevated for the last two visits. His physician prescribes niacin (nicotinic acid) to reduce his cholesterol level. Describe the data you will collect and how you will use it to individualize a teaching plan.

PRINCIPLES OF THERAPY

Drug Selection

Drug selection is based on the type of hyperlipidemia and its severity. For single-drug therapy to lower cholesterol, a statin is preferred. To lower both cholesterol and triglycerides, a statin, gemfibrozil, or niacin may be used. To lower triglycerides, gemfibrozil or niacin may be used. Gemfibrozil is usually preferred for people with diabetes because niacin increases blood sugar.

When monotherapy is not effective, combination therapy is rational because the drugs act by different mechanisms. In general, a statin and a bile acid sequestrant or niacin and a bile acid sequestrant are the most effective combinations in reducing total and LDL cholesterol. A fibrate or niacin may be included when a goal of therapy is to increase levels of HDL cholesterol. However, a

fibrate–statin combination should be avoided because of increased risks of severe myopathy, and a niacin–statin combination increases the risks of hepatotoxicity.

Use in Children

Hyperlipidemia occurs in children and may lead to atherosclerotic cardiovascular disease, including myocardial infarction, in early adulthood. Hyperlipidemia is diagnosed with total serum cholesterol levels of 200 mg/dL or above (desirable level, <170) and LDL cholesterol levels of 130 mg/dL or above (desirable level, <110). Early identification and treatment are needed. As with adults, initial treatment consists of diet therapy (for 6 to 12 months) and treatment of any secondary causes, especially with younger children. With additional risk factors or primary familial hypercholesterolemia (type IIa), however, these measures are not likely to be effective without drug therapy.

Antilipemic drugs are not recommended for children younger than 10 years of age. Bile acid sequestrants are considered the drugs of choice, and niacin also may be used. Despite considerable use of bile acid sequestrants, children's dosages have not been established. The statin drugs are not recommended in children younger than 18 years of age, and safety and effectiveness of the fibrates have not been established. The long-term consequences of antilipemic drug therapy in children are unknown.

Use in Older Adults

As with younger adults, diet, exercise, and weight control should be tried first. When drug therapy is required, statins are effective for lowering LDL cholesterol and usually are well tolerated by older adults. However, they are expensive. Niacin and bile acid sequestrants are effective, but older adults do not tolerate their adverse effects very well. In postmenopausal women, estrogen replacement therapy (alone or with a progestin) has beneficial antilipemic effects, lowering LDL cholesterol and raising HDL cholesterol.

Older adults often have diabetes, impaired liver function, or other conditions that raise blood lipid levels. Thus, treatment of secondary causes is especially important. They are also likely to have cardiovascular and other disorders that increase the adverse effects of antilipemic drugs. Overall, use of antilipemic drugs should be cautious, with close monitoring for therapeutic and adverse effects. Lower starting dosages are recommended for fenofibrate (67 mg/day), pravastatin (10 mg/day), and simvastatin (5 mg/day).

Use in Renal Impairment

Statins are metabolized by the liver and excreted partly through the kidneys (their main route of excretion is through bile). Drug plasma concentrations may be increased in clients with renal impairment and they should be used cautiously; some need reduced dosage.

- With *atorvastatin*, plasma levels are not affected and dosage reductions are not needed.
- With *cerivastatin*, half-life is increased with moderate to severe renal impairment and the recommended starting dose is 0.2 or 0.3 mg daily for creatinine clearance of 60 mL/minute or less.
- With *fluvastatin*, because it is cleared hepatically and less than 6% of the dose is excreted in urine, dosage reduction for mild to moderate renal impairment is unnecessary. Use caution with severe impairment.
- With *lovastatin*, plasma concentrations are increased in clients with severe renal impairment (creatinine clearance <30 mL/minute), and doses above 20 mg/day should be used with caution.
- With *pravastatin*, initiate therapy with 10 mg/day.
- With *simvastatin*, initiate therapy with 5 mg/day and monitor closely.

Fibrates are excreted mainly by the kidneys and therefore accumulate in the serum of clients with renal impairment. With *gemfibrozil*, there have been reports of worsening renal impairment in clients whose baseline serum creatinine levels were higher than 2 mg/dL. A different type of antilipemic drug may be preferred in these clients. *Fenofibrate* is contraindicated in clients with severe renal impairment, and the recommended starting dose is 67 mg/day in clients with a creatinine clearance of less than 50 mL/minute. Drug and dose effects on renal function and triglyceride levels should be evaluated before dosage is increased.

Use in Hepatic Impairment

Statins are metabolized in the liver and may accumulate in clients with impaired hepatic function. They are contraindicated in clients with active liver disease or unexplained elevations of serum aspartate or alanine aminotransferase. They should be used cautiously, in reduced dosages, for clients who ingest substantial amounts of alcohol or have a history of liver disease.

Liver function tests are recommended before starting a statin, at 6 and 12 weeks after starting the drug or increasing the dose, then every 6 months. Monitor clients who have increased serum aminotransferases until the abnormal values resolve. If the increases are more than three times the upper limit of normal levels and persist, reduce the dose or discontinue the statin drug.

Fibrates may cause hepatotoxicity. Abnormal elevations of serum aminotransferases have occurred with both gemfibrozil and fenofibrate, but they usually subside when the drug is discontinued. Fenofibrate is contraindicated in severe hepatic impairment, including clients with primary biliary cirrhosis, preexisting gallbladder disease, and persistent elevations in liver function test results. In addition, hepatitis (hepatocellular, chronic active, and cholestatic) has been reported after use of fenofibrate from a few weeks to several years. Liver function tests should be monitored during the first year of drug administration. The drug should be discontinued if elevated enzyme levels persist (at more than three times the normal limit).

Niacin may cause hepatotoxicity, especially with doses above 2 g daily, with timed-release preparations, and if given in combination with a statin or fibrate.

 Home Care

For a client with hyperlipidemia, the home care nurse may teach about the role of blood lipids in causing myocardial infarction, stroke, and peripheral arterial insufficiency; the prescribed treatment regimen and its goals; and the importance of improving hyperlipidemia in preventing or improving cardiovascular disorders. In addition, the client may need assistance in obtaining blood tests (eg, lipids and liver function tests) and dietary counseling.

NURSING ACTIONS   Drugs for Hyperlipidemia

NURSING ACTIONS	RATIONALE/EXPLANATION
1. Administer accurately **a.** Give lovastatin with food; give atorvastatin, cerivastatin, fluvastatin, pravastatin, or simvastatin in the evening, with or without food.	Food decreases gastrointestinal (GI) upset associated with lovastatin. These drugs are more effective if taken in the evening or at bedtime, because more cholesterol is produced by the liver at night and the drugs block cholesterol production.
b. Give fenofibrate with food.	Food increases drug absorption.
c. Give gemfibrozil on an empty stomach, approximately 30 min before morning and evening meals.	
d. Give immediate-release niacin with meals; give timed-release niacin without regard to meals.	The immediate-release formulation may cause gastric irritation.
e. Mix cholestyramine powder and colestipol granules with water or other fluids, soups, cereals, or fruits such as applesauce or crushed pineapple and follow with more fluid.	These drug forms should not be taken dry.
f. Do not give cholestyramine or colestipol with other drugs; instead, give them 1 h before or 4–6 h after cholestyramine or colestipol.	Cholestyramine and colestipol prevent absorption of many drugs.
g. Instruct clients to swallow colestipol tablets whole; do not cut, crush, or chew.	
2. Observe for therapeutic effects **a.** Decreased levels of total serum cholesterol, low-density lipoprotein cholesterol and triglycerides and increased levels of high-density lipoprotein cholesterol.	With statins, effects occur in 1–2 wk, with maximum effects in 4–6 wk. With fibrates and niacin, effects occur in approximately 1 mo. With cholestyramine and colestipol, maximum effects occur in approximately 1 mo.
3. Observe for adverse effects **a.** GI problems—nausea, vomiting, flatulence, constipation or diarrhea, abdominal discomfort	GI symptoms are the most common adverse effects of antilipemic drugs. Constipation is especially common with cholestyramine and colestipol.
b. With lovastatin and related drugs, observe for GI upset (see 3a), skin rash, pruritus, and myopathy	Adverse effects are usually mild and of short duration. A less common but potentially serious effect is liver dysfunction, usually manifested by increased levels of serum aminotransferases. Serum aminotransferases (aspartate and alanine aminotransferase) should be measured before starting the drug, every 4–6 wk during the first 3 mo, then every 6–12 wk or after dosage increases for 1 y, then every 6 mo.
c. With nicotinic acid, flushing of the face and neck, pruritus, and skin rash may occur, as well as tachycardia, hypotension, and dizziness.	These symptoms may be prominent when nicotinic acid is used to lower blood lipids because relatively high doses are required. Aspirin 325 mg, given 30 min before nicotinic acid, decreases the flushing reaction.

(continued)

NURSING ACTIONS	RATIONALE/EXPLANATION
4. Observe for drug interactions	
a. Drugs that *increase* effects of lovastatin and related drugs:	
(1) Azole antifungals (eg, itraconazole, keto-conazole)	Risk of myopathy is increased. It is recommended that statin therapy be interrupted temporarily if systemic azole antifungals are needed.
(2) Cyclosporine	Risk of severe myopathy or rhabdomyolysis is increased.
(3) Erythromycin	Risk of severe myopathy or rhabdomyolysis is increased.
(4) Fibrate antilipemics (eg, fenofibrate, gemfibrozil)	Risk of severe myopathy or rhabdomyolysis is increased. These drugs should not be given concurrently with statin antilipemic drugs.
(5) Niacin	Risk of severe myopathy or rhabdomyolysis is increased.
(6) Drugs that *increase* effects of fluvastatin:	
(a) Alcohol, cimetidine, ranitidine, omeprazole	Increased blood levels
b. Drugs that *decrease* effects of lovastatin and related drugs:	
(1) Bile acid sequestrant antilipemics	Decreased blood levels unless the drugs are taken 1–4 h apart
(2) Antacids	Decrease absorption of atorvastatin
(3) Isradipine	This calcium channel blocker may decrease blood levels of lovastatin and its metabolites by increasing their hepatic metabolism.
(4) Rifampin	Decreases blood levels of fluvastatin
c. Drugs that *decrease* effects of fibrate antilipemic drugs:	
(1) Bile acid sequestrant antilipemic drugs	Decrease absorption unless the fibrate is taken about 1 h before or 4–6 h after the bile acid sequestrant

How Can You Avoid This Medication Error?

Answer: Questran should not be administered at the same time as other oral medications because it interferes with the absorption of many other drugs, including digoxin. Give other drugs 1 hour before or 4 to 6 hours after Questran is administered.

Nursing Notes: Apply Your Knowledge

Answer: Mr. Dwyer will need teaching regarding lifestyle modifications to reduce his cholesterol level as well as information on the niacin that has been prescribed. First, ask what he knows about high cholesterol and methods that he has used to try to decrease his cholesterol level. Make sure you include a dietary assessment, especially his knowledge of foods high in cholesterol or fat. Explore together possible ways to reduce cholesterol and fat in the diet. If he is overweight, also talk about calorie reduction. Often, people have the correct knowledge about necessary changes, but compliance with lifestyle modification is difficult. Explore his supports and provide a list of referrals for long-term follow-up. Assess his exercise pattern. Provide positive reinforcement for any exercise that he does and together develop a reasonable exercise plan.

Mr. Dwyer also needs teaching about niacin to prevent unpleasant side effects. Gradually increasing the dose can possibly limit the unpleasant side effects of flushing and pruritus, as can premedicating with aspirin. Niacin should be taken with meals. Because niacin is a vitamin, many patients may feel it is safe to increase the dose. If side effects limit compliance, discuss this with the physician. Many newer, more expensive antilipid agents with fewer side effects can be prescribed to lower cholesterol. It is important to stress the importance of ongoing follow-up for clients with hyperlipidemia.

 ## REVIEW AND APPLICATION EXERCISES

1. How would you describe hyperlipidemia to a client?
2. What is the goal of treatment for hyperlipidemia?
3. Differentiate lipid-lowering drugs according to their mechanisms of action.
4. What are the main nonpharmacologic measures to decrease total and LDL cholesterol and increase HDL cholesterol?
5. What are the main nonpharmacologic measures to decrease serum triglyceride levels?

SELECTED REFERENCES

Drug facts and comparisons. (Updated monthly). St. Louis: Facts and Comparisons.

Ettinger, W.H. & Hazzard, W.R. (1997). Approach to the elderly patient with dyslipidemia. In W.N. Kelley (Ed.), *Textbook of internal medicine*, 3rd ed., pp. 2494–2497. Philadelphia: Lippincott-Raven.

Guyton, A.C. & Hall, J.E. (1996). *Textbook of medical physiology*, 9th ed. Philadelphia: W.B. Saunders.

Knopp, R.H. (1999). Drug treatment of lipid disorders. *New England Journal of Medicine, 341*, 498–511.

Porth, C.M. (Ed.). (1998). *Pathophysiology: Concepts of altered health states*, 5th ed. Philadelphia: Lippincott Williams & Wilkins.

Talbert, R.L. (1997). Hyperlipidemia. In J.T. DiPiro, R.L. Talbert, G.C. Yee, G.R. Matzke, B.G. Wells, & L.M. Posey (Eds.), *Pharmacotherapy: A pathophysiologic approach*, 3rd ed., pp. 459–489. Stamford, CT: Appleton & Lange.

Witztum, J.L. (1996). Drugs used in the treatment of hyperlipoproteinemias. In J.G. Hardman, L.E. Limbird, P.B. Molinoff, & R.W. Ruddon (Eds.), *Goodman & Gilman's The pharmacological basis of therapeutics*, 9th ed., pp. 875–897. New York: McGraw-Hill.

Drugs Affecting the Digestive System

59

Physiology of the Digestive System

Objectives

After studying this chapter, the student will be able to:

1. Review roles of the main digestive tract structures.

2. List common signs and symptoms affecting gastrointestinal functions.

3. Identify general categories of drugs used to treat gastrointestinal disorders.

4. Discuss the effects of nongastrointestinal drugs on gastrointestinal functioning.

THE DIGESTIVE SYSTEM

The digestive system consists of the alimentary canal (a tube extending from the oral cavity to the anus, approximately 25 to 30 feet [7.5 to 9 m] long) and the accessory organs (salivary glands, gallbladder, liver, and pancreas). The main function of the system is to provide the body with fluids, nutrients, and electrolytes in a form that can be used at the cellular level. The system also disposes of waste products that result from the digestive process.

The alimentary canal has the same basic structure throughout. The layers of the wall are mucosa, connective tissue, and muscle. Peristalsis propels food through the tract and mixes the food bolus with digestive juices. Stimulation of the parasympathetic nervous system (by vagus nerves) increases motility and secretions. The tract has an abundant blood supply, which increases cell regeneration and healing. Blood flow increases during digestion and absorption. Blood flow decreases with strenuous exercise, sympathetic nervous system stimulation (ie, "fight or flight"), aging (secondary to decreased cardiac output and atherosclerosis), and conditions that shunt blood away from the digestive tract (eg, heart failure, atherosclerosis).

ORGANS OF THE DIGESTIVE SYSTEM

Oral Cavity

In the oral cavity, chewing mechanically breaks food into smaller particles, which can be swallowed more easily and provide a larger surface area for enzyme action. Food is also mixed with saliva, which lubricates the food bolus for swallowing and initiates the digestion of starch.

Esophagus

The esophagus is a musculofibrous tube approximately 10 inches (25 cm) long; its main function is to convey food from the pharynx to the stomach. It secretes a small amount of mucus and has some peristaltic movement.

Stomach

The stomach is a dilated area that serves as a reservoir. It churns and mixes the food with digestive juices, secretes mucus and enzymes, starts protein breakdown, and secretes intrinsic factor, which is necessary for absorption of vitamin B_{12} from the ileum. Although there is much diffusion of water and electrolytes through the gastric mucosa in both directions, there is little absorption of these substances. Carbohydrates and amino acids are also poorly absorbed. Only a few highly lipid-soluble substances, such as alcohol and some drugs, are absorbed in moderate quantities from the stomach.

The inlet of the stomach is the end of the esophagus, and the outlet is the pyloric sphincter at the beginning of the duodenum. The stomach normally holds approximately 1000 mL comfortably and empties in approximately 4 hours. Numerous factors influence the rate of gastric emptying, including the size of the pylorus, gastric motility, type of food, fluidity of chyme (the material produced by gastric digestion of food), and the state of the duodenum. Factors that cause rapid emptying include carbohydrate foods, increased motility, fluid chyme, and an empty duodenum. The stomach empties more slowly with decreased gastric tone and motility, fatty foods, chyme of excessive acidity, and a duodenum that contains fats, proteins, or chyme of excessive acidity. When fats are present, the duodenal mucosa produces a hormone, enterogastrone, that inhibits gastric secretion and motility. This allows a longer time for the digestion of fats in the small intestine.

Small Intestine

The small intestine consists of the duodenum, jejunum, and ileum and is approximately 20 feet (6 m) long. The duodenum makes up the first 10 to 12 inches (25 to 30 cm) of the small intestine. The pancreatic and bile ducts empty into the duodenum at the papilla of Vater. The small intestine contains numerous glands that secrete digestive enzymes, hormones, and mucus. For the most part, digestion and absorption occur in the small intestine, including absorption of most orally administered drugs.

Large Intestine

The large intestine consists of the cecum, colon, rectum, and anus. The ileum opens into the cecum. The colon secretes mucus and absorbs water.

Pancreas

The pancreas secretes enzymes required for the digestion of carbohydrates, proteins, and fats. It also secretes insulin and glucagon, hormones that regulate glucose metabolism and blood sugar levels.

Gallbladder

The gallbladder is a small pouch attached to the underside of the liver that stores and concentrates bile. It has a capacity of approximately 50 to 60 mL. The gallbladder releases bile when fats are present in the duodenum.

Liver

The liver is a vital organ that performs numerous functions. It receives approximately 1500 mL of blood per minute, or 25% to 30% of the total cardiac output. Approximately three fourths of the blood flow is venous blood from the stomach, intestines, spleen, and pancreas (portal circulation); the remainder is arterial blood through the hepatic artery. The hepatic artery carries blood to the connective tissue of the liver and bile ducts, then empties into the hepatic sinuses. Arterial blood mixes with blood from the portal circulation. Venous blood from the liver flows into the inferior vena cava for return to the systemic circulation. The ample blood flow facilitates specific hepatic functions, which include the following:

1. **Blood reservoir**. The liver can eject approximately 500 to 1000 mL of blood into the general circulation in response to stress, decreased blood volume, and sympathetic nervous system stimulation (eg, hemorrhagic or hypovolemic shock).

2. **Blood filter and detoxifier**. Kupffer cells in the liver phagocytize bacteria carried from the intestines by the portal vein. They also break down worn-out erythrocytes, saving iron for reuse in hemoglobin synthesis, and form bilirubin, a waste product excreted in bile. The liver metabolizes many body secretions and most drugs to prevent accumulation and harmful effects on body tissues.

   Most drugs are active as the parent compound and are metabolized in the liver to an inactive metabolite, which is then excreted by the kidneys. However, some drugs become active only after formation of a metabolite in the liver.

   The liver detoxifies or alters substances by oxidation, hydrolysis, or conjugation. Conjugation involves combining a chemical substance with an endogenous substance to produce an inactive or harmless compound. Essentially all steroid hormones, including adrenal corticosteroids and sex hormones, are at least partially conjugated in the liver and secreted into the bile. When the liver is damaged, these hormones may accumulate in body fluids and cause symptoms of hormone excess.

3. **Metabolism of carbohydrate, fat, and protein**. In carbohydrate metabolism, the liver converts glucose to glycogen for storage and reconverts glycogen to glucose when needed to maintain an adequate blood sugar concentration. Excess glucose that cannot be converted to glycogen is converted to fat. The liver also changes fructose and galactose, which cannot be used by body cells, to glucose, which provides energy for cellular metabolism. Fats are synthesized and catabolized by the liver. Amino acids from protein breakdown may be used to form glycogen, plasma proteins, and enzymes.

4. **Storage of nutrients**. In addition to glycogen, the liver also stores fat-soluble vitamins (ie, vitamins A, D, E, K), vitamin B_{12}, iron, phospholipids, cholesterol, and small amounts of protein and fat.

5. **Synthesis** of bile; serum albumin and globulin; prothrombin; fibrinogen; blood coagulation factors V, VII, VIII, IX, XI, and XII; and urea. Formation of

urea removes ammonia from body fluids. Large amounts of ammonia are formed by intestinal bacteria and absorbed into the blood. If the ammonia is not converted to urea by the liver, plasma ammonia concentrations rise to toxic levels and cause hepatic coma and death.

6. **Production of body heat** by continuous cellular metabolism. The liver is the body organ with the highest rate of chemical activity during basal conditions, and it produces approximately 20% of total body heat.

SECRETIONS OF THE DIGESTIVE SYSTEM

Mucus

Mucus is secreted by mucous glands in every part of the gastrointestinal (GI) tract. The functions of mucus are to protect the lining of the tract from digestive juices, lubricate the food bolus for easier passage, promote adherence of the fecal mass, and neutralize acids and bases.

Saliva

Saliva consists of mucus and salivary amylase. It is produced by the salivary glands and totals approximately 1000 mL daily. Saliva has a slightly acidic to neutral pH (6 to 7); it lubricates the food bolus and starts starch digestion.

Gastric Juice

Gastric juice consists of mucus, digestive enzymes, hydrochloric acid, and electrolytes. The gastric glands secrete approximately 2000 mL of gastric juice daily. The pH is highly acidic (1 to 3). Secretion is stimulated by the parasympathetic nervous system (by the vagus nerve), the hormone gastrin, the presence of food in the mouth, and seeing, smelling, or thinking about food.

The major digestive enzyme in gastric juice is pepsin, a proteolytic enzyme that functions best at a pH of 2 to 3. Hydrochloric acid provides the acid medium to promote pepsin activity. The major function of gastric juice is to begin digestion of proteins. There is also a weak action on fats by gastric lipase and on carbohydrates by gastric amylase. A large amount of mucus is secreted in the stomach to protect the stomach wall from the proteolytic action of pepsin. When mucus is not secreted, gastric ulceration occurs within hours.

Pancreatic Juices

Pancreatic juices are alkaline (pH $\geq$ 8) secretions that contain amylase for carbohydrate digestion, lipase for fat digestion, and trypsin and chymotrypsin for protein digestion. They also contain large amounts of sodium bicarbonate, a base (alkali) that neutralizes the acid chyme from the stomach by reacting with hydrochloric acid. This protects the mucosa of the small intestine from the digestive properties of gastric juice. The daily amount of pancreatic secretion is approximately 1200 mL. The hormone cholecystokinin stimulates secretion of pancreatic juices.

Bile

Bile is an alkaline (pH of approximately 8) secretion that is formed continuously in the liver, carried to the gallbladder by the bile ducts, and stored there. The hormone cholecystokinin causes the gallbladder to contract and release bile into the small intestine when fats are present in intestinal contents. The liver secretes approximately 600 mL of bile daily. This amount is concentrated to the 50- to 60-mL capacity of the gallbladder. Bile contains bile salts, cholesterol, bilirubin, fatty acids, and electrolytes. Bile salts are required for digestion and absorption of fats, including fat-soluble vitamins. Most of the bile salts are reabsorbed and reused by the liver (enterohepatic circulation); some are excreted in feces.

EFFECTS OF DRUGS ON THE DIGESTIVE SYSTEM

The digestive system and drug therapy have a reciprocal relationship. Many common symptoms (ie, nausea, vomiting, constipation, diarrhea, abdominal pain) relate to GI dysfunction. These symptoms may result from a disorder in the digestive system, disorders in other body systems, or drug therapy. Many GI symptoms and disorders alter the ingestion, dissolution, absorption, and metabolism of drugs. Drugs may be administered to relieve these symptoms and disorders, but drugs administered for conditions unrelated to the digestive system may cause such symptoms and disorders. GI conditions may alter responses to drug therapy.

Drugs used in digestive disorders primarily alter GI secretion, absorption, or motility. They may act systemically or locally in the GI tract. The drug groups included in this section are drugs used for acid-peptic disorders, laxatives, antidiarrheals, and antiemetics. Other drug groups used in GI disorders include cholinergics (see Chap. 20), anticholinergics (see Chap. 21), corticosteroids (see Chap. 24), and anti-infective drugs (see Section VI).

 REVIEW AND APPLICATION EXERCISES

1. What is the main function of the GI system?
2. What is the role of the parasympathetic nervous system in GI function?
3. List factors affecting GI motility and secretions.
4. Describe important GI secretions and their functions.
5. What factors stimulate or inhibit GI secretions?
6. How does the GI tract affect oral medications?
7. How do oral medications affect the GI tract?

SELECTED REFERENCES

Guyton, A.C. & Hall, J.E. (1996). *Textbook of medical physiology*, 9th ed. Philadelphia: W.B. Saunders.
Porth, C.M. (Ed.). (1998). *Pathophysiology: Concepts of altered health states*, 5th ed., pp. 703–718. Philadelphia: Lippincott Williams & Wilkins.

60

Drugs Used in Peptic Ulcer Disease

Objectives

After studying this chapter, the student will be able to:

1. Describe the role of *Helicobacter pylori* and other etiologic factors in peptic ulcer disease.

2. Differentiate the types of antiulcer drugs in terms of their mechanisms of action, indications for use, common adverse effects, and nursing process implications.

3. Discuss the advantages and disadvantages of proton pump inhibitors.

4. Differentiate between prescription and over-the-counter uses of histamine-2 receptor blocking agents.

5. Discuss significant drug–drug interactions with cimetidine (Tagamet).

6. Describe characteristics, uses, and effects of selected antacids.

7. Discuss the rationale for using combination antacid products.

8. Teach clients nonpharmacologic measures to manage gastroesophageal reflux disease and peptic ulcer disease.

Mrs. Greenspan, a 26-year-old homemaker, has rheumatoid arthritis that has been treated with aspirin, nonsteroidal anti-inflammatory drugs, and prednisone for the last 10 years. During the past week, Mrs. Greenspan has been feeling increasingly weak. She is dizzy when getting up and has had one episode of syncope (fainting). A work-up indicates that she has a peptic ulcer. Omeprazole, a proton pump inhibitor, is ordered.

Reflect on:

▶ Mrs. Greenspan's risk factors that contributed to the development of her ulcer.

▶ How symptoms of weakness, dizziness, and syncope are associated with a peptic ulcer.

▶ How proton pump inhibitors work to heal ulcers.

▶ What therapies (drugs and nondrugs) can be used to prevent a recurrence of her ulcer.

PEPTIC ULCER DISEASE

Peptic ulcer disease is characterized by ulcer formation in areas of the gastrointestinal (GI) mucosa that are exposed to gastric acid and pepsin (ie, esophagus, stomach, and duodenum). Although esophageal ulcers are less common than gastric and duodenal ulcers, another esophageal disorder associated with exposure to gastric acid and pepsin is gastroesophageal reflux disease (GERD). This disorder is included here because antiulcer medications are used to prevent and treat GERD. Gastric ulcers (which may be preceded by less severe mucosal defects such as erosions or gastritis) may be acute ulcers associated with stress (eg, surgery, shock, head injury, severe burn injuries,

major medical illness), certain drugs (mainly aspirin and other nonsteroidal anti-inflammatory drugs [NSAIDs]), or *Helicobacter pylori* infection. Duodenal ulcers are usually chronic in nature and are also commonly associated with NSAID ingestion and *H. pylori* infection. Selected acid-peptic disorders for which antiulcer drugs are used are described further in Box 60-1.

Causes of Peptic Ulcer Disease

Peptic ulcer disease is attributed to an imbalance between cell-destructive and cell-protective effects. Cell-destructive effects include those of gastric acid (hydrochloric acid),

---

BOX 60–1	SELECTED UPPER GASTROINTESTINAL DISORDERS

Gastroesophageal Reflux Disease

Gastroesophageal reflux disease (GERD) is a common condition characterized by regurgitation of gastric contents into the esophagus and exposure of esophageal mucosa to gastric acid and pepsin. The main symptom is heartburn, which most people experience occasionally. Depending on the frequency and extent of acid-pepsin reflux, GERD may result in mild to severe esophagitis or esophageal ulceration. The main cause of GERD is thought to be an incompetent lower esophageal sphincter. GERD occurs in men, women, and children, but is especially common during pregnancy and after 40 years of age.

Nonsteroidal Anti-inflammatory Drug Gastropathy

Nonsteroidal anti-inflammatory drug (NSAID) gastropathy indicates damage to gastroduodenal mucosa by aspirin and other NSAIDs. The damage may range from minor superficial erosions to ulceration and bleeding. NSAID gastropathy is one of the most common causes of gastric ulcers, and it may cause duodenal ulcers as well. Many people take NSAIDs daily for pain, arthritis, and other conditions. Chronic ingestion of NSAIDs causes local irritation of gastroduodenal mucosa, inhibits the synthesis of protective prostaglandins, and increases the synthesis of leukotrienes and possibly other inflammatory substances that may contribute to mucosal injury.

Peptic Ulcer Disease

Peptic ulcer disease usually denotes gastric and duodenal ulcers. Although there is considerable overlap in etiology, clinical manifestations, and treatment of gastric and duodenal ulcers, there are differences as well. Gastric ulcers may be caused by severe physiologic stress, *Helicobacter pylori* infection, and NSAID ingestion. Stress ulcers may occur in any age group and are usually acute

in nature. Gastric ulcers associated with *H. pylori* infection or NSAID ingestion are more likely to occur in older adults, especially in the sixth and seventh decades, and to be chronic in nature. Duodenal ulcers are strongly associated with *H. pylori* infection, may occur at any age, and occur more often in men than women.

A gastric or duodenal ulcer may penetrate only the mucosal surface or it may extend into the smooth muscle layers. When superficial lesions heal, no defects remain. When smooth muscle heals, however, scar tissue remains and the mucosa that regenerates to cover the scarred muscle tissue may be defective. These defects contribute to repeated episodes of ulceration.

Overall, peptic ulcers are thought to result from an imbalance between gastric acid and pepsin production and the ability of the gastroduodenal mucosa to resist the destructive action of these digestive agents. *H. pylori* organisms colonize the mucus-secreting epithelial cells of the stomach and probably impair mucosal function. *H. pylori* infection is strongly associated with chronic gastritis and gastric and duodenal ulcers.

Stress Ulcers

Stress ulcers indicate gastric mucosal lesions that develop in patients who are critically ill from trauma, shock, hemorrhage, sepsis, burns, acute respiratory distress syndrome, major surgical procedures, or other severe illnesses. They are usually manifested by painless upper gastrointestinal (GI) bleeding. The frequency of occurrence has decreased, possibly because of prophylactic use of antiulcer drugs and improved management of sepsis, hypovolemia, and other disorders associated with critical illness.

Although the exact mechanisms of stress ulcer formation are unknown, several factors are thought to play a role, including mucosal ischemia, reflux of bile salts into the stomach, reduced GI tract motility, and

(continued)

systemic acidosis. Acidosis increases severity of lesions, and correction of acidosis decreases their formation. In addition, lesions do not form if the pH of gastric fluids is kept about 3.5 or above.

Zollinger-Ellison Syndrome

Zollinger-Ellison syndrome is a rare condition characterized by excessive secretion of gastric acid and

a high incidence of ulcers. It is caused by gastrin-secreting tumors in the pancreas, stomach, or duodenum. Approximately two thirds of the gastrinomas are malignant. Symptoms are those of peptic ulcer disease, and diagnosis is based on high levels of serum gastrin and gastric acid. Treatment may involve long-term use of a proton pump inhibitor to diminish gastric acid, or surgical excision.

---

pepsin, and *H. pylori* infection. Gastric acid, a strong acid that can digest the stomach wall, is secreted by the parietal cells in the mucosa of the stomach antrum, near the pylorus. The parietal cells contain receptors for acetylcholine, gastrin, and histamine, substances that stimulate gastric acid production. Acetylcholine is released by vagus nerve endings in response to stimuli, such as thinking about or ingesting food. Gastrin is a hormone released by cells in the stomach and duodenum in response to food ingestion and stretching of the stomach wall. It is secreted into the bloodstream and eventually circulated to the parietal cells. Histamine is released from cells in the gastric mucosa and diffuses into nearby parietal cells. Once produced, gastric acid is released by activation of an enzyme system (hydrogen–potassium adenosine triphosphatase, or H^+,K^+-ATPase) at the surface of parietal cells. This enzyme system acts as a gastric acid (proton) pump to move gastric acid from parietal cells in the mucosal lining of the stomach into the stomach lumen.

Pepsin is a proteolytic enzyme that also can digest the stomach wall. Pepsin is derived from a precursor called pepsinogen, which is secreted by chief cells in the gastric mucosa. Pepsinogen is converted to pepsin only in a highly acidic environment (ie, when the pH of gastric juices is approximately 3 or less).

H. pylori is a gram-negative bacterium found in the gastric mucosa of most clients with gastritis, approximately 75% of clients with gastric ulcers, and more than 90% of clients with duodenal ulcers. The mechanism by which *H. pylori* infection leads to gastritis or ulceration is unknown but may involve impairment of mucosal defense mechanisms. It is known, however, that eradication of the organism accelerates ulcer healing and significantly decreases the rate of ulcer recurrence.

Autodigestion of stomach and duodenal tissues and ulcer formation are normally prevented by the cell-protective effects of mucus, dilution of gastric acid by food and secretions, prevention of diffusion of hydrochloric acid from the stomach lumen back into the gastric mucosal lining, the presence of certain prostaglandins (eg, prostaglandin E), alkalinization of gastric secretions by pancreatic juices and bile, and perhaps other mechanisms. Overall, then, peptic ulcers form when cell-destructive elements exceed cell-protective elements. The main

pathophysiologic mechanism may reflect an abnormality in acid and pepsin secretion or impaired mucosal defense mechanisms.

TYPES OF ANTIULCER DRUGS

Drugs used in the treatment of acid-peptic disorders promote healing of lesions and prevent recurrence of lesions by decreasing cell-destructive effects or increasing cell-protective effects. Several types of drugs are used for this purpose, alone or in various combinations. Antacids neutralize gastric acid and decrease pepsin production; antimicrobials and bismuth can eliminate *H. pylori* infection; histamine-2 receptor antagonists (H₂RAs) and proton pump inhibitors (PPIs) decrease gastric acid secretion; sucralfate provides a barrier between mucosal erosions or ulcers and gastric secretions; and misoprostol restores prostaglandin activity. Types of drugs and individual agents are described in the following sections and listed in Tables 60-1 and 60-2.

Antacids

Antacids are alkaline substances that neutralize acids. They react with hydrochloric acid in the stomach to produce neutral, less acidic, or poorly absorbed salts and to raise the pH (alkalinity) of gastric secretions. Raising the pH to approximately 3.5 neutralizes more than 90% of gastric acid and inhibits conversion of pepsinogen to pepsin. Commonly used antacids are aluminum, magnesium, and calcium compounds. Small amounts of aluminum, magnesium, and calcium are absorbed from the GI tract. Normally insignificant, these small amounts may cause serious adverse effects in the presence of renal disease.

Antacids differ in the amounts needed to neutralize gastric acid (approximately 50 to 80 mEq of acid is produced hourly), in onset of action, and in adverse effects. *Aluminum compounds* have a low neutralizing capacity (ie, large doses are required) and a slow onset of action. They can cause constipation. In people who ingest large amounts

TABLE 60-1 **Representative Antacid Products**

	Components				
Trade Name	Magnesium Oxide or Hydroxide	Aluminum Hydroxide	Calcium Carbonate	Other	Route and Dosage Ranges (Adults)
Aludrox	103 mg/5 mL	307 mg/5 mL			PO 10 mL q4h, or as needed
Amphojel		300 or 600 mg/tab, 320 mg/5 mL			PO 10 mL or 600 mg five or six times daily
Di-Gel		200 mg/5 mL		Simethicone 20 mg/5 mL	PO 2 tsp liquid q2h, after meals or between meals, and at bedtime. Maximal dose, 20 tsp/24 h. Do not use maximal dose longer than 2 wk.
Gelusil	200 mg/tab	200 mg/tab		Simethicone 25 mg/tab	PO 10 or more mL or 2 or more tablets after meals and at bedtime or as directed by physician to a maximum of 12 tablets or tsp/24 h
Maalox suspension	200 mg/5 mL	225 mg/5 mL			PO 30 mL four times daily, after meals and at bedtime or as directed by physician; maximal dose, 16 tsp/24 h
Maalox tablets	200 mg/tab	200 mg/tab			PO 2–4 tablets, four times daily, after meals and at bedtime or as directed by physician; maximal dose, 16 tablets/24 h
Maalox Plus	200 mg/tab, 200 mg/5 mL	200 mg/tab, 225 mg/5 mL		Simethicone 25 mg/tab, 20 mg/5 mL	PO 2–4 tsp or tablets, four times daily after meals and at bedtime, or as directed by physician
Mylanta	200 mg/tab, 200 mg/5 mL	200 mg/tab, 200 mg/5 mL		Simethicone 25 mg/tab, 20 mg/5 mL	PO 5–10 mL or 1–2 tablets q2–4h, between meals and at bedtime or as directed by physician
Mylanta Double strength	400 mg/tab, 400 mg/5 mL	400 mg/tab, 400 mg/5 mL		Simethicone 30 mg/tab, 30 mg/5 mL	Same as Mylanta
Titralac			420 mg/tab, 1 g/5 mL	Glycine 180 mg/tab, 300 mg/5 mL	PO 1 tsp or 2 tablets, after meals or as directed by physician, to maximal dose of 19 tablets or 8 tsp/24 h

PO, oral.

of aluminum-based antacids over a long period, hypophosphatemia and osteomalacia may develop because aluminum combines with phosphates in the GI tract and prevents phosphate absorption. Aluminum compounds are rarely used alone for acid-peptic disorders. *Magnesium-based antacids* have a high neutralizing capacity and a rapid onset of action. They may cause diarrhea and hypermagnesemia. *Calcium compounds* have a rapid onset of action but may cause hypersecretion of gastric acid ("acid rebound") and the "milk-alkali syndrome," which includes alkalosis and azotemia. Consequently, calcium compounds are rarely used in peptic ulcer disease.

Commonly used antacids are mixtures of aluminum hydroxide and magnesium hydroxide (eg, Gelusil, Mylanta, Maalox). Some antacid mixtures contain other ingredients, such as simethicone or alginic acid. Simethicone is an antiflatulent drug available alone as Mylicon. When added to antacids, simethicone does not affect gastric acidity. It reportedly decreases gas bubbles, thereby reducing GI distention and abdominal discomfort. Alginic acid (eg, in Gaviscon) produces a foamy, viscous layer on top of gas-

tric acid and thereby decreases backflow of gastric acid onto esophageal mucosa.

Antacids act primarily in the stomach and are used to prevent or treat peptic ulcer disease, GERD, esophagitis, heartburn, gastritis, GI bleeding, and stress ulcers. Aluminum-based antacids also are given to clients with chronic renal failure and hyperphosphatemia to decrease absorption of phosphates in food.

Magnesium-based antacids are contraindicated in clients with renal failure.

Helicobacter pylori Agents

Multiple drugs are required to eradicate *H. pylori* organisms and heal related ulcers. Effective combinations include two antimicrobials and a PPI or an H₂RA. For the antimicrobial component, two of the following drugs—**amoxicillin**, **clarithromycin**, **metronidazole**, and **tetracycline**—are used. A single antimicrobial agent is not used because of concern about emergence of

TABLE 60-2	Antiulcer Drugs	
Generic/Trade Name	**Indications for Use**	**Routes and Dosage Ranges (Adults)**
Histamine-2 Receptor Antagonists	Treatment of gastric ulcer, duodenal ulcer, and erosive esophagitis, to promote healing, then maintenance to prevent recurrence Prevention of stress ulcers and GI bleeding; prevention of aspiration pneumonitis Treatment of Zollinger-Ellison syndrome Treatment of heartburn (over-the-counter only)	
Cimetidine (Tagamet)		PO 800 mg once daily at bedtime or 300 mg four times per day *Prophylaxis of recurrent ulcer*, PO 400 mg at bedtime *IV injection*, 300 mg, diluted in 20 mL of 5% dextrose or saline solution and infused over at least 2 min, q6–8h *IV intermittent infusion*, 300 mg diluted in at least 50 mL of dextrose or saline solution and infused over 15–20 min, q6h *IM* 300 q6–8h (undiluted) *GERD*, PO 1600 mg daily in divided doses (800 mg twice daily or 400 mg four times daily) Prevention of upper GI bleeding, IV continuous infusion, 50 mg/h *Impaired renal function*, PO, IV 300 mg q8–12h
Famotidine (Pepcid)		*Acute duodenal ulcer*, PO 40 mg once daily at bedtime or 20 mg twice daily for 4–8 wk; maintenance therapy, PO 20 mg once daily at bedtime *Zollinger-Ellison syndrome*, PO 20 mg q6h, increased if necessary *IV injection*, 20 mg q12h, diluted to 5 or 10 mL with 5% dextrose or 0.9% sodium chloride, and injected over at least 2 min *IV infusion*, 20 mg q12h, diluted with 100 mL of 5% dextrose or 0.9% sodium chloride, and infused over 15–30 min *Impaired renal function* (creatinine clearance <10 mL/min), PO, IV 20 mg q24–48h
Nizatidine (Axid)		*Acute duodenal ulcer*, PO 300 mg once daily at bedtime; maintenance therapy, PO 150 mg once daily at bedtime *Impaired renal function* (creatinine clearance 20–50 mL/min), PO 150 mg daily; (creatinine clearance <20 mL/min), PO 150 mg q48h
Ranitidine (Zantac)		PO 300 mg once daily at bedtime or 150 mg twice daily *IM* 50 mg q6–8h (undiluted) *IV injection*, 50 mg diluted in 20 mL of 5% dextrose or 0.9% sodium chloride solution and injected over at least 5 min q6–8h *IV intermittent infusion*, 50 mg diluted in 100 mL of 5% dextrose or 0.9% sodium chloride solution and infused over 15–20 min *Impaired renal function* (creatinine clearance <50 mL/min), PO 150 mg q24h; IV, IM 50 mg q18–24h
Proton Pump Inhibitors	Treatment of gastric and duodenal ulcers, for 4–8 wk Treatment of GERD for 4–8 wk to promote healing, then maintenance to prevent recurrence Treatment of Zollinger-Ellison syndrome	
Lansoprazole (Prevacid)		*Duodenal ulcer*, PO 15 mg daily for healing and maintenance *Gastric ulcer*, PO 30 mg once daily for approximately 8 wk

(continued)

TABLE 60-2　**Antiulcer Drugs** (*continued*)

Generic/Trade Name	Indications for Use	Routes and Dosage Ranges (Adults)
Omeprazole (Prilosec)		*Erosive esophagitis*, PO 30 mg daily for 8 wk; 15 mg daily for maintenance of healing *Helicobacter pylori infection*, PO 30 mg (with clarithromycin and amoxicillin) twice daily for 14 d *Hypersecretory conditions*, PO 60–90 mg daily, increased if necessary *Gastric ulcer*, PO 40 mg once daily for 4–8 wk *Duodenal ulcer*, PO 20 mg once daily for 4–8 wk *GERD*, PO 20 mg once daily *Zollinger-Ellison syndrome*, PO 60 mg once daily initially, increased if necessary
Pantoprazole (Protonix) **Rabeprazole** (Aciphex)		*GERD*, PO 40 mg once daily for 8 wk *Duodenal ulcer*, PO 20 mg once daily for 4 wk *GERD*, PO 20 mg once daily for healing and maintenance *Hypersecretory conditions*, PO 60 mg once daily initially, increased up to 60 mg twice daily if necessary
Misoprostol (Cytotec)	Prevention of aspirin and NSAID-induced gastric ulcers in selected clients	PO 100–200 mg four times daily with meals and at bedtime
Sucralfate (Carafate)	Treatment of active duodenal ulcer to promote healing, then maintenance to prevent recurrence	*Treatment of active ulcer*, PO 1 g four times daily before meals and at bedtime *Maintenance therapy*, PO 1 g two times daily
H. pylori Agents ANTIMICROBIALS **Amoxicillin** **Clarithromycin** **Metronidazole** **Tetracycline**	*H. pylori* infection causing gastric or duodenal ulcers	 PO 500 mg four times daily PO 500 mg two to three times daily PO 250 mg four times daily PO 500 mg four times daily
BISMUTH SUBSALICYLATE	*H. pylori* eradication and GI upset (abdominal cramping, indigestion, nausea, diarrhea)	*Adults:* PO 525 mg (2 tabs or 30 mL) four times daily *Children:* 9–12 y, PO 1 tab or 15 mL; 6–9 y, PO ⅔ tab or 10 mL; 3–6 y, PO ⅓ tab or 5 mL; <3 y, consult physician. Dosage may be repeated every 30–60 min, if needed, up to eight doses in 24 h.
COMBINATION REGIMENS **Bismuth subsalicylate, metronidazole, and tetracycline** (Helidac)		PO Bismuth 525 mg (2 tabs), metronidazole 250 mg (1 tab), tetracycline 500 mg (1 capsule) four times daily for 14 d
Amoxicillin, clarithromycin, and lansoprazole (Prevpac)		PO amoxicillin 1 g, clarithromycin 500 mg, lansoprazole 30 mg twice daily, morning and evening, for 14 d
Ranitidine and bismuth citrate (Tritec)		PO 400 mg twice daily for 4 wk, with clarithromycin 500 mg three times daily for the first 2 wk

GERD, gastroesophageal reflux disease, including erosive esophagitis; GI, gastrointestinal; IM, intramuscular; IV, intravenous; NSAID, nonsteroidal anti-inflammatory drug; PO, oral.

drug-resistant *H. pylori* organisms. For clients with an active ulcer, adding an antisecretory drug to an antimicrobial regimen accelerates symptom relief and ulcer healing. In addition, antimicrobial–antisecretory combinations are associated with low ulcer recurrence rates.

A bismuth preparation is added to some regimens. Bismuth exerts antibacterial effects against *H. pylori* by disrupting bacterial cell walls, preventing the organism from adhering to gastric epithelium, and inhibiting bacterial enzymatic and proteolytic activity. It also increases secretion of mucus and bicarbonate, inhibits pepsin activity, and accumulates in ulcer craters.

Because client compliance is a difficulty with all the *H. pylori* eradication regimens, some drug combinations are packaged as individual doses to increase convenience. For example, Helidac contains bismuth, metronidazole, and tetracycline (taken with an H$_2$RA); Prevpac contains amoxicillin, clarithromycin, and lansoprazole.

Nursing Notes: Apply Your Knowledge

Famotidine (Pepcid) 20 mg, IVPB, bid is ordered. The pharmacy sends up 20 mg of Pepcid diluted in a 100-mL bag of normal saline. Your tubing has a drip factor of 10 drops/mL. Calculate the IV drip rate in drops per minute.

Histamine-2 Receptor Antagonists

Histamine is a substance found in almost every body tissue and released in response to certain stimuli (eg, allergic reactions, tissue injury). Once released, histamine causes contraction of smooth muscle in the bronchi, GI tract, and uterus; dilation and increased permeability of capillaries; dilation of cerebral blood vessels; and stimulation of sensory nerve endings to produce pain and itching.

Histamine also causes strong stimulation of gastric acid secretion. Vagal stimulation causes release of histamine from cells in the gastric mucosa. The histamine then acts on receptors located on the parietal cells to increase production of hydrochloric acid. These receptors are called the H_2 receptors.

Traditional antihistamines or H_1 receptor antagonists prevent or reduce other effects of histamine but do not block histamine effects on gastric acid production. The H_2RAs inhibit secretion of gastric acid stimulated by histamine, acetylcholine, and gastrin. They decrease the amount, acidity, and pepsin content of gastric juices.

Clinical indications for use include prevention and treatment of peptic ulcer disease, esophagitis resulting from gastroesophageal reflux of gastric acid, GI bleeding due to acute stress ulcers, and Zollinger-Ellison syndrome. When used therapeutically for gastric or duodenal ulcers, H_2RAs promote healing within 6 to 8 weeks. Over-the-counter oral preparations are approved for the treatment of heartburn.

There are no known contraindications, but the drugs should be used with caution in children, pregnant women, older adults, and clients with impaired renal or hepatic function. Dosage should be reduced in the presence of impaired renal function.

Adverse effects occur infrequently with usual doses and duration of treatment. They are more likely to occur with prolonged use of high doses and in older adults or those with impaired renal or hepatic function.

Cimetidine, **ranitidine**, **famotidine**, and **nizatidine** are the four available H_2RAs. Cimetidine was the first, and it is still widely used. It is well absorbed after oral administration. After a single dose, peak blood level is reached in 1 to 1.5 hours, and an effective concentration is maintained approximately 4 hours. The drug is distributed in almost all body tissues. Cimetidine should be used with caution during pregnancy because it crosses the placenta, and it should not be taken during lactation because it is excreted in breast milk. Most of an oral dose is excreted unchanged in the urine within 24 hours; some is excreted in bile and eliminated in feces. For acutely ill clients, cimetidine is given intravenously. A major disadvantage of cimetidine is that it inhibits the hepatic metabolism of numerous other drugs, thereby increasing blood levels and risks of toxicity with the inhibited drug.

Ranitidine is more potent than cimetidine, and smaller doses can be given less frequently. In addition, ranitidine causes fewer drug interactions than cimetidine. Oral ranitidine reaches peak blood levels 1 to 3 hours after administration, and is metabolized in the liver; approximately 30% is excreted unchanged in the urine. Parenteral ranitidine reaches peak blood levels in approximately 15 minutes; approximately 65% to 80% is excreted unchanged in the urine. Famotidine and nizatidine are pharmacologically similar to cimetidine and ranitidine. They are more potent on a weight basis. The drugs cause similar adverse effects but are less likely to cause mental confusion and gynecomastia (antiandrogenic effects) than cimetidine. In addition, they do not affect the cytochrome P450 drug-metabolizing system in the liver and therefore do not interfere with the metabolism of other drugs, as does cimetidine.

Proton Pump Inhibitors

Proton pump inhibitors are strong inhibitors of gastric acid secretion. These drugs bind irreversibly to the gastric proton pump (ie, H^+,K^+-ATPase) to prevent the "pumping" or release of gastric acid into the stomach lumen and therefore block the final step of acid production. Inhibition of the proton pump suppresses gastric acid secretion in response to all primary stimuli, histamine, gastrin, and acetylcholine. Thus, the drugs inhibit both daytime (including meal-stimulated) and nocturnal (unstimulated) acid secretion.

Indications for use include treatment of peptic ulcer disease, erosive gastritis, GERD, and Zollinger-Ellison syndrome. PPIs are first-line agents for treatment of duodenal and gastric ulcers, including those that did not heal with H_2RA therapy. Compared with H_2RAs, PPIs suppress gastric acid more strongly and for a longer time, effects that are associated with faster symptom relief and healing in acid-related diseases. H_2RAs inhibit nocturnal acid secretion but have little effect on meal-stimulated acid production and thus on daytime acidity.

In peptic ulcer disease, PPIs and H_2RAs are similarly effective in maintenance therapy, with similar rates of ulcer recurrence. In clients with *H. pylori*-associated ulcers, eradication of the organism with antimicrobial drugs is preferable to long-term maintenance therapy with antisecretory drugs. In GERD, PPIs are reportedly more effective than H_2RAs in relieving symptoms, healing esophagitis, and maintaining esophageal healing. PPIs are the treatment of choice for Zollinger-Ellison syndrome.

The drugs usually are well tolerated. Nausea, diarrhea, and headache are the most frequently reported adverse effects. However, long-term consequences of profound gastric acid suppression are unknown.

Omeprazole, **lansoprazole**, **pantoprazole**, and **rabeprazole** are available PPIs. Omeprazole was the first and is still widely used. It is well absorbed after oral administration, highly bound to plasma proteins (approximately 95%), metabolized in the liver, and excreted in the urine (approximately 75%) and bile or feces. Acid-inhibiting effects occur within 2 hours and last 72 hours or longer. When the drug is discontinued, effects persist for 3 to 5 days, until the gastric parietal cells can synthesize additional H+,K+-ATPase. The other drugs are very similar to omeprazole.

Prostaglandin

Naturally occurring prostaglandin E, which is produced in mucosal cells of the stomach and duodenum, inhibits gastric acid secretion and increases mucus and bicarbonate secretion, mucosal blood flow, and perhaps mucosal repair. When synthesis of prostaglandin E is inhibited, erosion and ulceration of gastric mucosa may occur. This is the mechanism by which aspirin and other NSAIDs are thought to cause gastric and duodenal ulcers (see Chap. 7).

Misoprostol is a synthetic form of prostaglandin E approved for concurrent use with NSAIDs to protect gastric mucosa from NSAID-induced erosion and ulceration. It is indicated for clients at high risk of GI ulceration and bleeding, such as those taking high doses of NSAIDs for arthritis and older adults. It is contraindicated in women of childbearing potential, unless effective contraceptive methods are being used, and during pregnancy, because it may induce abortion. The most common adverse effects are diarrhea (occurs in 10% to 40% of recipients) and abdominal cramping. Older adults may be unable to tolerate misoprostol-induced diarrhea and abdominal discomfort.

Sucralfate

Sucralfate is a preparation of sulfated sucrose and aluminum hydroxide that binds to normal and ulcerated mucosa. It is used to prevent and treat peptic ulcer disease. When an ulcer is present, the drug combines with ulcer exudate, adheres to the ulcer site, and forms a protective barrier between the mucosa and gastric acid, pepsin, and bile salts. Sucralfate requires an acid pH for activation and should not be given with an antacid, H$_2$RA, or PPI.

Sucralfate is effective in healing duodenal ulcers and in maintenance therapy to prevent ulcer recurrence. Because sucralfate is not absorbed systemically, the incidence and severity of adverse effects are low; constipation and dry mouth are most often reported. However, the drug may bind other drugs and prevent their absorption. As a general rule, sucralfate should be given approximately 2 hours before or after other drugs.

> **How Can You Avoid This Medication Error?**
>
> Sucralfate (Carafate), 1 g PO, ac and hs is ordered for a patient with active peptic ulcer disease. The unit secretary transcribes the administration times as 0900, 1300, 1800, and 2200. You administer the morning dose at 0845.

NURSING PROCESS

Assessment

Assess the client's status in relation to peptic ulcer disease, GERD, and other conditions in which anti-ulcer drugs are used.

- Identify risk factors for peptic ulcer disease:
  - Cigarette smoking. Effects are thought to include stimulation of gastric acid secretion and decreased blood supply to gastric mucosa. Moreover, clients with peptic ulcers who continue to smoke heal more slowly and have more recurrent ulcers, despite usually adequate treatment, than those who stop smoking.
  - Stress, including physiologic stress (eg, shock, sepsis, burns, surgery, head injury, severe trauma, or medical illness) and psychological stress. One mechanism may be that stress activates the sympathetic nervous system, which then causes vasoconstriction in organs not needed for "fight or flight." Thus, stress may lead to ischemia in gastric mucosa, with ulceration if ischemia is severe or prolonged.
  - Genetic influences. Clients with blood type O are more likely to have duodenal ulcers; those with blood type A are more likely to have gastric ulcers. Also, close relatives of clients with peptic ulcer disease have an increased risk for development of ulcers.
  - Male sex. Men have a higher incidence of duodenal and gastric ulcers than women.
  - Drug therapy with aspirin and other NSAIDs, corticosteroids, and antineoplastics.
- Signs and symptoms depend on the type and location of the ulcer:
  - Periodic epigastric pain, which occurs 1 to 4 hours after eating or during the night and is often described as burning or gnawing, is a characteristic symptom of chronic duodenal ulcer.
  - Gastrointestinal bleeding occurs with acute or chronic ulcers when the ulcer erodes into a blood vessel. Clinical manifestations may range from mild (eg, occult blood in feces and eventual anemia) to severe (eg, hematemesis, melena, hypotension, and shock).

- Gastroesophageal reflux disease produces heartburn (a substernal burning sensation), which is caused by the backward flow of gastric acid onto esophageal mucosa.

Nursing Diagnoses

- Pain related to effects of gastric acid on peptic ulcers or inflamed esophageal tissues
- Ineffective Individual Coping related to acute and chronic manifestations of peptic ulcer disease or GERD
- Risk for Injury: GI bleeding, ulcer perforation, bowel obstruction
- Altered Nutrition: Less Than Body Requirements related to anorexia and abdominal discomfort
- Constipation related to aluminum- or calcium-containing antacids and sucralfate
- Diarrhea related to magnesium-containing antacids and misoprostol
- Risk for Injury: Adverse drug effects
- Knowledge Deficit related to disease processes
- Knowledge Deficit related to drug therapy for GERD and peptic ulcer disease

Planning/Goals

The client will:

- Take or receive antiulcer drugs accurately
- Experience relief of symptoms
- Avoid situations that cause or exacerbate symptoms, when possible
- Be observed for GI bleeding and other complications of peptic ulcer disease and GERD
- Maintain normal patterns of bowel function
- Avoid preventable adverse effects of drug therapy

Interventions

Use measures to prevent or minimize peptic ulcer disease and gastric acid–induced esophageal disorders.

- With peptic ulcer disease, helpful interventions may include the following:
  - General health measures such as a well-balanced diet, adequate rest, and regular exercise
  - Avoiding cigarette smoking and gastric irritants (eg, alcohol, aspirin and NSAIDs, caffeine)
  - Reducing psychological stress (eg, by changing environments) or learning healthful methods of handling it (eg, relaxation techniques, physical exercise). There is no practical way to avoid psychological stress, because it is part of everyday life.
  - Long-term drug therapy with small doses of H$_2$RAs, antacids, or sucralfate. With "active" peptic ulcer disease, helping the client follow the prescribed therapeutic regimen

helps to promote healing and prevent serious complications (ie, hemorrhage, perforation, obstruction).

  - Diet therapy is of minor importance in prevention or treatment of peptic ulcer disease. Some physicians prescribe no dietary restrictions, whereas others suggest avoiding or minimizing highly spiced foods, gas-forming foods, and caffeine-containing beverages.
- With heartburn and esophagitis, helpful measures are those that prevent or decrease gastroesophageal reflux of gastric contents (eg, elevating the head of the bed, avoiding gastric distention by eating small meals, not lying down for 1 to 2 hours after eating, and avoiding obesity, constipation, or other conditions that increase intra-abdominal pressure).

Evaluation

- Observe and interview regarding drug use.
- Observe and interview regarding relief of symptoms.
- Observe for signs and symptoms of complications.
- Observe and interview regarding adverse drug effects.

PRINCIPLES OF THERAPY

Drug Selection

All of the antiulcer drugs are effective for indicated uses; the choice of drugs may depend on etiology, acuity, severity of symptoms, cost, and convenience. General guidelines include the following:

- *Proton pump inhibitors* may be drugs of first choice in most situations. They may heal peptic ulcers more rapidly and be more effective in erosive gastritis and Zollinger-Ellison syndrome than H$_2$RAs. However, most are given orally only. If the drug must be injected for a client who is unable to take an oral medication, an H$_2$RA must be used. PPIs are more expensive than H$_2$RAs.
- *H. pylori* infection should be considered in most cases of peptic ulcer disease. If confirmed by appropriate diagnostic tests, agents to eradicate the organisms should be drugs of first choice.
- *H$_2$RAs* are widely used. Cimetidine may be less expensive but it may cause confusion and antiandrogenic effects. It also increases the risks of toxicity with several commonly used drugs. Compared with cimetidine, other H$_2$RAs are more potent on a weight basis and have a longer duration of action, so they can be given in smaller, less frequent doses. In addition, they do not alter the hepatic metabolism of other drugs.

CLIENT TEACHING GUIDELINES
Antiulcer Drugs

General Considerations

✔ Antiulcer drugs are commonly used to prevent and treat peptic ulcers and heartburn. Peptic ulcers usually form in the stomach or first part of the small bowel (duodenum), where tissues are exposed to stomach acid. Two common causes of peptic ulcer disease are stomach infection with a bacterium called *Helicobacter pylori* and taking nonsteroidal anti-inflammatory drugs (NSAIDs) such as ibuprofen and many others. Heartburn (also called gastroesophageal reflux disease) is caused by stomach acid splashing back onto the esophagus.

Peptic ulcer disease and heartburn are chronic conditions that are usually managed on an outpatient basis. Complications such as bleeding require hospitalization. Overall, these conditions can range from mild to serious, and it is important to seek information about the disease process, ways to prevent or minimize symptoms, and drug therapy.

✔ With heartburn, try to minimize acid reflux by elevating the head of the bed; avoiding stomach distention by eating small meals; not lying down for 1 to 2 hours after eating; avoiding or minimizing intake of coffee and alcohol; avoiding smoking (stimulates gastric acid production); and avoiding obesity, constipation, or other conditions that increase intra-abdominal pressure.

✔ Most medications for peptic ulcer disease and heartburn act to decrease stomach acid. An exception is the antibiotics used to treat ulcers caused by *H. pylori* infection. The strongest acid reducers are omeprazole (Prilosec), lansoprazole (Prevacid), pantoprazole (Protonix), and rabeprazole (Aciphex). These are prescription drugs. Histamine-blocking drugs such as cimetidine (Tagamet), famotidine (Pepcid), and others are available as both prescription and over-the-counter (OTC) preparations. OTC products are indicated for heartburn, and smaller doses are taken than for peptic ulcer disease. These drugs usually should not be taken longer than 2 weeks without the advice and supervision of a physician. The concern is that OTC drugs may delay diagnosis and treatment of potentially serious illness. In addition, cimetidine can increase toxic effects of numerous drugs and should be avoided if you are taking other medications.

Misoprostol (Cytotec) is given to prevent ulcers from NSAIDs, which are commonly used to relieve pain and inflammation with arthritis and other conditions. This drug should be taken only while taking a traditional NSAID such as ibuprofen. Newer, related drugs such as celecoxib (Celebrex) and rofecoxib (Vioxx) are less likely to cause peptic ulcer disease. Do not take misoprostol if pregnant and do not become pregnant while taking the drug. If pregnancy occurs during misoprostol therapy, stop the drug and notify your physician immediately. Misoprostol can cause miscarriage.

Numerous antacid preparations are available, but they are not equally safe in all people and should be selected carefully. For example, products that contain magnesium have a laxative effect and may cause diarrhea; those that contain aluminum or calcium may cause constipation. Some commonly used antacids (eg, Maalox, Mylanta) are a mixture of magnesium and aluminum preparations, an attempt to avoid both constipation and diarrhea. People with kidney disease should not take products that contain magnesium because magnesium can accumulate in the body and cause serious adverse effects. Thus, it is important to read product labels and, if you have a chronic illness or take other medications, ask your physician or pharmacist to help you select an antacid and an appropriate dose.

Self- or Caregiver Administration

✔ Take antiulcer drugs as directed. Underuse decreases therapeutic effectiveness; overuse increases adverse effects. For acute peptic ulcer disease or esophagitis, drugs are given in relatively high doses for 4 to 8 weeks to promote healing. For long-term maintenance therapy, dosage is usually reduced.

✔ With Prilosec, swallow the capsule whole; do not open, chew, or crush (to prevent destruction of the drug by stomach acid). With Prevacid, the capsule can be opened and the granules sprinkled on applesauce or other soft food for patients who are unable to swallow capsules. The granules should not be crushed or chewed.

✔ Take cimetidine with meals or at bedtime. Take famotidine, nizatidine, ranitidine, and ranitidine bismuth citrate (Tritec) with or without food. Do not take an antacid for approximately 1 hour before or after taking one of these drugs.

✔ Take sucralfate on an empty stomach at least 1 hour before meals and at bedtime. Also, do not take an antacid for approximately 1 hour before or after taking sucralfate.

✔ Take misoprostol with food.

✔ For treatment of peptic ulcer disease, take antacids 1 and 3 hours after meals and at bedtime (seven doses daily), 1 to 2 hours before or after other medications. Antacids decrease absorption of many medications if taken at the same time. Also, chew chewable tablets thoroughly before swallowing, then drink a glass of water; allow effervescent tablets to dissolve completely and almost stop bubbling before drinking; and shake liquids well before measuring the dose.

Over-the-counter H₂RAs are indicated for the treatment of heartburn. In some cases, clients may depend on self-medication with over-the-counter drugs and delay seeking treatment for peptic ulcer disease or GERD. For prescription or nonprescription uses, cimetidine should probably be taken only by clients who are taking no other medications.

- *Antacids* are often used as needed to relieve heartburn and abdominal discomfort. If used to treat peptic ulcer disease, they are more often used with other agents than alone and require a regular dosing schedule. The choice of antacid depends on characteristics of clients and drug preparations and should be individualized to find a preparation that is acceptable to the client in terms of taste, dosage, and convenience of administration. Some guidelines include the following:
  1. **Neutralizing capacity**. Use of an agent with high in vitro neutralizing capacity is probably better. However, the clinical or in vivo capacity may be different, depending on the amount of gastric acid and rate of gastric emptying. In a fasting state, for example, the antacid leaves the stomach in approximately 30 minutes and thereafter becomes ineffective. After a meal, acid-neutralizing effects last 3 hours or longer.
  2. **Side effects**. Calcium carbonate has a high neutralizing capacity, but doses large and frequent enough to maintain neutralization of gastric acid may cause hypercalcemia and impaired renal function owing to systemic absorption. Magnesium hydroxide has a higher buffering capacity than magnesium hydroxide–aluminum hydroxide mixtures, but it may cause diarrhea and hypermagnesemia. Aluminum hydroxide has the least buffering capacity and may cause constipation.
  3. **Rapid action**. Magnesium hydroxide, magnesium oxide, and calcium carbonate act rapidly. Effervescent antacids have a rapid onset but short duration of action because they leave the stomach quickly.
  4. **Dosage form**. Liquid suspensions usually act faster than chewable tablets, but they may not be more effective in neutralizing gastric acid. Chewable tablets may be more convenient.
  5. **Ingredients**. Combination products are commonly used. For example, combining aluminum hydroxide and magnesium oxide or hydroxide minimizes constipation and diarrhea; combining fast-acting and slow-acting antacids can prolong gastric acid neutralization.

    Antacids with magnesium are contraindicated in renal disease because hypermagnesemia may result; those with high sugar content are contraindicated in diabetes mellitus.

    Simethicone, which is added to several antacid mixtures, has no effect on intragastric pH but may be useful in relieving flatulence or gastroesophageal reflux. Alginic acid (eg, in Gaviscon and other products) creates a foam that helps keep gastric acid from reaching esophageal mucosa.

- *Sucralfate* must be taken before meals, and this is inconvenient for some clients.

Guidelines for Therapy With Proton Pump Inhibitors

1. Recommended doses of PPIs heal most gastric and duodenal ulcers in approximately 4 weeks. Large gastric ulcers may require 8 weeks.
2. The drugs may be used to maintain gastroduodenal ulcer healing and decrease risks of ulcer recurrence.
3. A PPI and two antimicrobial drugs is one of the most effective regimens for eradication of *H. pylori* organisms.
4. With GERD, higher doses or longer therapy may be needed for severe disease and esophagitis. Lower doses can maintain symptom relief and esophageal healing.

Guidelines for Therapy With Histamine-2 Receptor Antagonists

1. For an acute ulcer, full dosage may be given for up to 8 weeks. When the ulcer heals, the drug may be reduced in dosage for maintenance therapy to prevent recurrence. These drugs are effective and convenient in a single daily dose taken at bedtime to suppress nocturnal secretion of gastric acid. Dosage of all these drugs should be reduced in the presence of impaired renal function.
2. Antacids are often given concurrently with H₂RAs to relieve pain. They should not be given at the same time because the antacid reduces absorption of the other drug. H₂RAs relieve pain after approximately 1 week of administration.

Guidelines for Therapy With Sucralfate

1. When sucralfate is used to treat an ulcer, it should be administered for 4 to 8 weeks unless healing is confirmed by radiologic or endoscopic examination.
2. When used over the long term to prevent ulcer recurrence, dosage should be reduced.

Guidelines for Therapy With Antacids

1. Antacid dosage, including frequency of administration, depends primarily on the purpose for use, buffering capacity of the antacid, and client response.

2. To prevent stress ulcers in critically ill clients and to treat acute GI bleeding, nearly continuous neutralization of gastric acid is desirable. Dose and frequency of administration must be sufficient to neutralize approximately 50 to 80 mEq of gastric acid each hour. This can be accomplished by a continuous intragastric drip through a nasogastric tube or by hourly administration.
3. When a client has a nasogastric tube in place, antacid dosage may be titrated by aspirating stomach contents, determining pH with Nitrazine paper, and then basing the dose on the pH. (Most gastric acid is neutralized and most pepsin activity is eliminated at a pH above 3.5.)
4. When antacids are used to treat active ulcers, taking them 1 hour and 3 hours after meals and at bedtime is effective and rational.
5. When antacids are used to relieve pain, they usually may be taken as needed. However, they should not be taken in high doses or for prolonged periods because of potential adverse effects.

Effects of Antiulcer Drugs on Other Drugs

Antacids may prevent absorption of most drugs taken at the same time, including benzodiazepine antianxiety drugs, corticosteroids, digoxin, H$_2$RAs (eg, cimetidine), iron supplements, phenothiazine antipsychotic drugs, phenytoin, fluoroquinolone antibacterials, and tetracyclines. Antacids increase absorption of a few drugs, including levodopa, quinidine, and valproic acid. These interactions can be avoided or minimized by separating administration times by 1 to 2 hours.

H$_2$RAs may alter the effects of several drugs. Most significant effects occur with cimetidine, which interferes with the metabolism of several commonly used drugs. Consequently, the affected drugs are eliminated more slowly, their serum levels are increased, and they are more likely to cause adverse effects and toxicity unless dosage is reduced.

Interacting drugs include antiarrhythmics (lidocaine, propafenone, quinidine), the anticoagulant warfarin, anticonvulsants (carbamazepine, phenytoin), benzodiazepine antianxiety or hypnotic agents (alprazolam, diazepam, flurazepam, triazolam), beta-adrenergic blocking agents (labetalol, metoprolol, propranolol), the bronchodilator theophylline, calcium channel blocking agents (eg, verapamil), tricyclic antidepressants (eg, amitriptyline), and sulfonylurea antidiabetic drugs. In addition, cimetidine may increase serum levels (eg, fluorouracil, procainamide and its active metabolite) and pharmacologic effects of other drugs (eg, flecainide, respiratory depression with narcotic analgesics or succinylcholine) by unidentified mechanisms. Cimetidine also may decrease effects of several drugs, including drugs that require an acidic environment for absorption (eg, iron salts, indomethacin, fluconazole,

ketoconazole, tetracyclines) and miscellaneous drugs (eg, digoxin, tocainide) by unknown mechanisms.

Ranitidine, famotidine, and nizatidine do not inhibit the cytochrome P450 metabolizing enzymes. Ranitidine decreases absorption of diazepam if given at the same time and increases hypoglycemic effects of glipizide. Nizatidine increases serum salicylate levels in people taking high doses of aspirin.

PPIs have relatively few effects on other drugs. Omeprazole increases blood levels of diazepam, phenytoin, and warfarin, probably by inhibiting hepatic metabolism. These interactions have not been reported with lansoprazole.

Sucralfate decreases absorption of ciprofloxacin and other fluoroquinolones, digoxin, ketoconazole, phenytoin, and warfarin. Sucralfate binds to these drugs when both are present in the GI tract. This interaction can be avoided or minimized by giving the interacting drug 2 hours before sucralfate.

Effects of Antiulcer Drugs on Nutrients

Dietary folate, iron, and vitamin B$_{12}$ are better absorbed from an acidic environment. When gastric fluids are made less acidic by antacids, H$_2$RAs, or PPIs, deficiencies of these nutrients may occur. In addition, sucralfate interferes with absorption of fat-soluble vitamins, and magnesium-containing antacids interfere with absorption of vitamin A.

Use in Children

Antacids may be given to ambulatory children in doses of 5 to 15 mL every 3 to 6 hours or at 1 and 3 hours after meals and at bedtime, as for adults with acute peptic ulcer disease. For prevention of GI bleeding in critically ill children, 2 to 5 mL may be given to infants and 5 to 15 mL to children every 1 to 2 hours. Safety and effectiveness of other antiulcer drugs have not been established for children.

Although PPIs are not approved by the Food and Drug Administration for use in children and are not available in pediatric dosage formulations, they are widely used in the treatment of peptic ulcer and gastroesophageal disease. They are also used to eradicate *H. pylori* organisms, usually with 1 to 2 weeks of omeprazole or lansoprazole. Most published reports involve adult doses for children older than 3 years of age, such as 20 mg for those younger than 10 years and 30 or 40 mg in older, larger children. Some clinicians titrate dosage by client weight, such as an initial dose of 0.7 mg/kg/day.

Use in Older Adults

All of the antiulcer drugs may be used in older adults. With antacids, smaller doses may be effective because older adults usually secrete less gastric acid than younger adults.

Further, with decreased renal function, older adults are more likely to have adverse effects, such as neuromuscular effects with magnesium-containing antacids. The use of sodium-containing antacids in older adults with cardiovascular disorders has been a concern because of potential edema, hypertension, and heart failure. However, most of these have been reformulated to contain little sodium. Many physicians recommend calcium carbonate antacids (eg, Tums) as a calcium supplement to prevent osteoporosis in older women.

With H$_2$RAs, older adults are more likely to experience adverse effects, especially confusion, agitation, and disorientation with cimetidine. In addition, older adults often have decreased renal function, and doses need to be reduced.

Older adults often take large doses of NSAIDs for arthritis and therefore are at risk for development of acute gastric ulcers and GI bleeding. Thus, they may be candidates for treatment with misoprostol. Dosage of misoprostol may need to be reduced to prevent severe diarrhea and abdominal cramping.

PPIs and sucralfate seem to be well tolerated by older adults. A PPI is probably the drug of choice for treating symptomatic GERD because evidence suggests that clients 60 years of age and older require stronger antisecretory effects than younger adults. No dosage adjustment is recommended with omeprazole or lansoprazole.

Use in Renal Impairment

A major concern with antacids is the use of magnesium-containing preparations (eg, Mylanta, Maalox). These are contraindicated in clients with impaired renal function (creatinine clearance <30 mL/minute) because approximately 5% to 10% of the magnesium may be absorbed and accumulate to cause hypermagnesemia. In addition, antacids with calcium carbonate can cause alkalosis and raise urine pH; chronic use may cause renal stones, hypercalcemia, and renal failure.

Antacids containing aluminum hydroxide (eg, Amphogel, Rolaids) are the antacids of choice in clients with chronic renal failure. Aluminum tends not to accumulate and it binds with phosphate in the GI tract to prevent phosphate absorption and hyperphosphatemia.

With **omeprazole** and **lansoprazole**, no special precautions or dosage reductions are required in clients with renal impairment.

All of the available **H$_2$RAs** are eliminated through the kidneys, and dosage needs to be substantially reduced in clients with renal impairment to avoid adverse effects. Adverse effects are uncommon unless renal function is compromised. Cimetidine may cause mental confusion in clients with renal impairment. It also blocks secretion of creatinine in renal tubules, thereby decreasing creatinine clearance and increasing serum creatinine level. With moderate to severe renal impairment, recommended dosages include cimetidine 300 mg every 12 hours, raniti-

dine 150 mg orally once daily or intravenously every 18 to 24 hours, and famotidine 20 mg at bedtime or every 36 to 48 hours if indicated. Dosage may be cautiously increased if necessary and if renal function is closely monitored. For clients on hemodialysis, an H$_2$RA should be given at the end of dialysis.

Use in Hepatic Impairment

Proton pump inhibitors are metabolized in the liver and may cause transient elevations in liver function tests. With omeprazole, bioavailability is increased because of decreased first-pass metabolism, and plasma half-life is increased. However, dosage adjustments are not recommended. With lansoprazole, dosage should be reduced in clients with severe liver impairment.

Histamine-2 receptor antagonists are partly metabolized in the liver and may be eliminated more slowly in clients with impaired liver function. A major concern with cimetidine is that it can reduce hepatic blood flow and inhibit hepatic metabolism of many other drugs.

Use in Critical Illness

Gastric acid suppressant drugs, including PPIs, H$_2$RAs, and sucralfate, are commonly used in critically ill clients. The **PPIs** are the strongest gastric acid suppressants available for clinical use and are usually well tolerated. The **H$_2$RAs** are used to prevent stress-induced gastric ulceration in adults and children. Except for renal impairment, in which dosage must be reduced, information about the pharmacokinetics of these drugs in critically ill clients is limited and only cimetidine and ranitidine have been studied. Compared with healthy people, critically ill clients had a longer half-life and lower clearance rate for H$_2$RAs.

The drugs are usually given by intermittent intravenous infusion. Because they can be given parenterally, the H$_2$RAs are the drugs of choice in clients who are unable to take oral medications. However, cimetidine should be avoided because critically ill clients often require numerous other drugs with which cimetidine may interact and alter effects.

 Home Care

All of the antiulcer drugs are commonly taken in the home setting, usually by self-administration. The home care nurse can assist clients by providing information about taking the drugs correctly and monitoring responses. If cimetidine is being taken, the home care nurse needs to assess for potential drug–drug interactions. With over-the-counter H$_2$RAs, clients should be instructed to avoid daily use for longer than 2 weeks. If use of antacids or over-the-counter H$_2$RAs seems to be excessive or prolonged, the client should be assessed for peptic ulcer disease or GERD.

(*text continues on page 902*)

NURSING ACTIONS   Antiulcer Drugs

NURSING ACTIONS	RATIONALE/EXPLANATION
1. Administer accurately	
a. Give oral cimetidine with meals or at bedtime. Famotidine, nizatidine, and ranitidine may be given without regard to food intake.	When cimetidine is taken with meals, peak serum drug level coincides with gastric emptying, when gastric acidity is usually highest. When taken at bedtime, cimetidine prevents secretion of gastric acid for several hours. Thus, correct timing of drug administration may promote faster healing of the ulcer.
b. To give cimetidine or ranitidine intravenously, dilute in 20 mL of 5% dextrose or normal saline solution, and inject over at least 2 min. For intermittent infusion, dilute in at least 50 mL of 5% dextrose or 0.9% sodium chloride solution, and infuse over 15–20 min.	
c. To give famotidine intravenously, dilute with 5–10 mL of 0.9% sodium chloride injection, and inject over at least 2 min. For intermittent infusion, dilute in 100 mL of 5% dextrose or 0.9% sodium chloride, and infuse over 15–30 min.	
d. Do not give antacids within approximately 1 h of oral H$_2$ antagonists or sucralfate.	Antacids decrease absorption and therapeutic effectiveness of the other drugs.
e. Shake liquid antacids well before measuring the dose.	These preparations are suspensions. Drug particles settle to the bottom of the container on standing and must be mixed thoroughly to give the correct dose.
f. Instruct clients to chew antacid tablets thoroughly.	To increase the surface area of drug available to neutralize gastric acid
g. Give sucralfate 1 h before meals and at bedtime.	To allow the drug to form its protective coating over the ulcer before high levels of gastric acidity. Sucralfate requires an acidic environment. After it has adhered to the ulcer, antacids and food do not affect drug action.
h. Give omeprazole and lansoprazole before food intake, with instructions to swallow the capsules whole (without crushing or chewing).	The drugs are formulated in an enteric-coated (to prevent destruction by gastric acid), extended-release preparation.
	For clients who are unable to swallow the lansoprazole capsule, the capsule may be opened and the granules mixed with applesauce, yogurt, or apple, orange, or cranberry juice. These acidic substances preserve the enteric coating of the granules, allowing them to remain intact until they reach the small intestine. The granules should not be chewed.
i. Give misoprostol with food.	
2. Observe for therapeutic effects	Therapeutic effects depend on the reason for use.
a. Decreased epigastric pain	Antacids should relieve ulcer pain within a few minutes. H$_2$ antagonists relieve pain in approximately 1 wk by healing effects on the ulcer.

(*continued*)

NURSING ACTIONS	RATIONALE/EXPLANATION
b. Decreased gastrointestinal (GI) bleeding (eg absence of visible or occult blood in vomitus, gastric secretions, or feces)	
c. Higher pH of gastric contents	The minimum acceptable pH with antacid therapy is 3.5. In acute situations the goal may be a pH of 7 (neutral).
d. Radiologic or endoscopic reports of ulcer healing	
3. Observe for adverse effects	
a. With H$_2$ antagonists, observe for diarrhea or constipation, headache, dizziness, muscle aches, fatigue, skin rashes, mental confusion, delirium, coma, depression, fever.	Adverse effects are uncommon and usually mild with recommended doses and duration of drug therapy (8 wk). Central nervous system effects have been associated with high doses in elderly clients or those with impaired renal function. With long-term administration of cimetidine, other adverse effects have been observed. These include decreased sperm count and gynecomastia in men and galactorrhea in women.
b. With antacids containing magnesium, observe for diarrhea and hypermagnesemia.	Diarrhea may be prevented by combining these antacids with other antacids containing aluminum or calcium. Hypermagnesemia is unlikely in most clients but may occur in those with impaired renal function. These antacids should not be given to clients with renal failure.
c. With antacids containing aluminum or calcium, observe for constipation.	Constipation may be prevented by combining these antacids with other antacids containing magnesium. A high-fiber diet and adequate fluid intake (2000–3000 mL daily) also help prevent constipation.
d. With sucralfate, observe for constipation.	Thus far, adverse effects observed with sucralfate have been few and minor. (The drug is not absorbed systemically.) The most common one was constipation (4.7% in 2500 people).
e. With misoprostol, observe for diarrhea, abdominal pain, nausea, and vomiting, headache, uterine cramping, vaginal bleeding.	Diarrhea is the most commonly reported and may be severe enough to indicate dosage reduction or stopping the drug.
f. With omeprazole, observe for headache, diarrhea, abdominal pain, nausea, and vomiting.	These effects occur infrequently and are usually well tolerated.
g. With bismuth, observe for black stools.	This is a harmless discoloration of the stool; it does not indicate GI bleeding.
4. Observe for drug interactions	Most significant drug interactions alter the effect of the other drug rather than that of the antiulcer drug. For example, cimetidine may potentiate anticoagulants; antacids alter the absorption of many oral drugs.
a. Drugs that *decrease* effects of cimetidine and ranitidine: (1) Antacids	Antacids decrease absorption of cimetidine and probably ranitidine. The drugs should not be given at the same time.

(continued)

NURSING ACTIONS	RATIONALE/EXPLANATION
b. Drugs that *increase* effects of antacids: (1) Anticholinergic drugs (eg, atropine)	May increase effects by delaying gastric emptying and by decreasing acid secretion themselves
c. Drugs that *decrease* effects of antacids: (1) Cholinergic drugs (eg, dexpanthenol [Ilopan])	May decrease effects by increasing GI motility and rate of gastric emptying
d. Drugs that *decrease* effects of sucralfate: (1) Antacids	Antacids should not be given within ½ hour before or after administration of sucralfate.
e. Drug that *increases* effects of omeprazole: (1) Clarithromycin	May increase blood levels of omeprazole
f. Drug that *decreases* effects of lansoprazole: (1) Sucralfate	Decreases absorption of lansoprazole. Lansoprazole should be given about 30 min before sucralfate if both are being used.

Nursing Notes: Apply Your Knowledge

Answer: 100 mL/20 min × 10 drops/mL

$$5 \times 10 = 50 \text{ drops/min}$$

How Can You Avoid This Medication Error?

Answer: Carafate was ordered to be administered ac, which means before meals. Carafate works to heal the ulcer by binding with the normal and ulcerated mucosa, forming a protective barrier between the mucosa and digestive acids. If the drug is given at 0845, it is likely the protective barrier will not coat the stomach mucosa before high levels of gastric acidity. Also, the drug could bind with food or drugs in the stomach at the time of administration. Carafate should be given 1 hour before meals and at bedtime.

REVIEW AND APPLICATION EXERCISES

1. What are risk factors for peptic ulcer disease?
2. How are ulcers thought to develop? What roles do gastric acid, pepsin, *H. pylori* organisms, prostaglandins, and mucus play in ulcer occurrence?
3. How do the various antiulcer drugs heal ulcers or prevent their recurrence?
4. Compare H₂RAs and PPIs in indications for use and effectiveness.
5. Compare and contrast cimetidine with other H_2 blockers.
6. What is the rationale for taking H_2 blockers at bedtime, sucralfate before meals, and antacids after meals?
7. Why are aluminum and magnesium salts often combined in antacid preparations?
8. For a client who smokes cigarettes and is newly diagnosed with peptic ulcer disease, how would you explain that smoking cessation aids ulcer healing?
9. Compare and contrast peptic ulcer disease and GERD in terms of risk factors, drug therapy, and client teaching needs.

SELECTED REFERENCES

American Society of Health-System Pharmacists. (1999). Guidelines on stress ulcer prophylaxis. *American Journal of Health-System Pharmacy*, *56*, 347–379.

Aronson, B. (1998). Update on peptic ulcer drugs. *American Journal of Nursing*, *98*(1), 41–46.

Battle, E.H. & Peura, D.A. (1999). New guidelines for the detection and treatment of *H pylori* infection. *Infections in Medicine*, *16*, 337–341. [Online: Available http:www.medscape.com. Accessed December 10, 1999.]

Berardi, R.R. (1997). Peptic ulcer disease and Zollinger-Ellison syndrome. In J.T. DiPiro, R.L. Talbert, G.C. Yee, G.R. Matzke, B.G. Wells, & L.M. Posey (Eds.), *Pharmacotherapy: A pathophysiologic approach*, 3rd ed., pp. 697–721. Stamford, CT: Appleton & Lange.

Berardi, R.R. & Welage, L.S. (1998). Proton-pump inhibitors in acid-related diseases. *American Journal of Health-System Pharmacy*, *55*, 2289–2298.

Brunton, L.L. (1996). Agents for control of gastric acidity and treatment of peptic ulcers. In J.G. Hardman, L.E. Limbird, P.B. Molinoff, & R.W. Ruddon (Eds.), *Goodman & Gilman's The pharmacological basis of therapeutics*, 9th ed., pp. 901–915. New York: McGraw-Hill.

Buck, M.L. (1999). Using proton pump inhibitors in children. *Pediatric Pharmacotherapy*, *5*, 504. [Online: Available http://www.

medscape.com/UVA/PedPharm/1999/v05.n04/pp0504.
buck-01.html. Accessed August, 1999.]

Drug facts and comparisons. (Updated monthly). St. Louis: Facts and
Comparisons.

Guyton, A.C. & Hall, J.E. (1996). *Textbook of medical physiology*, 9th ed.
Philadelphia: W.B. Saunders.

Porth, C.M. (Ed.). (1998). *Pathophysiology: Concepts of altered health
states*, 5th ed., pp. 719–744. Philadelphia: Lippincott Williams & Wilkins.

Soll, A. (1998). Pathogenesis of nonsteroidal anti-inflammatory drug-
related upper gastrointestinal toxicity. *American Journal of Medicine*,
105(5A), 10S–16S.

Walsh, J.H. & Fass, R. (1997). Acid peptic disorders of the gastrointestinal tract. In W.N. Kelley (Ed.), *Textbook of internal medicine*, 3rd ed.,
pp. 684–702. Philadelphia: Lippincott-Raven.

Williams, D.B. & Welage, L.S. (1997). Gastroesophageal reflux disease.
In J.T. DiPiro, R.L. Talbert, G.C. Yee, G.R. Matzke, B.G. Wells, & L.M.
Posey (Eds.), *Pharmacotherapy: A pathophysiologic approach*, 3rd ed.,
pp. 675–696. Stamford, CT: Appleton & Lange

Willis, J. (1998). Gastrointestinal diseases. In C.F. Carey, H.H. Lee, & K.F.
Woeltje (Eds.), *The Washington manual of medical therapeutics*,
29th ed., pp. 302–328. Philadelphia: Lippincott Williams & Wilkins.

61

Laxatives and Cathartics

Objectives

After studying this chapter, the student will be able to:

1. Differentiate the major types of laxatives according to effects on the gastrointestinal tract.

2. Differentiate the consequences of occasional use from those of chronic use.

3. Discuss rational choices of laxatives for selected client populations or purposes.

4. Discuss bulk-forming laxatives as the most physiologic agents.

5. Discuss possible reasons for and hazards of overuse and abuse of laxatives.

Elmer Wong, a 67-year-old teacher, fractured his hip when he fell on a patch of ice. He is scheduled for hip surgery to repair the fracture; this will be followed by a period of rehabilitation as he regains his mobility. Mr. Wong's history reveals he usually has a bowel movement every 2 to 3 days and occasionally uses laxatives.

Reflect on:

▶ Factors that increase his risk for constipation during the postoperative period.

▶ Expectation for postoperative bowel elimination, considering his history.

▶ Nonpharmacologic interventions that can promote normal bowel function during the postoperative period.

▶ Appropriate use of laxatives to promote normal bowel function. What kinds of laxatives are usually used, and why?

DESCRIPTION

Laxatives and cathartics are drugs used to promote bowel elimination (defecation). The term *laxative* implies mild effects and elimination of soft, formed stool. The term *cathartic* implies strong effects and elimination of liquid or semiliquid stool. Because the different effects depend more on the dose than on the particular drug used, the terms often are used interchangeably.

DEFECATION

Defecation is normally stimulated by movements and reflexes in the gastrointestinal (GI) tract. When the stomach and duodenum are distended with food or fluids, gastro-colic and duodenocolic reflexes cause propulsive movements in the colon, which move feces into the rectum and arouse the urge to defecate. When sensory nerve fibers in the rectum are stimulated by the fecal mass, the defecation reflex causes strong peristalsis, deep breathing, closure of the glottis, contraction of abdominal muscles, contraction of the rectum, relaxation of anal sphincters, and expulsion of the fecal mass.

The cerebral cortex normally controls the defecation reflex so defecation can occur at acceptable times and places. Voluntary control inhibits the external anal sphincter to allow defecation or contracts the sphincter to prevent defecation. When the external sphincter remains contracted, the defecation reflex dissipates, and the urge to defecate usually does not recur until additional feces enter the rectum or several hours later.

In people who often inhibit the defecation reflex or fail to respond to the urge to defecate, constipation develops as the reflex weakens. *Constipation* is the infrequent and painful expulsion of hard, dry stools. Although there is no "normal" number of stools because of variations in diet and other factors, most people report more than three bowel movements per week. Normal bowel elimination should produce a soft, formed stool without pain.

LAXATIVES AND CATHARTICS

Laxatives and cathartics are somewhat arbitrarily classified as bulk-forming laxatives, surfactant laxatives or stool softeners, saline cathartics, stimulant cathartics, and lubricant or emollient laxatives. Individual drugs are listed in Table 61-1.

Bulk-Forming Laxatives

Bulk-forming laxatives (eg, polycarbophil, psyllium seed) are substances that are largely unabsorbed from the intestine. When water is added, these substances swell and become gel-like. The added bulk or size of the fecal mass stimulates peristalsis and defecation. The substances also may act by pulling water into the intestinal lumen. Bulk-forming laxatives are the most physiologic laxatives because their effect is similar to that of increased intake of dietary fiber.

Surfactant Laxatives (Stool Softeners)

Surfactant laxatives (eg, docusate sodium) decrease the surface tension of the fecal mass to allow water to penetrate into the stool. They also act as a detergent to facilitate admixing of fat and water in the stool. As a result, stools are softer and easier to expel. These agents have little if any laxative effect. Their main value is to prevent straining while expelling stool.

Saline Cathartics

Saline cathartics (eg, magnesium citrate, milk of magnesia, sodium phosphate) are not well absorbed from the intestine. Consequently, they increase osmotic pressure in the intestinal lumen and cause water to be retained. Distention of the bowel leads to increased peristalsis and decreased intestinal transit time for the fecal mass. The resultant stool is semifluid.

Irritant or Stimulant Cathartics

The irritant or stimulant cathartics are the strongest and most abused laxative products. These drugs act by irritating the GI mucosa and pulling water into the bowel lumen. As a result, feces are moved through the bowel too rapidly to allow colonic absorption of fecal water, so a watery stool is eliminated. These cathartics are subdivided into three groups, which differ in location and time of action but are similar in mechanism of action, pharmacokinetics, and adverse effects. The groups are castor oil, anthraquinones (senna products, cascara sagrada), and diphenylmethanes (bisacodyl, phenolphthalein). Phenolphthalein is the active ingredient in several over-the-counter laxatives (eg, Correctol, Dialose Plus, Doxidan, Feen-a-Mint).

In addition to the oral agents, glycerin is administered as a rectal suppository. Glycerin stimulates bowel evacuation by its irritant effects on rectal mucosa and hyperosmotic effects in the colon. Glycerin is not given orally for laxative effects.

Lubricant Laxatives

Mineral oil is the only lubricant laxative used clinically. It lubricates the intestine and is thought to soften stool by

TABLE 61-1   Laxatives and Cathartics

Generic/Trade Name	Routes and Dosage Ranges	
	Adults	Children
Bulk-forming Laxatives		
Methylcellulose (Citrucel)	PO 1 heaping tbsp one to three times daily with water (8 oz or more)	PO 1 level tbsp one to three times daily with water (4 oz)
Polycarbophil (FiberCon, Mitrolan)	PO 1 g four times daily or PRN with 8 oz of fluid; maximum dose, 6 g/24 h	6–12 y, PO 500 mg one to three times daily or PRN; maximum dose, 3 g/24 h 2–6 y, PO 500 mg one or two times daily or PRN; maximum dose, 1.5 g/24 h
Psyllium preparations (Metamucil, Effersyllium, Serutan, Perdiem Plain)	PO 4–10 g (1–2 tsp) one to three times daily, stirred in at least 8 oz of water or other liquid	
Surfactant Laxatives (Stool Softeners)		
Docusate sodium (Colace, Doxinate)	PO 50–200 mg daily	>12 y, same dosage as adults 3–12 y, 20–120 mg daily <3 y, 10–40 mg daily
Docusate calcium (Surfak)	PO 50–240 mg daily	>12 y, same dosage as adults 2–12 y, 50–150 mg daily <2 y, 25 mg daily
Docusate potassium (Dialose)	PO 100–300 mg daily	6–12 y, 100 mg at bedtime
Saline Cathartics		
Magnesium citrate solution	PO 200 mL at bedtime	
Magnesium hydroxide (milk of magnesia, magnesia magma)	Regular liquid, PO 15–60 mL at bedtime. Concentrated liquid, PO 10–20 mL at bedtime	Regular liquid, PO 2.5–5 mL
Polyethylene glycol–electrolyte solution (PEG 3350, sodium sulfate, sodium bicarbonate, sodium chloride, potassium chloride) (CoLyte, Colovage, GoLYTELY)	For bowel cleansing before gastrointestinal examination: PO 240 mL (8 oz) every 10 min until 4 L is consumed	No recommended children's dose
Sodium phosphate and sodium biphosphate (Fleet Phosphosoda, Fleet Enema)	PO 20–40 mL in 8 oz of water Rectal enema, 60–120 mL	≥10 y, PO 10–20 mL in 8 oz of water 5–10 y, PO 5–10 mL in 8 oz of water Rectal enema, 60 mL
Irritant or Stimulant Cathartics		
ANTHRAQUINONE		
Cascara sagrada (Cas-Evac)	PO, tablets, 325 mg; fluid extract, 0.5–1.5 mL; aromatic fluid extract, 5 mL	
Senna preparations (Senokot, Black Draught)	Granules, PO 1 level tsp once or twice daily; geriatric, obstetric, gynecologic clients, PO 0.5 level tsp once or twice daily Syrup, PO 2–3 tsp once or twice daily; geriatric, obstetric, gynecologic clients, 1–1½ tsp once or twice daily Tablets, PO 2 tablets once or twice daily; geriatric, obstetric, gynecologic clients, 1 tablet once or twice daily Suppositories, 1 suppository at bedtime	Weight >27 kg: granules, syrup, tablets, suppositories—½ adult dose
DIPHENYLMETHANE CATHARTICS		
Bisacodyl (Dulcolax)	PO 10–15 mg Rectal suppository, 10 mg	≥6 y, PO 5–10 mg <2 y, rectal suppository 5 mg
Phenolphthalein (Doxidan, Feen-a-Mint)	PO 30–194 mg daily	
OTHER IRRITANT CATHARTICS		
Castor oil (Neoloid)	PO 15–60 mL	5–15 y, PO 5–30 mL depending on strength of emulsion <2 y, PO 1.25–7.5 mL depending on strength of emulsion
Glycerin	Rectal suppository, 3 g	<6 y, rectal suppository 1–1.5 g

TABLE 61–1	Laxatives and Cathartics (*continued*)	
	Routes and Dosage Ranges	
Generic/Trade Name	**Adults**	**Children**
Lubricant Laxative		
Mineral oil (Agoral Plain, Milkinol, Fleet Mineral Oil Enema)	PO 15–30 mL at bedtime Rectal enema, 30–60 mL	>6 y, PO 5–15 mL at bedtime Rectal enema, 30–60 mL
Miscellaneous Laxatives		
Lactulose (Chronulac, Cephulac)	PO 15–30 mL daily; maximum dose, 60 mL daily Portal systemic encephalopathy, PO 30–45 mL three or four times daily, adjusted to produce two or three soft stools daily Rectally as retention enema, 300 mL with 700 mL water or normal saline, retained 30–60 min, q4–6h	Infants, PO 2.5–10 mL daily in divided doses Older children, PO 40–90 mL daily in divided doses
Sorbitol	PO 30–50 g daily	

PO, oral.

retarding colonic absorption of fecal water, but the exact mechanism of action is unknown. Mineral oil may cause several adverse effects and is not recommended for long-term use.

Miscellaneous Laxatives

Lactulose is a disaccharide that is not absorbed from the GI tract. It exerts laxative effects by pulling water into the intestinal lumen. It is used to treat constipation and hepatic encephalopathy. The latter condition usually results from alcoholic liver disease in which ammonia accumulates and causes stupor or coma. Ammonia is produced by metabolism of dietary protein and intestinal bacteria. Lactulose decreases production of ammonia in the intestine. The goal of treatment is usually to maintain two to three soft stools daily.

Polyethylene glycol–electrolyte solution (CoLyte, GoLYTELY) is a nonabsorbable oral solution that induces diarrhea within 30 to 60 minutes and rapidly evacuates the bowel, usually within 4 hours. It is used for bowel cleansing before GI examination (eg, colonoscopy) and is contraindicated with GI obstruction, gastric retention, colitis, or bowel perforation.

Sorbitol is a monosaccharide that pulls water into the intestinal lumen and has laxative effects. It is often given with sodium polystyrene sulfonate (Kayexalate), a potassium-removing resin used to treat hyperkalemia, to prevent constipation and aid expulsion of the potassium–resin complex.

Indications for Use

Laxatives and cathartics are widely available on a nonprescription basis. They are among the most frequently used

and abused drugs. One reason for overuse is the common misconception that a daily bowel movement is necessary for health and well-being. This notion may lead to a vicious cycle of events in which a person fails to have a bowel movement, takes a strong laxative, again fails to have a bowel movement, and takes another laxative before the fecal column has had time to become reestablished (2 to 3 days). Thus, a pattern of laxative dependence and abuse is established. Despite widespread abuse of laxatives and cathartics, there are several rational indications for use:

1. To relieve constipation in pregnant women, elderly clients whose abdominal and perineal muscles have become weak and atrophied, children with megacolon, and clients receiving drugs that decrease intestinal motility (eg, opioid analgesics, drugs with anticholinergic effects)
2. To prevent straining at stool in clients with coronary artery disease (eg, postmyocardial infarction), hypertension, cerebrovascular disease, and hemorrhoids and other rectal conditions
3. To empty the bowel in preparation for bowel surgery or diagnostic procedures (eg, colonoscopy, barium enema)

Nursing Notes: Apply Your Knowledge

You are a home health nurse visiting Gina Simboli, a 36-year-old client with cancer. Her disease has progressed to a point where she is taking large amounts of narcotics to control the pain and she spends most of the day in a recliner chair. Your assessment reveals complaints of feeling full and bloated. For over a week, Ms. Simboli has been incontinent of small amounts of liquid stool two to three times a day. What will you recommend to promote normal bowel function?

4. To accelerate elimination of potentially toxic substances from the GI tract (eg, orally ingested drugs or toxic compounds)

5. To prevent absorption of intestinal ammonia in clients with hepatic encephalopathy

6. To obtain a stool specimen for parasitologic examination

7. To accelerate excretion of parasites after anthelmintic drugs have been administered

Contraindications to Use

Laxatives and cathartics should not be used in the presence of undiagnosed abdominal pain. The danger is that the drugs may cause an inflamed organ (eg, the appendix) to rupture and spill GI contents into the abdominal cavity with subsequent peritonitis, a life-threatening condition. The drugs also are contraindicated with intestinal obstruction and fecal impaction.

NURSING PROCESS

Assessment

Assess clients for current or potential constipation.

- Identify risk factors:
  - Diet with minimal fiber (ie, small amounts of fruits, vegetables, and whole-grain products)
  - Low fluid intake (eg, <2000 mL daily)
  - Immobility or limited activity
  - Drug therapy with central nervous system depressant drugs (eg, opioid analgesics), anticholinergics, and others that reduce intestinal motility. Overuse of antidiarrheal agents also may cause constipation.
  - Hemorrhoids, anal fissures, or other conditions characterized by painful bowel elimination
  - Elderly or debilitated clients
- Signs and symptoms include the following:
  - Decreased number and frequency of stools
  - Passage of dry, hard stools
  - Abdominal distention and discomfort
  - Flatulence

Nursing Diagnoses

- Constipation related to decreased activity, inadequate dietary fiber, inadequate fluid intake, drugs, or disease processes
- Pain (abdominal cramping and distention) related to constipation or use of laxatives
- Impaired Tissue Integrity: Loss of normal bowel function related to overuse of laxatives

- Noncompliance with recommendations for nondrug measures to prevent or treat constipation
- Noncompliance with instructions for appropriate use of laxatives
- Risk for Fluid Volume Deficit related to diarrhea from frequent or large doses of laxatives
- Altered Nutrition: Poor absorption of nutrients during laxative-induced diarrhea
- Knowledge Deficit: Nondrug measures to prevent constipation
- Knowledge Deficit: Appropriate use of laxatives

Planning/Goals

The client will:

- Take laxative drugs appropriately
- Use nondrug measures to promote normal bowel function and prevent constipation
- Regain normal patterns of bowel elimination
- Avoid excessive losses of fluids and electrolytes from laxative use
- Be protected from excessive fluid loss, hypotension, and other adverse drug effects, when possible
- Be assisted to avoid constipation when at risk (ie, has illness or injury that prevents activity, food and fluid intake; has medically prescribed drugs that decrease GI function)

Interventions

Assist clients with constipation and caregivers to:

- Understand the importance of diet, exercise, and fluid intake in promoting normal bowel function and preventing constipation
- Increase activity and exercise
- Increase intake of dietary fiber (vegetables, fruits, cereal grains)
- Drink at least 2000 mL of fluid daily
- Establish and maintain a routine for bowel elimination (eg, going to the bathroom immediately after breakfast)

  Monitor client responses:

- Record number, amount, and type of bowel movements.
- Record vital signs. Hypotension and weak pulse may indicate fluid volume deficit.

Evaluation

- Observe and interview for improved patterns of bowel elimination.
- Observe for use of nondrug measures to promote bowel function.
- Observe for appropriate use of laxatives.
- Observe and interview regarding adverse effects of laxatives.

CLIENT TEACHING GUIDELINES
Laxatives

General Considerations

✔ Diet, exercise, and fluid intake are important in maintaining normal bowel function and preventing or treating constipation.

✔ Eat foods high in dietary fiber daily. Fiber is the portion of plant food that is not digested. It is contained in fruits, vegetables, and whole-grain cereals and breads. Bran, the outer coating of cereal grains, such as wheat or oats, is an excellent source of dietary fiber and is available in numerous cereal products.

✔ Drink at least 6 to 10 glasses (8 oz each) of fluid daily if not contraindicated.

✔ Exercise regularly. Walking and other activities aid movement of feces through the bowel.

✔ Establish a regular time and place for bowel elimination. The defecation urge is usually strongest after eating or drinking and the defecation reflex is weakened or lost if repeatedly ignored.

✔ Laxative use should be temporary and not regular, as a general rule. Regular use may prevent normal bowel function, cause adverse drug reactions, and delay treatment for conditions that cause constipation

✔ *Never* take laxatives when acute abdominal pain, nausea, or vomiting is present. Doing so may cause a ruptured appendix or other serious complication.

✔ After taking a strong laxative, it takes 2 to 3 days of normal eating to produce enough feces in the bowel for a bowel movement. Frequent use of a strong laxative promotes loss of normal bowel function, loss of fluids and electrolytes that your body needs, and laxative dependence.

✔ If you have chronic constipation and are unable or unwilling to eat enough fiber-containing foods in your diet, the next-best action is regular use of a bulk-forming laxative (eg, Metamucil) as a dietary supplement. These laxatives act the same way as increasing fiber in the diet and are usually best for long-term use. When taken daily, they can prevent constipation. However, they take 2 to 3 days to work and are not effective in relieving acute constipation.

✔ Your urine may be discolored if you take a laxative containing senna (eg, Senokot) or cascara sagrada. The color change is not harmful.

✔ Some people have used strong laxatives for weight control. This is a dangerous practice because it can lead to life-threatening fluid and electrolyte imbalances.

Self- or Caregiver Administration

✔ Take all laxatives as directed and do not exceed recommended doses to avoid adverse effects.

✔ With bulk-forming laxatives, mix in 8 oz of fluid immediately before taking and follow with additional fluid, if able. *Never* take the drug dry. Adequate fluid intake is essential with these drugs.

✔ With bisacodyl tablets, swallow whole (do not crush or chew), and do not take within 1 hour of an antacid or milk. This helps prevent stomach irritation, abdominal cramping, and possible vomiting.

✔ Take magnesium citrate or milk of magnesia on an empty stomach with 8 oz of fluid to increase effectiveness.

✔ Refrigerate magnesium citrate before taking to improve taste and retain effectiveness.

✔ Mix lactulose with fruit juice, water or milk, if desired, to improve taste.

PRINCIPLES OF THERAPY

Drug Selection

Choice of a laxative or cathartic depends on the reason for use and the client's condition.

1. For long-term use of laxatives or cathartics in clients who are elderly, unable or unwilling to eat an adequate diet, or debilitated, bulk-forming laxatives (eg, Metamucil) usually are preferred. However, because obstruction may occur, these agents should not be given to clients with difficulty in swallowing or adhesions or strictures in the GI tract, or to those who are unable or unwilling to drink adequate fluids.

2. For clients in whom straining is potentially harmful or painful, stool softeners (eg, docusate sodium) are the agents of choice.

3. For occasional use to cleanse the bowel for endoscopic or radiologic examinations, saline or stimulant cathartics are acceptable (eg, magnesium citrate, polyethylene glycol–electrolyte solution, bisacodyl). These drugs should not be used more than once per week. Frequent use is likely to produce laxative abuse.

4. Oral use of mineral oil may cause potentially serious adverse effects (decreased absorption of fat-soluble vitamins and some drugs, lipid pneumonia if aspirated into the lungs). Thus, mineral oil is not an oral laxative of choice in any condition, although occasional use in the alert client is unlikely to be harmful. Mineral oil is probably most useful as a retention enema to soften hard, dry feces and aid in their expulsion. Mineral oil should not be used regularly.

5. In fecal impaction, a rectal suppository (eg, bisacodyl) or an enema (eg, oil retention or Fleet enema) is preferred. Oral laxatives are contraindicated when fecal impaction is present but may be given after the rectal mass is removed. Once the impaction is relieved, measures should be taken to prevent recurrence. If dietary and other nonpharmacologic measures are ineffective or contraindicated, use of a bulk-forming agent daily or another laxative once or twice weekly may be necessary.

6. Saline cathartics containing magnesium, phosphate, or potassium salts are contraindicated in clients with renal failure because hypermagnesemia, hyperphosphatemia, or hyperkalemia may occur.

7. Saline cathartics containing sodium salts are contraindicated in clients with edema or congestive heart failure because enough sodium may be absorbed to cause further fluid retention and edema. They also should not be used in clients with impaired renal function or those following a sodium-restricted diet for hypertension.

8. Polyethylene glycol–electrolyte solution is formulated for rapid and effective bowel cleansing without significant changes in water or electrolyte balance.

Use in Children

As in adults, increasing fluids, high-fiber foods, and exercise is preferred when possible. For acute constipation, glycerin suppositories are often effective in infants and small children. Stool softeners may be given to older children. Children usually should not use strong, stimulant laxatives. Parents should be advised not to use any laxative more than once a week without consulting a health care provider. Polyethylene glycol–electrolyte solution is effective in treating acute iron overdose in children, although it is not approved by the Food and Drug Administration for this indication.

Use in Older Adults

Constipation is a common problem in older adults, and laxatives are often used or overused. Nondrug measures to prevent constipation (eg, increasing fluids, high-fiber foods, and exercise) are much preferred to laxatives. If

a laxative is required on a regular basis, a psyllium compound (eg, Metamucil) is best because it is most physiologic in its action. If taken, it should be accompanied by a full glass of fluid. There have been reports of obstruction in the GI tract when a psyllium compound is taken with insufficient fluid. Strong stimulant laxatives should be avoided.

Use in Clients With Cancer

Many clients with cancer require moderate to large amounts of opioid analgesics for pain control. The analgesics slow GI motility and cause constipation. These clients need a bowel management program that includes routine laxative administration. Stimulant laxatives (eg, a senna preparation or bisacodyl) increase intestinal motility, which is the action that opiates suppress. These drugs may cause abdominal cramping, which may be lessened by giving small doses three or four times daily.

Use in Renal Impairment

Saline cathartics containing phosphate, sodium, magnesium, or potassium salts are usually contraindicated or must be used cautiously in the presence of impaired renal function. Ten percent or more of the magnesium in magnesium salts may be absorbed and cause hypermagnesemia; sodium phosphate and sodium biphosphate may cause hyperphosphatemia, hypernatremia, acidosis, and hypocalcemia; potassium salts may cause hyperkalemia.

Use in Hepatic Impairment

Because most laxatives are not absorbed or metabolized extensively, they can usually be used without difficulty in clients with hepatic impairment. In fact, they are used therapeutically in hepatic encephalopathy to decrease absorption of ammonia from dietary protein in the GI tract. Lactulose is usually given, in dosages to produce two to three soft stools daily.

 ## Home Care

Laxatives are commonly self-prescribed and self-administered in the home setting. The home care nurse may become involved when visiting a client for other purposes. The role of the home care nurse may include assessing usual patterns of bowel elimination, identifying clients at risk for development of constipation, promoting lifestyle interventions to prevent constipation, obtaining laxatives when indicated, and counseling about rational use of laxatives.

Laxatives and Cathartics

NURSING ACTIONS	RATIONALE/EXPLANATION
1. Administer accurately	
a. Give bulk-forming laxatives with at least 8 oz of water or other fluid. Mix with fluid immediately before administration.	To prevent thickening and expansion in the gastrointestinal (GI) tract with possible obstruction. These substances absorb water rapidly and solidify into a gelatinous mass.
b. With bisacodyl tablets, instruct the client to swallow the tablets without chewing and not to take them within an hour after ingesting milk or gastric antacids or while receiving cimetidine therapy.	The tablets have an enteric coating to delay dissolution until they reach the alkaline environment of the small intestine. Chewing or giving the tablets close to antacid substances or to cimetidine-treated clients causes premature dissolution and gastric irritation and results in abdominal cramping and vomiting.
c. Give saline cathartics on an empty stomach with 240 mL of fluid.	To increase effectiveness
d. Refrigerate magnesium citrate and polyethylene glycol–electrolyte solution before giving.	To increase palatability and retain potency
e. Castor oil may be chilled and followed by fruit juice or other beverage.	To increase palatability
f. Insert rectal suppositories to the length of the index finger, next to rectal mucosa.	These drugs are not effective unless they are in contact with intestinal mucosa.
2. Observe for therapeutic effects	
a. Soft to semiliquid stool	Therapeutic effects occur in approximately 1–3 d with bulk-forming laxatives and stool softeners; 6–8 h with bisacodyl tablets, cascara sagrada, phenolphthalein, and senna products; 15–60 min with bisacodyl and glycerin suppositories.
b. Liquid to semiliquid stool	Effects occur in approximately 1–3 h with saline cathartics and castor oil
c. Decreased abdominal pain when used in irritable bowel syndrome or diverticulosis	
d. Decreased rectal pain when used in clients with hemorrhoids or anal fissures	Pain results from straining to expel hard, dry feces.
3. Observe for adverse effects	
a. Diarrhea—several liquid stools, abdominal cramping. Severe, prolonged diarrhea may cause hyponatremia, hypokalemia, dehydration, and other problems.	Diarrhea is most likely to result from strong, stimulant cathartics (eg, castor oil, bisacodyl, phenolphthalein, senna preparations) or large doses of saline cathartics (eg, milk of magnesia).
b. With bulk-forming agents, impaction or obstruction	Impaction or obstruction of the GI tract can be prevented by giving ample fluids with these agents and not giving the drugs to clients with known dysphagia or strictures anywhere in the alimentary canal.
c. With saline cathartics, hypermagnesemia, hyperkalemia, fluid retention, and edema	Hypermagnesemia and hyperkalemia are more likely to occur in clients with renal insufficiency

(continued)

NURSING ACTIONS	RATIONALE/EXPLANATION
	because of impaired ability to excrete magnesium and potassium. Fluid retention and edema are more likely to occur in clients with congestive heart failure or other conditions characterized by edema. Polyethylene glycol–electrolyte solution produces the least change in water and electrolyte balance.
d. With mineral oil, lipid pneumonia and decreased absorption of vitamins A, D, E, and K	Lipid pneumonia can be prevented by not giving mineral oil to clients with dysphagia or impaired consciousness. Decreased absorption of fat-soluble vitamins can be prevented by not giving mineral oil with or shortly after meals or for longer than 2 wk.
4. Observe for drug interactions	
a. Drugs that *increase* effects of laxatives and cathartics:	
(1) GI stimulants (eg, metoclopramide)	Additive stimulation of intestinal motility.
b. Drugs that *decrease* effects of laxatives and cathartics:	
(1) Anticholinergic drugs (eg, atropine) and other drugs with anticholinergic properties (eg, phenothiazine antipsychotic drugs, tricyclic antidepressants, some antihistamines, and antiparkinsonism drugs)	These drugs slow intestinal motility. Clients receiving these agents are at risk for development of constipation and requiring laxatives, perhaps on a long-term basis.
(2) Central nervous system depressants (eg, narcotic analgesics)	Narcotic analgesics commonly cause constipation.

Nursing Notes: Apply Your Knowledge

Answer: Abdominal fullness, bloating, and seepage of liquid stool are all symptoms of fecal impaction. Fecal impaction is likely in this patient because she is taking large amounts of narcotics and is inactive. To treat the impacted stool, oil retention enemas are helpful to soften the hardened stool. Oral laxatives are usually ineffective in moving the hardened plug of feces. Frequently, manual disimpaction is required, especially if the patient is weak. It is very important to institute an aggressive bowel program for any patient receiving long-term narcotics for pain control. Tolerance is never developed for the constipating side effect of opioids. Bulk-forming laxatives and stool softeners should be used on a daily basis. Saline or stimulant cathartics can be administered when 2 to 3 days elapse without a bowel movement. Because impaction can occur, enemas are also used. Teaching regarding increasing fluids, fiber, and activity, within individual limitations, is also important.

How Can You Avoid This Medication Error?

Answer: Never recommend laxatives for a patient who is experiencing acute abdominal pain. It is important to collect more data from this patient, including a complete description of the pain (onset, locations, pattern), temperature, and other symptoms. If the patient has appendicitis, taking a laxative could cause the appendix to rupture and result in serious complications.

 ## REVIEW AND APPLICATION EXERCISES

1. What are risk factors for development of constipation?
2. Describe nonpharmacologic strategies to prevent constipation.
3. Which type of laxative is in general the most desirable for long-term use? Which is the least desirable?
4. What are the most significant adverse effects of strong laxatives?

5. If an adult client asked you to recommend an over-the-counter laxative, what information about the client's condition would you need, and what would you recommend? Why?

SELECTED REFERENCES

Barnett, J.L. (1997). Approach to the patient with constipation and fecal incontinence. In W.N. Kelley (Ed.), *Textbook of internal medicine*, 3rd ed., pp. 632–637. Philadelphia: Lippincott-Raven.

Brunton, L.L. (1996). Agents affecting gastrointestinal water flux and motility; emesis and antiemetics; bile acids and pancreatic enzymes. In J.G. Hardman, L.E. Limbird, P.B. Molinoff, & R.W. Ruddon (Eds.), *Goodman & Gilman's The pharmacological basis of therapeutics*, 9th ed., pp. 917–936. New York: McGraw-Hill.

Drug facts and comparisons. (Updated monthly). St. Louis: Facts and Comparisons.

Longe, R.L. & DiPiro, J.T. (1997). Diarrhea and constipation. In J.T. DiPiro, R.L. Talbert, G.C. Yee, G.R. Matzke, B.G. Wells, & L.M. Posey (Eds.), *Pharmacotherapy: A pathophysiologic approach*, 3rd ed., pp. 767–783. Stamford, CT: Appleton & Lange.

McMillan, S.C. (1999). Assessing and managing narcotic-induced constipation in adults with cancer. [Online: Available http://www.medscape.com/Moffitt/CancerControl/1999/v06.n02.cc0602.12.mcmi/cc0602.12.mcmi-01.html. Accessed December, 1999.]

Porth, C.M. (1998). Alterations in gastrointestinal function. In C.M. Porth (Ed.). *Pathophysiology: Concepts of altered health states*, 5th ed., pp. 719–744. Philadelphia: Lippincott Williams & Wilkins.

Smeltzer, S.C. & Bare, B.G. (1996). *Brunner and Suddarth's Textbook of medical-surgical nursing*, 8th ed. Philadelphia: Lippincott-Raven.

62

Antidiarrheals

Objectives

After studying this chapter, the student will be able to:

1. Identify clients at risk for development of diarrhea.

2. Discuss guidelines for assessing diarrhea.

3. Describe types of diarrhea in which antidiarrheal drug therapy may be indicated.

4. Differentiate the major types of antidiarrheal drugs.

5. Discuss characteristics, effects, and nursing process implications of opiate-related antidiarrheal agents.

John Finney, a 32-year-old client with acquired immunodeficiency syndrome, is admitted to your medical unit for management of severe diarrhea. He reports having 12 to 20 liquid stools per day and feeling weak and dizzy when he gets up. This current bout of diarrhea has been continuing for 6 days, during which he has lost 18 pounds. Diphenoxylate (Lomotil) and IV fluids are ordered.

Reflect on:

▶ The physiologic effects of severe diarrhea.

▶ The impact of severe diarrhea on a person's ability to carry out normal activities.

▶ Appropriate nursing assessments and interventions while diarrhea continues.

▶ How diphenoxylate (Lomotil) works to decrease diarrhea.

DESCRIPTION

Antidiarrheal drugs are used to treat diarrhea, defined as the frequent expulsion of liquid or semiliquid stools. Diarrhea is a symptom of numerous conditions that increase bowel motility, cause secretion or retention of fluids in the intestinal lumen, and cause inflammation or irritation of the gastrointestinal (GI) tract. As a result, bowel contents are rapidly propelled toward the rectum, and absorption of fluids and electrolytes is limited. Some causes of diarrhea include the following:

1. Excessive use of laxatives
2. Intestinal infections with viruses, bacteria, or protozoa. A common source of infection is ingestion of food or fluid contaminated by *Salmonella, Shigella,* or *Staphylococcus* microorganisms. So-called *travelers' diarrhea* is usually caused by an enteropathogenic strain of *Escherichia coli.*
3. Undigested, coarse, or highly spiced food in the GI tract. The food acts as an irritant and attracts fluids in a defensive attempt to dilute the irritating agent. This may result from inadequate chewing of food or lack of digestive enzymes.
4. Lack of digestive enzymes. Deficiency of pancreatic enzymes inhibits digestion and absorption of carbohydrates, proteins, and fats. Deficiency of lactase, a sugar-splitting intestinal enzyme, inhibits digestion of milk and milk products.
5. Inflammatory bowel disorders, such as gastroenteritis, diverticulitis, ulcerative colitis, and Crohn's disease. In these disorders, the inflamed mucous membrane secretes large amounts of fluids into the intestinal lumen. In addition, when the ileum is diseased or a portion is surgically excised, large amounts of bile salts reach the colon, where they act as cathartics and cause diarrhea. Bile salts are normally reabsorbed from the ileum.
6. Drug therapy. Many oral drugs irritate the GI tract and may cause diarrhea. Antibacterial drugs often do so. Antibacterial drugs also may cause diarrhea by altering the normal bacterial flora in the intestine.

   Antibiotic-associated colitis (also called pseudomembranous colitis and *Clostridium difficile* colitis) is a serious condition that results from oral or parenteral antibiotic therapy. By suppressing normal flora, antibiotics allow gram-positive, anaerobic *C. difficile* organisms to proliferate. The organisms produce a toxin that causes fever, abdominal pain, inflammatory lesions of the colon, and severe diarrhea with stools containing mucus, pus, and sometimes blood. Symptoms may develop within a few days or several weeks after the causative antibiotic is discontinued. Antibiotic-associated colitis is more often associated with ampicillin, cephalosporins, and clindamycin, but may occur with any antibiotic or combination of antibiotics that alters intestinal microbial flora.
7. Intestinal neoplasms. Tumors may increase intestinal motility by occupying space and stretching the intestinal wall. Diarrhea sometimes alternates with constipation in colon cancer.
8. Functional disorders. Diarrhea may be a symptom of stress or anxiety in some clients. No organic disease process can be found in such circumstances.
9. Hyperthyroidism. This condition increases bowel motility.
10. Surgical excision of portions of the intestine, especially the small intestine. Such procedures decrease the absorptive area and increase fluidity of stools.
11. Human immunodeficiency virus (HIV) infection/ acquired immunodeficiency syndrome (AIDS). Diarrhea occurs in most clients with HIV infection, often as a chronic condition that contributes to malnutrition and weight loss. It may be caused by drug therapy, infection with a variety of microorganisms, or other factors.

Diarrhea may be acute or chronic and mild or severe. Most episodes of acute diarrhea are defensive mechanisms by which the body tries to rid itself of irritants, toxins, and infectious agents. These are usually self-limiting and subside within 24 to 48 hours without serious consequences. If severe or prolonged, acute diarrhea may lead to serious fluid and electrolyte depletion, especially in young children and elderly adults. Chronic diarrhea may cause malnutrition and anemia and is often characterized by remissions and exacerbations.

ANTIDIARRHEAL DRUGS

Antidiarrheal drugs include a variety of agents, most of which are discussed in other chapters. When used for treatment of diarrhea, the drugs may be given to relieve the symptom (nonspecific therapy) or the underlying cause of the symptom (specific therapy). Individual drugs are listed in Table 62-1.

Nonspecific Therapy

For symptomatic treatment of diarrhea, opiates and opiate derivatives (see Chap. 6) are the most effective. These drugs decrease diarrhea by slowing propulsive movements in the small and large intestines. Morphine, codeine, and related drugs are effective in relieving diarrhea but are rarely used for this purpose because of their adverse effects. Opiates have largely been replaced by the synthetic drugs diphenoxylate, loperamide, and difenoxin, which are used only for treatment of diarrhea and do not cause morphine-like adverse effects in recommended doses.

(text continues on page 919)

TABLE 62-1	Antidiarrheal Drugs

| Generic/Trade Name | Characteristics | Clinical Indications | Routes and Dosage Ranges | |
			Adults	Children
Opiates and Related Drugs				
Camphorated tincture of opium (paregoric)	Contains 0.04% morphine, alcohol, camphor, anise oil, and benzoic acid Antidiarrheal activity is caused by morphine content. Morphine slows propulsive movements in small and large intestines. Under Controlled Substances Act, a Schedule III drug when used alone and a Schedule V drug in the small amounts combined with other drugs. Recommended doses and short-term duration of administration do not produce euphoria, analgesia, or dependence.	Symptomatic treatment of acute diarrhea	PO 5–10 mL one to four times daily (maximum of four doses) until diarrhea is controlled	PO 0.25–0.5 mL/kg one to four times daily (maximum of four doses) until diarrhea is controlled
Difenoxin with atropine sulfate (Motofen)	It is the main active metabolite of diphenoxylate. It slows intestinal motility by a local effect on the GI wall. Overdose may cause severe respiratory depression and coma. Each tablet contains 1 mg of difenoxin and 0.025 mg of atropine. The subtherapeutic dose of atropine is added to discourage overdose and abuse for opiatelike effects Contraindicated in children <2 y of age, clients allergic to the ingredients, and clients with hepatic impairment. A Schedule IV drug under the Controlled Substances Act	Symptomatic treatment of acute or chronic diarrhea	PO 2 mg initially, then 1 mg after each loose stool or 1 mg q3–4h as needed; maximum dose, 8 mg (8 tablets)/24 h	Safety and effectiveness not established for children <12 y
Diphenoxylate with atropine sulfate (Lomotil)	A derivative of meperidine (Demerol) used only for treatment of diarrhea Most commonly prescribed antidiarrheal drug. Decreases intestinal motility. As effective as paregoric and more convenient to administer In recommended doses, does not produce euphoria, analgesia, or dependence. In high doses, produces morphine-like effects, including euphoria, dependence, and respiratory depression. Antidote for overdose is the narcotic antagonist naloxone (Narcan).	Symptomatic treatment of acute or chronic diarrhea	PO 5 mg (2 tablets or 10 mL of liquid) three or four times daily; maximal daily dose, 20 mg	Liquid preparation (2.5 mg diphenoxylate and 0.025 mg atropine per 5 mL), PO 4 times daily, as follows: 2 y, 11–14 kg: 1.5–3 mL; 3 y, 12–16 kg: 2–3 mL; 4 y, 14–20 kg: 2–4 mL; 5 y, 16–23 kg: 2.5–4.5 mL; 6–8 y, 17–32 kg: 2.5–5 mL; 9–12 y, 23–55 kg: 3.5–5 mL

| TABLE 62-1 | Antidiarrheal Drugs (*continued*) |

Generic/Trade Name	Characteristics	Clinical Indications	Routes and Dosage Ranges	
			Adults	Children
	Each tablet or 5 mL of liquid contains 2.5 mg of diphenoxylate and 0.025 mg of atropine. The subtherapeutic dose of atropine is added to discourage drug abuse by producing unpleasant anticholinergic side effects. Contraindicated in severe liver disease, glaucoma, and children <2 y of age. Safety during pregnancy and lactation has not been established. The drug is excreted in breast milk. A Schedule V drug under the Controlled Substances Act			
Loperamide (Imodium)	A derivative of meperidine (Demerol) used only for treatment of diarrhea Decreases intestinal motility Compared with diphenoxylate, loperamide is equally effective and may cause fewer adverse reactions in recommended doses. High doses may produce morphine-like effects. Safety has not been established for use in pregnancy, lactation, and in children <2 y of age. Antidote for overdose is the narcotic antagonist naloxone. Each capsule or 10 mL of liquid contains 2 mg of loperamide.	Symptomatic treatment of acute or chronic diarrhea	PO 4 mg initially, then 2 mg after each loose stool to a maximal daily dose of 16 mg. For chronic diarrhea, dosage should be reduced to the lowest effective amount (average 4–8 mg daily).	2–5 y, 13–20 kg: PO 1 mg three times daily; 6–8 y, 20–30 kg: PO 2 mg twice daily; 8–12 y, >30 kg: PO 2 mg three times daily
Antibacterial Agents				
Ampicillin (Omnipen, Penbriten, others)	A broad-spectrum penicillin	Bacillary dysentery caused by sensitive strains of *Shigella* Typhoid fever resistant to chloramphenicol Typhoid fever to eliminate the postinfective carrier state	PO, IM 2–4 g/d, in divided doses, q6h	PO, IM, IV 50–100 mg/ kg/d, in divided doses, q6h
Chloramphenicol (Chloromycetin)		Typhoid fever (gastroenteritis caused by *Salmonella typhi*)	PO, IV 50 mg/kg/d, in divided doses, q6h	PO 50 mg/kg/d, in divided doses, q6h
Neomycin		Bacillary dysentery caused by strains of *Shigella* that are resistant to other antibiotics but sensitive to neomycin	PO 4 g/d in divided doses, q6h	PO 50–100 mg/kg/d, in divided doses, q6h
Tetracycline		Cholera Bacillary dysentery caused by sensitive strains of *Shigella*	PO 2 g/d in divided doses, q6h	PO 40 mg/kg/d in divided doses, q6h

TABLE 62-1   **Antidiarrheal Drugs** (*continued*)

Generic/Trade Name	Characteristics	Clinical Indications	Routes and Dosage Ranges	
			Adults	Children
Trimethoprim-sulfamethoxazole (TMP-SMX) (Bactrim, Septra)		Bacillary dysentery caused by susceptible strains of *Shigella* Typhoid fever resistant to chloramphenicol and ampicillin Enteritis caused by susceptible strains of *Escherichia coli*	PO 160 mg of trimethoprim and 800 mg of sulfamethoxazole daily, in divided doses, q12h IV 8–10 mg/kg of trimethoprim and 50 mg/ kg sulfamethoxazole daily, in two to four divided doses	PO 8 mg/kg of trimethoprim and 40 mg/kg of sulfamethoxazole daily, in divided doses, q12h IV 8–10 mg/kg of trimethoprim and 50 mg/kg sulfamethoxazole daily, in two to four divided doses
Vancomycin (Vancocin)		Pseudomembranous colitis due to suppression of normal bacterial flora by antibiotics and overgrowth of *Clostridium* organisms Staphylococcal colitis due to broad-spectrum antibiotic therapy, combined with parenteral nafcillin (Unipen)	PO 2 g/d in divided doses, q6h	PO 44 mg/kg/d in divided doses, q6h
Miscellaneous Drugs				
Bismuth subsalicylate (Pepto-Bismol)	Has antimicrobial, antisecretory, and possibly anti-inflammatory effects	Control of diarrhea, including travelers' diarrhea, and relief of abdominal cramping	PO 2 tablets or 30 mL every 30–60 min, if needed, up to 8 doses in 24 h	9–12 y: PO 1 tablet or 15 mL; 6–9 y: PO ⅔ tablet or 10 mL; 3–6 y: PO ⅓ tablet or 5 mL; under <3 y, consult pediatrician
Cholestyramine (Questran)	Binds and inactivates bile salts in the intestine	Diarrhea due to bile salts reaching the colon and causing a cathartic effect. "Bile salt diarrhea" is associated with Crohn's disease or surgical excision of the ileum.	PO 16–32 g/d in 120–180 mL of water, in two to four divided doses before or during meals and at bedtime	
Colestipol (Colestid)	Same as cholestyramine, above	Same as cholestyramine	PO 15–30 g/d in 120–180 mL of water, in two to four divided doses before or during meals and at bedtime	
Octreotide (Sandostatin)	In GI tract, decreases secretions and motility	Control diarrhea associated with carcinoid tumors, vasoactive intestinal peptide tumors, acquired immunodeficiency syndrome, cancer chemotherapy, or radiation, or diarrhea that does not respond to other antidiarrheal agents	Subcutaneous, IV 50 μg two to three times daily initially, then adjusted according to response	Dosage not established

TABLE 62-1 **Antidiarrheal Drugs** (*continued*)

Generic/Trade Name	Characteristics	Clinical Indications	Routes and Dosage Ranges	
			Adults	Children
Pancreatin or pancrelipase (Viokase, Pancrease, Cotazym)	Pancreatic enzymes used only for replacement	Diarrhea and malabsorption due to deficiency of pancreatic enzymes	PO 1–3 tablets or capsules or 1–2 packets of powder with meals and snacks	PO 1–3 tablets or capsules or 1–2 packets of powder with each meal
Psyllium preparations (Metamucil, Effersyllium)	Absorbs water and decreases fluidity of stools	Possibly effective for symptomatic treatment of diarrhea	PO 6–10 g (1–2 tsp), two or three times daily, in a full glass of water or other fluid, mixed immediately before ingestion	

GI, gastrointestinal; IM, intramuscular; IV, intravenous; PO, oral.

Bismuth salts have antibacterial and antiviral activity; bismuth subsalicylate (Pepto-Bismol, a commonly used over-the-counter drug) also has antisecretory and possibly anti-inflammatory effects because of its salicylate component.

Octreotide acetate is a synthetic form of somatostatin, a hormone produced in the anterior pituitary gland and in the pancreas. The drug may be effective in diarrhea because it decreases GI secretion and motility. It is used for diarrhea associated with carcinoid syndrome, intestinal tumors, HIV/AIDS, and diarrhea that does not respond to other antidiarrheal drugs.

Other nonspecific agents sometimes used in diarrhea are anticholinergics (see Chap. 21) and polycarbophil and psyllium preparations (see Chap. 61). Anticholinergic drugs, of which atropine is the prototype, are infrequently used because doses large enough to decrease intestinal motility and secretions cause intolerable adverse effects. The drugs are occasionally used to decrease abdominal cramping and pain (antispasmodic effects) associated with acute nonspecific diarrhea and chronic diarrhea associated with inflammatory bowel disease.

Psyllium preparations (eg, Metamucil) are most often used as bulk-forming laxatives. They are occasionally used in diarrhea to decrease fluidity of stools. The preparations absorb large amounts of water and produce stools of gelatin-like consistency.

Specific Therapy

Specific drug therapy for diarrhea depends on the cause of the symptom and may include the use of antibacterial, enzymatic, and bile salt–binding drugs. Antibacterial drugs are recommended for use in selected cases of bacterial enteritis. Although effective in preventing travelers' diarrhea, antibiotics usually are not recommended because their use may promote the emergence of drug-resistant microorganisms. Although effective in reducing diarrhea due to *Salmonella* and *E. coli* intestinal infections, antibiotics may induce a prolonged carrier state during which the infection can be transmitted to other people.

Indications for Use

Despite the limitations of drug therapy in prevention and treatment of diarrhea, antidiarrheal drugs are indicated in the following circumstances:

1. Severe or prolonged diarrhea (>2 to 3 days), to prevent severe fluid and electrolyte loss
2. Relatively severe diarrhea in young children and elderly adults. These groups are less able to adapt to fluid and electrolyte losses.
3. In chronic inflammatory diseases of the bowel (ulcerative colitis and Crohn's disease), to allow a more nearly normal lifestyle
4. In ileostomies or surgical excision of portions of the ileum, to decrease fluidity and volume of stool
5. HIV/AIDS-associated diarrhea
6. When specific causes of diarrhea have been determined

How Can You Avoid This Medication Error?

Diphenoxylate (Lomotil), 1 tab after every bowel movement PRN, up to 20 mg/day, is ordered to manage severe diarrhea from Jan Howe's ulcerative colitis. Your stock supply contains 2.5-mg tablets of Lomotil. On the evening shift, Jan is still having diarrhea. You note she has already had 6 tablets during earlier shifts. Can you safely give her another dose of Lomotil?

Contraindications to Use

Contraindications to the use of antidiarrheal agents include diarrhea caused by toxic materials, microorganisms that penetrate intestinal mucosa (eg, pathogenic *E. coli*, *Salmonella*, *Shigella*), or antibiotic-associated colitis. In these circumstances, antidiarrheal agents that slow peristalsis may aggravate and prolong diarrhea. Opiates (morphine, codeine) usually are contraindicated in chronic diarrhea because of possible opiate dependence. Difenoxin, diphenoxylate, and loperamide are contraindicated in children younger than 2 years of age.

NURSING PROCESS

Assessment

Assess for acute or chronic diarrhea.

- Try to determine the duration of diarrhea; number of stools per day; amount, consistency, color, odor, and presence of abnormal components (eg, undigested food, blood, pus, mucus) in each stool; precipitating factors; accompanying signs and symptoms (ie, nausea, vomiting, fever, abdominal pain or cramping); and measures used to relieve diarrhea. When possible, look at stool specimens.
- Try to determine the cause of the diarrhea. This includes questioning about causes such as chronic inflammatory diseases of the bowel, food intake, possible exposure to contaminated food, living or traveling in areas of poor sanitation, and use of laxatives or other drugs that may cause diarrhea. When available, check laboratory reports on stool specimens (eg, culture reports).
- With severe or prolonged diarrhea, especially in young children and elderly adults, assess for dehydration, hypokalemia, and other fluid and electrolyte disorders.

Nursing Diagnoses

- Diarrhea related to GI infection or inflammatory disorders, other disease processes, dietary irritants, or overuse of laxatives
- Altered Nutrition: Less Than Body Requirements related to impaired absorption of nutrients with diarrhea
- Anxiety related to availability of bathroom facilities
- Body Image Disturbance with chronic diarrhea related to loss of control and possible incontinence of stool

- Social Isolation with chronic diarrhea related to frequent bowel movements
- Fluid Volume Deficit related to excessive losses in liquid stools
- Pain (abdominal cramping) related to intestinal hypermotility and spasm
- Impaired Tissue Integrity: Perianal skin excoriation related to irritants in liquid stools
- Self Care Deficit related to weakness
- Constipation related to use of antidiarrheal drugs
- Knowledge Deficit: Factors that cause or aggravate diarrhea
- Knowledge Deficit: Appropriate use of antidiarrheal drugs

Planning/Goals

The client will:

- Take antidiarrheal drugs appropriately
- Obtain relief from acute diarrhea (reduced number of liquid stools, reduced abdominal discomfort)
- Maintain fluid and electrolyte balance
- Maintain adequate nutritional intake
- Be assisted when weak from diarrhea
- Avoid adverse effects of antidiarrheal medications
- Reestablish normal bowel patterns after an episode of acute diarrhea
- Have fewer liquid stools with chronic diarrhea

Interventions

Use measures to prevent diarrhea:

- Prepare and store food properly and avoid improperly stored foods and those prepared under unsanitary conditions. Dairy products, cream pies, and other foods may cause diarrhea ("food poisoning") if not refrigerated.
- Wash hands before handling any foods, after handling raw poultry or meat, and always before eating.
- Chew food well.
- Do not overuse laxatives (ie, amount per dose or frequency of use). Many over-the-counter products contain senna or phenolphthalein, which are strong stimulant laxatives.

Regardless of whether antidiarrheal drugs are used, supportive therapy is required for the treatment of diarrhea. Elements of supportive care include the following:

- Replacement of fluids and electrolytes (approximately 2 to 3 quarts daily). Fluids such as weak tea, water, bouillon, clear soup, noncarbonated, caffeine-free beverages, and gelatin are usually

CLIENT TEACHING GUIDELINES
Antidiarrheal Medications

General Considerations

✔ Taking a medication to stop diarrhea is not always needed or desirable because diarrhea may mean the body is trying to rid itself of irritants or bacteria. Treatment is indicated if diarrhea is severe, prolonged, or occurs in young children or elderly adults, who are susceptible to excessive losses of body fluids and electrolytes.

✔ Try to drink approximately 2 to 3 quarts of fluid daily. This helps prevent dehydration from fluid loss in stools. Water, clear broths, and noncarbonated, caffeine-free beverages are recommended because they are unlikely to cause further diarrhea.

✔ Avoid highly spiced or "laxative" foods, such as fresh fruits and vegetables, until diarrhea is controlled.

✔ Frequent and thorough hand washing and careful food storage and preparation can help prevent diarrhea.

✔ Consult a health care provider if diarrhea is accompanied by severe abdominal pain or fever or lasts longer than 3 days, or if stools contain blood or mucus. These signs and symptoms may indicate more serious disorders for which other treatment measures are needed.

✔ Stop antidiarrheal drugs when diarrhea is controlled to avoid adverse effects such as constipation.

✔ Bismuth subsalicylate (Pepto-Bismol) and loperamide (Imodium A-D) are available over-the-counter; difenoxin (Motofen) and diphenoxylate (Lomotil) are prescription drugs.

✔ Difenoxin, diphenoxylate, and loperamide may cause dizziness or drowsiness and should be used with caution

if driving or performing other tasks requiring alertness, coordination, or physical dexterity. In addition, alcohol and other drugs that cause drowsiness should be avoided.

✔ Pepto-Bismol may temporarily discolor bowel movements a grayish-black.

✔ Keep antidiarrheal drugs out of reach of children. Accidental overdose of Motofen may cause fatal respiratory depression.

Self- or Caregiver Administration

✔ Take or give antidiarrheal drugs only as prescribed or directed on nonprescription drug labels.

✔ Do not exceed maximal daily doses of diphenoxylate (Lomotil), loperamide, difenoxin, or paregoric.

✔ With liquid diphenoxylate, use only the calibrated dropper furnished by the manufacturer for accurate measurement of dosages.

✔ With Pepto-Bismol liquid, shake the bottle well before measuring and swallowing the dose; with tablets, chew them well or allow them to dissolve in the mouth.

✔ Add at least 30 mL of water to each dose of paregoric to help the drug dose reach the stomach. The mixture appears milky.

✔ Take cholestyramine or colestipol with at least 4 oz of water. These drugs should never be taken without fluids because they may block the gastrointestinal tract. Also, do not take within approximately 4 hours of other drugs because they may combine with and inactivate other drugs.

---

tolerated and helpful. If the client cannot tolerate adequate amounts of oral liquids or if diarrhea is severe or prolonged, intravenous fluids may be needed (ie, solutions containing dextrose, sodium chloride, and potassium chloride).

• Avoid foods and fluids that may further irritate GI mucosa (eg, highly spiced foods or "laxative" foods, such as raw fruits and vegetables).

• Increase frequency and length of rest periods, and decrease activity. Exercise and activity stimulate peristalsis.

• If perianal irritation occurs because of frequent liquid stools, cleanse the area with mild soap and water after each bowel movement, then apply an emollient, such as white petrolatum (Vaseline).

Evaluation

• Observe and interview for decreased number of liquid or loose stools.

• Observe for signs of adequate food and fluid intake (eg, good skin turgor and urine output, stable weight).

• Observe for appropriate use of antidiarrheal drugs.

• Observe and interview for return of prediarrheal patterns of bowel elimination.

• Interview regarding knowledge and use of measures to prevent or minimize diarrhea.

PRINCIPLES OF THERAPY

Drug Selection

Choice of antidiarrheal agent depends largely on the cause, severity, and duration of diarrhea.

1. For symptomatic treatment of diarrhea, difenoxin with atropine (Motofen), diphenoxylate with atro-

pine (Lomotil), or loperamide (Imodium) is probably the drug of choice for most people.

2. In bacterial gastroenteritis or diarrhea, choice of antibacterial drug depends on the causative microorganism and susceptibility tests.

3. In ulcerative colitis, sulfonamides, adrenal corticosteroids, and other anti-inflammatory agents are the drugs of choice.

4. In antibiotic-associated colitis, stopping the causative drug is the initial treatment. If symptoms do not improve within 3 or 4 days, oral metronidazole or vancomycin is given for 7 to 10 days. Both are effective against *C. difficile*, but metronidazole is the drug of first choice and is much less expensive. Vancomycin may be given for severe disease or when metronidazole is ineffective. For approximately 6 weeks after recovery, relapse often occurs and requires retreatment. Because relapse is not due to emergence of drug-resistant strains, the same drug used for the initial bout may be used to treat the relapse.

5. In diarrhea caused by enzyme deficiency, pancreatic enzymes are given rather than antidiarrheal drugs.

6. In bile salt diarrhea, cholestyramine or colestipol may be effective.

7. Although morphine and codeine are contraindicated in chronic diarrhea, they may occasionally be used in the treatment of acute, severe diarrhea. Dosages required for antidiarrheal effects are smaller than those required for analgesia. The following oral drugs and dosages are approximately equivalent in antidiarrheal effectiveness: 4 mg morphine, 30 mg codeine, 10 mL paregoric, 5 mg diphenoxylate, and 2 mg loperamide.

Use in Children

Antidiarrheal drugs, including antibiotics, are often used in children to prevent excessive losses of fluids and electrolytes. In small children, fluid volume deficit may rapidly develop with diarrhea. Drug therapy should be accompanied by appropriate fluid replacement and efforts to decrease further stimuli.

Difenoxin and **diphenoxylate** contain atropine, and signs of atropine overdose may occur with usual doses. Difenoxin and diphenoxylate are contraindicated in children younger than 2 years of age; **loperamide** is contraindicated in children younger than 6 years. Loperamide is a nonprescription drug. See Table 62-1 for doses.

Use in Older Adults

Diarrhea is less common than constipation in older adults, but it may occur from laxative abuse and bowel

cleansing procedures before GI surgery or diagnostic tests. Fluid volume deficits may rapidly develop in older adults with diarrhea. General principles of fluid and electrolyte replacement, measures to decrease GI irritants, and drug therapy apply as for younger adults. Most antidiarrheal drugs may be given to older adults, but cautious use is indicated to avoid inducing constipation.

Use in Renal Impairment

Difenoxin and diphenoxylate should be used with extreme caution in clients with severe hepatorenal disease because hepatic coma may be precipitated.

Use in Hepatic Impairment

Difenoxin and diphenoxylate should be used with extreme caution in clients with abnormal liver function test results or severe hepatorenal disease because hepatic coma may be precipitated. With loperamide, monitor clients with hepatic impairment for signs of central nervous system toxicity. Loperamide normally undergoes extensive first-pass metabolism, which may be lessened by liver disease. As a result, a larger portion of a dose reaches the systemic circulation and may cause adverse effects. Dosage may need to be reduced.

Nursing Notes: Apply Your Knowledge

Mrs. Greta Riley, a 72-year-old resident of the retirement center where you work as the nurse, comes in to see you. She states, "My bowels have been in an uproar for over 3 weeks. First I had terrible constipation and had to use all sorts of laxatives to get me cleaned out. Now I seem to be having just the opposite problem. What kind of medication can I take for the diarrhea?"

 Home Care

Prescription and over-the-counter antidiarrheal aids are often taken in the home setting. The role of the home care nurse may include advising clients and caregivers about appropriate use of the drugs, trying to identify the cause and severity of the diarrhea (ie, risk of fluid and electrolyte deficit), and teaching strategies to manage the current episode and prevent future episodes. If octreotide is taken at home, the home care nurse may need to teach the client and a caregiver how to administer subcutaneous injections.

NURSING
ACTIONS **Antidiarrheals**

NURSING ACTIONS	RATIONALE/EXPLANATION
1. Administer accurately	
a. With liquid diphenoxylate, use only the calibrated dropper furnished by the manufacturer for measuring dosage.	For accurate measurement
b. Add at least 30 mL of water to each dose of paregoric. The mixture appears milky.	To add sufficient volume for the drug to reach the stomach
c. Do not exceed maximal daily doses of diphenoxylate, loperamide, difenoxin, and paregoric. Also, stop the drugs when diarrhea is controlled.	To decrease risks of adverse reactions, including drug dependence
d. Give cholestyramine and colestipol with at least 120 mL of water. Also, do not give within approximately 4 h of other drugs.	The drugs may cause obstruction of the gastrointestinal (GI) tract if swallowed in a dry state. They may combine with and inactivate other drugs.
2. Observe for therapeutic effects	
a. Decreased number, frequency, and fluidity of stools	Therapeutic effects are usually evident within 24 to 48 h.
b. Decreased or absent abdominal cramping pains	
c. Signs of normal fluid and electrolyte balance (adequate hydration, urine output, and skin turgor)	
d. Resumption of usual activities of daily living.	
3. Observe for adverse effects	
a. Constipation	Constipation is the most common adverse effect. It can be prevented by using antidiarrheal drugs only as prescribed and stopping the drugs when diarrhea is controlled.
b. Drug dependence	Dependence is unlikely with recommended doses but may occur with long-term use of large doses of paregoric, diphenoxylate, and difenoxin.
c. With diphenoxylate, anorexia, nausea, vomiting, dizziness, abdominal discomfort, paralytic ileus, toxic megacolon, hypersensitivity (pruritus, urticaria, angioneurotic edema), headache, and tachycardia	Although numerous adverse reactions have been reported, their incidence and severity are low when diphenoxylate is used appropriately.
With overdoses of a diphenoxylate-atropine or difenoxin–atropine combination, respiratory depression and coma may result from diphenoxylate or difenoxin content and anticholinergic effects (eg, dry mouth, blurred vision, urinary retention) from atropine content	Deliberate overdose and abuse are unlikely because of unpleasant anticholinergic effects. Overdose can be prevented by using the drug in recommended doses and only when required. Overdose can be treated with naloxone (Narcan) and supportive therapy.
d. With loperamide, abdominal cramps, dry mouth, dizziness, nausea, and vomiting	Abdominal cramps are the most common adverse effect. No serious adverse effects have been reported with recommended doses of loperamide. Overdose may be treated with naloxone, gastric lavage, and administration of activated charcoal.

(continued)

NURSING ACTIONS	RATIONALE/EXPLANATION
e. With cholestyramine and colestipol, constipation, nausea, and abdominal distention	Adverse effects are usually minor and transient because these drugs are not absorbed from the GI tract.
f. With octreotide, diarrhea, headache, cardiac dysrhythmias, and injection site pain	These are commonly reported adverse effects.
4. Observe for drug interactions	Few clinically significant drug interactions have been reported with commonly used antidiarrheal agents.
a. Drugs that *increase* effects of antidiarrheal agents:	
(1) Central nervous system (CNS) depressants (alcohol, sedative–hypnotics, opioid analgesics, antianxiety agents, antipsychotic agents)	Additive CNS depression with opiate and related antidiarrheals. Opioid analgesics have additive constipating effects.
(2) Anticholinergic agents (atropine and synthetic anticholinergic antispasmodics; antihistamines and antidepressants with anticholinergic effects)	Additive anticholinergic adverse effects (dry mouth, blurred vision, urinary retention) with diphenoxylate–atropine (Lomotil) and difenoxin–atropine (Motofen)

How Can You Avoid This Medication Error?

Answer: If Jan has received six 2.5-mg tablets of Lomotil she has had a total of 15 mg, which is still under the 24-hour limit of Lomotil that was ordered (20 mg). You can safely give her another dose as ordered. Clarify the frequency specified in this order (after every bowel movement). In following this order, you might repeat doses before the previous dose has had a chance to absorb and work.

Nursing Notes: *Apply Your Knowledge*

Answer: First ask Mrs. Riley about her normal bowel pattern and her usual management strategies. Sometimes people think it is very important to have a bowel movement every day; thus, they take laxatives when they perceive they are constipated. Overuse or inappropriate use of laxatives can cause diarrhea. Treatment of this diarrhea can cause constipation, creating a cycle of bowel dysfunction. Try education first, explaining the importance of exercise and fiber in the diet. A bulk-forming laxative can be helpful in re-establishing a more regular bowel pattern. Unless the diarrhea is severe, causing significant fluid loss and impaired ability to carry on daily activities, antidiarrheal medications should be avoided.

REVIEW AND APPLICATION EXERCISES

1. What are some common causes of diarrhea?
2. In which populations is diarrhea most likely to cause serious problems?
3. Which types of diarrhea do not require antidiarrheal drug therapy, and why?
4. How do antidiarrheal drugs decrease frequency or fluidity of stools?
5. What are adverse effects of commonly used antidiarrheal drugs?
6. If a client asked you to recommend an over-the-counter antidiarrheal agent, which would you recommend, and why?
7. Would your recommendation differ if the proposed recipient were a child? Why or why not?

SELECTED REFERENCES

Bonis, P.A. & Plaut, A.G. (1997). Gastrointestinal infections. In W.N. Kelley (Ed.), *Textbook of internal medicine*, 3rd ed., pp. 752–761. Philadelphia: Lippincott-Raven.

Brunton, L.L. (1996). Agents affecting gastrointestinal water flux and motility; emesis and antiemetics; bile acids and pancreatic enzymes. In J.G. Hardman, L.E. Limbird, P.B. Molinoff, & R.W. Ruddon (Eds.), *Goodman & Gilman's The pharmacological basis of therapeutics*, 9th ed., pp. 917–936. New York: McGraw-Hill.

Drug facts and comparisons. (Updated monthly). St. Louis: Facts and Comparisons.

George, W.L. & Finegold, S.M. (1997). Clostridial infections. In W.N. Kelley (Ed.), *Textbook of internal medicine*, 3rd ed., pp. 1673–1678. Philadelphia: Lippincott-Raven.

Longe, R.L. & DiPiro, J.T. (1997). Diarrhea and constipation. In J.T. DiPiro, R.L. Talbert, G.C. Yee, G.R. Matzke, B.G. Wells, & L.M. Posey (Eds.), *Pharmacotherapy: A pathophysiologic approach*, 3rd ed., pp. 767–783. Stamford, CT: Appleton & Lange.

McCray, W., Jr. & Krevsky, B. (1999). Diarrhea in adults: When is intervention necessary? *Hospital Medicine, 35*(1): 39–46. [On-line: Available http://www.medscape.com/quadrant/HospitalMedicine/1999/v35.n01/hm3501.03.mccr/hm3501.03.mccr-01.html. Accessed December, 1999.]

Porth, C.M. (1998). Alterations in gastrointestinal function. In C.M. Porth (Ed.). *Pathophysiology: Concepts of altered health states*, 5th ed., pp. 719–744. Philadelphia: Lippincott Williams & Wilkins.

Powell, D.W. (1997). Approach to the patient with diarrhea. In W.N. Kelley (Ed.), *Textbook of internal medicine*, 3rd ed., pp. 617–632. Philadelphia: Lippincott-Raven.

Smeltzer, S.C. & Bare, B.G. (1996). *Brunner and Suddarth's Textbook of medical-surgical nursing*, 8th ed. Philadelphia: Lippincott-Raven.

63

Antiemetics

Objectives

After studying this chapter, the student will be able to:

1. Identify clients at risk of developing nausea and vomiting.

2. Discuss guidelines for preventing, minimizing, or treating nausea and vomiting.

3. Differentiate the major types of antiemetic drugs.

4. Discuss characteristics, effects, and nursing process implications of selected antiemetic drugs.

Kelly Morgan, a 44-year-old woman, is having elective abdominal surgery. In the past, she has experienced significant postoperative nausea. Her physician orders lorazepam (Ativan), prochlorperazine (Compazine), and metoclopramide (Reglan) on a PRN basis to treat postoperative nausea and vomiting.

Reflect on:

▶ Factors that contribute to nausea and vomiting for the postoperative client.

▶ How each ordered antiemetic works to decrease nausea and vomiting.

▶ Why more than one antiemetic is ordered.

▶ How you will make decisions regarding what antiemetic medications to give Ms. Morgan.

NAUSEA AND VOMITING

Antiemetic drugs are used to prevent or treat nausea and vomiting. *Nausea* is an unpleasant sensation of abdominal discomfort accompanied by a desire to vomit. *Vomiting* is the expulsion of stomach contents through the mouth. Nausea may occur without vomiting, and vomiting may occur without prior nausea, but the two symptoms most often occur together.

Nausea and vomiting are common symptoms experienced by virtually everyone. These symptoms may accompany almost any illness or stress situation. Causes of nausea and vomiting include the following:

1. Systemic illness or infection
2. Gastrointestinal (GI) infection or inflammation (eg, any portion of the GI tract, liver, gallbladder, or pancreas)
3. Impaired GI motility and muscle tone (eg, gastroparesis)
4. Overeating or ingestion of foods or fluids that irritate the GI mucosa
5. Drug therapy. Nausea and vomiting are the most common adverse reactions to drug therapy. Although the symptoms may occur with most drugs, they are especially associated with alcohol, aspirin, digoxin, anticancer drugs, antimicrobials, estrogen preparations, and opioid analgesics.
6. Pain and other noxious stimuli, such as unpleasant sights and odors
7. Emotional disturbances, physical or mental stress
8. Radiation therapy
9. Motion sickness
10. Postoperative status, which may include pain, impaired GI motility, and receiving various medications

Vomiting occurs when the vomiting center in the medulla oblongata is stimulated. Stimuli may be relayed to the vomiting center from peripheral (eg, gastric mucosa, peritoneum, intestines, joints) and central (eg, cerebral cortex, vestibular apparatus of the ear, and neurons in the fourth ventricle, called the *chemoreceptor trigger zone* [CTZ]) sites. The vomiting center, CTZ, and GI tract contain benzodiazepine, cholinergic, dopamine, histamine, opiate, and serotonin receptors, which are stimulated by emetogenic drugs and toxins circulating in blood and cerebrospinal fluid. In motion sickness, rapid changes in body motion stimulate receptors in the inner ear (vestibular branch of the auditory nerve, which is concerned with equilibrium), and nerve impulses are transmitted to the CTZ and the vomiting center. When stimulated, the vomiting center initiates efferent impulses that cause closure of the glottis, contraction of abdominal muscles and the diaphragm, relaxation of the gastroesophageal sphincter, and reverse peristalsis, which moves stomach contents toward the mouth for ejection.

ANTIEMETIC DRUGS

Drugs used in nausea and vomiting belong to several different therapeutic classifications, and most have anticholinergic, antidopaminergic, antihistaminic, or antiserotonergic effects. In general, the drugs are more effective in prophylaxis than treatment. Most antiemetics prevent or relieve nausea and vomiting by acting on the vomiting center, CTZ, cerebral cortex, vestibular apparatus, or a combination of these. Major drugs are described in the following sections and in Table 63-1.

Phenothiazines

Phenothiazines, of which chlorpromazine (Thorazine) is the prototype, are central nervous system depressants used in the treatment of psychosis and psychotic symptoms in other disorders (see Chap. 9). These drugs have widespread effects on the body. Their therapeutic effects in psychosis and vomiting are attributed to their ability to block dopamine from receptor sites in the brain (antidopaminergic effects). When used as antiemetics, phenothiazines act on the CTZ and the vomiting center. Not all phenothiazines are effective antiemetics.

Phenothiazines are usually effective in preventing or treating nausea and vomiting induced by drugs, radiation therapy, surgery, and most other stimuli, but are usually ineffective in motion sickness. Drowsiness usually occurs with these drugs.

Antihistamines

Antihistamines (eg, hydroxyzine) are used primarily to prevent histamine from exerting its widespread effects on body tissues (see Chap. 48). Antihistamines used as antiemetic agents are the "classic" antihistamines or H_1 receptor blocking agents (as differentiated from cimetidine and related drugs, which are H_2 receptor blocking agents). The drugs are thought to relieve nausea and vomiting by blocking the action of acetylcholine in the brain (anticholinergic effects). Antihistamines are particularly effective in preventing and treating motion sickness. Not all antihistamines are effective as antiemetic agents.

Corticosteroids

Although corticosteroids are used mainly as antiallergic, anti-inflammatory, and antistress agents (see Chap. 24), they have antiemetic effects as well. The mechanism by which the drugs exert antiemetic effects is unknown. Dexamethasone and methylprednisolone are commonly used in the management of chemotherapy-induced emesis, usually in combination with one or more other antiemetic

TABLE 63-1   Antiemetic Drugs

Generic/Trade Name	Routes and Dosage Ranges	
	Adults	Children
Phenothiazines		
Chlorpromazine (Thorazine)	PO 10–25 mg q4–6h IM 25 mg q3–4h until vomiting stops, followed by oral administration if necessary Rectal suppository 50–100 mg q6–8h	PO, IM 0.5 mg/kg q4–6h as needed Rectal suppository 1 mg/kg q6–8h Not recommended for children <6 mo
Perphenazine (Trilafon)	PO 8–16 mg daily in divided doses IM 5 mg as a single dose	Dosage not established
Prochlorperazine (Compazine)	PO 5–10 mg three or four times daily (sustained-release capsule, 10 mg twice daily) IM 5–10 mg q3–4h to a maximum of 40 mg daily Rectal suppository 25 mg twice daily	>10 kg: PO 0.4 mg/kg/d, in three or four divided doses IM 0.2 mg/kg as a single dose Rectal suppository 0.4 mg/kg/d, in three or four divided doses
Promethazine (Phenergan)	PO, IM, rectal suppository 12.5-25 mg q4-6h	>3 mo: PO, IM, rectal suppository 0.25–0.5 mg/kg q4–6h
Thiethylperazine (Torecan)	PO, IM, rectal suppository 10–30 mg/d in divided doses	Dosage not established
Triflupromazine (Vesprin)	PO 20–30 mg/d IM 5–15 mg q4–6h; maximal dose, 60 mg/d IV 1–3 mg as a single dose	>2 y: PO, IM 0.2 mg/kg/d in three divided doses; maximal daily dose, 10 mg
Antihistamines		
Buclizine (Bucladin-S)	Motion sickness, PO 50 mg 30 min before departure and 4–6 h later, if needed; maintenance dose, 50 mg twice daily	Dosage not established
Cyclizine (Marezine)	Motion sickness, PO 50 mg 30 min before departure, then q4–6h as needed, to a maximal daily dose of 200 mg IM 50 mg q4–6h as needed	6–12 y: Motion sickness, PO 25 mg up to three times daily (maximal daily dose 75 mg)
Dimenhydrinate (Dramamine)	PO 50–100 mg q4–6h as needed (maximal dose, 400 mg in 24 h) IM 50 mg as needed IV 50 mg in 10 mL of sodium chloride injection, over 2 min	6–12 y: PO 25–50 mg q6–8h (maximal dose, 150 mg in 24 h) IM 1.25 mg/kg four times daily (maximal dose, 300 mg in 24 h)
Diphenhydramine (Benadryl)	PO 25–50 mg three or four times daily as needed IV, deep IM 10–50 mg (maximal single dose, 100 mg; maximal dose in 24 h, 400 mg)	>9 kg: PO 12.5–25 mg three or four times daily (maximal dose 300 mg in 24 h) IV, deep IM 5 mg/kg/24 h in four divided doses (maximal dose, 300 mg in 24 h)
Hydroxyzine (Vistaril)	IM 25–100 mg q4–6h as needed	IM 0.5 mg/lb q4–6h as needed
Meclizine (Antivert, Bonine)	Motion sickness, PO 25–50 mg 1 h before travel Vertigo, PO 25–100 mg daily in divided doses	Dosage not established
Prokinetic Agent		
Metoclopramide (Reglan)	PO 10 mg 30 min before meals and at bedtime for 2–8 wk IV 2 mg/kg 30 min before injection of cisplatin and 2 h after injection of cisplatin, then 1–2 mg/kg q2–3h if needed, up to four doses	Dosage not established
5-HT$_3$ (Serotonin) Receptor Antagonists		
Dolasetron (Anzemet)	Prevention of PONV, PO 100 mg 2 h before surgery Prevention or treatment of PONV, IV 12.5 mg as a single dose, 15 min before cessation of anesthesia or as soon as nausea or vomiting develops	2–16 y: Prevention of PONV, PO 1.2 mg/kg within 2 h before surgery. Maximum dose, 100 mg Prevention or treatment of PONV, IV 0.35 mg/kg as a single dose, 15 min before cessation of anesthesia or as soon

TABLE 63-1 **Antiemetic Drugs** (*continued*)

Generic/Trade Name	Routes and Dosage Ranges	
	Adults	Children
	Prevention of chemotherapy-induced nausea and vomiting, PO 100 mg within 1 h before chemotherapy; IV 1.8 mg/kg as a single dose approximately 30 min before chemotherapy	as nausea or vomiting develops. Maximum dose, 12.5 mg Prevention of chemotherapy-induced nausea and vomiting, PO 1.8 mg/kg within 1 h before chemotherapy, maximum dose, 100 mg; IV 1.8 mg/kg as a single dose approximately 30 min before chemotherapy, maximum dose 100 mg
Granisetron (Kytril)	Cancer chemotherapy, PO 1 mg twice daily, first dose approximately 1 h before emetogenic drug, second dose 12 h later, only on days receiving chemotherapy; IV 10 μ/kg infused over 5 min, 30 min before emetogenic drug, only on days receiving chemotherapy	2–16 y: IV 10 μg/kg
Ondansetron (Zofran)	Cancer chemotherapy, PO 8 mg 30 min before emetogenic drug, repeat in 8 h, then 8 mg q12h for 1–2 d IV 0.15 mg/kg for three doses (first 30 min before emetogenic drug, then at 4 and 8 h after the first dose) or a single dose of 32 mg 30 min before emetogenic drug PONV, PO 16 mg 1 h before anesthesia or IV 4 mg just before anesthesia or postoperatively	Cancer chemotherapy, ≥12 y: PO 8 mg; 4–11 y: PO 4 mg 30 min before emetogenic drug, repeat in 4 and 8 h, then q8h for 1–2 d 4–18 y: IV 0.15 mg/kg for three doses as for adults 2–12 y: ≤40 kg: IV 0.1 mg/kg; >40 kg: IV 4 mg as a single dose
Miscellaneous Agents		
Dronabinol (Marinol)	PO 5 mg/m² (square meter of body surface area) 1–3 h before chemotherapy, then q2–4h for a total of four to six doses daily. Dosage can be increased by 2.5 mg/m² increments to a maximal dose of 15 mg/m² if necessary.	Same as adults for treatment of chemotherapy-induced nausea and vomiting
Phosphorated carbohydrate solution (Emetrol)	PO 15–30 mL repeated at 15-min intervals until vomiting ceases	PO 5–10 mL repeated at 15-min intervals until vomiting ceases
Scopolamine (Transderm Scop)	Motion sickness, PO, SC, 0.6–1 mg/kg as a single dose Transdermal disc (1.5 mg scopolamine) placed behind the ear every 3 d if needed	Motion sickness, PO, SC 0.006 mg as a single dose

IM, intramuscular; IV, intravenous; PO, oral; PONV, postoperative nausea and vomiting; SC, subcutaneous.

agents. Regimens vary from a single dose before chemotherapy to doses every 4 to 6 hours for 24 to 48 hours. With this short-term use, adverse effects are mild (eg, euphoria, insomnia, mild fluid retention).

Benzodiazepine Antianxiety Drugs

These drugs (see Chap. 8) are not antiemetics, but they are often used in multidrug regimens to prevent nausea and vomiting associated with cancer chemotherapy. They produce sedation and relaxation, especially in clients who experience anticipatory nausea and vomiting before administration of anticancer drugs. Lorazepam (Ativan) is commonly used.

5-Hydroxytryptamine₃ (Serotonin) Receptor Antagonists

Ondansetron, **granisetron**, and **dolasetron** are used to prevent or treat postoperative and chemotherapy-induced nausea and vomiting. Some anticancer drugs apparently cause nausea and vomiting by combining with a subset of serotonin (5-hydroxytryptamine or 5-HT) receptors located centrally in the CTZ and peripherally on vagal nerve endings. The drugs antagonize 5-HT₃ receptors and prevent their activation by emetogenic anticancer drugs. It is unknown whether the drugs' antiemetic effects are central, peripheral, or both. The drugs may be given intravenously or orally, and are metabolized in the liver. Adverse effects are usually mild to moderate, and the most common ones reported in clinical trials were diarrhea, headache, constipation, and transient elevation of liver enzymes.

Miscellaneous Antiemetics

Dronabinol is a cannabinoid (derivative of marijuana) used in the management of nausea and vomiting associated with anticancer drugs and unrelieved by other drugs. Dronabinol may cause the same adverse effects as marijuana, including psychiatric symptoms, has a high potential for abuse, and may cause a withdrawal syndrome when abruptly discontinued. As a result, it is a Schedule II drug under federal narcotic laws.

Metoclopramide (Reglan) is a prokinetic agent that increases GI motility and the rate of gastric emptying by increasing the release of acetylcholine from nerve endings in the GI tract (peripheral cholinergic effects). As a result, it can decrease nausea and vomiting associated with gastroparesis and other nonobstructive disorders characterized by gastric retention of food and fluids. Metoclopramide also has central antiemetic effects; it antagonizes the action of dopamine, a catecholamine neurotransmitter. Metoclopramide is given orally in diabetic gastroparesis and esophageal reflux. Large doses of the drug are given intravenously during chemotherapy with cisplatin (Platinol) and other emetogenic antineoplastic drugs.

Phosphorated carbohydrate solutions (Emetrol, Nausetrol) are hyperosmolar carbohydrate solutions with phosphoric acid. They are thought to exert a direct local action on the wall of the GI tract, reducing smooth muscle contraction. These preparations are available over-the-counter.

Scopolamine, an anticholinergic drug (see Chap. 21), is effective in relieving nausea and vomiting associated with motion sickness. A transdermal patch is often used to prevent seasickness.

Indications for Use

Antiemetic drugs are indicated to prevent and treat nausea and vomiting associated with surgery, pain, motion sickness, cancer chemotherapy, radiation therapy, and other causes. Phenothiazines, because of their relatively high incidence and severity of adverse effects, are indicated only when other antiemetic drugs are ineffective or when only a few doses are expected to be required.

Contraindications to Use

Antiemetic drugs are usually contraindicated when their use may prevent or delay diagnosis, when signs and symptoms of drug toxicity may be masked, and for routine use to prevent postoperative vomiting.

NURSING PROCESS

Assessment

Assess for nausea and vomiting.

- Identify risk factors (eg, digestive or other disorders in which nausea and vomiting are symptoms; drugs associated with nausea and vomiting).
- Interview regarding frequency, duration, and precipitating causes of nausea and vomiting. Also, question the client about accompanying signs and symptoms, characteristics of vomitus (amount, color, odor, presence of abnormal components, such as blood), and any measures that relieve nausea and vomiting. When possible, observe and measure the vomitus.

Nursing Diagnoses

- Fluid Volume Deficit related to uncontrolled vomiting
- Altered Nutrition: Less Than Body Requirements related to impaired ability to ingest and digest food
- Altered Tissue Perfusion: Hypotension related to fluid volume depletion or antiemetic drug effect
- Risk for Injury related to adverse drug effects
- Knowledge Deficit related to nondrug measures to reduce nausea and vomiting
- Knowledge Deficit related to appropriate use of antiemetic drugs

Planning/Goals

The client will:

- Receive antiemetic drugs at appropriate times, by indicated routes
- Take antiemetic drugs as prescribed for outpatient use
- Obtain relief of nausea and vomiting
- Eat and retain food and fluids
- Have increased comfort
- Maintain body weight
- Maintain normal bowel elimination patterns
- Have fewer vomiting episodes and less discomfort with cancer chemotherapy

Interventions

Use measures to prevent or minimize nausea and vomiting:

- Assist clients to identify situations that cause or aggravate nausea and vomiting.
- Avoid exposure to stimuli when feasible (eg, unpleasant sights and odors; excessive ingestion of food, alcohol, or nonsteroidal anti-inflammatory drugs).

CLIENT TEACHING GUIDELINES
Antiemetic Drugs

General Considerations

✔ Try to identify the circumstances that cause or aggravate nausea and vomiting and avoid them when possible.

✔ Drugs are more effective in preventing nausea and vomiting than in stopping them. Thus, they should be taken before the causative event when possible.

✔ Do not eat, drink, or take oral medications during acute vomiting episodes to avoid aggravating the stomach upset.

✔ Lying down may help nausea and vomiting to subside; activity tends to increase stomach upset.

✔ Once your stomach has settled down, try to take enough fluids to prevent dehydration and potentially serious problems. Tea, broth, and Jello are usually tolerated.

✔ Do not drive an automobile or operate dangerous machinery if drowsy from antiemetic drugs to avoid injury.

✔ If taking antiemetic drugs regularly, do not drink alcohol or take other drugs without consulting a health care provider. Several drugs interact with antiemetic agents to increase adverse effects.

✔ Dronabinol, which is derived from marijuana and recommended only for nausea and vomiting unrelieved by other medications, can cause dizziness, drowsiness, mood changes, and other mind-altering effects. You should avoid alcohol and other drugs that cause drowsiness. Also, do not drive or perform hazardous tasks requiring alertness, coordination, or physical dexterity to decrease risks of injury.

Self- or Caregiver Administration

✔ Take the drugs as prescribed: do not increase dosage, take more often, or take when drowsy, dizzy, or unsteady on your feet. Several of the drugs cause sedation and other adverse effects, which are likely to be more severe if too much is taken.

✔ To prevent motion sickness, take medication approximately 30 minutes before travel and then every 4 to 6 hours, if necessary, to avoid or minimize adverse effects.

✔ Take or give antiemetic drugs approximately 30 to 60 minutes before a nausea-producing event, when possible. This includes cancer chemotherapy, radiation therapy, painful dressings, or other treatments.

✔ Take dronabinol only when you can be supervised by a responsible adult because of its sedative and mind-altering effects.

- Because pain may cause nausea and vomiting, administration of analgesics before painful diagnostic tests and dressing changes or other therapeutic measures may be helpful.

- Administer antiemetic drugs approximately 30 to 60 minutes before a nausea-producing event (eg, radiation therapy, cancer chemotherapy, or travel), when possible.

- Many oral drugs cause less gastric irritation, nausea, and vomiting if taken with or just after food. For any drug likely to cause nausea and vomiting, check reference sources to determine whether it can be given with food without altering beneficial effects.

- When nausea and vomiting occur, assess the client's condition and report to the physician. In some instances, a drug (eg, digoxin, an antibiotic) may need to be discontinued or reduced in dosage. In other instances (eg, paralytic ileus, GI obstruction), preferred treatment is restriction of oral intake and nasogastric intubation.

- Eating dry crackers before rising in the morning may help prevent nausea and vomiting associated with pregnancy.

- Avoid oral intake of food, fluids, and drugs during acute episodes of nausea and vomiting. Oral intake may increase vomiting and risks of fluid and electrolyte imbalances.

- Avoid activity during acute episodes of nausea and vomiting. Lying down and resting quietly are often helpful.

Give supportive care during vomiting episodes:

- Give replacement fluids and electrolytes. Offer small amounts of food and fluids orally when tolerated and according to client preference.

- Record vital signs, intake and output, and body weight at regular intervals if nausea or vomiting occurs frequently.

- Decrease environmental stimuli when possible (eg, noise, odors). Allow the client to lie quietly in bed when nauseated. Decreasing motion may decrease stimulation of the vomiting center in the brain.

- Help the client rinse his or her mouth after vomiting. This decreases the bad taste and corrosion of tooth enamel by gastric acid.

- Provide requested home remedies when possible (eg, a cool, wet washcloth to the face and neck).

Evaluation

- Observe and interview for decreased nausea and vomiting.
- Observe and interview regarding ability to maintain adequate intake of food and fluids.
- Compare current weight with baseline weight.
- Observe and interview regarding appropriate use of antiemetic drugs.

PRINCIPLES OF THERAPY

Drug Selection

Choice of an antiemetic drug depends largely on the cause of nausea and vomiting and the client's condition.

1. The 5-HT$_3$ receptor antagonists (ondansetron, granisetron, and dolasetron) are usually the drugs of first choice for clients with chemotherapy-induced or postoperative nausea and vomiting.
2. Drugs with anticholinergic and antihistaminic properties are preferred for motion sickness. Antihistamines such as meclizine and dimenhydrinate are also useful for vomiting caused by labyrinthitis, uremia, or postoperative status.
3. For ambulatory clients, drugs causing minimal sedation are preferred. However, most antiemetic drugs cause some sedation in usual therapeutic doses.
4. Promethazine, a phenothiazine, is often used clinically for its antihistaminic, antiemetic, and sedative effects.
5. Although phenothiazines are effective antiemetic agents, they may cause serious adverse effects (eg, hypotension, sedation, anticholinergic effects, extrapyramidal reactions that simulate signs and symptoms of Parkinson's disease). Consequently, phenothiazines other than promethazine usually should not be used, especially for pregnant, young, elderly, and postoperative clients, unless vomiting is severe and cannot be controlled by other measures.
6. A prokinetic drug is preferred when nausea and vomiting are associated with nonobstructive gastric retention.

Dosage and Administration Factors

Dosage and route of administration depend primarily on the reason for use.

1. Doses of phenothiazines are much smaller for antiemetic effects than for antipsychotic effects.
2. Most antiemetic agents are available in oral, parenteral, and rectal dosage forms. As a general rule, oral dosage forms are preferred for prophylactic use and rectal or parenteral forms are preferred for therapeutic use.
3. Antiemetic drugs are often ordered PRN (as needed). As for any PRN drug, the client's condition should be assessed before drug administration.
4. The use of antiemetic drugs is usually short term, from a single dose to a few days.

Timing of Drug Administration

When nausea and vomiting are likely to occur because of travel, administration of emetogenic anticancer drugs, diagnostic tests, or therapeutic procedures, an antiemetic drug should be given before the emetogenic event. Pretreatment usually increases client comfort and allows use of lower drug doses. It also may prevent aspiration and other potentially serious complications of vomiting.

Chemotherapy-Induced Nausea and Vomiting

Several anticancer drugs may cause severe nausea and vomiting and much discomfort for clients. Cisplatin is one of the most emetogenic drugs. For this reason, new antiemetics are usually compared with older drugs in the treatment of cisplatin-induced nausea and vomiting. Some general guidelines for managing this difficult problem include the following:

1. Chemotherapy may be given during sleeping hours.
2. Some clients may experience less nausea and vomiting if they avoid or decrease food intake for a few hours before scheduled chemotherapy.
3. Antiemetic drugs should be given before the emetogenic drug to prevent nausea and vomiting when possible. Most often, they are given intravenously for rapid effects and continued for 2 to 3 days. Continuous intravenous infusion may be more effective than intermittent bolus injections.
4. The 5-HT$_3$ receptor antagonists (eg, ondansetron) are usually considered the most effective antiemetics. They may be given in a single daily dose.
5. Metoclopramide, given intravenously in high doses, may be used alone or in combination with various other drugs. Diphenhydramine (Benadryl) or another drug with anticholinergic effects may be given at the same time or PRN because high doses of metoclopramide often cause extrapyramidal effects (see Chap. 9).
6. Various combinations of antiemetic and sedative-type drugs are used, and research continues in this area. A commonly used regimen for prophylaxis is a corticosteroid (eg, dexamethasone 8 to 10 mg)

and a 5-HT$_3$ receptor antagonist (eg, dolasetron 1.8 mg/kg, granisetron 10 μg/kg, or ondansetron 16 to 32 mg).

Use in Children

The use of antiemetics in children is not clearly defined. Thus, antiemetic drug therapy should be cautious and limited to prolonged vomiting of known etiology.

1. With the 5-HT$_3$ receptor antagonists, safety and efficacy of granisetron and dolasetron have not been established for children younger than 2 years of age, and there is little information available about the use of ondansetron in children 3 years of age and younger.
2. Phenothiazines (eg, chlorpromazine) are more likely to cause dystonias and other neuromuscular reactions in children than in adults. Promethazine is probably preferred because its action is more like that of the antihistamines than the phenothiazines. However, promethazine should not be used in children with hepatic disease, Reye's syndrome, a history of sleep apnea, or a family history of sudden infant death syndrome. Excessive doses may cause hallucinations, convulsions, and sudden death.
3. Several antiemetics are not recommended for use in children younger than 12 years of age (eg, buclizine, cyclizine, scopolamine).
4. Dronabinol may be used to prevent or treat chemotherapy-induced nausea and vomiting in children who do not respond to other antiemetic drugs. However, the drug should be used cautiously in children because of its psychoactive effects. Dosage is the same as for adults.

Use in Older Adults

Most antiemetic drugs cause drowsiness, especially in older adults, and therefore should be used cautiously.

Nursing Notes: Apply Your Knowledge

Sally Roberts is being treated in an outpatient chemotherapy unit. She will be receiving cisplatin, a very emetogenic chemotherapeutic drug. The following drugs have been ordered IV 30 minutes before her treatment: ondansetron (Zofran), metoclopramide (Reglan), and lorazepam (Ativan). Explain the rationale for these orders.

Efforts should be made to prevent nausea and vomiting when possible. Older adults are at risk of fluid volume depletion and electrolyte imbalances with vomiting.

Dronabinol should be used cautiously because older adults are usually more sensitive to the drug's psychoactive effects than young or middle-aged adults.

Use in Renal Impairment

Several drugs are commonly used for clients with renal impairment who have nausea and vomiting.

1. Metoclopramide dosage should be reduced in clients with severe renal impairment to decrease adverse effects. With metoclopramide, drowsiness and extrapyramidal effects commonly occur in clients with end-stage renal disease (ESRD).
2. Phenothiazines are metabolized primarily in the liver and dosage reductions are not usually needed for clients with renal impairment. However, these drugs have anticholinergic effects and can cause urinary retention and orthostatic hypotension. They also can cause extrapyramidal symptoms and sedation in clients with ESRD.

Use in Hepatic Impairment

Most antiemetic drugs are metabolized in the liver and should be used cautiously in clients with impaired hepatic function.

1. With oral ondansetron, do not exceed an 8-mg dose; with intravenous use, a single, maximal daily dose of 8 mg infused over 15 minutes is recommended. With granisetron, no dosage reduction is recommended for clients with hepatic impairment.
2. Phenothiazines are metabolized in the liver and eliminated in urine. In the presence of liver disease (eg, cirrhosis, hepatitis), metabolism may be slowed and drug elimination half-lives prolonged, with resultant accumulation and increased risk of adverse effects. Thus, the drugs should be used cautiously in clients with hepatic impairment. Cholestatic jaundice has been reported with promethazine.
3. Dronabinol normally undergoes extensive first-pass hepatic metabolism to active and inactive metabolites. Resultant plasma levels consist of approximately equal portions of the parent drug and the main active metabolite. In addition, the drug is eliminated mainly by biliary excretion, over several weeks. Thus, long-term use at recommended doses may lead to accumulation of toxic amounts of the drug and its metabolite, even in clients with normal liver function.

In clients with hepatic impairment, more of the parent drug and less of the active metabolite are likely to reach the bloodstream. Thus, therapeutic and adverse effects are less predictable. Also, impaired liver function can decrease metabolism and excretion in bile so that accumulation is likely and adverse effects may be increased and prolonged. The drug should be used very cautiously, if at all, in clients with moderate to severe hepatic impairment.

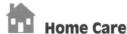 **Home Care**

Antiemetics are usually given orally or by rectal suppository in the home setting. The home care nurse may need to assess clients for possible causes of nausea and vomiting and assist clients and caregivers with appropriate use of the drugs and other interventions to prevent fluid and electrolyte depletion. Teaching safety precautions with sedating drugs may also be needed.

NURSING ACTIONS Antiemetics

NURSING ACTIONS	RATIONALE/EXPLANATION
1. Administer accurately	
a. For prevention of motion sickness, give antiemetics approximately 30 min before travel and q3–4h, if necessary.	To allow time for drug dissolution and absorption
b. For prevention of vomiting with cancer chemotherapy and radiation therapy, give antiemetic drugs 30–60 min before treatment.	Drugs are more effective in preventing than in aborting nausea and vomiting.
c. Inject intramuscular antiemetics deeply into a large muscle mass (eg, gluteal area).	To decrease tissue irritation.
d. As a general rule, do not mix parenteral antiemetics in a syringe with other drugs.	To avoid physical incompatibilities
e. Omit antiemetic agents and report to the physician if the client appears excessively drowsy or is hypotensive.	To avoid potentiating adverse effects and central nervous system (CNS) depression
f. Mix intravenous (IV) ondansetron in 50 mL of 5% dextrose or 0.9% sodium chloride injection and infuse over 15 min	
g. Mix granisetron in 20–50 mL of 5% dextrose or 0.9% sodium chloride injection and infuse over 5 min	
h. With dolasetron:	
(1) Give oral drug 1–2 h before chemotherapy; give IV drug about 30 min before chemotherapy	For oral administration to clients who cannot swallow tablets, dolasetron injection can be mixed in apple or apple–grape juice. Specific instructions should be obtained from a pharmacy. When kept at room temperature, the diluted product should be used within 2 h.
(2) Give IV drug (up to 100-mg dose) by direct injection over 30 sec or longer or dilute up to 50 mL with 0.9% sodium chloride, 5% dextrose, or 5% dextrose and 0.45% sodium chloride and infuse over 15 min	
2. Observe for therapeutic effects	
a. Verbal reports of decreased nausea	
b. Decreased frequency or absence of vomiting	

(continued)

NURSING ACTIONS	RATIONALE/EXPLANATION

3. Observe for adverse effects

a. Excessive sedation and drowsiness

Excessive sedation may occur with usual therapeutic doses of antiemetics and is more likely to occur with high doses. This may be minimized by avoiding high doses and assessing the client for responsiveness before each dose.

b. Anticholinergic effects—dry mouth, urinary retention

These effects are common to many antiemetic agents and are more likely to occur with large doses.

c. Hypotension, including orthostatic hypotension

Most likely to occur with phenothiazines

d. Extrapyramidal reactions—dyskinesia, dystonia, akathisia, parkinsonism

These disorders may occur with phenothiazines and metoclopramide. They are more likely to occur when phenothiazines are used as antipsychotics rather than as antiemetics.

e. With dronabinol, observe for alterations in mood, cognition, and perception of reality, depersonalization, dysphoria, drowsiness, dizziness, anxiety, tachycardia, and conjunctivitis. Also, a withdrawal syndrome (eg, irritability, insomnia, restlessness) may occur within 12 h of abruptly stopping the drug, with peak intensity within approximately 24 h (with hot flashes, sweating, rhinorrhea, loose stools, hiccups, anorexia) and dissipation within approximately 96 h.

According to the manufacturer, these adverse effects are well tolerated. Tachycardia may be prevented with a beta-adrenergic blocking drug, such as propranolol (Inderal).

Withdrawal symptoms are most likely to occur with high doses or prolonged use. Sleep disturbances may persist for several weeks.

4. Observe for drug interactions

a. Drugs that *increase* effects of antiemetic agents:

(1) CNS depressants (alcohol, sedative-hypnotics, anti-anxiety agents, other antihistamines or antipsychotic agents)

Additive CNS depression

(2) Anticholinergics (eg, atropine)

Additive anticholinergic effects. Some phenothiazines and antiemetic antihistamines have strong anticholinergic properties.

(3) Antihypertensive agents

Additive hypotension

Nursing Notes: Apply Your Knowledge

Answer: When giving very emetogenic drugs, it is important to use antiemetics preventively. The drugs are most effective when given before the onset of nausea. Because gastrointestinal absorption is often variable, the IV route is preferred in this situation to obtain adequate effects before treatment is started. The antiemetics work in different ways, so they can be used in combination aggressively to treat chemotherapy-induced nausea and vomiting.

 REVIEW AND APPLICATION EXERCISES

1. List common causes of nausea and vomiting or circumstances in which nausea and vomiting often occur.
2. How do antiemetic drugs prevent or relieve nausea and vomiting?
3. What are adverse effects of commonly used antiemetics?
4. Are antiemetics more effective if given before, during, or after nausea and vomiting?

5. Which antiemetics are often given to control nausea and vomiting that occur with certain antineoplastic drugs?

SELECTED REFERENCES

Brunton, L.L. (1996). Agents affecting gastrointestinal water flux and motility; emesis and antiemetics; bile acids and pancreatic enzymes. In J.G. Hardman, L.E. Limbird, P.B. Molinoff, & R.W. Ruddon (Eds.), *Goodman & Gilman's The pharmacological basis of therapeutics*, 9th ed., pp. 917–936. New York: McGraw-Hill.

Drug facts and comparisons. (Updated monthly). St. Louis: Facts and Comparisons.

Hasler, W.L. (1997). Approach to the patient with nausea and vomiting. In W.N. Kelley (Ed.), *Textbook of internal medicine*, 3rd ed., pp. 608–617. Philadelphia: Lippincott-Raven.

Miguel, R. (1999). Supportive care: Controlling chemotherapy-induced and postoperative nausea and vomiting. *Journal of the Moffitt Cancer Center, 6*, 393–397. [Online: Available http://www.medscape.com/moffitt/CancerControl/1999/v06.n04/cc0604.12.migu/cc0604.12.migu-01.html. Accessed December 1999.]

Porth, C.M. (1998). Alterations in gastrointestinal function. In C.M. Porth (Ed.), *Pathophysiology: Concepts of altered health states*, 5th ed., pp. 719–744. Philadelphia: Lippincott Williams & Wilkins.

Taylor, A.T. & Holland, E.G. (1997). Nausea and vomiting. In J.T. DiPiro, R.L. Talbert, G.C. Yee, G.R. Matzke, B.G. Wells, & L.M. Posey (Eds.), *Pharmacotherapy: A pathophysiologic approach*, 3rd ed., pp. 751–765. Stamford, CT: Appleton & Lange.

Wadibia, E.C. (1999). Antiemetics. *Southern Medical Journal, 92*, 161–165. [Online: Available http://www.medscape.com/SMA/SMJ/1999/v92.n02/smj9202.01.wadi/smj9202.01.wadi-01.html. Accessed December 1999.]

Drugs Used in Special Conditions

64

Drugs Used in Oncologic Disorders

Objectives

After studying this chapter, the student will be able to:

1. Contrast normal and malignant cells.

2. Describe major types of antineoplastic drugs in terms of mechanism of action, indications for use, administration, and nursing process implications.

3. Discuss the rationales for using chemotherapeutic drugs in combination with each other, with surgical treatment, and with radiation therapy.

4. Discuss common and potentially serious adverse drug effects.

5. Describe pharmacologic and nonpharmacologic interventions to prevent or minimize adverse drug effects.

6. Promote reduction of risk factors for development of cancer and early recognition of cancer signs and symptoms.

7. Manage or assist clients/caregivers in managing symptoms associated with chemotherapy regimens.

Georgia Sommers, a 39-year-old mother of four, is diagnosed with breast cancer that was detected by routine mammography. She is recovering from a modified radical mastectomy when she comes to your clinic to discuss additional chemotherapy treatment with the oncologist. He explains that she will receive combination therapy with three drugs on a cycle of every 4 weeks.

Reflect on:

▶ Possible reactions of Ms. Sommers to a diagnosis of cancer. What is the role of the nurse during the period of initial diagnosis?

▶ How will you assess Ms. Sommers' concerns regarding chemotherapy?

▶ What are the benefits of combination (using more than one drug) therapy?

▶ What impact do you think chemotherapy might have on Ms. Sommers' ability to function normally?

Oncology is the study of malignant neoplasms and their treatment. Drugs used in oncologic disorders include cytotoxic and hormonal antineoplastic agents, which are used to prevent or retard tumor growth. In addition, some drugs are used to prevent or treat adverse effects of cytotoxic chemotherapy (eg, myelosuppression, nausea and vomiting). The focus of this chapter is antineoplastic drugs; most others are discussed elsewhere and are included here only in relation to their use in oncology.

Antineoplastic drug therapy, commonly called *chemotherapy*, is a major treatment modality for cancer. It may cure some malignancies and is important in the treatment of many others. To participate effectively in cancer chemotherapy, nurses must know the characteristics of normal and malignant cells and of antineoplastic drugs.

CHARACTERISTICS OF NORMAL CELLS

Normal cells undergo an orderly process of replication and differentiation into cells that perform specialized functions:

- They reproduce in a predetermined sequence of events. The normal cell cycle is the interval between the "birth" of a cell and its division into two daughter cells (Fig. 64-1), which may then enter the resting phase (G_0) or proceed through the reproductive cycle.
- They reproduce in response to a need (eg, growth or tissue repair) and stop reproduction when the need has been met.
- They are well differentiated in appearance and function. Thus, they can be examined under a microscope and the tissue of origin can be determined.

CHARACTERISTICS OF MALIGNANT NEOPLASMS

Malignant neoplasms and *cancer* are terms used to describe many disease processes with a few common characteristics and many different etiologies, clinical manifestations, and treatments. In general, it takes years for malignant cells to produce a clinically detectable tumor. Factors influencing the growth rate include blood and nutrient supply, immune response, and hormonal stimulation (eg, in tumors of the breast, uterus, ovary, and prostate). Neoplastic disease can be described as a disorder of cell growth, replication, maturation, and death.

A cancer develops from a single normal cell that is transformed into a malignant cell. The transformation may begin with a random mutation (abnormal structural changes in the genetic material of a cell). A mutated cell

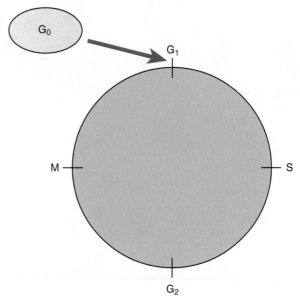

FIGURE 64–1 Normal cell cycle. The normal cell cycle (the interval between the birth of a cell and its division into two daughter cells) involves several phases. During the resting phase (G_0), cells perform all usual functions except replication; that is, they are not dividing but are capable of doing so when stimulated. Different types of cells spend different lengths of time in this phase, after which they either reenter the cell cycle and differentiate or die. During the first active phase (G_1), ribonucleic acid (RNA) and enzymes required for production of deoxyribonucleic acid (DNA) are developed. During the next phase (S), DNA is synthesized for chromosomes. During G_2, RNA is synthesized, and the mitotic spindle is formed. Mitosis occurs in the final phase (M). The resulting two daughter cells may then enter the resting phase (G_0) or proceed through the reproductive cycle.

may be destroyed by body defenses (eg, an immune response), or it may replicate. During succeeding cell divisions, additional changes and mutations may produce cells with progressively fewer normal and more malignant characteristics. Malignant cells differ from normal cells in several ways, including the following:

- Although they reproduce in the same sequence, the restraints (eg, contact with other cells) that stop the growth of normal cells are not effective with malignant cells and they grow in an uncontrolled fashion. They do not differentiate, mature, or function like normal cells, and they can proliferate indefinitely (ie, do not die when they normally would).
- They serve no useful purpose in the body. Instead, they occupy space and act as parasites by taking blood and nutrients away from normal tissues.
- They are anaplastic or undifferentiated, which means they have lost the structural and functional characteristics of the cells from which they originated. During diagnosis, malignant tumors are graded according to the degree of malignancy. Grades 1 and 2 are similar to the normal tissue of origin and show cellular differentiation. Grades 3 and 4 are unlike the normal tissue of origin, less differentiated, and more malignant.

- They cause disease when they destroy healthy tissues and eventually cause death unless effective treatment intervenes. Malignant cells grow in the tissue of origin and invade normal adjacent structures, including blood vessels and lymphatic channels, partly by producing enzymes that destroy host tissues.
- They also break away from the primary tumor, enter blood and lymph vessels, and circulate through the body. The cells cause new tumor growth when they lodge in a blood vessel and penetrate the blood vessel walls and surrounding tissues. Metastatic cells also spread from blood vessels to lymph channels, especially in tissues with a rich lymphatic network (eg, breast). During diagnosis, malignant tumors are staged according to tissue involvement (ie, whether localized or metastasized and which organs are involved), to identify tumors amenable to surgical or radiation therapy.

Etiology

Despite extensive study, the cause of cancer is not clear. Because cancer is actually many diseases, many etiologic factors are probably involved. The factors that initiate the transformation of a single normal cell into a malignant cell and allow tumor growth are complex and overlapping.

One theory of carcinogenesis involves abnormal genes and cells, in which cancer may be caused by mutation of genes (abnormal structural changes in cellular genetic material), abnormal activation of genes that regulate cell growth and mitosis, or lack of tumor suppressor genes. The abnormal genes, called *oncogenes*, are mutations of normal growth-regulating genes called protooncogenes, which are present in all body cells. Normally, proto-oncogenes are active for a brief period in the cell reproductive cycle. When exposed to carcinogens and genetically altered to oncogenes, however, they may operate continuously and cause abnormal, disordered, and unregulated cell growth. Unregulated cell growth and proliferation increases the probability of neoplastic transformation of the cell. Tumors of the breast, colon, lung, and bone have been linked to activation of oncogenes.

Tumor suppressor genes (antioncogenes) normally function to regulate and inhibit inappropriate cellular growth and proliferation. Abnormal tumor suppressor genes (ie, absent, damaged, mutated, or inactivated) may be inherited or result from exposure to carcinogens. When these genes are inactivated, a block to cellular proliferation is removed and the cells begin unregulated growth.

One tumor suppressor gene, p53, is present in virtually all normal tissues. When cellular deoxyribonucleic acid (DNA) is damaged, the p53 gene prevents cells from entering the S phase of the cell cycle. This action allows time for DNA repair and restricts proliferation of cells with abnormal DNA.

The p53 gene is deleted or mutated in most cases of colorectal cancer and often in cancers of the breast, lung, brain, and bone. Mutations of this gene are thought to be the most common genetic change in human cancers. Mutant p53 proteins can also form complexes with normal p53 proteins and thereby inactivate the function of the normal suppressor gene.

Thus, activation of oncogenes and inactivation of antioncogenes probably both play roles in cancer development. Multiple genetic abnormalities are usually characteristic of cancer cells and may occur concurrently or sequentially.

Most cancers (approximately 80%) are thought to be environmental in origin. Carcinogens and risk factors that predispose people to the development of cancer are described in Box 64-1.

Classification of Malignant Neoplasms

Malignant neoplasms are classified in several different ways according to the type of tissue involved, the rate of growth, and other characteristics. With the exception of the acute leukemias, they are considered chronic diseases. These diseases can be broadly categorized as hematologic or solid neoplasms.

Hematologic Malignancies
Hematologic malignancies involve the bone marrow and lymphoid tissues; they include leukemias, lymphomas, and multiple myeloma.

Leukemias are cancers of the bone marrow characterized by overproduction of abnormal white blood cells that range from very primitive and immature to nearly normal. The abnormal cells cannot defend the body against microorganisms and tissue injuries. They also decrease production of normal red blood cells, white blood cells, and platelets and infiltrate other organs.

Leukemias are classified according to the type of abnormal white blood cell. Acute leukemias involve more immature and less functional cells; chronic leukemias involve cells that are more nearly normal and somewhat functional. The four main types of leukemia are acute lymphocytic leukemia, which is more common in children; acute myelogenous leukemia, which occurs in all ages but more often in young adults; chronic lymphocytic leukemia, which is more common in elderly people; and chronic myelogenous leukemia, which is more common in middle age.

Lymphomas are tumors of lymphoid tissue characterized by abnormal proliferation of the white blood cells normally found in lymphoid tissue. They usually develop within lymph nodes and may occur anywhere, because virtually all body tissues contain lymphoid structures. They develop as a solid tumor mass, impair immunity, and

BOX 64–1   CARCINOGENS AND RISK FACTORS

Cancer development is thought to involve complex interactions among environmental factors and host factors in at least two stages. The initiation stage involves exposure of normal cells to carcinogens that cause a permanent change in cell structure and produce premalignant tissues (eg, cigarette smoke). The promotion stage involves agents that are not carcinogenic in themselves, but that cause additional damage to the cells altered by initiation (eg, hormones).

Overall, evidence indicates that neoplastic transformation is a progressive process involving several generations of cells, with each new generation becoming more like malignant cells. Thus, malignancy probably results from a combination of factors experienced over a person's lifetime. One factor may be a chance circumstance during which a cell mutation occurs. However, it seems clear that mutations and malignancies are increased in people exposed to certain chemical, physical, or biologic factors. In addition, carcinogenic effects are usually dose dependent, with larger amounts or longer exposure increasing the risk that cancer will develop.

Environmental Carcinogens

Physical carcinogens include radiation from x-rays and ultraviolet light from sunlight, sunlamps, and tanning beds. These agents form reactive ions that can rupture deoxyribonucleic acid (DNA) strands and cause mutations by changing cell structure or causing damage that interferes with transfer of genetic information during cell reproduction. For example, people exposed to large amounts of sunlight are at high risk for development of skin cancer. Skin cancer is more likely to develop in light-skinned people; in those with dark skins, melanin pigment absorbs ultraviolet radiation and protects the skin.

Biologic carcinogens include several viruses, which have been linked to the development of leukemia and cancers of the lymph nodes, liver, pharynx, and cervix and other genitalia. Viruses inject their genes into the genetic makeup of affected host cells. Oncogenes are also thought to be present. Then, the information carried by the tumor virus and the oncogenes is transmitted to new cells produced during cell division.

Almost 40 oncogenic viruses have been identified, including human immunodeficiency virus, human papilloma viruses, herpesviruses, hepatitis B and C viruses, and retroviruses. Overall, these viruses transform cells by coding for products that either activate protooncogene functions or inhibit tumor suppressor gene functions. These events may occur only when certain other environmental or host factors are also present.

Chemical carcinogens include numerous substances that are thought to form reactive ions that bind with DNA, ribonucleic acid (RNA), or cellular proteins. After binding, they can alter the synthesis of cellular enzymes and structural proteins, which then interferes with cell replication and regulatory controls.

Industrial carcinogens include benzene (bladder cancer), hydrocarbons (lung and skin cancer), polyvinyl chloride (liver cancer), and other substances used in the production of various products. Workers who manufacture the products and people who live in the plant vicinity are most likely to be affected.

Tobacco products include numerous carcinogens and are associated with cancers of the lungs, mouth, pharynx, larynx, esophagus, and bladder. Chemicals in cigarette smoke cause most lung cancer. Although the cigarette smoker is most likely to have a smoking-related cancer, other people exposed to cigarette smoke (ie, passive smoking or breathing smoke from other peoples' cigarettes) are also at increased risk for lung cancer, and children whose parents smoke have an increased risk of brain cancer, lymphomas, and acute lymphocytic leukemia. Smokeless tobacco products, which are often used by athletes and teenage boys, are also carcinogens.

Therapeutic drugs are associated with both hematologic and solid neoplasms.

- **Antineoplastic drugs**, mainly the alkylating agents, have been associated with leukemia, lymphoma, and other cancers. When given therapeutically, the drugs damage DNA and interfere with growth or replication of tumor cells. At the same time, they may damage the DNA of normal cells and transform some of them into malignant cells. Clients who are given these drugs and survive their illness have a relatively high risk for development of leukemia for approximately 15 to 20 years. Antineoplastic drugs that cause bone marrow suppression or immunosuppression may also lead to secondary cancer.
- **Immunosuppressants**, in relation to cancer causation, have been studied mainly in renal transplant recipients, most of whom received azathioprine and corticosteroids. The subsequent risk of non-Hodgkin's lymphoma is very high and may appear within months of transplantation. Clients are also at risk for later skin cancer (eg, squamous cell carcinoma and malignant melanoma) and Kaposi's sarcoma.

Other clients on immunosuppressant drugs are at risk for lymphomas, squamous cell carcinoma of skin, and soft tissue sarcomas, but at lower rates than transplant recipients. For example, leukemia and

(continued)

BOX 64–1 **CARCINOGENS AND RISK FACTORS** (*continued*)

solid tumors have been reported in clients who took azathioprine for rheumatoid arthritis.

Overall, malignancies after immunosuppressant therapy are more related to the intensity and duration of immunosuppression than the use of particular drugs.

- **Sex hormones** are growth factors for certain cells. They bind intracellular receptor proteins that, in turn, bind directly to genes and alter genetic transcription. Some of these genes specify differentiated functions and some are involved with growth. *Estrogens* have been associated with cancer of the vagina in daughters of women who took the drugs during pregnancy and with endometrial cancer in women who took the drugs for menopausal symptoms. With breast cancer, endogenous estrogens are clearly causative, but the role of exogenous estrogens is less clear. *Oral contraceptives*, most of which contain an estrogen and a progestin, have been related to endometrial cancer and possibly to breast cancer. A *progestin* taken to prevent estrogen-induced endometrial cancer may increase risks of breast cancer.

  Androgens and anabolic steroids, especially with high doses and prolonged use, have been associated with hepatic neoplasms. Anabolic steroids, sometimes taken in large amounts for body-building purposes, may also be involved in the development of angiosarcoma.

Host Factors

Host factors include a number of physiologic characteristics and lifestyle practices that increase risks for development of cancer, including the following:

- **Age**. Except for a few early childhood cancers, the risks for development of cancer increase with age.
- **Alcohol use**. Alcohol is thought to make carcinogens (eg, those in cigarette smoke) more soluble or enhance their tissue penetration. Cancers associated with alcohol use include those of the breast, head and neck, and liver.
- **Diet**. A high-fat diet is associated with breast, colon, and prostate cancer; a low-fiber diet may increase risks of colon cancer.
- **Sex**. Men are more likely to have leukemia and cancer of the urinary bladder, stomach, and

pancreas; women are at risk of cancer of the breast, cervix, and endometrium. Lung and colon cancer occur approximately equally in both sexes.

- **Geography and ethnicity** are considered more environmental than hereditary or racial. Immigrants who adopt dietary and lifestyle habits of people in industrialized countries have similar risks of particular cancers. In addition, people who live in cities are more likely to have cancer because of greater exposure to air pollutants and other carcinogens. In the United States, African Americans have higher rates of multiple myeloma and cancers of the lung, prostate, esophagus, and pancreas than white people.
- **Heredity**. In some families, there is a strong tendency toward development of cancer. For example, close relatives of premenopausal women with breast cancer are at high risk for breast cancer. A possible explanation is that because cancers require two or more gene mutations, some mutations have already occurred, so that few more are needed for cancer development.
- **Immunosuppression**, whether caused by disease or drug therapy, is associated with an increased risk of cancer. For example, clients with acquired immunodeficiency syndrome are at risk for Kaposi's sarcoma, and clients who undergo organ transplantation and receive immunosuppressant drugs are at risk for lymphomas and skin cancers. It is believed that tumors develop when a cancer cell eludes or escapes the immune system.
- **Obesity** has been associated with breast and endometrial cancers, probably related to hormonal and metabolic abnormalities.
- **Previous cancer**. Children who survive cancer have a higher risk of other cancers, and women with cancer in one breast have a higher risk of cancer in the other breast. Secondary cancers are usually attributed to treatment of the first cancer with radiation or chemotherapy, which can damage DNA and eventually transform normal cells into malignant cells.
- **Tobacco use** is a major lifestyle risk factor for cancers of the lung, esophagus, and head and neck.

increase susceptibility to infection. As the disease progresses, the liver, spleen, bone marrow, and other organs become functionally impaired. The two main types are Hodgkin's disease and non-Hodgkin's lymphoma.

Multiple myeloma is a tumor of the bone marrow in which abnormal plasma cells proliferate. Because normal

plasma cells produce antibodies and abnormal plasma cells cannot fulfill this function, the body's immune system is impaired. As the malignant cells expand, they crowd out normal cells, interfere with other bone marrow functions, infiltrate and destroy bone, and eventually metastasize to other tissues, such as the spleen, liver, and lymph nodes.

Solid Neoplasms

Solid tumors are composed of a mass of malignant cells (parenchyma) and a supporting structure of connective tissue, blood vessels, and lymphatics (stroma). The two major classifications are carcinomas and sarcomas.

Carcinomas are derived from epithelial tissues (skin, mucous membrane, linings and coverings of viscera) and are the most common type of malignant tumors. They are further classified by cell type, such as adenocarcinoma or basal cell carcinoma.

Sarcomas are derived from connective tissue (muscle, bone, cartilage, fibrous tissue, fat, blood vessels). They are subclassified by cell type (eg, osteogenic sarcoma, angiosarcoma).

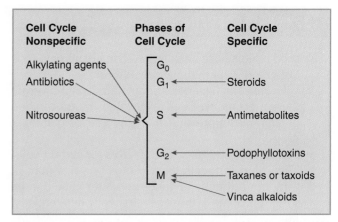

FIGURE 64–2 Cell cycle effects of cytotoxic antineoplastic drugs.

Effects of Cancer on the Host

Effects vary according to the extent and location of the disease process. There are few effects initially. As the neoplasm grows, effects occur when the tumor becomes large enough to cause pressure, distortion, or deficient blood supply in surrounding tissues; interfere with organ function; obstruct ducts and organs; and cause malnutrition of normal tissues. More specific effects include anemia, malnutrition, pain, infection, hemorrhagic tendencies, thromboembolism, hypercalcemia, cachexia, and various symptoms related to impaired function of affected organs and tissues.

ANTINEOPLASTIC DRUGS

General Characteristics

1. Many drugs damage body cells (ie, they are cytotoxic). They kill malignant cells by interfering with cell replication, which requires nutrients and genetic materials. Effective drugs interfere with the supply and use of nutrients (amino acids, purines, pyrimidines) or with the genetic materials in the cell nucleus (DNA or ribonucleic acid [RNA]).

2. The drugs act during the cell's reproductive cycle (Fig. 64-2). Some, called cell cycle specific, act mainly during specific phases such as DNA synthesis or formation of the mitotic spindle. Others act during any phase of the cell cycle and are called cell cycle nonspecific.

3. Cytotoxic drugs are most active against rapidly dividing cells, both normal and malignant. Commonly damaged normal cells are those of the bone marrow, the lining of the gastrointestinal (GI) tract, and the hair follicles.

4. Each drug dose kills a specific percentage of cells. If the drug destroys 99% of cells, it reduces 1 million cells to 10,000. Succeeding doses would destroy 99% of remaining cells. To achieve a cure, all malignant cells must be killed or reduced to a small number that can be killed by the person's immune system.

5. Antineoplastic drugs may induce drug-resistant malignant cells. Mechanisms may involve the ability of malignant cells to act on the drug (eg, by inhibiting drug uptake or activation, increasing the rate of drug inactivation, or pumping the drug out of the cell before it can act) or to act on themselves (eg, increase cellular repair of DNA damaged by the drugs or alter metabolic pathways and target enzymes of the drugs). Mutant cells also may emerge.

6. Most cytotoxic antineoplastic drugs are potential teratogens.

7. Most antineoplastic drugs are given orally or intravenously (IV); some are given topically, intrathecally, or by instillation into a body cavity.

Indications for Use

Cytotoxic antineoplastic drugs are used in the treatment of malignant neoplasms to cure the disease, relieve symptoms, or induce or maintain remissions (symptom-free periods that last for varying lengths of time). Chemotherapy is the treatment of choice for a few types of cancer, including Hodgkin's disease, leukemia, Wilms' tumor, and Ewing's sarcoma, but is less effective in cancers of the lung, colon, and prostate gland.

In hematologic neoplasms, drug therapy is the treatment of choice because the disease is systemic rather than localized. In solid tumors, drug therapy is often used before or after surgery or radiation therapy.

Antineoplastic drugs are sometimes used in the treatment of nonmalignant conditions. For example, small doses of methotrexate (MTX) are used for rheumatoid arthritis and psoriasis.

Classifications

Cytotoxic antineoplastic drugs are usually classified in terms of their mechanisms of action (alkylating agents and antimetabolites) or their sources (plant alkaloids, antibiotics). Other drugs used in chemotherapy are immunostimulants (see Chap. 44), hormones, antihormones, and cytoprotectants.

Alkylating Agents

Alkylating agents include nitrogen mustard derivatives, nitrosoureas, and platinum compounds. *Nitrogen mustard* is the prototype of the nitrogen mustard derivatives, but cyclophosphamide is the most commonly used. Because the drugs interfere with cell division and the structure of DNA during dividing and resting stages of the malignant cell cycle, they have a broad spectrum of activity. They are most effective in hematologic malignancies but also are used to treat breast, lung, and ovarian tumors. All of these drugs cause significant myelosuppression (bone marrow depression); all except nitrogen mustard may be given orally.

Nitrosoureas also interfere with DNA replication and RNA synthesis and may inhibit essential enzymatic reactions of cancer cells. They are cell cycle nonspecific and have been used in clients with GI, lung, and brain tumors. A unique feature of the drugs is their high lipid solubility, which allows them to enter the brain and cerebrospinal fluid more readily than most antineoplastic drugs. Another unique feature is that they cause delayed bone marrow depression, with maximum leukopenia and thrombocytopenia occurring approximately 5 to 6 weeks after drug administration. As a result, the drugs are given less often than other drugs, and complete blood counts (CBC) need to be done weekly for at least 6 weeks after a dose.

Platinum compounds are cell cycle–nonspecific agents that inhibit DNA, protein, and RNA synthesis. Cisplatin is widely used to treat both hematologic and solid cancers. Adverse effects are mainly GI, renal, neurologic, and otologic damage. Carboplatin is most often used to treat endometrial and ovarian carcinomas and it produces bone marrow depression as a major adverse effect.

Antimetabolites

Antimetabolites are allowed to enter cancer cells because they are similar to nutrients needed by the cells for reproduction. Once inside the cell, the drugs may substitute for a natural metabolite, occupy an enzyme-binding site, or inactivate an enzyme-binding site. These actions deprive

the cell of substances needed for formation of DNA or cause formation of abnormal DNA. The drugs are cell cycle specific because they exert their cytotoxic effects only during the S phase of the cell's reproductive cycle, when DNA is being synthesized.

This group includes a folic acid antagonist (eg, methotrexate), purine antagonists (eg, mercaptopurine), and pyrimidine antagonists (eg, fluorouracil). These drugs have been used to treat many types of cancers, but they are most effective against rapidly growing tumors, and individual drugs vary in their effectiveness with different kinds of cancer. Toxic effects mainly involve the bone marrow, GI tract, and hair follicles. Some antimetabolites can be given orally and parenterally; others are given only by one route.

Antitumor Antibiotics

These drugs (eg, doxorubicin) are active in all phases of the cell cycle and their cytotoxic effects are similar to those of the alkylating agents. They bind to DNA so that DNA and RNA transcription is blocked. Major toxicities are bone marrow depression and GI upset. Doxorubicin and related drugs also cause cardiotoxicity and tissue necrosis if extravasation occurs. Bleomycin may cause significant pulmonary toxicity. All of these drugs except bleomycin must be given IV.

Plant Alkaloids

Plant alkaloids include derivatives of camptothecin (eg, topotecan), podophyllotoxin (eg, etoposide), taxanes (eg, paclitaxel), and plants of the *Vinca* genus (eg, vincristine). These drugs vary in their characteristics and clinical uses.

Camptothecins (also called topoisomerase inhibitors) inhibit an enzyme required for DNA replication and repair. They have effects in several types of cancers, including colorectal, lung, and ovarian cancers. Dose-limiting toxicity is myelosuppression.

Podophyllotoxins act mainly in the G_2 phase of the cell cycle and prevent mitosis. Etoposide is used mainly to treat testicular and small cell lung cancer; teniposide is used mainly for childhood acute lymphocytic leukemia. Dose-limiting toxicity is myelosuppression.

Taxanes (also called taxoids) inhibit cell division (antimitotic effects). They are used mainly for advanced breast or ovarian cancers. Dose-limiting toxicity is neutropenia; other adverse effects include alopecia, mucositis, neurotoxicity, and hypersensitivity reactions.

Vinca alkaloids are cell cycle–specific agents that stop mitosis. These drugs have similar structures but different ranges of antineoplastic activity and adverse effects. Vincristine is used to treat Hodgkin's disease, acute lymphoblastic leukemia, non-Hodgkin's lymphomas, oat cell carcinoma of the lung, and Wilms' tumor. Vinblastine is used to treat Hodgkin's disease and choriocarcinoma; vinorelbine is used to treat non-small cell lung cancer. The drugs can cause severe tissue damage with extravasation (leaking of medication into soft tissues around the venipuncture site). In addition, vinblastine and vinorelbine

---

Nursing Notes: Apply Your Knowledge

Your client, Sally Moore, is receiving an antineoplastic drug that is known to cause bone marrow depression, with a nadir 12 days after administration. Discuss the effects of bone marrow depression and appropriate nursing assessments. What teaching would be appropriate for this patient?

are more likely to cause bone marrow depression, and vincristine is more likely to cause peripheral nerve toxicity.

Miscellaneous Cytotoxic Agents

Miscellaneous agents vary in their sources, mechanisms of action, indications for use, and toxic effects. L-*Asparaginase* is an enzyme that inhibits cellular protein synthesis and reproduction by depriving cells of required amino acids. The drug can cause allergic reactions and GI symptoms. *Hydroxyurea* acts in the S phase of the cell cycle to impair DNA synthesis. It is used mainly in myeloproliferative disorders such as leukemias. It may also be used to increase the sensitivity of some tumors (eg, cervix, head and neck, lung) to radiation therapy. A major adverse effect is myelosuppression. *Procarbazine* inhibits DNA, RNA, and protein synthesis. Its main use is treatment of Hodgkin's disease. It is a monoamine oxidase inhibitor and may cause hypertension if given with adrenergic drugs, tricyclic antidepressants, or foods with high tyramine content (see Chap. 10). Common adverse effects include leukopenia and thrombocytopenia.

Hormones and Hormone Inhibitors

Hormones used in cancer chemotherapy interfere with protein synthesis and attempt to stop tumor growth in hormone-dependent tissues. The goal of hormonal therapy is control of tumor growth and palliation of symptoms rather than cure. Hormones are not cytotoxic and adverse effects are usually mild.

Sex hormones (estrogens, progestins, androgens) are useful in cancers of the breast, prostate gland, and other reproductive organs. *Adrenal corticosteroids* suppress formation and function of lymphocytes and therefore are most useful in the treatment of leukemia and lymphoma. They are also used for complications of cancer (eg, intracranial metastases, hypercalcemia) and with radiation therapy to reduce radiation-related edema in the mediastinum, brain, and spinal cord. Dexamethasone is commonly used in neurologic disorders.

Hormone inhibitors include tamoxifen, an antiestrogen that competes with estrogen for binding sites in breast tissue; aminoglutethimide, an adrenocorticosteroid-inhibiting agent that produces a "medical adrenalectomy"; and goserelin and leuprolide, which inhibit testosterone secretion in advanced prostatic cancer.

INDIVIDUAL DRUGS

Cytotoxic antineoplastic drugs are listed in Table 64-1; hormones and hormone inhibitors are listed in Table 64-2.

(*text continues on page 951*)

TABLE 64-1 Cytotoxic Antineoplastic Drugs

Generic/Trade Name	Routes and Dosage Ranges*	Clinical Uses	Common or Potentially Severe Adverse Reactions
Alkylating Drugs			
NITROGEN MUSTARD DERIVATIVES			
Busulfan (Myleran)	PO 4–8 mg daily until white blood cell count decreases by half, then maintenance doses up to 4 mg daily	Chronic granulocytic leukemia	Bone marrow depression (leukopenia, thrombocytopenia, anemia), pulmonary toxicity
Chlorambucil (Leukeran)	PO 0.1–0.2 mg/kg/d for 3–6 wk. If maintenance therapy is required, 0.03–0.1 mg/kg/d	Chronic lymphocytic leukemia, non-Hodgkin's lymphomas, carcinomas of breast and ovary	Bone marrow depression, hyperuricemia
Cyclophosphamide (Cytoxan)	Induction of therapy, PO 1–5 mg/kg/d; IV 35–40 mg/kg over several days (20–30 mg/kg for clients with prior chemotherapy or radiation) Oral maintenance therapy, 1.5–2 mg/kg daily	Hodgkin's disease, non-Hodgkin's lymphomas, neuroblastoma. Often combined with other drugs for acute lymphoblastic leukemia in children, carcinomas of breast, ovary, and lung; multiple myeloma and other malignancies	Bone marrow depression, anorexia, nausea, vomiting, alopecia, hemorrhagic cystitis
Ifosfamide (Ifex)	IV 1.2 g/m^2/d for 5 consecutive d. Repeat every 3 wk or after white blood cell and platelet counts return to normal after a dose.	Germ cell testicular cancer	Bone marrow depression, hemorrhagic cystitis, nausea and vomiting
Mechlorethamine (nitrogen mustard) (Mustargen)	IV 0.4 mg/kg in one or two doses. Repeat in 3–6 wk. Intracavitary 0.4 mg/kg instilled into pleural or peritoneal cavities	Hodgkin's disease and non-Hodgkin's lymphomas, lung cancer, pleural and peritoneal malignant effusions	Bone marrow depression, nausea, vomiting. Extravasation may lead to tissue necrosis.

TABLE 64-1   **Cytotoxic Antineoplastic Drugs** (*continued*)

Generic/Trade Name	Routes and Dosage Ranges*	Clinical Uses	Common or Potentially Severe Adverse Reactions
Melphalan (Alkeran)	PO 0.25 mg/kg/d for 7 d, followed by 21 drug-free days, then maintenance dose of 2 mg daily	Multiple myeloma	Bone marrow depression, nausea and vomiting
NITROSOUREAS			
Carmustine (BCNU)	IV 200 mg/m² every 6 wk	Hodgkin's disease, malignant melanoma, multiple myeloma, brain tumors	Bone marrow depression, nausea, vomiting. Extravasation may lead to tissue necrosis.
Lomustine (CCNU)	PO 130 mg/m² every 6 wk	Hodgkin's disease, brain tumors	Bone marrow depression, nausea and vomiting
Streptozocin (Zanosar)	IV 500 mg/m² for 5 consecutive d every 6 wk	Metastatic islet cell carcinoma of pancreas	Nephrotoxicity, nausea, vomiting
PLATINUM COMPOUNDS			
Carboplatin (Paraplatin)	IV infusion 360 mg/m² over at least 15 min on day 1 every 4 wk	Palliation of ovarian cancer	Bone marrow depression, nausea and vomiting
Cisplatin (Platinol)	IV 100 mg/m² once every 4 wk	Carcinomas of testes, bladder, ovary, head and neck, and endometrium	Renal toxicity and ototoxicity
Antimetabolites			
Capecitabine (Xeloda)	PO 2500 mg/m²/d, in two divided doses, approximately 12 h apart, for 2 wk, followed by a rest period of 1 wk	Metastatic breast cancer	Anemia, lymphopenia, severe diarrhea
Cladribine (Leustatin)	IV infusion 0.09 mg/kg/d for 7 consecutive d	Hairy cell leukemia	Bone marrow depression, nausea, vomiting, fever
Cytarabine (ARA-C, cytosine arabinoside) (Cytosar-U)	IV 2 mg/kg/d for 10 d	Leukemias of adults and children	Bone marrow depression, nausea, vomiting, stomatitis, diarrhea
Floxuridine (FUDR)	Intra-arterial infusion, 0.1–0.6 mg/kg/d until toxicity occurs	Head and neck tumors, carcinomas of the GI tract, liver, pancreas, and biliary tract	Same as cytarabine, above
Fludarabine (Fludara)	IV 25 mg/m²/d for 5 consecutive d	Chronic lymphocytic leukemia	Bone marrow depression, fever, nausea, vomiting
Fluorouracil (5-FU) (Adrucil, Efudex, Fluoroplex)	IV 12 mg/kg/d for 5 d	Carcinomas of the breast, colon, rectum, stomach, and pancreas	Same as cytarabine, above
	Topical, apply to skin cancer lesion twice daily for several weeks	Solar keratoses, basal cell carcinoma	Pain, pruritus, burning at site of application
Gemcitabine (Gemzar)	IV 1000 mg/m² over 30 min once weekly. First cycle, up to 7 wk or toxicity occurs, then withhold for 1 wk. Later cycles, once weekly for 3 wk, then off for 1 wk	Pancreatic and lung cancer	Bone marrow depression, nausea, vomiting, fever, influenza-like symptoms, edema, skin rash, alopecia
Mercaptopurine (Purinethol)	PO 2.5 mg/kg/d	Acute and chronic leukemias	Bone marrow depression, nausea, hyperuricemia
Methotrexate (MTX, Amethopterin) (Mexate)	Induction of remission of acute leukemia in children PO, IV 3 mg/m²/d. Maintenance of remission, PO 30 mg/m² two times per week (combined with prednisone for induction and maintenance of remission) Choriocarcinoma, PO, IM 15 mg/m² daily for 5 d	Acute lymphoblastic leukemia in children, lymphocytic lymphoma, choriocarcinoma of the testes, osteogenic carcinoma, others	Bone marrow depression, nausea, diarrhea, stomatitis

(*continued*)

TABLE 64-1 **Cytotoxic Antineoplastic Drugs** (*continued*)

Generic/Trade Name	Routes and Dosage Ranges*	Clinical Uses	Common or Potentially Severe Adverse Reactions
Thioguanine	PO 2 mg/kg/d	Acute and chronic leukemias	Bone marrow depression, nausea
Antitumor Antibiotics			
Bleomycin (Blenoxane)	IV, IM 0.25–0.5 units/kg once or twice weekly	Squamous cell carcinoma, lymphomas, testicular carcinoma, Hodgkin's disease	Pulmonary toxicity, stomatitis, alopecia, hyperpigmentation and ulceration of skin
Dactinomycin (Actinomycin D) (Cosmegen)	IV 15 µg/kg/d for 5 d and repeated every 2–4 wk	Rhabdomyosarcoma, Wilms' tumor	Bone marrow depression, anorexia, nausea, vomiting. Extravasation may lead to tissue necrosis.
Daunorubicin hydrochloride	IV 60 mg/m² daily for 3 d every 3–4 wk	Acute granulocytic and acute lymphocytic leukemias, lymphomas	Same as doxorubicin, below
Daunorubicin (liposomal formulation) (DaunoXome)	IV infusion, 40 mg/m² over 1 h, every 2 wk, until disease progression or complications occur	AIDS-related Kaposi's sarcoma	Bone marrow depression, pain, nausea, vomiting, diarrhea, cough, fever, dyspnea, fatigue, headache
Doxorubicin (Adriamycin)	Adults, IV 60–75 mg/m² every 21 d Children, IV 30 mg/m² daily for 3 d, repeated every 4 wk	Acute leukemias, lymphomas, carcinomas of breast, lung, and ovary	Bone marrow depression, alopecia, stomatitis, GI upset, cardiomyopathy. Extravasation may lead to tissue necrosis.
Doxorubicin (liposomal formulation) (Doxil)	IV infusion, 20 mg/m² over 30 min, once every 3 wk, as long as client responds and tolerates	AIDS-related Kaposi's sarcoma	Bone marrow depression, nausea, vomiting, fever, alopecia, chest pain, weakness, skin eruptions of hands and feet
Epirubicin (Ellence)	IV infusion 120 mg/m² q 3–4 wk	Breast cancer	Cardiotoxicity
Idarubicin (Idamycin)	IV injection 12 mg/m² daily for 3 d, with concomitant cytarabine	Acute myelogenous leukemia in adults, with other antileukemic drugs	Same as doxorubicin, above
Mitomycin (Mutamycin)	IV 2 mg/m²/d or 50 µg/kg/d for 5 d, repeated after 2 d. This course of therapy may be repeated after recovery of the bone marrow.	Carcinomas of stomach, colon, rectum, pancreas, bladder, breast, lung, head and neck, and malignant melanoma	Bone marrow depression, nausea, vomiting, diarrhea, stomatitis. Extravasation may lead to tissue necrosis.
Mitoxantrone (Novantrone)	IV infusion 12 mg/m² on days 1–3, for induction	Acute nonlymphocytic leukemia	Fever, cough, dyspnea, congestive heart failure, cardiac arrhythmias, nausea, vomiting, diarrhea
Pentostatin (Nipent)	IV 4 mg/m² every other week	Hairy cell leukemia unresponsive to alpha-interferon	Bone marrow depression, hepatotoxicity, nausea, vomiting, fever, skin rash
Valrubicin (Valstar)	Intravesically, 800 mg once weekly for 6 wk	Bladder cancer	Bladder symptoms (dysuria, urgency, frequency, spasm, hematuria, pain)
Plant Alkaloids			
CAMPTOTHECINS			
Irinotecan (Camptosar)	IV infusion over 90 min, 125 mg/m² once weekly for 4 wk, followed by a 2-wk rest period	Advanced colorectal cancer that has relapsed or progressed with 5-fluorouracil therapy	Bone marrow depression, nausea, vomiting, diarrhea, abdominal cramping
Topetecan (Hycamtin)	IV infusion 1.5 mg/m² over 30 min daily for 5 consecutive days	Advanced ovarian cancer	Bone marrow depression, nausea, vomiting, diarrhea, constipation, abdominal pain, alopecia, fatigue, fever
PODOPHYLLOTOXINS			
Etoposide (VePesid)	IV 50–100 mg/m²/d on days 1–5, or 100 mg/m²/d on days 1, 3, and 5, every 3–4 wk	Testicular cancer, acute leukemias, lymphomas, small cell lung cancer	Bone marrow depression, anaphylaxis, nausea, vomiting, alopecia
Teniposide (Vumon)	IV infusion 165 mg/m² twice weekly (with cytarabine)	Acute lymphocytic leukemia in children	Same as etoposide, above

TABLE 64-1	**Cytotoxic Antineoplastic Drugs** (*continued*)		

Generic/Trade Name	Routes and Dosage Ranges*	Clinical Uses	Common or Potentially Severe Adverse Reactions
TAXANES			
Docetaxel (Taxotere)	IV 60–100 mg/m^2, infused over 1 h, every 3 wk	Advanced breast cancer	Bone marrow depression, nausea, vomiting, diarrhea, edema, hypotension, oral mucositis, changes in liver enzymes, skin rash, alopecia
Paclitaxel (Taxol)	IV 135 mg/m^2 every 3 wk	Advanced ovarian cancer	Bone marrow depression, allergic reactions, hypotension, bradycardia, peripheral neuropathy, nausea, vomiting, muscle and joint pain, alopecia
VINCA ALKALOIDS			
Vinblastine (Velban)	IV 0.1 mg/kg weekly, increased gradually by 0.05 mg/kg increments	Metastatic testicular carcinoma, Hodgkin's disease, carcinoma of breast	Bone marrow depression, especially leukopenia, neurotoxicity. Extravasation may lead to tissue necrosis.
Vincristine (Oncovin)	Adults, IV 0.01–0.03 mg/kg weekly Children, IV 0.4–1.4 mg/m^2 weekly	Hodgkin's disease and other lymphomas, acute leukemia	Neurotoxicity with possible foot drop from muscle weakness, paresthesias, constipation, and other manifestations. Extravasation may lead to tissue necrosis.
Vinorelbine (Navelbine)	IV injection 30 mg/m^2 once weekly, over 6-10 min, until disease progression or dose-limiting toxicity occurs	Non-small cell lung cancer	Bone marrow depression, peripheral neuropathy, chest pain, fatigue, nausea, alopecia
Miscellaneous Antineoplastic Agents			
L-Asparaginase (Elspar)	IV 1000 IU/kg/d for 10 d	Acute lymphocytic leukemia refractory to other drugs. Usually used in conjunction with other agents.	Abnormal functioning of the liver, kidneys, pancreas, central nervous system, and the blood clotting mechanism; hypersensitivity reactions
Hydroxyurea (Hydrea)	PO 80 mg/kg as single dose every third day or 20–30 mg/kg as a single dose daily	Chronic granulocytic leukemia, malignant melanoma	Bone marrow depression, GI upset
Levamisole (Ergamisol)	PO 50 mg every 8 h for 3 d every 2 wk for 1 y	Colon cancer, with fluorouracil	Nausea, vomiting, diarrhea, dermatitis
Mitotane (Lysodren)	PO 8–10 g daily in three to four divided doses. Maximal daily dose, 19 g	Inoperable carcinoma of the adrenal cortex	Anorexia, nausea, damage to adrenal cortex
Procarbazine (Matulane)	PO 100–200 mg/d for 1 wk, then 300 mg/d until maximal response or toxicity occurs	Hodgkin's disease	Bone marrow depression, nausea, vomiting
Rituximab (Rituxan)	IV infusion, 375 mg/m^2 once weekly for 4 doses (days 1, 8, 15, 22)	Non-Hodgkin's lymphoma	Hypersensitivity reactions, serious cardiac dysrhythmias
Temozolomide (Temodar)	PO 150 mg/m^2 once daily for 5 d, then 200 mg/m^2 every 21–28 d as tolerated	Brain tumors	Myelosuppression
Trastuzumab (Herceptin)	IV infusion, 4 mg/kg over 90 min initially, then 2 mg/kg over 30 min once weekly	Metastatic breast cancer in clients whose tumors express the HER2 protein	Cardiotoxicity (dyspnea, edema, heart failure)

* Dosages may vary significantly, according to use in different types of cancer and in different combinations. They also change frequently.
AIDS, acquired immunodeficiency syndrome; GI, gastrointestinal; IM, intramuscular; IV, intravenous; PO, oral.

TABLE 64-2 **Antineoplastic Hormones and Hormone Inhibitors**

Generic/Trade Name	Routes and Dosage Ranges	Clinical Uses	Common or Potentially Severe Adverse Reactions
Hormones			
ADRENOCORTICOSTEROID			
Prednisone (Meticorten, others)	PO 60–100 mg/m²/d for first few days, then gradual reduction to 20–40 mg/d	Used as adjunct for palliation of symptoms in acute leukemia, Hodgkin's disease, lymphomas, complications of cancer, such as thrombo-cytopenia, hypercalcemia, intracranial metastases	Potentially toxic to almost all body systems. See Chapter 24.
ANDROGENS			
Fluoxymesterone (Halotestin)	PO 10 mg three times daily (30 mg/d)	Advanced breast cancer in premenopausal women	Masculinizing effects, hyper-calcemia
Testolactone (Teslac)	PO 250 mg four times daily	Advanced breast cancer	Anorexia, nausea, vomiting, alopecia, paresthesias
ESTROGENS			
Diethylstilbestrol (DES) (Stilbestrol)	Breast cancer, PO 1–5 mg three times daily Prostate cancer, PO 1–3 mg daily	Carcinoma of prostate gland, carcinoma of breast in post-menopausal women	Feminizing effects in men, anorexia, nausea, vomiting, edema, hypercalcemia, and others. See Chapter 28.
Ethinyl estradiol (Estinyl, others)	Breast cancer, PO 0.5 mg/d ini-tially, gradually increased to 3 mg/d in three divided doses Prostate cancer, PO 0.15–2 mg daily	Carcinoma of prostate, advanced carcinoma of breast in postmenopausal women	Feminizing effects in men, anorexia, nausea, vomiting, edema, hypercalcemia, and others. See Chapter 28.
PROGESTINS			
Medroxyprogesterone (Provera, Depo-Provera)	Intramuscular 400–800 mg twice weekly PO 200–300 mg/d	Advanced endometrial carcinoma	Usually well tolerated. May cause edema and irritation at injection sites.
Megestrol (Megace)	PO 40–320 mg/d in divided doses	Advanced endometrial carci-noma, breast carcinoma	Usually produces minimal adverse reactions
Hormone Inhibitors			
ADRENOCORTICOSTEROID INHIBITOR			
Aminoglutethimide (Cytadren)	PO 250 mg four times daily	Advanced prostatic cancer	Adrenal insufficiency
ANTIANDROGENS			
Bicalutamide (Casodex)	PO 500 mg once daily (with goserelin or leuprolide)	Advanced prostatic cancer	Nausea, vomiting, diarrhea, con-stipation, hot flashes, gyneco-mastia, pain, weakness
Flutamide (Eulexin)	PO 250 mg every 8 h	Advanced prostatic cancer	Hot flashes, decreased libido, impotence, nausea, vomiting, diarrhea, hepatotoxicity
Nilutamide (Nilandron)	PO 300 mg daily for 30 d, then 150 mg daily	Advanced breast cancer in postmenopausal women with disease progression after tamoxifen therapy	Diarrhea, gastrointestinal bleed-ing, heart failure, cough, hyper-glycemia
ANTIESTROGENS			
Anastrazole (Arimidex)	PO 1 mg once daily	Advanced breast cancer in postmenopausal women with disease progression after tamoxifen therapy	Nausea, vomiting, diarrhea, con-stipation, hot flashes, gyneco-mastia, pain, weakness
Letrozole (Femara)	PO 2.5 mg once daily	Advanced breast cancer	Nausea, headache, muscle and joint discomfort
Tamoxifen (Nolvadex)	PO 20–40 mg/d in two divided doses	Advanced breast cancer in postmenopausal women	Hot flashes, nausea and vomiting, ocular toxicity
Toremifene (Fareston)	PO 60 mg once daily	Metastatic breast cancer	Hypercalcemia, tumor flare
GONADOTROPIN RELEASING HORMONE ANALOGUES (ANTITESTOSTERONE EFFECTS)			
Goserelin (Zoladex)	SC 3.6 mg every 28 d	Advanced prostatic cancer, advanced breast cancer, endometriosis	Worsening of symptoms during first few weeks, especially bone pain
Leuprolide (Lupron)	SC 1 mg/d	Advanced prostatic cancer	Same as for goserelin, above

PO, oral; SC, subcutaneous.

CYTOPROTECTANT DRUGS

Cytoprotectants reduce the adverse effects of cytotoxic drugs, which may be severe, debilitating, and life threatening to clients. Severe adverse effects may also limit drug dosage or frequency of administration, thereby limiting the effectiveness of chemotherapy.

Several cytoprotectants have been developed to protect certain body cells from one or more adverse effects and allow a more optimal dose and schedule of cytotoxic agents. To be effective, administration and scheduling must be precise in relation to administration of the cytotoxic agent. A cytoprotective agent does not prevent or treat all adverse effects of a particular cytotoxic agent and it may have adverse effects of its own.

Amifostine produces a metabolite that combines with cisplatin and ameliorates cisplatin-induced renal damage. **Dexrazoxane** decreases cardiac toxicity of doxorubicin. **Erythropoietin, filgrastim, oprelvekin,** and **sargramostim** are colony-stimulating factors (see Chap. 44) that stimulate the bone marrow to produce blood cells. Erythropoietin stimulates production of red blood cells and is used for anemia; oprelvekin stimulates production of platelets and is used to prevent thrombocytopenia; filgrastim and sargramostim stimulate production of white blood cells and are used to shorten neutropenia and the accompanying risk of severe infection. **Leucovorin** is used with high-dose MTX. **Mesna** is used with ifosfamide, which produces a metabolite that causes hemorrhagic cystitis. Mesna combines with and inactivates the metabolite and thereby decreases cystitis. Dosages and routes of administration for these medications are listed in Table 64-3.

NURSING PROCESS

Assessment

Assess the client's condition before chemotherapy is started and often during treatment. Useful information includes the type, grade, and stage of the tumor as well as the signs and symptoms of cancer. General manifestations include anemia, malnutrition, weight loss, pain, and infection; specific manifestations depend on the organs affected.

Assess for other diseases and organ dysfunctions (eg, cardiac, renal or hepatic) that influence response to chemotherapy.

Assess emotional status, coping mechanisms, family relationships, and financial resources. Anxiety and depression are common features during cancer diagnosis and treatment.

TABLE 64-3 **Cytoprotective Agents**		
Generic/Trade Name	**Clinical Uses**	**Routes and Dosage Ranges**
Amifostine (Ethyol)	Reduction of cisplatin-induced renal toxicity	IV infusion 910 mg/m^2 once daily, over 15 min, within 30 min of starting chemotherapy
Dexrazoxane (Zinecard)	Reduction of doxorubicin-induced cardiomyopathy in women with metastatic breast cancer who have received a cumulative dose of 300 mg/m^2 and would benefit from additional doxorubicin	IV 10 times the amount of doxorubicin (eg, dexrazoxane 500 mg/m^2 per doxorubicin 50 mg/m^2), then administer the doxorubicin dose within 30 min of completing administration of dexrazoxane
Erythropoietin (Epogen, Procrit)	Treatment of chemotherapy-induced anemia	SC 150 units/kg three times weekly, increased to 300 units/kg if necessary, adjusted to maintain desired hematocrit
Filgrastim (Neupogen)	Treatment of chemotherapy-induced neutropenia	SC, IV 5 μg/kg/d, at least 24 h after a dose of cytotoxic chemotherapy, up to 2 wk or an absolute neutrophil count of 10,000/mm^3
Leucovorin (Wellcovorin)	"Rescue" after high-dose methotrexate for osteosarcoma Advanced colorectal cancer, with 5-fluorouracil	"Rescue," PO, IV, IM 15 mg q6h for 10 doses, starting 24 h after methotrexate begun Colorectal cancer, IV injection, 20 mg/m^2 or 200 mg/m^2, followed by 5-fluorouracil injection, daily for 5 d, then repeated every 28 d
Mesna (Mesnex)	Prevention of ifosfamide-induced hemorrhagic cystitis	IV injection, 20% of ifosfamide dose for three doses; first dose at time of ifosfamide administration; repeat at 4 h and 8 h after ifosfamide dose (total dose, 60% of ifosfamide dose).
Oprelvekin (Neumega) Sargramostim (Leukine)	Prevention of thrombocytopenia To decrease neutropenia associated with induction chemotherapy for acute myelogenous leukemia in clients >55 y	SC 50 μg/kg once daily IV 250 μg/m^2/d, over 4 h, starting 4 d after completing induction chemotherapy

IM, intramuscular; IV, intravenous; PO, oral; SC, subcutaneous.

Assess laboratory test results before chemotherapy to establish baseline data and during chemotherapy to monitor drug effects:

- **Blood tests for tumor markers** (tumor specific antigens on cell surfaces). *Alpha-fetoprotein* is a fetal antigen normally present during intrauterine and early postnatal life but absent in adulthood. Increased amounts may indicate hepatic or testicular cancer. *Carcinoembryonic antigen (CEA)* is secreted by several types of malignant cells (eg, CEA is present in approximately 75% of people with colorectal cancer). A rising level may indicate tumor progression and levels that are elevated before surgery and disappear after surgery indicate adequate tumor excision. If CEA levels rise later, it probably indicates tumor recurrence. In chemotherapy, falling CEA levels indicate effectiveness. Other tumor markers are *immunoglobulins* (elevated levels may indicate multiple myeloma) and *prostate-specific antigen* (elevated levels may indicate prostatic cancer).
- **Complete blood cell count** to check for anemia, leukopenia, and thrombocytopenia because most cytotoxic antineoplastic drugs cause bone marrow depression. A CBC and white blood cell differential are done before each cycle of chemotherapy to determine dosage and frequency of drug administration, to monitor bone marrow function so fatal bone marrow depression does not occur, and to assist the nurse in planning care. For example, the client is very susceptible to infection when the leukocyte count is low, and bleeding is likely when the platelet count is low.
- **Other tests.** These include renal function tests, liver function tests, serum calcium, uric acid, and others, depending on the organs affected by the malignant disease or its treatment.

Nursing Diagnoses

- Pain, nausea and vomiting, and weakness related to disease process or chemotherapy
- Altered Nutrition: Less Than Body Requirements related to disease process or chemotherapy
- Activity Intolerance related to anemia and weakness from disease process or chemotherapy
- Self Care Deficit related to debilitation from disease process or chemotherapy
- Anxiety related to the disease, its possible progression, and its treatment
- Ineffective Individual Coping related to medical diagnosis of cancer
- Ineffective Family Coping related to illness and treatment of a family member
- Altered Tissue Perfusion related to anemia
- Fluid Volume Deficit related to chemotherapy-induced nausea, vomiting, and diarrhea

- Body Image Disturbance related to drug-induced alopecia
- Risk for Injury: Infection related to drug-induced neutropenia
- Risk for Injury: Bleeding related to drug-induced thrombocytopenia
- Risk for Injury: Stomatitis (mucositis) related to damage of oral mucosal cells
- Sexual Dysfunction related to adverse drug effects
- Knowledge Deficit about cancer chemotherapy

Planning/Goals

The client will:

- Receive assistance in coping with the diagnosis of cancer
- Experience reduced anxiety and fear
- Receive chemotherapy accurately
- Experience reduction of tumor size, change of laboratory values toward normal, or other therapeutic effects of chemotherapy
- Experience minimal bleeding, infection, nausea and vomiting, and other consequences of adverse drug effects
- Maintain adequate food intake and body weight
- Receive assistance in activities of daily living when needed
- Be informed about community resources for cancer care (eg, hospice, Reach to Recovery, other support groups)

Interventions

Participate in and promote efforts to prevent cancer.

- **Follow and promote the diet recommended by the American Cancer Society** (ie, decrease fat; eat five or more servings of fruits and vegetables daily; increase intake of dietary fiber; minimize intake of salt-cured or smoked foods).
- **Promote weight control in women.** Obesity may contribute to the development of breast and endometrial cancer.
- **Identify cancer-causing agents** and strategies to reduce exposure to them when possible.
- **Strengthen host defenses** by promoting a healthful lifestyle (eg, good nutrition, adequate rest and exercise, stress management techniques, avoiding or minimizing alcohol and tobacco use).
- **Avoid smoking cigarettes and being around smokers.** Passive smoking increases risk of lung cancer in spouses of smokers and risk of brain cancer, lymphomas, and acute lymphogenous leukemia in children of smokers.
- **Minimize exposure to sunlight**, use sunscreens liberally, and wear protective clothing to prevent skin cancer.

Participate in and promote cancer screening tests. Screening involves nonsymptomatic people, especially those at high risk, and the goal is to detect cancer before signs and symptoms occur. Screening tests include regular examination of breasts, testicles, and skin and tests for colon cancer such as hemoccult tests on stool, digital rectal examination, and sigmoidoscopy. The earliest possible recognition of risk factors, premalignant tissue changes (dysplasia), biochemical tumor markers, and beginning malignancies may be life saving. If not life saving, early recognition and appropriate treatment can greatly reduce the suffering and long-term consequences associated with advanced cancer.

For clients receiving cytotoxic anticancer drugs, try to prevent or minimize the incidence and severity of adverse reactions (Box 64-2).

Provide supportive care to clients and families.

- Physiologic care includes pain management, comfort measures, and assistance with nutrition, hygiene, ambulation, and other activities of daily living as needed.
- Psychological care includes allowing family members or significant others to be with the client and

participate in care when desired, and keeping clients and families informed. In addition, mental health professionals may be consulted to assist in coping with the distress that often accompanies cancer and its treatment.

Evaluation

- Monitor drug administration for accuracy.
- Observe and interview for therapeutic effects of chemotherapy.
- Compare current laboratory reports with baseline values for changes toward normal values.
- Compare weight and nutritional status with baseline values for maintenance or improvement.
- Observe and interview for adverse drug reactions and interventions to prevent or manage them.
- Observe and interview for adequate pain management and other symptom control.
- Observe and interview regarding mental and emotional status of the client and family members.
- Interview for knowledge of resources (eg, family, health care providers, hospice, others).

(text continues on page 956)

CLIENT TEACHING GUIDELINES
Managing Chemotherapy

Most chemotherapy is given intravenously, in outpatient clinics, by nurses who are specially trained to administer the medications and monitor your condition. The medications are usually given in cycles such as a few days every few weeks. There are many different chemotherapy drugs, and the ones used for a particular client depend on the type of malignancy, its location, and other factors.

The goal of chemotherapy is to be as effective as possible with tolerable side effects. Particular side effects vary with the medications used; some increase risks of infection, some cause anemia, nausea, or hair loss. All of these can be managed effectively, and several medications can help prevent or minimize side effects. Your oncologist can provide information about the specific medications planned for your treatment. In general, though, some things you can do to take care of yourself during chemotherapy are listed below.

✔ Keep all appointments for receiving chemotherapy, having blood tests, and having check-ups. This is extremely important. Chemotherapy effectiveness depends on its being given on time; blood tests help to determine when the drugs should be given and how the drugs affect your body tissues.

✔ You need to do everything you can to avoid infection, such as avoiding other people who have infections of any kind and washing your hands frequently and thoroughly. If you have a fever, chills, sore throat, or cough, notify your oncologist.

✔ Try to maintain or improve your intake of nutritious food and fluids; this will help you feel better. A dietitian can be helpful in designing a diet to meet your needs.

✔ If your chemotherapy may cause bleeding, you can decrease the likelihood by shaving with an electric razor, avoiding aspirin and other nonsteroidal anti-inflammatory drugs (including over-the-counter Advil, Aleve, and others), and avoiding injections, cuts, and other injuries when possible. If you notice excessive bruising, bleeding gums when you brush your teeth, or blood in your urine or bowel movement, notify your oncologist immediately.

✔ If hair loss is expected with the medications you take, you can use wigs, scarves, and hats. These should be purchased before starting chemotherapy, if possible. Hair loss is temporary; your hair will grow back!

✔ Inform any other physician, dentist, or health care provider that you are taking chemotherapy before any diagnostic test or treatment is begun. Some procedures may be contraindicated or require special precautions.

✔ If you are of childbearing age, effective contraceptive measures should be carried out during and a few months after chemotherapy.

✔ A few chemotherapy medications and medications to prevent or treat side effects are taken at home. Instructions for taking the drugs should be followed exactly for the most beneficial effects.

(continued)

CLIENT TEACHING GUIDELINES
Managing Chemotherapy *(continued)*

✔ Although specific instructions vary with the drugs you are taking, the following are a few precautions with some commonly used drugs:

   ✔ With **cyclophosphamide**, take the tablets on an empty stomach. If severe stomach upset occurs, take with food. Also, drink 2 or 3 quarts of fluid daily, if possible, and urinate often, especially at bedtime. If blood is seen in the urine or signs of cystitis occur (e g, burning with urination), report to a health care provider. The drug is irritating to the bladder lining and may cause cystitis. High fluid intake and frequent emptying of the bladder help to decrease bladder damage.

   ✔ With **doxorubicin**, the urine may turn red for 1 to 2 days after drug administration. This discoloration is

harmless; it does not indicate bleeding. Also, report to a health care provider if you have edema, shortness of breath, and excessive fatigue. Doxorubicin may need to be stopped if these symptoms occur.

✔ With **fluorouracil**, drink plenty of liquids while taking.

✔ With **methotrexate**, avoid alcohol, aspirin, and prolonged exposure to sunlight.

✔ With **vincristine**, eat high-fiber foods, such as raw fruits and vegetables and whole cereal grains, if you are able, to prevent constipation. Also try to maintain a high fluid intake. A stool softener or bulk laxative may be prescribed for daily use.

BOX 64–2   MANAGEMENT OF CHEMOTHERAPY COMPLICATIONS

Complications and adverse reactions may range from relatively minor to life threatening. If they cannot be prevented, they must be detected early so treatment can be started and damaging effects minimized.

■ **Nausea** and **vomiting** may occur with many antineoplastic drugs. They are usually treated with antiemetics (see Chap. 63), which are most effective when started before chemotherapy and continued on a regular schedule up to 48 hours afterward. The most effective regimen seems to be a serotonin receptor antagonist (eg, ondansetron) and a corticosteroid (eg, dexamethasone). The drugs are often given intravenously (IV), but some cancer centers are using oral drugs, which seem to be effective and are much less expensive.

   Other measures include a benzodiazepine (eg, lorazepam) for anticipatory nausea and vomiting and limiting oral intake for a few hours.

■ **Anorexia** and altered taste perception interfere with nutrition. Well-balanced meals, consisting of foods the client is able and willing to eat, are very important. Also, nutritional supplements can be used to increase intake of protein and calories. Consulting a nutritionist is advisable.

■ **Fatigue** may be profound. It is often caused or aggravated by anemia and can be prevented or treated with administration of erythropoietin. An adequate diet and light to moderate exercise, as tolerated, may also be helpful.

■ **Alopecia** occurs with several commonly used drugs, including cyclophosphamide, doxorubicin,

methotrexate, and vincristine. Complete hair loss can be psychologically devastating, especially for women. Helpful measures include the following:

   □ Warn clients before drug therapy is started. Reassure them that alopecia is temporary. Hair may grow back a different color and texture.

   □ Suggest the purchase of wigs, hats, and scarves before hair loss is expected to occur.

   □ Suggest that clients use a mild shampoo approximately twice a week and avoid rollers, hair dryers, permanent waves, hair coloring, and other hair treatments that damage the hair and may affect the degree of hair loss.

   □ Allow clients to express feelings about the altered body image.

■ **Mucositis** (stomatitis) occurs often with the antimetabolites, antibiotics, and plant alkaloids and usually lasts 7 to 10 days. It may interfere with nutrition; lead to oral ulcerations, infections, and bleeding; and cause pain. Nurse or client interventions to minimize or treat stomatitis include:

   □ Brush the teeth at least twice daily with a soft toothbrush. Stop if the platelet count drops below 20,000/mm^3 because gingival bleeding is likely. Teeth may then be cleaned with soft, sponge-tipped devices or cotton-tipped applicators.

   □ Floss teeth daily with unwaxed floss. Stop if the platelet count drops below 20,000/mm^3 to prevent gingival bleeding.

   □ Rinse the mouth several times daily, especially before meals (to decrease unpleasant taste and

(continued)

BOX 64–2   MANAGEMENT OF CHEMOTHERAPY COMPLICATIONS (*continued*)

increase appetite) and after meals (to remove food particles that promote growth of micro-organisms). One suggested solution is 1 tsp of table salt and 1 tsp of baking soda in 1 quart of water; others include chlorhexidine, 15 to 30 mL swish and spit three times daily, and the combination of equal parts of diphenhydramine elixir, normal saline, and 3% hydrogen peroxide.

- Encourage the client to drink fluids. Systemic dehydration and local dryness of the oral mucosa contribute to the development and progression of mucositis. Pain and soreness contribute to dehydration. Fluids usually tolerated include tea, carbonated beverages, ices (eg, popsicles), and plain gelatin desserts. Fruit juices may be diluted with water, ginger ale, Sprite, or 7-Up to decrease pain, burning, and further tissue irritation. Drinking fluids through a straw may be more comfortable, because this decreases contact of fluids with painful ulcerations.
- Encourage the client to eat soft, bland, cold, nonacidic foods. Although individual tolerances vary, it is usually better to avoid highly spiced or rough foods.
- Remove dentures entirely or for at least 8 hours daily because they may irritate oral mucosa.
- Inspect the mouth daily for signs of inflammation and lesions.
- Give medications for pain. Local anesthetic solutions, such as viscous lidocaine, can be used approximately 15 minutes before meals to make eating more comfortable. Because the mouth and throat are anesthetized, swallowing and detecting the temperature of hot foods may be difficult, and aspiration or burns may occur. Doses should not exceed 15 mL every 3 hours or 120 mL in 24 hours. If systemic analgesics are used, they should be given approximately 30 to 60 minutes before eating.
- In oral infections resulting from stomatitis, local or systemic antimicrobial drugs are used. Fungal infections with *Candida albicans*, which are common, can be treated with antifungal tablets, suspensions, or lozenges. Severe infections may require systemic antibiotics, depending on the causative organism as identified by cultures of mouth lesions.

■ **Infection** is common because the disease and its treatment lower host resistance to infection.

- Help the client maintain a well-balanced diet. Oral hygiene before meals and analgesics when appropriate may increase food intake. High-protein, high-calorie foods and fluids can be given between

meals. Several types of nutritional supplements are available commercially and can be taken with or between meals. Provide fluids with high nutritional value (eg, milkshakes or nutritional supplements) rather than coffee, tea, or carbonated beverages if the client can tolerate them and has an adequate intake of water and other fluids.

- Instruct and assist the client to avoid exposure to infection by avoiding crowds, anyone with a known infection, and contact with fresh flowers, soil, animals, or animal excrement.
- Frequent and thorough hand washing by the client and everyone involved in his or her care is probably the best way to reduce exposure to pathogenic microorganisms.
- The client should take a bath daily and put on clean clothes. In addition, the perineal area should be washed with soap and water after each urination or defecation.
- When venous access devices are used, take care to prevent them from becoming sources of infection. For implanted catheters, for example, inspect and cleanse around exit sites according to agency policies and procedures. Use strict sterile technique when changing dressings or flushing the catheters. For peripheral venous lines, the same principles of care apply, except that sites should be changed approximately every 3 days or if signs of phlebitis occur.
- Avoid indwelling urinary catheters when possible. If they are necessary, cleanse the perineal area with soap and water at least once daily and provide sufficient fluids to ensure an adequate urine output.
- If fever occurs, especially in a neutropenic client, possible sources of infection are usually cultured and antibiotics initiated immediately.
- Severe neutropenia can be prevented or its extent and duration minimized by administering filgrastim or sargramostim to stimulate the bone marrow to produce leukocytes. A protective environment may be needed to decrease exposure to pathogens.

■ **Bleeding** may be caused by thrombocytopenia and may occur spontaneously or with minor trauma. Precautions should be instituted if the platelet count drops to 50,000/mm^3 or below. Measures to avoid bleeding include:

- Giving oprelvekin to stimulate platelet production and prevent thrombocytopenia.
- Avoiding trauma, including venipuncture and injections when possible.
- Using an electric razor for shaving.

(continued)

BOX 64–2 MANAGEMENT OF CHEMOTHERAPY COMPLICATIONS (*continued*)

□ Checking skin, urine, and stool for blood.

□ For platelet counts less than 20,000/mm³, stop brushing the teeth.

□ Giving platelet transfusions. These are less likely to be needed if oprelvekin is used.

- **Extravasation.** Several cytotoxic drugs (called *vesicants*) cause severe inflammation, pain, ulceration, and tissue necrosis if extravasation occurs. Thus, efforts are needed to prevent extravasation if possible or to minimize tissue damage if it occurs.

□ Identify clients at risk for extravasation injuries, including those who are unable to communicate (eg, sedated clients, infants), have vascular impairment (eg, from multiple attempts at venipuncture), or have obstructed venous drainage after axillary node surgery.

□ Be especially cautious with the anthracyclines (doxorubicin and related drugs) and the vinca alkaloids (vincristine and related drugs). Choose peripheral IV sites carefully, avoiding veins that are small, located in an edematous extremity, or located near a joint. Inject the drugs slowly (1 to 2 mL at a time) into the tubing of a rapidly running IV infusion, for rapid dilution and detection of extravasation. Observe the venipuncture site for swelling and ask the client about pain or burning. After a drug has been injected, continue the rapid flow rate of the IV fluid for 2 to 5 minutes to flush the vein thoroughly.

If using a central IV line, do not give the drug unless patency is indicated by a blood return. Using a central line does not eliminate the risk of extravasation.

□ When extravasation occurs, the drug should be stopped immediately. Techniques to decrease tissue damage include aspirating the drug (approximately 5 mL of blood, if able) through the IV catheter before it is removed, elevating the involved extremity, and applying warm (with dacarbazine, etoposide, vinblastine, and vincristine) or cold compresses (with daunorubicin and doxorubicin). In addition, antidotes may be injected (hyaluronidase 1 to 6 mL, 150 units/mL, subcutaneously [SC] around the area for vincristine and related drugs; sodium thiosulfate, IV or SC, for cisplatin, dacarbazine, and paclitaxel). There is no antidote available for antibiotics such as doxorubicin. Nurses involved in chemotherapy must know the procedure to be followed if extravasation occurs so it can be instituted immediately.

- **Hyperuricemia** results from rapid breakdown or destruction of malignant cells, whether it occurs spontaneously or as a result of antineoplastic drugs. Uric acid crystals can cause kidney damage. Interventions to minimize nephropathy include a high fluid intake, with IV fluids if necessary, and a high urine output; alkalinizing the urine with sodium bicarbonate or other agents; and giving allopurinol to inhibit uric acid formation.

PRINCIPLES OF THERAPY

Overview of Cancer Treatment

Most cancer treatment is multimodal, involving surgery, radiation therapy, and chemotherapy, and using more than one modality effectively treats most cancers. Optimal treatment regimens, best designed by oncologists, should maximize effectiveness (eg, attempt to eradicate tumor cells at primary, regional, and systemic sites) and minimize morbidity (eg, pain, disfigurement, and treatment-associated toxicity).

Surgical Treatment

Surgical resection is often used to treat malignant disease. One use is excision of small, localized tumors, which may effect a cure. Another use is in conjunction with radiation therapy or chemotherapy. For example, tumors of the breast, lung, head and neck, and others that are locally advanced and not considered resectable may become resectable after treatment with radiation therapy, chemo-

therapy, or both. Such use may reduce the size of the primary tumor, allow less extensive tissue excision, and promote organ preservation and function. At the same time, however, radiation therapy may require that surgery be delayed until erythema and edema subside and chemotherapy may delay postoperative healing and increase postoperative complications. Thus, overall, surgical risks are greater in clients who have received preoperative radiation therapy or chemotherapy. Radiation therapy and chemotherapy are also used after surgery to eliminate or reduce systemic spread. A third use of surgery is to treat complications of cancer, such as bowel obstruction.

Radiation Therapy

Radiation therapy is used to treat most types of tumor and has become more important as increased knowledge and improved techniques have made it more effective and less toxic. It may be used alone to cure some malignancies such as Hodgkin's disease or cervical cancer. It may be used in combination with surgery to reduce the need for radical surgery. For example, in breast cancer, excision of the tumor (called a *lumpectomy*) plus radiation therapy is as effective as mastectomy. With soft tissue sarcomas of the limbs, wide excision plus radiation therapy can be used instead of amputation. Radiation is also used to eliminate local or regional malignant cells (eg, positive lymph nodes) that remain after surgery.

Radiation is also used with cytotoxic chemotherapy to cure or control growth of malignant tumors. Some drugs (eg, cisplatin, fluorouracil, hydroxyurea) increase the likelihood of cure with various neoplasms. Some cancers (eg, esophageal, bladder, unresectable lung cancers) can be more effectively treated with the combination than with radiation alone.

Finally, radiation therapy is often used as a palliative treatment in metastatic disease, such as relieving symptoms in clients with bone or brain involvement.

Cytotoxic Chemotherapy

Chemotherapy regimens should be managed by medical oncologists experienced in use of the drugs and knowledgeable about new drugs and treatment protocols. In addition, the consequences of inappropriate or erroneous drug therapy may be fatal for clients (from the disease or the treatment). Chemotherapy is most effective when started before extensive tumor growth or when the tumor burden has been reduced by surgical excision or radiation therapy.

Adjuvant and Palliative Chemotherapy

Chemotherapy used after surgery or radiation is called *adjuvant chemotherapy*, and is given to destroy or reduce microscopic metastases and prolong survival or decrease symptoms. Adjuvant therapy is often used in the treatment of clients with carcinomas of the breast, colon, lung, ovaries, or testes.

Drug therapy also is used in advanced malignant disease for palliation of symptoms and treatment or prevention of severe complications of cancer (eg, bowel obstruction). Once metastasized, solid tumors become systemic diseases and are not accessible to surgical excision or radiation therapy.

Drug Selection

Choice of antineoplastic drugs depends largely on which drugs have been effective in similar types of cancer. Other factors to be considered include primary tumor sites, presence and extent of metastases, physical status of the client, and other disease conditions that affect chemotherapy, such as liver or kidney disease.

Dosage Factors

Dosage must be calculated and regulated carefully to avoid unnecessary toxicity. The client's age, nutritional status, blood count, kidney and liver function, and previous chemotherapy or radiation therapy must be considered. Additional guidelines include the following:

1. High doses, to the limits of tolerance of normal tissues (eg, bone marrow), are most effective.
2. Doses are usually calculated according to body surface area, which includes both weight and height, and expressed as milligrams of drug per square meter of body surface area (mg/m^2). Doses also can be expressed as milligrams per kilogram of body weight (mg/kg). Because dosages based on body surface area consider the client's size, they are especially important for children receiving chemotherapy. If the client's weight changes more than a few pounds during treatment, dosages should be recalculated.
3. Dosage may be reduced for neutropenia, thrombocytopenia, stomatitis, diarrhea, and renal or hepatic impairment that reduces the client's ability to eliminate the drugs.
4. Total dose limits for doxorubicin ($550 mg/m^2$) and bleomycin (450 units) should not be exceeded.

Administration Factors

1. Dosage schedules are largely determined by clinical trials and should be followed as exactly as possible.
2. Antineoplastic drugs are usually given in relatively high doses, on an intermittent or cyclic schedule. This regimen seems more effective than low doses given continuously or massive doses given once. It also produces less immunosuppression and provides drug-free periods during which normal tissues can repair themselves from damage inflicted by the drugs. Fortunately, normal cells repair themselves faster than malignant cells. Succeeding doses are given as soon as tissue repair becomes evident, usually when leukocyte and platelet counts return to acceptable levels.
3. Each antineoplastic drug should be used in the schedule, route, and dosage judged to be most effective for a particular type of cancer. With combinations of drugs, the recommended schedule should be followed precisely because safety and effectiveness may be schedule dependent. When chemotherapy is used as an adjuvant to surgery, it usually should be started as soon as possible after surgery, given in maximal tolerated doses just as if advanced disease were present, and continued for several months (usually 1 year for breast cancer).
4. Intravenous drug administration should be performed by experienced personnel who ensure free flow of fluid to the vein and verify adequate blood return before a drug is injected. Infusion should be through a large, upper extremity vein. When possible, veins of the antecubital fossa, wrist, dorsum of the hand, and the arm where an axillary lymph node

dissection has been done should be avoided. An indwelling central venous catheter is often inserted for clients with poor peripheral venous access or who require many doses of chemotherapy.

5. With bleomycin, a test dose of 1 to 2 mg subcutaneously should be given before starting full doses. Severe allergic reactions with hypotension may occur.

6. With paclitaxel and docetaxel, premedication is needed to decrease severe hypersensitivity reactions with dyspnea, hypotension, angioedema, and urticaria. A few deaths have occurred despite premedication. With paclitaxel, one regimen is oral dexamethasone 20 mg approximately 12 and 6 hours before, with IV diphenhydramine 50 mg and cimetidine 300 mg, famotidine 20 mg, or ranitidine 50 mg 30 to 60 min before. Additional paclitaxel is contraindicated for clients who experience severe hypersensitivity reactions. With docetaxel, an oral corticosteroid (eg, dexamethasone 8 mg twice daily) is recommended for 3 days, starting 1 day before docetaxel administration. This reduces risk and severity of hypersensitivity reactions and fluid retention.

Combination Regimens

Combination chemotherapy is usually used because it is more effective, less toxic, and less likely to cause drug resistance than single agents. Numerous combinations have been developed for use in specific types of cancer. Selection and scheduling of individual drugs in a multidrug regimen are based on efforts to maximize effectiveness for the type of neoplasm being treated and to minimize adverse effects on the client. Some characteristics of effective drug combinations include the following:

1. Each drug should have activity against the type of tumor being treated.

2. Each drug should act by a different mechanism. Drugs can be combined to produce sequential or concurrent inhibition. For example, one drug can be chosen to damage the DNA, RNA, or proteins of the malignant cell, and another drug can be chosen to prevent their repair or synthesis.

3. Drugs should act at different times in the reproductive cycle of the malignant cell. For example, more malignant cells are likely to be destroyed by combining cell cycle–specific and cell cycle–nonspecific drugs. The first group kills only dividing cells; the second group kills cells during any part of the life cycle, including the resting phase.

4. Consecutive doses kill a percentage of the tumor cells remaining after earlier doses and further decrease the tumor burden.

5. Toxic reactions of the various drugs should not overlap so that maximal tolerated doses may be given. It is preferable to use drugs that are not toxic to the same organ system (eg, bone marrow, kidney) and

to use drugs that do not exert their toxic effects at the same time.

6. Bleomycin is often combined with myelosuppressive drugs because it rarely causes myelosuppression. However, it can cause severe allergic reactions with hypotension and pulmonary toxicity (eg, interstitial pneumonitis and pulmonary fibrosis).

Hormonal Therapy

Hormonal therapy is often used to treat breast or prostate cancer. Decreasing the hormones that stimulate tumor growth in these tissues can decrease symptoms and prolong survival.

In some clients with breast cancer, the presence of receptors for estrogen or progesterone may indicate a likely response to hormonal therapy. Tamoxifen is often used to treat breast cancers with estrogen receptors because it inhibits the interaction between estrogen and estrogen receptors. However, tumors may be resistant to hormonal therapy because of mutations in receptors that alter receptor functions. In clients with prostate cancer, hormonal therapy involves drugs that decrease androgens.

When both hormonal and cytotoxic drug therapies are needed, they are not given concurrently because hormonal antagonists decrease malignant cell growth, and cytotoxic agents are most effective when the cells are actively dividing. In clients with breast cancer, hormonal therapy is usually given before cytotoxic chemotherapy in metastatic disease and after chemotherapy when used for adjuvant treatment.

Planning With Client and Family

Clients with cancer and their families should be provided with information about their disease and their treatment options. For those with Internet access, helpful information can be obtained at:

CancerNet, http://wwwicic.nci.nih.gov
CancerNews on the Net, http://www.cancernews.com/quickload.htm
Oncolink, http://cancer.med.upenn.edu

When cytotoxic chemotherapy is the recommended treatment, additional factors must be discussed.

1. **What is the goal of chemotherapy?** Expected benefits may include curing the disease, decreasing tumor size, relieving symptoms, killing metastatic cells left after surgery or radiation therapy, or prolonging life. Chemotherapy cannot be justified unless expected benefits outweigh the potential hazards.

2. **What adverse reactions are likely to occur?** Which reactions should be reported to the physician? How will they be managed if they occur? Even if the realities of chemotherapy are unpleasant, it is usually better for the client to know what they are than to fear the unknown. Some specific

effects that should be discussed, depending on the drugs to be used, include alopecia, amenorrhea, oligospermia, and possibly permanent sterility. Because most of these drugs are teratogenic, clients in the reproductive years are advised to avoid pregnancy during treatment.

3. **Who will administer the drugs, where, and for how long?** Chemotherapy is highly specialized. Because the drugs are toxic and require meticulous administration, they are preferably given at a cancer treatment center. Some clients undergo chemotherapy at a cancer center far from home; others undergo treatment at a nearby hospital, clinic, physician's office, or even at home. The duration of treatment varies, depending on the type of tumor and response.

Clients should be informed about the frequent venipunctures required for blood tests and drug administration. When CBC indicates excessive leukopenia or thrombocytopenia, chemotherapy is postponed.

Guidelines for Handling Cytotoxic Antineoplastic Drugs

Exposure to chemotherapy drugs may lead to adverse effects such as contact dermatitis, cough, nausea, vomiting, diarrhea, and others. In addition, exposure during pregnancy increases risks of fetal abnormalities, ectopic pregnancy, and spontaneous abortions. Guidelines to avoid adverse effects include the following:

1. Avoid contact with solutions for injection by wearing gloves, eye protectors, and protective clothing (eg, disposable, liquid-impermeable gowns).
2. If handling a powder form of a drug, wear a mask to avoid inhaling the powder.
3. Do not prepare the drugs in eating areas (to decrease risks of oral ingestion).
4. Dispose of contaminated materials (eg, needles, syringes, ampules, vials, IV tubing and bags) in

---

Nursing Notes: Ethical/Legal Dilemma

You are working on an oncology unit and have recently become certified to administer antineoplastic medications. You read a new study that documents significant cancer with contact exposure to a new antineoplastic agent.

Reflect on:

- Does a nurse have the right to refuse to administer this new medication if he or she feels it poses a personal health risk?
- The nurse's responsibility for his or her own safety.
- The institution's responsibility for the safety of the workers in this situation.

---

puncture-proof containers labeled "Warning: Hazardous Material."

5. Wear gloves when handling clients' clothing, bed linens, or excreta. Blood and body fluids are contaminated with drugs or metabolites for approximately 48 hours after a dose.
6. Wash hands thoroughly after exposure or potential exposure.
7. Follow recommended procedures for cleaning up spills.

Use in Children

Children are at risk for a wide range of malignant diseases, including acute leukemias, lymphomas, brain tumors, Wilms' tumor, and sarcomas of muscle and bone. Although chemotherapy drugs have been widely used in children, few studies have been done and their safety and effectiveness are not established. Chemotherapy is often used in conjunction with surgical excision or radiation therapy.

Cancer care and chemotherapy should be designed and supervised by pediatric oncologists. Dosage of cytotoxic drugs should be based on body surface area because this takes size into account. Long-term effects on growth and development of survivors are not clear and special efforts are needed to maintain nutrition, organ function, psychological support, and other aspects of growth and development. After successful treatment, children should continue to be closely monitored because they are at increased risk for development of secondary malignancies.

Use in Older Adults

Older adults are at risk for development of a wide range of malignant diseases. Although they also are likely to have chronic cardiovascular, renal, and other disorders that increase their risks of serious adverse effects, they should not be denied the potential benefits of chemotherapy on the basis of age alone. Instead, greater vigilance is needed to maximize benefits and minimize hazards of chemotherapy. For example, older adults are more sensitive to the neurotoxic effects of vincristine and need reduced dosages of some drugs (eg, cyclophosphamide, MTX) if renal function is impaired. Creatinine clearance should be monitored; serum creatinine level is not a reliable indicator of renal function in older adults because of their decreased muscle mass.

Use in Renal Impairment

Some antineoplastic drugs are nephrotoxic (eg, cisplatin, MTX) and many are excreted through the kidneys. In the presence of impaired renal function, risks of further impairment or accumulation of toxic drug levels are increased.

Thus, renal function should be monitored carefully with chemotherapeutic agents and drug dosages are often reduced according to creatinine clearance levels. In advanced cancer, creatinine clearance may not be reliable because these clients are often in catabolic states characterized by increased production of creatinine (from breakdown of skeletal muscle and other proteins). Renal effects of selected drugs are as follows:

- **Carmustine** has been associated with azotemia and renal failure, most often with long-term IV administration and large cumulative doses.
- **Cisplatin** is nephrotoxic and acute overdosage can cause renal failure. Because nephrotoxicity is increased with repeated doses, cisplatin is given at 3- or 4-week intervals and renal function tests (eg, serum creatinine, blood urea nitrogen [BUN]) and serum electrolytes (eg, sodium, potassium, calcium) are measured before each course of therapy. Renal function is usually allowed to return to normal before another dose is given. Nephrotoxicity may be reduced by the use of amifostine or IV hydration and mannitol.
- **Cyclophosphamide** may cause hemorrhagic ureteritis and renal tubular necrosis with IV doses above 50 mg/kg. These effects usually subside when the drug is stopped.
- **Ifosfamide** may increase BUN and serum creatinine, but its major effect on the urinary tract is hemorrhagic cystitis, manifested by hematuria. Cystitis can be reduced by the use of mesna, vigorous hydration, and delaying drug administration if a predose urinalysis shows hematuria.
- **Irinotecan** has a longer plasma half-life and should be given in reduced dosage (0.75 mg/m^2) to clients with moderate impairment (creatinine clearance 20 to 39 mL/minute). No dosage reduction is recommended with mild impairment (creatinine clearance 40 to 60 mL/minute), and there are inadequate data for dosage recommendations in severe impairment.
- **Lomustine** is the same as carmustine, above.
- **Melphalan** should be reduced in dosage when given IV to reduce accumulation and increased bone marrow toxicity. It is unknown whether dosage reduction is needed with oral drug.
- **Mercaptopurine** should be given in smaller doses because the drug may be eliminated more slowly.
- **Methotrexate** is excreted mainly by the kidneys and its use in clients with impaired renal function may lead to accumulation of toxic amounts or additional renal damage. The client's renal status should be evaluated before and during MTX therapy. If significant renal impairment occurs, the drug should be discontinued or reduced in dosage until renal function improves.

In clients who receive high doses for treatment of osteosarcoma, MTX may cause renal damage leading to acute renal failure. Nephrotoxicity is attrib-uted to precipitation of MTX and a metabolite in renal tubules. Renal impairment may be reduced by monitoring renal function closely, ensuring adequate hydration, alkalinizing the urine, and measuring serum drug levels.

- **Procarbazine** may cause more severe adverse effects if given to clients with impaired renal function. Hospitalization is recommended for the first course of treatment.
- **Streptozocin** is nephrotoxic in approximately two thirds of clients treated. Toxicity is dose related and cumulative, and may be severe or fatal. It may be manifested by azotemia, anuria, hypophosphatemia, glycosuria, and renal tubular acidosis. Renal function tests (eg, BUN, serum creatinine, creatinine clearance, and serum electrolytes) should be performed before starting therapy, at least weekly during therapy, and for 4 weeks after drug administration. In addition, serial urinalyses are needed to detect proteinuria, an early sign of renal damage. If significant renal impairment occurs, streptozocin should be discontinued or its dosage reduced. Keeping the client well hydrated may reduce nephrotoxicity.

In clients with preexisting renal impairment, the risk of additional damage is great. Streptozocin should not be given unless expected benefits outweigh risks of serious renal damage. If used, concomitant use of other potential nephrotoxins should be avoided and renal function should be closely monitored for signs of additional impairment.

Many other drugs should be used with caution in clients with renal impairment. **Asparaginase** often causes azotemia (eg, increased BUN); acute renal failure and fatal renal insufficiency have been reported. **Bleomycin** is rarely associated with nephrotoxicity but its elimination half-life is prolonged in clients with a creatinine clearance of less than 35 mL/minute. **Cytarabine** is detoxified mainly by the liver. However, clients with renal impairment may have more central nervous system (CNS)-related adverse effects, and dosage reduction may be needed. **Gemcitabine** should be used with caution, although it has not been studied in clients with preexisting renal impairment. Mild proteinuria and hematuria were commonly reported during clinical trials, and hemolytic–uremic syndrome (HUS) was reported in a few clients. HUS may be manifested by anemia, indications of blood cell breakdown (eg, elevated bilirubin and reticulocyte counts), and renal failure. The drug should be stopped immediately if HUS occurs; hemodialysis may be required.

Use in Hepatic Impairment

Some antineoplastic drugs are hepatotoxic and many are metabolized in the liver. In the presence of impaired hepatic function, risks of further impairment or accumulation of toxic drug levels are increased. Dosage reduction is needed with some drugs and hepatic function should be monitored with most. However, abnormal values for the usual liver function tests (eg, serum aminotransferases such as aspartate aminotransferase [AST] and alanine aminotransferase [ALT], bilirubin, alkaline phosphatase) may indicate liver injury but do not indicate decreased ability to metabolize drugs. Clients with metastatic cancer often have impaired liver function.

Hepatotoxic drugs include the anthracyclines (eg, doxorubicin), mercaptopurine, MTX, paclitaxel, and vincristine. Hepatic effects of these and selected other drugs are as follows:

- **Asparaginase** is hepatotoxic in most clients and may increase preexisting hepatic impairment. It may also increase hepatotoxicity of other medications. Signs of liver impairment, which usually subside when the drug is discontinued, include increased AST, ALT, alkaline phosphatase, and bilirubin and decreased serum albumin, cholesterol, and plasma fibrinogen.
- **Carmustine** may increase AST, ALT, alkaline phosphatase, and bilirubin when given IV.
- **Capecitabine** blood levels are significantly increased with hepatic impairment and clients with mild to moderate impairment caused by liver metastases should be monitored closely. The effects of severe impairment have not been studied.
- **Chlorambucil** may be hepatotoxic and cause jaundice.
- **Cisplatin** may cause a transient increase in liver enzymes and bilirubin, which should be measured periodically during cisplatin therapy.
- **Cytarabine** is metabolized in the liver and clients with impaired liver function are more likely to have CNS-related adverse effects. The drug should be used with caution and dosage may need to be reduced.
- **Dacarbazine** is hepatotoxic and a few cases of hepatic vein thrombosis and fatal liver necrosis have been reported.
- **Daunorubicin**, liposomal formulation, should be reduced in dosage according to the serum bilirubin (eg, bilirubin 1.2 to 3 mg/dL, give three fourths the normal dose; bilirubin >3 mg/dL, give one half the normal dose).
- **Doxorubicin** is excreted primarily in bile and toxicity is increased with impaired hepatic function. Liver function tests should be done before drug administration, and dosage of both regular and liposomal formulations should be reduced according to the serum bilirubin (eg, bilirubin 1.2 to 3 mg/dL, give one half the normal dose; bilirubin >3 mg/dL, give one fourth the normal dose).
- **Gemcitabine** has not been studied in clients with significant hepatic impairment but should be used with caution. Transient increases in serum aminotransferases occurred in most clients during clinical trials.

- **Idarubicin** should not be given to clients with a serum bilirubin above 5 mg/dL.
- **Irinotecan** has been associated with abnormal liver function tests in clients with liver metastases.
- **Mercaptopurine** causes hepatotoxicity, especially with higher doses (>2.5 mg/kg/day) and in combination with doxorubicin. Encephalopathy and fatal liver necrosis have occurred. The drug should be discontinued if signs of hepatotoxicity occur (eg, jaundice, hepatomegaly, liver function tests indicating toxic hepatitis or biliary stasis). Serum aminotransferases, alkaline phosphatase, and bilirubin should be monitored weekly with initial therapy, then monthly. Liver function tests may be needed more often in clients who have preexisting liver impairment or are receiving other hepatotoxic drugs.
- **Methotrexate** may cause acute (increased serum aminotransferases, hepatitis) and chronic (fibrosis and cirrhosis) hepatotoxicity. Chronic toxicity is potentially fatal. It is more likely to occur after prolonged use (eg, 2 years or longer) and after a total dose of at least 1.5 g. Cautious use of MTX is especially indicated in clients with preexisting liver damage or impaired hepatic function. Liver function tests should be closely monitored.
- **Paclitaxel** is mainly metabolized by the liver and may cause more toxicity in clients with impaired hepatic function.
- **Procarbazine** causes more toxic effects in clients with hepatic impairment. Hospitalization is recommended for the first course of therapy.
- **Streptozocin** may cause hepatotoxicity manifested by increased liver enzymes (eg, AST, lactate dehydrogenase), hypoalbuminemia, and jaundice. The drug may need to be discontinued or reduced in dosage. Liver function tests should be monitored at least weekly.
- **Topotecan** is cleared from plasma more slowly in clients with hepatic impairment, but dosage reductions are not recommended.
- **Vinblastine** may cause more toxicity with hepatic impairment and dosage should be reduced 50% for clients with a direct serum bilirubin value above 3 mg/dL.
- **Vincristine** dosage should be reduced as for vinblastine.

Other drugs that should be used with caution because of their hepatic effects include the antineoplastic hormones and hormone antagonists. The antiandrogens include bicalutamide, flutamide, and nilutamide. **Bicalutamide** is extensively metabolized by the liver and has a long serum half-life in clients with severe hepatic impairment. Excretion may be delayed and the drug may accumulate. The drug should be used with caution in clients with moderate to severe hepatic impairment and liver function tests should be monitored periodically during long-term therapy. **Flutamide** has been associated with serum aminotransferase abnormalities, cholestatic jaundice, hepatic encephalopathy, hepatic necrosis, and a few deaths. Liver function tests should be performed periodically and at the first sign or symptom of liver dysfunction (eg, pruritus, dark urine, jaundice). Flutamide should be discontinued if jaundice develops in clients who do not have liver metastases or if serum aminotransferase levels increase more than two to three times the upper limit of normal. Liver damage usually subsides if flutamide is discontinued or if dosage is reduced. **Nilutamide** may cause hepatitis or increases in liver enzymes. Serum aminotransferases and other liver enzymes should be checked at baseline and approximately every 3 months. If symptoms of liver injury occur or if aminotransferases increase over two to three times the upper limits of normal, nilutamide should be discontinued.

Medroxyprogesterone should be discontinued with the development of any manifestations of impaired liver function. Tamoxifen and toremifene are antiestrogens. **Tamoxifen** has been associated with changes in liver enzyme levels and occasionally more severe liver damage, including fatty liver, cholestasis, hepatitis, and hepatic necrosis. **Toremifene's** elimination half-life is prolonged in clients with hepatic cirrhosis or fibrosis.

 Home Care

Clients may receive parenteral cytotoxic drugs as outpatients and return home, or the drugs may be administered at home by the client or a caregiver. The home care nurse may be involved in a wide range of activities associated with chemotherapy, including administering antineoplastic drugs, administering drugs to prevent or manage adverse effects, and assessing client and family responses to therapy. In addition, a major role involves teaching about the disease process, management of pain and other symptoms, the anticancer drugs, prevention or management of adverse drug effects, preventing infection, maintaining food and fluid intake, and other aspects of care. If a client is receiving erythropoietin or oprelvekin subcutaneously, the client or a caregiver may need to be taught injection technique.

The home care nurse also needs to teach clients and caregivers about safe handling of chemotherapeutic agents and items contaminated with the drugs or client body fluids or excreta. Precautions need to be similar to those used in health care agencies.

(*text continues on page 966*)

NURSING ACTIONS	RATIONALE/EXPLANATION
1. Administer accurately	
a. If not accustomed to giving cytotoxic antineoplastic drugs regularly, read package inserts, research protocols, or other recent drug references for specific instructions on administration of individual drugs.	Cancer chemotherapy is a highly specialized area of nursing practice, with most agencies requiring training and demonstration of competency. Obtaining current information is necessary because of the large number and varied characteristics of the drugs; differences in administration according to the type of neoplasm being treated and other client characteristics; and continuing development of new drugs, dosages, routes, schedules of administration, and combinations of drugs.
b. For cytotoxic drugs to be given intravenously (IV).	
(1) Compare labels on pre-prepared solutions to medication orders in terms of the drug, concentration, expiration date, and instructions for administration.	Many of the drugs must be reconstituted from a powder form and further diluted in an IV solution. Drug solutions should usually be prepared in the pharmacy to maintain sterility and avoid dispersing drug particles into the environment.
(2) A commonly used method is to inject the drug into the tubing of a rapidly flowing IV infusion.	To decrease tissue irritation and allow rapid detection of extravasation
(3) For clients with a long-term venous access device (eg, Hickman or Groshong	Long-term venous access devices are often desirable to decrease the number of venipunctures a

NURSING ACTIONS Antineoplastic Drugs

(continued)

NURSING ACTIONS	RATIONALE/EXPLANATION
catheter), follow agency protocols for drug administration and catheter care.	client must undergo. These devices require special care to maintain patency and prevent infection of the patient's bloodstream.
(4) Follow agency protocols for skin exposure or spills of cytotoxic drug solutions.	These solutions are considered hazardous materials that require special handling.
c. For drugs to be given orally, the total dose of most drugs can be given at one time. An exception is mitotane, which is given in three or four divided doses.	
2. Observe for therapeutic effects	Therapeutic effects depend to a large extent on the type of malignancy being treated. They may not become evident for several weeks after chemotherapy is begun. Some clients experience anorexia, nausea, and vomiting for 2 to 3 wk after each cycle of drug therapy.
a. Increased appetite	
b. Increased sense of well-being	
c. Improved mobility	
d. Decreased pain	
e. With busulfan, given for chronic myelogenous leukemia, also observe for decreased white blood cell count and decreased size of the spleen.	Decreased white blood cell count and splenomegaly usually become evident approximately the second or third week of drug therapy.
f. With melphalan, given for multiple myeloma, also observe for decreased amounts of abnormal proteins in urine and blood, decreased levels of serum calcium, and increased hemoglobin.	
3. Observe for adverse effects	Because they are toxic to both normal and malignant cells, cytotoxic antineoplastic drugs may have adverse effects on almost any body tissue. These adverse effects range from common to rare, from relatively mild to life threatening. Some are expected, such as bone marrow depression, and this is used to guide drug therapy. Most of the adverse effects occur with usual dosage ranges and are likely to be increased in incidence and severity with larger doses.
a. Hematologic effects:	
(1) Bone marrow depression with leukopenia (decreased white blood cell count), thrombocytopenia (decreased platelets), and anemia (decreased red blood cell count, hemoglobin, and hematocrit)	For most of these drugs, white blood cell count and platelet counts reach their lowest points approximately 7 to 14 d after drug administration and return toward normal after approximately 21 d. Normal leukocyte and platelet counts signify recovery of bone marrow function. Anemia may occur later because the red blood cell lives longer than white cells and platelets.
(2) Decreased antibodies and lymphocytes	Most of these drugs have immunosuppressant effects, which impair body defenses against infection.
b. Gastrointestinal (GI) effects—anorexia, nausea, vomiting, diarrhea, constipation, stomatitis and other mucosal ulcerations, oral candidiasis	Anorexia, nausea, and vomiting are very common. They usually occur within a few hours of drug administration. Nausea and vomiting often subside within approximately 12 to 24 h, but anorexia may persist. Constipation is most likely to occur with

(continued)

NURSING ACTIONS	RATIONALE/EXPLANATION
	vincristine. Mucosal ulcerations may occur anywhere in the GI tract and can lead to serious complications (infection, hemorrhage, perforation). Their occurrence is usually an indication to stop drug therapy, at least temporarily. Fungal and bacterial infections may interfere with nutrition. They may be relatively mild or severe.
c. Integumentary effects—alopecia, dermatitis, tissue irritation at injection sites.	Complete hair loss may take several weeks to occur. Alopecia is most significant in terms of altered body image, possible mental depression, and other psychological effects. Several drugs may cause phlebitis and sclerosis of veins used for injections, as well as pain and tissue necrosis if allowed to leak into subcutaneous tissues around the injection site.
d. Renal effects:	
(1) Hyperuricemia and uric acid nephropathy	When malignant cells are destroyed by drug therapy, they release uric acid into the bloodstream. Uric acid crystals may precipitate in the kidneys and cause impaired function or even renal failure. Adverse effects on the kidneys are especially associated with methotrexate and cisplatin. Hyperuricemia can be decreased by an ample fluid intake or by administration of allopurinol.
(2) With cyclophosphamide, hemorrhagic cystitis (blood in urine, dysuria, burning on urination)	Hemorrhagic cystitis is thought to occur in approximately 10% of the clients who receive cyclophosphamide and to result from irritating effects of drug metabolites on the bladder mucosa. The drug is stopped if this occurs. Cystitis can be decreased by an ample fluid intake.
e. Pulmonary effects—cough, dyspnea, chest x-ray changes	Adverse reactions affecting the lungs are associated mainly with bleomycin, busulfan, and methotrexate. With bleomycin particularly, pulmonary toxicity may be severe and progress to pulmonary fibrosis.
f. Cardiovascular effects—congestive heart failure (dyspnea, edema, fatigue), arrhythmias, electrocardiographic changes	Cardiomyopathy is associated primarily with daunorubicin and doxorubicin. This is a life-threatening adverse reaction. The heart failure may be unresponsive to digitalis preparations.
g. Central nervous system effects—peripheral neuropathy with vincristine, manifested by muscle weakness, numbness and tingling of extremities, foot drop, and decreased ability to walk	This fairly common effect of vincristine may worsen for several weeks after drug administration. There is usually some recovery of function eventually.
h. Endocrine effects—menstrual irregularities, sterility in men and women	
4. Observe for drug interactions	
a. Drugs that *increase* effects of cytotoxic antineoplastic drugs:	
(1) Allopurinol	Allopurinol is usually given to prevent or treat hyperuricemia, which may occur with cancer chemotherapy. When given with mercaptopurine, allopurinol facilitates the formation of the active metabolite.

(continued)

NURSING ACTIONS	RATIONALE/EXPLANATION
	Consequently, doses of mercaptopurine must be reduced to one third to one fourth the usual dose.
(2) Anticoagulants, oral	Increased risk of bleeding
(3) Bone marrow depressants	Increased bone marrow depression
(4) Other antineoplastic drugs	Additive cytotoxic effects, both therapeutic and adverse
b. Drugs that *increase* effects of cyclophosphamide:	
(1) Anesthetics, inhalation	Lethal combination. Discontinue cyclophosphamide at least 12 h before general inhalation anesthesia is to be given.
(2) Barbiturates	Potentiate cyclophosphamide by induction of liver enzymes, which accelerate transformation of the drug into its active metabolites
(3) Other alkylating antineoplastic drugs	Increased bone marrow depression
c. Drugs that *increase* effects of methotrexate:	
(1) Alcohol	Additive liver toxicity. Avoid concomitant use.
(2) Aspirin; analgesics and antipyretics containing aspirin or other salicylates; barbiturates; phenytoin; sulfonamides	Potentiate methotrexate by displacing it from protein-binding sites in plasma. Salicylates also block renal excretion of methotrexate. This may cause pancytopenia and liver toxicity.
(3) Other hepatotoxic drugs	Additive liver toxicity
(4) Other antineoplastic drugs	Additive cytotoxic effects, both therapeutic and adverse. Methotrexate is one component of several drug combinations used to treat breast cancer.
d. Drug that *decreases* effects of methotrexate:	
(1) Leucovorin (citrovorum factor, folinic acid)	Leucovorin antagonizes the toxic effects of methotrexate and is used as an antidote for high-dose methotrexate regimens or for overdose. It must be given exactly at the specified time, before affected cells become too damaged to respond.

Nursing Notes: Apply Your Knowledge

Answer: Platelets, red blood cells, and white blood cells (WBC) are produced in the bone marrow. The production of any of these cells can decrease when an antineoplastic agent with a side effect of bone marrow depression is given. The impact is greatest at nadir, when platelets decrease below 50,000/mm^3. When red blood cells decrease, as evidenced by a hemoglobin less than 9 g/dL, the client experiences anemia and fatigue. The WBC count is a measure of the body's ability to fight infection. Neutrophils are WBCs that are especially helpful in fighting infection; thus, when the WBC count is low, a neutrophil count is done. A client with neutrophil counts less than 500/mm^3 is at significant risk for infection. Common signs of infection are often mediated by neutrophils, so the signs and symptoms of infection may be low in the neutropenic client.

Client teaching should focus on avoiding infection (good hand washing, avoiding contact with infected people), especially if the neutrophil count is low. The client should report any fever, even low-grade fevers. Fatigue can be managed with frequent rest, energy conservation measures, and good nutrition. When platelets are low, clients should be taught to avoid trauma. The importance of keeping appointments for monitoring should be stressed so that blood products can be given if values are critically low.

REVIEW AND APPLICATION EXERCISES

1. Compare and contrast normal and malignant cells.

2. Which common cancers are attributed mainly to environmental factors? Which are attributed to genetic factors?

3. How do cytotoxic antineoplastic drugs destroy malignant cells?

4. Which cytotoxic antineoplastic drugs are associated with serious adverse effects (eg, bone marrow suppression, cardiotoxicity, hepatotoxicity, nephrotoxicity, neurotoxicity)?

5. Which drugs are associated with second malignancies?

6. What is the basis for the anticancer effects of hormones and antihormones?

7. For which cytotoxic drugs are cytoprotective drugs available?

8. List at least one intervention to prevent or minimize each of the following adverse effects of chemotherapy: alopecia, anemia, bleeding, infection, nausea and vomiting, stomatitis.

SELECTED REFERENCES

Balmer, C. & Valley, A.W. (1997). Basic principles of cancer treatment and cancer chemotherapy. In J.T. DiPiro, R.L. Talbert, G.C. Yee, G.R. Matzke, B.G. Wells, & L.M. Posey (Eds.), *Pharmacotherapy: A pathophysiologic approach*, 3rd ed., pp. 2403–2465. Stamford, CT: Appleton & Lange.

Blattner, W.A. (1997). Etiology of malignant disease. In W.N. Kelley (Ed.), *Textbook of internal medicine*, 3rd ed., pp. 129–133. Philadelphia: Lippincott-Raven.

Calabresi, P. & Chabner, B.A. (1996). Chemotherapy of neoplastic diseases: Introduction. In J.G. Hardman, L.E. Limbird, P.B. Molinoff, & R.W. Ruddon (Eds.), *Goodman & Gilman's The pharmacological basis of therapeutics*, 9th ed., pp. 1225–1232. New York: McGraw-Hill.

Cassell, G.H. (1998). Infectious causes of chronic inflammatory diseases and cancer. *Emerging Infectious Diseases, 4*, 475–487. [Online: Available http://www.medscape.com/govmt/CDC/EID/1998/v04.n03;e0403.21.cass/e0403.21.cass.01.html. Accessed October 1999.]

Caudell, K.A. (1998). Alterations in cell differentiation: Neoplasia. In C.M. Porth (Ed.), *Pathophysiology: Concepts of altered health states*, 5th ed., pp. 79–109. Philadelphia: Lippincott Williams & Wilkins.

Del Gaudio, D. & Menonna-Quinn, D. (1998). Chemotherapy: Potential occupational hazards. *American Journal of Nursing, 98*(11), 59–65.

Drug facts and comparisons. (Updated monthly). St. Louis: Facts and Comparisons.

Grochow, L.B. & Ames, M.M. (1998). *A clinician's guide to chemotherapy pharmacokinetics and pharmacodynamics*. Baltimore: Williams & Wilkins.

McEnroe, L.E. (1996). Role of the oncology nurse in home care: Family-centered practice. *Seminars in Oncology Nursing, 12*, 188–192.

Mortimer, J.E. & Arquette, M.A. (1998). Medical management of malignant disease. In C.F. Carey, H.H. Lee, & K.F. Woeltje (Eds.), *The Washington manual of medical therapeutics*, 29th ed., pp. 375–395. Philadelphia: Lippincott Williams & Wilkins.

Mrozek-Orlowske, M.E., Frye, D.K., & Sanborn, H.M. (1999). Capecitabine: Nursing implications of a new oral chemotherapeutic agent. *Oncology Nursing Forum, 26*, 753–762.

Navarro, T.M. (1998). Chemotherapy extravasation. *American Journal of Nursing 98*(11), 38.

Seiden, M., Urba, W., & Chabner, B.A. (1997). Principles of chemotherapy and hormonal therapy. In W.N. Kelley (Ed.), *Textbook of internal medicine*, 3rd ed., pp. 1508–1518. Philadelphia: Lippincott-Raven.

Stucky-Marshall, L. (1999). New agents in gastrointestinal malignancies: Part 2. Gemcitabine in clinical practice. *Cancer Nursing, 22*, 290–296.

Viele, C.S. & Holmes, B.C. (1998). Amifostine: Drug profile and nursing implications of the first pancytoprotectant. *Oncology Nursing Forum, 25*, 515–523.

65

Drugs Used in Ophthalmic Conditions

Objectives

After studying this chapter, the student will be able to:

1. Review characteristics of ocular structures that influence drug therapy of eye disorders.

2. Discuss autonomic nervous system, antimicrobial, anti-inflammatory, and selected miscellaneous drugs in relation to their use in ocular disorders.

3. Use correct techniques to administer ophthalmic medications.

4. Assess for ocular effects of systemic drugs and systemic effects of ophthalmic drugs.

5. Teach clients, family members, or caretakers correct administration of eye medications.

6. For a client with an eye disorder, teach about the importance of taking medications as prescribed to protect and preserve eyesight.

Jean Green, a 40-year-old accountant, has made an appointment to have her eyes examined because she has been having difficulty reading small print. She has not had her eyes tested for over 10 years. When she arrives at the office, you explain that the examination will include using medications to dilate her eyes and a test for glaucoma.

Reflect on:

▶ Age-related visual changes that often occur at midlife.

▶ Which drugs are used to dilate the eyes for examination, and how they work.

▶ Why glaucoma testing is important.

▶ What teaching is necessary for Mrs. Green.

STRUCTURES OF THE EYE

The eye is the major sensory organ through which the person receives information about the external environment. An in-depth discussion of vision and ocular anatomy is beyond the scope of this chapter, but some characteristics and functions are described to facilitate understanding of ocular drug therapy. These include the following:

- The eyelids and lacrimal system function to protect the eye. The *eyelid* is a covering that acts as a barrier to the entry of foreign bodies, strong light, dust, and other potential irritants. The *conjunctiva* is the mucous membrane lining of the eyelids. The *canthi* (singular, *canthus*) are the angles where the upper and lower eyelids meet. The *lacrimal system* produces a fluid that constantly moistens and cleanses the anterior surface of the eyeball. The fluid drains through two small openings in the inner canthus and flows through the nasolacrimal duct into the nasal cavity. When the conjunctiva is irritated or certain emotions are experienced (eg, sadness), the lacrimal gland produces more fluid than the drainage system can accommodate. The excess fluid overflows the eyelids and becomes *tears*.
- The eyeball is a spherical structure composed of the sclera, cornea, choroid, and retina, plus special refractive tissues. The *sclera* is a white, opaque, fibrous tissue that covers the posterior five sixths of the eyeball. The *cornea* is a transparent, special connective tissue that covers the anterior sixth of the eyeball. The cornea contains no blood vessels. The *choroid*, composed of blood vessels and connective tissue, continues forward to form the iris. The *iris* is composed of pigmented cells, the opening called the *pupil*, and muscles that control the size of the pupil by contracting or dilating in response to stimuli. The *retina* is the innermost layer of the eyeball.

  For vision to occur, light rays must enter the eye through the cornea; travel through the pupil, lens, and vitreous body (see later); and be focused on the retina. Light rays do not travel directly to the retina. Instead, they are deflected in various directions according to the density of the ocular structures through which they pass. This process, called *refraction*, is controlled by the aqueous humor, lens, and vitreous body. The *optic disk* is the area of the retina where ophthalmic blood vessels and the optic nerve enter the eyeball.

- The structure and function of the eyeball are further influenced by the lens, aqueous humor, and vitreous body. The *lens* is an elastic, transparent structure; its function is to focus light rays to form images on the retina. It is located behind the iris and held in place by suspensory ligaments attached to the ciliary body. The *aqueous humor* is a clear fluid produced by capillaries in the ciliary body. Most of the fluid flows through the pupil into the anterior chamber (between the cornea and the lens and anterior to the iris). A

small amount flows into a passage called Schlemm's canal, from which it enters the venous circulation. Under normal circumstances, production and drainage of aqueous humor are approximately equal, and normal intraocular pressure (approximately 10 to 20 mm Hg) is maintained. Impaired drainage of aqueous humor causes increased intraocular pressure. The *vitreous body* is a transparent, jelly-like mass located in the posterior portion of the eyeball. It functions to refract light rays and maintain the normal shape of the eyeball.

DISORDERS OF THE EYE

The eye is subject to the development of many disorders that threaten its structure, function, or both. Some disorders in which ophthalmic drugs play a prominent role are discussed in the following sections.

Refractive Errors

Refractive errors include myopia (nearsightedness), hyperopia (farsightedness), presbyopia, and astigmatism. These conditions impair vision by interfering with the eye's ability to focus light rays on the retina. Ophthalmic drugs are used only in the diagnosis of the conditions; treatment involves prescription of eyeglasses or contact lenses.

Glaucoma

Glaucoma, a common preventable cause of blindness, was formerly defined as increased intraocular pressure. The definition has changed because glaucoma may occur with normal intraocular pressure and because some people have increased intraocular pressure without having glaucoma. Thus, glaucoma is now described as a group of diseases characterized by optic nerve damage and changes in visual fields. Diagnostic tests for glaucoma include ophthalmoscopic examination of the optic disk, measurement of intraocular pressure (tonometry), and testing of visual fields.

The most common type of glaucoma is called primary open-angle glaucoma. It is a chronic disorder of unknown cause. A less common but more dramatic type is called narrow-angle glaucoma. Acute narrow-angle glaucoma, which occurs with a sudden, severe increase in intraocular pressure, causes progressive ocular damage and loss of vision unless promptly and effectively treated. Acute increases in intraocular pressure occur in people with narrow-angle glaucoma when pupils are dilated and the outflow of aqueous humor is blocked. Darkness and drugs with anticholinergic effects (eg, atropine, antihistamines, tricyclic antidepressants) may dilate the pupil, reduce outflow of aqueous humor, and precipitate acute glaucoma. Secondary glaucoma may follow traumatic or inflammatory conditions of the eye.

Inflammatory or Infectious Conditions

Inflammation may be caused by bacteria, viruses, allergic reactions, or irritating chemicals. Infections may result from foreign bodies, contaminated hands, contaminated eye medications, or infections in contiguous structures (eg, nose, face, sinuses). Common inflammatory and infectious disorders include the following:

- **Conjunctivitis** is a common eye disorder that may be caused by allergens (eg, pollens), bacterial or viral infection, or physical or chemical irritants. Symptoms include redness, tearing, itching, and burning or gritty sensations. Bacterial conjunctivitis is often caused by *Staphylococcus aureus*, *Streptococcus pneumoniae*, or *Hemophilus influenzae* and produces mucopurulent drainage. Conjunctivitis with a purulent discharge is most often caused by the gonococcus; corneal ulcers and scarring may result.
- **Blepharitis** is a chronic infection of glands and lash follicles on the margins of the eyelids characterized by burning, redness, and itching. A hordeolum (commonly called a sty) is often associated with blepharitis. The most common causes are seborrhea and staphylococcal infections.
- **Keratitis** (inflammation of the cornea) may be caused by microorganisms, trauma, allergy, ischemia, and drying of the cornea (eg, from inadequate lacrimation). The major symptom is pain, which ranges from mild to severe. Vision may not be affected initially. However, if not treated effectively, corneal ulceration, scarring, and impaired vision may result.
- Bacterial **corneal ulcers** are most often caused by pneumococci and staphylococci. Pseudomonal ulcers are less common but may rapidly progress to perforation. Fungal ulcers may follow topical corticosteroid therapy or injury with vegetable matter, such as a tree branch. Viral ulcers are usually caused by the herpesvirus.
- **Fungal infections** are being diagnosed more often than formerly. This is attributed to increased physician awareness and frequent use of ophthalmic antibiotics and corticosteroids.

TYPES OF OPHTHALMIC DRUGS

Drugs used to diagnose or treat ophthalmic disorders represent numerous therapeutic classifications, most of which are discussed in other chapters. Some drugs are used primarily by ophthalmologists. Major classes of drugs used in ophthalmology include the following:

- **Antihistamines** (H$_1$ receptor antagonists) and **mast cell stabilizers** are used to decrease redness and itching associated with allergic conjunctivitis.
- **Antimicrobials** are used to treat bacterial, viral, and fungal infections (see Chaps. 33 through 41). Bacterial infections include conjunctivitis, keratitis, blepharitis, and corneal ulcers. The drugs are usually applied topically but may be given orally or intravenously, or injected subconjunctivally in severe infections.
- **Autonomic drugs** are used extensively for diagnostic and therapeutic purposes (see Chaps. 17 through 21). Some are used to dilate the pupil before ophthalmologic examinations or surgical procedures; some are used to decrease intraocular pressure in glaucoma. Ophthalmic beta-adrenergic blocking agents are the most commonly used drugs for treatment of glaucoma, in which they decrease intraocular pressure by decreasing formation of aqueous humor. Adrenergic vasoconstricting drugs are commonly used to decrease redness associated with allergic conjunctivitis.

  Autonomic drugs indicated in one disorder may be contraindicated in another (eg, anticholinergic drugs may be contraindicated in glaucoma). In addition, adrenergic mydriatics (eg, epinephrine, phenylephrine) should be used cautiously in clients with hypertension, cardiac arrhythmias, arteriosclerotic heart disease, and hyperthyroidism. Ophthalmic beta blockers usually have the same contraindications and precautions as oral or injected drugs (eg, bradycardia, heart block, bronchospastic disorders).
- **Corticosteroids** (see Chap. 24) are often used to treat inflammatory conditions of the eye, thereby reducing scarring and preventing loss of vision. Corticosteroids are generally more effective in acute than chronic inflammatory conditions. Because these drugs are potentially toxic, they should not be used to treat minor disorders or disorders that can be effectively treated with safer drugs. When used, corticosteroids should be administered in the lowest effective dose and for the shortest effective time. Long-term use should be avoided when possible, because it may result in glaucoma, increased intraocular pressure, optic nerve damage, defects in visual acuity and fields of vision, cataract, or secondary ocular infections.

  Ophthalmologic corticosteroids may be administered topically, systemically, or both. They are contraindicated in eye infections caused by the herpesvirus because the drugs increase the severity of the infection.
- **Nonsteroidal anti-inflammatory drugs**, in ophthalmic formulations for topical use, may be used in eye disorders (see Table 65-3 and Chap. 7).
- **Carbonic anhydrase inhibitors** and **osmotic diuretics** are given to decrease intraocular pressure in glaucoma and before certain surgical procedures. Carbonic anhydrase inhibitors lower intraocular pressure by decreasing production of aqueous humor.
- **Fluorescein** is a dye used in diagnosing lesions or foreign bodies in the cornea, fitting contact lenses, and studying the lacrimal system and flow of aqueous humor.

OPHTHALMIC DRUG THERAPY

Drug therapy of ophthalmic conditions is unique because of the location, structure, and function of the eye. Many systemic drugs are unable to cross the blood–eye barrier and achieve therapeutic concentrations in ocular structures. Some drugs penetrate the eye better than others, however, depending on the serum drug concentration, size of drug molecules, solubility of the drug in fat, extent of drug protein binding, and whether inflammation is present in the eye. In general, penetration is greater if the drug achieves a high concentration in the blood, has small molecules, is fat soluble, and is poorly bound to serum proteins, and if inflammation is present.

Because of the difficulties associated with systemic therapy, various methods of administering drugs locally have been developed. The most common method is topical application of ophthalmic solutions (eye drops) to the conjunctiva. Drugs are distributed through the tear film covering the eye and may be used for superficial disorders (eg, conjunctivitis) or for relatively deep ocular disorders (eg, glaucoma). Other topical dosage forms include ophthalmic ointments and a specialized method of administering pilocarpine so the drug is slowly released over 1 week (Ocusert). Ocusert is a small plastic device inserted into the conjunctival area and replaced weekly by the client. It may be used for long-term management of glaucoma.

Other methods of local administration of drugs involve special injection techniques used by ophthalmologists. These include injections through the conjunctiva to subconjunctival tissues or under the fibrous capsule beneath the conjunctiva (sub-Tenon's injection). These injections are painful, and topical anesthetic solutions should be applied before the procedure. Antibiotics and corticosteroids are the drugs most likely to be administered by subconjunctival or sub-Tenon's injection. A third type of injection, called retrobulbar injection, involves injecting a drug behind the globe of the eyeball. Corticosteroids and preoperative local anesthetics may be administered this way.

INDIVIDUAL DRUGS

See Tables 65-1, 65-2, and 65-3.

(*text continues on page 974*)

TABLE 65-1 **Drugs Used in Ocular Disorders***

Ocular Effects	Clinical Indications	Generic/Trade Name	Routes and Dosage Ranges	
			Adults	Children
Autonomic Drugs				
ADRENERGICS				
Decreased production of aqueous humor	Glaucoma	**Dipivefrin (0.1% solution)** (Propine)	Topically, 1 drop in affected eye(s) twice daily q12h	
Mydriasis	Ophthalmoscopic examination	**Epinephrine hydrochloride (0.25%, 0.5%, 1%, and 2% solutions)** (Epifrin, Glaucon)	Topically 1 drop in each eye once or twice daily	Same as adults
Decreased intraocular pressure	Reduction of adhesion formation with uveitis			
Vasoconstriction	Preoperative and postoperative mydriasis	**Hydroxyamphetamine (1% solution)** (Paredrine)	Before ophthalmoscopy, topically, 1 drop in each eye	
Photophobia	Local hemostasis	**Phenylephrine (2.5% and 10% solutions)** (Neo-Synephrine)	Before ophthalmoscopy or refraction, topically, 1 drop of 2.5% or 10% solution	Refraction, topically, 1 drop of 2.5% solution
			Preoperatively, topically, 1 drop of 2.5% or 10% solution 30–60 min before surgery	
			Postoperatively, topically, 1 drop of 10% solution once or twice daily	
ANTIADRENERGIC (BETA-BLOCKING) DRUGS				
Decreased production of aqueous humor	Glaucoma	**Betaxolol** (Betoptic)	Topically to each eye, 1 drop q12h	
Reduced intraocular pressure		**Carteolol** (Ocupress)	Topically to affected eye(s), 1 drop q12h	
		Levobunolol (Betagan)	Topically to the affected eye, 1 drop once or twice daily	
		Metipranolol (OptiPranolol)	Topically to affected eye(s), 1 drop q12h	

TABLE 65-1) **Drugs Used in Ocular Disorders*** (*continued*)

Ocular Effects	Clinical Indications	Generic/Trade Name	Routes and Dosage Ranges	
			Adults	Children
		Timolol maleate (Timoptic)	Topically, 1 drop of 0.25% or 0.5% solution in each eye twice daily q12h	
CHOLINERGICS				
Increased outflow of aqueous humor Miosis	Glaucoma	**Pilocarpine (0.25%–10% solutions)** (Isopto Carpine, Pilocar)	Chronic glaucoma, topically, 1 drop of 1% or 2% solution instilled in each eye three to four times daily	
		Pilocarpine ocular therapeutic system (Ocusert Pilo-20, Ocusert Pilo-40)	One system placed into conjunctival sac per week, according to package directions. Each system releases 20 or 40 µg pilocarpine per hour for 1 wk.	
		Carbachol (Carboptic)	Topically, 2 drops of 0.75%–3% solution into eye(s) up to three times daily	
ANTICHOLINESTERASE AGENTS				
Increased outflow of aqueous humor Miosis	Glaucoma	**Demecarium bromide** (Humorsol)	Topically, 1 drop of 0.125%–0.25% solution in each eye twice a day to twice a week, depending on condition	
		Echothiopate iodide (Phospholine iodide)	Topically, 1 drop of solution (0.03%, 0.06%, 0.125%, or 0.25%) in each eye q12–48h	
ANTICHOLINERGICS				
Mydriasis Cycloplegia Photophobia	Mydriasis for refraction and other diagnostic purposes Before and after intraocular surgery Treatment of uveitis Treatment of some secondary glaucoma	**Atropine sulfate (0.5%–3% solutions)**	Before intraocular surgery, topically, 1 drop of solution After intraocular surgery, topically, 1 drop of solution once daily	
		Cyclopentolate hydrochloride (Cyclogyl)	For refraction, topically, 1 drop of 0.5% or 2% solution instilled once Before ophthalmoscopy, 1 drop of 0.5% solution	For refraction, topically, 1 drop of 0.5%, 1%, or 2% solution, repeated in 10 min
		Homatropine hydrobromide (2% and 5% solutions)	Refraction, topically, 1 drop of 5% solution every 5 min for two or three doses or 1–2 drops of 2% solution every 10–15 min for five doses Uveitis, topically, 1 drop of 2% or 5% solution two or three times daily	
		Scopolamine hydrobromide (0.25% solution) (Isopto Hyoscine)	Refraction, topically, 1–2 drops in affected eye(s) 1 h before examination	
		Tropicamide (0.5% and 1% solutions) (Mydriacyl)	Before refraction or ophthalmoscopy, topically, 1 drop of 0.5% or 1% solution, repeated in 5 min, then every 20–30 min as needed to maintain mydriasis	

Diuretics

CARBONIC ANHYDRASE INHIBITORS

Decreased production of aqueous humor	Glaucoma	**Acetazolamide** (Diamox)	PO 250 mg q6h	PO 10–15 mg/kg/d in divided doses

(*continued*)

TABLE 65-1 **Drugs Used in Ocular Disorders*** (*continued*)

Ocular Effects	Clinical Indications	Generic/Trade Name	Routes and Dosage Ranges	
			Adults	Children
Decreased intraocular pressure	Preoperatively in intraocular surgery		Sustained-release capsules (Diamox Sequels), PO 500 mg q12h IV, IM 5–10 mg/kg/d in divided doses, q6h	IV, IM 5–10 mg/kg/d in divided doses, q6h
		Brinzolamide (Azopt)	Topically, 1 drop in affected eye(s) three times daily	
		Dichlorphenamide (Daranide)	PO 50–200 mg q6–8h. Maintenance dosage, 25–50 mg one to three times daily	
		Dorzolamide (Trusopt)	Topically, 1 drop in affected eye(s) three times daily	
		Methazolamide (Neptazane)	PO 50–100 mg q8h	

OSMOTIC AGENTS

Ocular Effects	Clinical Indications	Generic/Trade Name	Adults	Children
Reduced volume of vitreous humor Decreased intraocular pressure	Before intraocular surgery Treatment of acute glaucoma	Glycerin (Osmoglyn)	PO 1–1.5 g/kg, usually given as a 50% or 75% solution 1–1½ h before surgery	Same as adults
		Isosorbide (Ismotic)	Emergency reduction of intraocular pressure (*eg,* acute angle-closure glaucoma), PO 1.5 g/kg up to four times daily if necessary	
		Mannitol (Osmitrol)	IV 1.5–2 g/kg given as a 20% solution over 30–60 min	Same as adults

Miscellaneous Agents

ALPHA₂-ADRENERGIC AGONISTS

Ocular Effects	Clinical Indications	Generic/Trade Name	Adults	Children
	Glaucoma Prevention of increased intraocular pressure after ocular surgery	Apraclonidine (Iopidine)	1–2 drops in affected eye(s) three times daily	
		Brimonidine (Alphagan)	Topically, 1 drop in affected eye(s) three times daily, q8h	

ANESTHETICS, LOCAL

Ocular Effects	Clinical Indications	Generic/Trade Name	Adults	Children
Surface anesthesia of conjunctiva and cornea	Tonometry Subconjunctival injections Removal of foreign bodies Removal of sutures	Proparacaine hydrochloride (Alcaine, Ophthaine)	Minor procedures, topically, 1–2 drops of 0.5% solution; instillation may be repeated for deeper anesthesia	
		Tetracaine hydrochloride (Pontocaine)	Minor procedures, topically, 1–2 drops of 0.5% solution; two to four instillations are required for deeper anesthesia	

LUBRICANTS

Ocular Effects	Clinical Indications	Generic/Trade Name	Adults	Children
Serve as "artificial tears"	Prevent damage to the cornea in clients with keratitis Protect the cornea during gonioscopy and other procedures Moisten contact lenses Lubricate artificial eyes	Methylcellulose (Methulose, Visculose, others)	Topically, 1–2 drops as needed	
		Polyvinyl alcohol (Liquifilm, others)	Topically, 1–2 drops as needed	

PROSTAGLANDIN

Ocular Effects	Clinical Indications	Generic/Trade Name	Adults	Children
	Glaucoma	Latanoprost (Xalatan)	Topically, 1 drop in affected eye(s) once daily in the evening	

IM, intramuscular; IV, intravenous; PO, oral.

* Antimicrobial agents are listed in Table 65-2; antiallergic and anti-inflammatory agents are listed in Table 65-3.

TABLE 65-2 **Ophthalmic Antimicrobial Agents**

Generic/Trade Name	Routes and Dosage Ranges	
	Adults	Children
Antibacterial Agents		
Bacitracin (Baciguent)	Ophthalmic ointment, topically, instill in infected eye one to three times daily	
Ciprofloxacin ophthalmic solution (Ciloxan)	Corneal ulcers, topically to affected eye. Day 1, 2 drops every 15 min for 6 h, then every 30 min for rest of day; day 2, 2 drops q1h; days 3–14, 2 drops q4h. Conjunctivitis, 1–2 drops q2h while awake for 2 d, then 1–2 drops q4h while awake for 5 d	Safety and effectiveness not established for children <12 y
Erythromycin (Ilotycin ophthalmic [0.5% ointment])		Prevention of neonatal gonococcal or chlamydial conjunctivitis, topically, 0.5–1 cm in each eye
Gentamicin sulfate (Garamycin)	Topically, ophthalmic solution (0.3%) 1 drop q1–4h; ophthalmic ointment (0.3%), instill two or three times daily	Topically, same as adults
Norfloxacin ophthalmic solution (Chibroxin)	Topically to affected eye(s), 1–2 drops four times daily, up to 7 d	Same as adults for children ≥1 y; safety not established for children <1 y
Ofloxacin (Ocuflox)	Bacterial conjunctivitis, topically, 1–2 drops of 0.3% solution q2–4h while awake for 2 d, then 1–2 drops four times daily for up to 5 more days	Same as adults for children ≥1 y
Polymyxin B sulfate	Corneal ulcers due to *Pseudomonas aeruginosa*: topically, 1 drop of a freshly prepared solution (20,000 units/mL), instilled two to ten times hourly	
Sulfacetamide sodium (Bleph-10 Liquifilm [10% solution or ointment], Isopto Cetamide [15% solution]) (Cetamide [10% ointment], Sodium Sulamyd (10% and 30% solution, 10% ointment]) (Also available generically as 10% and 30% solutions)	Acute catarrhal conjunctivitis caused by *Staphylococcus aureus, Diplococcus pneumoniae, Hemophilus influenzae, Neisseria catarrhalis*: topically, 1 drop of 10% or 15% solution every 10–30 min Chronic conjunctivitis due to *Proteus* organisms: topically, 10% ointment instilled three or four times daily Chronic blepharoconjunctivitis due to *S. aureus*: topically, 1 drop of 30% solution three or four times daily Corneal ulcers due to *Escherichia coli* or *Klebsiella pneumoniae*: 1 drop of 10% solution every 30 min or 10% ointment instilled three or four times daily	
Sulfisoxazole diolamine (Gantrisin [4% solution])	Topically, 2–3 drops in affected eye three or more times daily	
Tetracycline (Achromycin)	Inclusion conjunctivitis: topically, 1% solution or ointment instilled three or four times daily for 30 d	Conjunctivitis, same as adults Prevention of neonatal gonococcal or chlamydial conjunctivitis, 0.5–1 cm of ointment into each eye
Tobramycin (Tobrex [0.3% solution and ointment])	Topically, 1–2 drops two to six times daily or ointment two or three times daily	
Antiviral Agent		
Trifluridine (Viroptic)	Keratoconjunctivitis or corneal ulcers caused by herpes simplex virus: topically, 1 drop of 1% solution q2h while awake (maximal daily dose, 9 drops) until corneal ulcer heals, then 1 drop q4h (minimal dose, 5 drops daily for 7 d)	
Antifungal Agent		
Natamycin (Natacyn)	Topically, 1 drop of 5% suspension q1–2h	

TABLE 65-3	Topical Ophthalmic Antiallergic and Anti-inflammatory Agents	
Generic/Trade Name	**Indications for Use**	**Dosage Ranges**
Antiallergic Agents		
Cromolyn (Crolom, Opticrom)	Treatment of seasonal allergic conjunctivitis, keratitis, and keratoconjunctivitis	1–2 drops in each eye four to six times daily at regular intervals
Emedastine (Emadine)	Allergic conjunctivitis	1–2 drops twice daily
Ketotifen (Zaditor)	Allergic conjunctivitis	1 drop in affected eye(s) q8–12h
Levocabastine (Livostin)	Treatment of seasonal allergic conjunctivitis	1 drop in affected eyes four times daily, for up to 2 wk
Lodoxamide (Alomide)	Conjunctivitis Keratitis	1–2 drops in affected eye(s) four times daily, for up to 3 mo
Olopatadine (Patanol)	Allergic conjunctivitis	1–2 drops twice daily
Corticosteroids		
Dexamethasone (Decadron, Maxidex)	Inflammatory disorders of the conjunctiva, cornea, eyelid, and anterior eyeball (e.g. conjunctivitis, keratitis) Corneal injury from chemical, radiation or thermal burns, or penetration of foreign bodies Prevention of graft rejection after corneal transplant	Solution or suspension 1–2 drops q1h daytime, q2h nighttime until response; then 1 drop q4h Postoperative inflammation, 1–2 drops four times daily, starting 24 h after surgery, for 2 wk Ointment thin strip three to four times daily until response, then once or twice daily
Fluorometholone (FML)	Inflammatory disorders	Solution 1 drop q1–2h until response, then less often Ointment thin strip three to four times daily until response, then once or twice daily
Loteprednol (Lotemax, Alrex)	Allergic conjunctivitis Keratitis Treatment of inflammation after ocular surgery	Allergic conjunctivitis, 0.2%, 1 drop in affected eye(s) four times daily Keratitis, 0.5%, 1–2 drops in affected eye(s) four times daily Postoperative inflammation, 0.5%, 1–2 drops in affected eye(s) four times daily starting 24 h after surgery and continuing for 2 wk
Medrysone (HMS)	Inflammatory disorders	1 drop q1–2h until response obtained, then less frequently
Prednisolone (Econopred, others)	Inflammatory disorders	Solution or suspension 1–2 drops q1–2h until response, then 1 drop q4h, then less frequently Ointment thin strip three to four times daily until response, then once or twice daily
Rimexolone (Vexol)	Treatment of anterior uveitis Treatment of inflammation after ocular surgery	Uveitis, 1–2 drops in affected eye q1h during waking hours for 1 wk, then 1 drop q2h for 1 wk, then taper until uveitis resolved Postoperative inflammation, 1–2 drops in affected eye(s) four times daily starting 24 h after surgery and continuing for 2 wk
Nonsteroidal Anti-inflammatory Drugs		
Diclofenac (Voltaren)	Treatment of inflammation after cataract surgery	1 drop to affected eye four times daily, starting 24 h after surgery, for 2 wk
Flurbiprofen (Ocufen)	Inhibition of pupil constriction during eye surgery	1 drop every 30 min for four doses, starting 2 h before surgery
Ketorolac (Acular)	Treatment of ocular itching due to seasonal allergic conjunctivitis	1 drop four times daily for approximately 1 wk
Suprofen (Profenal)	Inhibition of pupil constriction during eye surgery	2 drops at 3, 2, and 1 h before surgery or q4h while awake the day before surgery

NURSING PROCESS

Assessment

Assess the client's condition in relation to ophthalmic disorders.

- Determine whether the client has impaired vision and, if so, the extent or severity of the impairment. Minimal assessment includes the vision-impaired client's ability to participate in activities of daily living, including safe ambulation. Maximal assessment depends on the nurse's ability and

working situation. Some nurses do complete vision testing and ophthalmoscopic examinations.
- Identify risk factors for eye disorders. These include trauma, allergies, infection in one eye (a risk factor for infection in the other eye), use of contact lenses, infections of facial structures or skin, and occupational exposure to chemical irritants or foreign bodies.
- Signs and symptoms vary with particular disorders:
  - Pain is usually associated with corneal abrasions or inflammation. Sudden, severe pain may indicate acute narrow-angle glaucoma. Acute narrow-angle glaucoma requires immediate treatment to lower intraocular pressure and minimize damage to the optic nerve.
  - Signs of inflammation (redness, edema, heat, tenderness) are especially evident with infection or inflammation of external ocular structures, such as the eyelids and conjunctiva. A watery or mucoid discharge also often occurs.
  - Pruritus is most often associated with allergic conjunctivitis.
  - Photosensitivity commonly occurs with keratitis.

Nursing Diagnoses

- Sensory-Perceptual Alteration: Impaired vision
- Pain in eyes related to infection, inflammation, or increased intraocular pressure (glaucoma)
- Risk for Injury: Blindness related to inadequately treated glaucoma or ophthalmic infections
- Risk for Injury: Trauma related to blurred vision from disease process or drug therapy
- Impaired Physical Mobility related to impaired vision
- Body Image Disturbance related to impaired vision and chronic illness
- Anxiety related to acute and chronic disturbances in vision
- Knowledge Deficit related to prevention and treatment of ocular disorders

Planning/Goals

The client will:

- Take ophthalmic medications as prescribed
- Follow safety precautions to protect eyes from trauma and disease
- Experience improvement in signs and symptoms (eg, decreased drainage with infections, decreased eye pain with glaucoma)
- Avoid injury from impaired vision (eg, falls)
- Avoid systemic effects of ophthalmic drugs
- Have regular eye examinations to monitor effects of antiglaucoma drugs

Interventions

Use measures to minimize ocular disorders.

- Promote regular eye examinations. This is especially important among middle-aged and older adults, who are more likely to have several ocular disorders. They are also more likely to experience ocular disorders as adverse effects of drugs taken for nonocular disorders.
- Assist clients at risk of eye damage from increased intraocular pressure (eg, those with glaucoma; those who have had intraocular surgery, such as cataract removal) to avoid straining at stool (use laxatives or stool softeners if needed), heavy lifting, bending over, coughing, and vomiting when possible.
- Promote hand washing and keeping hands away from eyes to prevent eye infections.
- Cleanse contact lenses or assist clients in lens care, when needed.
- Treat eye injuries appropriately:
  - For chemical burns, irrigate the eyes with copious amounts of water as soon as possible (ie, near the area where the injury occurred). Do not wait for transport to a first aid station, hospital, or other health care facility. Damage continues as long as the chemical is in contact with the eye.
  - For thermal burns, apply cold compresses to the area.
  - Superficial foreign bodies may be removed by irrigation with water. Foreign bodies embedded in ocular structures must be removed by a physician.
- Warm, wet compresses are often useful in ophthalmic inflammation or infections. They relieve pain and promote healing by increasing the blood supply to the affected area.

Evaluation

- Observe and interview for compliance with instructions regarding drug therapy and follow-up care.
- Observe and interview for relief of symptoms.
- Observe for systemic adverse effects of ophthalmic drugs (eg, tachycardia and arrhythmias with adrenergics; bradycardia with beta blockers).

PRINCIPLES OF THERAPY

General Guidelines

1. Topical application is the most common route of administration for ophthalmic drugs, and correct administration is essential for optimal therapeutic effects.

CLIENT TEACHING GUIDELINES
Topical Eye Medications

General Considerations

✔ Prevent eye disorders, when possible. For example, try to avoid long periods of reading and computer work; minimize exposure to dust, smog, cigarette smoke, and other eye irritants; wash hands often and avoid touching the eyes to decrease risks of infection.

✔ Do not use nonprescription eye drops (eg, Murine, Visine) on a regular basis for longer than 48 to 72 hours. Persistent eye irritation and redness should be reported to a physician.

✔ Have regular eye examinations and testing for glaucoma after 40 years of age.

✔ Eye drop preparations often contain sulfites, which can cause allergic reactions in some people.

✔ If you have glaucoma, do not take any drugs without the ophthalmologist's knowledge and consent. Many drugs given for purposes other than eye disorders may cause or aggravate glaucoma. Also, wear a medical alert bracelet or carry identification that states you have glaucoma. This helps to avoid administration of drugs that aggravate glaucoma or to maintain treatment of glaucoma, in emergencies.

✔ If you have an eye infection, wash hands before and after contact with the infected eye to avoid spreading the infection to the unaffected eye or to other people. Also, avoid touching the unaffected eye.

✔ If you wear contact lenses, wash your hands before inserting them and follow instructions for care (eg, cleaning, inserting or removing, and duration of wear). Improper or infrequent cleaning may lead to infection. Overwearing is a common cause of corneal abrasion and may cause corneal ulceration. The lens wearer should consult a physician when eye pain occurs. Antibiotics are often prescribed for corneal abrasions to prevent development of ulcers.

✔ If you wear soft contact lenses, do not use any eye medication without consulting a specialist in eye care. Some eye drops contain benzalkonium hydrochloride, a preservative, which is absorbed by soft contacts. The medication should not be applied while wearing soft contacts and should be instilled 15 minutes or longer before inserting soft contacts.

✔ Never use eye medications used by someone else and never allow your eye medications to be used by anyone

else. These preparations should be used by one person only and they are dispensed in small amounts for this purpose. Single-person use minimizes cross-contamination and risks of infection.

✔ Many eye drops and ointments cause temporary blurring of vision. Do not use such medications just before driving or operating potentially hazardous machinery.

✔ Avoid straining at stool (use laxatives or stool softeners if necessary), heavy lifting, bending over, coughing, and vomiting when possible. These activities increase intraocular pressure, which may cause eye damage in glaucoma and after eye surgery.

Self-administration

✔ If using more than one eye medication, be sure to administer the correct one at the correct time. Benefits depend on accurate administration.

✔ Check expiration dates; do not use any eye medication after the expiration date and do not use any liquid medications that have changed color or contain particles.

✔ Shake the container if instructed to do so on the label. Solutions do not need to be shaken; suspensions should be shaken well to ensure the drug is evenly dispersed in the liquid and not settled in the bottom of the container.

✔ Wash hands thoroughly.

✔ Tilt head back or lie down and look up.

✔ Grasp the lower eyelid and pull it gently away from the eye to form a pouch.

✔ Place the dropper directly over the eye. Avoid contact of the dropper with the eye, finger, or any other surface. Such contact contaminates the solution and using contaminated solutions can cause eye infections and serious damage to the eye, with possible loss of vision.

✔ Look up just before applying a drop; look down for several seconds after applying a drop.

✔ Release the eyelid, close the eyes, and press on the inside corner of the eye with a finger for 3 to 5 minutes. The finger pressure helps the medication be more effective by slowing its drainage out of the eye into the tear duct.

✔ Do not rub the eye; do not rinse the dropper.

✔ If more than one eye drop is ordered, wait at least 5 minutes before instilling the second medication.

✔ Use the same basic procedure to insert eye ointments.

---

2. The value of more than one drop is questionable because the normal eye retains only a very small amount.

3. Systemic absorption of eye drops can be decreased by applying pressure over the tear duct for 3 to 5 minutes after instillation.

4. When multiple eye drops are required, there should be an interval of at least 5 minutes between

drops because of limited eye capacity and rapid drainage into tear ducts.

5. Absorption of eye medications is increased in eye disorders associated with hyperemia and inflammation.

6. Many ophthalmic drugs are available as eye drops (solutions or suspensions) and ointments. Ointments do not need to be administered as fre-

quently and often produce higher concentrations of drug in target tissues. However, ointments also cause blurred vision, which limits their daytime use, at least for ambulatory clients. In some situations, drops may be used during waking hours and ointments at bedtime. However, the two formulations are not interchangeable.

7. Topical ophthalmic medications should not be used after the expiration date and cloudy, discolored solutions should be discarded.

8. Topical eye medications contain a number of inactive ingredients, such as preservatives, buffers, tonicity agents, antioxidants, and so forth. Some contain sulfites, to which some people may have allergic reactions.

9. Contact lens wearers should be meticulous in cleaning, disinfecting, and handling lenses to prevent infection and corneal abrasions. They should also consult a physician when eye pain occurs, preferably an ophthalmologist. In addition, wearers of soft contact lenses should not use any eye medication without consulting a specialist in eye care. Some eye drops contain benzalkonium hydrochloride, a preservative, which is absorbed by soft contacts. The medication should not be applied while wearing soft contacts and should be instilled 15 minutes or longer before inserting soft contacts.

10. To increase safety and accuracy of ophthalmic drug therapy, the labels and caps of eye medications are color coded.

Ocular Infections

Guidelines for drug therapy of ocular infections include the following:

1. Drug therapy is usually initiated as soon as culture material (eye secretions) has been obtained, often with a broad-spectrum antibacterial agent or a combination of two or more antibiotics.

2. Topical administration is used most often, and recommended drugs include bacitracin, polymyxin B, and sulfacetamide. These agents are rarely given systemically. They do not cause sensitization to commonly used systemic antibiotics and do not promote growth of drug-resistant microorganisms.

Other antibacterial drugs available in ophthalmic formulations include erythromycin, gentamicin, tobramycin, ciprofloxacin, norfloxacin, ofloxacin, and combination products.

3. In severe infections, antibacterial drugs may be given both topically and systemically. Because systemic antibiotics penetrate the eye poorly, large doses are required to attain therapeutic drug concentrations in ocular structures. Drugs that reach therapeutic levels in the eye when given in proper dosage include ampicillin and dicloxacillin. Gentamicin and other antibiotics penetrate the eye when inflammation is present.

4. Combination products containing two or more antibacterials are available for topical treatment of external ocular infections. These products are most useful when therapy must be initiated before the infecting microorganism is identified. Mixtures provide a broader spectrum of antibacterial activity than a single drug. Some of the available combinations are polymyxin B and bacitracin. Some combinations also contain neomycin, which may cause sensitization with even short-term topical use.

5. Fixed-dose combinations of an antibacterial agent and corticosteroid are available for topical use in selected conditions (eg, staphylococcal keratitis, blepharoconjunctivitis, allergic conjunctivitis, and some postoperative inflammatory reactions). Neomycin and corticosteroid mixtures include Neo-Decadron. Neomycin, polymyxin B, and corticosteroid mixtures include Poly-Pred and Maxitrol. Neomycin, polymyxin B, bacitracin, and corticosteroid mixtures include Cortisporin. Sulfacetamide and corticosteroid mixtures include Blephamide, Cetapred, Metimyd, and Vasocidin.

6. Trifluridine (Viroptic) is the drug of choice in eye infections caused by the herpes simplex virus.

7. In fungal infections, natamycin (Natacyn) may be preferred because it has a broad spectrum of antifungal activity and is nonirritating and nontoxic. It is the only drug approved by the Food and Drug Administration for fungal keratitis.

Glaucoma

For drug therapy of chronic, primary open-angle glaucoma, beta-adrenergic blocking agents are the most commonly used drugs. Several beta blockers are available for ophthalmic use. Most adverse effects occurring with systemic beta blockers also have been reported with ophthalmic preparations.

Use in Children

Topical ophthalmic drug therapy in children differs little from that in adults. Few studies of ophthalmic drug therapy in children have been reported, and many conditions for which adults need therapy (eg, cataract, glaucoma) rarely occur in children. A major use of topical ophthalmic drugs in children is to dilate the pupil and paralyze accommodation for ophthalmoscopic examination. As a general rule, the short-acting mydriatics and cycloplegics (eg, cyclopentolate, tropicamide) are preferred because they cause fewer systemic adverse effects than atropine and scopolamine. In addition, lower drug concentrations are usually given empirically because of the smaller size of children and the potential risk of systemic adverse effects.

Use in Older Adults

Older adults are at risk for development of ocular disorders, especially glaucoma and cataracts. General principles of ophthalmic drug therapy are the same as for younger adults. In addition, older adults are likely to have cardiovascular disorders, which may be aggravated by systemic absorption of topical eye medication. Thus, accurate dosage and occlusion of the nasolacrimal duct in the inner canthus of the eye are needed to prevent adverse drug effects (eg, hypertension, tachycardia, or arrhythmias with adrenergic drugs and bradycardia or heart block with beta blockers).

Home Care

The home care nurse may be involved in the care of clients with acute or chronic eye disorders. As with other drug therapy, the nurse may need to teach clients and caregivers reasons for use, accurate administration, and assessment of therapeutic and adverse responses to eye medications. The nurse may also need to encourage periodic eye examinations to promote optimal vision and prevent blindness.

(*text continues on page 982*)

NURSING ACTIONS **Ophthalmic Drugs**

NURSING ACTIONS	RATIONALE/EXPLANATION
1. Administer accurately	
a. Read labels of ophthalmic medications carefully.	To avoid error. For example, many drugs are available in several concentrations. The correct concentration and the correct drug must be given.
b. Read medication orders carefully and accurately.	To avoid error. Abbreviations (eg, OS, OD, OU) are often used in physicians' orders and must be interpreted accurately.
c. For hospitalized clients, keep eye medications at the bedside when possible.	Eye medications should be ordered for and used by one person only. They are dispensed in small amounts for this purpose. This minimizes cross-contamination and risk of infection.
d. Wash hands before approaching the client for instillation of eye medications.	To reduce risks of infection
e. To administer eye drops, have the client lie down or tilt the head backward and look upward. Then, pull down the lower lid to expose the conjunctival sac, and drop the medication into the sac. Alternate method: gently grasp the lower lid and pull it outward to form a pouch into which medication is instilled.	Absorption of the drug and its concentration in ocular tissues depend partly on the length of time the medication is in contact with ocular tissues. Contact time is increased by the "pouch" method of administration, closing the eyes (delays outflow into the nasolacrimal duct), and pressure on the inner canthus (delays outflow and decreases side effects resulting from systemic absorption).

(continued)

NURSING ACTIONS	**RATIONALE/EXPLANATION**
After instillation, have the client close the eyes gently, and apply pressure to the inner canthus briefly (nurse or client).	
f. When instilling ophthalmic ointments, position the client as above, and apply a ¼-inch to ½-inch strip of ointment to the conjunctiva.	
g. Do not touch the dropper tip or ointment top to the eye or anything else.	To avoid contamination of the medication and infection
h. When crusts or secretions are present, cleanse the eye before administering medication.	If the eye is not cleansed, the drug may not be absorbed.
i. When two or more eye drops are scheduled for the same time, they should be instilled approximately 5 min apart.	To avoid drug loss by dilution and outflow into the nasolacrimal duct
2. Observe for therapeutic effects	Therapeutic effects depend on the reason for use.
a. With beta-blocking agents, observe for decreased intraocular pressure.	Lowering of intraocular pressure usually occurs within a month; periodic measurements should be done.
b. With mydriatics, observe for dilation of the pupil.	Mydriasis begins within 5 to 15 min after instillation.
c. With miotics, observe for constriction of the pupil.	
d. With antimicrobial drugs, observe for decreased redness, edema, and drainage.	
e. With osmotic agents, observe for decreased intraocular pressure.	With oral glycerin, maximal decrease in intraocular pressure occurs approximately 1 h after administration, and effects persist for about 5 h. With intravenous (IV) mannitol, maximal decrease in intraocular pressure occurs within 30 to 60 min, and effects last 6 to 8 h.
3. Observe for adverse effects	
a. Local effects:	
(1) Irritation, burning, stinging, blurred vision, discomfort, redness, itching, tearing, conjunctivitis, keratitis, allergic reactions	These effects may occur with any topical ophthalmic agents. Burning and stinging discomfort occur with instillation and are usually transient. Allergic reactions may occur with the active ingredient, preservatives, or other components.
(2) With antibacterial agents—superinfection or sensitization	Superinfection caused by drug-resistant organisms may occur. Sensitization means that topical application induces antibody formation. Therefore, if the same or a related drug is subsequently administered systemically, an allergic reaction may occur. The allergic reaction most often involves dermatitis; occasionally urticaria or anaphylaxis occurs. Penicillin is the most frequently involved drug. Other drugs include streptomycin, neomycin, gentamicin, and sulfonamides (with the exception of sulfacetamide sodium). Sensitization can be prevented or minimized by avoiding topical administration of antibacterial agents that are commonly given systemically.

(continued)

NURSING ACTIONS	RATIONALE/EXPLANATION
(3) With anticholinergics, adrenergics, topical corticosteroids—glaucoma	Mydriatic drugs (anticholinergics and adrenergics) may cause an acute attack of angle closure in clients with narrow-angle glaucoma by blocking outflow of aqueous humor. Topical corticosteroids raise intraocular pressure in some clients. The "glaucomatous" response occurs most often in clients with chronic, primary open-angle glaucoma and their relatives. It also may occur in clients with myopia or diabetes mellitus. The magnitude of increased intraocular pressure depends on the concentration, frequency of administration, duration of therapy, and anti-inflammatory potency of the corticosteroid. Increased intraocular pressure has been reported most often with 0.1% dexamethasone (Decadron). This adverse effect can be minimized by checking intraocular pressure every 2 mo in clients receiving long-term therapy with topical corticosteroids.
(4) Cataract formation	This is most likely to occur with long-term use of anticholinesterase agents.
(5) With miotic drugs—decreased vision in dim light	These agents prevent pupil dilation, which normally occurs in dim light or darkness.
b. Systemic effects:	Systemic absorption and adverse effects of eye drops can be prevented or minimized by applying pressure to the inner canthus during and after instillation of the medications. Pressure may be applied by the nurse or the client.
(1) With beta-blocking agents—bradycardia, congestive heart failure, bronchospasm, and others (see Chap. 19)	These agents may be absorbed systematically and cause all the adverse effects associated with oral or injected drugs.
(2) With miotics—sweating, nausea, vomiting, diarrhea, abdominal pain, bradycardia, hypotension, bronchoconstriction. Toxic doses produce ataxia, confusion, convulsions, coma, respiratory failure, and death	These cholinergic or parasympathomimetic effects occur rarely with pilocarpine or carbachol. They are more likely to occur with the long-acting anticholinesterase agents, especially echothiophate (Phospholine iodide). Acute toxicity may be reversed by an anticholinergic agent, atropine, given IV.
(3) With anticholinergic mydriatics—dryness of the mouth and skin, fever, rash, tachycardia, confusion, hallucinations, delirium	These effects are most likely to occur with atropine and in children and older adults. Tropicamide (Mydriacyl) rarely causes systemic reactions.
(4) With adrenergic mydriatics—tachycardia, hypertension, premature ventricular contractions, tremors, headache	Systemic effects are uncommon. They are more likely to occur with repeated instillations of high drug concentrations (eg, epinephrine 2%, phenylephrine [Neo-Synephrine] 10%).
(5) With carbonic anhydrase inhibitors—anorexia, nausea, vomiting, diarrhea, paresthesias, weakness, lethargy	Nausea, malaise, and paresthesias (numbness and tingling of extremities) commonly occur with oral drugs.
(6) With osmotic diuretics—dehydration, nausea, vomiting, headache, hyperglycemia and glycosuria with glycerin (Osmoglyn)	These agents may produce profound diuresis and dehydration. Oral agents (eg, glycerin) are less likely to cause severe systemic effects than IV agents *(continued)*

NURSING ACTIONS	RATIONALE/EXPLANATION
	(eg, mannitol). These agents are usually given in a single dose, which decreases the risks of serious adverse reactions unless large doses are given.
(7) With corticosteroids, see Chapter 24.	Serious adverse effects may occur with long-term use of corticosteroids.
(8) With antibacterial agents, see Chapter 33 and the chapter on the individual drug group.	Adverse effects may occur with all antibacterial agents.
(9) With apraclonidine—bradycardia, orthostatic hypotension, headache, insomnia	This drug is related to clonidine, an alpha-adrenergic agonist antihypertensive agent (see Chaps. 19 and 55).
(10) With latanoprost—common cold or flu-like upper respiratory infection, muscle and joint pain, angina pectoris, skin rash	These were the most commonly reported systemic adverse effects in clinical trials.
(11) With ophthalmic nonsteroidal anti-inflammatory drugs—potential for increased bleeding	Systemic absorption may interfere with platelet function and increase risks of bleeding with surgery or anticoagulant therapy.
4. Observe for drug interactions	
a. Drugs that *increase* effects of adrenergic (sympathomimetic) ophthalmic drugs:	
(1) Anticholinergic ophthalmic drugs	The combination (eg, atropine and phenylephrine) produces additive mydriasis
(2) Systemic adrenergic drugs	Additive risks of adverse effects (eg, tachycardia, cardiac arrhythmias, hypertension)
b. Drugs that *decrease* effects of adrenergic ophthalmic preparations:	
(1) Cholinergic and anticholinesterase ophthalmic drugs	Antagonize mydriatic effects of adrenergic drugs
c. Drugs that *increase* effects of antiadrenergic ophthalmic preparations:	
(1) Systemic antiadrenergics (eg, propranolol, atenolol, metoprolol, nadolol, timolol)	When the client is receiving a topical beta blocker in ocular disorders, administration of systemic beta-blocking agents in cardiovascular disorders may cause additive systemic toxicity.
d. Drugs that *increase* effects of anticholinergic ophthalmic drugs:	
(1) Adrenergic ophthalmic agents	Additive mydriasis
(2) Systemic anticholinergic drugs (eg, atropine) and other drugs with anticholinergic effects (eg, some antihistamines, antipsychotic agents, and tricyclic antidepressants)	Additive anticholinergic effects (mydriasis, blurred vision, tachycardia). These drugs are hazardous in narrow-angle glaucoma.
e. Drugs that *decrease* effects of cholinergic and anticholinesterase ophthalmic drugs:	
(1) Anticholinergics and drugs with anticholinergic effects (eg, atropine, antipsychotic agents, tricyclic antidepressants, some antihistamines)	Antagonize antiglaucoma (miotic) effects of cholinergic and anticholinesterase drugs

(continued)

NURSING ACTIONS	RATIONALE/EXPLANATION
(2) Corticosteroids	Long-term use of corticosteroids, topically or systemically, raises intraocular pressure and may cause glaucoma. Therefore, corticosteroids decrease effects of all drugs used for glaucoma
(3) Sympathomimetic drugs	Antagonize miotic (antiglaucoma) effects

How Can You Avoid This Medication Error?

Answer: The order indicates that this patient should receive 1 drop of Chloromycetin in her left eye. The abbreviations for ocular medications include OS, left eye; OD, right eye; and OU, both eyes. Chloromycetin is used to treat infection that may have been present only in the left eye.

Nursing Notes: Apply Your Knowledge

Answer: Start by assessing what Mrs. Jetson knows about glaucoma and providing basic information about the condition. Review and write down the order for eye drops. Sometimes the small print on the medication container is difficult to read. Ask Mrs. Jetson if she has taken eye drops before. If so, watch her demonstrate this procedure, reinforcing proper technique (tilt head back, pull down lower lid, drop medication into sac, close eyes). Good aseptic technique should be stressed (wash hands, keep container clean, do not let dropper touch eye). Also caution Mrs. Jetson to notify her doctor before taking any medications or remedies.

REVIEW AND APPLICATION EXERCISES

1. What is the main function of the eye?

2. List common disorders of the eye for which drug therapy is indicated.

3. Do ophthalmic medications need to be sterile? Why or why not?

4. What are important principles and techniques related to the nurse's administration of ophthalmic drugs?

5. For a client with newly prescribed eye drops, how would you teach self-administration principles and techniques?

SELECTED REFERENCES

Cioffi, G.A. & VanBuskirk, E.M. (1997). Glaucoma therapy. In K.W. Wright (Ed.), *Textbook of ophthalmology*, pp. 627–645. Baltimore: Williams & Wilkins.

Curtis, S.M. & Carroll, E.M. (1998). Alterations in vision. In C.M. Porth (Ed.), *Pathophysiology: Concepts of altered health states*, 5th ed., pp. 1025–1052. Philadelphia: Lippincott Williams & Wilkins.

Drug facts and comparisons. (Updated monthly). St. Louis: Facts and Comparisons.

Fechner, P.U. & Teichmann, K.D. (1998). *Ocular therapeutics: Pharmacology and clinical application*. Thorofare, NJ: Slack.

Lesar, T.S. (1997). Glaucoma. In J.T. DiPiro, R.L. Talbert, G.C. Yee, G.R. Matzke, B.G. Wells, & L.M. Posey (Eds.), *Pharmacotherapy: A pathophysiologic approach*, 3rd ed., pp. 1783–1799. Stamford, CT: Appleton & Lange.

Liesegang, T.J. (1996). Glaucoma: Changing concepts and future directions. *Mayo Clinic Proceedings, 71*, 689–694.

Moroi, S.E. & Lichter, P.R. (1996). Ocular pharmacology. In J.G. Hardman, L.E. Limbird, P.B. Molinoff, & R.W. Ruddon (Eds.), *Goodman & Gilman's The pharmacological basis of therapeutics*, 9th ed., pp. 1619–1645. New York: McGraw-Hill.

Wallace, D.K. & Steinkuller, P.G. (1998). Ocular medications in children. *Clinical Pediatrics, 37*, 645–652.

66

Drugs Used in Dermatologic Conditions

Objectives

After studying this chapter, the student will be able to:

1. Review characteristics of skin structures that influence drug therapy of dermatologic disorders.

2. Discuss antimicrobial, anti-inflammatory, and selected miscellaneous drugs in relation to their use in dermatologic disorders.

3. Use correct techniques to administer dermatologic medications.

4. Teach clients, family members, or caregivers correct administration of dermatologic medications.

5. For clients with "open lesion" skin disorders, teach about the importance and techniques of preventing infection.

6. Practice and teach measures to protect the skin from the damaging effects of sun exposure.

Fifteen-year-old Shawn Kelly stops by to talk when you are working in the teen clinic. For the last 6 months, he has had a severe problem with acne and his face is currently spotted with pimples and pustules.

Reflect on:

▶ Why acne is so common during adolescence.

▶ The impact acne has on the psychosocial development of an adolescent.

▶ How you will structure your intervention to be most therapeutic.

▶ Plan appropriate teaching for Shawn related to his acne.

CHARACTERISTICS OF THE SKIN

The skin, the largest organ of the body, is the interface between the body's internal and external environments. The skin is composed of the epidermis and dermis. Epidermal or epithelial cells begin in the basal layer of the epidermis and migrate outward, undergoing degenerative changes in each layer. The outer layer, called the *stratum corneum*, is composed of dead cells and keratin. The dead cells are constantly being shed (desquamated) and replaced by newer cells. Normally, approximately 1 month is required for cell formation, migration, and desquamation. When dead cells are discarded, keratin remains on the skin. Keratin is a tough protein substance that is insoluble in water, weak acids, and weak bases. Hair and nails, which are composed of keratin, are referred to as appendages of the skin.

Melanocytes are pigment-producing cells located at the junction of the epidermis and the dermis. These cells produce yellow, brown, or black skin coloring in response to genetic influences, melanocyte-stimulating hormone released from the anterior pituitary gland, and exposure to ultraviolet (UV) light (eg, sunlight).

The dermis is composed of elastic and fibrous connective tissue. Dermal structures include blood vessels, lymphatic channels, nerves and nerve endings, sweat glands, sebaceous glands, and hair follicles. The dermis is supported underneath by subcutaneous tissue, which is composed primarily of fat cells.

The skin has numerous functions, most of which are protective, including the following:

- Serves as a physical barrier against loss of fluids and electrolytes and against entry of microorganisms, foreign bodies, and other potentially harmful substances
- Detects sensations of pain, pressure, touch, and temperature through sensory nerve endings
- Assists in regulating body temperature through production and elimination of sweat
- Serves as a source of vitamin D when exposed to sunlight or other sources of UV light. Skin contains a precursor for vitamin D.
- Serves as an excretory organ. Water, sodium, chloride, lactate, and urea are excreted in sweat.
- Inhibits growth of many microorganisms by its acidic pH (approximately 4.5 to 6.5)

Mucous membranes are composed of a surface layer of epithelial cells, a basement membrane, and a layer of connective tissue. They line body cavities that communicate with the external environment (ie, mouth, vagina, anus). They receive an abundant blood supply because capillaries lie just beneath the epithelial cells.

Dermatologic disorders may be primary (ie, originate in the skin or mucous membranes) or secondary (ie, result from a systemic condition, such as measles or adverse drug reactions). This chapter emphasizes selected primary skin disorders and the topical medications used to prevent or treat them.

DISORDERS OF THE SKIN

Because the skin is constantly exposed to the external environment, it is susceptible to numerous disorders, including those described in the following sections.

Inflammatory Disorders

Dermatitis

Dermatitis is a general term denoting an inflammatory response of the skin to injuries from irritants, allergens, or trauma. *Eczema* is often used as a synonym for dermatitis. Whatever the cause, dermatitis is usually characterized by erythema, pruritus, and skin lesions. It may be acute or chronic.

- **Atopic dermatitis** is a common disorder characterized mainly by pruritus and lesions that vary according to the extent of inflammation, stages of healing, and scratching. Scratching damages the skin and increases the risks of secondary infection. Acute lesions are reddened skin areas containing papules and vesicles; chronic lesions are often thick, fibrotic, and nodular.

  The cause is uncertain but may involve allergic, hereditary, or psychological elements. Approximately 50% to 80% of clients have asthma or allergic rhinitis; some have a family history of these disorders. Thus, exposure to possible causes or exacerbating factors such as allergens, irritating chemicals, foods, and emotional stress should be considered. The condition may occur in all age groups but is more common in children.

- **Contact dermatitis** results from direct contact with irritants (eg, strong soaps, detergents, acids, alkalis) or allergens (eg, clothing materials or dyes, jewelry, cosmetics, hair dyes) that stimulate inflammation. Irritants cause tissue damage and dermatitis in anyone with sufficient contact or exposure. Allergens cause dermatitis only in sensitized or hypersensitive people. The location of the dermatitis may indicate the cause (eg, facial dermatitis may indicate an allergy to cosmetics).

- **Seborrheic dermatitis** is a disease of the sebaceous glands characterized by excessive production of sebum. A simple form of seborrheic dermatitis involving the scalp is dandruff, which is characterized by flaking and itching of the skin. More severe forms of seborrheic dermatitis are characterized by greasy, yellow scales or crusts with variable amounts of erythema and itching. Seborrheic dermatitis may occur on the scalp, face, or trunk.

- **Urticaria** ("hives") is an inflammatory response characterized by a skin lesion called a wheal, a raised edematous area with a pale center and red border, which itches intensely. Histamine is the most common mediator of urticaria and it causes vasodilation, increased vascular permeability, and pruritus.

  Histamine is released from mast cells and basophils by both allergic (eg, insect bites, foods, drugs) and nonallergic (eg, radiocontrast media, opiates, and some antibiotics as well as heat, cold, pressure, UV light) stimuli. An important difference between allergic and nonallergic reactions is that many allergic reactions require prior exposure to the stimulus, whereas nonallergic reactions can occur with the first exposure.

- **Drug-induced skin reactions** vary widely and can imitate the signs and symptoms of virtually any skin disorder. Topical drugs usually cause a localized, contact dermatitis type of reaction and systemic drugs cause generalized skin lesions. These reactions most often occur within the first or second week of drug administration and usually subside when the drug is discontinued.

Psoriasis

Psoriasis is a chronic skin disorder characterized by erythematous, dry, scaling lesions. The lesions may occur anywhere on the body but commonly involve the skin covering bony prominences, such as the elbows and knees. The disease is characterized by remissions and exacerbations. Exacerbating factors include infections, winter weather, some drugs (eg, beta blockers, lithium) and possibly stress, obesity, and alcoholism.

The cause of psoriasis is thought to be an inflammatory process. The pathophysiology involves excessively rapid turnover of epidermal cells. Instead of approximately 30 days from formation to elimination of normal epidermal cells, epidermal cells involved in psoriasis are abnormal in structure and have a life span of approximately 4 days.

Skin lesions may be tender, but they do not usually cause severe pain or itching. However, the lesions are unsightly and usually cause embarrassment and mental distress.

Rosacea

Rosacea is characterized by erythema and pustules of facial skin and hyperplasia of the soft tissues of the nose (rhinophyma). It is a chronic disease of unknown etiology that usually occurs in middle-aged and older people, more often in men than women.

Dermatologic Infections

Bacterial Infections

Bacterial infections of the skin are common; they are most often caused by streptococci or staphylococci.

- **Cellulitis** is characterized by erythema, tenderness, and edema, which may spread to subcutaneous tissue. Generalized malaise, chills, and fever may occur.
- **Folliculitis** is an infection of the hair follicles that most often occurs on the scalp or bearded areas of the face.
- **Furuncles** and **carbuncles** are infections usually caused by staphylococci. Furuncles (boils) may result from folliculitis. They usually occur in the neck, face, axillae, buttocks, thighs, and perineum. Furuncles tend to recur. Carbuncles involve many hair follicles and include multiple pustules. Carbuncles may cause fever, malaise, leukocytosis, and bacteremia. Healing of carbuncles often produces scar tissue.
- **Impetigo** is a superficial skin infection caused by streptococci or staphylococci. An especially contagious form is caused by group A beta-hemolytic streptococci. This form occurs most often in children.

Fungal Infections

Fungal infections of the skin and mucous membranes are most often caused by *Candida albicans*.

- Oral candidiasis (thrush) involves mucous membranes of the mouth. It often occurs as a superinfection after the use of broad-spectrum systemic antibiotics.
- **Candidiasis of the vagina and vulva** occurs with systemic antibiotic therapy and in women with diabetes mellitus.
- **Intertrigo** involves skin folds or areas where two skin surfaces are in contact (eg, groin, pendulous breasts).
- **Tinea** infections (ringworm) are caused by fungi (dermatophytes). These infections may involve the scalp (tinea capitis), the body (tinea corporis), the foot (tinea pedis), and other areas of the body. Tinea pedis, commonly called *athlete's foot*, is the most common type of ringworm infection.

Viral Infections

Viral infections of the skin include veruccal (warts) and herpes infections. There are two types of herpes simplex infections. Type 1 infections usually involve the face or neck (eg, fever blisters or cold sores on the lips), and type 2 infections involve the genital organs. Other herpes infections include herpes zoster (shingles) and varicella (chickenpox).

Trauma

Trauma refers to a physical injury that disrupts the skin. When the skin is broken, it may not be able to function properly. The major problem associated with skin wounds is infection. Common wounds include lacerations (cuts or tears), abrasions (shearing or scraping of the skin), and puncture wounds; surgical incisions; and burn wounds.

Ulcerations

Cutaneous ulcerations are usually caused by trauma and impaired circulation. They may become inflamed or infected.

- **Pressure ulcers** (also called decubitus ulcers) may occur anywhere on the body where external pressure decreases blood flow. Common sites include the sacrum, trochanters, ankles, and heels. Cutaneous ulcers also may result from improper moving and lifting techniques. For example, when a person is pulled across bed linens rather than lifted, friction and shearing force may cause skin abrasions. Abraded skin is susceptible to infection and ulcer formation.

    Pressure ulcers are most likely to develop in clients who are immobilized, incontinent, malnourished, and debilitated.
- **Venous stasis ulcers** are commonly located on the lower extremities.

Acne

Acne is a common disorder characterized by excessive production of sebum and obstruction of hair follicles, which normally carry sebum to the skin surface. As a result, hair follicles expand and form comedones (blackheads and whiteheads). Acne lesions vary from small comedones to acne vulgaris, the most severe form, in which follicles become infected and irritating secretions leak into surrounding tissues to form inflammatory pustules, cysts, and abscesses. Most clients have a variety of lesion types at one time.

Acne occurs most often on the face, upper back, and chest because large numbers of sebaceous glands are located in these areas. One etiologic factor is increased secretion of male hormones (androgens), which occurs at puberty in both sexes. This leads to increased production of sebum and proliferation of *Propionibacterium acnes* bacteria, which depend on sebum for survival. The *P. acnes* organisms contain lipase enzymes that break down free fatty acids and produce inflammation in acne lesions. Other causative factors may include medications (eg, phenytoin, corticosteroids) and stress, whose mechanism may involve stimulation of androgen secretion. There is no evidence that lack of cleanliness or certain foods (eg, chocolate) cause acne.

External Otitis

External otitis is an infection of the external ear characterized by pain, itching, and drainage. The external ear, including the meatus, canal, and tympanic membrane (eardrum), is lined with epidermal tissue. The epidermal tissue is susceptible to the same skin disorders that affect other parts of the body. External otitis is most often caused by *Pseudomonas aeruginosa* and *Staphylococcus aureus*

organisms and may be treated with antimicrobial ear drops for approximately 7 to 10 days.

Anorectal Disorders

Hemorrhoids and anal fissures are common anorectal disorders characterized by pruritus, bleeding, and pain. Inflammation and infection may occur.

TYPES OF DERMATOLOGIC DRUGS

Many different agents are used to prevent or treat dermatologic disorders. Most agents fit into one or more of the following categories:

- **Antiseptics** kill or inhibit the growth of bacteria, viruses, or fungi. They are used primarily to prevent infection. They are occasionally used to treat dermatologic infections. Skin surfaces should be clean before application of antiseptics.
- **Antimicrobial drugs** are used to treat infections caused by bacteria, fungi, and viruses (see Chaps. 33 through 41). When used in dermatologic infections, antimicrobials may be administered locally (topically) or systemically (orally or parenterally).
- **Anti-inflammatory agents** are used to treat the inflammation present in many dermatologic conditions. The major anti-inflammatory agents are the adrenal corticosteroids (see Chap. 24). When used in dermatologic conditions, corticosteroids are most often applied topically, but also may be given orally or parenterally.
- **Retinoids** are vitamin A derivatives that are active in proliferation and differentiation of skin cells. These agents are commonly used to treat acne, psoriasis, aging and wrinkling of skin from sunlight exposure, and skin cancers. Retinoids (eg, etretinate and isotretinoin) are contraindicated in women of childbearing potential unless the women have negative pregnancy tests; agree to use effective contraception before, during, and after drug therapy; and agree to take the drugs as prescribed. These drugs have been associated with severe fetal abnormalities.
- **Astringents** (eg, dilute solutions of aluminum salts) are used for their drying effects on exudative lesions.
- **Emollients** or lubricants (eg, mineral oil, lanolin) are used to relieve pruritus and dryness of the skin.
- **Enzymes** are used to débride burn wounds, decubitus ulcers, and venous stasis ulcers. They promote healing by removing necrotic tissue.
- **Keratolytic agents** (eg, salicylic acid) are used to remove warts, corns, calluses, and other keratin-containing skin lesions.
- **Sunscreens** are used to protect the skin from the damaging effects of UV radiation, thereby decreasing

skin cancer and signs of aging, including wrinkles. Dermatologists recommend sunscreen preparations that block both UVA and UVB and have a "sun protection factor" value of 30 or higher. These highly protective sunscreens are especially needed by people who are fair skinned, allergic to sunlight, or using medications that increase skin sensitivity to sunlight (eg, estrogens, tetracycline).

Application of Dermatologic Drugs

Most dermatologic medications are applied topically. To be effective, topical agents must be in contact with the underlying skin or mucous membrane. Numerous dosage forms have been developed for topical application of drugs to various parts of the body and for various therapeutic purposes. Basic components of topical agents are one or more active ingredients and a usually inactive vehicle. The vehicle is a major determinant of the drug's ability to reach affected skin and mucous membranes. Many topical preparations contain other additives (eg, emollients, dispersing agents) that further facilitate application to skin and mucous membranes. Commonly used vehicles and dosage forms include ointments, creams, lotions, aerosols, gels, otic solutions, and vaginal and rectal suppositories. Many topical drug preparations are available in several dosage forms.

Topical medications are used primarily for local effects when systemic absorption is undesirable. Factors that influence percutaneous absorption of topical agents include the following:

- **Degree of skin hydration**. Drug penetration and percutaneous absorption are increased when keratin in the outermost layer of the epidermis is well hydrated.
- **Drug concentration**. Because percutaneous absorption occurs by passive diffusion, higher concentrations increase the amount of drug absorbed.
- **Skin condition**. Absorption from abraded, damaged, or inflamed skin is much greater than from intact skin.
- **Length of contact time**. Absorption is increased when drugs are left in place for prolonged periods.
- **Size of area**. Absorption is increased when topical medications are applied to large areas of the body.
- **Location of area**. Absorption from mucous membranes and facial skin is comparatively rapid. Absorption from thick-skinned areas (eg, palms of hands and soles of feet) is comparatively slow.

INDIVIDUAL DRUGS

See Tables 66-1, 66-2, and 66-3.

TABLE 66-1 Topical Antimicrobial Agents

Generic/Trade Name	Indications for Use	Application
Antibacterial Agents		
Azelaic acid (Azelex)	Acne	To lesions, twice daily
Bacitracin (Baciguent)	Bacterial skin infections	To affected area, after cleansing, one to three times daily, small amount. Cover with a sterile dressing, if desired. Do not use longer than 1 wk.
Benzoyl Peroxide	Acne	To affected areas, after cleansing, one to three times daily
Clindamycin (Cleocin T)	Acne vulgaris	To affected areas, twice daily
Erythromycin (Aknemycin)	Acne vulgaris	To affected areas, after cleansing, twice daily, morning and evening
Gentamicin (Garamycin)	Skin infections caused by susceptible strains of streptococci, staphylococci, and gram-negative organisms	To infected areas, three to four times daily. Cover with dressing if desired.
Mafenide (Sulfamylon)	Treatment of burn wounds	To affected area, after cleansing, once or twice daily, using sterile technique
Metronidazole (MetroLotion)	Rosacea	To affected areas, after cleansing, twice daily, morning and evening
Mupirocin (Bactroban)	Impetigo caused by *Staphylococcus aureus,* beta-hemolytic streptococci, or *Streptococcus pyogenes* Eradication of nasal colonization with methicillin-resistant *S. aureus*	Impetigo: Ointment, to affected areas, three times daily. Cover with dressing, if desired. Other skin lesions: Cream, three times daily for 10 days. Cover with dressing, if desired. Eradication of nasal colonization: Ointment from single-use tube, one half in each nostril, morning and evening for 5 d

(continued)

TABLE 66-1   **Topical Antimicrobial Agents** (*continued*)

Generic/Trade Name	Indications for Use	Application
Neomycin (Myciguent)	Bacterial skin infections	To affected area, after cleansing, one to three times daily, small, fingertip-size amount. Cover with a sterile dressing, if desired. Do not use longer than 1 wk.
Silver sulfadiazine (Silvadene)	Prevent or treat infection in burn wounds caused by *Pseudomonas* and many other organisms	To affected area, after cleansing, once or twice daily, using sterile technique
Sulfacetamide sodium (Sebizon)	Bacterial skin infections Seborrheic dermatitis	Skin infections: two to four times daily until infection clears Seborrhea: to scalp and adjacent skin areas, at bedtime
Tetracycline (Topicycline)	Acne vulgaris	To affected areas, twice daily, morning and evening
Combination Products		
Bacitracin and polymyxin B (Polysporin)	Bacterial skin infections	To lesions, two to three times daily
Erythromycin/benzoyl peroxide (Benzamycin)	Acne	To affected areas, after cleansing, twice daily, morning and evening
Neomycin, polymyxin B and bacitracin (Neosporin)	Bacterial skin infections	To lesions, two to three times daily
Antifungal Agents		
Amphotericin B (Fungizone)	Cutaneous candidiasis	To affected areas, two to four times daily
Butenafine (Mentax)	Tinea pedis	To affected area, once daily for 4 wk
Ciclopirox (Loprox)	Tinea infections Cutaneous candidiasis	To affected area, twice daily for 2–4 wk
Clioquinol (Vioform)	Fungal skin infection and inflammation	To affected areas, two to three times daily. Do not use for >1 wk.
Clotrimazole (Lotrimin, Mycelex)	Tinea infections Cutaneous candidiasis	To affected areas, twice daily, morning and evening
Econazole (Spectazole)	Tinea infections Cutaneous candidiasis	Tinea infections: To affected areas, once daily Cutaneous candidiasis: To affected areas, twice daily
Haloprogin (Halotex)	Tinea infections	To affected area, twice daily for 2–4 wk
Ketoconazole (Nizoral)	Tinea infections Cutaneous candidiasis Seborrheic dermatitis	Tinea infections and cutaneous candidiasis: To affected areas, once daily for 2–4 wk Seborrheic dermatitis: To affected areas twice daily for 4 wk or until clinical clearing
Miconazole (Micatin)	Tinea infections Cutaneous candidiasis	To affected areas, twice daily for 2–4 wk
Naftifine (Naftin)	Tinea infections	To affected areas, once daily with cream, twice daily with gel
Nystatin (Mycostatin)	Candidiasis of skin and mucous membranes	To affected areas, after cleansing, two to three times daily until healing is complete
Oxiconazole (Oxistat)	Tinea infections	To affected areas, once or twice daily for 2–4 wk
Sulconazole (Exelderm)	Tinea infections	To affected areas, once or twice daily
Terbinafine (Lamisil)	Tinea infections	To affected areas, twice daily for 1–4 wk
Antiviral Agents		
Acyclovir (Zovirax)	Herpes genitalis Herpes labialis in immunosuppressed clients	To lesions, q3h six times daily for 7 d
Penciclovir (Denavir)	Herpes labialis	To lesions, q2h while awake for 4 d

NURSING PROCESS

Assessment

Assess the client's skin for characteristics or lesions that may indicate current or potential dermatologic disorders.

- When a skin rash is present, interview the client and inspect the area to determine the following:
  - **Appearance of individual lesions**. Lesions should be described as specifically as possible so changes can be identified. Terms commonly used in dermatology include macule (flat spot), papule (raised spot), nodule (small,

TABLE 66-2 **Topical Corticosteroids**

Generic/Trade Names	Dosage Forms	Potency
Alclometasone (Aclovate)	Cream, ointment	Low
Amcinonide (Cyclocort)	Cream, lotion, ointment	High
Augmented betamethasone dipropionate (Diprolene)	Cream, gel, lotion, ointment	Ointment very high; cream high
Betamethasone dipropionate (Alphatrex, others)	Aerosol, cream, lotion, ointment	Cream and ointment high; lotion medium
Betamethasone valerate (Valisone, others)	Cream, foam, lotion, ointment	Ointment high; cream medium
Clobetasol (Temovate)	Cream, gel, ointment, scalp application	Very high
Clocortolone (Cloderm)	Cream	Medium
Desonide (Tridesilon)	Cream, lotion, ointment	Low
Desoximetasone (Topicort)	Cream, gel, ointment	Medium
Dexamethasone (Decaderm, Decadron)	Aerosol, cream	Low
Diflorasone (Florone, Maxiflor)	Cream, ointment	Ointment, very high; cream, high
Fluocinolone (Synalar, others)	Cream, oil, ointment, shampoo, solution	High
Fluocinonide (Lidex)	Cream, gel, ointment, solution	High
Flurandrenolide (Cordran)	Cream, lotion, ointment, tape	Medium
Fluticasone (Cutivate)	Cream, ointment	Medium
Halcinonide (Halog)	Cream, ointment, solution	High
Halobetasol (Ultravate)	Cream, ointment	Very high
Hydrocortisone (Cortril, Hydrocortone, others)	Cream, lotion, ointment, solution, spray, roll-on stick	Medium or low
Mometasone (Elocon)	Cream, lotion, ointment	Medium
Triamcinolone acetonide (Aristocort, Kenalog, others)	Aerosol, cream, lotion, ointment	0.5% cream and ointment, high; lower concentrations, medium

solid swelling), vesicle (blister), pustule (pus-containing lesion), petechia (flat, round, purplish-red spot the size of a pinpoint, caused by intradermal or submucosal bleeding), and erythema (redness). Lesions also may be described as weeping, dry and scaly, or crusty.

○ **Location or distribution.** Some skin rashes occur exclusively or primarily on certain parts of the body (eg, face, extremities, trunk), and distribution may indicate the cause.

○ **Accompanying symptoms.** Pruritus occurs with most dermatologic conditions. Fever, malaise, and other symptoms may occur as well.

○ **Historic development.** Appropriate questions include
○ When and where did the skin rash appear?
○ How long has it been present?
○ Has it changed in appearance or location?
○ Has it occurred previously?

○ **Etiologic factors.** In many instances, appropriate treatment is determined by the cause. Some etiologic factors include the following:

○ **Drug therapy.** Many commonly used drugs may cause skin lesions, including antibiotics (eg, penicillins, sulfonamides, tetracyclines), narcotic analgesics, phenothiazine antipsychotic agents (eg, chlorpromazine), and thiazide diuretics. Skin rashes due to drug therapy are usually generalized and appear abruptly.

○ **Irritants or allergens** may cause contact dermatitis. For example, dermatitis involving the hands may be caused by soaps, detergents, or various other cleansing agents. Dermatitis involving the trunk may result from allergic reactions to clothing.

○ **Communicable diseases** (ie, measles, chickenpox) cause characteristic skin rashes and systemic signs and symptoms.

• When skin lesions other than rashes are present, assess appearance, size or extent, amount and character of any drainage, and whether the lesion appears infected or contains necrotic material. Bleeding into the skin is usually described as *petechiae* (pinpoint hemorrhages) or *ecchymoses* (bruises). Burn wounds are usually described in terms of depth (partial or full thickness of skin) and percentage of body surface area. Burn wounds with extensive skin damage are rapidly colonized with potentially pathogenic microorganisms. Venous stasis, pressure, and other cutaneous ulcers are usually described in terms of diameter and depth.

• When assessing the skin, consider the age of the client. Infants are likely to have "diaper" dermatitis, miliaria (heat rash), and tinea capitis (ringworm infection of the scalp). School-aged children have a relatively high incidence of measles, chickenpox, and tinea infections. Adolescents often have acne. Older adults are more likely to have dry skin, actinic keratoses (premalignant lesions that occur on sun-exposed skin), and skin neoplasms.

- Assess for skin neoplasms. *Basal cell carcinoma* is the most common type of skin cancer. It may initially appear as a pale nodule, most often on the head and neck. *Squamous cell carcinomas* may appear as ulcerated areas. These lesions may occur anywhere on the body but are more common on sun-exposed parts, such as the face and hands. Malignant melanoma is the most serious skin cancer. It involves melanocytes, the pigment-producing cells of the skin. *Malignant melanoma* may occur in pigmented nevi (moles) or previously normal skin. In nevi, malignant melanoma may be manifested by enlargement and ulceration. In previously normal skin, lesions appear as irregularly shaped pigmented areas. Although it can occur in almost any area, malignant melanoma is most likely to be located on the back in white people and in toe webs and soles of the feet in African-American or Asian people.
- When assessing dark-skinned clients, color changes and skin rashes are more difficult to detect. Some guidelines include the following:
  - Adequate lighting is required; nonglare daylight is best. The illumination provided by overbed lights or flashlights is inadequate for most purposes.
  - Some skin rashes may be visible on oral mucous membranes.
  - Petechiae are not visible on dark brown or black skin, but they may be visible on oral mucous membranes or the conjunctiva.
- When skin disorders are present, assess the client's psychological response to the condition. Many clients, especially those with chronic disorders, feel self-conscious and depressed.

Nursing Diagnoses

- Body Image Disturbance related to visible skin lesions
- Anxiety related to potential for permanent scarring or disfigurement
- Pain related to skin lesions and pruritus
- Risk for Injury: Infection related to entry of microbes through damaged skin
- Knowledge Deficit related to prevention and treatment of skin disorders

Planning/Goals

The client will:

- Apply topical drugs correctly
- Experience relief of symptoms
- Use techniques to prevent or minimize skin damage and disorders
- Avoid scarring and disfigurement when possible

- Be encouraged to express concerns about acute and chronic body image changes

Interventions

Use measures to prevent or minimize skin disorders.

- Use general measures to promote health and increase resistance to disease (ie, maintain nutrition, rest, and exercise).
- Practice good personal hygiene, with at least once-daily cleansing of skin areas with high bacterial counts, such as underarms and perineum.
- Practice safety measures to avoid injury to the skin. Any injury, especially one that disrupts the integrity of the skin (eg, lacerations, puncture wounds, scratching of skin lesions) increases the likelihood of skin infections.
- Avoid known irritants or allergens. Have the client substitute nonirritating soaps or cleaning supplies for irritating ones; use hypoallergenic jewelry and cosmetics if indicated; wear cotton clothing if indicated.
- Use measures to relieve dry skin and pruritus. Dry skin causes itching, and itching promotes scratching. Scratching relieves itching only if it is strong enough to damage the skin and serve as a counterirritant. Skin damaged or disrupted by scratching is susceptible to invasion by pathogenic microorganisms. Thus, dry skin may lead to serious skin disorders. Older adults are especially likely to have dry, flaky skin. Measures to decrease skin dryness include the following:
  - Alternating complete and partial baths. For example, the client may alternate a shower or tub bath with a sponge bath (of face, hands, underarms, and perineal areas). Warm water, mild soaps, and patting dry are recommended because hot water, harsh soaps, and rubbing with a towel have drying effects on the skin.
  - Liberal use of lubricating creams, lotions, and oils. Bath oils, which usually contain mineral oil or lanolin oil and a perfume, are widely available. If bath oils are used, precautions against falls are necessary because the oils make bathtubs and shower floors slippery. Creams and lotions may be applied several times daily.
- Prevent pressure ulcers by avoiding trauma to the skin and prolonged pressure on any part of the body. In clients at high risk for development of pressure ulcers, major preventive measures include frequent changes of position and correct lifting techniques. Various pressure-relieving devices also are useful. These include special beds and mattresses. Daily inspection of the skin is needed for early detection and treatment of beginning pressure ulcers.
- Avoid excessive exposure to sunlight and other sources of UV light. Although controlled amounts of UV light are beneficial in some dermatologic

disorders (ie, acne, psoriasis), excessive amounts cause wrinkling, dryness, and malignancies. If prolonged exposure is necessary, protective clothing and sunscreening lotions decrease skin damage.

- When skin rashes are present, cool, wet compresses or baths are often effective in relieving pruritus. Water or normal saline may be used alone or with additives, such as colloidal oatmeal (Aveeno) or baking soda. A cool environment also tends to decrease pruritus. The client's fingernails should be cut short and kept clean to avoid skin damage and infection from scratching.

For severe itching, a systemic antihistamine may be needed. Topical antihistamines are not recommended because they may sensitize the skin and cause allergic reactions with later exposures.

Evaluation
- Observe and interview regarding use of dermatologic drugs.
- Observe for improvement in skin lesions and symptoms.
- Interview regarding use of measures to promote healthy skin and prevent skin disorders.

TABLE 66-3 Miscellaneous Dermatologic Agents

Generic/Trade Name	Dermatologic Effects	Clinical Indications	Method of Administration
Enzymes			
Collagenase (Santyl)	Débriding effects	Enzymatic debridement of infected wounds (eg, burn wounds, decubitus ulcers)	Topically once daily until the wound is cleansed of necrotic material
Papain (Panafil)	Débriding effects	Débridement of surface lesions	Topically one or two times daily
Trypsin (Granulex)	Débriding effects	Débridement of infected wounds (eg, decubitus and varicose ulcers)	Topically by spray twice daily
Retinoids			
Acitretin (Soriatane)	A metabolite of etretinate	Severe psoriasis	PO 25–50 mg/d
Adapalene (Differin)	Reportedly causes less burning, itching, redness, and dryness than tretinoin	Acne vulgaris	Topically to skin lesions once daily
Etretinate (Tegison)	Anti-inflammatory and anti-keratinizing effects	Severe psoriasis	PO 0.75–1 mg/kg/d in divided doses
Isotretinoin (Accutane)	Inhibits sebum production and keratinization	Severe cystic acne. Disorders characterized by excessive keratinization (eg, pityriasis, ichthyosis). Mycosis fungoides	PO 1–2 mg/kg/d, in two divided doses, for 15–20 wk
Tazarotene (Tazorac)	A prodrug, mechanism of action is unknown	Acne. Psoriasis	Topically to skin, after cleansing, once daily in the evening
Tretinoin (Retin-A)	Irritant	Acne vulgaris	Topically to skin lesions once daily
Other Agents			
Anthralin (Anthra-Derm, others)	Slows the rate of skin cell growth and replication	Psoriasis	Topically to lesions once daily or as directed
Becaplermin (Regranex)	A recombinant human platelet-derived growth factor	Diabetic skin ulcers	Topically to ulcer, amount calculated according to size of the ulcer
Calcipotriene (Dovonex)	Synthetic analogue of vitamin D that helps to regulate skin cell production and development	Psoriasis	Topically to lesions twice daily
Capsaicin (Zostrix)	Depletes substance P (which transmits pain impulses) in sensory nerves of the skin	Relief of pain associated with rheumatoid arthritis, osteoarthritis, and neuralgias	Topically to affected area, up to three to four times daily
Coal tar (Balnetar, Zetar, others)	Irritant	Psoriasis. Dermatitis	Topically to skin, in various concentrations and preparations (eg, creams, lotions, shampoos, bath emulsion). Also available in combination with hydrocortisone and other substances

(continued)

TABLE 66-3 **Miscellaneous Dermatologic Agents** (*continued*)

Generic/Trade Name	Dermatologic Effects	Clinical Indications	Method of Administration
Colloidal oatmeal (Aveeno)	Antipruritic	Pruritus	Topically as a bath solution (1 cup in bathtub of water)
Dextranomer (Debrisan)	Absorbs exudates from wound surfaces	Cleansing of ulcers (eg, venous stasis, decubitus) and wounds (eg, burn, surgical, traumatic)	Apply to a clean, moist wound surface q12h initially, then less often as exudate decreases
Fluorouracil (Efudex)	Antineoplastic	Actinic keratoses Superficial basal cell carcinomas	Topically to skin lesions twice daily for 2–6 wk
Masoprocol (Actinex)	Inhibits proliferation of keratin-containing cells	Actinic keratoses	Topically to skin lesions morning and evening for 28 d
Salicylic acid	Keratolytic, antifungal	Removal of warts, corns, calluses Superficial fungal infections Seborrheic dermatitis Acne Psoriasis	Topically to lesions
Selenium sulfide (Selsun)	Antifungal, antidandruff	Dandruff Tinea versicolor	Topically to scalp as shampoo once or twice weekly

PO, oral.

CLIENT TEACHING GUIDELINES
Topical Medications for Skin Disorders

General Considerations

✔ Severe dermatologic disorders should be treated by a dermatologist.

✔ Promote healthy skin by a balanced diet, personal hygiene measures, avoiding excessive exposure to sunlight, avoiding skin injuries, and lubricating dry skin. Healthy skin is less susceptible to inflammation, infections, and other disorders. It also heals more rapidly when disorders or injuries occur.

✔ Common symptoms of skin disorders are inflammation, infection, and itching and the goal of most drug therapy is to relieve these symptoms and promote healing. Systemic medications (eg, oral antihistamines, antibiotics and corticosteroids) may be used for severe disorders, at least initially, but most medications are applied directly to the skin. There is a wide array of topical products, both prescription and over-the-counter.

✔ It is extremely important to use the correct topical medication and the correct amount for the condition being treated. Topical corticosteroids, for example, come in many vehicles (eg, creams, lotions, ointments). These products cannot be used interchangeably. In addition, they should not be combined (ie, using a prescription and a nonprescription product) and should not be covered with occlusive dressings unless specifically instructed to do so. Correct use increases beneficial effects, decreases risks of worsening the condition being treated, and decreases risks of adverse effects.

✔ Adverse effects of topical medications may involve the skin (eg, irritation, excessive drying, infection) where the drug is applied or the entire body, when the drug is absorbed into the bloodstream. Systemic absorption is increased when the drug is strong; applied to inflamed skin, over a large surface area, or frequently; or covered with an occlusive dressing (eg, plastic wrap). Systemic absorption is of most concern with corticosteroid preparations.

✔ Some ways to prevent or decrease skin disorders include:
  ✔ Identifying and avoiding, when possible, substances that cause skin irritation and inflammation (eg, harsh cleaning products, latex gloves, cosmetics, wool fabrics, pet dander)
  ✔ Bathing in warm water with a mild cleanser (eg, Dove, Basis, Cetaphil), patting skin dry, and applying lotions or oils (eg, Aquaphor, Eucerin, mineral oil or baby oil) to lubricate skin and decrease dryness
  ✔ Avoiding scratching, squeezing, or rubbing skin lesions. These behaviors cause additional skin damage and increase risks of infection. Fingernails should be cut short; cotton gloves can be worn at night.
  ✔ Maintaining a cool environment; preventing sweating
  ✔ Applying cold compresses to inflamed, itchy skin
  ✔ Using baking soda or colloidal oatmeal (Aveeno) in bath water to relieve itching

✔ If you are taking an oral antihistamine to relieve itching, it should be taken on a regular schedule, around the clock, for greater effectiveness.

✔ Misinformation about acne is common. Acne is not caused by dirt, washing does not improve acne, and vigorous scrubbing and squeezing may worsen acne lesions. There is also no evidence that acne is caused by eating chocolate or other foods.

(*continued*)

Topical Medications for Skin Disorders *(continued)*

✔ People with psoriasis can obtain information and support from:

  National Psoriasis Foundation (NPF)
  6600 SW 92nd Avenue, Suite 300
  Portland, OR 97223
  Telephone: 1-800-723-9166
  E-mail: getinfo@npfusa.org
  Web site:http//www.psoriasis.org

✔ Unavoidable skin lesions or scars can often be hidden or rendered less noticeable with makeup or clothing.

✔ Women can wear cosmetics over most topical medications. If unclear, ask a physician or pharmacist whether makeup is permissible.

✔ If taking an oral retinoid (eg, Accutane), avoid vitamin supplements containing vitamin A and excessive exposure to sunlight, to decrease risks of excessive vitamin A intake and photosensitivity.

Self-administration

✔ Use topical medications only as prescribed or according to the manufacturer's instructions (for over-the-counter products). Use the correct preparation for the intended area of application (ie, skin, ear, vagina).

✔ For topical application to skin lesions, cleanse the skin and remove previously applied medication to promote drug contact with the affected area of the skin.
  ✔ Wash the skin and pat it dry.
  ✔ Apply a small amount of the drug preparation and rub it in well. A thin layer of medication is effective and decreases the incidence and severity of adverse effects.
  ✔ For burn wounds, broken skin, or open lesions, apply

the drug with sterile gloves or sterile cotton-tipped applicators to prevent infection.

✔ Wash hands before and after application. Wash before to avoid infection; wash afterward to avoid transferring the drug to the face or eyes and causing adverse reactions.

✔ For minor wounds and abrasions, cleansing with soap and water is usually adequate. If an antiseptic is used, an iodine preparation (eg, aqueous iodine solution 1%) is preferred. Alcohol should not be applied to open wounds. Hydrogen peroxide may help with cleansing but it is a weak antiseptic.

✔ With azelaic acid (Azelex) for acne, use for the full prescribed period; do not use occlusive dressings or wrappings; and keep away from mouth, eyes, and other mucous membranes (if it gets into eyes, wash eyes with a large amount of water).

✔ With benzoyl peroxide for acne:
  ✔ With cleansing solutions, wash affected areas once or twice daily. Wet skin areas to be treated before applying the cleanser. Rinse thoroughly and pat dry. Reduce use if excessive drying or peeling occurs.
  ✔ With other dosage forms, apply once daily initially and gradually increase to two or three times daily if needed. Cleanse skin and apply a small amount over the affected area. Reduce dosage if excessive drying, redness, or discomfort occurs. If excessive stinging or burning occurs after any single application, remove with mild soap and water and resume use the next day. Keep away from eyes, mouth, and inside of nose. Rinse with water if contact occurs with these areas. Avoid other sources of skin irritation (eg, sunlight, sunlamps, other topical acne medications).

How Can You Avoid This Medication Error?

You are working in the operating room. A surgeon asks for acetic acid for irrigation of a wound. You go to the stock supply and locate where acetic acid is usually stored. The bottle has been previously used and the label is difficult to read. What should you do?

PRINCIPLES OF THERAPY

Goals

General treatment goals for many skin disorders are to relieve symptoms (eg, dryness, pruritus, inflammation, infection), eradicate or improve lesions, promote healing

and repair, restore skin integrity, and prevent recurrence. Specific goals often depend on the condition being treated.

General Aspects of Dermatologic Drug Therapy

1. Pharmacologic therapy may include a single drug or multiple agents used concurrently or sequentially.

2. For severe skin conditions, a dermatologist is best qualified to prescribe medications and other treatments. Because many skin conditions are so visible, early and aggressive treatment may be needed to prevent additional tissue damage, repeated infections, scarring, and mental anguish.

3. Topical medications are preferred, when effective, and many preparations are available. Astringents

and lotions are usually used as drying agents for "wet," oozing lesions, and ointments and creams are used as "wetting" agents for dry, scaling lesions.

4. To relieve pruritus, a common symptom of inflammatory skin disorders, skin lubricants, systemic antihistamines, and topical corticosteroids are important elements.

5. Topical corticosteroids are used for both acute and chronic inflammatory and pruritic lesions. However, when acute lesions involve extensive areas or chronic lesions are resistant to topical drugs, systemic corticosteroid therapy may be needed. Prednisone 0.5 to 1 mg/kg/day is often used, for approximately 1 to 3 weeks.

Use of Topical Corticosteroids

Because of the extensive use of topical corticosteroids and the risks of potentially serious adverse effects, numerous precautions, guidelines, and recommendations have evolved to increase safety and effectiveness of these drugs.

Drug Selection
Choice of drug depends mainly on the acuity, severity, location, and extent of the condition being treated. For acute lesions, a more potent corticosteroid may be needed, at least initially; for chronic lesions, the least potent preparation that is effective is indicated (see Table 66-2).

- Low-potency drugs (eg, hydrocortisone) are preferred when likely to be effective. They are especially recommended for use in children, on large areas, and on body sites especially prone to corticosteroid damage (eg, face, scrotum, axillae, flexures and skin folds).
- Mid-potency drugs (eg, flurandreolide) are usually effective in nonintertriginous areas in children and adults.
- High-potency drugs (eg, amcinonide) usually are used for more acute or severe disorders and areas resistant to lower-potency agents. Short-term or intermittent use (eg, every other day, 3 or 4 consecutive days per week, once per week) may be more effective and cause fewer adverse effects than continuous use of lower-potency products. These drugs may also be alternated with lower-potency agents.
- Very–high-potency drugs (eg, clobetasol, halobetasol) usually are used for less absorptive areas such as soles of feet, palms of hands, and thick skin plaques. Usage should not exceed 2 consecutive weeks and total dosage should not exceed 50 g/week because of the potential for these drugs to suppress the hypothalamic–pituitary–adrenal (HPA) axis. Clobetasol suppresses the HPA axis at doses as low as 2 g/day.

These drugs should not be used with occlusive dressings or for children younger than 12 years of age.
- Drug potency and clinical use vary with the dosage form, and many topical corticosteroids are available in creams, ointments, and other preparations. Creams are usually the most acceptable to clients; ointments penetrate the epidermis better and are often used for chronic dry or scaly lesions; lotions are recommended for intertriginous areas and the scalp. Some preparations are available in aerosol sprays, gels, and other dosage forms.

Dosage
Dosage depends on the drug concentration, the area of application, and the method of application.

- The skin covering the face, scalp, scrotum, and axillae is more permeable to corticosteroids than other skin surfaces, and these areas can usually be treated with less potent formulations, smaller amounts, or less frequent applications.
- Drug absorption and risks of systemic toxicity are significantly increased when the drug is applied to inflamed skin or covered by an occlusive dressing. Application should be less frequent and limited to isolated, resistant areas when occlusive dressings are used.
- The drug should be applied sparingly. Some clinicians recommend twice-daily applications until a clinical response is obtained, then decreasing to the least-frequent schedule needed to control the condition.
- With continuous use, one or two applications daily may be as effective as three or four applications, because the drugs have a repository effect.
- If an occlusive dressing is applied, leave it on overnight or at least 6 hours. However, do not leave it in place for more than 12 hours in a 24-hour period.
- After long-term use or after using a potent drug, taper dosage by switching to a less potent agent or applying the drug less frequently. Discontinuing the drug abruptly can cause a rebound effect, in which the skin condition worsens.

Drug Selection in Selected Skin Conditions

The choice of topical dermatologic agents depends primarily on the reason for use and client response.

Acne
Numerous prescription and nonprescription antiacne products are available.

- **Antimicrobial drugs** include both topical and systemic agents. Topical drugs usually are used for mild to moderate acne, often in combination with a topical retinoid to maximize effects. *Benzoyl peroxide* is an effective topical bactericidal agent that is available in numerous preparations (eg, gel, lotion, cream, wash) and concentrations (eg, 2.5% to 10%). Lotion and cream preparations are the least irritating. *Clindamycin* and *erythromycin* are also available in topical dosage forms. These drugs reduce *P. acnes* bacteria and are approximately equally effective. A prescription product combining benzoyl peroxide and erythromycin in a gel form (Benzamycin) is reportedly more effective than either agent alone.

  Oral antimicrobials are useful with widespread or severe, disfiguring acne or when a rapid response is needed. Tetracyclines, which have both antibacterial and anti-inflammatory activity, are commonly used for long-term treatment. These drugs are usually given twice daily to increase compliance. Therapeutic effects usually occur within a few weeks, but maximal effects may require 2 to 3 months.

- **Retinoids**, in both systemic and topical forms, are commonly used for moderate to severe acne. When used alone, topical tretinoin may take several months to decrease acne lesions significantly. Thus, it is usually used in combination with other products. Adapalene and tazarotene are newer topical retinoids.

  Isotretinoin is usually given to clients with severe acne who do not respond to safer drugs. Its antiacne effects include suppression of sebum production, inhibition of comedone formation, and inhibition of inflammation. Approximately 70% to 80% of clients treated appropriately (usually approximately 1 mg/kg/day for 5 months) have a long-term remission. The main drawbacks are teratogenic and other adverse effects. This oral drug must never be given to a woman of childbearing age unless she agrees to practice adequate contraceptive measures.

Anorectal Disorders

In anorectal disorders, most preparations contain a local anesthetic, emollients, and perhaps a corticosteroid. These preparations relieve pruritus and pain but do not cure the underlying condition. Some preparations contain ingredients of questionable value, such as vasoconstrictors, astringents, and weak antiseptics. No particular mixture is clearly superior.

Dermatitis

Both systemic and topical agents are usually needed. Sedating, systemic antihistamines such as diphenhydramine or hydroxyzine are often used to relieve itching and promote rest and sleep. An oral antibiotic such as clindamycin, dicloxacillin, a cephalosporin, or a macrolide may be given for approximately a week to treat secondary infections. An oral corticosteroid such as prednisone may be needed initially for severe inflammation, but topical corticosteroids are most often used.

Coal tar preparations have anti-inflammatory and antipruritic actions and can be used alone or with topical corticosteroids. However, these agents have an unpleasant odor and they stain clothing. They are usually applied at bedtime.

Additional preparations include moisturizers and lubricants (eg, Aquaphor) for dry skin and itching; mild skin cleansers (eg, Basis, Cetaphil) to avoid further skin irritation; and baking soda or colloidal oatmeal (Aveeno) in baths or soaks for pruritus.

External Otitis

Otic preparations of various dermatologic medications are used. Hydrocortisone is the corticosteroid most often included in topical otic preparations. It relieves pruritus and inflammation in chronic external otitis. Systemic analgesics are usually required.

Pressure Ulcers

In pressure ulcers, the only clear-cut guideline for treatment is avoiding further pressure on the affected area. Many topical agents are used, most often with specific procedures for dressing changes, skin cleansing, and so on. No one agent or procedure is clearly superior. Consistent implementation of a protocol (ie, position changes, inspection of current or potential pressure areas, dressing changes, use of alternating, pressure-relieving mattresses) may be more effective than drug therapy.

Psoriasis

Localized lesions are usually treated by a combination of topical agents, such as a corticosteroid during daytime hours and a coal tar ointment at night. Newer antipsoriasis drugs such as calcipotriene or tazarotene may also be used. Calcipotriene is reportedly as effective as topical fluocinonide. However, its onset of action is slower than that of a topical corticosteroid. A combination of calcipotriene and a topical corticosteroid may be used initially for rapid improvement, after which the calcipotriene can be continued as monotherapy. Tazarotene is a new topical retinoid that may cause cutaneous irritation.

Generalized psoriasis, which requires systemic treatment or body light therapy, should be managed mainly by dermatologists. Systemic therapy often involves oral retinoids or methotrexate. Acitretin has replaced etretinate as the oral retinoid of choice for treatment of severe psoriasis. Acitretin is a metabolite of etretinate that can be converted back to etretinate, especially in the presence of alcohol. The drug, like other oral retinoids, is teratogenic. Thus, women of childbearing potential who take acitretin should be instructed to avoid ingesting alcohol and to use adequate contraception while taking the drug and for at least 3 years thereafter. Methotrexate is an antineoplastic drug that may cause significant adverse effects.

Phototherapy can involve natural sunlight, which is highly effective. Most clients with psoriasis notice some remission during summer months. A sunscreen should be used on uninvolved areas to decrease risk of skin cancer. Office phototherapy treatments are usually performed three to five times weekly.

Rosacea

Mild skin cleansers (eg, Cetaphil), oral tetracycline, and topical metronidazole are commonly used; oral isotretinoin and topical metronidazole are also effective.

Urticaria

Systemic drug therapy with antihistamines (H_1 receptor antagonists) is the major element of drug therapy. In addition, an epinephrine injection may be used initially and topical medications may be applied to relieve itching.

With chronic urticaria, the goal of treatment is symptom relief. Antihistamines are most effective when given before histamine-induced urticaria occurs and should be given around the clock, not just when lesions appear.

Dosage Forms

The choice of dosage form for topical drug therapy depends largely on the reason for use. Guidelines include the following:

- **Ointments** are oil-based substances that usually contain a medication in an emollient vehicle, such as petrolatum or lanolin. Ointments occlude the skin and promote retention of moisture. Thus, they are especially useful in chronic skin disorders characterized by dry lesions. Ointments should usually be avoided in hairy, moist, and intertriginous areas of the body because of potential maceration, irritation, and secondary infection.
- **Creams** (emulsions of oil in water, which may be greasy or nongreasy) and **gels** (transparent colloids, which dry and leave a film over the area) retain moisture in the skin but are less occlusive than ointments. These preparations are cosmetically acceptable for use on the face and other visible areas of the body. They also may be used in hairy, moist, intertriginous areas. Creams and gels are especially useful in subacute dermatologic disorders.
- **Lotions** are suspensions of insoluble substances in water. They cool, dry, and protect the skin. They are most useful in subacute dermatologic disorders. **Sprays** and **aerosols** are similar to lotions.

- **Powders** have absorbent, cooling, and protective effects. Powders usually should not be applied in acute, exudative disorders or on denuded areas because they tend to cake, occlude the lesions, and retard healing. Also, some powders (eg, cornstarch) may lead to secondary infections by promoting growth of bacteria and fungi.
- **Topical otic medications** are usually liquids. However, creams or ointments may be used for dry, crusted lesions, and powders may be used for drying effects.
- **Topical vaginal medications** may be applied as douche solutions, vaginal tablets, or vaginal creams used with an applicator.
- **Anorectal medications** may be applied as ointments, creams, foams, and rectal suppositories.

Use in Children

Children are at risk for development of a wide range of dermatologic disorders, including dermatitis and skin rashes in younger children and acne in adolescents. Few guidelines have been developed for drug therapy of these disorders. Infants, and perhaps older children, have more permeable skin and are more likely to absorb topical drugs than adults. In addition, absorption is increased in the presence of broken or damaged skin. Therefore, cautious use of topical agents is advised.

With topical corticosteroids, suppression of the HPA axis (see Chap. 24), Cushing's disease, and intracranial hypertension have been reported in children. Signs of impaired adrenal function may include delayed growth and low plasma cortisol levels. Signs of intracranial hypertension may include headaches and swelling of the optic nerve (papilledema) on ophthalmoscopic examination. The latter may lead to blindness if pressure on the optic nerve is not relieved.

Because children are at high risk for development of systemic adverse effects with topical corticosteroids, these drugs should be used only if clearly indicated, in the least effective dose, for the shortest effective time, and usually without occlusive dressings or wraps. In addition, a low-potency agent should be used initially in infants and in intertriginous areas of older children. If a more potent drug is required for severe dermatitis, the child should be examined often and the strength of the drug reduced as skin lesions improve.

Use in Older Adults

Older adults often have dry skin and are at risk of pressure ulcers if mobility, nutrition, or elimination is impaired. Principles of topical drug therapy are the same as for younger adults.

Nursing Notes: Apply Your Knowledge

You are making a home visit to young parents of a 6-month-old baby. The teenage mother is home alone with the baby when you visit. You ask if she has any concerns. She states that the baby has had a severe diaper rash for the last 2 weeks. What assessment data do you need to collect? What general principles should you include in your teaching about diaper rash?

 Home Care

Skin disorders are commonly treated at home by clients or caregivers. When a home care nurse is involved, responsibilities may include assessing clients, other members of the household, and the home environment for risks of skin disorders; teaching preventive or treatment measures; assisting with treatment; and assessing response to treatment.

NURSING ACTIONS — Dermatologic Drugs

NURSING ACTIONS	RATIONALE/EXPLANATION
1. Administer accurately	
a. Use the correct preparation for the intended use (ie, dermatologic, otic, vaginal, anorectal)	Preparations may differ in drug contents and concentrations.
b. For topical application to skin lesions:	
(1) Wash the skin, and pat it dry.	To cleanse the skin and remove previously applied medication. This facilitates drug contact with the affected area of the skin.
(2) Apply a small amount of the drug preparation, and rub it in well.	A thin layer of medication is effective and decreases the incidence and severity of adverse effects.
(3) For burn wounds, broken skin, or open lesions, apply the drug with sterile gloves or sterile cotton-tipped applicators.	To prevent infection
(4) Use the drug only for the individual client (ie, do not use the same tube for more than one client).	To avoid bacterial cross-contamination between clients
(5) Wash hands before and after application.	Wash hands before to avoid exposing the client to infection; wash hands afterward to avoid transferring the drug to your own face or eyes and causing adverse reactions.
2. Observe for therapeutic effects	Therapeutic effects depend on the medication being used and the disorder being treated.
a. With dermatologic conditions, observe for healing of skin lesions.	
b. With external otitis, observe for decreased pain and pruritus.	
c. With vaginal disorders, observe for decreased vaginal discharge and pruritus.	
d. With anorectal disorders, observe for decreased pain and pruritus.	
3. Observe for adverse effects	Incidence of adverse effects is low with topical agents. Local adverse effects may occur with most topical agents but may be more likely with antiseptics, local anesthetics, and antimicrobials.
a. Local irritation or inflammation—burning on application, erythema, skin rash, pruritus	

(continued)

NURSING ACTIONS	RATIONALE/EXPLANATION
b. With topical corticosteroids, observe for local and systemic effects.	
(1) Local effects include skin atrophy, striae, telangiectasia, hypopigmentation, rosacea, dermatitis, and acne.	These effects commonly occur with prolonged use. Atrophy is more likely in the face, groin and axillae.
(2) Systemic effects include suppression of adrenal function, cataracts, glaucoma, and growth retardation in children.	Systemic effects are more likely with more potent agents (eg, clobetasol can cause suppression of the hypothalamic–pituitary–adrenal axis with as little as 2 g daily), application over large areas of skin, prolonged use, and the use of occlusive dressings. In addition, children are at higher risk because they may absorb proportionally larger amounts and be more sensitive to systemic toxicity. Little adrenal suppression is likely to occur with doses less than 50 g weekly for an adult and 15 g weekly for a small child, unless occlusive dressings are used.
c. With topical antibiotics, superinfection and sensitization may occur.	Superinfection with drug-resistant organisms may occur with any antibacterial agent. It is less likely to occur with mixtures that have a broad spectrum of antibacterial activity. Sensitization may cause serious allergic reactions if the same drug is given systemically at a later time.
d. With oral retinoids, observe for hypervitaminosis A (nausea, vomiting, headache, blurred vision, eye irritation, conjunctivitis, skin disorders, abnormal liver function, musculoskeletal pain, increased plasma triglycerides, others).	Adverse effects commonly occur with usual doses but are more severe with higher doses.
4. Observe for drug interactions	Clinically significant drug interactions rarely occur with topical agents.

How Can You Avoid This Medication Error?

Answer: Never use a drug that is not labeled clearly. Even topical agents can cause serious adverse effects. When pouring liquids, always pour away from the label, so that accidental spillage will not impair the written drug label. Another concern in this situation is sterility. Using previously opened bottles, where sterility cannot be guaranteed, is not acceptable practice.

the baby's skin for the severity of diaper rash and other skin irritation. Observe for any sign of fungal infection.

Stress the importance of keeping the baby clean and dry by changing the diaper frequently and washing with gentle soap and water. If the area is excoriated, a protective barrier can be achieved by applying a thin coat of many commercially available products such as Desitin.

Nursing Notes: Apply Your Knowledge

Answer: Ask the mother to describe when the rash appeared and if its occurrence corresponded with diarrhea or new foods being introduced in the diet. Question the mother regarding the types of diapers she uses and how often the baby is changed. Inspect

 REVIEW AND APPLICATION EXERCISES

1. What are the main functions of the skin?

2. Describe interventions to promote skin health and integrity.

3. During initial assessment of a client, what signs and symptoms may indicate common skin disorders?

4. Which client groups are at risk for development of common skin disorders (eg, skin infections, pressure ulcers)?

5. Compare topical and systemic corticosteroids in terms of adverse effects.

6. If an adolescent client with acne asks your advice about over-the-counter topical drugs, which would you recommend, and why?

7. List general principles of using topical agents for common skin disorders.

SELECTED REFERENCES

Allman, R.M. (1997). Approach to the elderly patient with pressure ulcers. In W.N. Kelley (Ed.), *Textbook of internal medicine*, 3rd ed., pp. 2530–2532. Philadelphia: Lippincott-Raven.

Barnard, C.M., Kim, Y.H., & Bauer, E.A. (1997). Approach to the patient with skin lesions. In W.N. Kelley (Ed.), *Textbook of internal medicine*, 3rd ed., pp. 1215–1222. Philadelphia: Lippincott-Raven.

Beltrani, V.S. (1998). Allergic dermatoses. *Medical Clinics of North America, 82*, 1105–1133.

Correale, C.E., Walker, C., Murphy, L., & Craig, T.J. (1999). Atopic dermatitis: A review of diagnosis and treatment. *American Family Physician, 60*, 1191–1198.

Deters, G.E. (1996). Management of patients with dermatologic problems. In S.C. Smeltzer & B.G. Bare (Eds.), *Brunner and Suddarth's Textbook of medical-surgical nursing*, 8th ed., pp. 1493–1543. Philadelphia: Lippincott-Raven.

Drug facts and comparisons. (Updated monthly). St. Louis: Facts and Comparisons.

Feldman, S.R. & Clark, A.R. (1998). Psoriasis. *Medical Clinics of North America, 82*, 1135–1144.

Guzzo, C.A., Lazarus, G.S., & Werth, V.P. (1996). Dermatological pharmacology. In J.G. Hardman, L.E. Limbird, P.B. Molinoff, & R.W. Ruddon (Eds.), *Goodman & Gilman's The pharmacological basis of therapeutics*, 9th ed., pp. 1593–1616. New York: McGraw-Hill.

Nowakowski, P.A., Rumsfield, J.A., & West, D.P. (1997). Common skin disorders: Acne and psoriasis. In J.T. DiPiro, R.L. Talbert, G.C. Yee, G.R. Matzke, B.G. Wells, & L.M. Posey (Eds.), *Pharmacotherapy: A pathophysiologic approach*, 3rd ed., pp. 1815–1833. Stamford, CT: Appleton & Lange.

Simandl, G. (1998). Alterations in skin function and integrity. In C.M. Porth (Ed.), *Pathophysiology: Concepts of altered health states*, 5th ed., pp. 259–300. Philadelphia: Lippincott Williams & Wilkins.

Thiers, B.H. (1998). Dermatology therapy update. *Medical Clinics of North America, 82*, 1405–1414.

Webster, G.F. (1998). Acne and rosacea. *Medical Clinics of North America, 82*, 1145–1154.

67

Drug Use During Pregnancy and Lactation

Objectives

After studying this chapter, the student will be able to:

1. Discuss reasons for avoiding or minimizing drug therapy during pregnancy and lactation.

2. Describe selected teratogenic drugs.

3. Discuss guidelines for drug therapy of pregnancy-associated signs and symptoms.

4. Discuss guidelines for drug therapy of chronic disorders during pregnancy and lactation.

5. Discuss the safety of immunizations given during pregnancy.

6. Teach adolescent and young adult women to avoid prescribed and over-the-counter drugs when possible and to inform physicians and dentists if there is a possibility of pregnancy.

7. Discuss the role of the home care nurse working with the pregnant mother.

8. Discuss drugs used during labor and delivery in terms of their effects on the mother and newborn infant.

9. Describe abortifacients in terms of characteristics and nursing process implications.

Thirty-eight-year-old Susan Williams comes in for her first prenatal visit. Susan works as a corporate lawyer and is married to a university professor. Susan is very excited about this planned pregnancy, but seems somewhat anxious as she asks lots of questions.

Reflect on:

▶ The effects of drug use by the mother on the fetus during pregnancy.

▶ Do you make any assumptions about Susan's knowledge level based on her profession and class?

▶ How might such judgments assist you to individualize teaching? How might such judgments impair the teaching process?

▶ Essential information to provide Susan regarding the use of any prescription, nonprescription, or herbal drugs during pregnancy.

Drug use during pregnancy and lactation requires special consideration because both the mother and the fetus or nursing infant are affected. Few drugs are considered safe, and drug use is in general contraindicated. However, many pregnant or lactating women take drugs for various reasons, including acute disorders that may or may not be associated with pregnancy, chronic disorders that require continued treatment during pregnancy or lactation, and habitual use of nontherapeutic drugs (eg, alcohol, tobacco, others). The main purpose of this chapter is to describe potential drug effects on the fetus and maternal drug therapy to protect the fetus while providing therapeutic effects to the pregnant woman.

PREGNANCY AND LACTATION

Pregnancy is a dynamic state: mother and fetus undergo physiologic changes that influence drug effects. In the pregnant woman, physiologic changes alter drug pharmacokinetics (Table 67-1), and drug effects are less predictable than in the nonpregnant state. Most of the drugs in this chapter are described more fully elsewhere; they are discussed here in relation to pregnancy and lactation. Other drugs are used mainly to influence some aspect of pregnancy. These drugs are discussed in greater detail and include those used to induce abortion (abortifacients), drugs used to stop preterm labor (tocolytics), and drugs used during labor and delivery.

MATERNAL–PLACENTAL–FETAL CIRCULATION

Drugs ingested by the pregnant woman reach the fetus through the maternal–placental–fetal circulation, which is completed approximately the third week after conception. On the maternal side, arterial blood pressure carries blood and drugs to the placenta. In the placenta, maternal and fetal blood are separated by a few thin layers of tissue over a large surface area. Drugs readily cross the placenta, mainly by passive diffusion. This process, called placental transfer, begins approximately the fifth week after conception. When drugs are given on a regular schedule, serum levels reach equilibrium, with fetal blood containing 50% to 100% of the amount in maternal blood.

After drugs enter the fetal circulation, relatively large amounts are pharmacologically active because the fetus has low levels of serum albumin and thus low levels of drug binding. Drug molecules are distributed in two ways. Most are transported to the liver, where they are metabolized. Metabolism occurs slowly because the fetal liver is immature in quantity and quality of drug-metabolizing enzymes. Drugs metabolized by the fetal liver are excreted by fetal kidneys into amniotic fluid. Excretion also is slow and inefficient owing to immature development of fetal kidneys. In addition, the fetus swallows some amniotic fluid, and some drug molecules are recirculated.

Other drug molecules are transported directly to the heart, which then distributes them to the brain and coronary arteries. Drugs enter the brain easily because the

TABLE 67-1	Pregnancy: Physiologic and Pharmacokinetic Changes
Physiologic Change	**Pharmacokinetic Change**
Increased plasma volume and body water, approximately 50% in a normal pregnancy	Once absorbed into the bloodstream, a drug (especially if water soluble) is distributed and "diluted" more than in the nonpregnant state. Drug dosage requirements may increase. However, this effect may be offset by other pharmacokinetic changes of pregnancy.
Increased weight (average 25 lb) and body fat	Drugs (especially fat-soluble ones) are distributed more widely. Drugs that are distributed to fatty tissues tend to linger in the body because they are slowly released from storage sites into the bloodstream.
Decreased serum albumin. The rate of albumin production is increased. However, serum levels fall because of plasma volume expansion. Also, many plasma protein-binding sites are occupied by hormones and other endogenous substances that increase during pregnancy.	The decreased capacity for drug binding leaves more free or unbound drug available for therapeutic or adverse effects on the mother and for placental transfer to the fetus. Thus, a given dose of a drug is likely to produce greater effects than it would in the nonpregnant state. Some commonly used drugs with higher unbound amounts during pregnancy include dexamethasone (Decadron), diazepam (Valium), lidocaine (Xylocaine), meperidine (Demerol), phenobarbital, phenytoin (Dilantin), propranolol (Inderal), and sulfisoxazole (Gantrisin).
Increased renal blood flow and glomerular filtration rate secondary to increased cardiac output	Increased excretion of drugs by the kidneys, especially those excreted primarily unchanged in the urine. These include penicillins, digoxin (Lanoxin), and lithium.
	In late pregnancy, the increased size and weight of the uterus may decrease renal blood flow when the woman assumes a supine position. This may result in decreased excretion and prolonged effects of renally excreted drugs.

blood–brain barrier is poorly developed in the fetus. Approximately half of the drug-containing blood is then transported through the umbilical arteries to the placenta, where it reenters the maternal circulation. Thus, the mother can metabolize and excrete some drug molecules for the fetus.

DRUG EFFECTS ON THE FETUS

The fetus, which is exposed to any drugs circulating in maternal blood, is very sensitive to drug effects because it is small, has few plasma proteins that can bind drug molecules, and has a weak capacity for metabolizing and excreting drugs. Once drug molecules reach the fetus, they may cause teratogenicity (anatomic malformations) or other adverse effects. The teratogenicity of many drugs is unknown. However, since 1984, the U.S. Food and Drug Administration (FDA) has required that new drugs be assigned a risk category (Box 67-1).

Drug teratogenicity is most likely to occur when drugs are taken during the first trimester of pregnancy, when fetal organs are formed (Fig. 67-1). For drugs taken during the second and third trimesters, adverse effects are usually manifested in the neonate (birth to 1 month) or infant (1 month to 1 year) as growth retardation, respiratory problems, infection, or bleeding. Overall, effects are determined mainly by the type and amount of drugs, the duration of exposure, and the level of fetal growth and development when exposed to the drugs. Therapeutic and nontherapeutic drugs may affect the fetus.

Fetal effects of commonly used *therapeutic* drugs are listed in Table 67-2. Effects of *nontherapeutic* drugs are described in the following paragraphs.

Alcohol is contraindicated during pregnancy; no amount is considered safe. Heavy intake may cause fetal

(*text continues on page 1006*)

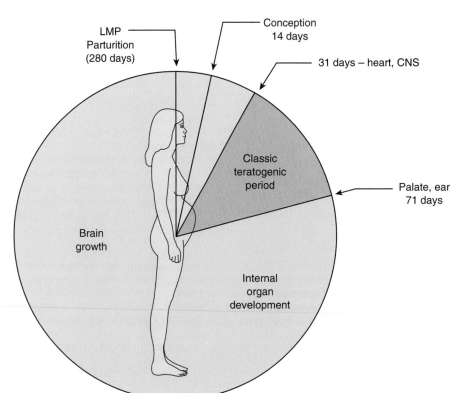

FIGURE 67–1 The gestational clock showing the classic teratogenic risk assessment. (Adapted from Niebyl, J. [1999]. Drugs and related areas in pregnancy. In J. Sciarra [Ed.], Obstetrics and gynecology. Philadelphia: Lippincott Williams & Wilkins.)

TABLE 67-2   **Drug Effects in Pregnancy**

Adrenergics	These drugs stimulate the heart to increase rate and force of contractions. They also may increase blood pressure. Several are teratogenic and embryocidal in animal studies, but no adequate studies have been done in pregnant women. These drugs are common ingredients in over-the-counter decongestants, cold remedies, and appetite suppressants.
	Oral and parenteral adrenergics may inhibit uterine contractions during labor; cause hypokalemia, hypoglycemia, and pulmonary edema in the mother; and cause hypoglycemia in the neonate. These effects are unlikely with inhaled adrenergics. Oral *albuterol* (Proventil, Ventolin) and oral or intravenous *terbutaline* (Brethine) relax uterine muscles and inhibit preterm labor.
Analgesics, Opioid	Safety is not established. The drugs rapidly cross the placenta and reach the fetus. Maternal addiction and neonatal withdrawal symptoms result from regular use. Use of codeine during the first trimester has been associated with congenital defects. *Alfentanil* (Alfenta) and *sufentanil* (Sufenta) had embryocidal effects in animal studies.
	When given to women in labor, opioid analgesics may decrease uterine contractility and slow progress toward delivery. They may also cause respiratory depression in the neonate. *Meperidine* (Demerol) reportedly causes less neonatal respiratory depression than other opioids. *Butorphanol* (Stadol) is also used. If respiratory depression occurs, it can be reversed by administration of *naloxone* (Narcan), an opioid antagonist.
Angiotensin-Converting Enzyme (ACE) Inhibitors	Considered potentially fatal to fetus. Should be discontinued in the second and third trimesters if used.
Angiotensin II Receptor Antagonists	Should be discontinued if pregnancy is detected. Can cause fetal and neonatal morbidity and death. The drugs are considered category C in the first trimester and D in the second and third trimesters. Inadequate studies are reported regarding safe use during pregnancy. *Losartan* (Cozaar) and *valsartan* (Diovan) are examples of this classification of drugs.
Antianginal Agents (Nitrates)	Animal studies have not been conducted and safety for use has not been established. Because the drugs lower blood pressure and may decrease blood supply to the fetus, use only if necessary.
Antianxiety and Sedative-Hypnotic Agents (Benzodiazepines)	These drugs should generally be avoided. The benzodiazepines and their metabolites cross the placenta freely and accumulate in fetal blood. If taken during the first trimester, they may cause physical malformations. If taken during labor, they may cause sedation, respiratory depression, hypotonia, lethargy, and sucking difficulties in the neonate. Neonatal tremors and irritability also have been attributed to maternal use of the drugs.
Antiarrhythmics	*Quinidine* (Quinaglute) crosses the placenta and reaches fetal serum levels similar to maternal levels with no reported congenital defects. Neonatal thrombocytopenia has been reported. *Disopyramide* (Norpace) has been found in human fetal blood, and it may cause uterine contractions. Adequate studies have not been done to support safety. *Lidocaine* (Xylocaine) has not been established as safe. *Tocainide* (Tonocard) was not teratogenic in animal studies but did increase the incidence of abortions and still births. *Mexilitene* (Mexitil) has not been studied. *Flecainide* (Tambocor) had teratogenic and embryotoxic effects in animal studies.
	Ibutilide (Convert) is teratogenic. *Propafenone* (Rhythmol) is not recommended because of inadequate reported studies. *Adenosine* (Adenocard) is also not recommended because of unreported studies in pregnant women. Toxicity in rats reported.
Antibiotics	
BETA LACTAMS	*Penicillins* cross the placenta but apparently produce no adverse effects on the fetus. They are considered safer than other antibiotics. *Cephalosporins* cross the placenta and seem to be safe, although they have not been studied extensively in pregnancy. They apparently have shorter half-lives, lower serum concentrations, and a faster rate of elimination during pregnancy. *Aztreonam* (Azactam) crosses the placenta and enters fetal blood, but fetal effects are unknown. *Imipenem/cilastatin* (Primaxin) showed no teratogenicity in animal studies but has not been studied in pregnant women.
AMINOGLYCOSIDES	*Aminoglycosides* cross the placenta and fetal serum levels may reach 15% to 50% of maternal levels. Serious adverse effects on the fetus or neonate have not been reported, but there is potential harm because the drugs are nephrotoxic and ototoxic.
CLINDAMYCIN	*Clindamycin* (Cleocin) should be used only when infection with *Bacteroides fragilis* is suspected.
FLUOROQUINOLONES	*Ciprofloxacin* (Cipro) and others are contraindicated in pregnancy. Safer alternatives are available.
MACROLIDES	*Erythromycin* (E-Mycin, others) crosses the placenta to reach fetal serum levels up to 20% of maternal levels, but no fetal abnormalities have been reported.
	Clarithromycin (Biaxin) and related drugs should be used with caution because of inadequate reported studies in pregnant women.
NITROFURANTOIN	*Nitrofurantoin* (Macrodantin) should not be used during late pregnancy because of possible hemolytic anemia in the neonate.
SULFONAMIDES	Sulfonamides should not be used during the last 2 weeks of pregnancy because they displace bilirubin from binding sites on serum albumin and may cause kernicterus in the neonate.

(continued)

TABLE 67-2	**Drug Effects in Pregnancy** (*continued*)
TETRACYCLINES	Tetracyclines are contraindicated during pregnancy. They cross the placenta and interfere with development of teeth and bone in the fetus. Animal studies indicate embryotoxicity.
Antifungals	Teratogenic in rats. Systemic antifungals are in general contraindicated in pregnancy. They should be used only if potential benefit justifies potential harm to the fetus.
Antitubercular Drugs	*Isoniazid* (INH) was embryocidal in some animal studies and should be used only if necessary. *Ethambutol* (Myambutol) was teratogenic in animal studies, but administration to pregnant women produced no detectable effects on the fetus. The effects of combination with other antitubercular drugs are unknown. *Rifampin* (Rifadin) was teratogenic in animal studies.
Antivirals	Most systemic antivirals were teratogenic in animal studies. None of these drugs should be given unless clearly necessary. No well-controlled studies to support use in pregnancy, except for *zidovudine* (Retrovir) to prevent transmission of human immunodeficiency virus infection to the fetus.
Miscellaneous Antimicrobials	*Vancomycin* (Vancocin) is not recommended because of inadequate studies to support use in pregnancy. *Trimethoprim* (Proloprim), often given in combination with *sulfamethoxazole* (Bactrim, Septra), was teratogenic in small animals. It crosses the placenta to reach levels in fetal serum and amniotic fluid that are similar to those in maternal serum. It may interfere with folic acid metabolism in the fetus. A few studies in pregnant women have not indicated teratogenic effects.
Anticholinergics	*Atropine* crosses the placenta rapidly with intravenous injection; effects on the fetus depend on the maturity of its parasympathetic nervous system. *Scopolamine* may cause respiratory depression in the neonate and may contribute to neonatal hemorrhage by reducing vitamin K–dependent clotting factors in the neonate.
Anticoagulants	*Heparin* does not cross the placenta and has not been associated with congenital defects. However, its use during pregnancy has been associated with 13% to 22% unfavorable outcomes, including stillbirths and prematurity. *Warfarin* (Coumadin) crosses the placenta and fetal hemorrhage, spontaneous abortion, prematurity, stillbirth, and congenital anomalies may occur. Approximately 31% of fetuses exposed to warfarin may experience a problem related to the anticoagulant. If a woman becomes pregnant during warfarin therapy, inform her of the potential risks to the fetus, and discuss the possibility of terminating the pregnancy.
Anticonvulsants	Although most women receiving antiseizure drugs deliver normal infants, reports suggest an increased incidence of birth defects. Data are more extensive with *phenytoin* (Dilantin) and *phenobarbital*. The drugs may be discontinued before and during pregnancy when the type, frequency, and severity of seizures do not seriously threaten the client's well-being. They should not be discontinued when given for major seizures because of the risk of precipitating status epilepticus with resultant hypoxia and risk to mother and fetus. It is not known whether minor seizures cause fetal risk. Maternal ingestion of these drugs, especially barbiturates, may cause neonatal bleeding during the first 24 h after birth. This neonatal coagulation defect is characterized by decreased levels of vitamin K–dependent clotting factors and prolongation of either the prothrombin time or partial thromboplastin time, or both. This may be prevented by giving vitamin K to the mother 1 mo before delivery and during delivery and to the infant immediately after birth. Newer drugs such as *gabapentin* (Neurontin), *lamotrigine* (Lamictal), and *topiramate* (Topamax) are FDA category C and should be used only if potential benefits to the mother outweigh potential adverse effects on the fetus.
Antidepressants	Tricyclic antidepressants such as *amitriptyline* (Elavil) have been associated with teratogenicity and embryotoxicity when given in large doses, and there have been reports of congenital malformations and neonatal withdrawal syndrome. *Trazodone* (Desyrel), in animal studies with large doses, caused increased fetal resorption and congenital anomalies. Monoamine oxidase inhibitors, such as *phenelzine* (Nardil), were associated with fewer viable offspring and growth retardation in animal studies with large doses. Overall, clinical experience with these drugs in pregnant women is limited. The selective serotonin reuptake inhibitors such as *fluoxetine* (Prozac) and others are FDA category C and should be used only if potential benefits to the mother outweigh potential adverse effects on the fetus.
Antidiabetic Drugs	Insulin is the only antidiabetic drug recommended for use during pregnancy. Dosage requirements generally increase during the second and third trimesters and blood glucose levels must be monitored closely. None of the oral antidiabetic drugs has been adequately studied in relation to pregnancy, and their use is not recommended.

TABLE 67-2 Drug Effects in Pregnancy (*continued*)

Antidiarrheals	*Diphenoxylate* (Lomotil) has been used without reported teratogenic or other adverse effects. *Loperamide* (Imodium) has not been studied in relation to pregnancy.
Antiemetics	None of the available antiemetic drugs has been proven safe for use. Nondrug measures are preferred for controlling nausea and vomiting because of possible drug effects on the fetus.
Antihistamines	Histamine-1 receptor blocking agents, such as *diphenhydramine* (Benadryl), have been associated with teratogenic effects, but the extent and significance are unknown. Safety has not been established. The drugs should not be used during the third trimester because of possible convulsions and other adverse effects in the neonate. Histamine-2 receptor blocking agents, such as *cimetidine* (Tagamet), have not been established as safe. Animal studies indicated no harmful effects on the fetus, but studies in pregnant women have not been done.
Antihypertensives	Beta-blocking agents, such as *propranolol* (Inderal) and others, apparently improve fetal survival. *Methyldopa* (Aldomet) crosses the placenta and reaches fetal concentrations similar to those of maternal serum. However, no teratogenic effects have been reported despite widespread use during pregnancy. Neonates of mothers receiving methyldopa may have decreased blood pressure for approximately 48 h. *Hydralazine* (Apresoline) is often used and is generally considered safe. *Clonidine* (Catapres), *guanabenz* (Wytensin), and *guanfacine* (Tenex) are not recommended because effects in pregnant women are unknown.
Antilipemics	*Cholestyramine* (Questran) and *colestipol* (Colestid) are FDA category C, but are considered safe because they are not absorbed systemically. *Lovastatin* (Mevacor) and related drugs (HMG-CoA reductase inhibitors or "statins") are FDA category X and contraindicated during pregnancy. They should be given to women of childbearing age only if they are highly unlikely to become pregnant and are informed of potential hazards. If a woman becomes pregnant while taking one of these drugs, the drug should be stopped and the patient informed of possible adverse drug effects on the fetus.
Antimanic Agent	*Lithium* crosses the placenta. Approximately 11% of infants exposed to lithium during the first trimester had major congenital defects, 72% of which were cardiovascular. In the neonate, lithium has a prolonged half-life because of slow elimination and has caused bradycardia, cyanosis, diabetes insipidus, hypotonia, hypothyroidism, and electrocardiographic abnormalities. Most of these effects resolve within 1 to 2 wk.
Antipsychotics	Phenothiazines, such as *chlorpromazine* (Thorazine) and related drugs, readily cross the placenta. Several studies indicate that the drugs are not teratogenic, but animal studies indicate potential embryotoxicity, increased neonatal mortality, and decreased performance. The possibility of permanent neurologic damage cannot be excluded. Use near term may cause abnormal movements, abnormal reflexes, and jaundice in the neonate and hypotension in the mother. Newer drugs have not been studied in relation to pregnancy.
Antithyroid Drugs	The drugs readily cross the placenta and can cause fetal goiter and cretinism. If given, dosage must be carefully regulated so sufficient but not excessive amounts are given. In some women, thyroid function decreases as pregnancy progresses, and dosage must be reduced. Propylthiouracil is the preferred antithyroid drug. Neonatal goiter occurs in approximately 10% of cases.
Aspirin	*Aspirin* is usually contraindicated because of potential adverse effects on the mother and fetus. Maternal effects include prolonged gestation, prolonged labor, and antepartum and postpartum hemorrhage. Fetal effects include constriction of the ductus arteriosus, low birth weight, and increased incidence of stillbirth and neonatal death. However, for the pregnant client with rheumatoid arthritis, aspirin is considered the nonsteroidal anti-inflammatory drug of choice. The lowest possible doses should be given. For analgesic and antipyretic effects during pregnancy, acetaminophen (Tylenol) is preferred.
Beta-adrenergic Blocking Agents	Safety for use of *propranolol* (Inderal) and related drugs has not been established. Animal studies with large doses indicated embryotoxicity. Teratogenicity has not been reported in humans. However, problems have been reported during delivery. These include maternal bradycardia and neonatal bradycardia, hypoglycemia, apnea, low Apgar scores, and low birth weight. Neonatal effects may last up to 72 h.
Bronchodilators (Xanthine)	*Theophylline* (Theo-Dur, Aminophylline) has not been associated with teratogenic effects, but adequate studies have not been done in animals or humans. Thus, drug effects during pregnancy are unknown. Theophylline crosses the placenta, and therapeutic serum levels have been found in neonates. There have been reports of tachycardia and irritability in neonates whose mothers took the drug until labor and delivery.
Calcium Channel Blocking Agents	Teratogenic and embryotoxic effects occurred in small animals given large doses. *Diltiazem* (Cardizem) caused fetal death, skeletal abnormalities, and increased incidence of stillbirths. *Verapamil* (Calan) crosses the placenta, but effects are unknown. Adequate studies have not

(continued)

TABLE 67-2 **Drug Effects in Pregnancy** (*continued*)

	been done in pregnant women. Because the drugs decrease blood pressure, there is a potential risk of inadequate blood flow to the placenta and the fetus. *Nifedipine* (Procardia) is sometimes used as a tocolytic. Developmental toxicity demonstrated in animal studies; human risk is undetermined.
Corticosteroids	These drugs cross the placenta. Animal studies indicate that large doses of cortisol early in pregnancy may produce cleft palate, stillborn fetuses, and decreased fetal size. Chronic maternal ingestion during the first trimester has shown a 1% incidence of cleft palate in humans. Adequate human reproduction studies have not been done. Infants of mothers who received substantial amounts of corticosteroids during pregnancy should be closely observed for signs of adrenal insufficiency. *Betamethasone* (Celestone) is used to promote fetal production of surfactant to increase lung maturity in the premature infant.
Digoxin	*Digoxin* (Lanoxin) is apparently safe for use during pregnancy. It crosses the placenta to reach fetal serum levels that are 50% to 80% those of maternal serum. Fetal toxicity and neonatal death have occurred with maternal overdose. Dosage requirements may be less predictable during pregnancy, and serum drug levels and other assessment parameters must be closely monitored. Digoxin also has been administered to the mother for treatment of fetal tachycardia and congestive heart failure.
Diuretics	Thiazide diuretics such as *hydrochlorothiazide* (HydroDIURIL) cross the placenta. They are not associated with teratogenesis, but they may cause other adverse effects. Because the drugs decrease plasma volume, decreased blood flow to the uterus and placenta may occur with resultant impairment of fetal nutrition and growth. Other adverse effects may include fetal or neonatal jaundice, thrombocytopenia, hyperbilirubinemia, hemolytic jaundice, fluid and electrolyte imbalances, and impaired carbohydrate metabolism. These drugs are not indicated for treatment of dependent edema caused by uterine enlargement and restriction of venous blood flow. They also are not effective in prevention or treatment of pregnancy-induced hypertension (pre-eclampsia). They may be used for treatment of pathologic edema from cardiovascular and other conditions. Loop diuretics such as *furosemide* (Lasix) have not been studied adequately in pregnant women. Teratogenesis has not been reported, but animal studies indicated fetal toxicity and death. Like the thiazides, loop diuretics may decrease plasma volume and blood flow to the placenta and fetus. Potassium-conserving diuretics, such as *triamterene* (an ingredient in Dyazide and Maxide), cross the placenta in animal studies, but effects on the human fetus are unknown.
Laxatives	If a laxative is required, a bulk-forming agent, such as Metamucil, is preferred. It is more physiologic than other laxatives and is not absorbed systemically. It is unlikely to harm the fetus.
Nonsteroidal Anti-inflammatory Drugs (NSAIDs)	Use of *ibuprofen* (Motrin, Advil) and other NSAIDs has not been established as safe during pregnancy and should be avoided. There are no adequate studies in pregnant women. In animal studies, delayed delivery occurred. These drugs may cause fatal fetal kidney disease and are FDA category C. Because the drugs inhibit prostaglandin synthesis, they may cause premature closure of the ductus arteriosus and other adverse effects on the fetus. If taken during the third trimester, they may delay onset of labor and delivery. If taken within 1 week before delivery, they increase the risk of extensive maternal bleeding. The newer drugs *celecoxib* (Celebrex) and *rofecoxib* (Vioxx) have not been studied in pregnant women. *Diclofenac* (Voltaren) is contraindicated in pregnant women.
Thyroid Hormones	These drugs do not readily cross the placenta. No adverse effects have been reported in human fetuses. The drugs are apparently safe to use in appropriate dosages, but may cause tachycardia in the fetus. When given as replacement therapy in hypothyroid women, the drug should be continued through pregnancy. *Levothyroxine* (Synthroid) also has been given to the mother to treat hypothyroidism in the fetus. Thyroxine is an FDA category A drug.

FDA, Food and Drug Administration.

alcohol syndrome, a condition characterized by multiple congenital defects and mental retardation.

Cigarette smoking (nicotine and carbon monoxide ingestion) also is contraindicated. It interferes with fetal growth (decreases infant birth weight and size) and increases the incidence of preterm delivery. Nicotine causes vasoconstriction and decreases blood flow to the fetus;

carbon monoxide decreases the oxygen available to the fetus. Chronic fetal hypoxia from heavy smoking has been associated with mental retardation.

Cocaine, **marijuana**, and **heroin** are illegal drugs of abuse. Use of these drugs during pregnancy is particularly serious. **Cocaine** may cause maternal vasoconstriction, tachycardia, hypertension, cardiac arrhythmias, and seizures. These effects increase the risk of spontaneous abortion during the first and second trimesters. During the third trimester, cocaine causes increased uterine contractility, vasoconstriction and decreased blood flow in the placenta, fetal tachycardia, and increased risk of fetal distress and abruptio placentae. These life-threatening effects on mother and fetus are even more likely to occur with "crack" cocaine, a highly purified and potent form.

Marijuana impairs formation of deoxyribonucleic acid and ribonucleic acid, the basic genetic material of body cells. It also may decrease the oxygen supply of mother and fetus. **Heroin** ingestion increases the risks of pregnancy-induced hypertension, third trimester bleeding, complications of labor and delivery, and postpartum morbidity.

Caffeine in high quantities is associated with an increased incidence of spontaneous abortion, preterm labor, and small-for-gestational age infants. Caffeine is present in coffee, tea, cola drinks, over-the-counter analgesics, anti-sleep preparations, and chocolate.

Herbal supplements are not recommended during pregnancy. Safety with their use has not been established.

FETAL THERAPEUTICS

Although the major concern about drugs ingested during pregnancy is adverse effects on the fetus, a few drugs are given to the mother specifically for their therapeutic effects on the fetus. These include digoxin (Lanoxin) for fetal tachycardia or heart failure, levothyroxine (Synthroid) for hypothyroidism, penicillin for exposure to maternal syphilis, and corticosteroids to promote surfactant production to improve lung function and decrease respiratory distress syndrome in preterm infants.

MATERNAL THERAPEUTICS

Thus far, the main emphasis on drug use during pregnancy has related to actual or potential adverse effects on the fetus. Despite the general principle that drug use should be avoided when possible, pregnant women may require drug therapy for increased nutritional needs, pregnancy-associated problems, chronic disease processes, treatment of preterm labor, induction of labor, and pain management during labor.

Pregnancy-Associated Symptoms and Their Management

Anemias

Three types of anemia are common during pregnancy. One is physiologic anemia, which results from expanded blood volume. A second is iron-deficiency anemia, which is often related to long-term nutritional deficiencies. Iron supplements are usually given for prophylaxis (eg, ferrous sulfate 300 mg or ferrous gluconate 600 mg three times daily). Iron preparations should be given with food to decrease gastric irritation. Citrus juices enhance absorption. A third type is megaloblastic anemia, caused by folic acid deficiency. A folic acid supplement (0.8 mg daily) is often prescribed for prophylaxis.

Constipation

Constipation often occurs during pregnancy, probably from decreased peristalsis. Preferred treatment, if effective, is to increase intake of fluids and high-fiber foods. If a laxative is required, a bulk-producing agent (eg, Metamucil) is the most physiologic for the mother and safest for the fetus because it is not absorbed systemically. A stool softener, such as docusate (Colace), may be used occasionally. Mineral oil should be avoided because it interferes with absorption of fat-soluble vitamins. Strong laxatives or any laxative used in excess may initiate uterine contractions and labor.

Heartburn

Heartburn (pyrosis) often occurs in the later months of pregnancy, when increased abdominal pressure and a relaxed cardiac sphincter allow gastric acid to reflux into the esophagus and cause irritation and discomfort. Interventions to decrease abdominal pressure (eg, eating small meals, sitting in an upright position, avoiding gas-producing foods and constipation) may be helpful. Antacids may be used if necessary. Because little systemic absorption occurs, the drugs are unlikely to harm the fetus if used in recommended doses.

Nausea and Vomiting

Nausea and vomiting often occur, especially during early pregnancy. Dietary management (eg, eating a few crackers when awakening and waiting a few minutes before arising) and maintaining fluid and electrolyte balance are recommended. Antiemetic drugs should be given only if nausea and vomiting are severe enough to threaten the mother's nutritional or metabolic status. Meclizine (Antivert), 25 to 50 mg daily, and dimenhydrinate (Dramamine), 50 mg every 3 to 4 hours, are thought to have low teratogenic risks. However, possible teratogenesis cannot be ruled out. Pyridoxine (vitamin B_6) has also been found helpful in reducing symptoms. Recommended dosage is 10 to 25 mg daily. Use of promethazine (Phenergan) is questioned.

Pregnancy-Induced Hypertension

Pregnancy-induced hypertension includes preeclampsia and eclampsia. These serious complications endanger the lives of mother and fetus. Preeclampsia is most likely to occur during the last 10 weeks of pregnancy, during labor, or within the first 48 hours after delivery. The occurrence of edema, hypertension, and proteinuria characterizes the disease. Nonpharmacologic management includes bed rest in a left lateral position and a high-protein, high-carbohydrate, low-fat diet with a sodium content that does not exceed 6 g/day. The left lateral position increases blood flow to the kidneys and placenta, promotes diuresis, and lowers blood pressure. Drug therapy includes intravenous hydralazine (Apresoline) or methyldopa (Aldomet), which do not cause adverse fetal effects.

Eclampsia, characterized by severe symptoms and convulsions, occurs if preeclampsia is not treated effectively. Intravenous magnesium sulfate is the drug of choice to prevent or treat convulsive seizures. Delivery of the fetus is the only known cure for preeclampsia or eclampsia.

Selected Infections

Group B streptococcal infections may affect the pregnant woman and the neonate. During late pregnancy, urinary tract infections (UTIs) or amnionitis may occur. After delivery, endometritis, bacteremia, or wound infection may occur after cesarean section. In the infant, sepsis, meningitis, or pneumonia may occur.

Because of the potentially serious consequences of infection with the group B streptococcus, pregnant women should have a vaginal culture at 35 to 37 weeks of gestation for detection. A positive culture indicates infection that should be treated. However, antibiotics given at this time may not provide coverage during labor and delivery. Treatment should be initiated during labor, often with ampicillin 2 g intravenously (IV) as a loading dose, then 1 g IV every 4 hours until delivery.

Human immunodeficiency virus (HIV) infection and **acquired immunodeficiency syndrome (AIDS)** can be transmitted to the fetus and neonate, and treatment is needed to reduce the risk of transmission. Zidovudine (Retrovir, AZT) is approved for administration after 14 weeks of gestation, with oral doses of 100 mg five times daily. During labor, IV AZT is given in a 1-hour loading dose of 2 mg/kg, followed by 1 mg/kg/hour until delivery. After delivery, the infant should be given AZT syrup, 2 mg/kg every 6 hours, starting 8 to 12 hours after birth and continuing for the first 6 weeks of life.

Women with HIV infection or AIDS should be encouraged to avoid pregnancy. Those who are taking antiretroviral drugs when they become pregnant may be advised to suspend drug therapy during the first trimester.

Urinary tract infections commonly occur during pregnancy and may include asymptomatic bacteriuria, cystitis, and pyelonephritis. Although treatment of asymptomatic bacteriuria is controversial in some populations, the condition should be treated in pregnant women because of its association with pyelonephritis. UTIs are also associated with premature onset of labor. Amoxicillin (Amoxil), cephalexin (Keflex), and nitrofurantoin (Macrodantin) are commonly used drugs.

Management of Chronic Diseases During Pregnancy

Asthma

Pharmacologic treatment of pregnant women with asthma is similar to treatment of nonpregnant women. For mild symptoms or infrequent attacks, inhaled adrenergic bronchodilators, such as albuterol (Proventil, Ventolin) or metaproterenol (Alupent), are the drugs of choice. For more severe or more frequent attacks, oral theophylline, oral terbutaline, or an inhaled corticosteroid, such as beclomethasone (Vanceril), may be required. Severe episodes or status asthmaticus are managed as in nonpregnant women. Although large doses of corticosteroids in early pregnancy are teratogenic, cautious use of smaller amounts may benefit the mother sufficiently to risk adverse effects on the fetus.

Cromolyn and nedocromil, which are prophylactic agents, may be effective, but there are no pregnancy-related data to support their use. The antileukotrienes (eg, zafirlukast) are rated pregnancy category B and should be given with caution during pregnancy. Breastfeeding is not recommended while on the drugs.

Pregnancy is an indication for effective therapy because the best fetal and maternal outcomes are achieved when antiasthma treatment is optimized.

Diabetes Mellitus

For diabetic women who become pregnant, maintaining normal or near-normal blood sugar levels is required for successful outcomes because poor glycemic control increases the risks of birth defects. Pregnancy causes significant metabolic changes, and insulin is the only hypoglycemic drug acceptable for use during pregnancy. Human insulin should be used because it is least likely to cause an allergic response. Because insulin requirements vary according to the stage of pregnancy, the diabetic client's condition must be monitored very closely and insulin therapy individualized. At the same time, careful dietary control and other treatment measures are necessary. Some guidelines for insulin therapy during the antepartum, intrapartum, and postpartum periods are as follows.

Antepartum Period

Pregnancy has a diabetogenic effect because of several hormonal changes. First, human placental lactogen (HPL) exerts an increasing diabetogenic effect throughout pregnancy. This hormone increases mobilization of free fatty acids and decreases effects of maternal insulin. Second, estrogen levels increase as pregnancy advances; estrogen is thought to be an insulin antagonist. Third, progesterone may decrease insulin effectiveness. Fourth, cortisol from the adrenal cortex is thought to increase gluconeogenesis and thus cause maternal hyperglycemia.

Some women first show signs of diabetes during pregnancy. This is called *gestational diabetes*. These women may revert to a nondiabetic state when pregnancy ends, but they are at increased risk for later development of diabetes. Other women, who were previously able to control diabetes with diet alone, may become insulin dependent during pregnancy. Still other women, already insulin dependent, are likely to need larger doses as pregnancy advances. A mixture of NPH and regular insulin is usually effective.

More specifically, insulin requirements usually decrease during the first trimester and increase during the second and third trimesters. During the first trimester, decreased need for insulin is attributed to fetal use of maternal glucose for growth and development. This lowers maternal blood glucose levels and may cause hypoglycemia. During the second trimester, insulin requirements increase along with increasing blood levels of HPL, estrogen, progesterone, and cortisol. It is recommended that women be screened for diabetes between 24 and 28 weeks (by measuring blood sugar after an oral glucose dose of 50 or 100 g). During the third trimester, insulin requirements increase still further, and the largest amounts are likely to be needed near term.

It is especially important that sufficient insulin is given to prevent maternal acidosis. Uncontrolled acidosis is likely to interfere with neurologic development of the fetus.

Intrapartum Period

Women with diabetes are usually delivered at 37 to 38 weeks of gestation because of increased incidence of fetal death closer to full term. Early delivery is usually induced by oxytocin (Pitocin) or accomplished by cesarean section. Either method precipitates a high-risk situation. During labor, for example, strenuous muscular contractions increase cellular use of glucose and deplete glycogen stores. Thus, less insulin is needed, and hypoglycemia may occur. If a cesarean section is done, the stress of surgery may increase insulin requirements. Regular, short-acting insulin and frequent blood sugar tests are used to control diabetes during labor and delivery, as during other acute situations.

Postpartum Period

Insulin requirements continue to fluctuate during the immediate postpartum period because stress, trauma, infection, surgery, or other factors associated with delivery tend to increase blood glucose levels and insulin requirements. At the same time, termination of the pregnancy reverses the diabetogenic hormonal changes and decreases insulin requirements. Usually, women are at higher risk for hypoglycemia during the first 24 to 48 hours after delivery, and some may require no insulin during this time. As during the intrapartum period, regular, short-acting insulin is given, and dosage is based on frequent

measurements of blood sugar. Once the insulin requirement is stabilized, the client can return to the prepregnancy treatment regimen unless she is breastfeeding. Insulin does not enter breast milk; however, breastfeeding may decrease insulin requirements. Gestational diabetes usually subsides within 6 weeks after delivery.

Oral antidiabetic drugs are contraindicated in pregnancy and lactation. In pregnancy, sulfonylureas cross the placenta, stimulate the fetal pancreas, and may cause fetal hypoglycemia or death. They also increase the risk of congenital anomalies and may cause overt diabetes in women with gestational diabetes because they stimulate an already overstimulated pancreas. If these drugs are taken by a woman of childbearing potential, they should be discontinued before conception if possible or as soon as pregnancy is suspected. In lactation, some oral hypoglycemics are excreted in breast milk, and there is a risk of hypoglycemia in the nursing infant.

There is little information about the use of newer drugs (eg, repaglinide, rosiglitazone) in pregnancy and lactation, and none is recommended.

Hypertension

Chronic hypertension (hypertension beginning before conception or up to 20 weeks of pregnancy) is associated with increased maternal and fetal risks. Thus, appropriate management is mandatory. Nonpharmacologic interventions (avoiding excessive weight gain, sodium restriction, increased rest) should be emphasized. If drug therapy is required, methyldopa (Aldomet) is the drug of first choice because it has not been associated with adverse effects on the fetus or neonate. Nifedipine (Procardia) should be reserved for women with severe hypertension uncontrolled by other agents. Further studies are needed to confirm safety. Angiotensin-converting enzyme inhibitors are contraindicated during pregnancy. Long-term use of atenolol has been linked with intrauterine growth retardation. The reduced fetal growth appears to be related to increased vascular resistance in both mother and fetus.

Although diuretics are commonly used in the treatment of hypertension, they should not be given during pregnancy. They decrease blood volume, cardiac output, and blood pressure and may cause fluid and electrolyte imbalances, all of which may have adverse effects on the fetus.

Seizure Disorders

Women with seizure disorders, regardless of whether receiving anticonvulsant drugs, are more likely to have children with congenital defects and mental retardation than women who do not have epilepsy. Thus, the disease and anticonvulsant drugs have potential teratogenic effects, and none of the drugs has been proven safe for use. Despite this, however, women on medication have a 90% chance of having a normal child. Because seizures adversely affect the fetus, the goal of drug therapy is to prevent seizures with the fewest possible effects on the fetus. Women should be counseled that the risk of seizures outweighs the chance of fetal anomalies.

If a client has been seizure free for several years, it may be possible to discontinue drug therapy before pregnancy. If drug therapy is required, phenobarbital or phenytoin (Dilantin) may be preferred. Because dosage requirements may be altered during pregnancy, serum drug levels should be measured monthly and the dosage adjusted accordingly. Folic acid should be taken before conception and during pregnancy to decrease the occurrence of neural tube defects.

The effects of gabapentin (Neurontin) and lamotrigine (Lamictal) during pregnancy and lactation are largely unknown. They are assigned to FDA risk category C and are not recommended for use during pregnancy or lactation. Valproic acid (Depakene) is considered the most teratogenic and should not be given to women of childbearing potential.

Thyroid Disease

Propylthiouracil is the drug of choice for treatment of hyperthyroid disease in the pregnant woman. It is considered safe but may cross the placenta and cause fetal goiter. The goal of antithyroid therapy during pregnancy is to keep the mother slightly hyperthyroid and thus minimize fetal drug exposure. The management of chronic hypothyroidism includes thyroid hormone replacement therapy with levothyroxine (Synthroid), which can be used safely.

ABORTIFACIENTS

Abortion is the termination of pregnancy before 20 weeks. It may occur spontaneously or be intentionally induced. Medical abortion may be induced by prostaglandins and an antiprogestin (Table 67-3). Prostaglandins may be used to terminate pregnancy during the second trimester.

TABLE 67-3	Abortifacients, Tocolytics, and Oxytocics
Generic/Trade Name	**Routes and Dosage Ranges**
Abortifaciens	
Progesterone antagonist Mifepristone (RU-486)	PO 600 mg as a single dose or smaller amounts for 4–7 d
Prostaglandins	
Carboprost tromethamine (Hemabate)	IM 250 µg q1.5–3.5h, depending on uterine response, increased to 500 µg per dose if uterine contractility is inadequate after several 250-µg doses
Dinoprostone (Prostin E₂)	Intravaginally 20 mg, repeated q3–5h until abortion occurs
Misoprostol (Cytotec)	PO or intravaginally 200–400 µg q12h for second trimester termination. Termination usually complete within 48 h.
Tocolytics	
Ritodrine (Yutopar)	IV infusion 0.1 mg/min initially, increased by 50 µg/min every 10 min to a maximal dose of 350 µg/min if necessary to stop labor. The infusion should be continued for 12 h after uterine contractions cease. PO 10 mg 30 min before discontinuing the IV infusion, then 10 mg q2h for 24 h, then 10–20 mg q4–6h as long as necessary to maintain the pregnancy. Maximal oral dose, 120 mg daily.
Terbutaline (Brethine)	IV infusion 10 µg/min, titrated up to a maximum dose of 80 µg/min until contractions cease PO 2.5 mg q4–6h as maintenance therapy until term
Magnesium sulfate	IV infusion, loading dose 3–4 g mixed in 5% dextrose injection and administered over 15–20 min. Maintenance dose 1–2 g/h, according to serum magnesium levels and deep tendon reflexes. PO 250–450 mg q3h, to maintain a serum level of 2.0–2.5 mEq/L.
Nifedipine (Procardia)	PO 10 mg every 20 min for two to three doses; maximum dose 40 mg in 1 h.
Oxytocic	
Oxytocin (Pitocin)	During labor and delivery, IV 2 milliunits/min, gradually increased to 20 milliunits/min, if necessary, to produce three or four contractions within 10-min periods. Prepare solution by adding 10 units (1 mL) of oxytocin to 1000 mL of 0.9% sodium chloride or 5% dextrose in 0.45% sodium chloride. To control postpartum hemorrhage, IV 10–40 units added to 1000 mL of 0.9% sodium chloride, infused at a rate to control bleeding To prevent postpartum bleeding, IM 3–10 units (0.3–1 mL) as a single dose To promote milk ejection, topically, 1 spray of nasal solution to one or both nostrils 2–3 min before nursing
Methylergonovine maleate (Methergine)	After delivery of the placenta, IM 0.2 mg; repeat in 2–4 h if bleeding is severe. Severe uterine bleeding, IV, 0.2 mg To prevent excessive postpartum bleeding, PO 0.2 mg 2–4 times daily for 2–7 d, if necessary

IM, intramuscular; IV, intravenous; PO, oral.

In the female reproductive system, prostaglandins E and F are found in the ovaries, myometrium, and menstrual fluid. They stimulate uterine contraction and are probably important in initiating and maintaining the normal birth process. Drug preparations of prostaglandins are capable of inducing labor at any time during pregnancy. Misoprostol (Cytotec), a prostaglandin developed to prevent nonsteroidal anti-inflammatory drug–induced gastric ulcers (see Chap. 60), is being given orally or intravaginally for first or second trimester termination. It is not FDA approved for this use.

Mifepristone (RU-486) is a progesterone antagonist used in several countries to terminate pregnancy during the first trimester. A prostaglandin is usually given approximately 48 hours after the mifepristone to augment uterine contractions and ensure expulsion of the conceptus. Mifepristone has not been approved or marketed for use in the United States.

TOCOLYTICS

Drugs given to inhibit labor and maintain the pregnancy are called *tocolytics*. Uterine contractions with cervical changes between 20 and 37 weeks of gestation are considered premature labor. Nonpharmacologic treatment includes bed rest, hydration, and sedation. Drug therapy is most effective when the cervix is dilated less than 4 cm and membranes are intact.

Ritodrine (Yutopar), terbutaline (Brethine), magnesium sulfate, and nifedipine (Procardia) are used as tocolytics (see Table 67-3). Ritodrine and terbutaline are beta-adrenergic agents that relax uterine smooth muscle and thereby slow or stop uterine contractions. Terbutaline is not FDA approved for use in premature labor, but is used widely for that purpose. Magnesium sulfate is most often used as an anticonvulsant in the treatment of pregnancy-induced hypertension (preeclampsia), but it also inhibits preterm labor. Hypermagnesemia may occur because tocolytic serum levels (approximately 4 to 7 mEq/L) are higher than normal levels (1.5 to 2.5 mEq/L). Close monitoring of serum levels and signs of hypermagnesemia (eg, decreased respiratory rate and hypotonia) is required.

> ### *Nursing Notes: Ethical/Legal Dilemma*
>
> As a nursing student, you are assigned to a unit where abortions are performed. Your religious and family upbringing has taught you that abortion is an immoral act. Do you have a right to refuse to participate in an experience involving abortion as a student? If so, how might you approach your instructor about this issue? Would this situation be different if you were a regular employee on a unit that performs abortions?

DRUGS USED DURING LABOR AND DELIVERY AT TERM

At the end of gestation, labor usually begins spontaneously and proceeds through delivery of the neonate. Drugs often used during labor, delivery, and the immediate postpartum period include oxytocics, analgesics, and anesthetics.

Oxytocics

Oxytocic drugs include oxytocin (Pitocin) and methylergonovine (Methergine) (see Table 67-3). Oxytocin is a hormone produced in the hypothalamus and released by the posterior pituitary gland (see Chap. 23). Oxytocin stimulates uterine contractions to initiate labor and promotes letdown of breast milk to the nipples in lactation. Pitocin is a synthetic form used to induce labor at or near full-term gestation and to augment labor when uterine contractions are weak and ineffective. It also can be used to prevent or control uterine bleeding after delivery or to complete an incomplete abortion. It is contraindicated for antepartum use in the presence of fetal distress, cephalopelvic disproportion, preterm labor, placenta previa, previous uterine surgery, and severe preeclampsia. Methergine is used for management of postpartum hemorrhage related to uterine atony.

Analgesics

Parenteral opioid analgesics are used to control discomfort and pain during labor and delivery. They may prolong labor and cause sedation and respiratory depression in the mother and neonate. Meperidine (Demerol) may cause less neonatal depression than other opioid analgesics. Butorphanol (Stadol) is becoming more widely used and has been proven safe for the fetus. If neonatal respiratory depression does occur, it can be reversed by the opioid antagonist naloxone (Narcan).

Duramorph is a long-acting form of morphine that provides analgesia up to 24 hours after injection into the epidural catheter at the completion of a cesarean section.

Regional analgesia is achieved by the epidural injection of opioids (eg, fentanyl) or preservative-free morphine. Possible side effects include maternal urinary retention, but no significant effects on the fetus.

Anesthetics

Local anesthetics also are used to control discomfort and pain. They are injected by physicians for regional anesthesia in the pelvic area. Epidural blocks involve injection into the epidural space of the spinal cord. The most commonly used agents are lidocaine and bupivacaine. With regional anesthesia, the mother is usually conscious and comfortable, and the neonate is rarely depressed. Fentanyl is also commonly combined with a small amount of an anesthetic drug for both analgesia and anesthesia. No significant effects on the fetus have been demonstrated in clinical studies.

NEONATAL THERAPEUTICS

In the neonate, any drug must be used cautiously. Drugs are usually given less often because they are metabolized and excreted slowly. Immature liver and kidney function prolongs drug action and increases risks of toxicity. Also, drug therapy should be initiated with low doses, especially with drugs that are highly bound to plasma proteins. Neonates have few binding proteins, which leads to increased amounts of free, active drug and increased risk of toxicity. When assessing the neonate, drugs received by the mother during pregnancy, labor and delivery, and lactation must be considered.

At birth, some drugs are routinely administered to prevent hemorrhagic disease of the newborn and ophthalmia neonatorum. Hemorrhagic disease of the newborn occurs because the intestinal tract lacks the bacteria that normally synthesize vitamin K. Vitamin K is required for liver production of several clotting factors, including prothrombin. Thus, the neonate is at increased risk of bleeding during approximately the first week of life. One dose of phytonadione (AquaMEPHYTON) 0.5 to 1 mg is given intramuscularly in the thigh at delivery or on admission to the nursery.

Ophthalmia neonatorum, an eye infection that may cause ulceration and blindness, is usually caused by exposure to *Neisseria gonorrhoeae* during passage through the birth canal. It is a sexually transmitted disease for which prophylaxis is legally required. Another serious eye infection is caused by *Chlamydia trachomatis*, also a sexually transmitted microorganism. Erythromycin 0.5% or tetracycline 1% is applied to each eye at delivery. The drugs are effective against gonorrheal and chlamydial infections.

NURSING PROCESS

Assessment

Assess each female client of reproductive age for possible pregnancy. If the client is known to be pregnant, assess status in relation to pregnancy, as follows:

- Length of gestation
- Use of prescription, over-the-counter, nontherapeutic, and illegal drugs
- Acute and chronic health problems that may influence the pregnancy or require drug therapy

- With premature labor, assess length of gestation, the frequency and quality of uterine contractions, the amount of vaginal bleeding or discharge, and the length of labor. Also determine whether any tissue has been expelled from the vagina. When abortion is inevitable, oxytocics may be given. When stopping labor is possible or desired, a tocolytic may be given.
- When spontaneous labor occurs in normal, full-term pregnancy, assess frequency and quality of uterine contractions, amount of cervical dilatation, fetal heart rate and quality, and maternal blood pressure.
- Assess antepartum women for intention to breastfeed.

Nursing Diagnoses

- Risk for injury: Damage to fetus or neonate from maternal ingestion of drugs
- Risk for injury: Damage to the pregnant client from acute and chronic health problems
- Altered Nutrition: Less Than Body Requirements related to pregnancy-induced anemia and nausea and vomiting
- Altered Nutrition: More Than Body Requirements related to excessive weight gain with pregnancy
- Anxiety related to the outcome of pregnancy
- Noncompliance related to ingestion of nonessential drugs during actual or potential pregnancy
- Pain related to uterine contractions
- Risk for injury related to possible damage to mother or infant during the birth process
- Knowledge Deficit: Drug effects during pregnancy and lactation

Planning/Goals

The client will:

- Avoid unnecessary drug ingestion when pregnant or likely to become pregnant
- Use nonpharmacologic measures to relieve symptoms associated with pregnancy or other health problems when possible
- Maintain nutritional status and appropriate weight gain to support maternal health and fetal growth and development
- Obtain optimal care during pregnancy, labor and delivery, and the postpartum period
- Avoid behaviors that may lead to complications of pregnancy and labor and delivery
- Breastfeed safely and successfully if desired

Interventions

- Use nondrug measures to prevent the need for drug therapy during actual or potential pregnancy.
- Provide optimal prenatal care and counseling to promote a healthy pregnancy (eg, regular moni-

CLIENT TEACHING GUIDELINES
Drug Use During Pregnancy and Lactation

✔ Any drug taken by a pregnant woman reaches the fetus and may interfere with fetal growth and development. For most drugs, safety during pregnancy has not been established, and all drugs are relatively contraindicated. Therefore, any drug use (including prescription drugs) must be cautious and minimal to avoid potential damage to the fetus.

✔ Avoid drugs when possible and use them very cautiously when necessary. If women who are sexually active and not using contraception take *any* drugs, there is a high risk that potentially harmful agents may be ingested before pregnancy is suspected or confirmed.

✔ Measures to prevent the need for drug therapy include a healthful lifestyle (adequate nutrition, exercise, rest and sleep; avoiding alcohol and cigarette smoking) and avoiding infection (personal hygiene, avoiding contact with people known to have infections, maintaining indicated immunizations).

✔ Nondrug measures to relieve common health problems include positioning, adequate food and fluid intake, and deep breathing.

✔ See a health care provider as soon as pregnancy is suspected.

✔ Inform any health care provider from whom treatment is sought if there is a possibility of pregnancy.

✔ Many drugs are excreted in breast milk to some extent and reach the nursing infant.

---

toring of blood pressure, weight, blood sugar, urine protein, and counseling about nutrition and other health-promoting activities).

• Help clients and families cope with complications of pregnancy, including therapeutic abortion.

• Counsel candidates for therapeutic abortion about methods and expected outcomes; counsel abortion clients about contraceptive techniques.

Evaluation

• The pregnant woman takes actions to promote reproductive and general health.

• The pregnant woman complies with instructions for promoting and maintaining a healthy pregnancy.

• The prepregnant, pregnant, and lactating woman avoids ingestion of therapeutic and nontherapeutic drugs when possible.

• The mother and neonate achieve optimal health status.

• If chosen, breastfeeding is accomplished safely and successfully.

available drug information (see Box 67-1 and Table 67-2). During the first trimester, for example, an older drug that has not been associated with teratogenic effects is usually preferred over a newer drug of unknown teratogenicity.

3. Any drugs used during pregnancy should be given in the lowest effective doses and for the shortest effective time.

4. Counsel pregnant women about the use of immunizations during pregnancy. Live virus vaccines (eg, measles, mumps, polio, rubella, yellow fever) should be avoided because of possible harmful effects to the fetus.

   Inactive virus vaccines, such as influenza, rabies, and hepatitis B (if the mother is high risk and negative for hepatitis B antigen) and toxoids (eg, diphtheria, tetanus) are considered safe for use. In addition, hyperimmune globulins can be given to pregnant women who are exposed to hepatitis B, rabies, tetanus, or varicella, and some inactive vaccines (eg, cholera, pneumococcal, plague, typhoid) can be given if exposure has occurred or travel to endemic areas is required.

PRINCIPLES OF THERAPY

General Guidelines: Pregnancy

1. Give medications only when clearly indicated, weighing anticipated benefits to the mother against the risk of harm to the fetus.

2. When drug therapy is required, the choice of drug should be based on the stage of pregnancy and

Nursing Notes: Apply Your Knowledge

Rosa Sanchez is breastfeeding her 6-month-old son when she develops a cold. After she has started taking over-the-counter cold remedies, she calls the consulting nurse to see if these medications will affect her ability to breastfeed her son. If you were the consulting nurse, how would you respond?

General Guidelines: Lactation

1. Many drugs given to the mother reach the infant in breast milk. For some, the amount of drug is too small to cause significant effects; for others, effects on the nursing infant are unknown or potentially adverse. For the latter drugs, it is usually recommended that the mother stop the drug or stop breastfeeding. Effects of commonly used therapeutic drugs are listed in Table 67-4.

2. Give medications only when clearly indicated, weighing potential benefit to the mother against possible harm to the nursing infant.

3. Any drugs used during lactation should be given in the lowest effective dose for the shortest effective time.

4. Mothers should be encouraged to pump and discard breast milk while on drugs, to maintain lactation.

Use of Oxytocin

Oxytocin is the drug of choice for induction or augmentation of labor because physiologic doses produce a rhythmic uterine contraction–relaxation pattern that approx-

(*text continues on page 1016*)

TABLE 67-4	Drug Effects in Lactation
Adrenergics	Parenteral *epinephrine* (Adrenalin) is excreted in breast milk; the status of other adrenergic bronchodilators is not known. *Albuterol* (Proventil, Ventolin) had tumorigenic effects in animals; if considered necessary, breastfeeding should be discontinued. Oral drugs used as nasal decongestants (eg, *pseudoephedrine* [Sudafed]) are contraindicated in nursing mothers because of higher than usual risks to infants from sympathomimetic drugs.
Analgesics	*Acetaminophen* (Tylenol) is excreted in breast milk in low concentrations. No adverse effects have been reported, and it is probably the analgesic-antipyretic drug of choice for nursing mothers. Salicylates (eg, *aspirin*) are excreted in breast milk in small amounts. Adverse effects on nursing infants have not been reported but are a potential risk. Opioid analgesics such as *meperidine* (Demerol) are excreted in breast milk, but amounts may not be enough to cause adverse effects in the nursing infant. Some authorities recommend waiting 4 to 6 h after a dose before nursing. *Alfentanil* (Alfenta) was found in breast milk, but significance is unknown or nil. American Academy of Pediatrics supports use during lactation. Butorphanol (Stadol) is considered safe during lactation.
Angiotensin-converting Enzyme (ACE) Inhibitors	*Captopril* (Capoten) is excreted in breast milk, but minimal effects on the infant are documented. *Enalapril* (Vasotec) and *lisinopril* (Prinivil, Zestril) are excreted in small amounts in breast milk. American Academy of Pediatrics supports breastfeeding while taking these drugs.
Angiotensin II Receptor Antagonists	*Losartan* (Cozaar) and *valsartan* (Diovan) are not recommended for use during lactation because of inadequate studies.
Antianginal Agents (Nitrates)	Safety for use in the nursing mother has not been established.
Antianxiety and Sedative-hypnotic Agents (Benzodiazepines)	*Diazepam* (Valium) and other benzodiazepines should in general be avoided. They are excreted in breast milk and may cause lethargy and weight loss in the infant. The drugs and their metabolites may accumulate to toxic levels in neonates because of slow drug metabolism.
Antiarrhythmics	*Quinidine* (Quinaglute) can be safely used during lactation. *Disopyramide* (Norpace) and *mexiletine* (Mexitil) are secreted in breast milk and not recommended for use because no documented studies have been reported. There is a potential for serious adverse effects on infants with the use of *flecainide* (Tambocor). Newer drugs have not been studied in relation to lactation.
Antibiotics	*Penicillins* are excreted in breast milk in low concentrations and may cause diarrhea, candidiasis, or allergic responses in nursing infants. *Cephalosporins* are excreted in small amounts and may alter bowel flora, cause pharmacologic effects, and interfere with interpretation of culture reports with fever or infection. *Aztreonam* (Azactam) is excreted in small amounts; discontinuing breastfeeding temporarily is probably indicated. *Imipenem/cilastatin* (Primaxin) is secreted in breast milk but considered safe for use. The aminoglycoside *netilmicin* (Netromycin) is excreted in small amounts. Because these drugs are nephrotoxic and ototoxic, the immature kidney function of neonates and infants should be considered. *Tetracyclines* are excreted in breast milk and should be avoided. *Sulfonamides* are excreted and are acceptable for breastfeeding the term

TABLE 67-4	**Drug Effects in Lactation** (*continued*)

	infant, but not the premature infant. They may cause kernicterus in the neonate and diarrhea and skin rash in the nursing infant. *Erythromycin* is excreted and may become concentrated in breast milk. No adverse effects on nursing infants have been reported. However, the potential exists for alteration in bowel flora, pharmacologic effects, and interference with fever workup. *Nitrofurantoin* (Macrodantin) is excreted in very small amounts. However, safety for use in nursing mothers has not been established, and infants with glucose-6-phosphate dehydrogenase deficiency may be adversely affected. *Clindamycin* (Cleocin) is excreted. Breastfeeding is probably best discontinued if the drug is necessary, to avoid potential problems in the infant. *Ciprofloxacin* (Cipro) and other fluoroquinolones are not recommended because they are transferred through breast milk and may lead to serious toxicity in the infant. *Isoniazid* (INH) and *rifampin* (Rifadin) are excreted in breast milk, and nursing infants should be observed for adverse drug effects. *Trimethoprim* (Proloprim, Bactrim) is excreted and may interfere with folic acid metabolism in the infant. It is not recommended for use.
Anticholinergics	*Atropine* and others are excreted and may cause infant toxicity or decreased breast milk production. Safety for use is not established.
Anticoagulants	*Heparin* is not excreted in breast milk; *warfarin* (Coumadin) is excreted, but some evidence suggests no harm to the nursing infant. More data are needed, and heparin is preferred if anticoagulant therapy is required.
Anticonvulsants	*Phenytoin* (Dilantin) and other hydantoins are excreted and may cause serious adverse effects in nursing infants. The drug or breastfeeding should be discontinued. *Phenobarbital* is excreted in small amounts and may cause drowsiness in the infant. Newer drugs have not been studied and are not recommended for use.
Antidepressants	Tricyclic antidepressants such as *amitriptyline* (Elavil) and others are excreted in small amounts; effects on nursing infants are not known. Other antidepressants have not been established as safe for use, including newer drugs such as *fluoxetine* (Prozac).
Antidiabetic Drugs	Insulin does not enter breast milk and is not known to affect the nursing infant. However, insulin requirements of the mother may be decreased while breastfeeding. Oral agents such as *rosiglitazone* (Avandia), *metformin* (Glucophage), *meglitinide* (Prandin) are not considered safe for breastfeeding mothers because of a lack of controlled studies.
Antidiarrheals	*Diphenoxylate* (Lomotil) and *loperamide* (Imodium) should be used cautiously during lactation; effects on the nursing infant are unknown.
Antiemetics	Although information is limited, most of the drugs (*eg*, phenothiazines such as *promethazine* [Phenergan] and antihistamines such as *dimenhydrinate* [Dramamine]) are apparently excreted in breast milk and may cause drowsiness and possibly other effects in nursing infants. Antihistamines used for antiemetic effects also may inhibit lactation. *Metoclopramide* (Reglan) is excreted and concentrated in breast milk; it should be used cautiously, if at all.
Antifungals	Safety for use of systemic drugs has not been established.
Antihistamines	Histamine-1 receptor antagonists such as *diphenhydramine* (Benadryl) may inhibit lactation by their drying effects and may cause drowsiness in nursing infants. For most of the commonly used drugs, including over-the-counter allergy and cold remedies, little information is available about excretion in breast milk or effects on nursing infants. Histamine-2 receptor antagonists such as *cimetidine* (Tagamet) and *ranitidine* (Zantac) are excreted in breast milk. *Famotidine* (Pepcid) was excreted in animals, but it is not known whether it is excreted in human breast milk. It is generally recommended that either the drug or nursing be discontinued.
Antihypertensives	Beta-adrenergic blocking agents should in general be avoided by nursing mothers. *Propranolol* (Inderal) and *metoprolol* (Lopressor) are excreted in low concentrations; *acebutolol* (Sectral) and its major metabolite are excreted; it is unknown whether *nadolol* (Corgard) and *timolol* (Blocadren) are excreted. *Methyldopa* (Aldomet) is excreted; effects on nursing infants are unknown. It is unknown whether *hydralazine* (Apresoline) is excreted; safety for use is not established. *Captopril* (Capoten), *clonidine* (Catapres), *guanabenz* (Wytensin), and *guanfacine* (Tenex) are not usually recommended because information about effects on nursing infants is limited. Calcium channel blocking drugs should not be given to nursing mothers. *Verapamil* (Calan) and *diltiazem* (Cardizem) are excreted in breast milk.

(*continued*)

TABLE 67-4	Drug Effects in Lactation (*continued*)
Antilipemics	*Cholestyramine* (Questran) should be used with caution because of severe constipation in the infant. *Lovastatin* (Mevacor) and related drugs should be used with caution in the lactating woman because of the presence in breast milk. American Academy of Pediatrics supports the use during lactation with monitoring.
Antimanic Agent	*Lithium* is excreted in breast milk and reaches approximately 40% of the mother's serum level. Infant serum and milk levels are approximately equal. If the drug is required, nursing should be discontinued.
Antipsychotic Drugs	Little information is available considering the extensive use of these drugs. *Chlorpromazine* (Thorazine) and *haloperidol* (Haldol) have been detected in breast milk in small amounts. Safety has not been established.
Antithyroid Drugs	Nursing is contraindicated for clients on the antithyroid drugs *propylthiouracil* and *methimazole* (Tapazole).
Antivirals	The protease inhibitors such as *indinavir* (Crixivan) should be avoided during lactation. Mothers should be encouraged not to breastfeed. Inadequate studies support safety.
Beta-adrenergic Blocking Agents	See **Antihypertensives**
Bronchodilators (Xanthine)	Theophyline (Theo-Dur) enters breast milk readily; use with caution.
Calcium Channel Blocking Agents	See **Antihypertensives**
Corticosteroids	*Prednisone* (Deltasone), *dexamethasone* (Decadron), and others appear in breast milk and could suppress growth, interfere with endogenous corticosteroid production, or cause other adverse effects in nursing infants. Advise mothers taking pharmacologic doses not to breastfeed.
Digoxin	*Digoxin* (Lanoxin) is excreted. However, infants receive very small amounts, and no adverse effects have been reported.
Diuretics	If diuretic drug therapy is required, nursing mothers should discontinue breastfeeding. Thiazide diuretics such as *hydrochlorothiazide* (HydroDIURIL) and the loop diuretic *furosemide* (Lasix) are excreted in breast milk. It is unknown whether *bumetanide* (Bumex) and *ethacrynic acid* (Edecrin) are excreted. Little information is available about potassium-sparing diuretics, such as *amiloride* (Midamor), *triamterene* (Dyrenium, Dyazide, Maxzide), and *spironolactone* (Aldactone). They are not recommended for use.
Laxatives	*Cascara sagrada* is excreted in breast milk and may cause diarrhea in the nursing infant. It is not known whether *docusate* (Colace) is excreted.
Nonsteroidal Anti-inflammatory Drugs	Most of the drugs, such as *ibuprofen* (Motrin, Advil) are secreted in breast milk, but considered safe. The use of *celecoxib* (Celebrex) and *rofecoxib* (Vioxx) is not considered safe because no controlled studies have supported their safety.
Thyroid Hormones	Small amounts are excreted in breast milk. The drugs are not associated with adverse effects on nursing infants but should be used with caution in nursing mothers.

imates the normal labor process. It is also the drug of choice for prevention or control of postpartum uterine bleeding because it is less likely to cause hypertension than the ergot alkaloids.

 Home Care

Many obstetric clients with conditions such as premature labor, hyperemesis, and elevated blood pressure are now being managed in the home. The home care nurse who assists in managing these clients should be an obstetrical specialist who is knowledgeable about normal pregnancy and potential complications. The nurse should be aware of the drugs being used to treat the complicated obstetric client. Assessment of the client and her fetus' response to the prescribed drugs should be made in a consistent and

organized fashion on each visit through the use of a care plan or care map.

Home care visits also allow for assessment of compliance with the proposed medical plan. Understanding of previous teaching should be evaluated on each visit to ensure that instructions have been understood. Especially important is the need for the client to demonstrate an understanding of the danger signs and symptoms that may necessitate notifying the home care nurse or physician.

The overall goal of home care is that the pregnancy will be maintained to the most advanced gestational age possible. Home care, to be effective, should be done in the safest and most cost-efficient manner. Frequent home care follow-up by a nurse has been demonstrated to positively affect the outcome of a high-risk pregnancy.

(*text continues on page 1019*)

NURSING ACTIONS Abortifacients, Tocolytics, and Oxytocics

NURSING ACTIONS	RATIONALE/EXPLANATION
1. Administer accurately	
a. Give abortifacients orally (PO), intramuscularly (IM), or intravaginally.	Physicians administer intra-amniotic agents.
b. Give tocolytics intravenously (IV) initially, then PO. With IV ritodrine, have the client lie in the left lateral position.	The side-lying position decreases risks of hypotension.
c. For IV oxytocin, dilute the drug in an IV sodium chloride solution, and piggyback the solution into a primary IV line. Use an infusion pump to administer.	Oxytocin has an antidiuretic effect and may cause water intoxication. This is less likely to occur if the drug is given in a saline solution rather than a water solution, such as 5% dextrose in water. Piggybacking allows regulation of the oxytocin drip without interrupting the main IV line. Infusion pumps deliver more accurate doses and minimize the possibility of overdosage.
d. Give IM oxytocin immediately after delivery of the placenta.	To prevent excessive postpartum bleeding
2. Observe for therapeutic effects	
a. When an abortifacient is given, observe for the onset of uterine bleeding and the expulsion of the fetus and placenta.	Abortion usually occurs within 24 h after a prostaglandin is given and approximately 5 d after mifepristone administration. Uterine contractions may be perceived by the client as abdominal cramping or low back pain.
b. When a tocolytic drug is given in threatened abortion or premature labor, observe for absent or decreased uterine contractions.	The goal of drug therapy is to stop the labor process.
c. When oxytocin is given to induce or augment labor, observe for firm uterine contractions at a rate of three to four per 10 min. Each contraction should be followed by a palpable relaxation period. Examine periodically for cervical dilatation and effacement.	Oxytocin is given to stimulate the normal labor process. Contractions should become regular and increase in duration and intensity.
d. When oxytocin or an ergot alkaloid is given to prevent or control postpartum bleeding, observe for a small, firm uterus and minimal vaginal bleeding.	These agents control bleeding by causing strong uterine contractions. The uterus can be palpated in the lower abdomen.
3. Observe for adverse effects	
a. With mifepristone, observe for excessive uterine bleeding and abdominal pain	These effects are uncommon but may occur.
b. With prostaglandins, observe for:	
(1) Nausea, vomiting, diarrhea	These are the most common adverse effects. They occur with all routes of prostaglandin administration and result from drug-induced stimulation of gastrointestinal smooth muscle.
(2) Fever, cardiac arrhythmias, bronchospasm, convulsive seizures, chest pain, muscle aches	These effects occur less frequently and are not clearly related to prostaglandin administration. Bronchospasm is more likely to occur in clients with asthma; seizures are more likely in clients with known epilepsy.

(continued)

NURSING ACTIONS	RATIONALE/EXPLANATION
c. With ritodrine, observe for:	
(1) Change in fetal heart rate	This is a common adverse effect and may be significant if changes are extreme or prolonged.
(2) Maternal effects, such as changes in heart rate, arrhythmias, palpitations, nausea and vomiting, tremors, hypokalemia, hyperglycemia, dyspnea, chest pain and anaphylactic shock.	
d. With oxytocin, observe for:	
(1) Excessive stimulation of uterine contractility (hypertonicity, tetany, rupture, cervical and perineal lacerations, fetal hypoxia, arrhythmias, death or damage from rapid, forceful propulsion through the birth canal)	Most likely to occur when excessive doses are given to initiate or augment labor
(2) Hypotension or hypertension	Usual obstetric doses do not cause significant change in blood pressure. Large doses may cause an initial drop in blood pressure, followed by a sustained elevation.
(3) Water intoxication (convulsions, coma)	
(4) Allergic reactions, including anaphylactic shock	Unlikely with usual doses but may occur with prolonged administration of large doses (>20 milliunits/min)
(5) Nausea and vomiting	
e. With ergot preparations, observe for:	
(1) Nausea, vomiting, diarrhea	These drugs have a direct effect on the vomiting center of the brain and stimulate contraction of gastrointestinal smooth muscle.
(2) Symptoms of ergot poisoning—coolness, numbness and tingling of extremities, headache, vomiting, dizziness, thirst, convulsions, weak pulse, confusion, chest pain, tachycardia or bradycardia, muscle weakness and pain, cyanosis, gangrene of the extremities	The ergot alkaloids are highly toxic; poisoning may be acute or chronic. Acute poisoning is rare; chronic poisoning usually results from overdosage. Circulatory impairments may result from vasoconstriction and vascular insufficiency. Large doses also damage capillary endothelium and may cause thrombosis and occlusion. Gangrene of extremities rarely occurs with usual doses unless peripheral vascular disease or other contraindications also are present.
(3) Hypertension	Blood pressure may rise as a result of generalized vasoconstriction induced by the ergot preparation. Hypertension is most likely to occur when methylergonovine is given to postpartum women with previous hypertension or to those who have had regional anesthesia with vasoconstrictive agents (eg, epinephrine).
(4) Allergic reactions—local edema, pruritus, anaphylactic shock	Allergic reactions are relatively uncommon.
4. Observe for drug interactions	
a. Drugs that alter effects of prostaglandins:	
(1) Aspirin and other nonsteroidal anti-inflammatory agents, such as ibuprofen (Motrin)	These drugs inhibit effects of prostaglandins. When given concurrently with abortifacient prostaglandins, the abortive process is prolonged.

(continued)

NURSING ACTIONS	RATIONALE/EXPLANATION
b. Drugs that alter effects of ritodrine: (1) Beta-adrenergic blocking agents, such as propranolol (Inderal) (2) Corticosteroids	Decreased effectiveness of ritodrine, which is a beta-adrenergic stimulating (agonist) agent Increased risk of pulmonary edema
c. Drugs that alter effects of oxytocin: (1) Vasoconstrictors, such as epinephrine (Adrenalin) and other adrenergic drugs	Additive vasoconstriction with risks of severe, persistent hypertension and intracranial hemorrhage
d. Drugs that alter effects of ergot alkaloids: (1) Propranolol (Inderal) (2) Vasoconstrictors	Additive vasoconstriction See oxytocin, above.

Nursing Notes: Apply Your Knowledge

Answer: Many drugs given to the mother are excreted into breast milk. An increasing number of studies are being conducted to try to quantify drug effects during lactation, so use current resources to get the most up-to-date information. To determine possible effects on her son, the mother should consult her pediatrician regarding any medications she is taking. At times, it is best for the mother to pump her breast and discard the milk until she is no longer taking medication. Antihistamines, which often are found in cold remedies, may dry up milk production and cause drowsiness in the infant.

 ## REVIEW AND APPLICATION EXERCISES

1. Why should drugs be avoided during pregnancy and lactation when possible?

2. How does insulin therapy for diabetes mellitus differ during pregnancy?

3. What is the rationale for using methyldopa and hydralazine to treat hypertension during pregnancy?

4. Which antiseizure agents are preferred during pregnancy? Which should not be given during pregnancy?

5. In a client receiving a tocolytic to inhibit uterine contractions, how and when would you assess the client for adverse drug effects?

6. In a client receiving an oxytocin infusion to induce or augment labor, what interventions are needed to increase safety and decrease adverse drug effects?

7. Which drugs may be used to increase uterine muscle tone and decrease postpartum hemorrhage?

8. Which immunizations are safe to be administered during pregnancy? Which are contraindicated?

SELECTED REFERENCES

Briggs, G., Freeman, R., & Yaffe, S. (1998). *Drugs in pregnancy and lactation*, 5th ed. Baltimore: Williams & Wilkins.

Centers for Disease Control and Prevention. (1998). U.S. Public Health Service Task Force recommendations for the use of antiretroviral drugs in pregnant women for maternal health and reducing perinatal HIV-1 transmission in the United States. *Morbidity and Mortality Weekly Report 47* (RR-2).

Creinin, M. (1999). Medical termination of pregnancy. In J. Sciarra (Ed.), *Obstetrics and gynecology*. Philadelphia: Lippincott Williams & Wilkins.

Drug facts and comparisons. (Updated monthly). St. Louis: Facts and Comparisons.

Harding, J. (1999). The use of psychotropic medications during pregnancy and lactation. In J. Sciarra (Ed.), *Obstetrics and gynecology*. Philadelphia: Lippincott Williams & Wilkins.

Kain, J., et al. (1999). A comparison of two dosing regimens of intravaginal misoprostol for second trimester pregnancy termination. *Obstetrics and Gynecology, 93*, 571–575.

Moore, M.L. & Freda, M. (1998). Reducing preterm and low birthweight births: Still a nursing challenge. *MCN American Journal of Maternal Child Nursing, 23*, 200–208.

Niebyl, J. (1999). Drugs and related areas in pregnancy. In J. Sciarra (Ed.), *Obstetrics and gynecology*. Philadelphia: Lippincott Williams & Wilkins.

Olds, S., London, M., Ladewig, P. (2000). *Maternal-newborn nursing*, 6th ed. Upper Saddle River, NJ: Prentice Hall.

Reece, A. & Hobbins, J. (1999). *Medicine of the fetus and mother*, 2nd ed. Philadelphia: Lippincott Williams & Wilkins.

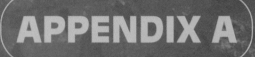
Recently Approved and Miscellaneous Drugs

Generic/Trade Name	Clinical Use	Characteristics	Routes and Dosage Ranges
Alprostadil (Caverject, Muse)	Treatment of impotence	A form of prostaglandin E Induces erection within 5–20 min	Injection into penis (Caverject) or insertion into urethra with applicator (Muse). Dosage individualized to lowest dose effective for sexual intercourse
Antithrombin III, Human (Thrombate III)	Treatment of hereditary antithrombin III deficiency in patients with thrombotic disorders	A replacement product for a substance normally found in plasma	Dosage individualized according to pretreatment plasma levels of antithrombin III
Entacapone (Comtan)	Parkinson's disease, with levodopa/carbidopa	Inhibits catechol-*O*-methyltransferase, an enzyme that normally metabolizes dopamine and levodopa	PO 200 mg with each dose of levodopa/carbidopa, to a maximum of 8 doses (1600 mg) daily
Epoprostenol (Flolan)	Pulmonary hypertension	Adverse effects include hypotension, nausea, vomiting, diarrhea, anxiety, influenza-like symptoms	Continuous IV infusion via central venous catheter See manufacturer's instructions re: dosage titration
Eprosartan (Teveten)	Hypertension	An angiotensin receptor antagonist (see Chap. 55)	PO 600 mg once daily
Levetiracetam (Keppra)	Antiseizure drug	Chemically unrelated to other antiepileptic drugs	PO 1000 mg daily, increased to 3000 mg daily, if necessary
Linezolid (Zyvox)	Pneumonia Skin and soft tissue infections Serious infections caused by vancomycin-resistant *Enterococcus faecium* (VRE) or methicillin-resistant *Staphylococcus aureus* (MRSA)	A new type of antibacterial drug Adverse effects include headache, nausea, vomiting, diarrhea, thrombocytopenia May interact with adrenergic drugs to increase blood pressure	PO, IV 400–600 mg q12h
Midodrine (ProAmatine)	Severe orthostatic hypotension	Recommended only when orthostatic hypotension seriously interferes with activities of daily living	PO 10 mg three times daily
Pentosan polysulfate sodium (Elmiron)	Relieves bladder pain associated with interstitial cystitis	Mechanism unknown; it may adhere to bladder mucosa and prevent mucosal irritation by urine	PO 100 mg three times daily

Generic/Trade Name	Clinical Use	Characteristics	Routes and Dosage Ranges
Quinupristin/dalfopristin (Synercid)	Complicated skin and soft tissue infections Serious infections caused by vancomycin-resistant *Enterococcus faecium* (VRE)	Common adverse effects are pain, edema, and inflammation at infusion sites	VRE, IV infusion, 7.5 mg/kg q8h Other infections, IV infusion, 7.5 mg/kg q12h
Rapacuronium (Raplon)	Adjunct to anesthesia to aid endotracheal intubation and provide muscle relaxation during surgery	A neuromuscular blocking agent (see Chap. 14) Rapid onset and short duration of action (15–20 min)	Given by anesthesiologist
Riluzole (Rilutek)	Amyotrophic lateral sclerosis (ALS)	Mechanism unknown. Adverse effects include drowsiness, nausea, and increased liver enzymes	PO 50 mg q12h
Sevelamer (Renagel)	Hyperphosphatemia in patients with end-stage renal disease	Reduces serum phosphorus levels	PO 2–4 capsules three times daily with meals
Sildenafil (Viagra)	Treatment of impotence	Has been associated with adverse cardiovascular effects (eg, myocardial infarction)	PO 50 mg about 1 h before sexual activity
Sirolimus (Rapamune)	Prevent renal transplant rejection	Hypersensitivity	PO 6 mg initially, then 2 mg daily
Sodium ferric gluconate complex (Ferrlecit)	Treatment of iron deficiency anemia in patients on hemodialysis who are receiving erythropoietin	Injectable iron supplement 2 mL given initially as test dose for hypersensitivity reactions	IV infusion, 10 mL (125 mg elemental iron) in 100 mL 0.9% sodium chloride, over 1 h
Zaleplon (Sonata)	Short-term treatment of insomnia	Chemically different from other hypnotic agents Adverse effects include nausea, dizziness, and headache	PO 10 mg at bedtime Elderly or low-weight adults, PO 5 mg at bedtime

APPENDIX B

The International System of Units

The International System of Units (Système International d'Unités or SI units), which is based on the metric system, has been adopted by many countries in an attempt to standardize reports of clinical laboratory data among nations and disciplines. A major reason for using SI units is that biologic substances react in the human body on a molar basis.

The international system, like the conventional system, uses the kilogram for measurement of mass or weight and the meter for measurement of length. The major difference is that the international system uses the mole for measurement of amounts per volume of a substance. A mole is the amount of a chemical compound of which its weight in grams equals its molecular weight. Thus, the concentration of solutions is expressed in moles, millimoles, or micromoles per liter (mol/L, mmol/L, μmol/L) rather than the conventional measurement of mass per volume, such as grams or milligrams per 100 mL or dL. A few laboratory values are the same in conventional and SI units, but many differ dramatically. Moreover, "normal values" in both systems often vary, depending on laboratory methodologies and reference sources. Thus, laboratory data should be interpreted in light of the client's clinical status and with knowledge of the "normal values" of the laboratory performing the test.

In addition to other laboratory tests, measuring the amount of a drug in blood plasma or serum is often useful in the clinical management of various disorders. For example, serum drug levels may be used to guide drug dosage (eg, aminoglycoside antibiotics such as gentamicin), to evaluate an inadequate therapeutic response, and to diagnose drug toxicity.

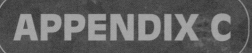

APPENDIX C

Therapeutic Serum Drug Concentrations for Selected Drugs

Listed below are generally accepted therapeutic serum drug concentrations, in conventional and SI units, for several commonly used drugs. In addition, toxic concentrations are listed for selected drugs. SI units have not been established for some drugs.

Drug	Conventional Units	SI units
Acetaminophen	0.2–0.6 mg/dL	13–40 µmol/L
	Toxic >5 mg/dL	>300 µmol/L
Amikacin	(peak) 16–32 µg/mL	20–30 mg/L
	(trough) 8 µg/mL	
	or less	
Amitriptyline	110–250 ng/mL	375–900 nmol/L
Carbamazepine	4–12 µg/mL	17–50 µmol/L
Desipramine	125–300 ng/mL	470–825 nmol/L
Digoxin	0.5–2.2 ng/mL	1–2.6 nmol/L
Disopyramide	2–8 µg/mL	6–18 µmol/L
Ethosuximide	40–110 µg/mL	280–780 µmol/L
Gentamicin	(peak) 4–8 µg/mL	5–10 mg/L
	(trough) 2 µg/mL	
	or less	
Imipramine	200–350 ng/ml	530–950 nmol/L
Lidocaine	1.5–6 µg/mL	6–21 µmol/L
Lithium	0.5–1.5 mEq/L	0.5–1.5 mmol/L
Maprotiline	50–200 ng/mL	180–270 nmol/L
Netilmicin	(peak) 6–10 µg/mL	5–10 mg/L
	(trough) 2 µg/mL	
	or less	

Drug	Conventional Units	SI units
Nortriptyline	50–150 ng/mL	190–570 nmol/L
Phenobarbital	15–50 µg/mL	65–170 µmol/L
Phenytoin	10–20 µg/mL	40–80 µmol/L
Primidone	5–12 µg/mL	25–45 µmol/L
Procainamide	4–8 µg/mL	17–40 µmol/L
Propranolol	50–200 ng/mL	190–770 nmol/L
Protriptyline	100–300 ng/mL	380–1140 nmol/L
Quinidine	2–6 µg/mL	4.6–9.2 µmol/L
Salicylate	100–200 mg/L	724–1448 µmol/L
	Toxic >200 mg/L	>1450 µmol/L
Theophylline	10–20 µg/mL	55–110 µmol/L
Tobramycin	(peak) 4–8 µg/mL	5–10 mg/L
	(trough) 2 µg/mL	
	or less	
Valproic acid	50–100 µg/mL	350–700 µmol/L
Vancomycin	(peak) 30–40 mg/mL	(peak) 20–
	(trough) 5–10 mg/mL	40 mg/L
		(trough)
		5–10 mg/L

µg, microgram; ng, nanogram; µmol, micromole.

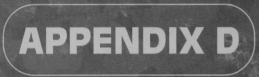

APPENDIX D

Canadian Drug Laws and Standards

Two national laws, with their amendments, regulate drug-related standards and practices. The Health Protection Branch of the Department of National Health and Welfare is responsible for administering and enforcing the laws, which are described below.

The Food and Drugs Act, initially passed in 1953 and amended periodically since then, regulates the manufacture, distribution, advertising, labeling, and use of drugs. Specific provisions:

- Empower the government to control the marketing of drugs according to proof of safety and effectiveness
- Require that drugs comply with the standards under which the drugs are approved for sale or the standards listed in "specific pharmacopeiae"
- Direct the government to supervise the manufacturing processes of some drugs
- Classify drugs (eg, antihypertensives, antimicrobials, hormones) that require a prescription and specify that refills must be designated on the original prescription and obtained within 6 months (Schedule F)
- Specify symbols to be placed on containers of the different classifications of drugs
- Require proof of appropriate drug release from oral dosage formulations
- Prohibit advertising of prescription and controlled drugs to the public
- Prohibit the sale of contaminated, adulterated, or unsafe drugs
- Establish requirements for labeling
- Prohibit false, misleading, or deceptive labeling of drug products

The Narcotic Control Act, originally passed in 1961 and amended periodically since then, restricts the sale, pos-session, and use of opiates, cocaine, marijuana, and methadone. Additional provisions:

- Restrict possession of the above drugs to authorized people
- Require people possessing the drugs to keep them in a secure place, maintain strict dispensing records, and promptly report any thefts or other losses
- Require prescriptions for dispensing narcotics
- Require that containers with prescribed narcotics be labeled with the symbol N
- Specify four levels of controlled drugs. The first level, narcotics, includes single drugs and preparations containing cocaine, codeine, heroin, hydrocodone, hydromorphone, methadone, morphine, oxycodone, and pentazocine. The second level, controlled drugs or Schedule G, includes non-narcotic prescription drugs, the use of which is restricted to treatment of certain disorders (eg, amphetamines, methylphenidate, pentobarbital, and secobarbital). The third level restricts anabolic steroids, amobarbital, phenobarbital, diethylpropion, and nalbuphine. The fourth level (Schedule H) includes substances with no recognized medicinal uses (eg, hallucinogens such as LSD).

Nurses in Canada are governed by these national laws; there also may be local and provincial laws. Legal possession of a narcotic by a nurse is restricted to the following circumstances:

- When administering to a client according to a physician's order
- When performing custodial care of narcotics as an agent of a health care facility
- When receiving a prescribed narcotic for medical treatment

Canadian Drug Names

Many drugs are distributed by international pharmaceutical companies, and most names (generic and trade) are the same in the United States and Canada. To assist the Canadian reader in identifying the drugs discussed in this book, generic names, relevant chapter number(s), and Canadian trade names are listed below. Generic names used in Canada but not in the United States are designated by an asterisk.

Canadian trade names that include Alti, Apo, Novo, or Nu are drugs manufactured by Altimed, Apotex, Novo-

Pharm, and Nu-Pharm companies, respectively. Some trade names consist of a company prefix and a generic name (eg, Alti-Ibuprofen, Apo-Cimetidine, Novo-Acebutolol, Nu-Clonidine). Because these names are easy to identify, they are not included in the accompanying list. However, some trade names consisting of a company prefix and a shortened version of the generic name (eg, Apo-Alpraz for alprazolam) are included.

Generic/Canadian Trade Names

Abciximab (57)
ReoPro
Acarbose (27)
Prandase
Acebutolol (19)
Monitan, Rhotral, Sectral
Acetaminophen (7), Paracetamol*
APAP, Abenol, Atasol, Tempra, Tylenol
Acetazolamide (65)
Diamox
Acetohexamide (27)
Dimelor
Acetylcysteine (49)
Mucomyst
Acyclovir (39, 66)
Avirax, Zovirax
Adenosine (52)
Adenocard
Albuterol (18, 47), Salbutamol*
Airomir, Asmavent, Novo-Salmol, Ventodisc, Ventolin
Alendronate (26)
Fosamax
Alfentanil (6)
Alfenta
Allopurinol (7)
Zyloprim

Alprazolam (8)
Apo-Alpraz, Novo-Alprazol, Nu-Alpraz, Xanax
Alteplase (57)
Activase rt-PA
Aluminum hydroxide (60)
Amphojel
Aluminum hydroxide gel/magnesium hydroxide (60)
Diovol, Maalox, Mylanta
Amantadine (12, 39)
Endantadine, Symmetrel
Amcinonide (66)
Cyclocort
Amifostine (64)
Ethyol
Amikacin (35)
Amikin
Amiloride (56)
Midamor
Aminocaproic acid (57)
Amicar
Aminoglutethimide (64)
Cytadren
Aminophylline (16, 47)
Phyllocontin
Amiodarone (52)
Cordarone

Amitriptyline (10)
Elavil
Amlodipine (53)
Norvasc
Amobarbital (8), Amylobarbitone*
Amytal
Amoxapine (10)
Asendin
Amoxicillin (34)
Amoxil, Apo-Amoxi, Novamoxin, Nu-Amoxi
Amoxicillin/clavulanate (34)
Clavulin
Amphotericin B (40)
Fungizone
Ampicillin (34)
Ampicin, Apo-Ampi, Nu-Ampi
Amrinone (51)
Inocor
Anagrelide (57)
Agrylin
Antithymocyte globulin (45)
Atgam
Asparaginase, Colaspase*
Kidrolase
Atenolol (19, 53, 55)
Apo-Atenol, Novo-Atenol, Nu-Atenol, Tenormin

(continued)

Generic/Canadian Trade Names

Atracurium (14)
  Tracium
Atropine sulfate (21, 65)
  Atropisol, Isopto Atropine
Azatadine (48)
  Optimine
Azathioprine (45)
  Imuran
Azithromycin (37)
  Zithromax
Bacampicillin (34)
  Penglobe
Bacitracin (65, 66)
  Baciguent
Baclofen (13)
  Lioresal, Liotec, Nu-Baclo
Beclomethasone (24, 47)
  Beclodisk, Becloforte, Beclovent,
    Beconase, Propaderm, Vancenase,
    Vanceril
Benzocaine (14)
  Topicaine
Benzoyl peroxide (66)
  Acetoxyl, Benoxyl, Benzac, Benzagel,
    Desquam-X, Panoxyl, Solugel
Benztropine (12, 21)
  Cogentin
Betamethasone (24, 66)
  Beben, Betaderm, Betnesol, Betnovate,
    Celestoderm, Celestone, Tara-Sone,
    Valisone
Betaxolol (19, 65)
  Betoptic
Bethanechol (20)
  Duvoid, Myotonachol, Urecholine
Biperiden (12, 21)
  Akineton
Bisacodyl (61)
  Dulcolax
Bleomycin (64)
  Blenoxane
Bretylium (52)
  Bretylate
Brimonidine (65)
  Alphagan
Bromocriptine (12)
  Parlodel
Brompheniramine (48),
  Parabromdylamine*
  Dimetane
Bumetanide (56)
  Burinex
Bupivacaine (14)
  Marcaine, Sensorcaine
Bupropion (10, 15)
  Wellbutrin, Zyban
Buspirone (8)
  Buspar, Buspirex, Bustab
Busulfan (64)
  Myleran
Calcitonin-salmon (26), Salcatonin*
  Calcimar, Caltine
Calcitriol (26)
  Calcijex, Rocaltrol
Calcium carbonate (26)
  Apo-Cal, Calsan, Caltrate, Os-Cal

Captopril (55)
  Apo-Capto, Capoten, Captril,
    Novo-Captoril, Nu-Capto
Carbachol (65)
  Carbostat, Isopto Carbachol, Miostat
Carbamazepine (11)
  Novo-Carbamaz, Tegretol
Carboplatin (64)
  Paraplatin
Carisoprodol (13), Isomeprobamate*
  Soma
Carmustine (64)
  BiCNU
Cefaclor (34)
  Ceclor
Cefadroxil (34)
  Duricef
Cefazolin (34)
  Ancef, Kefzol
Cefepime (34)
  Maxipime
Cefixime (34)
  Suprax
Cefoperazone (34)
  Cefobid
Cefotaxime (34)
  Claforan
Cefotetan (34)
  Cefotan
Cefoxitin (34)
  Mefoxin
Cefprozil (34)
  Cefzil
Ceftazidime (34)
  Ceptaz, Fortaz, Tazidime
Ceftizoxime (34)
  Cefizox
Ceftriaxone (34)
  Rocephin
Cefuroxime (34)
  Ceftin, Kefurox, Zinacef
Cephalexin (34)
  Apo-Cephalex, Keflex, Novo-Lexin,
    Nu-Cephalex
Cephalothin (34)
  Ceporacin, Keflin
Cerivistatin (58)
  Baycol
Chlorambucil (64)
  Leukeran
Chloramphenicol (37, 65)
  Chloromycetin, Diochloram,
    Ophtho-Chloram, Pentamycetin
Chlordiazepoxide (8)
  Novo-Poxide
Chlorhexidine (66)
  Hibidil, Hibitane
Chlorpheniramine (48),
  Chlorphenamine*
  Chlor-Tripolon
Chloroprocaine (14)
  Nesacaine
Chloroquine (41)
  Aralen
Chlorpromazine (9, 63)
  Chlorpromanyl, Largactil

Chlorpropamide (27)
  Diabinese
Chlorthalidone (56)
  Hygroton
Cholestyramine (58)
  Novo-Cholamine, Questran
Ciclopirox (66)
  Loprox
Cilazapril (55)
  Inhibace
Cimetidine (60)
  Novo-Cimetine, Nu-Cimet, Peptol,
    Tagamet
Ciprofloxacin (35, 65)
  Ciloxan, Cipro
Cisplatin, cis-platinum (64)
  Platinol AQ
Clarithromycin (37)
  Biaxin
Clemastine (48)
  Tavist
Clindamycin (37)
  Dalacin
Clomipramine (8)
  Anafranil, Novo-Clopamine
Clonazepam (8)
  Clonapam, Rivotril
Clonidine (55)
  Catapres, Dixarit
Clopidogrel (57)
  Plavix
Clorazepate (8)
  Novo-Clopate, Tranxene
Clotrimazole (40)
  Canesten, Clotrimaderm
Cloxacillin (34)
  Apo-Cloxi, Novo-Cloxin, Nu-Cloxi,
    Tegopen
Clozapine (9)
  Clozaril
Colestipol (58)
  Colestid
Cortisone (24)
  Cortone
Cromolyn (47), Sodium cromoglycate*
  Intal, Opticrom
Cyanocobalamin (31)
  Rubramin
Cyclobenzaprine (13)
  Flexeril, Novo-Cycloprine
Cyclopentolate (65)
  Cyclogyl, Diopentolate
Cyclophosphamide (64)
  Cytoxan, Procytox
Cyclosporine (45)
  Neoral, Sandimmune
Cyproheptadine (48)
  Periactin
Cytarabine, cytosine arabinoside (64)
  Cytosar
Dacarbazine (64)
  DTIC
Dactinomycin (Actinomycin D) (64)
  Cosmegen
Dalteparin (57)
  Fragmin

Generic/Canadian Trade Names

Danaparoid (57)
Orgaran
Danazol (29)
Cyclomen
Dantrolene (13)
Dantrium
Daunorubicin (daunomycin) (64)
Cerubidine
Deferoxamine (32)
Desferal
Demeclocycline (36)
Declomycin
Desipramine (10)
Norpramin
Desonide (66)
Desocort
Desoximetasone (66)
Topicort
Dexamethasone (24, 65, 66)
Decadron, Dexasone, Maxidex
Dexchlorpheniramine (48)
Polaramine
Dextroamphetamine (16),
Dexamphetamine*
Dexedrine
Dextromethorphan (49)
Balminil DM, Benylin DM, Delsym,
Koffex DM
Diazepam (8)
Diazemuls, Valium, Vivol
Dibucaine (14)
Nupercainal
Diclofenac (7)
Apo-Diclo, Diclotec, Novo-Difenac,
Nu-Diclo, Voltaren
Dicyclomine (21)
Bentylol
Didanosine (39)
Videx
Diethylpropion (30)
Tenuate
Diflunisal (7)
Dolobid
Digoxin (51)
Lanoxin
Digoxin immune Fab (51),
Digoxin-specific antibody
fragments*
Digibind
Dihydrotachysterol (26)
Hytakerol
Diltiazem (52, 53, 55)
Apo-Diltiaz, Cardizem, Novo-Diltiazem,
Nu-Diltiaz, Tiazac
Dimenhydrinate (48, 63)
Gravol, Traveltabs
Dinoprostone (prostaglandin E$_2$) (67)
Cervidil, Prepidil, Prostin E$_2$
Diphenhydramine (12, 48, 63)
Allerdryl, Benadryl, Nytol
Diphenoxylate (62)
Lomotil
Dipivefrin (65)
Propine
Dipyridamole (57)
Novo-Dipiradol, Persantine

Disopyramide (52)
Rythmodan
Dobutamine (18, 54)
Dobutrex
Docetaxel (64)
Taxotere
Docusate (61)
Colace, Surfak
Dopamine (18, 54)
Intropin
Doxacurium (14)
Nuromax
Doxazosin (19, 55)
Cardura
Doxepin (9)
Sinequan, Zonalon
Doxorubicin (64)
Adriamycin
Doxycycline (36)
Apo-Doxy, Doxycin, Doxytec,
Novo-Doxylin, Vibra-Tabs
Econazole (40)
Ecostatin
Edrophonium (20)
Enlon, Tensilon
Enalapril (55)
Vasotec
Enflurane (14)
Ethrane
Enoxaparin (57)
Lovenox
Epinephrine (18, 47, 54), Adrenaline
Bronkaid Mistometer, EpiPen,
Vaponefrin
Epoetin alfa (44)
Eprex
Ergocalciferol (26)
Drisdol, Ostoforte
Ergotamine (7)
Ergomar
Erythromycin (37, 65)
Apo-Erythro, Diomycin, Erybid, Eryc,
Erythromid, Novo-Rythro
Esmolol (52)
Brevibloc
Estradiol (28)
Climara, Delestrogen, Estraderm,
Estrace
Estrogens, conjugated (28)
Congest, Premarin
Estropipate (28), Piperazine estrone
sulfate*
Ogen
Ethacrynic acid (56)
Edecrin
Ethambutol (38)
Etibi, Myambutol
Ethinyl estradiol (28)
Estinyl
Ethinyl estradiol/ethynodiol (28)
Demulen
Ethinyl estradiol/levonorgestrel (28)
Alesse, Min-Ovral, Triphasil, Triquilar
Ethinyl estradiol/norethindrone (28)
Brevicon, Loestrin, Minestrin, Ortho,
Synphasic

Ethinyl estradicol/norgestrel (28)
Ovral
Ethosuximide (11)
Zarontin
Etidronate (26)
Didronel
Etodolac (7)
Ultradol
Etoposide (64)
Vepesid
Famciclovir (39)
Famvir
Famotidine (60)
Pepcid
Felodipine (53)
Plendil, Renedil
Fenofibrate (58)
Lipidil
Fenoprofen (7)
Nalfon
Fentanyl (6)
Duragesic
Ferrous sulfate (32)
Fer-In-Sol, Fero-Grad, Slow-Fe
Filgrastim (44)
Neupogen
Flavoxate (21)
Urispas
Flecainide (52)
Tambocor
Fluconazole (40)
Diflucan
Fludarabine (64)
Fludara
Fludrocortisone (24)
Florinef
Flumazenil (8)
Anexate
Flunisolide (24, 47)
Bronalide, Rhinalar
Fluocinolone (66)
Lidemol, Lidex, Synalar, Tiamol, Topsyn
Fluorometholone (65)
Flarex
Fluorouracil, 5-FU (64)
Adrucil, Efudex, Fluoroplex
Fluoxetine (10)
Prozac
Fluoxymesterone (29)
Halostestin
Fluphenazine (9)
Moditen
Flurazepam (8)
Dalmane, Somnol
Flurbiprofen (7, 65)
Ansaid, Froben, Ocufen
Flutamide (64)
Euflex
Fluticasone (24)
Flonase, Flovent
Fluvastatin (58)
Lescol
Fluvoxamine (10)
Luvox
Fosinopril (55)
Monopril

(continued)

Generic/Canadian Trade Names

Fosphenytoin (11)
Cerebyx
Furosemide (26, 56), Frusemide*
Lasix
Gabapentin (11)
Neurontin
Gallamine (14)
Flaxedil
Ganciclovir (39)
Cytovene
Gemcitabine (64)
Gemzar
Gemfibrozil (58)
Gen-Fibro, Lopid
Gentamicin (35, 65)
Cidomycin, Diogent, Garamycin
Glyburide (27), Glibenclamide*
DiaBeta, Euglucon, Gen-Glybe
Glycopyrrolate (21), Glycopyrronium*
Robinul
Goserelin (64)
Zoladex
Granisetron (63)
Kytril
Guaifenesin (49), Glyceryl guaiacolate*
Balminil Expectorant, Benylin-E,
Robitussin
Griseofulvin (40)
Fulvicin, Grisovin
Halcinonide (66)
Halog
Haloperidol (9)
Haldol, Peridol
Heparin sodium (57)
Hepalean
Hydralazine (55)
Apresoline, Novo-Hylazin, Nu-Hydral
Hydrochlorothiazide (56)
Apo-Hydro, HydroDiuril
Hydrocodone (6, 49)
Hycodan, Robidone
Hydrocortisone (24, 47, 66)
Aquacort, Cortate, Cortef, Cortenema
Hydromorphone (6, 49)
Dilaudid, Hydromorph Contin
Hydroxychloroquine (41)
Plaquenil
Hydroxyurea (64)
Hydrea
Hydroxyzine (8, 48, 63)
Atarax, Multipax
Ibuprofen (7)
Actiprofen, Advil, Motrin, Novo-Profen
Idarubicin (64)
Idamycin
Ifosfamide (64)
Ifex
Imipenem/cilastatin (34)
Primaxin
Imipramine (10)
Tofranil
Indapamide (56)
Lozide

Indomethacin (7)
Indocid, Indotec, Novo-methacin,
Nu-Indo
Insulins (27)
Humalog, Humulin, Iletin, Novolin
Interferons (44)
Alfa-2a (Roferon A); alfa-2b (Intron A);
alpha-n1 (Wellferon); beta-1a
(Avonex, Rebif); beta-1b (Betaseron)
Ipratropium (47)
Atrovent
Irbesartan (55)
Avapro
Irinotecan (64)
Camptosar
Isoflurane (14)
Forane
Isoproterenol (18, 47), Isoprenaline*
Isuprel
**Isosorbide dinitrate (53), Sorbide
nitrate***
Apo-ISDN, Cedocard-SR, Isordil
Isosorbide mononitrate (53)
Imdur, Ismo
Isotretinoin, (66)
Accutane, Isotrex
Ketoconazole (40)
Nizoral
Ketoprofen (7)
Apo-Keto, Novo-Keto, Orafen, Orudis,
Oruvail, Rhodis
Ketorolac (7)
Acular, Toradol
Labetalol (19, 55)
Trandate
Lactulose (61)
Duphalac
Lamotrigine (11)
Lamictal
Lansoprazole (60)
Prevacid
Leuprolide (64)
Lupron
Levobunolol (19, 65)
Betagan
Levofloxacin (35)
Levaquin
Levothyroxine (25)
Eltroxin, Levotec, Synthroid
Lidocaine (14, 52), Lignocaine*
Xylocaine, Xylocard
Lisinopril (55)
Prinivil, Zestril
Lithium (10)
Carbolith, Duralith, Lithane
Loperamide (62)
Imodium
Loratadine (48)
Claritin
Lorazepam (8)
Ativan, Novo-Lorazem, Nu-Loraz
Losartan (55)
Cozaar
Lovastatin (58)
Mevacor

Loxapine (9), Oxilapine*
Loxapac
Magnesium citrate (61)
Citro-Mag
Mannitol (56, 65)
Osmitrol
Maprotiline (10)
Ludiomil
Mazindol (30)
Sanorex
Mebendazole (41)
Vermox
Meclizine (48, 63), Histamethizine*
Bonamine
**Mechlorethamine (nitrogen mustard),
chlormethine (64)**
Mustargen
Medroxyprogesterone (28)
Depo-Provera, Novo-Medrone, Provera
Megestrol (28)
Megace
Melphalan (64)
Alkeran
Meperidine (6), Pethidine*
Demerol
Mepivacaine (14)
Carbocaine, Polocaine
Mercaptopurine (64)
Purinethol
Mesoridazine (9)
Serentil
Mestranol/norethindrone (28)
Norinyl, Ortho-Novum
Metaproterenol (18, 47), Orciprenaline*
Alupent
Metformin (27)
Glucophage
Methazolamide (65)
Neptazane
Methenamine (36)
Hip-Rex, Urasal
Methimazole (25), Thiamazole*
Tapazole
Methocarbamol (13)
Robaxin
Methotrexate (45, 64), Amethopterin*
Rheumatrex
Methyldopa (55)
Aldomet, Novo-Medopa, Nu-Medopa
Methylphenidate (16)
Ritalin
Methylprednisolone (24, 47, 66)
Depo-Medrol, Medrol, Solu-Medrol
Methysergide (7)
Sansert
Metoclopramide (63)
Apo-Metoclop, Maxeran, Reglan
Metolazone (56)
Zaroxolyn
Metoprolol (19, 55)
Betaloc, Lopressor, Novo-Metoprol,
Nu-Metop
Metronidazole (37, 41)
Flagyl, Metrogel, Novo-Nidazol,
Noritate

Generic/Canadian Trade Names

Mexiletine (52)
Mexitil
Miconazole (40, 66)
Micatin, Monistat, Micozole
Midazolam (8)
Versed
Minocycline (36)
Minocin
Minoxidil (55)
Apo-Gain, Loniten, Rogaine
Misoprostol (7, 60)
Cytotec
Mitomycin (64)
Mutamycin
Montelukast (47)
Singulair
Morphine (6)
Morphitec, MOS, MS Contin, MSIR,
Oramorph, Statex
Muromonab-CD3 (45)
Orthoclone OKT 3
Nabumetone (7)
Relafen
Nadolol (19, 53, 55)
Apo-Nadol, Corgard
Nalbuphine (6)
Nubain
Naloxone (6)
Narcan
Naphazoline (18, 49)
Naphcon, Vasocon
Naproxen (7)
Anaprox, Naprosyn, Naxen,
Novo-Naprox, Nu-Naprox, Synflex
Naratriptan (7)
Amerge
Nedocromil (47)
Mireze, Tilade
Nefazodone (10)
Serzone
Neostigmine (20)
Prostigmin
Netilmicin (35)
Netromycin
Nevirapine (39)
Viramune
Nicardipine (53)
Cardene
Nifedipine (53)
Adalat, Apo-Nifed, Novo-Nifedin,
Nu-Nifed
Nilutamide (64)
Anandron
Nimodipine (53)
Nimotop
Nitrofurantoin (36)
Macrodantin
Nitroprusside (55)
Nipride
Nitroglycerin (53), Glyceryl trinitrate*
Minitran, Nitro-Dur, Nitrol, Nitrolingual,
Nitrong, Nitrostat, Transderm-Nitro,
Trinipatch
Nizatidine (60)
Axid

Norepinephrine (18, 54),
Noradrenaline*
Levophed
Norethindrone (28)
Norlutate
Norfloxacin (35, 65)
Apo-Norflox, Noroxin
Nortriptyline (10)
Aventyl, Norventyl
Nystatin (40, 66)
Mycostatin, Nadostine, Nilstat, Nyaderm
Ofloxacin (35, 65)
Apo-Oflox, Floxin, Ocuflox
Olanzapine (9)
Zyprexa
Omeprazole (60)
Losec
Ondansetron (63)
Zofran
Orphenadrine (12, 13)
Disipal, Norflex
Oxaprozin (7)
Daypro
Oxazepam (8)
Serax
Oxycodone (6)
OxyContin, Supeudol
Paclitaxel (64)
Taxol
Pamidronate (26)
Aredia
Pancrelipase (30)
Cotazym, Creon, Pancrease, Viokase
Pantoprazole (60)
Pantoloc
Paroxetine (10)
Paxil
Penicillamine (32)
Cuprimine, Depen
Penicillin G benzathine (34)
Bicillin L-A
Penicillin V (34), Phenoxymethyl
penicillin*
Apo-Pen VK, Ledercillin VK, Nadopen-V,
Novo-Pen-VK, Nu-Pen-VK
Pentamidine (41)
Pentacarinat
Pentobarbital (8)
Nembutal
Perphenazine (9)
Trilafon
Phenelzine (10)
Nardil
Phenobarbital (8, 11),
Phenobarbitone*
Phenylephrine (18, 49)
Dionephrine, Mydfrin, Neo-Synephrine
Phenytoin (11)
Dilantin
Pilocarpine (65)
Diocarpine, Isopto Carpine, Miocarpine,
Pilopine, Salagen
Pindolol (19, 55)
Apo-Pindol, Novo-Pindol, Nu-Pindol,
Visken

Piperacillin (34)
Pipracil
Piperacillin/tazobactam (34)
Tazocin
Piroxicam (7)
Feldene, Fexicam, Novo-Pirocam,
Nu-Pirox
Polycarbophil (61)
Replens
Potassium chloride (32)
Apo-K, Kaochlor, K-Dur, Micro-K,
Roychlor, Slow-K
Pramipexole (12)
Mirapex
Pravastatin (58)
Pravachol
Prazosin (55)
Apo-Prazo, Minipress, Novo-Prazin,
Nu-Prazo
Prednisolone (24),
Deltahydrocortisone*
Diopred, Inflamase, Ophtho-Tate,
Pediapred
Prednisone (24), Deltacortisone*
Deltasone, Winpred
Prilocaine (14)
Citanest
Probenecid (6)
Benemid
Procainamide (52)
Procan-SR, Pronestyl
Procaine (14)
Novocain
Prochlorperazine (9)
Stemetil
Procyclidine (12)
Kemadrin, Procyclid
Promethazine (9, 48, 63)
Phenergan
Propafenone (52)
Rythmol
Propantheline (21)
Pro-Banthine
Proparacaine (14), Proxymetacaine*
Alcaine, Diocaine, Ophthetic
Propofol (14)
Diprivan
Propranolol (19, 52, 53, 55)
Inderal
Propylthiouracil (25)
Propyl-Thyracil
Protriptyline (10)
Triptil
Pseudoephedrine (49)
Eltor, Sudafed
Psyllium hydrophilic muciloid (61)
Metamucil, Novo-Mucilax, Prodiem
Plain
Pyrazinamide (38)
Tebrazid
Pyridostigmine (20)
Mestinon
Quetiapine (9)
Seroquel

(continued)

Generic/Canadian Trade Names

Quinapril (55)
Accupril
Quinidine (52)
Biquin, Cardioquin, Quinidex
Raloxifene (26)
Evista
Ramipril (55)
Altace
Ranitidine (60)
Novo-Ranidine, Nu-Ranit, Zantac
Ribavirin (39)
Virazole
Rifampin (38)
Rifadin, Rimactane, Rofact
Risperidone (9)
Risperdal
Ritodrine (67)
Yutopar
Ropinirole (12)
Requip
Salmeterol (47)
Serevent
Saquinavir (39)
Invirase
Scopolamine (21, 63)
Transderm-V
Selegiline (12)
Eldepryl
Sertraline (10)
Zoloft
Simvastatin (58)
Zocor
Sodium polystyrene sulfonate (32)
Kayexelate
Sotalol (19, 52)
Sotacor
Spironolactone (56)
Aldactone, Novo-Spiroton
Stavudine (39)
Zerit
Streptokinase (57)
Kabikinase, Streptase
Streptozocin (64)
Zanosar
Succinylcholine (14), Suxamethonium*
Anectine, Quelicin
Sucralfate (60)
Sulcrate
Sufentanil (6)
Sufenta
Sulfacetamide (65)
Cetamide, Diosulf, Sodium Sulamyd
Sulfamethoxazole/trimethoprim (36)
Apo-Sulfatrim, Bactrim, Novo-Trimel, Nu-Cotrimix, Septra
Sulindac (7)
Apo-Sulin, Novo-Sundac
Sumatriptan (7)
Imitrex

Tamoxifen (64)
Apo-Tamox, Nolvadex, Tamofen, Tamone
Temazepam (8)
Restoril
Teniposide (64)
Vumon
Terazosin (19, 55)
Hytrin
Terbutaline (18, 47)
Bricanyl
Terconazole (40)
Terazol
Testosterone (29)
Andriol, Delatestryl
Tetracaine (14)
Pontocaine, Supracaine
Tetracycline (36, 65)
Apo-Tetra, Novo-Tetra, Nu-Tetra
Theophylline (16, 47)
Slo-Bid, Theochron, Theo-Dur, Theolair, Theo-SR, Uniphyl
Thiabendazole (41)
Mintezol
Thiopental (14)
Pentothal
Thioridazine (9)
Mellaril
Thiothixene (9)
Navane
Ticarcillin/clavulanate (34)
Timentin
Ticlopidine (57)
Ticlid
Timolol (19, 55, 65)
Apo-Timol, Apo-Timop, Blocadren, Novo-Timol, Timoptic
Tioconazole (40)
Gynecure, Trosyd
Tobramycin (35, 65)
Nebcin, Tobrex
Tocainide (52)
Tonocard
Tolcapone (12)
Tasmar
Tolmetin (7)
Tolectin
Tolnaftate (40, 66)
Pitrex, Tinactin
Topiramate (11)
Topamax
Topotecan (64)
Hycamtin
Torsemide (56)
Demadex
Trandolapril (55)
Mavik

Tranexamic acid (57)
Cyklokapron
Trazodone (10)
Desyrel
Tretinoin (retinoic acid) (66)
Rejuva-A, Renova, Retin-A, Retisol-A
Triamcinolone (24, 47, 66)
Aristocort, Azmacort, Kenalog, Nasacort, Triaderm
Triamterene (56)
Dyrenium
Triazolam (8)
Apo-Triazo, Halcion
Trifluoperazine (9)
Stelazine
Trifluridine (39, 65)
Viroptic
Trihexyphenidyl (12), Benzhexol*
Apo-Trihex
Trimeprazine (48), Alimemazine*
Panectyl
Trimethoprim (36)
Proloprim
Trimipramine (10)
Apo-Trimip, Novo-Tripramine, Surmontil
Tripelennamine (48)
Pyribenzamine
Tropicamide (65)
Diotrope, Mydriacyl
Urokinase (57)
Abbokinase
Valproic acid (11)
Depakene, Deproic, Epiject
Valsartan (55)
Diovan
Vancomycin (37)
Vancocin
Venlafaxine (10)
Effexor
Verapamil (52, 53, 55)
Apo-Verap, Chronovera, Isoptin, Novo-Veramil, Verelan
Vinblastine (64)
Velbe
Vincristine (64)
Warfarin (57)
Warfarin (57)
Coumadin, Warfilone
Xylometazoline (18, 49)
Otrivin
Zafirlukast (47)
Accolate
Zalcitabine (39)
Hivid
Zidovudine (39) Azidothymidine, AZT
Novo-AZT, Retrovir
Zolmitriptan (7)
Zomig

Gillis, M.C. (Ed.) (1999). *Compendium of pharmaceuticals and specialities*, 34th ed. Ottawa, Ontario: Canadian Pharmacists Association.

INDEX

Note: Page numbers followed by b indicate boxes; those followed by f indicate figures; and those followed by t indicate tables.

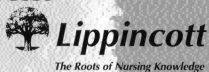